W9-APL-414

Krause's FOOD, NUTRITION & DIET THERAPY

Krause's FOOD, NUTRITION & DIET THERAPY

L. Kathleen Mahan, R.D., C.D., M.S.

Clinical Associate
Department of Pediatrics
School of Medicine
University of Washington
Seattle, Washington
and
Nutritionist
Children's Bellevue
Bellevue, Washington

Marian T. Arlin, R.D., M.S.

Formerly Assistant Professor
School of Home Economics
University of Washington
Seattle, Washington
and
Instructor
University of Alaska
Anchorage, Alaska

8th Edition

W. B. SAUNDERS COMPANY
Harcourt Brace Jovanovich, Inc.
Philadelphia ■ London ■ Toronto ■ Montreal ■ Sydney ■ Tokyo

W. B. SAUNDERS COMPANY
Harcourt Brace Jovanovich, Inc.

The Curtis Center
Independence Square West
Philadelphia, PA 19106

Library of Congress Cataloging-in-Publication Data

Mahan, L. Kathleen.
Krause's food, nutrition and diet therapy. —8th ed. / L. Kathleen Mahan, Marian T. Arlin.
p. cm.
Rev. ed. of: Food, nutrition, and diet therapy / Marie V. Krause, L. Kathleen Mahan. 7th ed. 1984.

Includes bibliographical references and index.

ISBN 0-7216-5508-4

1. Diet therapy. 2. Nutrition. 3. Food. I. Krause, Marie V. Food, nutrition and diet therapy. II. Arlin, Marian T. (Marian Thompson) III. Title.

[DNLM: WB 400 M214k]
RM216.M285 1992
615.8′54—dc20
DNLM/DLC 91-27885

5th Edition (French) Les Editions HRW Ltee. Montreal, Quebec, Canada

Listed here is the latest translated edition of this book together with the language of the translation and the publisher. 12-4-84; 7th ed., Portugues Livraria Roca, Sao Paulo, Brazil.

Editors: Daniel T. Ruth, Ilze Rader, and Michael J. Brown
Developmental Editor: Robin Richman
Designer: Dorothy Chattin
Cover Designer: Joan Wendt
Production Manager: Ken Neimeister
Manuscript Editors: Marjory I. Fraser and Linda Weinerman
Illustration Specialist: Lisa Lambert
Indexer: Roger Wall

KRAUSE'S FOOD, NUTRITION & DIET THERAPY 0-7216-5508-4

Printed in the United States of America

Last digit is the print number: 9 8 7 6 5 4 3 2 1

Dedication

To Ana, who was three when we started the "book" and who does not remember life without it; to Robert and Carlin for whom this was "oh no, not the book again"; and for Elsa and Richard who are always supportive, no matter what.

L. Kathleen Mahan

PREFACE

The eighth edition of this popular and highly respected text continues to recognize the increasing importance of nutrition in achieving and maintaining health and fitness and as a component of appropriate and effective health care. Its purpose is to furnish theoretical knowledge and clinical information in a form that will be useful to students from nursing, dietetics, and other allied health professions, many of whom are receiving education and training in an interdisciplinary clinical setting. Many features make it valuable as an auxiliary text for use in other disciplines such as medicine, dentistry, child development, and physical education. As always, with its extensive appendices, tables, illustrations, and figures providing practical hands-on procedures and clinical tools, it continues to be the textbook that can accompany the graduating student into clinical practice as a treasured reference source.

Many of the most popular features have been retained in this edition, but all material has been updated and referenced extensively to reflect the most current information available. In addition, significant changes have been made to simultaneously streamline and expand the content. These changes include modifications in organization as well as additions to both subject matter and interpretation.

TITLE

New to this revision is the addition of the original author's name to the title, which now becomes *Krause's Food, Nutrition and Diet Therapy.* Since Marie Krause authored the first edition in 1952, the text has enjoyed enduring popularity with students and teachers alike, among whom it has always been known as *Krause.* The new title will guarantee that her contributions will continue to be recognized in this and future editions.

AUTHORS

This edition introduces a new coauthor as well as several new guest authors who join those who participated in preparation of the last revision. The contributions of guest authors, all of whom are experts in their particular fields, reflect the increasing sophistication of nutritional education and care in specific areas of growth, development, and disease.

ORGANIZATION AND CONTENT

The text has been reorganized into four sections. Three of these — Nutrition Basics, Nutrition in the Life Cycle, and Nutrition for Health and Fitness — are appropriate for use together as the text for a basic nutrition course. The fourth section, Nutritional Care in Disease, provides the basis for training in diet therapy and adds the background information and hands-on tools necessary for successful clinical practice.

Part I — Nutrition Basics — continues to furnish material appropriate for teaching basic nutrition. Hands-on information is provided by many tables with useful clinical applications such as calculation of energy requirements and expenditure, and the levels of dietary fiber and omega-3 fatty acids in foods.

In Part II — Nutrition in the Life Cycle — an expert group of guest authors presents in-depth information on the importance of nutrition from pregnancy through the aging process. The chapter on Nutritional Care of the Low-Birthweight Infant has been placed in this section. Because increasing survival rates now permit diseases once specific to infancy and childhood to continue into adolescence and adulthood, this information has been incorporated into appropriate chapters in Part IV, rather than covered in a specific pediatric disease chapter.

Part III — Nutrition for Health and Fitness — is a new section that brings together nutrition concepts that have particular meaning in the achievement and maintenance of health and fitness and the delay or prevention of nutrition-related problems. Chapters on dental and bone health, atherosclerotic heart disease, hypertension, and weight control focus on the role of nutrition in the incidence and course of problems in these areas. Although theories of cancer prevention would also be appropriate to this section, these are discussed in the chapter on Nutritional Care in Neoplastic Disease that appears in Part IV.

A new chapter in this section addresses the requirements and issues of Nutrition for Athletic Training and Performance, from top-flight young athletes to adults who are trying to stay in shape. Also new to this section is a chapter on Guidelines for Dietary Planning that brings the 1989 Recommended Dietary Allowances together with the other major recommendations currently in effect, both in the United States and Canada. Other information in Section III includes techniques for assessing nutritional status, as well as issues affecting the community, such as food safety and federal nutrition programs. An expanded treatment of ethnic food practices is included as an Appendix.

Part IV — Nutritional Care in Disease — is appropriately introduced by a discussion of the nutritional care process. Many of the 27 chapters in this section have been contributed by guest authors who are specialists in the nutritional aspects of conditions such as renal disease, neoplastic disease, physiologic stress, and metabolic disorders. New to this edition are chapters on Nutritional Care in Pulmonary Disease, Acquired Immunodeficiency Syndrome (AIDS), Arthritic Disease, and Diseases of the Nervous System. The chapter on Nutritional Care in Cardiovascular Disease, which appeared in the previous edition, has been separated into Atherosclerotic Heart Disease, which appears in Part III, and Nutritional Care in Congestive Heart Disease, which is covered in Part IV. Discussion of Methods of Nutritional Support appears in this section as a separate chapter.

FEATURES NEW TO THIS EDITION

Several features new to this edition contribute to the teaching potential of the text. Each chapter is introduced by a list of Key Terms, which define terminology unique to the subject matter that follows. These terms provide a "road map" for the student beginning the chapter as well as a basis for review of understanding.

Inserts in the categories of Clinical Insight, New Directions, and Further Reading expand the information presented in each chapter. These provide the student and teacher with additional "nice-to-know" information and suggest areas for discussion, further study, or research. A list of Abbreviations summarizes all of the abbreviations encountered in the text. A Glossary defines terms common to the fields of nutrition and medicine.

The extensive Appendices continue to include the tools that have always been a valued feature of this text for clinicians. New to this edition are tables on the omega-3 fatty acid content of food, determination of body mass index, arm anthropometry for the elderly, and a nomogram for determining waist/hip circumference ratio.

INSTRUCTOR'S MANUAL AND AUXILIARY AIDS

The instructor's manual accompanying this edition, written by Dorice Czajka-Narins, Ph.D., is greatly expanded. In addition to learning objectives and strategies, it also includes teaching resources, case studies, and test questions, as well as transparencies for instructor use to enhance teaching and learning.

L. Kathleen Mahan, R.D., C.D., M.S.

Marian T. Arlin, R.D., M.S.

ACKNOWLEDGMENTS

A book of this scope is usually written with the help of many people "behind the scenes," and this book is no exception. We would like to extend our most sincere thanks to the following individuals who reviewed various sections of the manuscript and gave their thoughtful and insightful comments:

Roberta H. Anding, M.S., R.D., L.D., C.D.E.; Donna S. Bacon, M.S., R.D., L.D.; Vickeri J. Barton, R.D.; Jackie Berning, R.D.; Judith A. Beto, Ph.D., R.D., M.H.P.E.; Leah Bonovich, R.N., Sc.D.; Eileen Monahan Chopnick, M.B.A., R.D.; Marcia Cauley Costello, M.S., R.D.; Dorice Czajka-Narins, Ph.D., R.D.; Gene H. Evans, Ph.D., R.D.; Sharon Feucht, R.D., M.S.; Marion Franz, R.D., M.S.; James M. Gerber, M.S., D.C.; Sally Gleason, M.S., R.D.; Barbara F. Harland, Ph.D., R.D., L. D.; Elaine Hartsook, R.D., Ph.D.; R. Jean Hine, Ph.D., R.D.; Carolyn Holbrook Jenkins, B.S., M.S.N.; David B. Jones, D.D.S.; Mary Ann Klie; Anne Klijanowicz, R.N.; Carolyn Knutson, R.D., M.S.; Kathy Kraus, B.S.N., M.S.; Mary Elizabeth Kunkel, Ph.D., R.D.; Nancy A. Markin, R.N., P.N.A., B.S.N., M.S.N.; Ann McMullen, R.N., M.S.; Nancy Merlino, R.D., L.D., Ph.D., M.S.; Eileen P. Nee, M.S., R.D.; Elizabeth Nobmann, R.D., M.P.H.; Mary Beth Paradowski, M.S.N., R.N.; Louise Peck, R.D.; Gloria Petit, B.S., M.A.; Barbara Retzlaff, R.D., M.P.H.; Bonnie Worthington-Roberts, Ph.D.; Robert Schwartz, M.D.; Cynthia A. Tabor, R.D., Ed.D.; Megan Veldee, R.D., M.S.; Karen Voter, M.D.; Kendra S. Weaver, M.S., R.D.; and Joan Zerzan, R.D., M.S.

We would also like to thank Rhonda Hicken, R.D., M.S., and Amy Gresens who helped with research.

Lastly, we would like to thank Michael J. Brown, Ilze Rader, Daniel T. Ruth, Robin Richman, and Marjory I. Fraser at W. B. Saunders who stuck with us through this long and massive revision.

CONTRIBUTORS

MARY JO ADAM, R.N., M.N.
Formerly ALS Nurse Consultant, ALS Health Support Services, Kirkland, Washington.
Chapter 39. Nutritional Care in Diseases of the Nervous System

ELIZABETH J. ADAMS, M.S., R.D.
Teaching Associate, Department of Pediatrics; Nutrition Coordinator, Pediatric Pulmonary Center, University of Washington, Seattle, Washington.
Chapter 34. Nutritional Care in Pulmonary Disease; *Chapter 38.* Nutritional Care in Food Allergy and Food Intolerance

SAUNDRA N. AKER, R.D.
Clinical Instructor, Department of Physiological Nursing, University of Washington, Seattle, Washington; Director, Clinical Nutrition Program, Division of Clinical Research, Fred Hutchinson Cancer Research Center, Seattle, Washington.
Chapter 36. Nutritional Care in Neoplastic Disease

CAROL ASBECK, M.S., R.D., L.D.
Formerly Neuroscience Specialist, Clinical Nutrition, The Cleveland Clinic Foundation, Cleveland, Ohio.
Chapter 39. Nutritional Care in Diseases of the Nervous System

BERRI L. BURNS, R.D., L.D.
Neuroscience Specialist, Clinical Nutrition, The Cleveland Clinic Foundation, Cleveland, Ohio.
Chapter 39. Nutritional Care in Diseases of the Nervous System

CARRIE L. CHENEY, PH.D., R.D.
Affiliate Assistant Professor, Department of Epidemiology, University of Washington, Seattle, Washington; Research Associate, Cancer Prevention Research Program, Fred Hutchinson Cancer Research Center, Seattle, Washington.
Chapter 36. Nutritional Care in Neoplastic Disease

DORICE M. CZAJKA-NARINS, Ph.D.
Professor and Chairperson, Department of Nutrition and Food Sciences, Texas Woman's University, Denton, Texas.
Chapter 7. Minerals; *Chapter 8.* Water, Electrolytes, and Acid-Base Balance; *Chapter 17.* The Assessment of Nutritional Status

BARBARA ELDRIDGE, R.D., C.D.
Clinical Nutrition Specialist, Swedish Hospital Medical Center, Tumor Institute, Seattle, Washington.
Chapter 37. Nutritional Care in AIDS

SHARON FEUCHT, M.A., R.D., C.D.
Nutrition Consultant, Renton, Washington.
Appendix 33. Enteral Nutrition Products

SHARON CAMERON FURRER, M.S., R.D.
Outpatient Clinical Dietitian, Good Samaritan Hospital, Puyallup, Washington.
Chapter 37. Nutritional Care in AIDS

BETTY LUCAS, M.P.H., R.D.
Lecturer, Parent Child Nursing, School of Nursing, University of Washington, Seattle, Washington; Nutritionist, Child Development and Mental Retardation Center, University of Washington, Seattle, Washington.
Chapter 12. Nutrition in Childhood

CAROLYN NEARY, R.D., M.S., C.D.
Caremark Connection (HIV Healthcare Management), Affiliate of Baxter Healthcare Corporation, Seattle, Washington.
Chapter 37. Nutritional Care in AIDS

MARY J. O'LEARY, M.S., R.D.
Formerly Coordinator, Neonatal Nutrition Services and Training; Teaching Associate, Department of Pediatrics, University of Washington, Seattle, Washington.
Chapter 11. Nutritional Care of the Low-Birthweight Infant

PEGGY L. PIPES, M.A., M.P.H., R.D.
Assistant Chief Nutritionist, Child Development and Mental Retardation Center, University of Washington, Seattle, Washington.
Chapter 10. Nutrition in Infancy

MARY PODRABSKY, R.D.
Assistant Director, Nutrition Projects, Senior Services of Seattle/King County, Seattle, Washington.
Chapter 14. Nutrition in Aging

CHARLES J. PRUCHNO, M.D.
Assistant Professor, Department of Internal Medicine, University of Iowa and University of Iowa Hospital, Iowa City, Iowa.
Chapter 35. Nutritional Care in Renal Disease

JANE MITCHELL REES, M.S., R.D.
Teaching Associate, Department of Pediatrics, University of Washington, Seattle, Washington; Director, Nutrition Services and Education, Division of Adolescent Medicine, University of Washington, Seattle, Washington.
Chapter 13. Nutrition in Adolescence; *Chapter 18.* Section on Management of Eating Disorders *in* Weight Management

KRIS W. SCHROEDER, R.D., C.D.
Clinical Services Manager, Nutrition Services Department, Swedish Hospital Medical Center, Seattle, Washington.
Chapter 35. Nutritional Care in Renal Disease

CRISTINE M. TRAHMS, M.S., R.D.
Teaching Associate, Division of Pediatric Genetics, Department of Pediatrics, University of Washington; Coordinator, PKU Program and Nutritionist Biochemical Genetics Clinic, Child Development and Mental Retardation Center, University of Washington, Seattle, Washington.
Chapter 41. Nutritional Care in Metabolic Disorders

KATY G. WILKENS, M.S., R.D.
Manager, Nutrition Services Department, Northwest Kidney Center, Seattle, Washington.
Chapter 35. Nutritional Care in Renal Disease

JAYNE WILLIAMSON, R.D., C.D.
Research Dietitian, Nutrition Information Network, University of Washington, Seattle, Washington.
Chapter 29. Physiologic Stress: Trauma, Sepsis, Burns, and Surgery

BONNIE S. WORTHINGTON-ROBERTS, Ph.D.
Professor and Director, Nutritional Sciences and Chief Nutritionist, Child Development and Mental Retardation Center, University of Washington, Seattle, Washington.
Chapter 9. Nutrition During Pregnancy and Lactation

CONTENTS IN BRIEF

CONTENTS IN FULL

PART 1: NUTRITION BASICS

Chapter 4

Chapter 5

Chapter 6

Chapter 8

PART 2: NUTRITION IN THE LIFE CYCLE

Chapter 9

PART 3: NUTRITION FOR HEALTH AND FITNESS

Chapter 16

Chapter 17

Chapter 18

Chapter 22

Chapter 23

PART 4: NUTRITIONAL CARE IN DISEASE

Chapter 24

Chapter 30

Chapter 31

Chapter 32

Chapter 36

Chapter 37

Chapter 38

PART 1

NUTRITION BASICS

Life is nourished by food, and the substances in food on which life depends are the nutrients. These provide the energy and building materials for the countless substances that are essential to the growth and survival of living things. The manner in which nutrients become integral parts of the body and contribute to its function is dependent on the physiologic and biochemical processes that govern their actions.

This section opens with an overview of the processes of digestion, absorption, transportation, and excretion, because these functions determine the fate of the food after it enters the body. Foods invite consumption for a variety of reasons, including form, texture, and flavor and a host of psychosocial factors. Once inside the alimentary tract, however, their relative attractiveness is no longer an issue, since processes of digestion reduce them all to the same common denominators and make them available in size and form capable of absorption and transportation to the individual cells.

Proteins, fats, and carbohydrates all contribute in varying amounts to the total energy pool, but the energy that they yield is all in the same form. Utilization and conservation of this energy in order to build and maintain the body requires the involvement of vitamins and minerals. They function as coenzymes, catalysts, and buffers in the miraculous watery arena of metabolism.

CHAPTER 1

DIGESTION, ABSORPTION, TRANSPORT, AND EXCRETION OF NUTRIENTS

CHAPTER OUTLINE

Alimentary System
Digestion and Absorption
Role of the Large Intestine

KEY TERMS

ACTIVE TRANSPORT—the movement of particles in combination with a carrier protein across cell membranes and epithelial layers requiring expenditure of energy

AMYLASE—an enzyme found in the saliva (ptyalin) that catalyzes the hydrolysis of starch

BRUSH BORDER—the microvilli that greatly increase the surface area of the intestinal mucosal cell

CHOLECYSTOKININ—secreted by the duodenal mucosa, a hormone that acts to stimulate the pancreas to secrete enzymes and to a lesser extent bicarbonate and water, to stimulate gallbladder contraction, and to slow gastric emptying and possibly regulate appetite

CHYME—the semifluid, homogeneous, gruel-like material produced by the gastric digestion of food

ENTEROGASTRONE—a hormone whose secretion by the duodenal mucosa is stimulated by the presence of fat in the duodenum, which acts to inhibit gastric secretion and motility, thus slowing the delivery of further lipid into the duodenum

FACILITATED DIFFUSION—movement of particles across a membrane in which a carrier protein is involved

GASTRIC INHIBITORY POLYPEPTIDE—a hormone released from the intestinal mucosa in the presence of fat and glucose that inhibits gastric acid secretion and stimulates insulin release

GASTRIC LIPASE—an enzyme in the stomach that hydrolyzes the short-chain triglycerides into fatty acids and glycerol

GASTRIN—a hormone that is produced by the antral mucosa of the stomach that stimulates gastric secretions and motility

LACTASE—the intestinal enzyme that hydrolyzes lactose to glucose and galactose

MALTASE—the intestinal enzyme that hydrolyzes maltose into glucose units

MICELLE—a complex of free fatty acids, monoglycerides, and bile salts that allows for the absorption of lipid products into the intestinal mucosal cell

MICROVILLI—minute cylindrical processes on the surface of the intestinal cells that greatly increase the absorptive surface area of the cells

PANCREATIC LIPASE—an enzyme in pancreatic juice that hydrolyzes the ester linkages between fatty acids and glycerol

PARIETAL CELLS—large cells scattered along the walls of the stomach that secrete the hydrochloric acid in gastric juice

PERISTALSIS—the movement by which the alimentary canal propels its contents

PROTEOLYTIC ENZYMES—trypsin, chymotrypsin, and carboxypolypeptidase that break down protein into proteoses, peptones, peptides, and amino acids

SECRETIN—a hormone released from the duodenal wall into the blood stream, which stimulates the pancreas to secrete water and bicarbonate and which inhibits gastrin secretion

SIMPLE DIFFUSION—the random movement of particles through openings in cellular membranes

SUCRASE—the intestinal enzyme that hydrolyzes sucrose to glucose and fructose

VILLI—the multitudinous thread-like projections that cover the surface of the mucosa of the small intestine

Most of the major nutrients in foods are bound in large molecules that cannot be absorbed from the intestine because of their size or because they are not water-soluble. The digestive system is responsible for the reduction of these large molecules into smaller, readily absorbed units and the conversion of the insoluble molecules into soluble forms. Proper function of the absorptive and transport mechanisms is crucial to delivering the products of digestion to the individual cells. Derangements of any of these systems can result in malnutrition in the presence of an adequate diet.

ALIMENTARY SYSTEM

The *alimentary tract,* extending from the mouth to the anus, consists of the alimentary canal and its appendage organs, the liver and biliary tree and the pancreas (Fig. 1–1).

Functions of the alimentary system include receipt, maceration, and transport of ingested substances; secretion of digestive enzymes, acid, mucus, bile, and other materials; digestion of ingested foodstuffs; absorption and transport of products of digestion; and

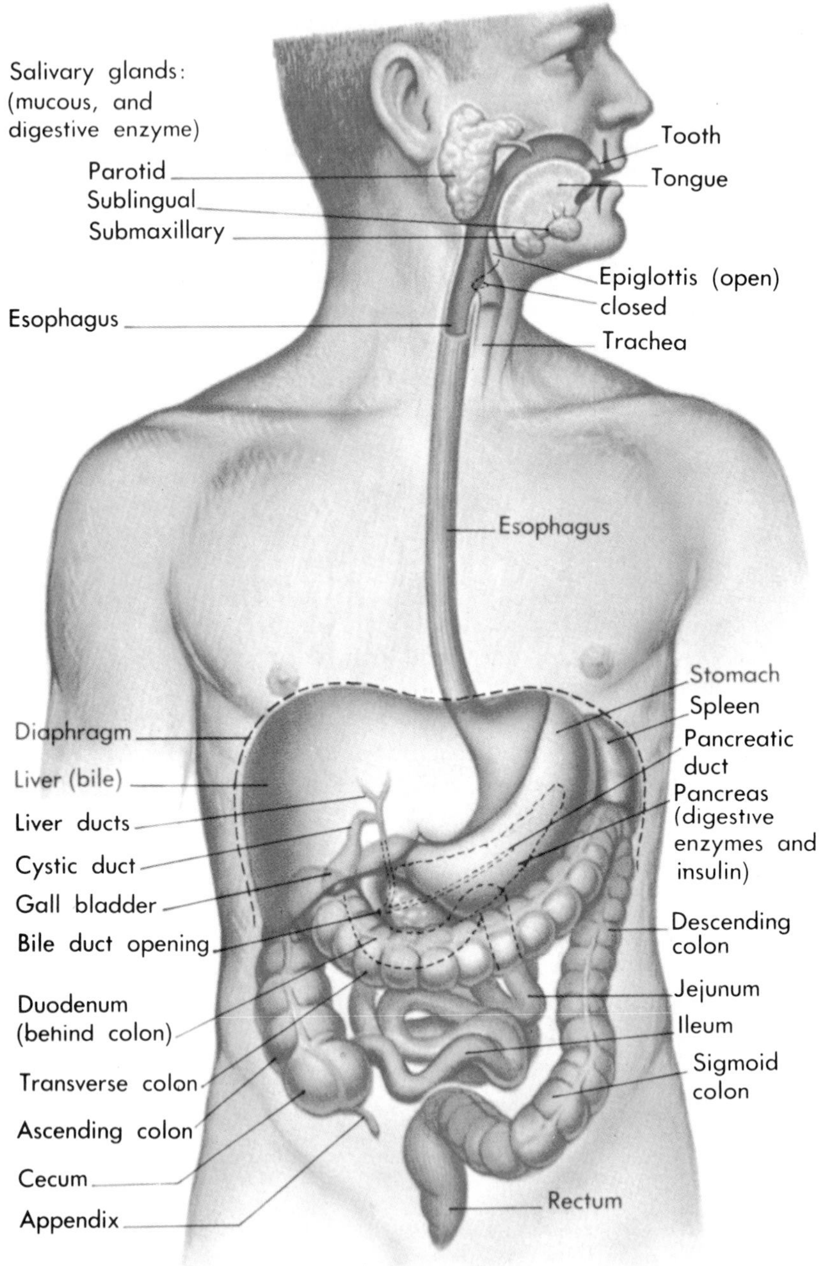

FIGURE 1–1. *The digestive system.*

transport, storage, and excretion of waste products.

The *mouth* receives food into the alimentary canal, reduces particle size by chewing, and mixes it with saliva. The *esophagus* transports food and liquids from the oral cavity and pharynx to the stomach. The *stomach* participates in the temporary storage and digestion of ingested materials. The *small intestine* receives the secretions of the *pancreas* and *liver* and functions in hydrolysis, transport, and absorption. The *large intestine* and the *rectum* absorb water, electrolytes, and, in reduced amounts, some of the final products of digestion. They also provide temporary storage for waste products that serve as a medium for bacterial synthesis of some vitamins. The *anus* controls defecation.

DIGESTION AND ABSORPTION

Digestion of foodstuffs is accomplished by hydrolysis under the direction of enzymes. Co-factors such as bile and hydrochloric acid support the digestive and absorptive processes. The digestive enzymes, which are primarily *exoenzymes,* are synthesized within specialized cells in the mouth, stomach, pancreas, and small intestine and are released to catalyze hydrolysis of nutrients in areas external to the cell. *Endoenzymes* are localized in the lipoprotein membranes of the mucosal cells and attach to their substrates as they enter the cell. The enzymes and their functions are summarized in Table 1-1.

Normally, 92 to 97% of the mixed American diet is digested and absorbed. Water, monosaccharides, vitamins, minerals, and alcohol are usually absorbed in their original form. The disaccharides and polysaccharides, lipids, and proteins must be converted for the most part to their simple constituents before they are absorbed.

Regulators of Gastrointestinal Activity

Neural Mechanisms

The neural control of gastrointestinal contractile and secretory activity consists of a local system located in the gut wall—the *enteric nervous system*—and an external system of nerve fibers from the autonomic nervous system. Mucosal receptors sensitive to the composition of chyme (e.g., acidity) and lumen stretch (e.g., fullness) send impulses to muscle and secretory cells of the intestinal tract via transmitters of the submucosal and myenteric plexuses. These transmitters include enkephalin, somatostatin, serotonin, bombesin, and neurotensin.

Autonomic innervation is supplied by the sympathetic fibers that run along blood vessels and by the parasympathetic fibers in the vagus nerve. In general the parasympathetic nerves innervate specific areas of the alimentary tract, while the sympathetic system inhibits activity. Acid secretion from parietal cells in the stomach is stimulated by vagal activity in response to the sight or smell of food. Thus the vagus nerve is sometimes cut to control the constant hyperacidity of peptic ulcer disease (see Chapter 26).

Hormonal Mechanisms

Regulation of the gastrointestinal system involves the action of many hormones, of which only gastrin, secretin, cholecystokinin, and gastric inhibitory polypeptide are well understood.

Gastrin, a hormone that stimulates gastric secretions and motility, is secreted from cells in the antral mucosa of the stomach. Secretion is initiated by (1) distention of the antrum, such as after a meal; (2) impulses from the vagus nerve, such as at the thought of food; and (3) the presence in the antrum of secretagogues, such as partially digested proteins, alcohol, caffeine, and food extracts (e.g., bouillon). When the lumen pH gets too low, a feedback mechanism reduces acid secretion by inhibiting gastrin release.

Secretin, a hormone released from the duodenal wall into the blood stream, opposes the action of gastrin. Secreted in response to duodenal acidity, it stimulates the pancreas to secrete water and bicarbonate into the duodenum. Neutralization of the acidity protects the duodenal mucosa from prolonged exposure to acid and provides the appropriate environment for the activity of duodenal enzymes. Secretin also inhibits gastrin secretion.

Other cells of the duodenal mucosa secrete *cholecystokinin (CCK),* whose release is stimulated by the amino acids and fatty acids resulting from protein and fat digestion. The functions of this hormone are (1) stimulation of the pancreas to secrete enzymes and to a lesser extent bicarbonate and water; (2) stimulation of gallbladder contraction; (3) slowing of gastric emptying; and (4) a possible role in appetite regulation (see Chapter 18).

Gastric inhibitory polypeptide (GIP), which is released from the intestinal mucosa in the presence of fat and glucose, inhibits gastric acid secretion and stimulates insulin release. Because of this hormone, an oral glucose load stimulates the release of more insulin and is metabolized more quickly than an equal amount of glucose given intravenously.

Table 1-2 summarizes additional functions of these hormones as well as functions of several GIPs that do not qualify as hormones because they are not released into the general circulation. Among these is *histamine,* which stimulates the parietal cells to secrete gastrin.

TABLE 1–1. Summary of Enzymatic Digestion and Absorption

Secretion and Source of Secretion	Enzyme	Substrate	Action and Products of Action	Absorption
Saliva from salivary glands in mouth	Ptyalin (salivary amylase)	Starch	Hydrolysis to form disaccharides (dextrins and maltose) and branched oligosaccharides	
Gastric juice from gastric glands in stomach mucosa	Rennin	Casein (milk protein)	Curdles casein to prepare it for pepsin action	
	Pepsin	Protein (presence of HCl)	Hydrolysis of peptide bonds to form polypeptides and amino acids	
	Lipase (tributyrinase)	Fat (tributyrin)	Hydrolysis to form free fatty acids	
Exocrine secretion from pancreas	Trypsin (activated trypsinogen)	Protein and polypeptides	Hydrolysis of interior peptide bonds to form polypeptides	
	Chymotrypsin (activated chymotrypsinogen)	Proteins and peptides	Hydrolysis of interior peptide bonds to form polypeptides	Pinocytosis of small peptides
	Carboxypolypeptidase	Polypeptides	Hydrolysis of terminal peptide bonds (carboxyl end) to form amino acids	Amino acids absorbed into blood
	Ribonuclease	Ribonucleic acids	Hydrolysis to form mononucleotides	
	Deoxyribonuclease	Deoxyribonucleic acids		
	Elastase	Fibrous protein	Hydrolysis to form peptides and amino acids	
	Lipase	Fat (presence of bile salts)	Hydrolysis to form simple glycerides, fatty acids and glycerol	
	Cholesterol esterase	Cholesterol	Hydrolysis to form esters of cholesterol and fatty acids	Micelles → mucosal cells → chylomicrons → lymph
	α-Amylase	Starch and dextrins	Hydrolysis to form dextrins and maltose	
Small intestine enzymes, most of which located in the "brush border"	Carboxypeptidase Aminopeptidase Dipeptidase	Polypeptides	Hydrolysis of peptide bonds to form amino acids	Amino acids absorbed into blood
	Nucleosidase	Nucleotides	Hydrolysis to form nucleosides and H_3PO_4	
	Nucleosidase	Nucleosides	Hydrolysis to form purines, pyrimidines and pentose	
	Enterokinase	Trypsinogen	Activates to trypsin	
	Lipase (enteric)	Monoglycerides	Hydrolysis to fatty acids and glycerol	Micelles → mucosal cell → chylomicrons → lymph
	Sucrase	Sucrose	Hydrolysis to glucose and fructose	Glucose, galactose, and fructose absorbed into blood
	α-Dextrinase (isomaltase)	Dextrin (isomaltose)	Hydrolysis to glucose	
	Maltase	Maltose		
	Lactase	Lactose	Hydrolysis to glucose and galactose	

There are no digestive enzymes in the large intestine. Digestion and absorption are completed by the time the colon is reached. Only water, salt, vitamins, and minerals are absorbed thereafter.

Digestive Process

Digestion in the Mouth

In the mouth, the teeth function to grind and crush food into small particles. The food mass is simultaneously moistened and lubricated by saliva, about 1.5 liters of which is produced daily by three pairs of salivary glands—the parotid, submaxillary, and sublingual glands. A serous secretion containing *alpha-amylase (ptyalin)* begins the digestion of starch. Another type of saliva contains mucus, a protein that causes particles of food to stick together and lubricates the mass for easier swallowing.

The masticated food mass, called a *bolus,* passes back to the pharynx under voluntary control, but from there on and through the esophagus the process of swallowing *(deglutition)* is involuntary. *Peristalsis* then

TABLE 1–2. Important Functions of Gastrointestinal Hormones

Hormone	Site of Release	Stimulant of Release	Organ Affected	Effect on Organ
Gastrin	Antral mucosa of stomach Duodenum Jejunum	Polypeptides Amino acids Caffeine Alcohol Food extracts Distention of stomach antrum Vagal nerve	Esophagus	Increases resting pressure of lower esophageal sphincter
			Stomach	Stimulates secretion of HCl and pepsinogen by parietal and chief cells, respectively Increases gastric antral motility
			Gallbladder	Weakly stimulates contraction of gallbladder
			Pancreas	Weakly stimulates pancreatic secretion of bicarbonate
Secretin	Duodenal mucosa	Gut acidity (pH $< 4-5$)	Esophagus	Reduces resting pressure of lower esophageal sphincter
			Stomach	Reduces gastric and duodenal motility Stimulates pepsinogen secretion Inhibits gastrin-stimulated gastric acid secretion
			Duodenum	Decreases motility Increases mucous output of Brunner's glands
			Pancreas	Increases output of H_2O and bicarbonate Increases some enzyme secretion from the pancreas as well as insulin release
			Liver	Increases volume and electrolyte output of bile
Cholecystokinin-pancreozymin (CCK-PZ)	Duodenal mucosa	Amino acids (esp. tryptophan) HCl Fatty acids ($<$9c) Food	Small bowel	Increases motility
			Gallbladder	Causes contraction of gallbladder
			Pancreas	Stimulates enzyme secretion of pancreas Potentiates effect of secretin on pancreas Slows gastric emptying May mediate feeding behavior
Gastric inhibitory polypeptide (GIP)	Small intestine	Glucose Fat	Stomach	Inhibits gastrin-stimulated gastric acid secretion
			Pancreas	Stimulates insulin secretion
Enteroglucagon and glucagon	Duodenum Jejunum	Carbohydrate Long-chain triglycerides	Liver	Stimulates glycogenolysis
			Pancreas	Inhibits pancreatic enzyme secretion
			Small intestine	Inhibits motility
Vasoactive intestinal polypeptide (VIP)	Neurons in small intestine	Fat Ethanol Increased gut acidity (?)	Liver	Increases glycogenolysis
			Pancreas	Increases output of H_2O and bicarbonate Releases insulin and glucagon
			Small intestine	Increases intestinal secretions
			Stomach	Inhibits gastric acid output
			Other	Vasodilates with hypotensive effect
Motilin	Duodenum Jejunum	Alkalinity in the duodenum	Stomach	Decreases gastric emptying Regulates gut motility (?)
Somatostatin	Antrum of stomach Upper small intestine Hypothalamus primarily	Gastric and duodenal acidity Amino acids Fat (?)	Pancreas	Inhibits release of insulin and glucagon Decreases pancreatic enzyme production
			Stomach	Inhibits gastrin release
			Gallbladder	Inhibits contraction
			Other	Suppresses secretion of growth hormone Suppresses secretion of thyroid-stimulating hormone
Pancreatic polypeptide	Pancreas	Ingestion of a meal—vagal stimulation	Pancreas	Decreases secretion of trypsin

moves the food rapidly into the stomach. (Swallowing is discussed further in Chapter 39.)

Digestion in the Stomach

Food particles are propelled forward and mixed with gastric secretions by wave-like contractions that progress forward from the fundus to the antrum and pylorus. Active chemical digestion begins in the middle portion of the stomach, where an average of 2,000 to 2,500 ml of gastric juice is secreted daily. This contains hydrochloric acid, intrinsic factor, the inactive protease pepsinogen, gastric lipase, mucus, and the gastrointestinal hormone gastrin. In the process of gastric digestion the food becomes semiliquid *(chyme)*, containing approximately 50% water.

The stomach is normally emptied in from 1 to 4 hours, depending on the amount and kinds of food eaten. When eaten alone, carbohydrates leave the stomach most rapidly, followed by protein and then by fat. However in a mixed diet, emptying of the stomach is prolonged.

The valves guarding the entrance to and the exit from the stomach prevent backflow of the mixture from the stomach into the pharynx and from the duodenum into the stomach. These sphincters can become excessively stimulated during emotional upsets; when the exit *pyloric valve* tightens or goes into spasms, the pain can be excruciating. Irritation from nearby ulcers may also alter the performance of this structure.

Digestion in the Small Intestine

The small intestine is divided into the duodenum, the jejunum, and the ileum, as shown in Figure 1–1. Most of the digestive process is completed in the duodenum, and the remainder functions principally in the absorption of nutrients.

The acidic chyme moves slowly in spurts of a few milliliters through the pyloric valve into the duodenum, where it is mixed with duodenal juices and the secretions from the pancreas and biliary tract. Chyme moves down the small intestine at a rate of 1 cm/min and takes from 3 to 10 hours to travel the entire length to the ileocecal valve.

Bile, a mixture consisting predominantly of bile salts, is collected and concentrated in the gallbladder and is secreted into the intestinal tract under the stimulus of *cholecystokinin,* which in turn responds primarily to the presence of fats in the intestinal tract. Through their emulsifying properties, the bile salts facilitate the digestion and absorption of lipids.

The pancreas secretes enzymes capable of digesting all of the major nutrients. Proteolytic enzymes include trypsin and chymotrypsin, carboxypolypeptidase, ribonuclease, and deoxyribonuclease. Trypsin and chymotrypsin are secreted in their inactive forms and are activated by *enterokinase,* which is secreted in response to contact of chyme with the intestinal mucosa. Fluids containing large amounts of bicarbonate ion, secreted under the influence of *secretin,* neutralize the highly acidic chyme.

Absorptive Mechanisms

Small Intestine

The primary organ of absorption is the small intestine, which is characterized by its enormous absorptive area. This is a product of the extensive length (22 feet) as well as the ordering of the mucosal lining into convolutions *(valvulae conniventes).* These folds are covered with finger-like projections called *villi,* which in turn are covered by *microvilli,* or the *brush border.* The combination produces an enormous absorptive surface of about 250 square meters. This rests on a supporting

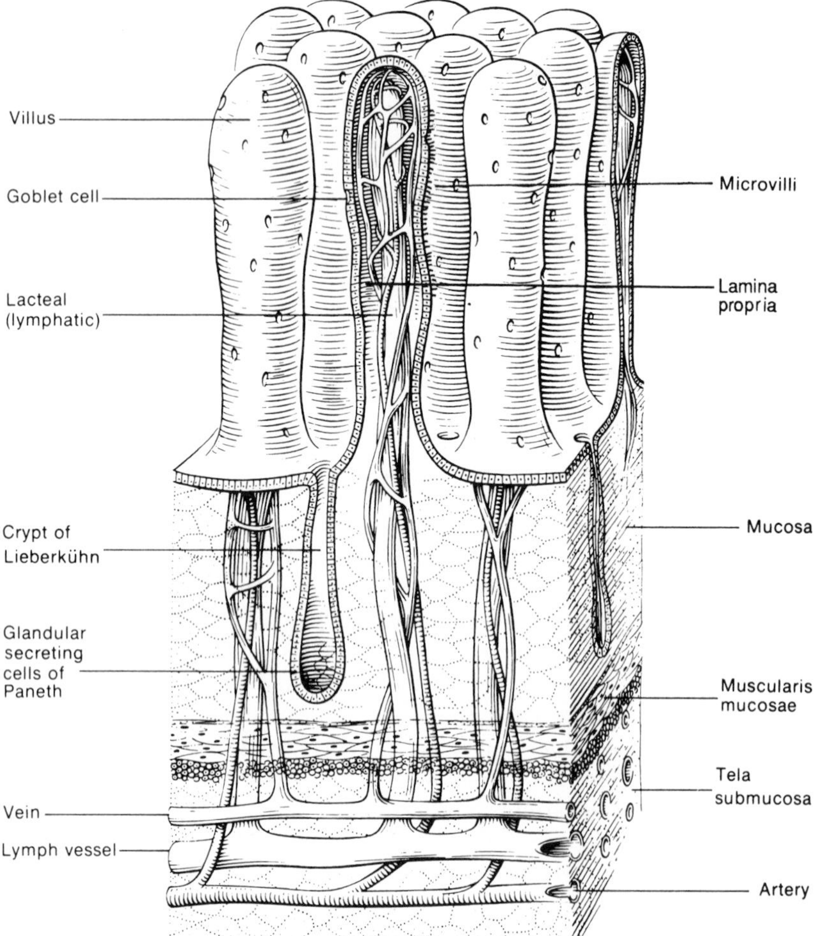

FIGURE 1–2. *Diagram of villi of human intestine showing their structure and blood and lymph vessels. (From Villee CA and Dethier VG: Biological Principles and Processes, 2nd ed. Philadelphia, WB Saunders, 1976.)*

structure called the *lamina propria,* composed of connective tissue in which the blood and lymph vessels that receive the products of digestion are suspended (Fig. 1–2). Each day the small intestine absorbs several hundred grams of carbohydrate, 100 grams or more of fat, 50 to 100 grams of amino acids, 50 to 100 grams of ions and 7 to 8 liters of water, and this does not represent its full capacity (Guyton, 1987).

Diffusion and Active Transport

Absorption is an extremely complex process, combining the relatively simple process of *diffusion,* where nutrients pass through the mucosal cells into the blood stream, with the more intricate process of *active transport.*

Diffusion involves random movement through openings in the membrane using channel proteins *(simple diffusion)* or in combination with a carrier protein *(facilitated diffusion)* (Fig. 1–3).

Active transport requires the input of energy for the movement of ions or other substances in combination with a carrier protein across a membrane against an energy gradient. Some nutrients may share the same carrier and thus compete for absorption. Carrier systems can also become saturated, and the absorption of the nutrient is thus slowed. The best-known carrier is the *intrinsic factor* that is responsible for the absorption of vitamin B_{12}.

Some molecules are moved from the intestinal lumen into the mucosal cell by means of *pumps,* which require adenosine triphosphate (ATP) and a carrier. The absorption of glucose, sodium, galactose, potassium, magnesium, phosphate, iodide, calcium, iron, and amino acids is thought to occur in this manner.

Pinocytosis has been described as a "drinking in" or engulfing of a small drop of intestinal contents by the epithelial cell membrane. In this manner, large particles such as whole proteins may be absorbed in a small quantity. The movement of foreign proteins across the gastrointestinal tract into the blood stream, where they cause allergic reactions, may be the result of pinocytosis.

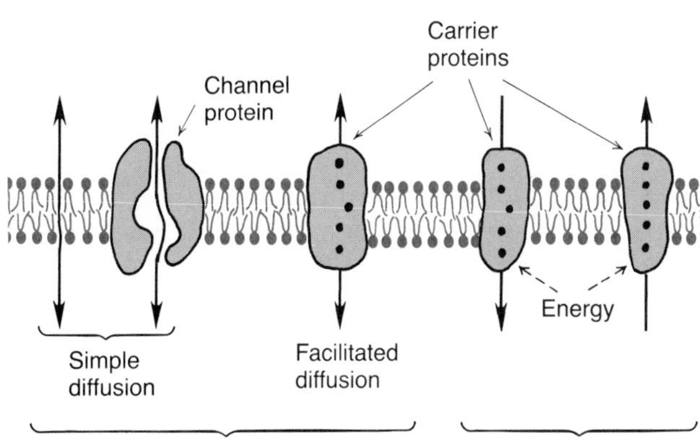

FIGURE 1–3. *Transport pathways through the cell membrane, and the basic mechanisms of transport. (From Guyton AC: Textbook of Medical Physiology, 8th ed. Philadelphia, WB Saunders, 1991.)*

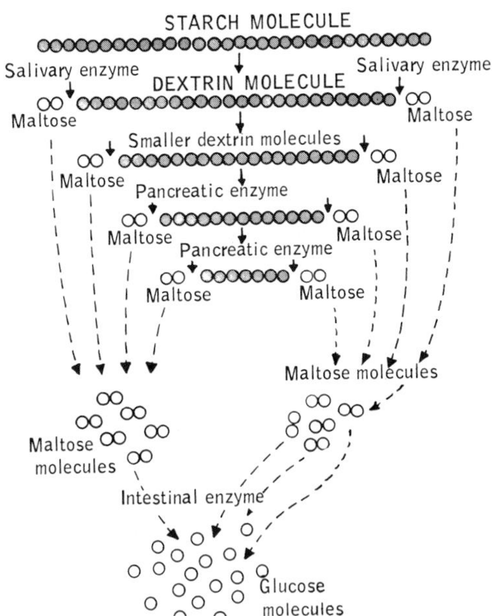

FIGURE 1–4. *Breakdown of starch molecule to glucose. Gradual breaking down of large starch molecules by enzymes in digestion. (From Briggs GM and Calloway DH: Bogert's Nutrition and Physical Fitness, 10th ed. Philadelphia, WB Saunders, 1979.)*

Digestion and Absorption of Nutrients

Carbohydrates

In the mouth, the enzyme *salivary amylase (ptyalin),* which is neutral or slightly alkaline, starts the digestive action on starch, hydrolyzing it to dextrins (or isomaltose) and maltose (Fig. 1–4). The activity of amylase continues in the stomach until it is halted by contact with hydrochloric acid. If the digestible carbohydrate remained in the stomach long enough, the acid hydrolysis could reduce much of it to the monosaccharide stage. However the stomach usually empties itself before this can take place, and carbohydrate digestion occurs almost entirely in the small intestine, with the greatest activity in the duodenum. *Pancreatic amylase* breaks the starches into dextrins and maltose, and *maltase* from the mucosal cells changes maltose to glucose. This action occurs in the brush border on the surfaces of the epithelial cells lining the intestines. These outer cell membranes contain the enzymes *sucrase, lactase, maltase,* and *isomaltase* (or *alpha-dextrinase*), which act on sucrose, lactose, maltose, and isomaltose, respectively (Fig. 1–5).

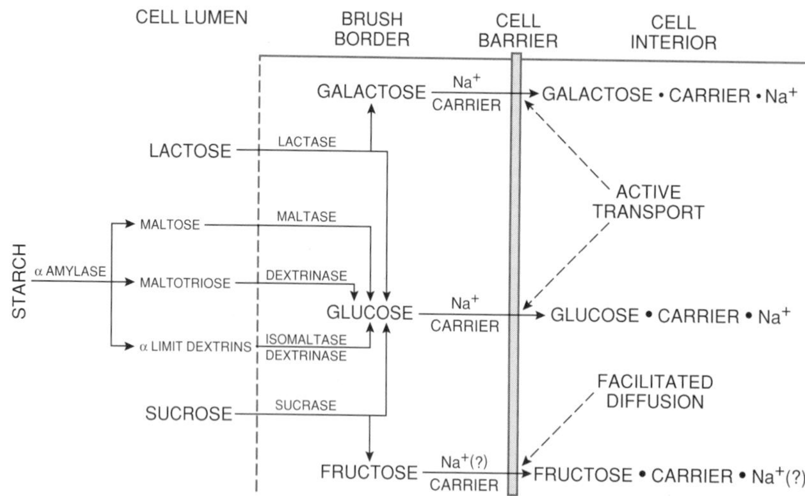

FIGURE 1–5. *Digestion and absorption of carbohydrates. Sodium and either glucose or galactose combine with carrier. The sugar-carrier-sodium ion complex is transported across the cell membrane into the interior of the cell. Once inside the cell, the glucose diffuses passively across the serosal membrane, and the sodium is actively pumped back out of the cell. The driving force for glucose transport against a concentration gradient is the gradient of sodium ion across the membrane that contains the glucose carrier. (Modified from Greene HL: Developmental Nutrition: Carbohydrate Absorption. No. 12. ©1976 Ross Laboratories. Reprinted with permission of Ross Laboratories, Columbus, OH 43216.)*

The resultant monosaccharides—glucose, galactose, and fructose—pass through the mucosal cell and, via the capillary of the villus into the blood stream, whence they are carried by the portal vein to the liver. Glucose and galactose are absorbed by active transport, presumably by a carrier that is sodium-dependent; fructose is absorbed by facilitated diffusion. Glucose is transported from the liver to the tissues, although some glucose is stored in the liver and muscles as glycogen. A small amount of fructose may be converted to glucose before it passes from the intestinal cell into the blood, but most is transported as fructose to the liver where, like galactose, it is converted to glucose.

Some forms of carbohydrate cannot be digested by humans. Cellulose, hemicellulose, lignin, and other forms of fiber are excreted unchanged in the feces (see Chapter 3). Neither salivary nor pancreatic amylase has the ability to split the cellulose bond. The cow and other ruminants, however, are able to subsist on high-fiber feeds because of the bacterial digestion that takes place in the rumen.

Proteins

Protein digestion begins in the stomach, where proteins are split into proteoses, peptones, and large polypeptides. The inactive *pepsinogen* is converted to the enzyme *pepsin* when it comes in contact with hydrochloric acid and other pepsin molecules. Unlike any of the other proteolytic enzymes, pepsin is able to digest collagen, the major protein of connective tissue. However, most protein digestion takes place in the duodenum, and the contribution of the stomach to the total process is small.

Contact of chyme with the intestinal mucosa stimulates release of *enterokinase,* an enzyme that transforms inactive pancreatic *trypsinogen* into active *trypsin,* which in turn activates the other pancreatic proteolytic enzymes. Pancreatic *trypsin, chymotrypsin,* and *carboxypolypeptidase* break down intact protein and continue the breakdown started in the stomach until small polypeptides and amino acids are formed.

Proteolytic *peptidases* located on the brush border also act on polypeptides, changing them to amino acids, dipeptides, and tripeptides. The final phase of protein digestion takes place in the brush border, where dipeptides and tripeptides are hydrolyzed to their constituent amino acids by peptide hydrolases. However, the presence of antibodies to many food proteins in the circulation of healthy individuals indicates that immunologically significant amounts of intact peptides escape hydrolysis and enter the portal circulation (Gardner, 1988).

Amino acids are absorbed via four distinct active transport systems: one each for neutral, basic, and acidic amino acids, and one for proline and hydroxyproline. Amino acid transport is thought to be by the same type of sodium co-transport mechanism that has been identified for glucose. Absorbed peptides and amino acids are transported to the liver via the portal vein for release into the general circulation.

Almost all of the protein is absorbed by the time it reaches the end of the jejunum, and only 1% of ingested protein is found in the feces. Some amino acids may remain in the epithelial cell and are used in the synthesis of intestinal enzymes and new cells. Endogenous protein from intestinal secretions and desquamated epithelial cells is also digested and absorbed from the small intestine.

Lipids

Fat digestion is initiated in the stomach with the action of gastric lipase (tributyrinase), which hydrolyzes the short-chain triglycerides (as in butter) into fatty acids and glycerol. However, the major portion of fat digestion takes place in the small intestine. Entrance of fat stimulates the release of *enterogastrone,* which acts to inhibit gastric secretion and motility, thus slowing the delivery of lipids into the duodenum. Products of fat digestion inhibit the digestive process; thus, it is necessary to allow sufficient time for removal of digested material from the duodenum so that digestion can proceed. As a result, a fatty meal may remain in the stomach up to 4 hours or longer.

The peristaltic action of the small intestine breaks larger fat globules into smaller particles, and the emulsifying action of the bile keeps them separated and thus more accessible to digestion by *pancreatic lipase. Bile* is a secretion of the liver composed of bile acids (glycocholic and taurocholic acids), bile pigments (which color the feces), inorganic salts, some protein, cholesterol, lecithin, and many compounds metabolized and secreted by the liver, such as detoxified drugs. From its storage organ, the gallbladder, about 2 pints of bile are secreted daily in response to the stimulus of food in the duodenum and stomach.

The free fatty acids and monoglycerides produced by digestion form complexes with bile salts called *micelles.* The micelles facilitate passage of the lipids through the watery environment of the intestinal lumen to the brush border (Further Reading, see below, and Fig. 1–6). The bile salts are then released from their lipid components and return to the lumen of the gut. Most of the bile salts are actively reabsorbed in the terminal ileum and are recycled back to the liver to enter the gut via the gallbladder. This efficient recycling is known as the *enterohepatic circulation.* The pool of bile acids may circulate anywhere from 3 to 15 times per day, depending on the amount of food ingested.

In the mucosal cell, the fatty acids and monoglycerides are reassembled into new triglycerides. A few are further digested into free fatty acids and glycerol and then reassembled to form triglycerides. These triglycerides, along with cholesterol and phospholipids, are surrounded by a beta-lipoprotein coat forming *chylomicrons,* as shown in Figure 1–6. The globules pass into the lacteals of the villi by a process of exocytosis. Chylomicrons are transported by the lymphatic vessels to the thoracic duct and are emptied into the blood stream at the junction of the left internal jugular and left subclavian veins. The chylomicrons are then carried to the liver, where the triglycerides are repackaged into lipoproteins and transported to the adipose tissue for metabolism and storage.

Cholesterol is absorbed in a similar manner after being hydrolyzed from the ester form by *pancreatic cholesterol esterase.* The fat-soluble vitamins A, D, E, and K are also absorbed in a micellar fashion, although some forms of vitamins A, E, and K and carotene can be absorbed in the absence of bile acids.

Under normal conditions about 97% of ingested fat

FURTHER READING: Unstirred Water Layer

The unstirred water layer (UWL) is a collection of watery plates that form a boundary between the intestinal lumen and the brush border membranes.

Emulsification of fats in the small intestine is followed by digestion, primarily by pancreatic lipase, into beta-monoglycerides (one fatty acid attached to the middle glycerol carbon) and free fatty acids. When the concentration of bile salts reaches a certain level, they combine to form micelles that are organized with the polar ends of the molecules oriented toward the watery lumen of the intestine. The lipid breakdown products of the fat digestion are rapidly solubilized in the central portion of the micelles and carried to the area of the brush border (see Fig. 1–6).

At the surface of the UWL, the micelles detach from their lipid passengers and return to the lumen for further transport. The monoglycerides and fatty acids are thus left to make their way across the lipophobic UWL to the more lipid-friendly membrane cells of the brush border. Once arrived, they are rapidly taken up for processing and entry into the transport system.

Because the UWL slows the progress of lipids from the lumen into the mucosal cell, it may be the major rate-limiting factor in the speed of lipid absorption (Thompson, 1989).

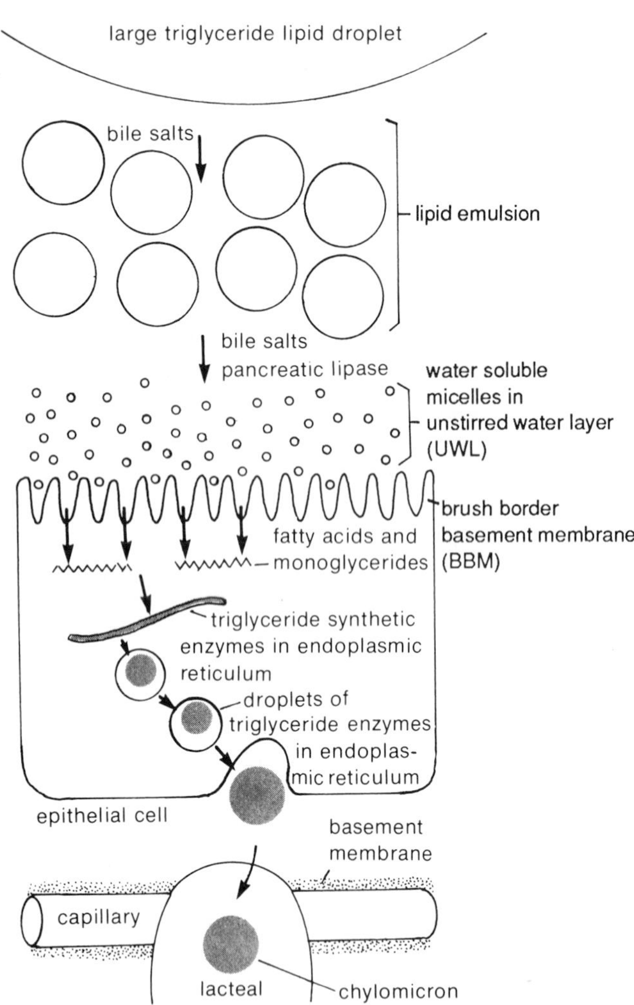

FIGURE 1–6. *Summary of fat absorption. (Redrawn from an adaptation from Vander AJ, Sherman JH, and Luciano DS: Human Physiology: The Mechanisms of Body Function, 3rd ed. Copyright © 1980 by McGraw-Hill, Inc. Used by permission of McGraw-Hill Book Company.)*

is absorbed into lymph vessels. Because of their shorter length and thus increased solubility, fatty acids of 10 carbons or less can be absorbed directly into the mucosal cell without the presence of bile and micelle formation. After entering the mucosal cell, they go directly without esterification into the portal vein by which they are carried to the liver.

This capability of medium-chain fatty acids is of clinical usefulness. Some individuals cannot efficiently absorb the usual types of dietary fat (long-chain triglycerides), because they lack necessary bile salts for micellar formation or the means for transporting triglycerides out of the intestinal epithelial cells into the lymphatics, as in abetalipoproteinemia. In these cases medium-chain triglycerides, with fatty acid chain length C8 and C10, which bypass micellar and chylomicron formation, are used for the fat in the diet (see Chapter 27).

Increased motility, intestinal mucosal changes, and the absence of bile decrease absorption of fat, and undigested fat appears in the feces in a condition known as *steatorrhea*.

Other Nutrients

Vitamins, minerals, and fluids are absorbed simultaneously through the intestinal mucosa. Each day about 8 liters of fluid from the body pass back and forth across the membrane of the gut to keep the nutrients in solution. Figure 1–7 illustrates the present understanding of the sites and routes of absorption of nutrients.

Vitamins and water pass unchanged from the small intestine into the blood by passive diffusion.

Mineral absorption is more complex and proceeds in three stages. The *intraluminal* stage consists of the chemical reactions and interactions that take place in the stomach and intestines. These reactions, which are dominated by the pH of the luminal contents and the composition of the food entering from the stomach, primarily affect the cations. The small anionic elements, such as fluoride, are not influenced by either pH or the composition of the diet and are absorbed quite freely. Cations, which are soluble in the acidic pH of the stomach, form insoluble hydroxides when the chyme passes into the higher pH of the small intestine. These cations are frequently kept available for absorption by ligands such as amino acids and other organic acids and sugars that form coordination or chelation compounds with the elements.

The *translocation stage* involves passage across the membrane into the intestinal mucosal cell. Transport of small anions may be by simple diffusion. For most cationic elements, the mechanism is either facilitated diffusion or active transport. For many minerals, more than one method of translocation may be operable depending on the concentration of a particular trace element in the intestinal contents.

During the *mobilization* stage, minerals are either transported across the serosal surfaces of the intestinal cells into the blood stream or are sequestered within the cell. Iron and zinc, for example, are either bound to proteins within the intestinal cell or added to the intracellular pool. The ions in the pool are then mobilized and transported across the serosal surface, while the protein-bound ions are either released to become part of the pool or remain bound, in which case they are lost with the cell during desquamation.

The gastrointestinal tract is the site of important interactions between minerals. Medication with iron may depress the absorption of copper. Copper in turn may lower iron and molybdenum absorption. Cobalt absorption is increased in patients with iron deficiency, but cobalt and iron compete and inhibit absorption of

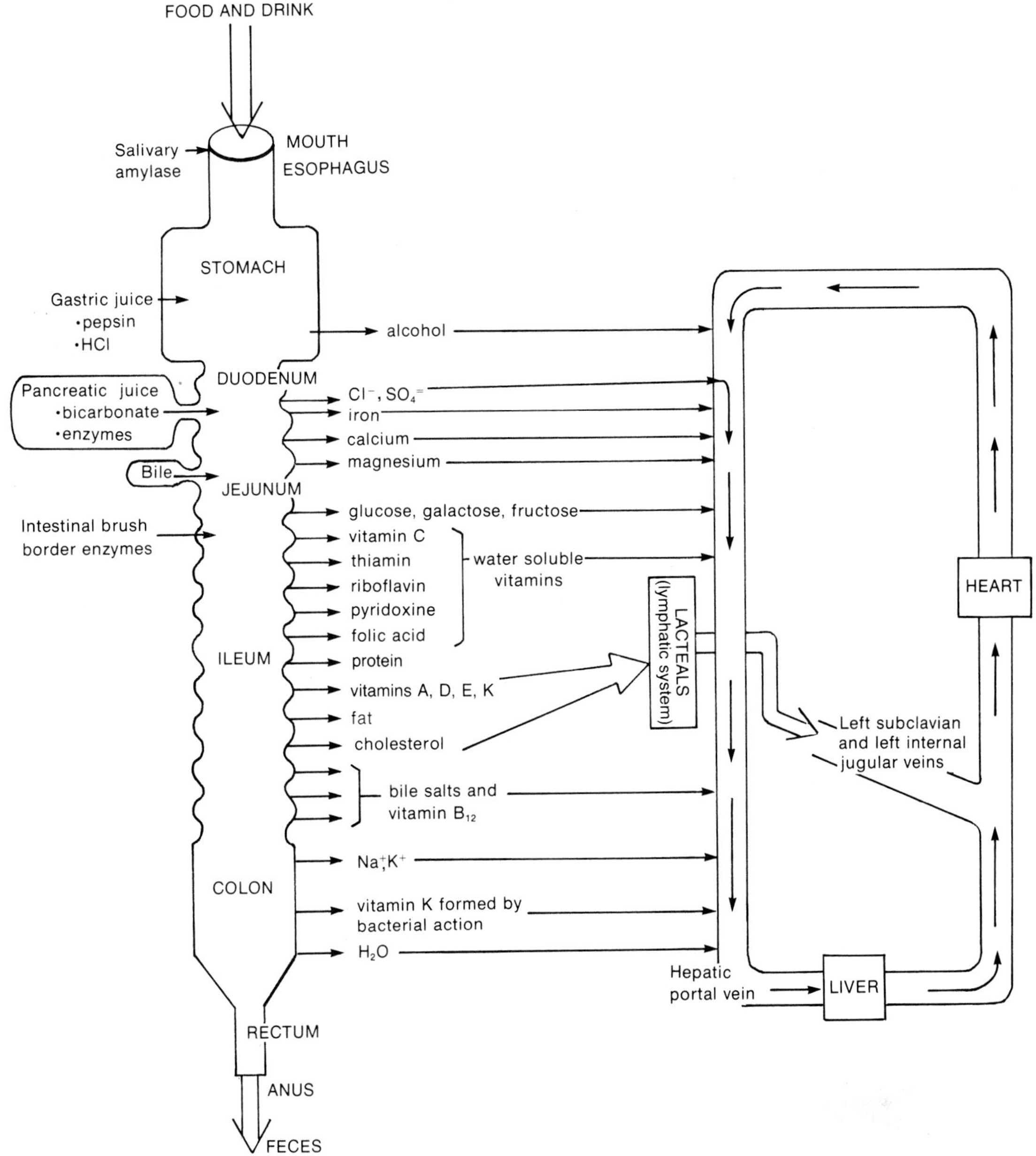

FIGURE 1–7. *Sites of secretion and absorption in the gastrointestinal tract.*

each other. These interactions probably reflect a lack of complete specificity of the absorption mechanism.

Metals are transported bound to protein carriers. The proteins are either specific, such as transferrin which binds with iron, or general, such as albumin which binds a variety of minerals. A fraction of each mineral is also carried in the serum in the form of amino acid or peptide complexes. Specific protein carriers are usually undersaturated, and the reserve capacity may be a buffer against excessive exposure. Toxicity from minerals usually results only after this buffering capacity is exceeded.

Factors Affecting Digestion

Psychologic Factors

The appearance, smell, and taste of food as it is served, along with the prevailing emotional climate, have an impact on the digestion of food. Sight, smell, taste, and even the thought of food increase secretions of saliva and the stomach juices and increase muscular activity of the gastrointestinal tract. Emotions of fear, anger, and worry stimulate the hypothalamus to activate the autonomic nervous system, which in turn depresses secretions, inhibits peristalsis, and slows propulsion of food by increasing sphincter tone.

Bacterial Action

The gut microflora make up a complex community in which about 100 species have been identified. At birth the gastrointestinal tract is essentially sterile, but implantation of various microorganisms soon takes place. *Lactobacillus* is the chief component of the flora until the infant begins to eat solid foods. *Escherichia coli* become predominant in the distal ileum, and the primary colonic flora appear to be anaerobic, with species of the genus *Bacteroides* being most frequent. *Lactobacilli* are also present in the stools of most persons on an ordinary mixed diet.

Normally there is very little bacterial action in the stomach, because the hydrochloric acid acts as a germicidal agent. However, in conditions marked by decreased secretion of hydrochloric acid, resistance to bacterial action is lowered and may lead occasionally to gastritis, an inflammation of the gastric mucosa.

Bacterial action is most intense in the large intestine. Colonic bacteria contribute to the formation of gases (hydrogen, carbon dioxide, oxygen, ammonia, methane), acids (e.g., lactic, acetic), and various toxic substances (e.g., indole, phenol), many of which contribute to the odor of feces.

Although dietary intake alters the fecal flora, the response is highly individual and variable. The ingestion of carbohydrate, in general, leads to increased fermentation in the large intestine; protein yields increased putrefaction. If faulty absorption in the small intestine allows large amounts of carbohydrate or protein to reach the large intestine, bacterial action may lead to the formation of excessive gas and also of certain toxic substances, some of which have been suspected in the etiology of colonic cancer.

Effects of Food Processing

In general, properly cooked foods are more digestible than raw foods. Cooking of meat, for example, loosens the connective tissue, aids chewing, and makes the meat more accessible to the digestive juices. Small frequent meals may sometimes be more easily digested than fewer large meals.

In some circumstances, chemical reactions take place between food and the secretions of the digestive system. *Acrolein,* a decomposition product produced by frying foods at excessive temperatures, retards the flow of digestive juices. Meat extracts, on the other hand, stimulate digestion.

Personal idiosyncrasy or an allergy may account for the fact that some foods agree with many people and disagree with others. Some people may be peculiarly sensitive to some chemical substances or to their physical states; for example, some people have distress from drinking orange juice, especially if it is ice cold and ingested when the stomach is empty.

ROLE OF THE LARGE INTESTINE

The large intestine is the site of the absorption of water, salts, and the vitamins synthesized in that organ by bacterial action. It is approximately 5 feet long and consists of the cecum, colon, and rectum. Most of the water in the 500 to 1,000 ml of chyme entering the colon each day is absorbed, leaving 50 to 200 ml to be excreted in the feces. Normally as the colonic contents move forward slowly at a rate of 5 cm/hr, almost everything of nutritional value is absorbed.

Large amounts of mucus secreted by the mucosa of the large intestine protect the intestinal wall from excoriation and bacterial activity and provide the medium for holding the feces together. Bicarbonate ions secreted in exchange for absorbed chloride ions help to neutralize the acidic end products of bacterial action.

Colonic bacteria continue digestion of some materials that have resisted previous digestive activity. In the process, several nutrients are formed by bacterial synthesis that are available for absorption and contribute to the nutrient intake in varying degrees. These nutrients include vitamin K, vitamin B_{12}, thiamin, and riboflavin. Vitamin K in particular contributes significantly to the available supply.

The feces consist of 75% water and 25% solids. About one third of the solid matter consists of dead bacteria. Inorganic materials and fats make up 20 to 40%, and protein constitutes approximately 2 to 3%. The remainder includes undigested dietary fiber, sloughed epithelial cells, and dried components of digestive juices such as bile pigments.

Defecation, or expulsion of feces through the anus, occurs with varying frequency, ranging from after every meal to once every 3 or more days.

CITED REFERENCES

Gardner MIG: Gastrointestinal absorption of intact proteins. Ann Rev Nutr 8:329, 1988.

Guyton AC: Human Physiology and Mechanisms of Disease, 4th ed. Philadelphia, WB Saunders, 1987.

Thompson ABR: Intestinal aspects of lipid absorption. Nutr Today 24(4):16, 1989.

ADDITIONAL REFERENCES

Furness JB and Costa M: The Enteric Nervous System. Edinburgh, Churchill Livingstone, 1987.

Guyton AC: Textbook of Medical Physiology, 8th ed. Philadelphia, WB Saunders, 1991.

Johnson LR: Gastrointestinal Physiology, 3rd ed. St Louis, CV Mosby, 1985.

Johnson LR et al: Physiology of the Gastrointestinal Tract, Vols 1 and 2, 2nd ed. New York, Raven Press, 1987.

McGarry JD et al: From dietary glucose to liver glycogen: The full circle round. Annu Rev Nutr 7:51, 1987.

Orten JM and Neuhaus OW: Human Biochemistry, 10th ed. St Louis, CV Mosby, 1982.

Wolfe MM and Soll AH: The physiology of gastric acid secretion. N Engl J Med 319:1707, 1988.

CHAPTER 2

ENERGY

CHAPTER OUTLINE

KEY TERMS

ADAPTIVE THERMOGENESIS (FACULTATIVE THERMOGENESIS)—a portion of the thermic effect of food; an increase in metabolic rate that is stimulated by eating and may serve the purpose of burning off excess energy in the form of heat

BASAL ENERGY EXPENDITURE—the amount of energy used in 24 hours by a person who is lying quietly, 12 hours after the last meal, in a comfortable temperature and environment

BASAL METABOLIC RATE—the basal energy expenditure expressed as kcal/kg body weight/hr

CALORIE—the amount of energy required to raise the temperature of 1 ml of water at a standard initial temperature by 1° C

DIRECT CALORIMETRY—measurement of the amount of energy expended by monitoring the amount of heat produced by a person placed inside a structure large enough to permit moderate amounts of activity

INDIRECT CALORIMETRY—measurement of the amount of energy expended by monitoring the oxygen consumption and carbon dioxide production of the body over a period of time

JOULE—the measure of energy in terms of mechanical work; 1 kilocalorie is equal to 4.184 kilojoules

KILOCALORIE (KCAL OR CAL)—1,000 calories; sometimes written as Calorie

METABOLIC RATE—an expression of the rate at which oxygen is utilized by the body

OBLIGATORY THERMOGENESIS—a portion of the thermic effect of food; the energy required to digest, absorb, and metabolize nutrients

RESTING ENERGY EXPENDITURE—the amount of energy used by a person in 24 hours when at rest, 3 to 4 hours after a meal

RESTING METABOLIC RATE—the resting energy expenditure expressed as kcal/kg body weight/hr

RESPIRATORY QUOTIENT—the ratio of moles of CO_2 expired/moles O_2 consumed

THERMIC EFFECT OF FOOD—the fraction of the total energy expenditure contributed by the processes of digestion, absorption, and metabolism of food; the increase in metabolism that is stimulated by eating

TOTAL ENERGY EXPENDITURE—the sum of the resting energy expenditure, energy expended in physical activity, and the thermic effect of food; the energy expended by an individual in 24 hours

Energy is defined as the capacity to do work. In the study of nutrition, it refers to the manner in which the body makes use of the energy locked in the chemical bonding within food.

The ultimate source of all energy in living organisms is the sun. Through the process of *photosynthesis,* green plants intercept a portion of the sunlight reaching their leaves and capture it within the chemical bonds of glucose (see Fig. 3–1). Proteins, fats, and other carbohydrates are synthesized from this basic carbohydrate to meet the needs of the plant. Animals and humans obtain these nutrients and the energy they contain by consuming plants and the flesh of other animals.

Energy is released by the metabolism of food, which must be supplied regularly to meet the energy needs for the body's survival. Although all energy appears eventually in the form of heat, which is dissipated into the atmosphere, the unique processes within the cells first make possible its use for all of the tasks required to maintain life. Among these processes are chemical reactions that accomplish synthesis and maintenance of body tissues, electrical conduction of nerve activity, the mechanical work of muscle effort, and the production of heat to maintain body temperature.

COMPONENTS OF ENERGY EXPENDITURE

Energy is expended by the human body in the form of *resting energy expenditure (REE), voluntary activity,* and the *thermic effect of food (TEF).* Except in extremely active subjects, the REE constitutes the largest portion of the *total energy expenditure (TEE).* The contribution of physical activity varies highly among individuals.

Resting (or Basal) Metabolic Rate

In the resting state, energy is expended in the mechanical activities necessary to the sustenance of life processes, such as respiration and circulation, synthesis of organic constituents, pumping ions across membranes, and maintaining body temperature. Half of the energy expended is used in meeting the metabolic requirements of the nervous system. Of the total, 27% is used by the liver, much of which is involved in synthesizing glucose and ketone bodies as fuels for the brain (WHO, 1985) (Table 2–1).

TABLE 2–1. Approximate Energy Expenditure of Organs in Human Adults*

Organ	% of REE†
Liver	29
Brain	19
Heart	10
Kidney	7
Skeletal muscles (at rest)	18
Remainder	17
	100

* Adapted from Grande F: Energy expenditure of organs and tissues. *In* Kinney JM (ed): Assessment of Energy Metabolism in Health and Disease. Columbus, Ross Laboratories, 1980, pp 88–92.
† REE = resting energy expenditure.

Measurement of Metabolic Rate

Energy used by the body at rest is defined in terms of either the *basal energy expenditure* (BEE) or the REE. These are measured as *basal metabolic rate (BMR)* or *resting metabolic rate (RMR).* The terms tend to be used interchangeably.

The measurement is made with the body at complete physical and mental rest, relaxed but not asleep, several hours after any strenuous exercise or activity and in a comfortable temperature and environment. Measurements of BMR and RMR differ only in the time of day when the test is administered and the length of time elapsed since the last meal. The BMR is measured in the morning after the subject awakens and is in the postabsorptive state (10 to 12 hours after the last meal). The RMR may be measured at any time of day and 3 to 4 hours after the last meal (Fig. 2–1).

The TEF reaches a maximum at 1 hour after a person has eaten and is virtually dissipated after 4 hours. However, some traces may persist from 8 to 18 hours after eating. In recognition of this fact, although most measurements are made according to the protocol governing the BMR, they are called RMR because the condition of 10 to 12 hours after a meal governing the BMR has not been met precisely (Bursztein et al, 1989).

Factors Affecting the Metabolic Rate

A number of factors cause the metabolic rate to vary among individuals. Among these factors are body size and composition, which are associated with heat loss and with energy required to maintain lean muscle mass at rest.

The *body surface area* is related closely to the BMR. It has been used as the basis for calculating the BMR with the assumption that, because of the need to maintain body temperature, the metabolic rate is affected significantly by the amount of heat lost to the atmosphere by evaporation from the skin, an effect determined to a large degree by the extent of body surface area. However, the observed relationship between surface area and BMR may not be the result of heat production but of the correlation between the surface area and the size of the actively metabolizing tissues of the body.

Although the original work on energy measurement

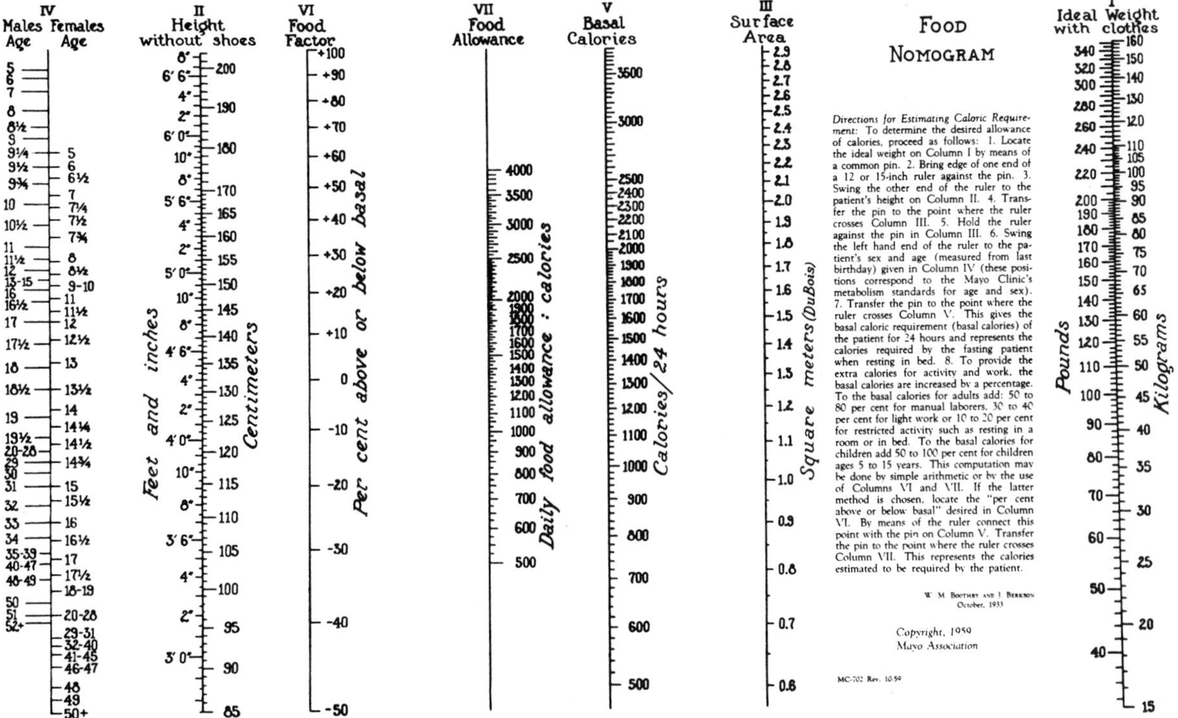

FIGURE 2–1. *Place the chart on a flat, smooth table. Use only a ruler with a true straight edge. Do not draw lines on the chart but merely indicate their positions by the straight edge of the ruler. Locate the various points by means of pins. Locate the patient's normal weight in Column I, and his or her height in Column II. A ruler joining these two points intersects Column III and gives the surface area. Mark this with a pin. Locate the age and sex of the patient in Column IV. A ruler joining this point with the point already determined for the patient's surface area crosses the scale third from the left at the basal energy requirement. To provide the additional calories for activity the basal calories are increased by a percentage given in Column VI. This can be determined from Table 2–2 or Table 2–3, or add 50 to 80% for manual laborers, 30 to 40% for moderately active adults, and 10 to 20% for those with restricted activity. To basal calories for children aged 5 to 15 years add 50 to 100%. The point is marked on Column VI, and where the ruler crosses Column VII is the total energy requirement. (Modified from Boothby WM and Sandiford RB: Nomographic charts for the calculation of the metabolic rate by the gasometer method. Boston Med Surg J 185:337, 1921 and Pemberton CM, Moxress KE, German MJ, et al [eds]: Mayo Clinic Diet Manual: A Handbook of Dietary Practices, 6th ed. Philadelphia, BC Decker, 1988, p. 547. By permission of Mayo Foundation.)*

was based on body surface area, more recent studies have shown that the RMR is determined primarily by the extent of *fat-free mass* or *lean body mass (LBM)*, which can be measured most accurately by underwater weighing or by total body potassium counting. Other newer techniques are also available (see Chapter 17). Estimates based on *body weight* produce results acceptably close to those obtained with body surface area. Sex and age do not add significantly to the estimate (Burzstein et al, 1989).

Almost one fifth of the resting metabolism is expended by the skeletal muscles. The proportion of lean body mass to adipose tissue is a function of both *sex* and *age* as well as *muscle development*. Athletes with greater muscular development show approximately a 5% increase in basal metabolism over nonathletic individuals. Women, who have more fat in proportion to muscle than men, have metabolic rates around 5 to 10% lower than men of the same weight and height. However, when based on lean body mass, the BMR for males and females is similar (Cunningham, 1982) (Fig. 2–2). Similarly, the shift in proportion of muscle to fat that occurs with aging is associated with decreases in resting energy expenditure amounting to about 2 to 3% per decade after early adulthood (Tzankoff and Norris, 1978).

The metabolic rate is highest during the periods of rapid *growth*, chiefly during the first and second years, and reaches a lesser peak through the ages of puberty and adolescence in both sexes (see Fig. 2–1). The additional energy required to cover the cost of synthesizing and depositing body tissue is about 5 kcal/g of tissue gained (Roberts and Young, 1988). Growing infants may store as much as 12 to 15% of the energy value of their food intake in the form of new tissue. As a child becomes older, the caloric requirement for growth is reduced to about 1% of the total energy requirement.

The secretions of the *endocrine glands*, particularly thyroxine and norepinephrine, are the principal regulators of the metabolic rate. When the supply of thyroxine is inadequate, the basal metabolism may fall by 30 to 50%. A hyperactive thyroid gland may increase the BMR to almost twice the normal amount. Stimulation of the sympathetic nervous system, such as during

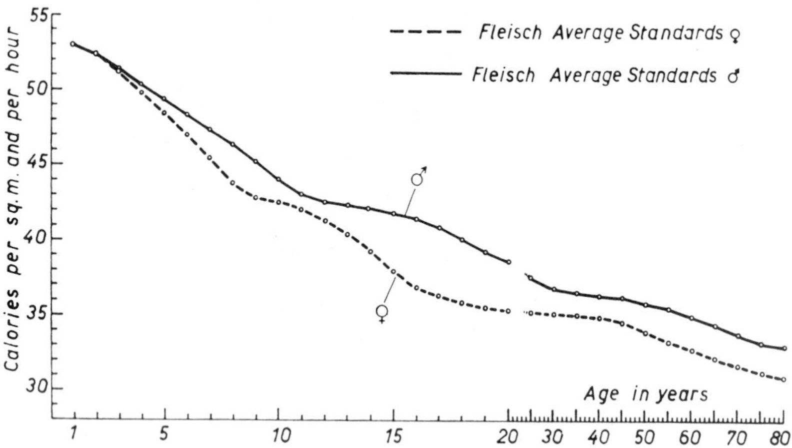

FIGURE 2–2. *Average basal metabolic rates per m^2 of surface area for males and females at different ages. (From Fleisch A: New Methods of Studying Gaseous Exchange and Pulmonary Function. 1960. Courtesy of Charles C Thomas, Publisher, Springfield, IL.)*

emotional excitement or stress, increases cellular activity by the release of epinephrine, which acts directly to promote glycogenolysis. Other hormones such as cortisol, growth hormone, and insulin also influence metabolic rate.

During *sleep* the metabolic rate falls approximately 10% below that of levels measured while the person is awake and reclining. This drop is caused by muscular relaxation and by decreased activity of the sympathetic nervous system.

Fevers increase the metabolic rate about 7% for each degree rise in body temperature above 98.6° F or 13% for each degree above 37° C.

The REE is affected by extremes in *environmental temperature.* People living in a tropical climate usually have REEs 5 to 20% higher than those in a temperate area. Exercise in temperatures greater than 86° F also imposes a small additional metabolic load of about 5% owing to increased sweat gland activity. The extent to which energy metabolism is increased in extremely cold environments depends on the insulation available from body fat and protective clothing.

The REE in adult females fluctuates with the *menstrual cycle.* An average of 359 kcal/day difference in the BMR has been measured between its low point about 1 week before ovulation at day 14 and its high point just before the onset of menstruation (Solomon et al, 1982). The mean increase in energy expenditure is about 150 kcal/day during the second half of the menstrual cycle (Webb, 1986). During *pregnancy,* the metabolic rate is increased by the processes of uterine, placental, and fetal growth and by the mother's increased cardiac work.

Physical Activity

The contribution of physical activity to TEE is highly variable. It may range from as little as 10% in the bedridden invalid to as much as 50% in the athlete. Energy expenditure can also vary considerably depending on *body size* and the *efficiency* of individual habits of motion. The level of *fitness* also affects the energy expenditure of voluntary activity, probably owing to increased muscle mass. Table 2–2 categorizes activity into five general levels as multiples of the REE and energy expenditure in kcal/min. The higher level of energy expenditure in each category represents a male with greater LBM.

Table 2–3 gives the factors to use for determining total daily energy requirements if the general level of activity of the individual is known. Activity patterns vary with age (Figs. 2–3, 2–4, and 2–5). Unless constrained, children typically are active and have daily energy expenditures of 1.7–2.0 × REE, compared with

TABLE 2–2. Approximate Energy Expenditure for Levels of Activity as Multiples of Resting Energy Expenditure*

Activity Category	Energy as Multiple of REE	kcal/min
Resting Sleeping, reclining	REE × 1.0	1–1.2
Very light Seated and standing activities, painting trades, driving, laboratory work, typing, sewing, ironing, cooking, playing cards, playing a musical instrument	REE × 1.5	Up to 2.5
Light Walking on a level surface at 2.5 to 3 mph, garage work, electrical trades, carpentry, restaurant trades, house cleaning, child care, golf, sailing, table tennis	REE × 2.5	2.5–4.9
Moderate Walking 3.5 to 4 mph, weeding and hoeing, carrying a load, cycling, skiing, tennis, dancing	REE × 5.0	5.0–7.4
Heavy Walking with load uphill, tree felling, heavy manual digging, basketball, climbing, football, soccer	REE × 7.0	7.5–12.0

* From Food and Nutrition Board, National Research Council, NAS: Recommended Dietary Allowances, 10th ed. Washington, DC, National Academy Press, 1989, p 27.

TABLE 2-3. Factors for Estimating Total Daily Energy Needs at Various Levels of General Activity for Men and Women (Aged 19 to 50)*

Level of General Activity	Activity Factor (×REE†)	Energy Expenditure (kcal/kg day)
Very light		
Men	1.3	31
Women	1.3	30
Light		
Men	1.6	38
Women	1.5	35
Moderate		
Men	1.7	41
Women	1.6	37
Heavy		
Men	2.1	50
Women	1.9	44
Exceptional		
Men	2.4	58
Women	2.2	51

* From Food and Nutrition Board, National Research Council, NAS: Recommended Dietary Allowances, 10th ed. Washington, DC, National Academy Press, 1989, p 29.
† REE = resting energy expenditure.

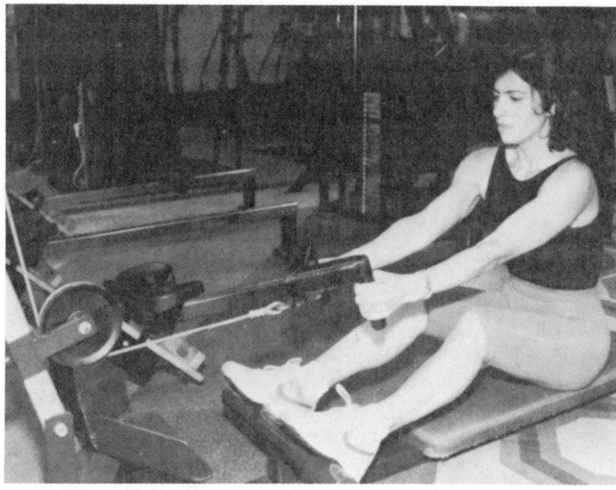

FIGURE 2-4. *The level of fitness affects the energy expenditure of voluntary activity, probably due to increased muscle mass. Calisthenics is considered moderate activity. (From DiNubile NA: Strength training, in the exercise prescription. Clin Sports Med 10[1]:49, 1991.)*

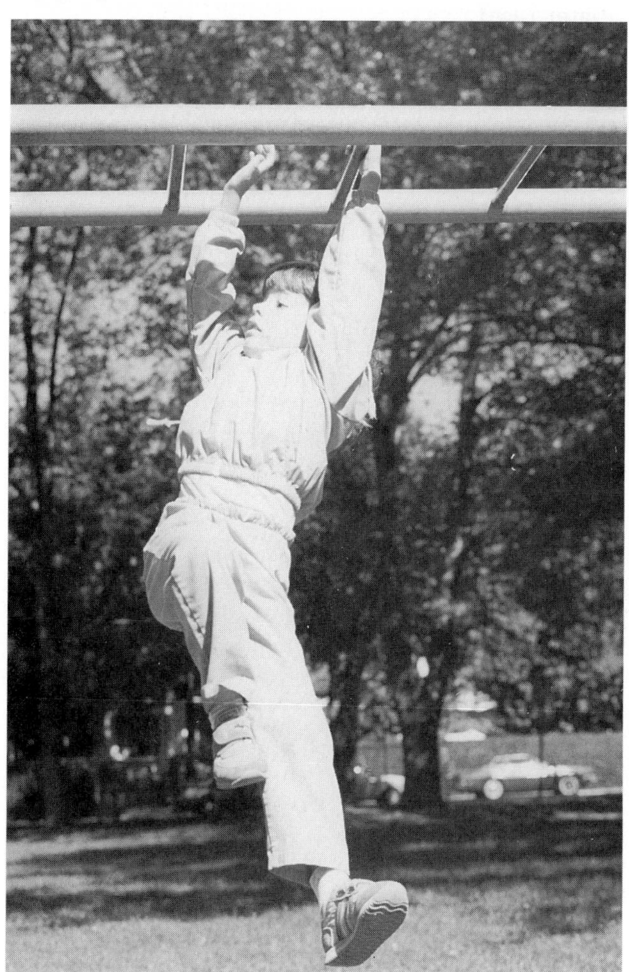

FIGURE 2-3. *A typically active child expends energy at a high rate.*

1.4–1.5 × REE for the less active elderly (Food and Nutrition Board, 1989).

Mental activity does not appreciably affect the energy requirement. Table 2-4 shows the amount of energy expended in specific activities.

Thermic Effect of Food

A small fraction of the TEE is contributed by the processes attendant on the consumption of food. This increase is called the thermic effect of food (TEF). It is sometimes called *diet-induced thermogenesis* (DIT). Some classifications separate the TEF into *obligatory* and *adaptive* (or *facultative*) components.

Obligatory thermogenesis is the energy required to digest, absorb, and metabolize nutrients. (The traditional terminology of *specific dynamic action [SDA]* is seldom used.) Although at one time it was thought that this energy was primarily involved in the synthesis of urea from amino acids, it now appears that much of obligatory thermogenesis is the result of synthesizing fat and glycogen from carbohydrate.

Consumption of carbohydrate or fat increases the metabolic rate by about 5% of the total calories consumed. If the food intake consists solely of protein, the increase may be as much as 25%. However, the effects of individual nutrients are decreased when these nutrients are mixed with other foods. An additional 10% of the total of energy requirements for basal metabolism and voluntary activity should be added to cover the TEF of a liberal mixed diet. If the food intake is very high in protein, about 15% should be added.

Adaptive or *facultative thermogenesis* is an increase

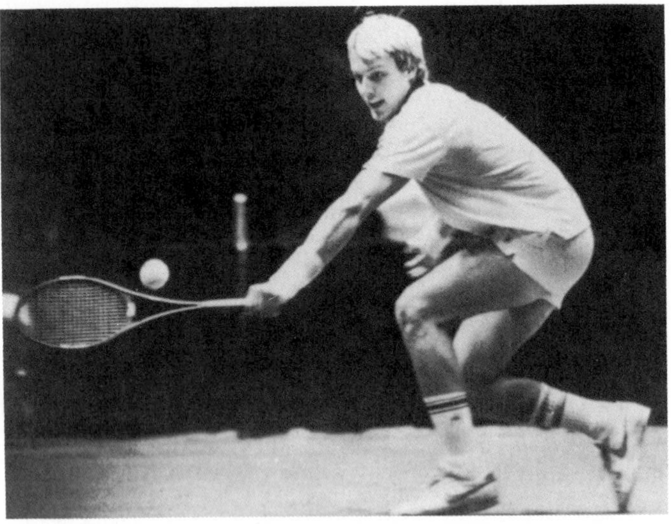

FIGURE 2–5. *A higher level of energy is expended by men, who generally have greater lean body mass. (From Leach RE and Miller JK: Lateral and medial epicondylitis of the elbow, in overuse injuries. Clin Sports Med 6[2]:261, 1987.)*

in metabolic rate that is stimulated by eating and that appears to serve the purpose of burning off excess calories in the form of heat. When eating is followed by exercise, the TEF is almost doubled (Bray, 1974). Adaptive thermogenesis is also stimulated by cold, caffeine, and nicotine. The amount of caffeine in one cup of coffee (100 mg) given every 2 hours for 12 hours has been shown to increase the TEF by 8 to 11% (Dulloo et al, 1989). Nicotine has a similar effect (Hofstetter, 1986).

The role of TEF in weight management is discussed further in Chapter 18.

ENERGY MEASUREMENTS

Units of Measurement

The standard unit for measuring energy is the *calorie,* which is the amount of heat energy required to raise the temperature of 1 ml of water at a standard initial temperature by 1° C. Because the amounts of energy involved in the metabolism of foodstuffs are fairly large, the *kilocalorie,* equal to 1,000 calories, is commonly used. A popular convention permits the designation of "Calorie" with a capital letter to represent a kilocalorie. In this text the kilocalorie, abbreviated as *kcal,* is used.

The *joule,* which measures energy in terms of mechanical work, is widely used in countries other than the United States. One kilocalorie is equivalent to 4.184 *kilojoules* (Clinical Insight, see below).

Calorimetry

Measuring Human Energy Expenditure

The amount of energy generated by the body can be assessed by direct or indirect methods.

DIRECT CALORIMETRY. Direct calorimetry requires monitoring the amount of heat produced by a subject placed inside a structure large enough to permit moder-

CLINICAL INSIGHT: The Joule

The joule, a unit of energy based on mechanical energy, is defined as the work done by a force of 1 newton acting through a distance of 1 meter.

The International Organization for Standardization has recommended the adoption of the joule (J) as the preferred unit for energy measurement in all branches of science. This recommendation was adopted by the US National Bureau of Standards in 1964, and in 1970 the Committee on Nomenclature of the American Institute of Nutrition recommended that replacement be effected as soon as the mechanics of the transition could be established. Although the joule has been in use internationally for a number of years, the United States and Canada have not made the change to date.

The multiplier recommended by the Committee on Nomenclature, International Union of Nutritional Sciences, to convert kilocalories to kilojoules (kJ) is 4.184 (4.2 may be used). Energy values per gram of each nutrient in kJ are as follows: carbohydrate, 17 kJ; protein, 17 kJ; and fat, 38 kJ. Because the energy content of diets is usually greater than 1,000 kJ, the megajoule (mJ), equivalent to 1,000 kJ, is often used.

TABLE 2–4. Caloric Expenditure During Various Activities*†

Activity	kcal/min	Activity	kcal/min	Activity	kcal/min
Sleeping	1.2	Mopping floors	4.9	Handball and squash	10.0
Resting in bed	1.3	Repaving roads	5.0	Mountain climbing	10.0
Sitting, normally	1.3	Gardening, weeding	5.6	Skipping rope	10.0–15.0
Sitting, reading	1.3	Stacking lumber	5.8	Judo and karate	13.0
Lying, quietly	1.3	Chain saw	6.2	Football (while active)	13.3
Sitting, eating	1.5	Stone, masonry	6.3	Wrestling	14.4
Sitting, playing cards	1.5	Pick-and-shovel work	6.7	Skiing:	
Standing, normally	1.5	Farming, haying, plowing with horse	6.7	Moderate to steep	8.0–12.0
Classwork, lecture (listen to)	1.7	Shoveling (miners)	6.8	Downhill racing	16.5
Conversing	1.8	Walking downstairs	7.1	Cross-country: 3–8 mph	9.0–17.0
Personal toilet	2.0	Chopping wood	7.5	Swimming:	
Sitting, writing	2.6	Crosscut saw	7.5–10.5	Pleasure	6.0
Standing, light activity	2.6	Tree felling (axe)	8.4–12.7	Crawl: 25–50 yd/min	6.0–12.5
Washing and dressing	2.6	Gardening, digging	8.6	Butterfly: 50 yd/min	14.0
Washing and shaving	2.6	Walking upstairs	10.0–18.0	Backstroke: 25–50 yd/min	6.0–12.5
Driving a car	2.8	Pool or billiards	1.8	Breaststroke: 25–50 yd/min	6.0–12.5
Washing clothes	3.1	Canoeing: 2.5 mph–4.0 mph	3.0–7.0	Sidestroke: 40 yd/min	11.0
Walking indoors	3.1	Volleyball: recreational—competitive	3.5–8.0	Dancing:	
Shining shoes	3.2	Golf: foursome—twosome	3.7–5.0	Modern: moderate—vigorous	4.2–5.7
Making bed	3.4	Horseshoes	3.8	Ballroom: waltz—rhumba	5.7–7.0
Dressing	3.4	Baseball (except pitcher)	4.7	Square	7.7
Showering	3.4	Ping pong—table tennis	4.9–7.0	Walking:	
Driving motorcycle	3.4	Calisthenics	5.0	Road—Field (3.5 mph)	5.6–7.0
Metal working	3.5	Rowing: pleasure—vigorous	5.0–15.0	Snow: hard—soft (3.5–2.5 mph)	10.0–20.0
House painting	3.5	Cycling: 5–15 mph (10 speed)	5.0–12.0	Uphill: 5–10–15% (3.5 mph)	8.0–11.0–15.0
Cleaning windows	3.7	Skating: recreation—vigorous	5.0–15.0	Downhill: 5–10% (2.5 mph)	3.6–3.5
Carpentry	3.8	Archery	5.2	15–20% (2.5 mph)	3.7–4.3
Farming chores	3.8	Badminton: recreational—competitive	5.2–10.0	Hiking: 40-lb pack (3.0 mph)	6.8
Sweeping floors	3.9	Basketball: half—full court (more for fast break)	6.0–9.0	Running:	
Plastering walls	4.1	Bowling (while active)	7.0	12-min mile (5 mph)	10.0
Truck and automobile repair	4.2	Tennis: recreational—competitive	7.0–11.0	8-min mile (7.5 mph)	15.0
Ironing clothes	4.2	Water skiing	8.0	6-min mile (10 mph)	20.0
Farming, planting, hoeing, raking	4.7	Soccer	9.0	5-min mile (12 mph)	25.0
Mixing cement	4.7	Snowshoeing (2.5 mph)	9.0		

* From Sharkey BJ: Physiology of Fitness. Champaign, IL, Human Kinetics Publishers, 1979.
† Depends on efficiency and body size. Add 10% for each 15 lb over 150, subtract 10% for each 15 lb under 150.

ate amounts of activity. This method provides a measure of energy expended in the form of heat but provides no information on the kind of fuel being oxidized. Its use is also limited by expense and by a lack of appropriate facilities.

INDIRECT CALORIMETRY. The indirect method measures the metabolic rate by determining with a spirometer the oxygen consumption and carbon dioxide production of the body over a given period of time. (In practice, an estimated value is usually used for CO_2 production, and only oxygen intake is measured.) This procedure has the advantage of mobility and low equipment cost and may be applied when the subject is lying at rest or engaged in various activities (Fig. 2–6). Metabolic carts are used at the hospital bedside to assess patients' energy requirements.

Data are obtained in a form that permits calculation of the *respiratory quotient (RQ):*

$$RQ = \text{moles } CO_2 \text{ expired/moles } O_2 \text{ consumed}$$

This determination is converted into kilocalories of heat produced per square meter of body surface per hour and is extrapolated to energy expenditure in 24 hours.

The RQ depends on the fuel mixture being metabolized. The RQ for carbohydrate is 1.00, because the same number of CO_2 molecules are produced as O_2 molecules consumed. The approximate RQ for fat is 0.7 and for protein 0.82. The RQ for a mixed diet is generally accepted to be 0.85. The energy value of 4.825 kcal/l of oxygen consumed (5 kcal/l for ease of calculation) is used as the factor for estimating the energy expenditure based on oxygen consumption. This unit is called a *metabolic equivalent (MET)* (see Clinical Insight, p. 351).

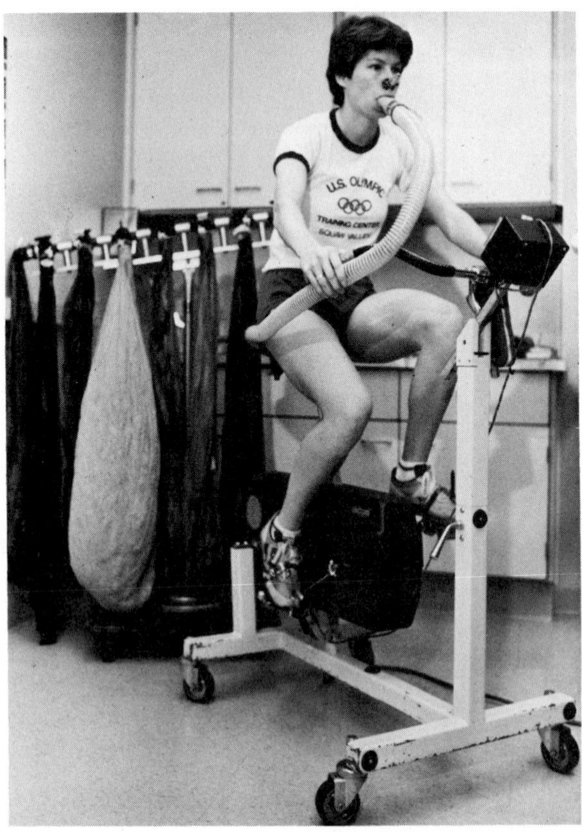

FIGURE 2–6. *Indirect calorimetry using open-circuit spirometry to determine energy expenditure of woman riding a bicycle.*

Measuring Food Energy

The total energy available from a food is measured by means of a *bomb calorimeter.* This device consists of a closed container in which a weighed food sample is burned in an oxygen atmosphere by ignition with an electric spark. The container is immersed in a known volume of water, and the rise in temperature of the water after ignition of food is used to calculate the heat energy generated.

Not all of the energy in foods and alcohol is available to the cells. The processes of digestion and absorption are not completely efficient, and the nitrogenous portion of amino acids is not oxidized but is excreted in the form of urea. Therefore, the biologically available energy from foods and alcohol is expressed in values rounded off slightly below those obtained in the calorimeter. These values for protein, fat, carbohydrate, and alcohol are 4, 9, 4, and 7 kcal/g, respectively, which are summarized in Figure 2–7. The kilocalorie content of various foods is given in Appendix Table 1.

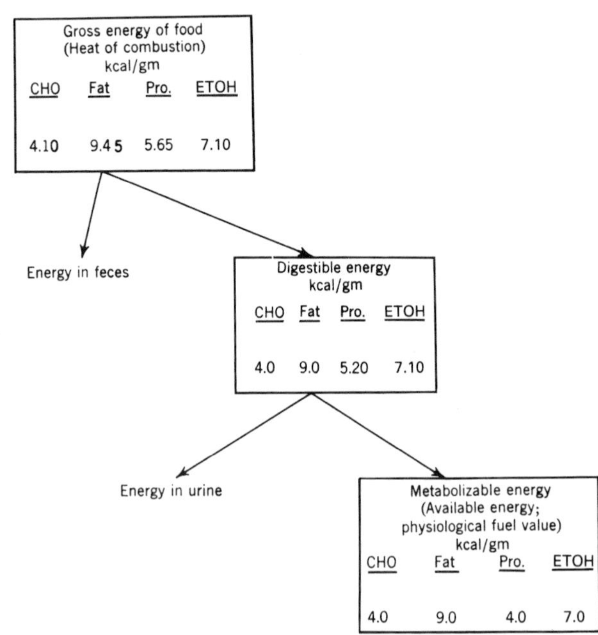

FIGURE 2–7. *Energy value of food. (Adapted from Pike RL, and Brown ML: Nutrition: An Integrated Approach, 2nd ed. New York, John Wiley, 1975.)*

ENERGY CALCULATIONS

Calculating Human Energy Requirements

The total daily energy requirement is commonly estimated by adding together the REE, the energy requirement for physical activity, and the TEF.

Resting Energy Expenditure

The method used for obtaining the REE depends on the degree of accuracy desired. When accurate knowledge of the REE is an important feature of treatment, it should be obtained by calorimetry. If a general estimate of the REE is sufficient, it is usually obtained by reference to standard tables and equations (Table 2–5).

With the use of more modern techniques, the widely used Harris-Benedict formulas developed in 1919 have been found to overestimate the BEE or REE by 7 to 24% (Daly et al, 1985; Owen et al, 1986 and 1987). The Mifflin-St. Jeor equations correct for this overestimation. However, their use results in an unexplained variability of 30% among individuals of the same sex, height, and weight, possibly owing to individual differences in metabolic efficiency (Mifflin et al, 1990). The World Health Organization (WHO) has decided on the equations using body weight presented in Table 2–6.

TABLE 2–5. Methods for Predicting Resting Energy Expenditure (REE)

Harris and Benedict (1919)

For children and adults, all ages

Women: REE (kcal) = 655.1 + 9.56 W + 1.85 H − 4.68 A

REE (kJ) + 2741 + 40 W + 7.74 H − 28.35 A

Men: REE (kcal) = 66.5 + 13.75 W + 5.0 H − 6.78 A

REE (kJ) + 278 + 57.5 W + 7.74 H − 19.56

(A = age; W = weight in kilograms; H = height in centimeters)

Boothby et al (1921)

Nomogram shown in Figure 2–1.
For children and adults, all ages

Mifflin-St. Jeor (Mifflin et al, 1990)

For adults 19 to 78 years of age

REE (female) = 10 W + 6.25 H − 5A − 161

REE (male) = 10 W + 6.25 H − 5A + 5

(A = age; W = weight in kilograms; H = height in centimeters)

REE based on age and body weight

See Table 2–6.

Abbreviated version for persons of normal height and weight

REE (female) = weight (kg) × 0.95 kcal/kg × 24 hr

REE (male) = weight (kg) × 1 kcal/kg × 24 hr

TABLE 2–6. Equations for Predicting Resting Energy Expenditure (REE) from Body Weight Alone*

Sex and Age Range (Yr)	Equation to Derive REE in kcal/day	SD†
Males		
0–3	(60.9 × wt‡) − 54	53
3–10	(22.7 × wt) + 495	62
10–18	(17.5 × wt) + 651	100
18–30	(15.3 × wt) + 679	151
30–60	(11.6 × wt) + 879	164
>60	(13.5 × wt) + 487	148
Females		
0–3	(61.0 × wt) − 51	61
3–10	(22.5 × wt) + 499	63
10–18	(12.2 × wt) + 746	117
18–30	(14.7 × wt) × 496	121
30–60	(8.7 × wt) + 829	108
>60	(10.5 × wt) + 596	108

* Adapted from Food and Nutrition Board, National Research Council, NAS: Recommended Dietary Allowances, 10th ed. Washington, DC, National Academy Press, 1989.

† Standard deviation (SD) of the differences between actual and computed values.

‡ Weight of person in kilograms.

Calculating REE in the obese involves the question of whether the increased surface area related to excessive fatness does in fact increase the REE, because adipose tissue is not as metabolically active as fat-free mass. Using actual body weight of a person who is more than 125% of ideal body weight (IBW) results in an REE that is too high. On the other hand, using IBW for the calculations does not allow for the increased LBM needed for structural support of the extra adipose tissue or for the increased energy expenditure required to move the excess weight.

Ideally, REE of the obese should be determined on the basis of LBM as determined from underwater weighing or other method (Cunningham, 1982; Webb, 1981) (see Chapter 17). However, when it is necessary to estimate energy requirements of the obese, the following formula has been recommended (Wilkens, 1986):

(ABW − IBW) × 0.25 + IBW = weight to be used for calculating REE

ABW = actual body weight

IBW = ideal body weight

0.25 = percentage of excess body weight that is metabolically active

Physical Activity

Energy expended in physical activity is usually calculated with the use of tables such as Table 2–4. The

TABLE 2–7. Methods for Estimating Total Energy Expenditure (TEE)

Method I:

1. Determine IBW in kilograms. This can be determined from (1) a record of the individual's constant weight, (2) Appendix Table 17, or (3) a formula presented in Chapter 18
2. Determine basal energy expenditure:

   male = 1 kcal/kg of IBW/hr × 24 hr

   female = 0.95 kcal/kg IBM/hr × 24 hr
3. Subtract 0.1 kcal/kg IBW/hr of sleep
4. Add activity increment (30, 50, 75, or 100%)
5. Add TEF (10% of BEE plus activity increment)
6. Sum equals the approximate daily energy requirement

Method II:

Multiply the IBW in kilograms by one of the factors presented in Table 2–3, which includes basal, activity, and TEF.

BEE = basal energy expenditure; IBW = ideal body weight; TEF = thermic effect of food.

calculation should include a factor for body size or weight to allow for the extra energy expended by the heavier person.

Thermic Effect of Food

Actual measurement of TEF is appropriate only for research purposes. For practical purposes, it is determined as 10% of the sum of the REE and energy expended in physical activity.

Total Energy Expenditure

Calculations for determining TEE for an individual using two different methods are given in Table 2–7. Application of those methods to an example, as seen in Table 2–8, shows that the results are very similar.

Calculating Food Energy

Although the energy value of each nutrient is known precisely, only a few foods, such as oils and sugars, are made up of a single nutrient. More commonly foods contain a mixture of protein, fat, and carbohydrate. The energy value of one medium egg (50 g), for example, when calculated in terms of weight, is derived from protein (13%), fat (12%), and carbohydrate (1%) as follows:

Protein:	13% × 50 g = 6.5 g × 4 kcal/g =	26 kcal
Fat:	12% × 50 g = 6 g × 9 kcal/g =	54 kcal
Carbohydrate:	1% × 50 g = 0.5 g × 4 kcal/g =	2 kcal
	Total	82 kcal

Energy values of foods based on chemical analyses may be found in the Agriculture Handbook No. 8 series, published by the US Department of Agriculture. Sources of composition values for common serving sizes of foods are (1) Bowes and Church: Food Values of Portions Commonly Used, 15th ed, 1989, (2) Agriculture Handbook No. 456, Nutritive Value of American Foods in Common Units, Agricultural Research Service, US Department of Agriculture, 1988, and (3) Home and Garden Bulletin No. 72, Nutritive Value of Foods, Human Nutrition Information Service, US Department of Agriculture, 1981. The approximate energy content of any diet can be estimated from Appendix Table 1.

Kilocalories in alcoholic beverages may be calculated as shown in Clinical Insight (see below).

RECOMMENDED ENERGY ALLOWANCES

The recommendations for energy intake for adults, revised in 1989 by the Food and Nutrition Board, National Research Council, National Academy of Sciences, are given in Table 2–9.

The recommended allowances are based on a light-to-moderate activity level and are calculated by using

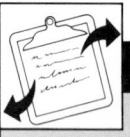

CLINICAL INSIGHT: Calculation of Energy Content of Alcoholic Beverages

The energy value of alcoholic beverages in kilocalories can be determined by the following equation (Gastineau, 1976):

kilocalories = ounces of beverage × proof × 0.8 kcal/proof/oz

proof: the proportion of alcohol to water or other liquids in an alcoholic beverage. The standard in the United States defines "100 proof" as equal to 50% of ethyl alcohol by volume.

To determine the percentage of ethyl alcohol in a beverage, divide the "proof" by 2. For example, a volume of whiskey that is "86 proof" will contain 43% ethyl alcohol.

0.8 kcal/proof/oz = the factor necessary to account for the caloric density of alcohol (7 kcal/g) and the fact that not all of the alcohol in liquor is available for energy.

For example, the number of kilocalories in 1½ oz of 86 proof whiskey would be determined as follows:

1½ oz × 86 proof × 0.8 kcal/proof/oz = 103 kcal

TABLE 2–8. Calculation of Total Energy Expenditure (TEE)

Example:	20-year-old woman, 165 cm tall and weighing 55 kg Activity: light
Method I:	a. Determine IBW—55 kg is IBW for this woman b. Basal needs = 0.95 kcal/kg IBW/hr × 55 kg × 24 hr = 1,254 kcal (5,250 kJ) c. Sleep = 0.1 kcal/kg IBW/hr × 55 kg × 8 hr = 45 kcal 1,254 kcal − 45 kcal = 1,209 kcal d. Activity: light = 50% above basal = 627 kcal (2,600 kJ) 1,209 kcal + 627 kcal = 1,836 kcal (7,850 kJ) e. TEF = 10% above energy requirement = 186 kcal 1836 kcal + 186 kcal = **2,024** *kcal/day (8500 kJ/day)*
Method 2:	Factor for light activity from Table 2–3 = 35 kcal/kg/day 55 kg × 35 kcal/kg/day = **1,925** kcal/day

The difference of 99 kcal/day between these two calculations is a minor one (5%). This calculation of TEE is only a guideline and should be adjusted depending on whether the individual maintains her weight on this level of energy intake. (IBW = ideal body weight; kJ = kilojoule; TEE = total energy expenditure; TEF = thermic effect of food.)

TABLE 2–9. Recommended Dietary Allowances for Energy*

		Weight		Height			Average Energy Allowance (kcal)†		
Category	**Age (Yr) or Condition**	*(kg)*	*(lb)*	*(cm)*	*(in)*	**REE‡ (kcal/day)**	***Multiples of REE***	***Per kg***	***Per day§***
Infants	0.0–0.5	6	13	60	24	320		108	650
	0.5–1.0	9	20	71	28	500		98	850
Children	1–3	13	29	90	35	740		102	1,300
	4–6	20	44	112	44	950		90	1,800
	7–10	28	62	132	52	1,130		70	2,000
Males	11–14	45	99	157	62	1,440	1.70	55	2,500
	15–18	66	145	176	69	1,760	1.67	45	3,000
	19–24	72	160	177	70	1,780	1.67	40	2,900
	25–50	79	174	176	70	1,800	1.60	37	2,900
	51+	77	170	173	68	1,530	1.50	30	2,300
Females	11–14	46	101	157	62	1,310	1.67	47	2,200
	15–18	55	120	163	64	1,370	1.60	40	2,200
	19–24	58	128	164	65	1,350	1.60	38	2,200
	25–50	63	138	163	64	1,380	1.55	36	2,200
	51+	65	143	160	63	1,280	1.50	30	1,900
Pregnant	1st trimester								+0
	2nd trimester								+300
	3rd trimester								+300
Lactating	1st 6 months								+500
	2nd 6 months								+500

* From Food and Nutrition Board. National Research Council, NAS: Recommended Dietary Allowances, 10th ed. National Academy Press, 1989.
† In the range of light to moderate activity, the coefficient of variation is ±20%.
‡ Calculation based on FAO equations (see Table 2–6), then rounded.
§ Figure is rounded.

the WHO (1985) equations for the calculation of REE. REE are multiplied by an activity factor appropriate to age and sex. The activity factors for men aged 19 to 24, 25 to 50, and 51 to 75 are 1.67, 1.6, and 1.5, respectively. Factors for women of the same age groups are 1.6, 1.55, and 1.5. Allowances for persons with heavy activity patterns should be adjusted to 2.0 × REE or higher.

The average daily energy allowances for the reference man (79 kg) and woman (63 kg) are 2,900 kcal and 2,200 kcal, respectively. The coefficient of variation in energy requirements of adults is approximately 20% (Food and Nutrition Board, 1989).

CITED REFERENCES

Boothby WM and Sandiford RB: Nomographic charts for the calculation of the metabolic rate by the gasometer method. Boston Med Surg J 185:337, 1921.

Bray G: The acute effects of food intake on energy expenditure during cycle ergometry. Am J Clin Nutr 27:254, 1974.

Bursztein S et al: Energy Metabolism: Indirect Calorimetry and Nutrition. Baltimore, MD, Williams & Wilkins, 1989.

Cunningham JJ: An individualization of dietary requirements for energy in adults. J Am Diet Assoc 80:335, 1982.

Daly JM et al: Human energy requirements: Overestimation by widely used prediction equation. Am J Clin Nutr 42:1170, 1985.

Dulloo AG et al: Normal caffeine consumption: Influence on thermogenesis and daily energy expenditure in lean and post-obese human volunteers. Am J Clin Nutr 49:44, 1989.

Food and Nutrition Board, National Research Council, National

Academy of Sciences: Recommended Dietary Allowances, 10th ed. Washington, DC, National Academy Press, 1989.
Gastineau CF: Alcohol and calories. Mayo Clin Proc 51(2):88, 1976.
Harris JA and Benedict FG: A Biometric Study of Basal Metabolism in Man. Washington, Carnegie Institute of Washington, Publ No 279, 1919.
Hofstetter A: Increased 24-hour energy expenditure in cigarette smokers. N Engl J Med 314:79, 1986.
Mifflin MD et al: A new predictive equation for resting energy expenditure in healthy individuals. Am J Clin Nutr 51:241, 1990.
Owen OE et al: A reappraisal of caloric requirements in healthy women. Am J Clin Nutr 44:1, 1986.
Owen OE et al: A reappraisal of the caloric requirements of men. Am J Clin Nutr 46:875, 1987.
Roberts SB and Young VR: Energy costs of fat and protein deposition in the human infant. Am J Clin Nutr 48:951, 1988.
Solomon SJ et al: Menstrual cycle and basal metabolic rate in women. Am J Clin Nutr 36:611, 1982.
Tzankoff SP and Norris AH: Longitudinal changes in basal metabolism in man. J Appl Physiol 45:536, 1978.
Webb P: 24 hour energy expenditure and the menstrual cycle. Am J Clin Nutr 44:614, 1986.
WHO: Energy and Protein Requirements. Report of a Joint FAO/WHO/UNU Expert Consultation. Technical Report Series 724. Geneva, World Health Organization, 1985.
Wilkens K (ed): Suggested Guidelines for Nutrition Care of Renal Patients. Chicago, American Dietetic Association, 1986, p 34.

ADDITIONAL REFERENCES

Du Bois EF: Basal Metabolism in Health and Disease. Philadelphia, Lea & Febiger, 1927, pp 141–147.
Fleisch A: New Methods of Studying Gaseous Exchange and Pulmonary Function. Springfield, IL, Charles C Thomas, 1960.
Foster GD et al: Resting energy expenditure, body composition and excess weight in the obese. Metabolism 37:467, 1988.
Haycock GB et al: Geometric method for measuring body surface area: A height-weight formula validated in infants, children and adults. J Pediatr 93:62, 1978.
McArdle WD, Katch FI, and Katch VL: Exercise Physiology, 2nd ed. Philadelphia, Lea & Febiger, 1986, p 131.
Owen OE: Resting metabolic requirements of men and women. Mayo Clin Proc 63:503, 1988.
Sukhatme PV and Margen S: Autoregulatory homeostatic nature of energy balance. Am J Clin Nutr 35:355, 1982.
Turcotte G: Erroneous nomogram for body surface area (Letter to the Editor). N Engl J Med 300:1339, 1979.
Webb P: Energy expenditure and fat-free mass in men and women. Am J Clin Nutr 34:1816, 1981.

CHAPTER 3

CARBOHYDRATES

CHAPTER OUTLINE

KEY TERMS

AMYLOPECTIN—a form of starch; branched chains of glucose units

AMYLOSE—a form of starch; long straight chains of glucose units

CELLULOSE—a structural carbohydrate in plants that resists hydrolysis in the human digestive tract

CRUDE FIBER—the amount of plant material remaining after being subjected to treatment with acid and alkali

DEXTRIN—an intermediate product of starch hydrolysis

DEXTROSE—glucose produced by the hydrolysis of corn starch

DIETARY FIBER—the amount of plant material remaining after treatment with digestive enzymes and reduction with acid and alkali

DISACCHARIDE—a sugar capable of being hydrolyzed to two monosaccharide molecules

FIBER (ROUGHAGE)—compounds of plant origin that are not capable of hydrolysis by enzymes in the human gut

FRUCTOSE—a monosaccharide occurring in fruit, honey and some vegetables; the sweetest of the monosaccharides

GALACTOSE—a monosaccharide produced by the hydrolysis of lactose by digestive enzymes

GLUCONEOGENESIS—the formation of glucose from noncarbohydrate molecules, such as glycerol and the carbon skeletons of amino acids

GLUCOSE—the main monosaccharide in blood and an important source of energy for living organisms; plentiful in fruits, sweet corn, corn syrup, honey, and certain roots

GLYCOGEN—storage form of carbohydrate in animals

GLYCOGENOLYSIS—the hydrolysis of glycogen to yield glucose

HEMICELLULOSES (NONCELLULOSE POLYSACCHARIDES)—a group of high molecular polysaccharides that resemble cellulose but are more soluble and more easily decomposed

INSOLUBLE FIBER—cellulose and some hemicelluloses that do not dissolve in water

LACTOSE—a disaccharide composed of glucose and galactose; the principal sugar found in mammalian milk

LIGNIN—a noncarbohydrate material sometimes included in fiber determination that is a major component of the woody portion of plants

MALTOSE (MALT SUGAR)—a disaccharide composed of two glucose units

MANNITOL—a sugar alcohol that exists in fruit, is poorly digested, and yields about half as many calories as glucose

MODIFIED FOOD STARCH—starch that has been treated with a variety of chemicals so that it can still function as a thickening agent but can also form solutions with cold water that maintain stability in the presence of acid, freezing, and thawing

MONOSACCHARIDE—a sugar incapable of being hydrolyzed to a simpler form

OLIGOSACCHARIDE—a carbohydrate that upon hydrolysis yields 3 to 10 monosaccharide units

PECTIN—a noncellulose polysaccharide made up of units of a derivative of galactose that is found in fruit

POLYSACCHARIDE—a carbohydrate that upon hydrolysis yields more than 10 monosaccharide units

SOLUBLE FIBER—pectins, gums, mucilages, and some hemicelluloses that form gels with water

SORBITOL—a sugar alcohol occurring naturally in fruits; in mammals is found in some tissues such as the lens of the eye

SUCROSE—ordinary table sugar; a disaccharide composed of glucose and fructose found in sugar cane, sugar beets, molasses, maple syrup, maple sugar, fruit, vegetables, and honey

XYLITOL—a noncariogenic sugar alcohol absorbed one fifth as fast as glucose and often used in sugarless chewing gum

Most of the energy that is needed to move, perform work, and live is consumed in the form of carbohydrates. As grains they have the highest yield of energy per acre of land and constitute the major source of food for the people of the world. Carbohydrates, primarily starches, are the least expensive, the most easily obtained, and the most readily digested form of fuel.

DEFINITION AND COMPOSITION

Carbohydrates are organic compounds that consist of carbon, hydrogen, and oxygen. In their simplest form the general formula is $C_n H_{2n} O_n$. They vary from simple sugars containing from three to seven carbon atoms to very complex polymers. Only the *hexoses* (six-carbon sugars) and *pentoses* (five-carbon sugars) and their polymers play important roles in nutrition.

Photosynthesis

Plants manufacture and store carbohydrates as their chief source of energy. Carbon dioxide from the air and water from the soil are brought together in green leaves where, in the presence of chlorophyll acting as a catalyst, they incorporate the energy of sunlight to form glucose, an elementary carbohydrate. Oxygen is released into the atmosphere as a by-product (Fig. 3–1).

The carbohydrate synthesized in the leaves is used as the basis for more complex forms of carbohydrate and other organic compounds. When consumed by animals, these forms also constitute the basis for animal life. Thus it can be said that the sun furnishes the energy for all living matter. To recover this locked-in energy, the carbohydrates and other organic compounds are eventually metabolized with the input of oxygen. The by-products of carbon dioxide and water

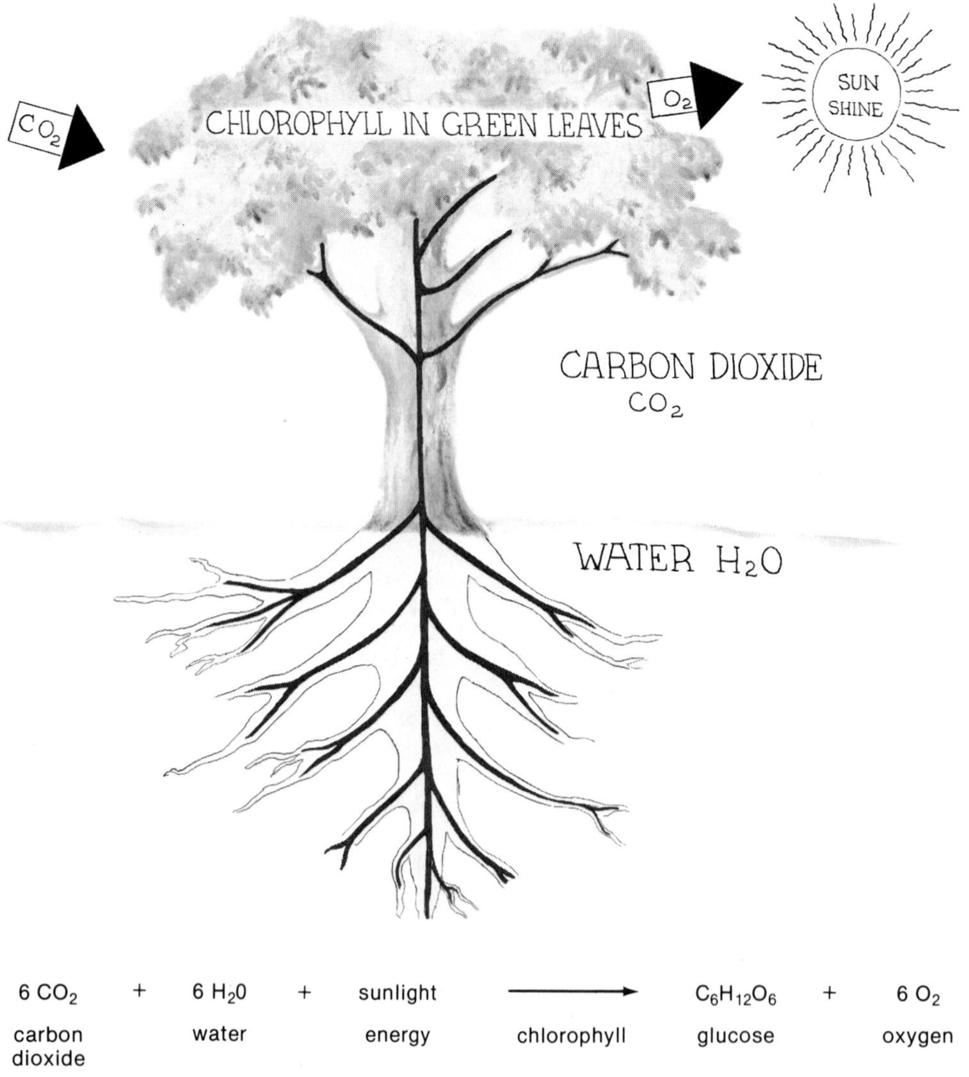

$$6\,CO_2 + 6\,H_2O + \text{sunlight} \xrightarrow{\text{chlorophyll}} C_6H_{12}O_6 + 6\,O_2$$

carbon dioxide — water — energy — chlorophyll — glucose — oxygen

FIGURE 3–1. *Synthesis of carbohydrates in plant life. Light from the sun is harnessed by the green chlorophyll of plant leaves. Cells in green leaves utilize this energy in synthesizing carbohydrates from the carbon dioxide in the air and the water in the soil. Carbohydrates are the chief form in which plants store potential energy.*

are then available to be taken up by the leaves and once more initiate the cycle.

CLASSIFICATION

Carbohydrate classification reflects the fact that all forms, from glucose to those of increasing complexity, are related to the simple sugars or "saccharides." *Monosaccharides* are incapable of being hydrolyzed to a simpler form. *Disaccharides* may be hydrolyzed to give two monosaccharide molecules. *Oligosaccharides* yield from three to ten monosaccharide units, and *polysaccharides* yield from ten units to 10,000 or more.

Monosaccharides

The principal monosaccharides that occur free in foods are *glucose* and *fructose.* They may exist in either an open-chain structure or a ring structure as shown in Figure 3–2. When linked together as disaccharides or polysaccharides they are held in the cyclic form. *Galactose* and *mannose* have the same structure as glucose, except for the orientation of the hydroxyl groups around the six carbon atoms.

Glucose (dextrose) is abundant in fruits, sweet corn, corn syrup, honey, and certain roots (Table 3–1). It is the principal product formed by hydrolysis of more complex carbohydrates in the process of digestion and is the form of sugar normally found in the blood stream. It is oxidized in the cells as a source of energy and is stored in the liver and muscles in the form of *glycogen.* Under normal conditions the central nervous system can use only glucose as a major fuel source.

Fructose (levulose, fruit sugar) is found together with glucose and sucrose in honey and fruit (Further Reading, p. 33). As shown in Table 3–2, it is the sweetest of the sugars. Large quantities of fructose can be manufactured relatively inexpensively from starch, and it is used commercially in sweeteners, such as high-fructose corn syrup. Soft drinks, for example, are now almost completely sweetened with high-fructose corn syrup rather than sucrose.

Galactose is not found free in nature but is produced from lactose (milk sugar) by hydrolysis in the digestive process.

Disaccharides

Each of the three common disaccharides consists of two monosaccharide molecules, at least one of which is glucose.

Sucrose = glucose and fructose

Maltose = glucose and glucose

Lactose = glucose and galactose

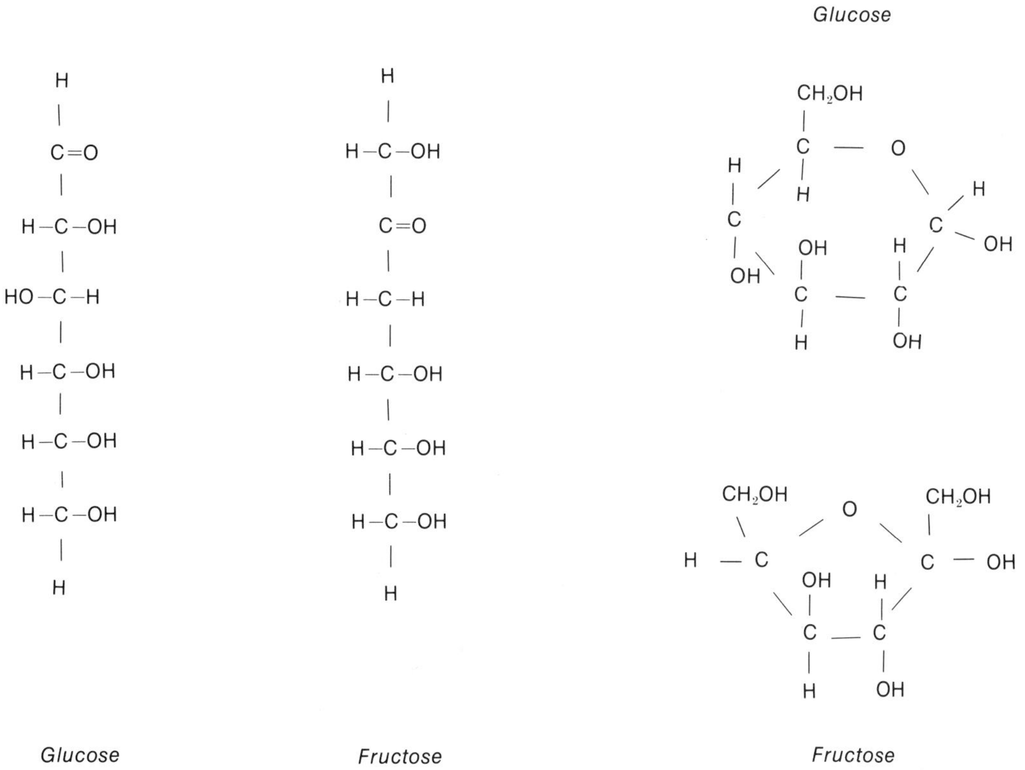

```
    H                 H
    |                 |
   C=O             H-C-OH
    |                 |
  H-C-OH             C=O
    |                 |
 HO-C-H             H-C-H
    |                 |
  H-C-OH            H-C-OH
    |                 |
  H-C-OH            H-C-OH
    |                 |
  H-C-OH            H-C-OH
    |                 |
    H                 H

 Glucose           Fructose
```

Glucose (ring form): CH_2OH, C, O, H, C, OH, H, OH, C, C, H, OH

Fructose (ring form): CH_2OH, O, CH_2OH, H — C, C — OH, OH, H, C, C, H, OH

FIGURE 3–2. *Structure of glucose and fructose.*

TABLE 3–1. Types, Sources and End-Products of Carbohydrates

Carbohydrates	Chief Food Sources	End-Products of Digestion	Remarks
Polysaccharides:			
Indigestible			
1. Cellulose	Stalks and leaves of vegetables; outer covering of seeds	—	May be partially split to glucose by bacterial action in large bowel
2. Hemicelluloses			
3. Pectins	Fruits	—	These substances have an affinity for water, form bulk, and slow gastric emptying time and may bind bile acids
4. Gums and mucilages	Plant secretions and seeds		
5. Algal substances	Seaweeds and algae	—	
Partially digestible			
1. Inulin	Jerusalem artichokes, onions, garlic, and mushrooms	Fructose	Digestion is incomplete; further splitting by bacteria may occur in the large bowel; may be production of flatus from raffinose and stachyose
2. Galactogens	Snails	Galactose	
3. Mannosans	Legumes	Mannose	
4. Raffinose	Sugar beets, kidney beans, lentils, and navy beans	Glucose, fructose, and galactose	
5. Stachyose	Beans	Pentoses	
6. Pentosans	Fruits and gums		
Digestible			
1. Starch and dextrins	Grains; vegetables (especially tubers and legumes)	Glucose	The most important group quantitatively; usually accompanied by some maltose
2. Glycogen	Meat products and seafood	Glucose	
Disaccharides and Oligosaccharides:			
1. Sucrose	Cane and beet sugars, molasses, and maple syrup	Glucose and fructose	
2. Lactose	Milk and milk products	Glucose and galactose	
3. Lactulose	Synthetic products	Not metabolized	Does not appear in foods; is synthetic, not digested; and is used as a laxative
4. Maltose and maltotriose	Malt products, some breakfast cereals	Glucose	
5. Trehalose	Mushrooms, insects, yeast	Glucose	
Monosaccharides:			
Hexoses:			
1. Glucose	Fruits; honey; corn syrup	Glucose	In fruits and vegetables the contents of glucose and fructose depend on species, ripeness, and state of preservation
Sorbitol	Fruits, vegetables, dietetic products		
2. Fructose	Fruits; honey	Fructose	
3. Galactose	—	Galactose	These monosaccharides do not occur in free form in foods
4. Mannose	—	Mannose	
Mannitol	Pineapples, olives, asparagus, sweet potatoes, carrots, and dietetic products		
Pentoses:			
1. Ribose	—	Ribose	Ribose, xylose and arabinose do not occur in free form in foods. They are derived from pentosans of fruits and from the nucleic acids of meat products and seafood
2. Xylose	Fruits, vegetables, cereals, mushrooms, seaweed, dietetic chewing gum, and other dietetic products	Xylose	
Xylitol			
3. Arabinose	—	Arabinose	
Carbohydrate Derivatives:			
1. Ethyl alcohol	Fermented liquors		
2. Lactic acid	Milk and milk products	Absorbed as same	These substances are the products of natural or induced carbohydrate breakdown
3. Malic acid	Fruits		
4. Citric acid	Fruits		

Sucrose is ordinary table sugar. It is found mainly in sugar cane, sugar beets, molasses, maple syrup, and maple sugar as well as in fruit, vegetables, and honey. When sucrose is hydrolyzed by digestive enzymes or boiled with acid, it is converted to a mixture of equal parts of glucose and fructose. Because the monosaccharide molecules are smaller, this mixture, called *invert sugar,* is frequently used in commercial sugar mixtures such as candies and icings to prevent the formation of coarse sugar crystals.

Maltose (malt sugar) does not ordinarily occur free in nature. It is created during the process of digestion by enzymes that break down large starch molecules to disaccharide fragments, which can then be split into two glucose molecules for easy absorption. This occurs in nature when the seed of a cereal grain sprouts and its

TABLE 3–2. Sweetness of Sugars

Sugar or Sugar Product	Sweetness Value
Levulose, fructose	173
Invert sugar	130
Sucrose	100
Glucose	74
Sorbitol	60
Mannitol	50
Galactose	32
Maltose	32
Lactose	16

enzymes convert the grain's starch into maltose. Barley malt, for example, is used as a sweetener in some products. A similar reaction occurs in beer manufacture when starch is hydrolyzed by diastase, a plant enzyme obtained from sprouting grain.

Lactose (milk sugar) is the principal sugar found in milk. It does not occur in plants and is limited almost exclusively to the mammary glands of lactating animals. It is less soluble than the other disaccharides and is only about one sixth as sweet as glucose. Upon hydrolysis it yields glucose and galactose. This sugar is of clinical significance in persons who lack sufficient digestive enzyme (lactase) for efficient hydrolysis and in young children who are born without the liver enzyme that converts galactose to glucose.

Polyhydroxy Alcohols

The alcohol forms of sucrose, mannose, and xylose (*sorbitol, mannitol,* and *xylitol,* respectively) retain some of the sweetness of the original sugars. Because they are absorbed more slowly from the digestive tract and thus inhibit a rapid rise in blood sugar, they are often used in products designed for persons who are unable to tolerate high-sugar intakes. The slow absorption of sugar alcohols can also lead to soft stools and diarrhea when they are consumed in amounts of 1 oz or more.

Sorbitol, which occurs naturally in fruits, has a sweetening power similar to glucose. It is absorbed eventually with relative efficiency from the digestive tract and thus has the same energy value as glucose. *Mannitol,* which also exists in fruit, is poorly digested and yields about one half as many calories per gram as glucose. *Xylitol* is absorbed only one fifth as fast as glucose. It is often used in sugarless chewing gums, because cariogenic bacteria are unable to use it as a substrate.

FURTHER READING: Honey

Honey is a unique carbohydrate food. It begins, of course, as the nectar of a flower, which is harvested by the honeybee and transported to the hive. The sweetness that attracts the bee consists mostly of sucrose at this point. During the journey back to the hive and while it is being deposited in the comb, the bee invests the nectar with the enzyme invertase, which hydrolyzes most of the sucrose into glucose and fructose. The unripe honey is deposited in the comb in a manner that permits maximum evaporation, and after several hours of ripening the concentrated product is stored in sealed cells of the honeycomb. The final composition of mature honey varies, but a typical analysis is given as glucose, 34%; fructose, 41%; sucrose, 2.4%; and water, 18.3%.

The sweetness of honey varies with the concentration and the degree of crystallization. It is generally thought to be sweeter than sugar, but there is considerable variation in individual perception of sweetness, which may rank it from 57 to 122% that of sucrose.

Most honey available commercially has been heated to a temperature of 150 to 160° F to prevent the crystallization and yeast fermentation that may occur during storage. So-called "organic" products are usually raw honeys that have not been processed.

The low temperatures used in processing honey are not sufficient to destroy the spores of *Clostridium botulinum.* These spores, which are widely distributed in soils and agricultural products, are normally a hazard only when they are permitted to germinate and form the deadly botulinum toxin, a circumstance that does not occur in the high sugar concentration of honey. However, conditions in the gastrointestinal tracts of very young infants sometimes favor spore germination and toxin production with the consequent development of infant botulism. It has therefore been recommended that honey—commonly used to sweeten infant pacifiers—should not be fed to infants under 1 year of age.

Contrary to popular belief, there are no nutritional advantages in the choice of honey, and because of its concentrated form it is actually higher in sucrose than table sugar. One tablespoon of honey contains 64 kcal compared with 46 kcal in an equal amount of sugar. Although honey contains vitamins and minerals that are not available in refined sugars, the trace amounts involved are inconsequential in terms of daily needs. Because sucrose is rapidly hydrolyzed to glucose and fructose in the small intestine, there is little difference in absorption time between sugar and honey.

The unique feature of honey is its high fructose content. Fructose in the blood is converted primarily to glycogen in the liver, a process that does not require insulin. However, its high content of glucose means that honey must still be a controlled food for persons with diabetes.

Polysaccharides

Most of the polysaccharides of interest in nutrition (starch, dextrin, glycogen, and cellulose) are assembled from glucose units, differing only in the kind of linkage. Other polysaccharides may contain monosaccharides other than glucose, either singly or in combination. As a group, polysaccharides are less soluble and more stable than the simpler sugars. Starch and glycogen are completely digestible; other polysaccharides are partly and sometimes completely indigestible.

Starch is found only in plants. It occurs in both the *amylose* form (long straight chains of glucose units) and the *amylopectin* form (branched chains of glucose units). The proportion of each form determines the nature of the starch, which is typical for each plant species. Starch granules of varying sizes and shapes are encased within the plant cells by cellulose walls. They are insoluble in cold water. Cooking causes the granules to swell and the mixture to gel. Cooking also softens and ruptures the cell to make the starch available for enzymatic digestive processes.

Modified food starch is a popular thickening agent used in commercially prepared foods, such as salad dressings, pie fillings, canned soups, gravies, canned puddings, and baby food. Although it differs structurally, the energy value is the same as for natural starch. The modification process permits the retention of desirable thickening properties after cooling and storage that are lost in ordinary starch.

Dextrins are intermediate products that occur in the hydrolysis of starch. These are formed during the process of digestion and also as the result of a variety of commercial processes using acid, enzymes, or dry heat. As they decrease in size, saccharide molecules increase in solubility and sweetness. These properties find commercial applications in products such as corn syrup, which is high in dextrins.

Glycogen is the storage form of carbohydrate in humans and animals and is the primary and most readily available source of glucose and energy. It consists of branched chains of glucose units similar to those in plant starch (Fig. 3–3). Normally about ¾ lb of glyco-

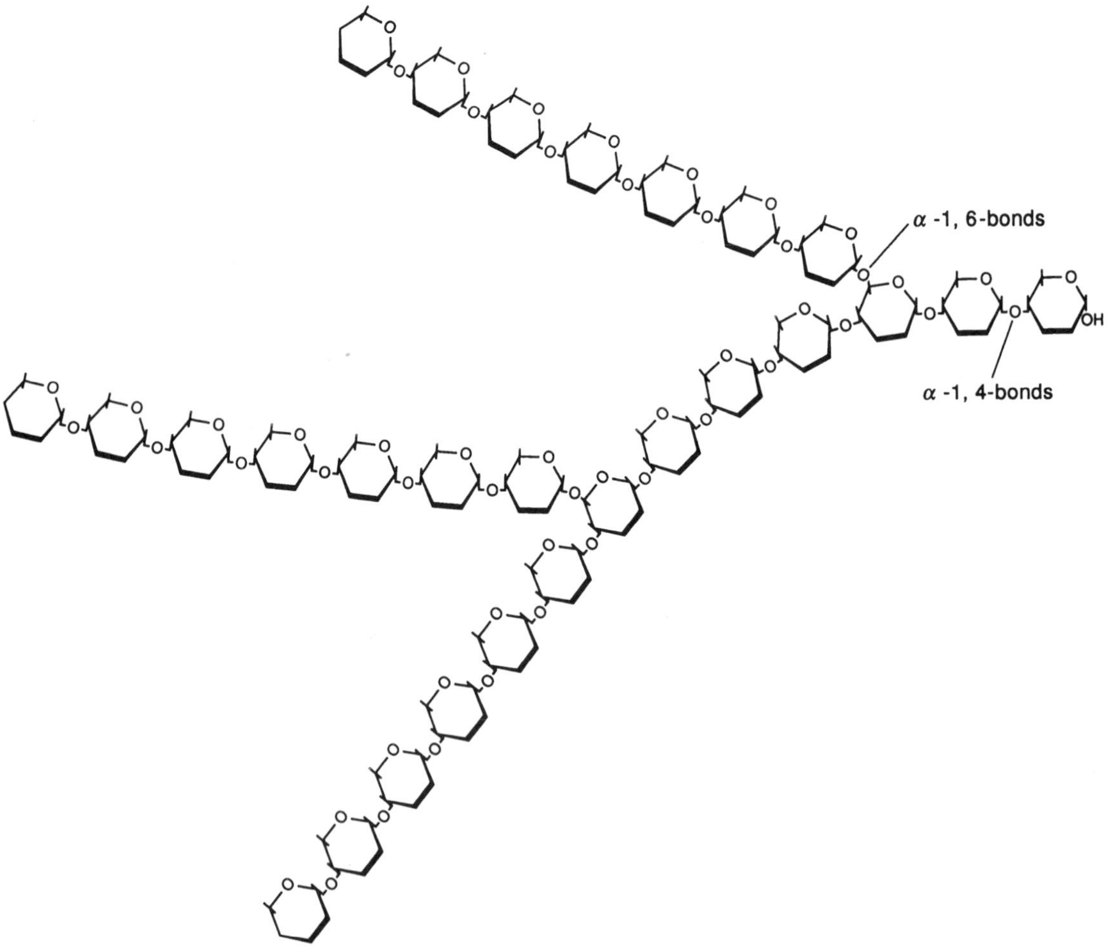

α -1, 6-bonds

α -1, 4-bonds

FIGURE 3–3. *Branched nature of glycogen. As seen, the branches are at least seven glucose units long and are separated by at least three glucose units. The bonds involved are α-1, 4-glucosidic linkages between glucose units and 6-glucosidic units at the branch points. (Redrawn from Orten JM and Neuhaus OW: Human Biochemistry, 10th ed. St. Louis, CV Mosby, 1982, p 248.)*

gen, or 340 grams, is stored in liver and muscle. The small amounts of glycogen in animal foods are largely converted to lactic acid before they are available for consumption.

Cellulose and *hemicellulose* constitute the cellular framework of plants. *Cellulose* resembles starch in that it is made up of many glucose molecules in an unbranched form similar to amylose. However, the glucose molecules in cellulose are linked in a form of bonding that resists the action of the enzymes that readily hydrolyze starch (Further Reading, p. 37). Cellulose occurs only in plant materials: fruit and vegetable pulp, skins, stalks, leaves, and in the outer covering of grains, nuts, seeds, and legumes. *Hemicelluloses* or *noncellulose polysaccharides* differ structurally from celluloses in that they have fewer glucose units. They may consist of hexoses, pentoses, and the acid forms of these compounds. Synthetic fiber products, *methyl cellulose* and *carboxymethylcellulose,* are used in laxatives as well as in the production of low-calorie foods because of their ability to produce bulk and a feeling of satiety.

Pectin, a noncellulose polysaccharide, is made up of units of a derivative of galactose. Because it absorbs water and forms a gel, it is widely used for making jams and jellies. It is found in apples, citrus fruits, strawberries, and other fruits to a lesser degree.

Gums and *mucilages* are similar to pectin except that the galactose units are combined with other polysaccharides. They are found in plant secretions or seeds and are often added to processed foods to confer specific qualities. *Algal polysaccharides* are found in seaweeds and algae. *Carageenan* is added as a thickening agent to many processed foods.

CARBOHYDRATE METABOLISM

Monosaccharides

Carbohydrates are delivered to the cells primarily in the form of glucose, along with minor quantities of other monosaccharides. Fructose and galactose are converted to glucose in the liver (Fig. 3–4).

Much of the glucose is oxidized via the citric acid cycle to meet immediate energy needs of all tissues. Some glucose is converted to other necessary carbohydrates, such as ribose, fructose (for spermatozoa), deoxyribose, glucosamine, and galactosamine and to carbon skeletons necessary for the production of nonessential amino acids. Excess carbohydrate is converted to glycogen or fatty acids, which are stored subsequently as triglyceride in adipose tissue.

Galactose is easily converted in the liver to uridine diphosphoglucose, which can either be incorporated into glycogen or can be converted to glucose-1-phosphate and metabolized via the glucose pathways.

The cellular entry of fructose is not insulin-dependent. However, fructose can be converted eventually to glucose, leading to a rise in blood glucose if present in a large amount.

Gluconeogenesis

The blood glucose level is maintained within normal limits through release of glucose from liver glycogen (Fig. 3–5). When necessary, glucose can be made available by the liver through the process of *gluconeogenesis* in which glucose is synthesized from noncarbohydrate carbon chains.

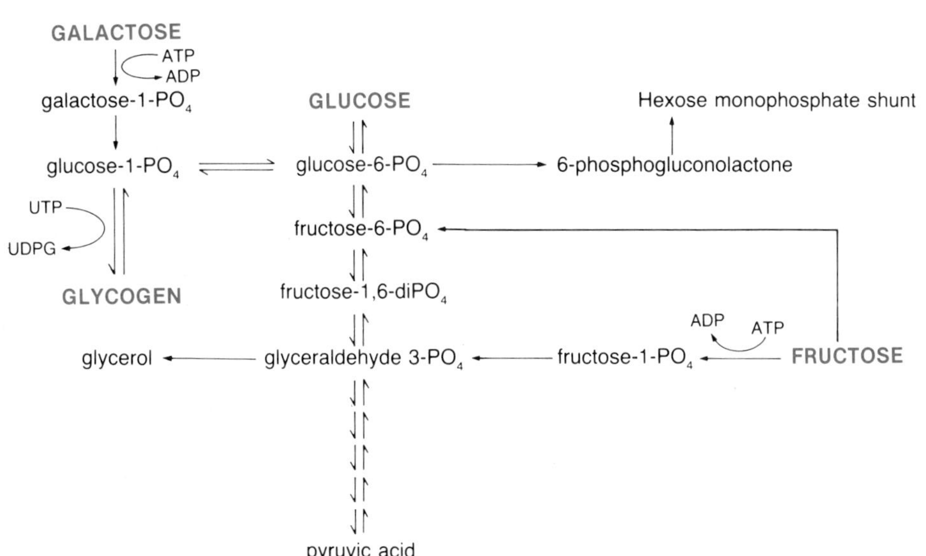

FIGURE 3–4. *Metabolism of fructose, galactose and glucose. UTP = uridine triphosphate; UDPG = uridine diphosphoglucose.*

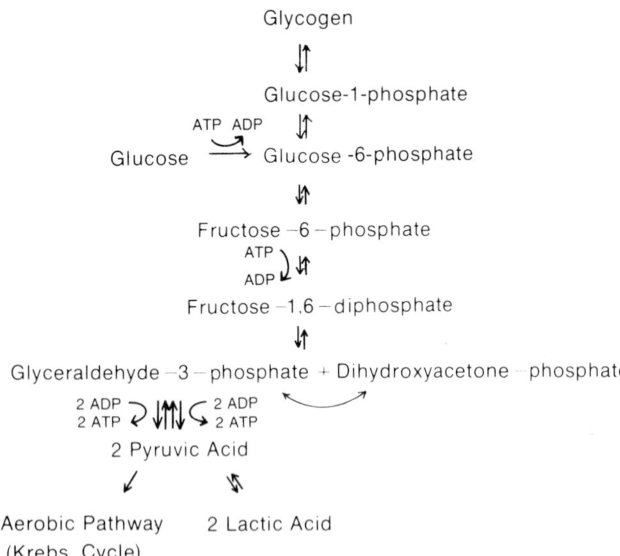

FIGURE 3–5. *Glycogenesis, glycogenolysis, and glycolysis.*

Regulation of Blood Sugar

A number of mechanisms function to maintain blood glucose at a remarkably constant level, 70 to 100 mg/100 ml under fasting conditions. As glucose in the blood is taken up by the tissues, liver glycogen is continually converted to glucose (glycogenolysis) and diffuses into the blood. Muscle glycogen is used for energy only by the muscle and cannot be returned to the blood as glucose; however, lactic acid produced from muscle glycogen oxidation is carried to the liver, where it can be converted to glucose and glycogen (Cori cycle) (Fig. 3–6). When adequate glucose is not available, such as in fasting or prolonged high-level energy expenditure, amino acids are converted to glucose through the process of *gluconeogenesis.*

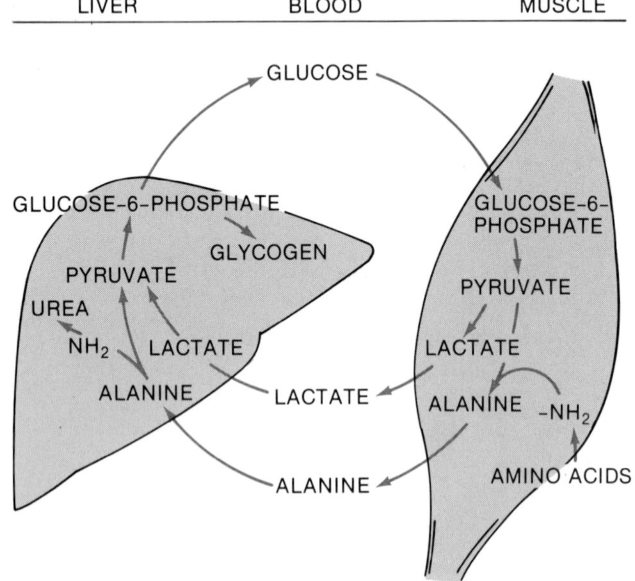

FIGURE 3–6. *The Cori and alanine cycles. The Cori cycle rids the muscle of lactic acid, and the alanine cycle represents the major pathway by which the amino groups from muscle amino acids are conveyed to the liver for conversion to urea.*

Hormonal Controls

A battery of hormones is involved in the regulation of these reactions. *Insulin* is produced by the beta cells of the islets of Langerhans in the pancreas. It has been called the "feasting hormone" because its liberation is enhanced by a high glucose level in the blood and to a lesser extent by the ingestion of protein or infusion of amino acids or ketone bodies. Insulin release is also stimulated by the action of glucagon and the gastrointestinal hormones, as well as by the vagus nerve and certain drugs (e.g., tolbutamide, which is an oral hypoglycemic agent). The mechanism by which insulin lowers blood glucose involves an increase in the rate of glucose utilization for oxidation, glycogenesis, and lipogenesis. Facilitated diffusion of glucose into muscle and adipose cells is increased, glucose is stored as glycogen in the liver and muscle cells, and the uptake of glucose by adipose and liver cells for conversion into fat is enhanced.

Glucagon, produced by the alpha cells of the islets of Langerhans, has an effect exactly opposite to that of insulin. It causes a rise in the amount of sugar in the blood by increasing glycogenolysis and gluconeogenesis and stimulates the release of insulin from the pancreas. Insulin and glucagon may thus be considered antagonists, and it is at least in part through their opposing effects that carbohydrate metabolism is maintained in a steady state.

Epinephrine, a hormone produced by the adrenal medulla, favors the breakdown of liver and muscle glycogen to yield blood glucose (glycogenolysis) and decreases the release of insulin from the pancreas, thus raising the blood sugar. The secretion of epinephrine is increased during anger or fear, and the subsequent glucose formation provides extra energy for crisis response.

Glucocorticoids, steroid hormones elaborated by the adrenal cortex, also influence blood glucose levels by stimulating gluconeogenesis. These hormones reduce glucose utilization and also increase the rate at which protein is converted into glucose, thus counteracting the action of insulin.

Severe lowering of blood glucose concentration increases *thyroxine* secretion. Hepatic glycogenolysis and gluconeogenesis are increased, leading to a rise in blood glucose concentration. Thyroxine also increases the rate of hexose absorption from the intestine.

Growth hormone, elaborated by the anterior pituitary gland, also raises the blood glucose by increasing amino acid uptake and protein synthesis by all cells,

FURTHER READING: Starch Versus Cellulose

The unique structure of cellulose is particularly significant in terms of the food supply. Although cellulose consists entirely of glucose, the human digestive tract is unable to reduce it to a form in which it can be absorbed into the blood. Digestive enzymes are available to hydrolyze the bonds joining chains of glucose molecules in starch and glycogen, but the glucose-to-glucose bonds in cellulose are of a structure that does not fit any of the enzymes in the human digestive tract. As cellulose passes through the digestive tract to excretion, it serves the useful purpose of providing bulk in the large intestine. However, no energy is derived from all those glucose molecules.

Some bacteria produce enzymes capable of reducing cellulose to its glucose components. The digestive systems of ruminants include temporary storage compartments in the form of divided stomachs where food lingers while extensive bacterial action takes place. This is a very important source of glucose production because these animals are thus able to include edibles such as hay and grass as dietary staples, and the energy stored in cellulose is then made available to us indirectly through animal products in the diet.

diminishing cellular uptake of glucose, and increasing the mobilization of fat for energy.

Figure 3–7 summarizes the means by which the processes adding glucose to the blood and removing glucose from the blood exist in dynamic equilibrium, depending on the body's need for energy and the time since the last meal.

FUNCTION OF CARBOHYDRATES IN THE BODY

Carbohydrates in the body function primarily in the form of glucose, although a few have structural roles. Carbohydrate is a major source of energy; each gram yields approximately 4 kcal, regardless of the source.

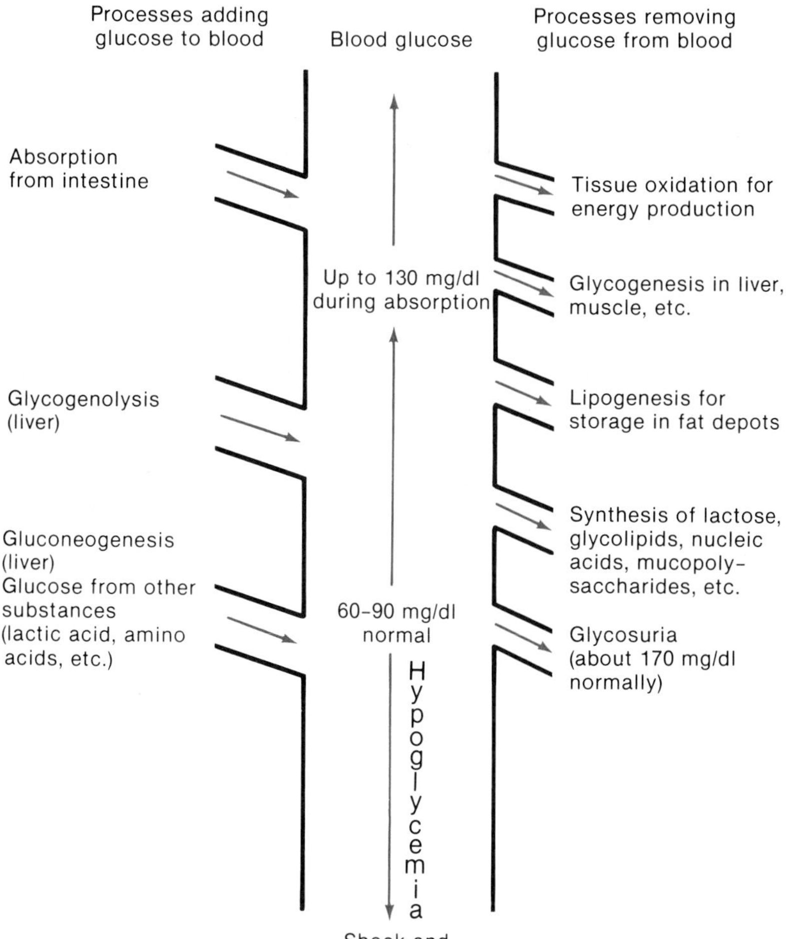

FIGURE 3–7. *Blood glucose maintenance. (Adapted by permission of Macmillan Publishing Company from West, ES et al: Textbook of Biochemistry, 4th ed. Copyright © 1966 by Macmillan Publishing Company.)*

Glucose is indispensable for the maintenance of functional integrity of the nerve tissue and under normal circumstances is the sole source of energy for the brain. The presence of carbohydrates is necessary for normal fat metabolism. In the absence of sufficient carbohydrate, larger amounts of fat are used for energy than the body is equipped to handle, and oxidation is incomplete. The resultant accumulation of acidic intermediates may lead to acidosis and eventually to sodium imbalance and dehydration.

Lactose remains in the intestines longer than the other disaccharides and thus encourages the growth of beneficial bacteria, resulting in a laxative action. One of the functions of these bacteria is believed to be the synthesis of certain vitamins in the large intestine.

Glucuronic acid, a metabolite of glucose, functions in the liver to combine with chemical and bacterial toxins as well as with some normal metabolites to convert them into a form in which they may be excreted.

Carbohydrates and their derivatives serve as precursors to compounds such as nucleic acids, connective tissue matrix, and galactosides of nerve tissue.

DIETARY FIBER

Definition

Substances commonly referred to as *roughage* or *fiber* are compounds of plant origin that are not available as energy sources because they are not capable of hydrolysis by enzymes in the human gut. A more precise definition of fiber is not available because indigestible material includes heterogeneous and complex mixtures of substances, and agreement has not been reached as to which of these constitute a part of "fiber."

Indigestible plant materials include components of the plant cell wall—cellulose, hemicellulose, and pectin—as well as substances from the intracellular cement and others secreted by the plant in response to injury—gums, mucilages, and algal polysaccharides. Not all of these are fibrous (see Table 3–1).

Most of the substances classified as fiber are nonstarch polysaccharides (NSP). However, lignin, a woody substance that occurs in stems and seeds of fruits and vegetables and in the bran layer of cereals, is not even a carbohydrate but a polymer of phenylpropyl alcohols and acids.

Furthermore, depending on the definition, all of the carbohydrate in fiber is not made up of NSP. Some starches that have been modified by processing, both home and commercial, resist enzyme action and are called *resistant starches.* These occur usually at very small levels in foods (less than 1% in bread flour and 3% in cornflakes) although, depending on the extent and nature of various processing methods, this level can be increased to as much as 20% of the total starch in a food (Englyst et al, 1987). Some believe that because the resistant starches are subject to bacterial action in the colon and their end-products affect the nutritional milieu, they should also be considered to be a part of total fiber.

Assay and Food Composition Data

Traditionally, the fiber content of foods has been described in terms of *crude fiber,* determined by subjecting materials to digestion by acid and alkali. Because the actual action of digestive enzymes is less rigorous, the amount of fiber remaining after digestion in the human alimentary tract is considerably greater than that estimated by the crude fiber process. Values obtained for *dietary fiber* as presently measured are usually from two to five times higher than those for crude fiber. However, no correction factors can be applied because the relationship between the two kinds of fiber varies depending on the composition of particular foods. Bran flakes, for example, contain six times as much dietary fiber as crude fiber, but in strawberries the amount of dietary fiber is only 1.6 times greater than crude fiber (Slavin, 1987).

Although it is universally agreed that dietary fiber is the more realistic and informative measurement, such consensus does not as yet extend to methods of assay. The principle area of disagreement is whether lignin and resistant starches should be included in the total.

Because of the relatively recent interest in fiber composition and because of the failure to standardize assay methods, tables of food composition contain fiber information in a variety of different forms. Some are still based on crude fiber, although the proliferation of new dietary fiber data is gradually eliminating these values. The Southgate method for determining dietary fiber was widely used for a time, and the results that appear in many tables of food composition data are currently the most comprehensive (Southgate et al, 1976). The data obtained by the Englyst method are based specifically on nonstarch polysaccharides (Englyst and Hudson, 1987). The method of the Association of Official Analytical Chemists, which is used in the United States, includes both lignin and resistant starches (Prosky et al, 1984).

Characteristics of Fiber

Physical Properties

Components of dietary fiber can be categorized on the basis of physical properties and physiologic roles as *soluble fiber* and *insoluble fiber* (Table 3–3).

TABLE 3–3. Sources of Fiber Components

Insoluble		
Cellulose	*Hemicellulose*	*Lignin*
Whole-wheat flour	Bran	Mature vegetables
Bran	Whole grains	Wheat
Vegetables		Fruits with edible seeds, such as strawberries
Soluble		
Gums	*Pectin*	
Oats	Apples	
Legumes	Citrus fruits	
Guar	Strawberries	
Barley		

SOLUBLE FIBERS. These fibers include pectins, gums, mucilages, and some hemicelluloses. Pectins are found primarily in fruits and vegetables, especially apples, oranges, and carrots. Other forms of soluble fiber occur in oat bran, barley, and legumes. The influence of soluble fibers on events in the alimentary tract is related to their ability to hold water and form gels and also to their role as substrate for fermentation by colonic bacteria.

INSOLUBLE FIBERS. These fibers consist primarily of cellulose and some hemicelluloses. They lend structure to plant cells and are found in all kinds of plant material; however, their major source is in the bran layers of cereal grains. **Lignin,** a noncarbohydrate material that is sometimes included in fiber determinations, is a major component of trees and provides structure to the woody portions of plants. It constitutes a very small part of the diet (1 g/day) and occurs mostly in fruits with edible skins and seeds.

Physiologic Properties

During their transit through the alimentary tract, dietary fibers have ample opportunity to interact with the substrates, effectors, and products of digestion as well as a variety of other substances progressing toward absorption or evacuation. Considering the complexity and continuing variability that characterize what is a relatively recent field of study, it is understandable that the outcomes of these associations cannot as yet be described with any degree of precision. However, what has been learned has implications for various disease states (Table 3–4).

TABLE 3–4. Physiologic Effects of Dietary Fiber

Stimulates chewing and thus saliva flow and gastric juice secretion
Fills the stomach and provides a sense of satiety
Increases fecal bulk, which decreases colon intraluminal pressure
"Normalizes" intestinal transit time
Becomes a substrate for colonic fermentation
Soluble fiber delays gastric emptying and slows the rate of digestion and absorption of nutrients
Soluble fiber lowers serum cholesterol

DISEASES OF THE COLON. Some diseases of the colon appear to be favorably affected by increased levels of dietary fiber, namely constipation and diarrhea, diverticulitis, and colorectal cancer.

Adequate dietary cellulose has long been recognized as a factor in preventing *constipation.* Both soluble and insoluble fibers contribute to increased fecal bulking through absorption of water and by the addition of undigestible material. Gas produced during fermentation of soluble fibers contributes to moving fecal material through the colon. Without sufficient water, cellulose tends to produce dry stools; therefore, the combination of cellulose and pectin is recommended as a superior bulk-forming laxative. Fiber, particularly insoluble fiber, seems to "normalize" intestinal transit time, hastening it in persons with constipation and prolonging it in those with rapid transit or diarrhea (Council on Scientific Affairs, 1989).

The observations of Burkitt and associates (1974) focused attention on the lack of dietary fiber as a possible cause of colon cancer. A proposed mechanism is the reduction of exposure to carcinogens passing through the colon by dilution of their concentration and by reduction in the transit time. Another theory states that any effect is due to the influence of specific components of fiber rather than to total intake (National Research Council, 1989). This possibility continues to attract interest and research.

In addition to fiber, fruits and vegetables also contribute vitamins A and C as well as the phenols and indoles of cruciferous vegetables, all of which have been associated with lowering the risk of colon cancer.

CARDIOVASCULAR DISEASE. The soluble fractions of dietary fiber, when given in large amounts, may reduce blood cholesterol. Bacteria reduce soluble fibers to short-chain fatty acids that appear to eventually block cholesterol synthesis in the liver (see Chapter 20).

DIABETES. Water-soluble fibers, primarily pectins and gums, exert a hypoglycemic effect by delaying gastric emptying, shortening intestinal transit, and reducing glucose absorption. They may also slow starch hydrolysis (see Chapter 31).

Occurrence in Foods

Dietary fiber is found only in plant products—fruits, vegetables, nuts, and grains. The most concentrated sources of dietary fibers are whole grains, especially wheat bran. Because of their higher water content, fruits and vegetables provide less dietary fiber than the drier grains and cereals per gram of ingested material.

The effect of cooking on fiber content of foods is unclear. Browning reactions that occur during cooking of foods can cause an increase in the apparent fiber content of the food, because these browning products are analyzed as lignin. Table 3–5 gives a range of fiber content for some foods (see also Fig. 3–8). Bran cereals providing 6 to 13 grams of fiber per serving are the most concentrated fiber sources that are generally consumed by Americans.

Recommendations and Intake

Which dietary fiber components are important physiologically in the long term remains to be identified, but the consumption of diets rich in plant foods appears to be related inversely to the incidence of cardiovascular disease, colon cancer, diabetes, and gastrointestinal disorders (Council on Scientific Affairs, 1989). However, it is impossible to increase the dietary fiber in the diet without also changing the fat and protein content, a modification that also has health implications. Although no specific recommendations for the amount of dietary fiber have been made, several groups have recommended that there should be an increase in the intake of dietary fiber and that this increase should come from a wide variety of whole-grain products, fruits, and vegetables, including legumes (Physiological Effects . . . , 1987; Surgeon General's Report on Nutrition and Health, 1988). The National Cancer Institute recommends a daily intake of 20 to 30 grams, with a maximum of 35 grams. Excessive fiber may interfere with the absorption of calcium and zinc, especially in children and the elderly.

Fiber intake should consist of equal amounts of soluble and insoluble fiber. This intake can be obtained with five servings or more of fruits and vegetables and six servings daily of whole-grain breads, cereals, and legumes. It is not possible to obtain adequate amounts and varieties of fiber simply by eating large amounts of fruits and vegetables.

The mean fiber intake for adults in the United States is estimated to be about 11 to 13 g/day or about 6 g/1,000 kcal (Bright-See, 1988; Lanza et al, 1987; Murphy and Calloway, 1986). It can range widely (up to 100%), depending on the method used to determine the fiber content of foods.

CARBOHYDRATE IN THE AMERICAN DIET

Recommended Dietary Allowance

There is no recommended dietary allowance for carbohydrate. In the absence of this nutrient, amino acids and glycerol from fats can be converted to glucose for nourishment of the brain and central nervous system. However, a diet without at least 50 to 100 grams of carbohydrate per day is likely to lead to ketosis, excessive breakdown of tissue protein, loss of sodium and other cations, and involuntary dehydration. The Na-

TABLE 3–5. Dietary Fiber Content of Foods in Commonly Served Portions*

Food Group	<1 g	1–1.9 g	2–2.9 g	3–3.9 g	4–4.9 g	5–5.9 g	>6 g
Breads (1 slice)	Bagel White French	Whole-wheat	Bran muffin (1)	NA†	NA	NA	NA
Cereals (1 oz)	Rice Krispies Special K Cornflakes	Oatmeal Nutri-Grain Cheerios	Wheaties Shredded Wheat	Most Honey Bran	Bran Chex 40% Bran Flakes Raisin Bran	Corn Bran	All-Bran Bran Buds 100% Bran
Pasta (1 cup)	NA	Macaroni Spaghetti	NA	Whole-wheat spaghetti	NA	NA	NA
Rice (½ cup)	White	Brown	NA	NA	NA	NA	NA
Legumes (½ cup) cooked	NA	NA	NA	Lentils	Lima beans Dried peas	NA	Kidney beans Baked beans Navy beans
Vegetables (½ cup unless stated)	Cucumber Lettuce (1 cup) Green pepper	Asparagus Green beans Cabbage Cauliflower Potato w/out skin (1) Celery	Broccoli Brussels sprouts Carrots Corn Potato w/ skin (1) Spinach	Peas	NA	NA	NA
Fruits (1 medium fruit unless stated)	Grapes (20) Watermelon (1 cup)	Apricots (3) Grapefruit (½) Peach w/ skin Pineapple (½ cup)	Apple, w/out skin Banana Orange	Apple, w/ skin Pear, w/ skin Raspberries (½ cup)	NA	NA	NA

* From Slavin JL: Dietary fiber: Classification, chemical analyses, and food sources. J Am Diet Assoc 87:1164, 1987.
† Not applicable.

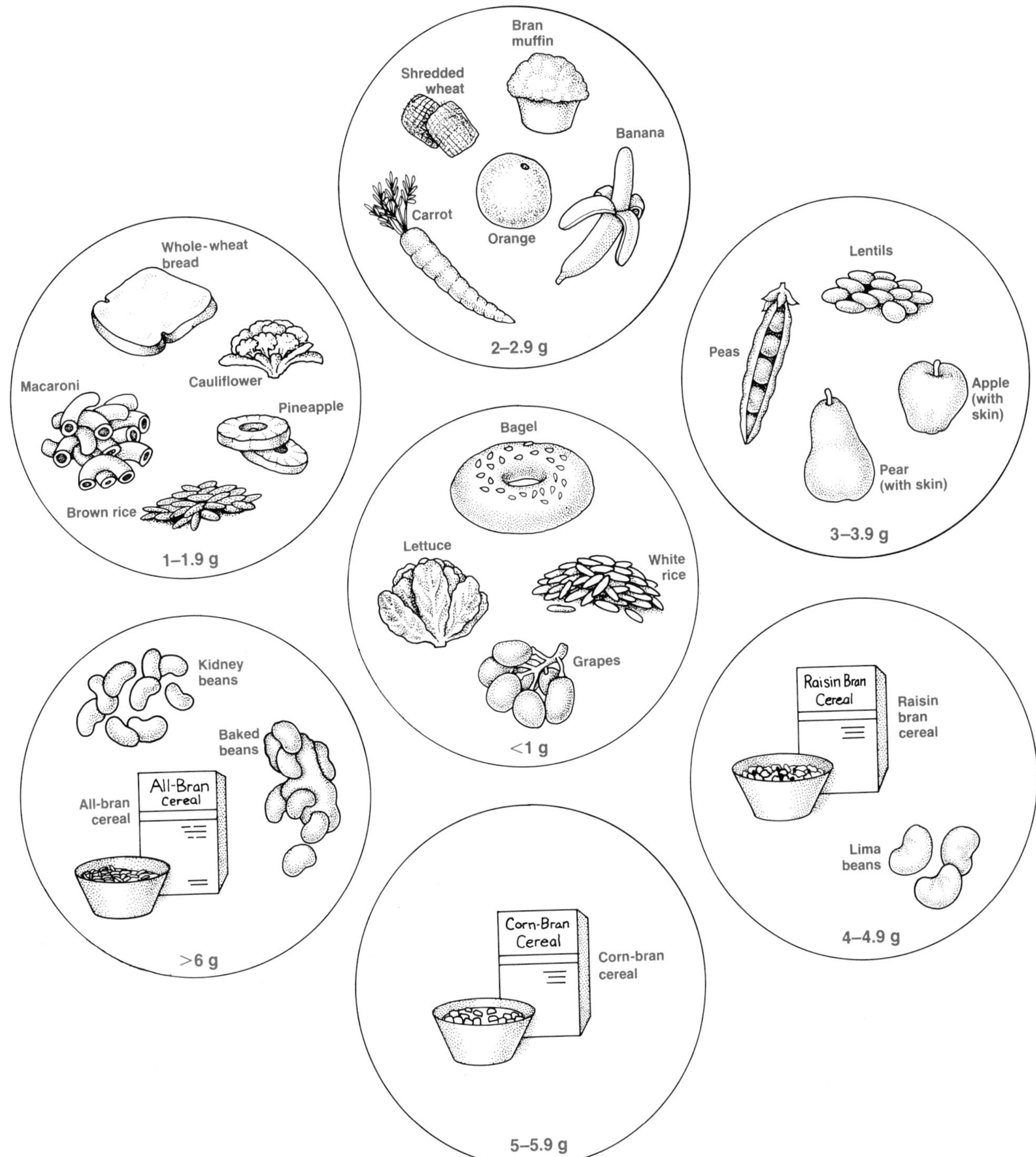

FIGURE 3–8. *Fiber content in food. See Table 3–5 for serving size.*

tional Research Council recommends that at least one half of the energy requirement after infancy be provided by carbohydrate, especially complex carbohydrate. This is an increase from the present consumption by adult men and women of 45 to 46% of their energy requirement from carbohydrate (Food and Nutrition Board, 1989).

Food Sources of Carbohydrates

Most dietary carbohydrates originate in foods of plant origin. The single major exception is lactose, the disaccharide that occurs in milk and products made from milk. Although glycogen is stored in muscle tissue, only trace amounts are available from meat as it is con-

TABLE 3–6. Carbohydrate Content of Foods

Sugar	Carbohydrate (%)	Starch	Carbohydrate (%)
Concentrated Sweets		*Grain Products*	
Sugar: Cane, beet, powdered,	99.5	Starches: Corn, tapioca, arrowroot	86–88
brown, maple	90–96	Cereals (dry): Corn, wheat, oat, bran	68–85
Candies	70–95	Flour: Corn, wheat (sifted)	70–80
Honey (extracted)	82	Popcorn (popped)	77
Syrup: Table blends, molasses	55–75	Cookies: Plain, assorted	71
Jams, jellies, marmalades	70	Crackers, saltines	72
Carbonated, sweetened beverages	10–12	Cakes: Plain, without icing	56
Fruits		Bread: White, rye, whole wheat	48–52
Prunes, apricots, figs (cooked, unsweet)	12–31	Macaroni, spaghetti, noodles, rice (cooked)	23–30
Bananas, grapes, cherries, apples, pears	15–23	Cereals (cooked): Oat, wheat, grits	10–16
Fresh: Pineapples, grapefruits, oranges, apricots, strawberries	8–14	*Vegetables*	
Milk		Boiled: Corn, white and sweet potatoes, lima, dried beans, peas	15–26
Skim	6	Beets, carrots, onions, tomatoes	5–7
Whole	5	Leafy: Lettuce, asparagus, cabbage, greens, spinach	3–4

TABLE 3–7. Carbohydrate in the US Diet in the 20th Century*

Years	Total Kilocalories	Grams of Carbohydrate	% of Total Kilocalories
1909–1913	3,400	494	58
1925–1929	3,400	478	56
1935–1939	3,200	437	55
1947–1949	3,200	405	51
1957–1959	3,100	376	49
1967–1969	3,200	379	47
1975	3,200	381	48
1980	3,400	392	46
1985	3,500	413	47

* Data from Nutrient Content of the US Food Supply. HNIS Adm. Report No. 299–21. Washington, Human Nutrition Information Service, USDA, 1988.

sumed. Even liver, in which much larger quantities are stored, contains only 5 grams of glycogen in a 3-oz serving.

Plants such as cereal grains, in which significant amounts of carbohydrate are stored for energy, are the major sources of starches. Fruits and vegetables contain varying amounts of monosaccharides and disaccharides. Table sugar is obtained primarily from sugar cane and sugar beets. Corn syrup is derived from corn by hydrolysis of the vegetable starch, and the further enzymatic processing of dextrins into simple sugars results in the production of high-fructose corn syrups. See Table 3–6 for the carbohydrate content of various foods.

Trends in Consumption of Carbohydrates

At the turn of the century, over half of the total calories consumed in the United States came from carbohydrates, most of it in the form of starch (Table 3–7). Sugars and sweeteners constituted less than one fourth of the total carbohydrate intake. By 1975, total carbohydrate calories were reduced 10%, but the proportion of carbohydrate furnished from sugars and sweeteners had risen to almost 40% of the total (Table 3–8). In 1985 about 18% of the total energy in the diet came from refined sugar, syrups, and other sweeteners, which is a per capita increase of 13% since the time period 1909 to 1913.

TABLE 3–8. Sources of Carbohydrate in the US Diet*

Year	% from Sugars, Sweeteners	% from Dairy Products	% from Fruit	% from Vegetables Including Potatoes	% from Legumes, Nuts and Soy	% from Grain Products	Other
1909–1913	21.9	4.0	5.1	10.6	2.2	55.9	0.3
1925–1929	30.6	4.4	5.7	9.4	2.0	47.1	0.8
1935–1939	31.1	5.1	6.3	9.9	2.5	44.2	0.9
1947–1949	33.7	6.7	6.6	9.6	2.2	40.1	1.1
1957–1959	35.7	7.2	6.5	9.7	2.3	37.5	1.1
1967–1969	38.5	6.7	5.9	9.6	2.1	36.2	1.0
1975	38.2	6.4	6.5	9.6	2.2	36.0	1.1
1980	39.7	6.0	6.4	8.9	1.7	36.3	1.0
1985	39.6	5.7	6.6	9.2	2.0	35.8	1.0

* Data from Nutrient Content of the US Food Supply, HNIS Adm. Report No. 299-21. Human Nutrition Information Service, USDA, 1988.

The form of sugar has also changed during the last 50 years. Whereas in 1949 the majority of sugar was used from the 5-, 10-, or 50-lb bag of sugar in the home, today most is eaten in commercially prepared foods to which sugar or sweetener has been added in the processing. For example, the consumption of high-fructose corn syrup has increased from 4.9 lb per capita in 1975 to 48 lb per capita in 1988 (Barry, 1990).

CITED REFERENCES

Barry RD: The U.S. sugar program in the 1980's. Nat Food Rev 13(1):55, 1990.
Bright-See E: Dietary fiber and cancer. Nutr Today 23(4):4, 1988.
Burkitt DP et al: Dietary fiber and disease. JAMA 229:1068, 1974.
Council on Scientific Affairs: Dietary fiber and health. JAMA 262:542, 1989.
Englyst HN and Hudson GJ: Colorimetric method for routine measurement of dietary fibre as non-starch polysaccharides: A comparison with gas-liquid chromatography. Food Chem 24:63, 1987.
Englyst HN et al: Dietary fiber and resistant starch (Editorial). Am J Clin Nutr 46:873, 1987.
Food and Nutrition Board, National Research Council, NAS: Recommended Dietary Allowances, 10th ed. Washington, DC, National Academy Press, 1989.
Lanza E et al: Dietary fiber intake in the U.S. population. Am J Clin Nutr 46:790, 1987.
Murphy SP and Calloway DH: Nutrient intakes of women in NHANES II, emphasizing trace minerals, fiber, and phytate. J Am Diet Assoc 86:1366, 1986.
National Research Council: Diet and Health: Implications for Reducing Chronic Disease Risk. Report of the Committee on Diet and Health, Food and Nutrition Board. Washington, DC, National Academy Press, 1989.
Physiological Effects and Health Consequences of Dietary Fiber. Washington, DC, Life Sciences Research Office, Federation of American Societies for Experimental Biology, 1987.
Prosky L et al: Determination of total dietary fiber in foods, food products and total diets: Interlaboratory study. J Assoc Off Anal Chem 67:1044, 1984.
Slavin JL: Dietary fiber: Classification, chemical analyses, and food sources. J Am Diet Assoc 87:1164, 1987.
Southgate DAT et al: A guide to calculating intakes of dietary fiber. J Hum Nutr 30:303, 1976.
Surgeon General's Report on Nutrition and Health. USDHHS Publ. No. 88-50210, Washington, DC, Public Health Service, 1988.

ADDITIONAL REFERENCES

Filer LJ: Modified food starch—an update. J Am Diet Assoc 88:342, 1988.
Lanza E and Butrum RR: A critical review of food fiber analysis and data. J Am Diet Assoc 86:732, 1986.
Position of The American Dietetic Association: Health implications of dietary fiber. J Am Diet Assoc 88:216, 1988.
Trowell H: Definition of dietary fiber and hypothesis that it is a protective factor in certain diseases. Am J Clin Nutr 29:417, 1976.
Trowell H: Dietary fiber definitions (Letter). Am J Clin Nutr 48:1079, 1988.

CHAPTER 4

LIPIDS

CHAPTER OUTLINE

Classification, Composition, and Function
Lipid Transport and Storage
Lipid Metabolism
Dietary Intakes

KEY TERMS

CARNITINE—an amino acid formed from methionine and lysine which, by forming an ester with the fatty acyl CoA form, facilitates the transfer of long-chain triglycerides across mitochondria membranes

CHOLESTEROL—a substance found in cell membranes of animal tissues, especially bile, gallstones, brain, blood, liver, adrenal glands, kidneys, myelin sheaths of nerve fibers, and egg yolk

CHYLOMICRONS—droplets consisting of triglyceride, cholesterol, phospholipids, and protein that are the form by which absorbed long-chain triglycerides and cholesterol are transported from the intestine into the intestinal blood or lymphatic system

DIGLYCERIDE—a lipid with two fatty acid chains attached to the glycerol molecule

ESSENTIAL FATTY ACIDS—linoleic and alpha-linolenic acids, which cannot be produced by the body and must be provided in the diet

FATTY ACID—a straight carbon chain terminating in a carboxyl and a methyl group and having the general formula $C_n H_{2n} O_2$ when fully saturated

GLYCOLIPID—a lipid containing carbohydrate groups, usually galactose

HYDROGENATION—the process of adding hydrogen to the double bonds and thus increasing the saturation of fatty acids

KETONE BODIES—acetoacetic acid, acetone and beta-hydroxybutyric acid

LECITHIN (PHOSPHATIDYLCHOLINE)—a choline-containing phospholipid that is found in all plant and animal tissues, and frequently functions as an emulsifier

LONG-CHAIN FATTY ACID—a fatty acid containing 13 to 27 carbons; 16 to 18 are most common

MEDIUM-CHAIN FATTY ACID—a fatty acid with 8 to 12 carbons

MEDIUM-CHAIN TRIGLYCERIDES—triacylglycerols with fatty acids of 8 to 12 carbons in length that are short enough to be absorbed directly into the portal blood

MONOGLYCERIDE—a lipid with one fatty acid attached to the glycerol molecule

MONOUNSATURATED FATTY ACID—a fatty acid containing one double bond

OMEGA NUMBER—the number of the carbon molecule with the first double bond, as counted from the methyl end of the fatty acid

OMEGA-3 FATTY ACIDS—fatty acids with the first double bond located at the third carbon from the methyl end of the hydrocarbon chain; most important are alpha-linolenic acid (LNA) and its derivatives eicosapentaenoic acid (EPA) and docosahexaenoic acid (DHA)

PHOSPHOLIPID—a triglyceride in which one of the fatty acids is replaced by a phosphorus-containing substance

POLYUNSATURATED FATTY ACID—a fatty acid containing two or more double bonds

SATURATED FATTY ACID—a fatty acid with the formula $C_n H_{2n} O_2$ that has no double bonds and that contains all the hydrogen it can hold

SHORT-CHAIN FATTY ACID—a fatty acid with 6 carbons or less

TRIGLYCERIDE (TRIACYLGLYCEROL)—a lipid consisting of three fatty acid chains esterified to a glycerol molecule

The general term of "lipid" embraces a heterogeneous group of compounds including the ordinary fats and oils, waxes, and related compounds found in foods and in the human body. They have the common properties of being (1) insoluble in water; (2) soluble in organic solvents, such as ether and chloroform; and (3) capable of use by living organisms.

CLASSIFICATION, COMPOSITION, AND FUNCTION

Most natural fats consist of 98 to 99% triglycerides, which in turn consist primarily of fatty acids. The remaining 1 or 2% include traces of monodiglycerides and diglycerides, free fatty acids, phospholipids, and unsaponifiable matter containing sterols. The fat-soluble vitamins are also included in this group (Table 4–1).

Fatty Acids

Fatty acids are straight hydrocarbon chains terminating in a carboxyl group at one end and a methyl group at the other end. There are 24 common fatty acids, differing in chain length as well as in degree and nature of saturation (Table 4–2).

TABLE 4–1. Classification of Lipids Important to Nutrition

Simple Lipids
Neutral fats: monoglycerides, diglycerides, triglycerides (esters of fatty acids and glycerol)
Esters of fatty acids with high molecular weight alcohols
1. Waxes
2. Sterol esters
3. Nonsterol esters—vitamin A esters, vitamin D esters

Compound Lipids
Phospholipids: Compounds of fatty acids, phosphoric acid and nitrogenous base
1. Lecithins
2. Cephalins
3. Sphingomyelins

Glycolipids: Compounds of fatty acid combined with carbohydrate and a nitrogenous base
1. Cerebrosides
2. Gangliosides

Sulfolipids: Sulfur-containing lipids
Lipoproteins: Lipids in combination with protein
1. Apolipoproteins

Lipopolysaccharides: polysaccharide-containing lipids

Derived Lipids
Fatty acids and their derivatives such as prostaglandins
Mono and diglycerides
Sterols
1. Cholesterol, ergosterol
2. Steroid hormones
3. Vitamin D
4. Bile salts

Miscellaneous lipids
1. Carotenoids and vitamin A
2. Vitamin E
3. Vitamin K

Designation

A convenient shorthand describes the structure of individual fatty acids with respect to the number of carbon atoms and the number and location of double bonds. The location of the first double bond, as counted from the methyl end of the fatty acid, is designated by the *omega ("ω")* number. Linoleic acid, for example, is designated as C18:2 ω-6 to indicate that it has 18 carbons and 2 double bonds, with the first double bond at the sixth carbon.

Chain Length

Chain length may vary from 4 to 30 carbon atoms. *Short chain* refers to fatty acids with 6 carbons or less, such as the butyric acid found in butter. *Medium-chain* fatty acids contain between 8 and 12 carbons and are usually encountered in synthetic fats. *Long-chain* fatty acids contain up to 27 carbons with chain length of 16 or 18 being the most common. Most natural fats consist mainly of long-chain fatty acids or triglycerides.

Degree of Saturation

A fatty acid with a carbon chain containing all the hydrogen it can hold is called a *saturated fatty acid.* An *unsaturated fatty acid* contains one or more double bonds where it is possible to attach additional hydrogen atoms. *Monounsaturated fatty acids* contain only one double bond. *Polyunsaturated fatty acids* contain two or more double bonds, as shown in Figure 4–1.

Essential Fatty Acids

There are two classes of essential polyunsaturated fatty acids (PUFA): *omega-6* (18:2) and *omega-3* (18:3). Linoleic, alpha-linolenic and arachidonic acids were originally designated "essential" because it was thought they could not be synthesized in the human body and therefore must be provided as a part of the diet. However, it is now known that arachidonic acid can be synthesized from linoleic acid.

Fatty acids with essential fatty acid (EFA) activity occur in cholesterol esters and phospholipids in plasma and in mitochondrial lipoproteins. They are also precursors of *prostaglandins, thromboxanes,* and *prostacyclins,* a group of hormone-like compounds that participate in the regulation of blood pressure, heart rate, vascular dilation, blood clotting, lipolysis, immune response, and the central nervous system. All PUFA have important roles in fat transport and metabolism, immune function, and maintaining the function and integrity of cellular membranes.

Linoleic acid is common in the vegetable kingdom, especially in vegetable seeds and the oils produced from these seeds. Nonseed oils such as coconut oil, palm oil, and cocoa butter are not good sources of linoleic acid.

TABLE 4–2. Common Fatty Acids*

Common Name	Systematic Name	No. of Carbon Atoms†	No. of Double Bonds	Typical Fat Source
Saturated Fatty Acids				
Butyric	Butanoic	4	0	Butterfat
Caproic	Hexanoic	6	0	Butterfat
Caprylic	Octanoic	8	0	Coconut oil
Capric	Decanoic	10	0	Coconut oil
Lauric	Dodecanoic	12	0	Coconut oil
Myristic	Tetradecanoic	14	0	Butterfat, coconut oil
Palmitic	Hexadecanoic	16	0	Most fats and oils
Stearic	Octadecanoic	18	0	Most fats and oils
Arachidic	Eicosanoic	20	0	Peanut oil
Behenic	Docosanoic	22	0	Peanut oil
Unsaturated Fatty Acids				
Caproleic	9-Decenoic	10	1	Butterfat
Lauroleic	9-Dodecenoic	12	1	Butterfat
Myristoleic	9-Tetradecenoic	14	1	Butterfat
Palmitoleic	9-Hexadecenoic	16	1	Some fish oils, beef fat
Oleic	9-Octadecenoic	18	1	Most fats and oils esp. olive oil
Elaidic	9-Octadecenoic	18	1	Butterfat
Vaccenic	11-Octadecenoic	18	1	Butterfat
Linoleic	9, 12-Octadecadienoic	18	2	Most vegetable oils esp. safflower, corn, soybean, cottonseed
Linolenic	9, 12, 15-Octadecatrienoic	18	3	Soybean oil, canola oil
Gadoleic	9-Eicosenoic	20	1	Some fish oils
Arachidonic	5, 8, 11, 14-Eicosatetraenoic	20	4	Lard
—	5, 8, 11, 14, 17-Eicosapentaenoic (EPA)	20	5	Some fish oils
Erucic	13-Docosenoic	22	1	Canola oil
—	4, 7, 10, 13, 16, 19-Docosahexaenoic (DHA)	22	6	Some fish oils

* Adapted from ISEO: Food Fats and Oils, 6th ed. Washington, DC, Institute of Shortening and Edible Oils, 1988.
† All double bonds are in the *cis* configuration except for elaidic acid and vaccenic acid, which are *trans*.

OMEGA-3 FATTY ACIDS. The omega-3 fatty acids of nutritional interest include alpha-linolenic acid (C18:3ω-3) (LNA) and its derivatives *eicosapentaenoic acid (EPA)* (C20:5ω-3) and *docosahexaenoic acid (DHA)* (C22:6ω-3) (see Table 4–2). LNA occurs in plant leaves and a few vegetable seed oils, including linseed, rapeseed (canola), and soybean. Fish oils, particularly those from deep, cold-water fish, are rich in EPA and DHA (see Appendix Table 40). Plankton contains omega-3 fatty acids; fish convert the alpha-LNA to EPA and DHA by elongation and desaturation. Although alpha-LNA can be similarly converted in humans, it is an inefficient process (Simopolous, 1988).

Omega-3 fatty acids appear to function as a balance to the action of arachidonic acid, which can cause inflammation leading to states such as thrombosis and arthritis when its metabolites are produced to excess. Omega-3 fatty acids increase the clearance of chylomicrons and probably very low density lipoproteins (VLDL) from the plasma. Metabolically they decrease the hepatic production of triglycerides and apolipoprotein B, the main lipid and protein constituents of VLDLs. The association of the ω-3 fatty acids with risk of cardiovascular disease is discussed in Chapter 20 and with inflammation and the management of arthritis in Chapter 40.

ESSENTIAL FATTY ACID DEFICIENCY. Infants fed a fat-free diet will develop a characteristic dermatitis (eczema) that can be prevented or cured by the addition of linoleic acid to the diet (Hansen et al, 1963). The only reported instances of EFA deficiency in adults are associated with long-term fat-free intravenous feedings. Some of the manifestations of EFA deficiency may result from a failure to produce adequate prostaglandins.

$CH_3(CH_2)_{16}COOH$ Stearic Acid (Saturated)

$CH_3(CH_2)_7CH{=}CH(CH_2)_7COOH$ Oleic Acid (Monounsaturated)

$CH_3(CH_2)_4CH{=}CHCH_2CH{=}CH(CH_2)_7COOH$ Linoleic Acid (Polyunsaturated)

$CH_3CH_2CH{=}CHCH_2CH{=}CH{-}CH_2{-}CH{=}CH(CH_2)_7COOH$ Linolenic Acid (Polyunsaturated)

FIGURE 4–1. *18-Carbon fatty acids.*

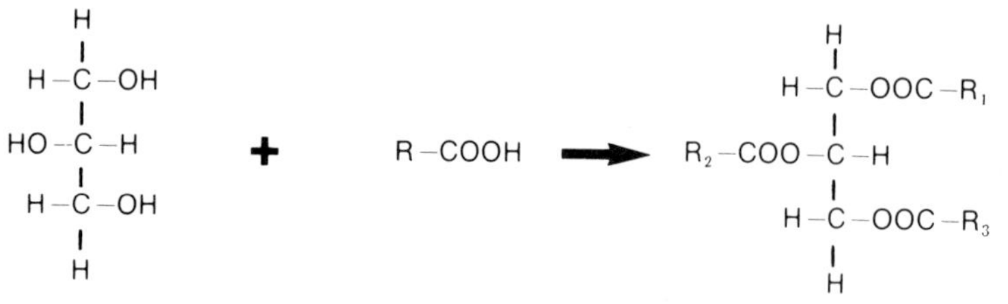

```
    H                                          H
    |                                          |
 H—C—OH                                     H—C—OOC—R1
    |                                          |
HO—C—H        +      R—COOH    ——>    R2—COO—C—H
    |                                          |
 H—C—OH                                     H—C—OOC—R3
    |                                          |
    H                                          H

 Glycerol           Fatty Acid              Triglyceride
```

FIGURE 4–2. *Structure of a triglyceride or triacylglycerol.*

Triglycerides (Triacylglycerols)

As esters of *glycerol,* a trihydric alcohol, and *fatty acids, triglycerides* are more correctly called *triacylglycerols* (Fig. 4–2).

Physical Properties

The properties of triglycerides are determined by the proportion and chemical structure of their constituent fatty acids. Shorter and more unsaturated fatty acids characterize fats that are soft or liquid oils at room temperature. Solid fats such as beef fat contain large amounts of long-chain fatty acids, such as palmitic (C16:0) and stearic (C18:0). Glyceride properties are also influenced by the ω-number and by the position of the fatty acids on the glycerol molecule.

Reactions of Triglycerides

SAPONIFICATION. When a fat is hydrolyzed with alkali, salts of the fatty acids are formed as soaps. Formation of insoluble soaps in the intestinal tract may be of concern in some abnormal conditions characterized by poor fat absorption.

HYDROGENATION. The degree of saturation of an unsaturated fat can be increased by adding hydrogen at the double bonds (Fig. 4–3). This process of *hydrogenation* is used commercially in processing liquid vegetable oils into table and cooking fats such as margarines and shortenings, which are solid at room temperature (Further Reading, p. 49).

RANCIDITY. Exposure to air over a period of time results in chemical changes in lipids known as *rancidity.*

```
                          H   H
                          |   |
—C=C—  +  H2  →          —C—C—
 |  |                     |   |
 H  H                     H   H
```

FIGURE 4–3. *Hydrogenation.*

Oxygen attaches at the double bonds to form *peroxides,* which are disagreeable in odor and flavor, destructive of vitamins A and E, and toxic in large amounts. Partial hydrogenation of oils decreases their tendency to oxidize and thus increases their stability.

Oxidation of vitamin E, which is present in large amounts in vegetable oils, prevents peroxidation; however, the vitamin is inactivated in the process. Fortification of fats or fatty foods with antioxidants such as butylated hydroxyanisole (BHA) and butylated hydroxytoluene (BHT) extends storage time and protects essential nutrients.

Functions of Triglycerides

ENERGY. Because of their high energy density and low solubility, the triglycerides in the adipose tissue are the major storage form of energy. Up to two thirds of the total energy of the cells may be supplied in this form. Each gram of fat supplies 9 kcal, more than twice the amount of energy supplied by each gram of carbohydrate. Fat spares protein for tissue synthesis that might otherwise be used for energy.

OTHER FUNCTIONS. Adipose tissue helps to hold the body organs and nerves in position and to protect them against traumatic injury and shock. The subcutaneous layer of fat insulates the body, serving to preserve body heat and maintain body temperature. Fats aid in transport and absorption of the fat-soluble vitamins. They depress gastric secretions and slow the emptying time of the stomach. In addition, fats add to the palatability of the diet and produce a feeling of satiety after a meal.

Characteristics of Animal and Vegetable Fats

Although all food fats contain a mixture of fatty acids, animal fats tend to be more saturated whereas, except for tropical plant oils such as palm and coconut oils, vegetable fats are primarily unsaturated. The fat of food products from herbivorous animals (beef, cow's milk, and lamb) is more saturated and thus harder than fats from pork and poultry. Flavors of different fats determine the unique flavors of different kinds of meat.

Fatty acids in fish fats are predominantly 20 and 22 carbons in length and are highly unsaturated with a majority of fatty acids in the omega-3 form.

Formulated and Substitute Fats

Medium-chain triglycerides (MCT) consist of fatty acids that are short enough to be absorbed directly into the portal blood. They have been formulated to provide a source of dietary fat that can be utilized effectively in the presence of malabsorption problems. MCT oils provide only 7 kcal/g. Their metabolism and use are discussed in Chapter 27.

Two fat substitutes have recently been developed which will facilitate reduction of dietary fat (New Directions, p. 50).

Derived and Compound Lipids

Derived lipids consist of triglycerides in which other compounds are substituted for one or more of the fatty acids making up the triacylglycerol molecule.

Monoglycerides and Diglycerides

Monoglycerides are lipids in which only one of the hydroxyl groups of the glycerol molecule has been replaced by a fatty acid. Diglycerides contain two fatty acids and one hydroxyl group. Because the remaining alcohol portion of glycerol is water-soluble, these lipids possess emulsifying properties useful both in digestion and in commercial processing.

Phospholipids

Phospholipids, which make up the second largest lipid component of the body, are triglycerides in which one of the fatty acids is replaced by a phosphorus-containing substance such as phosphoric acid. Because of their strong affinity for both water-soluble and fat-soluble substances, they are effective structural materials. Large concentrations are found in combination with protein in cell membranes where they facilitate the passage of fat in and out of the cell, and in the blood where they also function in the transport of lipids. The nature of the fatty acids in phospholipids is influenced by the fatty acid content of the diet (Berdanier, 1988).

LECITHIN. *Lecithin* (phosphatidylcholine) contains phosphoric acid and the nitrogen-containing base *choline.* It functions in the transport and utilization of fatty acids through the enzyme *lecithin-cholesterol acyltransferase.* Lecithin is the most widely distributed of the phospholipids; liver, egg yolk, and soybeans are especially rich sources. Because of its emulsifying properties, it is often added to food products, such as cheese, margarine, and confections.

OTHER PHOSPHOLIPIDS. Phospholipids such as *cephalins* (similar in structure to lecithins), *lipontols* (which contain inositol, a compound with vitamin-like activity), and *sphingomyelins* (which contain a complex amino alcohol in place of glycerol) are found in high concentrations in nerve tissue. A cephalin is needed to form thromboplastin for the blood clotting process. Sphingomyelin is found in the brain and other nerve tissue as a component of the myelin sheath.

Glycolipids

The glycolipids include the *cerebrosides* and *angliosides,* which contain the base sphingosine and very long chain fatty acids with 22 and 24 carbons. The carbohydrate component of the cerebrosides is galactose; the gangliosides also contain glucose and a complex compound containing an amino sugar. Structurally, both

FURTHER READING: Hydrogenation of Fats

Manufacturers add hydrogen to liquid oils to increase their level of saturation, thus making them semisolid. The level of saturation determines the consistency of a fat at room temperature. Vegetable oils used in margarines and shortenings are hydrogenated to increase resistance to oxidation and to imitate the hardness of more saturated animal fats. However, because the hydrogenation process primarily changes polyunsaturated to monounsaturated fatty acids, the saturation levels of the final products are not high. High-PUFA margarines combine a small amount of partially hydrogenated vegetable oil with large amounts of oil that have not been processed and therefore retain the original levels of PUFA. Margarines made in this fashion contain 17 to 20% SFA compared with 66% SFA in butter.

The monounsaturated fatty acids produced during the hydrogenation process occur in both the natural *cis* form and the unnatural stereoisomeric *trans* form. *Trans* fatty acids have been suspected of a possible relationship to the incidence of atherosclerosis, but studies over a number of years have failed to support this hypothesis. More recent suggestions that *trans* fatty acids may be cancer-promoting have not held up under study (Blume, 1988; Schaub and Green, 1988).

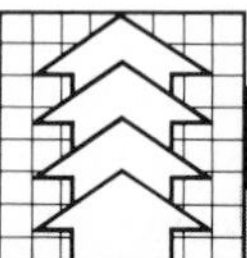

NEW DIRECTIONS: Commercial Fat Substitutes

Olestra and Simplesse are the first fat substitutes developed for the retail market.

Simplesse is formulated from egg white or milk protein by changing the physical form of the molecules to produce a texture so fine that the tongue perceives the product as a fluid. The process of *microparticulation,* which involves blending and heating similar to that of coagulating egg whites, results in a material with the creamy richness normally associated with fat.

Simplesse is digestible and is absorbed; however, because water molecules are incorporated during processing, 1 gram furnishes only 1 ⅓ kcal rather than the 4 kcal normally furnished by protein. Because 1 gram of Simplesse replaces 1 gram of fat at 9 kcal/g, the total kilocalorie saving is considerable.

Simplesse cannot be used for frying or as an ingredient in cooked foods because it coagulates and becomes rubbery when heated. Anticipated uses are as a substitute for part of the fat in uncooked diet foods, making possible such foods as salad dressing reduced from 100 kcal to 21 kcal per tablespoon, or ice cream reduced from 272 to 129 kcal per serving (Kroger, 1988).

Sucrose polyesters are a large class of fat-like substances, one of which is *Olestra.* They are formulated by heating soybean oil and sucrose in the presence of methyl alcohol to produce a sucrose molecule with 6 to 8 fatty acids attached. The product, which resembles a fat, is then cleaned to remove residual alcohol and is bleached and deodorized in the same fashion as vegetable oils.

The resultant molecule cannot be digested, and because of its large size cannot be absorbed through the intestinal wall. In safety studies in which Olestra was fed to animals in amounts up to 15% of the daily diet and to human volunteers at 100 g/day (the equivalent of 900 kcal), all that was consumed was excreted unchanged. Fat-soluble substances such as cholesterol and vitamin E are trapped to some degree and excreted; however, other fat-soluble vitamins are not affected. The product will presumably be fortified with vitamin E.

Olestra can be used safely in cooking. However, it probably will not be available in the pure form but will be mixed with cooking oils at the level of 35% for home use and 75% for commercial use. Because Olestra is calorie-free, its presence in a 50/50 mixture with oil will reduce calories from fat by 50% (Kroger, 1988).

compounds are components of nerve tissue and certain cell membranes where they play a role in lipid transport.

Sterols

Classification and Structure

A large group of compounds called *sterols* is characterized by the complex ring structure (Fig. 4–4) with individual variations. In addition to *cholesterol,* which is found only in animal tissues, other common sterols include *ergosterol,* which occurs in yeast, and *beta-sitosterol,* which is found in plant foods.

Cholesterol

Cholesterol is an essential component of the structural membranes of all cells and is a major component of brain and nerve cells. It is found in high concentrations in glandular tissues and in the liver, where it is synthesized and stored. It is a key intermediate in the biosynthesis of a number of important steroids, including the bile acids, adrenocortical hormones, estrogens, androgens, and progesterone. Cholesterol is found only in animal foods. Its relationship to fat in foods and to atherosclerosis is discussed further in Chapter 20.

FIGURE 4–4. *Cholesterol.*

Vitamin D Activity

Cholesterol and ergosterol are both precursors of vitamin D. Cholesterol is converted in the intestinal mucosa to *7-dehydrocholesterol,* the provitamin of *cholecalciferol* (vitamin D_3), and deposited in the subcutaneous fat layer. The transformation to the active form is accomplished upon exposure of skin to ultraviolet light from the sun.

Irradiated ergosterol is the form in which vitamin D is used in the fortification of milk. This is discussed further in Chapter 6.

LIPID TRANSPORT AND STORAGE

Almost all of the lipids of the diet are absorbed from the intestinal mucosa into the lymphatic system (see Chapter 1). Only the medium-chain fatty acids are absorbed directly into the portal blood, thus bypassing the lymphatic system. Lipids are carried in the lymph as *chylomicrons*—droplets of triglyceride, cholesterol, and phospholipids—with a small amount of protein (mainly *apolipoproteins* A and B) adsorbed to their outer surface. They empty into the venous blood at the thoracic duct and are carried to the liver or removed from the blood by the adipose tissue. Chylomicrons are so large that after a high-fat meal they cause the plasma to appear milky.

In the liver lipids may be metabolized, stored, or converted to *lipoproteins,* in which form they are carried in the blood to the tissues for immediate use for energy or special functions (see Chapter 20).

Within a few hours after eating, chylomicrons have been removed from the blood by the action of *lipoprotein lipase,* an enzyme located on endothelial cells lining the capillaries in the adipose tissue. Lipoprotein lipase hydrolyzes the triglycerides and phospholipids into fatty acids, glycerol, and phosphorus-containing substances, all of which are small enough to pass into the adipose cell. There they are re-esterified into triglycerides and phospholipids for storage.

Energy reserves of lipids are stored in adipose tissue. Most human adipose cells occur in the form of *white fat,* which accumulates in subcutaneous tissue (50%), around the internal organs in the abdominal cavity (45%) and in the intramuscular tissue (5%). These fat cells can store up to 95% of their volume as triglycerides. Fat storage is not static; even though the total remains the same, triglycerides are in a constant state of turnover. (See Chapter 18 for further discussion of fat storage and mobilization.)

Brown fat is much less abundant and occurs primarily in the interscapular region and on the back of the neck. The amount of this fat is higher in the neonate and decreases with age, but it can increase with extended exposure to cold. In *nonshivering thermogenesis,* brown fat cells produce heat from fatty acids by uncoupling the mitochondrial mechanism of oxidative phosphorylation, thus dissipating energy in the form of heat rather than entrapping it as ATP. This mechanism is important to hibernating animals and is especially active in maintaining body temperature of the neonate. Whether it is a significant part of human adult metabolism is not known (see Chapter 18).

LIPID METABOLISM

Almost all tissues can utilize fatty acids for energy. They constitute a major source of energy for muscular tissue, even when glucose is available. Glycerol can be oxidized in only a few tissues; thus, most of it is carried to the liver where it can be oxidized for energy or used in the synthesis of new triglycerides.

The liver is a major center of lipid metabolism and is largely responsible for regulation of lipid levels in the body. Among its important functions are (1) synthesis of triglycerides from carbohydrate and, to a smaller extent, from protein; (2) synthesis of other lipids, such as phospholipids and cholesterol from triglycerides; (3) desaturation of fatty acids (the monounsaturated oleic acid is the predominant acid in human adipose tissue); and (4) degredation of triglycerides for use as energy.

Catabolism of Fatty Acids and Triglycerides

When fatty acids are needed for energy, triglycerides —primarily in the adipose tissue—are hydrolyzed to fatty acids and glycerol under the direction of *lipoprotein lipase.* Free fatty acids (FFA) are released from the adipose cell by the action of *hormone-sensitive lipase.* In the blood stream, the FFA bind to albumin for transport. Although a great deal of fatty acid is transported in this form, its level in the plasma remains low because it is picked up by the liver very rapidly.

Glycerol diffuses back into the plasma because it can only be oxidized for energy in the liver and kidney cells. There it is converted to glycerophosphate and is either reincorporated into triacylglycerols or (more likely) converted to glucose.

In the liver, fatty acids are metabolized by beta oxidation (the beta carbon is the second from the carboxyl carbon), in which the chain is shortened by two carbons at a time, forming acetic acid and a shorter fatty acid chain (Fig. 4-5). The final product of the reaction is acetyl-CoA, which then combines with oxaloacetic acid

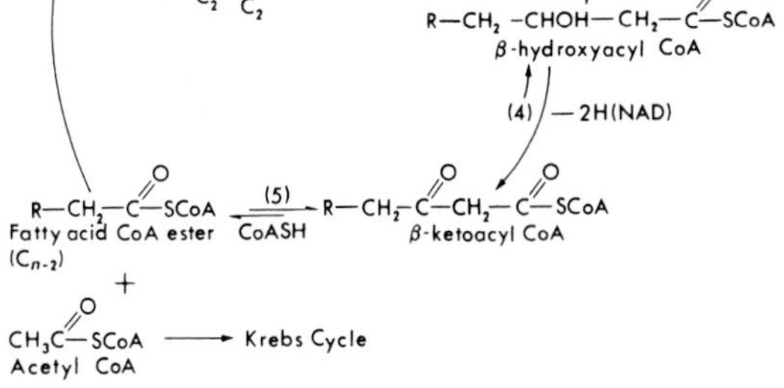

FIGURE 4-5. *Fatty acid oxidation. Enzymes are: (1) acyl CoA synthetase, (2) acyl CoA dehydrogenase, (3) enoyl CoA hydrase, (4) beta-hydroxyacyl CoA dehydrogenase and (5) beta-ketoacyl thiolase. (From Pike RL and Brown ML: Nutrition: An Integrated Approach, 3rd ed. New York, John Wiley, 1984, p 465.)*

and is oxidized via the citric acid cycle. Oxygen must be available for beta oxidation. In an anaerobic situation, such as in very strenuous exercise, fat catabolism is halted.

Carnitine is necessary for the oxidation of long-chain fatty acids, facilitating the transfer of the fatty acyl CoA from across the membrane of the mitochondrion by combining with the ester. Once inside, the fatty acyl CoA is regenerated enzymatically and proceeds through β-oxidation. Carnitine is released and passes out of the mitochondrion to continue with the transport process.

Fatty acids of C12:0 (lauric) chain length and shorter (MCT) are not carnitine-dependent and therefore are preferred fuel for infant feeding and for adults with difficulties in utilizing fat (Blackburn and Babayan, 1989).

Ketone Bodies

Even under normal conditions, the liver produces more acetyl-CoA than it can oxidize completely, and the excess is condensed in two-molecule units to form *acetoacetic acid.* The acetoacetic acid diffuses through the liver cell membranes and is carried to the peripheral tissues where it is converted once again to acetyl-CoA and is oxidized.

When the body is relying almost entirely on stored fat for energy, such as in uncontrolled diabetes mellitus or prolonged fasting or starvation, large quantities of fatty acids appear in the liver, and the production of acetoacetic acid greatly outstrips the oxidizing ability of the peripheral tissues. Part of the excess acetoacetic acid is converted to *beta-hydroxybutyric acid* and to *acetone.* The three compounds are known collectively as *ketone bodies.*

Both acetoacetic acid and beta-hydroxybutyric acid must be carried in the blood and excreted in the urine in combination with a base (sodium ion). This reduces the available base in the body, and the condition, if unchecked, leads to a lowering of the pH of body fluids *(ketoacidosis),* a condition that may be fatal if left untreated.

The breakdown of fatty acids depends on an adequate supply of oxaloacetic acid, which is generated primarily from carbohydrate metabolism. The acetyl-CoA from beta oxidation must combine with oxaloacetic acid to form citric acid in the citric acid cycle. Thus, complete fatty acid catabolism requires a continual background of glucose catabolism in order to provide the pyruvic acid to make the necessary oxaloacetic acid. In cases of severe carbohydrate limitation, the acetate fragments produced from beta oxidation cannot be accommodated in the Krebs cycle and build up in extracellular fluids. They are readily converted to ketones and excreted in the urine *(ketonuria)* and expired air.

Triglyceride Synthesis

Fatty acids in the adipose tissue cells are resynthesized into triglycerides for storage in adipose cells. The glycerol for this resynthesis comes from glucose, which also enters the adipose cell when insulin is present.

Hormonal Regulation

The hormones that have marked effects on the carbohydrate metabolism also affect fat metabolism. *Insulin* increases fat synthesis and inhibits fat utilization and uptake of the resultant fatty acids by adipose tissue. It also decreases activity of *hormone sensitive lipase (HSL),* which directs breakdown of adipose triglyceride and release of the free fatty acids thus formed into the circulation. By increasing the rate of cellular metabolism, *thyroxine* indirectly increases fat mobilization. *Glucocorticoids* increase the rate of fat mobilization by increasing permeability of the fat cell membrane. *Epinephrine, norepinephrine,* and *adrenocorticoids* (especially adrenocorticotropic hormone [ACTH]) also increase the rate of fat mobilization by stimulating HSL activity, and thus the release of free fatty acids for metabolism by tissue cells.

DIETARY INTAKES

Recommended Dietary Allowances

Although no Recommended Dietary Allowances (RDA) whave been established, the human requirement for linoleic acid has been estimated to be approximately 1 to 2% of the total energy intake (2.7% for infants). This requirement can be met by a daily intake of approximately 15 to 25 grams of the kinds of fat that characterize the American diet. It has been proposed that ω-3 fatty acids should be equal to 10 to 15% of the linoleic acid intake, particularly during pregnancy, lactation, and infancy. However, as yet no RDA has been established for these fatty acids (Food and Nutrition Board, 1989).

Accumulating evidence has associated intake of total fat as well as proportionate intakes of fatty acids at different levels of saturation to the incidence of cardiovascular disease and cancer. Recommendations for both quantity and quality of dietary fat are discussed in detail in Chapters 16 and 20.

TABLE 4–3. Fat Content of Some Common Foods*

0 Grams of Fat	7–10 Grams of Fat
Most fruits and vegetables	Cheese, cheddar, 1 oz
Nonfat milk	Milk, whole, 1 cup
Nonfat yogurt	Bologna, beef, 1 slice
Plain pasta and rice	Sausage, 1 patty
Angel food cake	Steak, sirloin, broiled, 3 oz
Popcorn, air-popped, unbuttered	Potatoes, French fried, 10
Soft drinks	Chow mein, chicken, 1 cup
Jam, jelly	Chocolate candy bar, 1 oz
1–3 Grams of Fat	Corn chips, 1 oz
Popcorn, oil-popped, unbuttered, 1 cup	Doughnut, cake type, plain, 1
Low-calorie salad dressing, 1 T†	Mayonnaise, 1 T
Baked beans, ½ cup	**15 Grams of Fat**
Soup, chicken noodle, canned, 1 cup	Hot dog, beef, 2 oz
Whole wheat bread, 1 slice	McDonald's Chicken McNuggets, 6 pieces
Dinner roll, 1	Peanut butter, 2 T
Waffle, frozen, 4″, 1	Pork chop, broiled, 3 oz
Coleslaw, ½ cup	Sunflower seeds, dry roasted, ¼ cup
Flounder or sole, baked, 3 oz	Avocado, ½ medium
Chicken, without skin, roasted, 3 oz	Chop suey, beef and pork, 1 cup
Tuna, canned in water, 3 oz	Cinnamon roll, 1
Cheese, cottage, 2% fat, ½ cup	**20 Grams of Fat**
Ice milk, soft serve, ½ cup	Cheesecake, 1/12 cake
4–6 Grams of Fat	Lasagna with meat, 1 medium piece
Low-fat yogurt, 1 cup	Macaroni and cheese, homemade, 1 cup
Cheese, mozarella, part-skim, 1 oz	Peanuts, dry roasted, ¼ cup
Chicken, roasted with skin, 3 oz	Ground beef, broiled, 3 oz
Egg, scrambled, 1	**25+ Grams of Fat**
Turkey, roasted, 3 oz	Polish sausage, 3 oz
Granola, 1 oz	Cheeseburger, large
Muffin, bran, 1 small	Pie, pecan, 1/8th 9″
Pizza, cheese, ¼ of 12″	Chicken pot pie, frozen, baked, 1 pie
Burrito, bean, 1	Quiche, bacon, 1/8 pie
Brownie, with nuts, 1 small	
Margarine or butter, 1 tsp	
Popcorn, oil popped, buttered, 1 cup	
French dressing, regular, 1 T	

* Data from Healthy Dividends, Rosemont, IL, National Dairy Council, 1990.
† T = tablespoon.

Food Sources of Fats

Animal products are the major source of fats in the American diet, providing most of the saturated fat and all of the cholesterol. According to the NHANES II survey, ground beef contributed the most fat. Other animal sources are dairy products and eggs. Fruits, vegetables, and cereal grains are relatively low in fat. However significant amounts of fat are provided by the concentrated seed oils such as safflower, corn, and cottonseed oils. Safflower oil contains the most linoleic acid, although most vegetable oils are good sources. Olive, canola (modified rapeseed), and peanut oil are high in monounsaturated oleic acid. The tropical oils (palm oil, palm kernel oil, and coconut oil) that are semisolid at room temperature are high in saturated fatty acids.

The amount of fat in dairy products can be adjusted to levels that meet the requirements of consumers. Whole milk, for example, contains 10 gm of butterfat in 8 oz, or the equivalent of 2 tsp. The same amount of low fat or 2% milk contains 1 tsp, whereas nonfat or skim milk is fat-free.

Pork and beef are being bred and raised to yield lower fat meats that better serve the needs of a diet-conscious public. For the fat content of selected foods see Table 4–3, Figure 4–6, and Appendix Tables 1 and 40.

Trends in Fat Consumption

Data from USDA surveys of food consumption in American households indicate that consumption of fat as a percentage of total kilocalories has decreased from 41% in 1977 to 36.4% in 1985 and 1986 (USDA, 1986, 1987). This represents the reversal of a trend that has seen increased consumption of total fat since the beginning of the century.

The Nationwide Food Consumption Survey of 1985 indicated that the mean consumption of fat by women aged 19 to 50 years was 63 g/day, of which one fifth was polyunsaturated fat and the remainder was divided equally between saturated and monounsaturated fats (Rizek et al, 1988).

Food supply data ("disappearance" data) reveal that

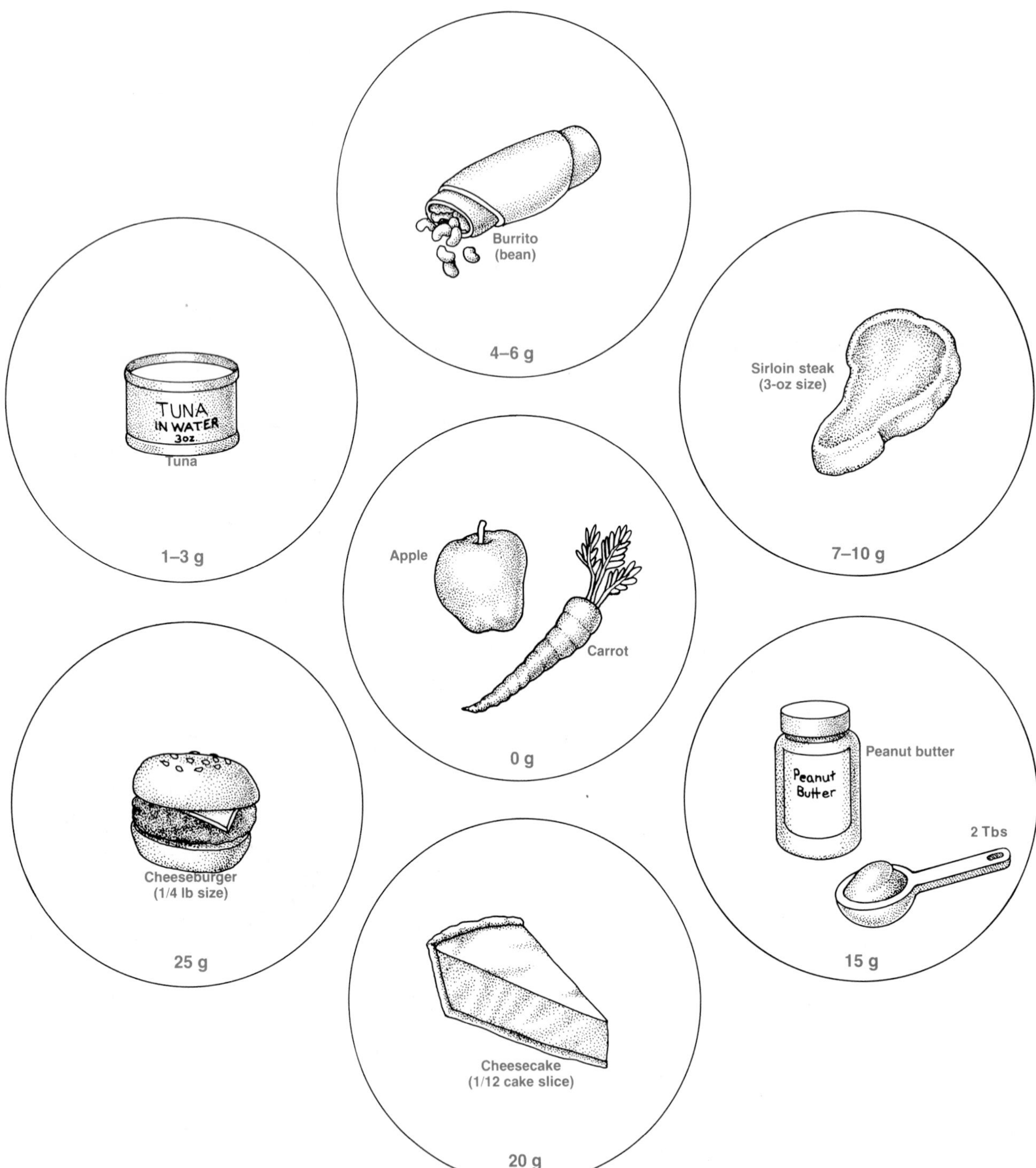

FIGURE 4–6. *Fat content of common serving sizes of food.*

TABLE 4–4. Composition of Fat in the American Diet during the 20th Century*

Year	% of Saturated Fat	% of Monounsaturated Fat	% of Polyunsaturated Fat
1909–1913	45	40	11
1925–1929	45	40	11
1935–1939	45	39	12
1947–1949	44	40	12
1957–1959	42	40	14
1967–1969	40	41	16
1975	36	41	18
1980	37	40	20
1985	36	40	20

* Data from Nutrient Content of the U.S. Food Supply, HNIS Admin. Report No. 299-21. Human Nutrition Information Service, USDA, 1988.

TABLE 4–5. U.S. Food Supply: Quantities of Fats and Oils Available for Consumption Per Capita*

Year	Butter	Margarine	Shortening	Lard†	Edible Beef Fat†	Oils
1950	10.7	6.1	11.0	12.6	0	8.5
1955	9.0	8.2	11.5	10.1	0	10.5
1960	7.5	9.3	12.5	7.5	0	11.4
1965	6.4	9.7	14.2	6.3	0	14.1
1970	5.3	10.9	17.3	4.6	0	17.7
1975	4.7	11.0	17.0	2.9	0	19.9
1980	4.5	11.4	18.2	2.6	1.1	22.5
1985	4.9	10.7	22.8	1.8	1.9	25.1

* In pounds.
† Excludes use in margarine and shortening.

for fat available for consumption (not counting waste and portions not consumed) there is a distinct trend toward greater use of vegetable fats in place of animal fats. Table 4–4 shows that the percentage of total fat in the form of saturated fat has consistently dropped from 45% in 1909 to 36% in 1985, whereas the amount of polyunsaturated fat has almost doubled during the same period, from 9% to 20%. Table 4–5 shows how this change is reflected in the use of fats and oils from 1950 to 1985.

CITED REFERENCES

Berdanier CD: Role of membrane lipids in metabolic regulation. Nutr Rev 46:145, 1988.

Blackburn GL and Babayan VK: Letter to the Editor. J Am Coll Nutr 8:253, 1989.

Blume E: The truth about trans. Nutr Action 15(2):8, 1988.

Food and Nutrition Board, National Research Council, NAS: Recommended Dietary Allowances, 10th ed. Washington, DC, National Academy Press, 1989.

Hansen AE et al: Role of linoleic acid in infant nutrition. Pediatrics 31:171, 1963.

Kroger F: Food lure: The sweet, the fat and the roasted. Presented at the Annual Meeting, American Dietetic Association, San Francisco, October, 1988.

Rizek RL, Raper NL, and Tippett KS: Trends in U.S. fat and oil consumption. J Am Oil Chem Soc 65:722, 1988.

Schaub M and Green NR: Effects of dietary trans fatty acids on mutagenesis of known carcinogens. J Food Protection 51:117, 1988.

Simopoulos AP: Omega-3 fatty acids in growth and development and in health and disease. Nutr Today 23(2):10, 1988.

USDA: Nationwide Food Consumption Survey. Continuing Survey of Food Intakes of Individuals: Men 19–50 Years, 1 day, 1985. Report No. 85-3. Hyattsville, MD, Nutrition Monitoring Division, Human Nutrition Information Service, US Department of Agriculture, 1986.

USDA: Nationwide Food Consumption Survey. Continuing Survey of Food Intakes of Individuals: Women 19–50 Years and Their Children 1–5 Years, 4 days, 1985. Report No. 85-4. Hyattsville, MD, Nutrition Monitoring Division, Human Nutrition Information Service, US Department of Agriculture, 1987.

ADDITIONAL REFERENCES

Dziezak JD: Fats, oils, and fat substitutes. Food Tech 43:65, 1989.

Enig MG et al: Fatty acid composition of the fat in selected food items with emphasis on trans components. J Am Oil Chem Soc 60:1788, 1983.

Feller AG and Rudman D: Role of carnitine in human nutrition. J Nutr 118:541, 1988.

Fischer S et al: Dietary docosahexaenoic acid is retroconverted in man to eicosapentaenoic acid, which can be quickly transformed to prostaglandin I3. Prostaglandins 34:367, 1987.

Harris WS: Fish oils and plasma lipid and lipoprotein metabolism in humans: A critical review. J Lipid Res 30:785, 1989.

Hwang D: Essential fatty acids and immune response. FASEB J 3:2052, 1989.

Lands WEM: Renewed questions about polyunsaturated fatty acids. Nutr Rev 44:189, 1986.

Nettleton JA: ω-3 fatty acids: Composition of plant and seafood sources in human nutrition. J Am Diet Assoc 91:331, 1991.

Orten JM and Neuhaus OW: Human Biochemistry, 10th ed. St Louis, CV Mosby, 1982.

Popkin BM et al: Food consumption trends of US women: Patterns and determinants between 1977 and 1985. Am J Clin Nutr 49:1307, 1989.

Sacks FM: Current and potential clinical indications of fish oil. Cardiovasc Rev Rep 9(8):20, 1988.

Simopoulos AP: Summary of the NATO Advanced Research Workshop on dietary omega 3 and omega 6 fatty acids: Biological effects and nutritional essentiality. J Nutr 119:521, 1989.

Some calories count more than others. Tufts Univ Diet Nutr Letter 6(9):2, 1988.

CHAPTER 5

PROTEINS

CHAPTER OUTLINE

KEY TERMS

AMINO ACID—an organic compound containing an amino (NH_2) group and a carboxyl (COOH) group, which functions as one of the building blocks of protein

AMINO ACID SCORE—a method of protein evaluation in which the milligrams of the limiting indispensable amino acid in the test protein is divided by the milligrams of the same indispensable amino acid in the reference protein

CONDITIONALLY DISPENSABLE AMINO ACIDS—amino acids that become indispensable under certain conditions

DENATURATION—"unraveling" or breaking down of the tertiary structure of proteins by mechanical agitation, heat, cold, acidity, or alkalinity

DISPENSABLE AMINO ACIDS (NONESSENTIAL AMINO ACIDS)—amino acids the body is able to synthesize to meet metabolic requirements

FIBROUS PROTEINS—proteins characterized by several helical peptide chains twisted together to form stiff rods with high mechanical strength

GLOBULAR PROTEINS—proteins characterized by tertiary structure and are thus very soluble and easily denatured

INDISPENSABLE AMINO ACIDS (ESSENTIAL AMINO ACIDS)—amino acids for which synthesis is inadequate to meet metabolic needs and that must be supplied in the diet; threonine, tryptophan, histidine, lysine, leucine, isoleucine, methionine, valine, and phenylalanine

KWASHIORKOR—a form of protein-energy malnutrition associated with extreme dietary protein deficiency and characterized by hypoalbuminemia, edema, and enlarged fatty liver; subcutaneous fat is usually preserved, and muscle wasting may be masked by edema

MARASMIC KWASHIORKOR—a form of protein-energy malnutrition that is characterized by loss of subcutaneous fat and edema; reflects a deficiency of both energy and protein

MARASMUS—a chronic form of protein-energy malnutrition in which the deficiency is primarily of energy; in advanced stages, it is characterized by muscular wasting and by absence of subcutaneous fat

PEPTIDE—any compound of low molecular weight that yields two or more amino acids on hydrolysis; constituent part of proteins

POLYPEPTIDE—a peptide that contains from a few up to as many as 300 amino acids

PROTEIN—a complex nitrogenous compound made up of amino acids in peptide linkages

PROTEIN ENERGY MALNUTRITION—a class of clinical disorders resulting from varying combinations and degrees of protein and energy deficiency

SIMPLE PROTEINS—proteins such as globulins and albumins that yield only amino acids on hydrolysis

TRANSAMINATION—the reversible transfer of an amino group from an amino acid to a keto acid, forming a new keto acid and a new amino acid without the appearance of ammonia

UREA—the chief nitrogenous end-product of protein metabolism and the chief nitrogenous constituent of urine

Protein was the first substance to be recognized as a vital part of living tissue. The name was derived more than a century ago from a Greek word meaning "of first importance."

COMPOSITION

Proteins, like fats and carbohydrates, contain carbon, hydrogen, and oxygen. They are unique because they also contain about 16% nitrogen, along with sulfur and sometimes other elements such as phosphorus, iron, and cobalt. The presence of nitrogen permits proteins to assume the hundreds of different forms that characterize life.

Plants synthesize protein from nitrogen, which they obtain from the nitrates and ammonia in the soil and, in the unique circumstance of the legumes, nitrates made available symbiotically from atmospheric nitrogen by bacteria in the root nodules (Further Reading, p. 60). Animals, in turn, obtain the nitrogen that they require from protein foods of either plant or animal origin. Animal metabolism, excretion, and death finally return the nitrogen to the soil in a continuation of the *nitrogen cycle.*

STRUCTURE AND CLASSIFICATION

The basis of protein structure is the amino acid, of which 20 have been recognized as constituents of most protein. Except for proline, all are alpha-amino carboxylic acids, in which a basic amino group and an acid carboxyl group are attached to the same carbon atom. They are differentiated by the remainder of the molecule (R) as shown in Figure 5-1.

Amino acids combine to form proteins by means of a *peptide bond* that joins the carboxylic carbon of one amino acid to the nitrogen of another (Fig. 5-2). The resultant compound has a free carboxyl group at one end and a free amino group at the other, enabling the chain to continue adding other amino acids at either end.

Proteins vary in size from relatively small polypeptides such as adrenocorticotropin (ACTH) with 23 amino acid units to very complex molecules with several hundred thousand amino acid units. *Polypeptides,* which constitute the *primary structure* of proteins, may contain from a few to as many as 300 amino acids. Several polypeptide chains may be linked together, usually through the sulfur-sulfur link of cystine, in a helical, pleated, or random coil form called the *secondary structure.* More complex proteins feature a *tertiary structure* in which the polypeptide chain is wound upon itself into a globular form, with the whole structure being held rigid by interatomic forces such as hydrogen bonds. The extensive possibilities of variation offered by these structures result in millions of different proteins with specific properties and biologic functions.

Proteins exist in either fibrous or globular forms. *Fibrous* proteins feature several helical peptide chains twisted together to form a stiff rod. They are characterized by low solubility and by high mechanical strength, and they appear in structural elements such as collagen of connective tissue, keratin of hair and nails, and myosin of muscle tissue. *Globular* proteins occur in tissue fluids. They are very soluble and are easily denatured (Further Reading, p. 60). Globular proteins of interest in nutrition are casein in milk, egg albumin, and the albumins and globulins of blood, plasma, and hemoglobin. In conjugated form, they constitute most of the intracellular enzymes.

Simple proteins yield only amino acids upon hydrolysis. They include albumins, globulins, glutelins, prolamins, and albuminoids. Proteins that are soluble in water and dilute salt solution, such as albumins and globulins, are present in animal fluids, whereas less soluble ones such as myosin and muscle protein are present in tissues.

Conjugated proteins are combinations in which a nonprotein substance is attached to a simple protein molecule as a prosthetic group, thus facilitating functions that neither constituent could properly perform by itself. These include the *nucleoproteins* found in ribonucleic acid (RNA) and deoxyribonucleic acid (DNA), which combine simple proteins and nucleic acid; *mucoproteins* and *glycoproteins,* combining proteins with variable quantities of complex polysaccharides, such as in mucin found in gastric secretions; *lipoproteins,* as found in blood plasma, which combine protein with lipids such as triglycerides, cholesterol, and phospholipids; *phosphoproteins,* in which phosphoric acid is joined by ester linkages to protein, such as in milk casein; and *metalloproteins,* such as ferritin and hemosiderin in which metals such as iron, copper, and zinc are attached to proteins.

Derived proteins—proteoses, peptones, and peptides—are formed in the various stages of protein metabolism.

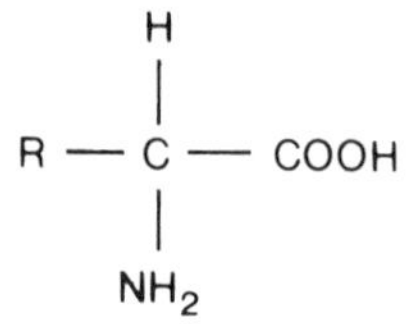

```
        H
        |
R — C — COOH
        |
       NH2
```

FIGURE 5-1. *Basic structure of an amino acid.*

FUNCTIONS OF PROTEINS

Dietary proteins are involved in the synthesis of tissue protein and other special metabolic functions. In *anabolic processes* they furnish the amino acids required to build and maintain body tissues. As an *energy source,*

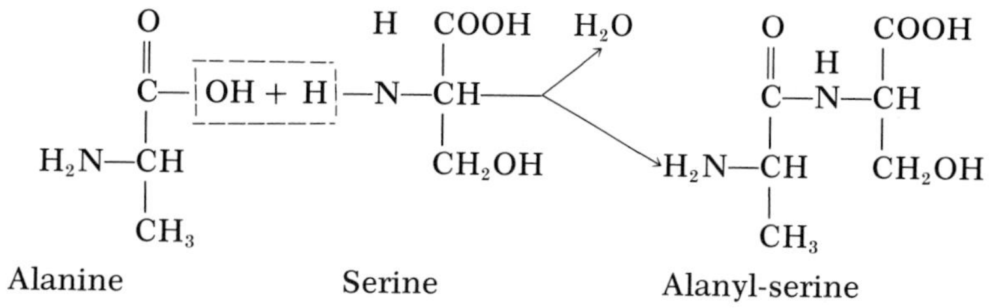

$$\underset{\text{Alanine}}{H_2N-\overset{\overset{O}{\|}}{\underset{\underset{CH_3}{|}}{CH}}\!-\!C-OH} + \underset{\text{Serine}}{H-N(H)-\underset{\underset{CH_2OH}{|}}{CH}-COOH} \rightarrow H_2O + \underset{\text{Alanyl-serine}}{H_2N-\underset{\underset{CH_3}{|}}{CH}-\overset{\overset{O}{\|}}{C}-\overset{H}{N}-\underset{\underset{CH_2OH}{|}}{CH}-COOH}$$

FIGURE 5–2. *Formation of a dipeptide.*

proteins are equivalent to carbohydrates in providing 4 kcal/g. However, they are considerably more expensive, both in terms of purchase and in the amount of energy required for their metabolism.

Proteins perform a major *structural role* not only in all body tissues but also in the formation of enzymes, hormones, and various fluids and body secretions (Further Reading, p. 67). As *antibodies,* they are involved in the function of the immune system.

In the form of lipoproteins, proteins participate in the *transportation* of triglyceride, cholesterol, phospholipid, and fat-soluble vitamins. Many vitamins and minerals are bound to specific protein carriers for transport. Albumin carries free fatty acids and bilirubin as well as many drugs.

Proteins also contribute to *homeostasis* by maintaining normal osmotic relations among body fluids, as evidenced by the appearance of edema as a consequence of hypoproteinemia. Albumin is particularly important to this function. Because of their unique structure, proteins are able to combine with either acidic or basic substances, thus maintaining the acid-base balance of blood and tissues.

AMINO ACIDS

Indispensable and Dispensable Amino Acids

Nine amino acids are classified as *indispensable (essential)* amino acids (IDAA) because body synthesis is inadequate to meet metabolic needs, and they must therefore be supplied as a part of the diet. These amino acids are threonine, tryptophan, histidine, lysine, leucine, isoleucine, methionine, valine, and phenylalanine (Table 5–1). Absence or inadequate intake of any one of these amino acids leads to negative nitrogen balance, weight loss, impaired growth in infants and children, and clinical symptoms. The estimated requirements of indispensable amino acids are given in Table 5–2. Data derived from studies with stable isotope tracers of lysine, leucine, valine, and threonine have suggested that requirements for these indispensable amino acids may be two to three times as high as those established previously by nitrogen balance studies (Young and Bier, 1987).

The remaining *dispensable (nonessential)* amino acids (DAA) are equally important to protein structure; however, if adequate amounts of particular dispensable amino acids are not present at the time of protein synthesis, they can either be synthesized from indispensable amino acids or from appropriate carbon skeletons readily manufactured in the cell.

Conditionally dispensable amino acids are those that can become indispensable under certain clinical condi-

TABLE 5–1. Classification of Amino Acids Based on Dispensability*

Indispensable	Conditionally Indispensable	Dispensable
Leucine	Proline	Glutamate
Isoleucine	Serine	Alanine
Valine	Arginine	Asparate
Tryptophan	Tyrosine	Glutamine
Phenylalanine	Cysteine	
Methionine	Taurine	
Threonine	Glycine	
Lysine		
Histidine		

* Adapted from Laidlaw AS and Kopple JD: Newer concepts of the indispensable amino acids. Am J Clin Nutr 46:593, 1987.

TABLE 5–2. Estimates of Amino Acid Requirements*

	Requirements (mg/kg/day) by Age Group			
Amino Acid	*Infants, Age 3–4 Mo*†	*Children, Age ~2 Yr*‡	*Children, Age 10–12 Yr*§	*Adults*‖
Histidine	28	?	?	8–12
Isoleucine	70	31	28	10
Leucine	161	73	44	14
Lysine	103	64	44	12
Methionine plus cystine	58	27	22	13
Phenylalanine plus tyrosine	125	69	22	14
Threonine	87	37	28	7
Tryptophan	17	12.5	3.3	3.5
Valine	93	38	25	10
Total without histidine	714	352	216	84

* Adapted, by permission from WHO: Energy and Protein Requirements Report of a Joint FAO/WHO/UNU Expert Consultation. Technical Report Series 724. Geneva, World Health Organization, 1985, p. 65.

† Based on amounts of amino acids in human milk or cow's milk formulas fed at levels that supported good growth.

‡ Based on achievement of nitrogen balance sufficient to support adequate lean tissue gain (16 mg N/kg/day).

§ Based on upper range of requirement for positive nitrogen balance.

‖ Based on highest estimate of requirement to achieve nitrogen balance.

FURTHER READING: Legumes as Sources of Protein

Legumes are unique in the vegetable kingdom because of their seeds, which are high in protein and low in starch, unlike the seeds of cereal grains, which are low in protein and high in starch. Furthermore, their content of essential amino acids is more like that of animal proteins. If supplemented with a small amount of methionine from cereal or animal sources, their amino acid pattern is adequate to support both life and growth in humans. Soybeans are unique in that a product of their processing, soy protein isolate, is a protein with an amino acid pattern capable of supporting life and growth (WHO, 1985).

This unusual nature is presumably the adventitious outcome of a rare ability of the leguminous plant to fix gaseous nitrogen from the air and put it to its own use. Actually, the plant itself does not have this capability, and like all other plants must take in nitrogen via the roots in the form of either nitrate or ammonium ions. However, located in nodules on leguminous roots are *Rhizobium* bacteria that are able to fix atmospheric nitrogen. In a symbiotic relationship, bacteria furnish nitrogen in the form of amino acids and amides in return for energy supplied by the plant via photosynthesis.

Whether this apparent profusion of protein simply spills over into the seeds of the plant or whether the high levels of amino acids in beans, peas, and peanuts is of some evolutionary advantage as yet remains a secret, the answer of which is known only to the plant.

tions. Taurine, cysteine, and possibly tyrosine are thought to be conditionally dispensable in preterm infants (Laidlaw and Kopple, 1987). Arginine may become indispensable in those who are malnourished, septic, or recovering from injury or surgery (Barbul et al, 1981). (See specific chapters for further discussion of amino acid requirements particular to disease states.)

Metabolic Pool of Amino Acids

There is no large reserve of free amino acids in the body, and any amount above that needed for synthesis of tissue protein and the various nonprotein nitrogen-containing compounds is metabolized. However, there does exist in the cellular proteins themselves a metabolic pool of amino acids in a state of dynamic equilibrium that may be called on at any given time to meet an appropriate need. The continuous turnover of protein in the adult is probably necessary for maintaining an amino acid pool and the capability to meet the demand for amino acids by various cells and tissues when they are stimulated to make necessary proteins (Young and Bier, 1987). The most active tissues for protein turnover are the plasma proteins, intestinal mucosa, pancreas, liver, and kidney, whereas the muscle, skin, and brain are much less active (Fig. 5–3).

Special Functions of Amino Acids

Almost all of the amino acids have certain unique functions in the body. *Tryptophan,* the most complex amino acid, is a precursor of the vitamin niacin and of the neurotransmitter serotonin. *Methionine* is a principal donor of methyl groups for the synthesis of compounds such as choline and creatinine. It is also a precursor of *cystine* and many other sulfur-containing compounds. *Phenylalanine* is a precursor of *tyrosine,* and together they lead to the formation of *thyroxine* and *epinephrine. Tyrosine* is the precursor from which the pigment

FURTHER READING: Denaturation of Proteins

The three-dimensional structure of a protein is significant in terms of its function. The bonds maintaining the three-dimensional shape are relatively weak and are easily disrupted by mechanical agitation or extremes of temperature, acidity, or alkalinity. When this occurs, the protein loses its characteristic shape and is no longer able to function in its particular role. This irreversible "unraveling" of the protein molecule is called *denaturation,* an event that is usually detrimental and sometimes even disastrous to the organism depending on how many protein molecules have been affected. While an egg is frying, the egg white gradually thickens and turns white as the protein is denatured by the heat. Similarly, a severe burn denatures and thus destroys protein in the skin and blood vessels.

It is actually the susceptibility of proteins to rather moderate excesses of heat, cold, acid, or alkali that determines the limitation of environment within which humans are able to survive and function.

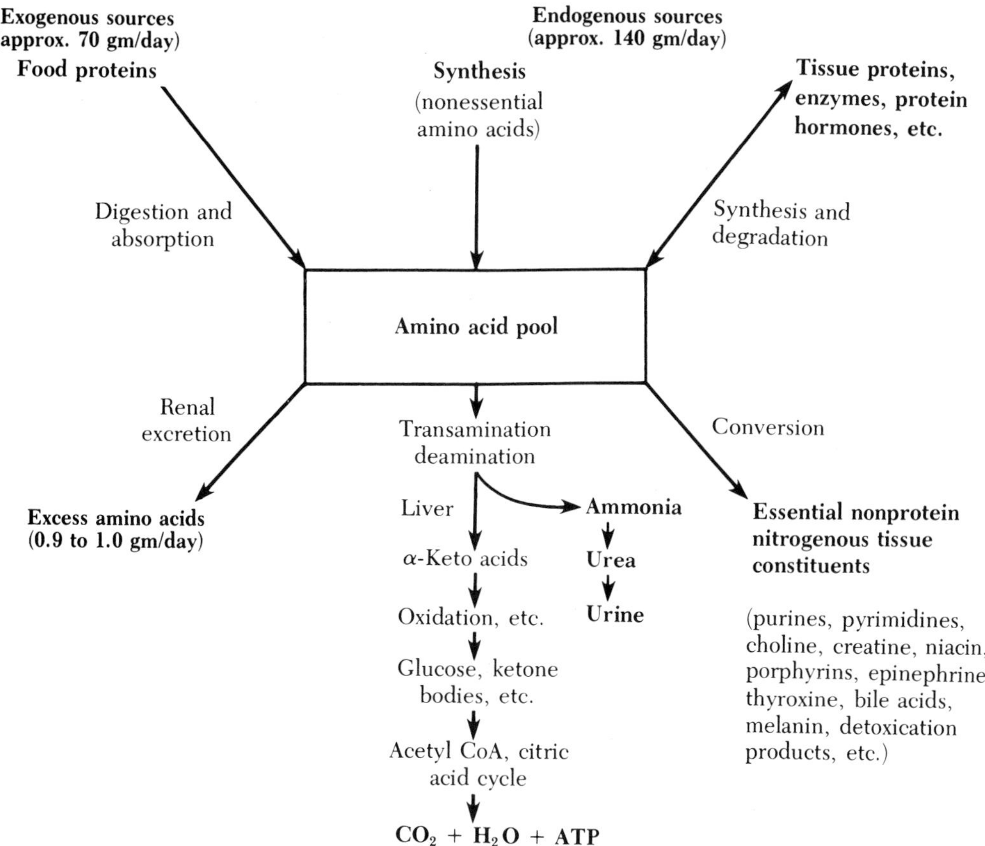

FIGURE 5–3. *Protein and amino acid metabolism. (From Orten JM and Neuhaus OW: Human Biochemistry, 10th ed. St. Louis, CV Mosby, 1982, p 327.)*

of skin and hair is made. *Arginine* and *citrulline* are specifically involved in the synthesis of urea in the liver. *Glycine,* the simplest and most ubiquitous of the amino acids, combines with many toxic substances and converts them to harmless forms that are then excreted. It is also used in the synthesis of the porphyrin nucleus of hemoglobin and is a constituent of one of the bile acids. *Histidine* is essential for the synthesis of *histamine,* which causes vasodilatation in the circulatory system. *Creatinine,* synthesized from *arginine, glycine,* and *methionine,* combines with phosphate to form creatine phosphate, an important reservoir of high-energy phosphate in the cell. *Glutamine,* formed from *glutamic acid,* and *asparagine,* from *aspartic acid,* have important roles as reservoirs of amino groups throughout the body. In addition, *glutamic acid* is a precursor of the neurotransmitter *gamma-amino butyric acid.*

PROTEIN METABOLISM

Amino Acid Catabolism

Before oxidation of the carbon skeleton of the amino acid molecule can take place, the amino group must be detached. This is accomplished by oxidative deamination, with the formation of a keto acid (Fig. 5–4). This process takes place mainly in the liver.

The carbon skeletons are converted into some of the same intermediates formed during glucose and fatty acid catabolism. These can be carried to the peripheral tissues where they enter into the citric acid cycle to produce adenosine triphosphate (ATP). These fragments can also be used in synthetic processes to make glucose or fats. Approximately 58% of the protein consumed can be converted into glucose in this manner.

Most amino acids, particularly alanine, are potentially glucogenic. Pyruvate from glucose oxidation in muscle is aminated to form alanine, which in turn is transported to the liver where it is deaminated and the carbon skeleton reconverted to glucose. This *alanine cycle* is important as a source of glucose during periods of low exogenous supply (see Fig. 3–6). It is also a method of moving nitrogen from the muscle to the liver without the formation of ammonia.

The amino group is released in deamination chiefly as ammonia, which is used in synthetic processes or is carried to the liver for conversion to *urea,* the form in which most of it is excreted. Because ammonia is highly toxic, it is transported in combination with glutamic acid as glutamine.

Synthesis of urea occurs through the *ornithine cycle,* which is presented in condensed form in Figure 5–5. Carbon dioxide and ammonia (with energy from ATP) combine with ornithine through a series of steps to

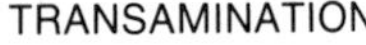

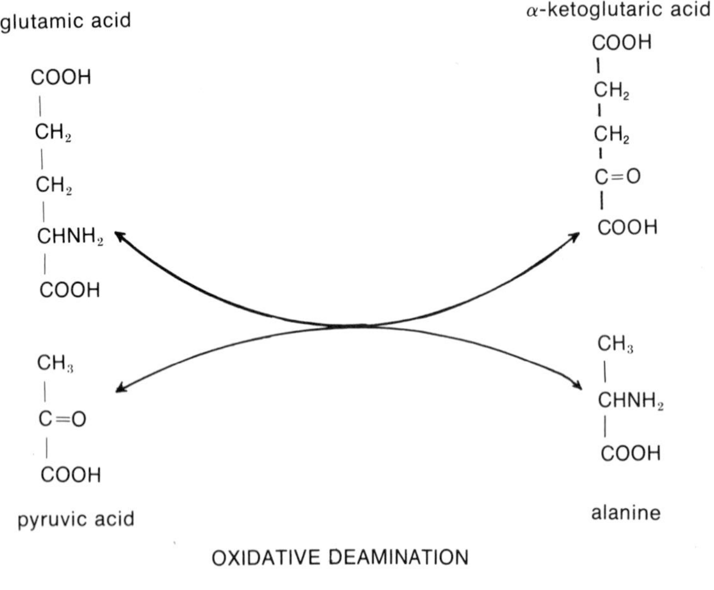

OXIDATIVE DEAMINATION

$$\underset{\alpha\text{-amino acid}}{R{-}\underset{NH_2}{\underset{|}{CH}}{-}COOH} \xrightarrow[\text{enzyme}]{\text{flavin}} \underset{\alpha\text{-amino acid}}{R{-}\underset{NH}{\underset{\|}{C}}{-}COOH} \xrightarrow[H_2O]{NH_3} \underset{\alpha\text{-ketoacid}}{R{-}\underset{O}{\underset{\|}{C}}{-}COOH}$$

FIGURE 5–4. *Transamination and deamination.*

form arginine, which is then hydrolyzed to yield urea and ornithine. Thus an ornithine molecule is used repeatedly in the formation of arginine and urea.

Protein Synthesis

The fundamental use of the amino acid is as a building block for body proteins, such as enzymes, hormones, vitamins, and structural proteins. Each cell has the capacity to synthesize an enormous number of specific proteins.

Protein synthesis requires that all of the necessary amino acids must be available. All of the indispensable amino acids must be present. The dispensable amino acids must either be supplied as such, or suitable carbon skeletons and amino groups from other amino acids must be available for the process of *transamination* (see Fig. 5–4).

Synthesis of the characteristic proteins of each cell is controlled by DNA, the genetic material in the cell nucleus. DNA functions as a template for the synthesis of the various forms of RNA, which then participate in protein synthesis. Energy for synthesis is supplied by ATP, which is itself a nucleotide.

Hormonal Regulation

Hormones have both anabolic and catabolic effects on protein metabolism. *Growth hormone* stimulates pro-

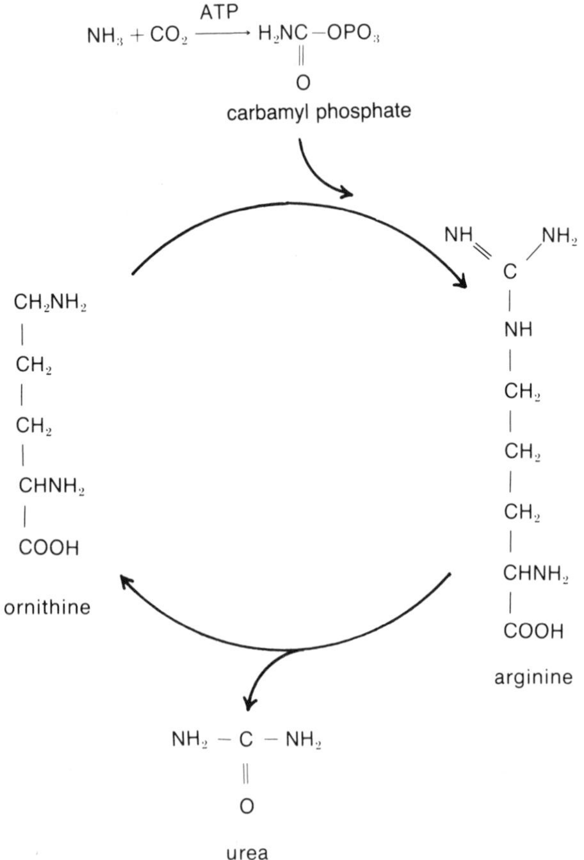

FIGURE 5–5. *Ornithine cycle.*

tein synthesis, thus increasing tissue concentration. *Insulin* also stimulates protein synthesis by accelerating amino acid transport across the cell membrane. Lack of insulin reduces protein synthesis. *Testosterone* also stimulates protein synthesis during growth periods. The *glucocorticoids* stimulate gluconeogenesis and ketogenesis from proteins. *Thyroxine* indirectly affects protein metabolism by increasing the rate of metabolism in all cells, thus increasing the rate of normal anabolic and catabolic reactions of protein. In physiologic doses and in the presence of adequate energy intake and amino acids, thyroxine promotes protein synthesis. However, with inadequate energy or in unphysiologically large doses, thyroxine has a catabolic effect.

PROTEIN DEFICIENCY

Low-protein intakes can be tolerated by both adults and children, depending on the quality of protein ingested and the level of energy intake. The urinary nitrogen output falls drastically on a low-protein intake, indicating the compensating effect of an adaptation process taking place within the body. After 4 or 5 days of negative nitrogen balance, equilibrium is re-established at a lower level. Beyond a critical point, however, the body can no longer adapt, and protein deficiency with edema, wasting of body tissues, fatty liver, dermatosis, diminished immune response, weakness, and loss of vigor develop.

Protein deficiency is seen more often in children because of their higher requirements for protein and energy per kilogram of body weight, their greater susceptibility to factors such as infections that increase protein requirements, and their inability to obtain food by their own means.

Protein-Energy Malnutrition

Protein-energy malnutrition (PEM) is a term describing a class of clinical disorders resulting from varying combinations and degrees of protein and energy deficiency, usually accompanied by additional physiologic and environmental insults and stresses. These disorders are often aggravated by infectious processes and are accompanied by other nutritional deficiencies, such as severe vitamin A deficiency.

The major forms of PEM are *marasmus,* in which the deficiency is primarily of energy-providing foods; *kwashiorkor,* characterized by protein deficiency; and *marasmic kwashiorkor* in which deficiencies of both protein and energy are present (Torun and Viteri, 1988). Although PEM can be found in all parts of the world and can occur at all ages, it is primarily a disease that occurs in young children who live in poverty in underdeveloped countries. The World Health Organization estimates that 300 million children in the world have growth retardation as a result of malnutrition. Severe PEM can result in a mortality rate of 40%, usually as the result of infection.

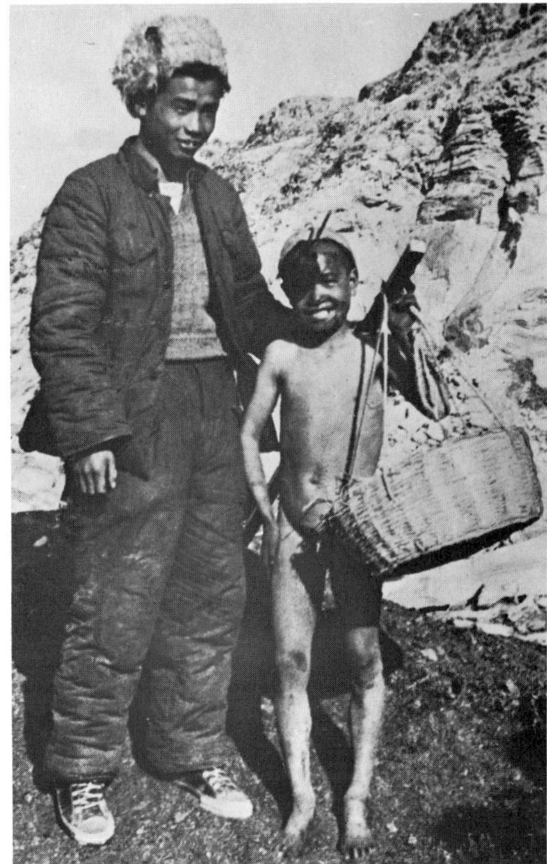

FIGURE 5–6. *Two Asian boys of the same age who illustrate growth differences due to diet. The boy on the right worked in a mine and received ordinary protein-poor local food. The other boy spent 4 years in a boarding school where he was well fed. (Courtesy of Food and Agriculture Organization of the United Nations.)*

Marasmus is a chronic condition of semistarvation, to which the child adjusts to some extent by reduced growth (Fig. 5–6). In advanced stages, it is characterized by muscular wasting and absence of subcutaneous fat. It is usually found in children of all ages and often results from failure of breast-feeding and the use of overdiluted formula. It is associated increasingly with the food shortages that occur typically with wars, droughts, and extreme poverty.

Kwashiorkor appears among infants and young children in the late breast-feeding, weaning, and post-weaning phases, usually between the ages of 1 and 4 years. It is associated with extreme protein deficiency, which leads to hypoalbuminemia, pitting edema, and enlarged fatty liver. Subcutaneous fat is usually preserved, but muscle wasting is often masked by the edema (Fig. 5–7). In *marasmic kwashiorkor,* which

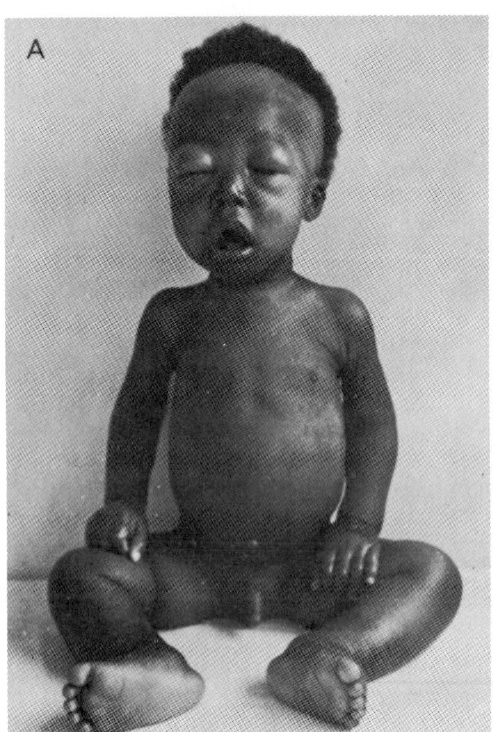

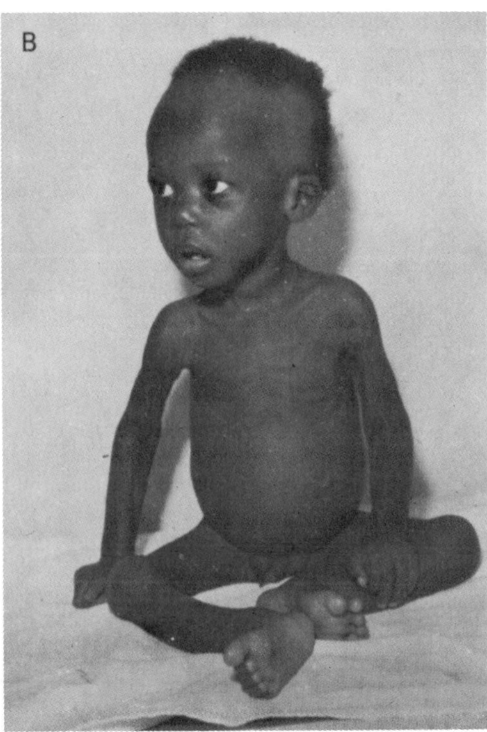

FIGURE 5–7. *Child with kwashiorkor (A) on admission and (B) after loss of edema with refeeding. (From McLaren DS and Burman D: Textbook of Paediatric Nutrition, 2nd ed. Edinburgh, Churchill Livingstone, 1982, p. 122.)*

combines symptoms of both deficiency states, the loss of subcutaneous fat becomes very apparent when edema is reduced in the early stages of treatment.

The condition of kwashiorkor was first described in 1933 by Cicely Williams, a pediatrician working among native children of the African Gold Coast (Ghana) (Williams, 1933). In the dialect of the region, "kwashiorkor" means "the disease of the deposed baby when the next one is born." The disease is associated with diets high in carbohydrate in which protein is inadequate and of low quality. Starchy gruels or vegetable diets of high bulk and low nutrient density are often fed as a result of poverty and ignorance.

In developed countries, PEM most often occurs secondary to trauma, disease, psychologic problems, or medical treatment. Management of this type of PEM is discussed in Chapter 29. Methods for assessing protein nutriture are given in Chapter 17.

EVALUATION OF PROTEIN QUALITY

Measurement Techniques

A variety of methods have been used to determine the quality of protein foods and food combinations in studies with laboratory animals. The simplest is the *protein efficiency ratio (PER),* which is equal to the gain in weight of a growing animal divided by its protein intake during the study period. The *biologic value (BV)* uses nitrogen balance techniques to determine the fraction of absorbed nitrogen retained in the body for growth or maintenance. *Net protein utilization (NPU)* compares the nitrogen intake over a period of time with the carcass nitrogen content. In addition to the percentage of absorbed nitrogen utilized (BV), this measure also includes the digestibility of the protein in question. Table 5–3 gives the digestibility values for various proteins.

The Food and Agriculture Organization of the United Nations has established an *amino acid requirement pattern* based on the requirements for indispensable amino acids for each age group (Table 5–4). This pattern can be used as a standard of comparison in roughly assessing the quality of food proteins and protein mixtures by calculating an *amino acid score.* The amino acid with the lowest score is designated as the *limiting amino acid.* Only tryptophan, threonine, lysine, and methionine plus cystine need to be calculated, because one of these is usually the limiting amino acid in most common foods. The formula for calculating this score is as follows:

$$\text{Amino acid score} = \frac{\text{milligrams of IDAA per gram of test protein}}{\text{milligrams of IDAA per gram of reference protein}}$$

in which IDAA = indispensable amino acid.

TABLE 5–3. Values for the Digestibility of Protein in Humans*

Protein Source	True Digestibility (mean % + SD)		Digestibility Relative to Reference Proteins
Eggs	97 ± 3	95	100
Milk and cheese	95 ± 3		
Meat and fish	94 ± 3		
Maize	85 ± 6		89
Rice, polished	88 ± 4		93
Wheat, whole	86 ± 5		90
Wheat, refined	96 ± 4		101
Oatmeal	86 ± 7		90
Peanut butter	95		100
Soy flour	86 ± 7		90
Beans	78		82
Mixed American diet	96†		101

* Reprinted with permission from *Recommended Dietary Allowances*, 10th ed., c. 1989 by the National Academy of Sciences. Published by National Academy Press.

Apparent protein digestibility is the percentage of nitrogen intake that does not appear in the feces, that is, $[(I - F) \times 100]/I$, where I = intake and F = fecal content. Estimates of true protein digestibility take into account the amount of nitrogen in feces when none is present in the diet plus the endogenous or obligatory loss, that is, $[I - (F - F_o) \times 100]/I$, where F_o = obligatory fecal nitrogen. If F_o is not measured, 12 mg/kg body weight may be used for the calculation.

† Recalculated from apparent digestibility, using F_o = 12 mg of nitrogen per kilogram of body weight.

Table 5–4 illustrates the high quality of proteins in foods from animal sources compared with the requirement pattern.

Complementarity of Food Proteins

A diet high in animal protein will obviously provide adequate indispensable amino acids to ensure efficient protein synthesis. Such a preponderance of animal protein is not necessary, however. Most people tend to ingest a mixture of foods in a meal, and when available in sufficient quantity, the various proteins tend to complement or supplement each other by providing a total mixture containing all of the indispensable amino acids.

The principle of protein *complementarity* applies particularly to diets in which cultural, religious, or economic factors restrict the amount of animal protein available. A variety of combinations will effectively provide protein of sufficient quality under these circumstances. Eating large amounts of cereal proteins, such as the protein in rice, which contain all of the essential amino acids but in less than adequate proportion, will provide enough of the limiting amino acids to allow for adequate protein synthesis. Adding small amounts of meat or fish to a primarily cereal diet will supplement an otherwise inadequate amino acid pattern. Combining cereals and legumes, which are low in

TABLE 5–4. Amino Acid Requirement Patterns* Compared with the Composition of High-Quality Proteins† and the US Diet‡§

	Amino Acid Requirement Pattern by Age (mg/g of protein)				Reported Composition (mg/g of protein)					
		Children‖							US Diet by Age Group	
Amino Acid	*Infants 3–4 Mo*	*~2 Yr*	*10–12 Yr*	*Adults*	*Human Milk*	*Chicken Egg*	*Cow's Milk*	*Beef*	*1–3 Yr*	*All Ages*
Histidine	16	(19)¶	(19)¶	(11)¶	26	22	27	34		
Isoleucine	40	28	28	13	46	54	47	48	54	52
Leucine	93	66	44	19	93	86	95	81	80	77
Lysine	60	58	44	16	66	70	78	89	70	68
Methionine plus cystine	33	25	22	17	42	57	33	40	35	35
Phenylalanine plus tyrosine	72	63	22	19	72	93	102	80	81	78
Threonine	50	34	28	9	43	47	44	46	40	39
Tryptophan	10	11	(9)	5	17	17	14	12	12	12
Valine	54	35	25	13	55	66	64	50	57	54
Total without histidine	412	320	222	111	434	490	477	445	429	415

* Requirement pattern is calculated from amino acid requirements (Table 5–2) divided by the recommended allowance of reference protein. Protein allowance (in g/kg) is 1.73 for infants 3–4 months of age, 1.10 for children at 2 years of age, 0.99 for children 10–12 years of age, and 0.75 for adults. Except for infants, for whom the difference is trivial, and histidine for adults, patterns are identical with those reported by WHO (1985).

† From WHO: Energy and Protein Requirements. Report of a Joint FAO/WHO/UNU Expert Consultation. Technical Report Series 724. Geneva, World Health Organization, 1985.

‡ From the 1977–1978 USDA Nationwide Food Consumption Survey (USDA, 1984).

§Reprinted with permission from *Recommended Dietary Allowances*, 10th ed., c. 1989 by the National Academy of Sciences. Published by National Academy Press.

‖ Values in parentheses are imputed.

¶ The pattern for children 2 yrs old should be applied to children age 2 to 6 years and that shown for children 10 to 12 years old should be applied to children age 6 to 13 years. The adult pattern is applicable to children above 13 years of age.

TABLE 5–5. Amino Acid Composition of Some Foods*

Indispensable Amino Acid	Cheese, Eggs, Milk, and Meat	Corn	Cereal	Legumes	Whole Grains (With Germ)	Nuts Seed Oils Soybeans	Sesame and Sunflower Seeds	Peanuts	Green Leafy Vegetables	Gelatin	Yeast
Methionine			x	—	x	—	x	—	—	—	x
Isoleucine	x										
Leucine	x										
Lysine	x	—	—	x	x	x	—	—		—	
Phenylalanine											—
Threonine	x	—	—	x	—	x		—			x
Tryptophan		—		—			x			—	
Valine	x										

* Adapted from Erhard D: Nutrition education for the "now" generation. J Nutr Educ 3:135, 1971.
X = high amount of amino acid present in that food; — = low amount of amino acid present in that food. Blank spaces indicate a general good balance of amino acids in the food.

lysine and methionine, respectively, will result in an adequate mixture for protein synthesis (Table 5–5. Adding milk to a cereal-based meal will also increase efficiency of the cereal protein. See also Further Reading, p. 290).

More total protein will be required in a vegetable protein diet than in a diet of mixed vegetable and animal proteins because more of the lower-quality protein will be needed to meet the minimum requirements for amino acids and nitrogen. Because of their lower digestibility values, vegetable proteins are less available.

DIETARY INTAKES

Recommended Dietary Allowances

The RDA for protein is based on evidence from nitrogen balance studies that determined the requirements of young male adults for *reference proteins* (i.e., highly digestible, high-quality protein, such as egg, meat, milk, or fish) to be 0.61 g/kg of body weight per day (WHO, 1985). Adjusting for differences in body weight indicated that needs of young women were similar to those of men. Also, it was judged that the requirements based on the quantity, quality, and digestibility of protein in the average American diet were similar to those determined on reference proteins (see Tables 5–3 and 5–4). Accordingly, after addition of a factor of 25% (2 standard deviations) to account for variability and thus meet the needs of 97.5% of the population, an RDA of 0.75 g/kg was established for adults in the United States. Few data are available on which to base recommendations for the elderly; however, it was believed that because inefficient use of dietary protein in this age group would be balanced by diminished levels of protein tissue, the RDA would not be dissimilar from that of all adults. The RDA Committee also recommended an upper limit of protein intake at no more than twice the RDA (Food and Nutrition Board, 1989), reflecting concern that a lifetime of excessive protein intake may accelerate the age-associated process of renal glomerular sclerosis and potentially influence the development of osteoporosis (National Research Council, 1989) (see Chapter 22).

Recommended allowances of protein for all age/sex groups, pregnancy, and lactation are listed in Table 5–6.

TABLE 5–6. Recommended Dietary Allowances for Protein*

Category	Age (Years) or Condition	Weight (kg)	Recommended Dietary Allowance (g/kg)	Recommended Dietary Allowance (g/day)
Both sexes	0–0.5	6	2.2	13
	0.5–1	9	1.6	14
	1–3	13	1.2	16
	4–6	20	1.1	24
	7–10	28	1.0	28
Males	11–14	45	1.0	45
	15–18	66	0.9	59
	19–24	72	0.8	58
	25–50	79	0.8	63
	51+	77	0.8	63
Females	11–14	46	1.0	46
	15–18	55	0.8	44
	19–24	58	0.8	46
	25–50	63	0.8	50
	51+	65	0.8	50
Pregnancy	1st trimester			+10
	2nd trimester			+10
	3rd trimester			+10
Lactation	1st 6 months			+15
	2nd 6 months			+12

* Reprinted with permission from *Recommended Dietary Allowances,* 10th ed., c. 1989 by the National Academy of Sciences. Published by National Academy Press.

† Amino acid score of typical American diet is 100 for all age groups, except for young infants. Digestibility is equal to reference proteins.

For infants from birth to 3 months of age, breast-feeding that meets energy needs also meets protein needs. Formula substitutes should have the same amount and amino acid composition as human milk, corrected for digestibility if appropriate.

Food Sources of Protein

From the United States Department of Agriculture (USDA) food consumption data of 1977 to 1978 and 1985, it is apparent that the average consumption levels of protein in the United States are quite generous. Foods of animal origin, such as meat, poultry, fish, eggs, milk, and milk products, supply 65% of the protein (Block et al, 1985; USDA 1983, 1984, 1986, and 1987). Plant products richest in protein are the legumes—soybeans, peanuts, peas, beans, and lentils—but because of their limited consumption in the United States they contribute only 3% of the protein. Cereals contain lesser amounts of protein of varying quality, but because of the large amounts in which they are consumed, they contribute 18% of the protein in the American diet. Fruits and vegetables provide protein of reasonable quality, but because it is diluted by large amounts of water and fiber, and, in the case of roots and tubers, by starch, it is only 7 to 8% of the protein in the diet (USDA 1983, 1984). Table 5–7 gives the protein content of some common foods (Fig. 5–8).

Food processing alters the nutritive value of protein. Overheating, particularly in the absence of water (e.g., in frying or "puffing" of dry cereals), may destroy heat labile amino acids such as lysine or may alter them in a manner that causes the protein to become resistant to digestive enzymes. Most cooking processes, however, exert a positive effect by softening connective tissue, thus increasing digestibility and favoring the release of amino acids.

TABLE 5–7. Protein Content of Some Foods

0–1 g
Butter, margarine, 1 tsp
Pear, 1 medium
Cake, 1 piece
2–3 g
Milk chocolate, 1 oz
Cereal, refined, 1 oz
Bread, 1 slice
Corn, canned, ½ cup
Chicken noodle soup, 1 cup
French fries, 1 regular serving
4–6 g
Cereal, bran, 1 oz
Baked potato, 1 large
Peas, ½ cup
7–8 g
Navy beans, cooked, ½ cup
Egg, 1 medium
Cheese, 1 oz
Tuna, 1 oz
Tofu, 3½ oz
Milk, 1 cup
9–10 g
Peanuts, roasted, 1 oz
Macaroni and cheese, ¾ cup
Pizza, cheese, ⅛ of a 12-in. slice
12–15 g
Taco, 1
Hamburger, 1
Chili with meat, 1 cup
22–26 g
Meat, lean, 3 oz
Big Mac, 1

Trends in Consumption of Protein

Protein deficiency is not a problem in the healthy American population. The 1985 Food Consumption Surveys showed that the average proportion of energy from protein was 16.6%, a level more than adequate based on the RDA. The protein intake of all individuals

FURTHER READING: Enzymes as Proteins

The fact that *all enzymes are proteins* and thus susceptible to denaturation is a significant circumstance with respect to the environmental demands of the human body. Enzymes function by attaching themselves to molecules of a very characteristic shape and size; thus, the importance of maintaining the original form of a particular enzyme is obvious. Because denaturation changes the form of enzymes and thus renders them nonfunctional, most living organisms cannot tolerate extremes of temperature and pH. A few exceptions occur, such as the minute forms of plant life that survive at the near-boiling temperatures of hot springs or in the frigid environment of snow banks. Because of the rigid requirements of enzyme function for optimal pH, a number of mechanisms exist for eliminating excess of acid or alkaline materials from the blood.

Among the physiologic examples of enzyme denaturation is the effect of lactic acid that accumulates during vigorous exercise, eventually reaching a level sufficient to interfere with normal enzyme action, thus contributing to the resultant fatigue. Enzymes in uncooked foods are denatured by the hydrochloric acid of the stomach. Papain—a papaya fruit enzyme used to tenderize meats—is rapidly denatured as meat temperatures rise during cooking. If not destroyed in this manner, it is later denatured and partially digested when it reaches the stomach. The same fate occurs with enzymes that are taken orally and that are advertised erroneously as cures for various human illnesses and diseases.

Occasionally, enzymes are legitimately given orally to supplement inadequate amounts secreted into the gut. In this case, however, the enzymes are packaged in capsules that do not dissolve until they have reached the small intestine.

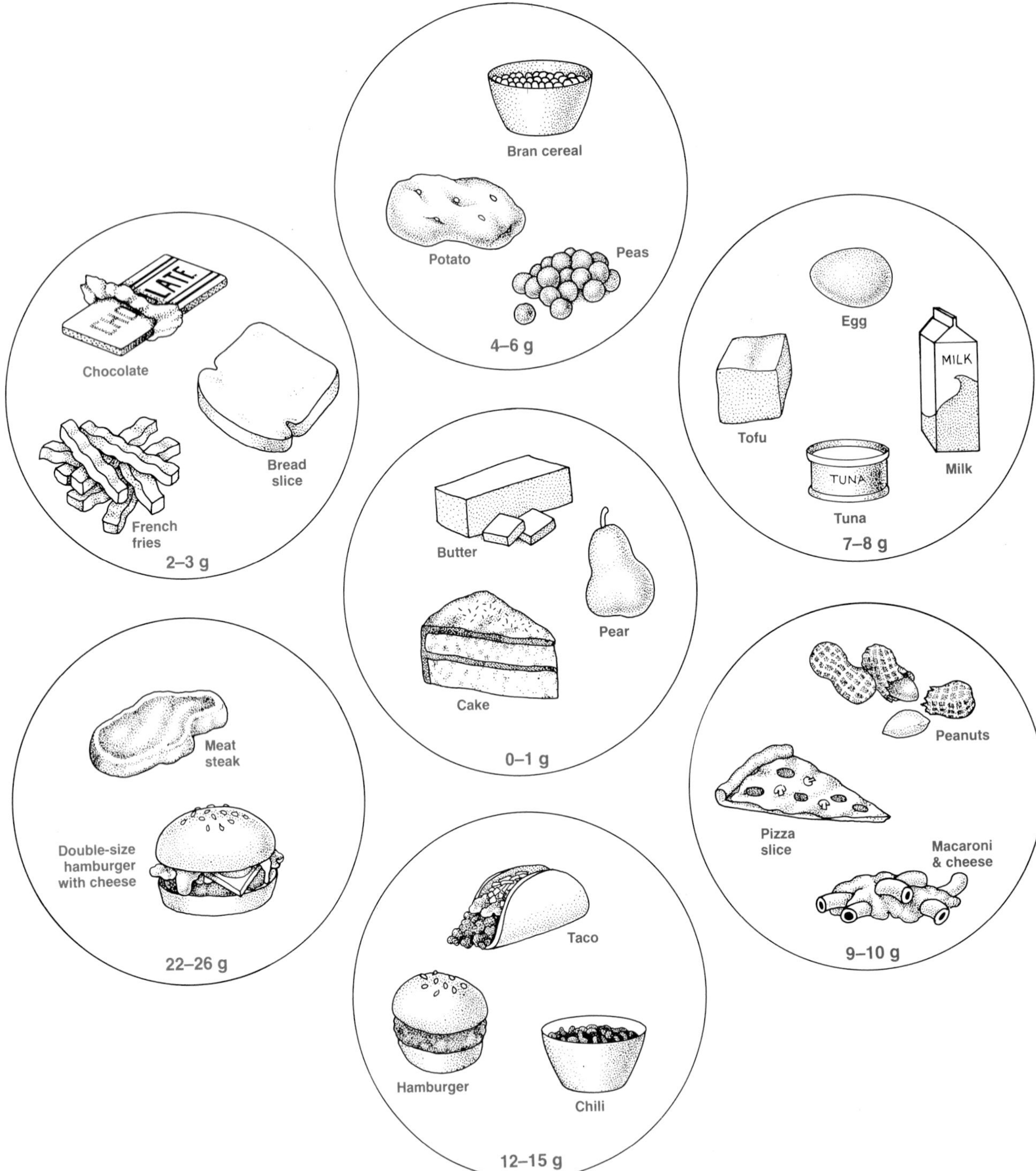

FIGURE 5–8. *Protein in some foods. (See Table 5–7 for serving sizes.)*

was 15 to 16% of energy intake for children 1 to 5 years of age, 16% for women 19 to 50 years of age, and 16.5% for men 19 to 50 years of age, regardless of income. All groups consumed amounts of protein well above the RDA, and some groups (preschoolers and adolescent males) had intakes close to twice the RDA (USDA 1986, 1987).

CITED REFERENCES

Barbul A et al: Metabolic and immune effects of arginine in post injury hyperalimentation. J Trauma 21:970, 1981.

Block G et al: Nutrient sources in the American diet: Quantitative data from the NHANES II Survey. II: Macronutrients and fats. Am J Epidemiol 122:27, 1985.

Food and Nutrition Board, National Research Council, NAS: Recommended Dietary Allowances, 10th ed. Washington, DC, National Academy Press, 1989.

Laidlaw SA and Kopple JD: New concepts of the indispensable amino acids. Am J Clin Nutr 46:593, 1987.

National Research Council: Diet and Health: Implications for Reducing Chronic Disease Risk. Washington, DC, National Academy Press, 1989.

Torun B and Viteri FE: Protein-energy malnutrition. *In* Shils ME and Young VE (eds): Modern Nutrition in Health and Disease, 7th ed. Philadelphia, Lea & Febiger, 1988.

USDA: Nationwide Food Consumption Survey 1977–78. Food Intakes: Individuals in 48 States, Year 1977–78. Report I-1, Consumer Nutrition Division, Human Nutrition Information Service. Hyattsville, MD, USDA, 1983.

USDA: Nationwide Food Consumption Survey 1977–78. Food Intakes: Individuals in 48 States, Year 1977–78. Report I-2, Consumer Nutrition Division, Human Nutrition Information Service. Hyattsville, MD, USDA, 1984.

USDA: Nationwide Food Consumption Survey. Continuing Survey of Food Intakes by Individuals. Men 19–50 Years, 1 Day, 1985, Report No. 85-3, Nutrition Monitoring Division, Human Nutrition Information Service. Hyattsville, MD, USDA, 1986.

USDA: Nationwide Food Consumption Survey. Continuing Survey of Food Intakes by Individuals. Women 19–50 Years and Their Children 1–5 Years, 4 Days, 1985, Report No. 85-4, Nutrition Monitoring Division, Human Nutrition Information Service. Hyattsville, MD, USDA, 1987.

WHO: Energy and Protein Requirements. Report of a Joint FAO/WHO/UNU Expert Consultation. Technical Report Series 724. Geneva, World Health Organization, 1985.

Williams CD: A nutritional disease of childhood associated with a maize diet. Arch Dis Child 8:423, 1933.

Young VR and Bier DM: A kinetic approach to the determination of human amino acid requirements. Nutr Rev 45:289, 1987.

ADDITIONAL REFERENCES

Butterfield GE: Whole-body protein utilization in humans. Med Sci Sports Exer 19:S157, 1987.

Christensen HN: Role of amino acid transport and countertransport in nutrition and metabolism. Physiol Rev 70:43, 1990.

Energy and protein requirements revisited. Lancet 2:1279, 1985.

Energy and Protein Requirements: Joint FAO/WHO Ad Hoc Committee, Tech. Report No. 522. Geneva, World Health Organization, 1973.

Harper AE and Peters JC: Protein intake, brain amino acid and serotonin concentrations and protein self-selection. J Nutr 119:677, 1989.

Hegsted DM: Protein needs and possible modification of the American diet. J Am Diet Assoc 68:317, 1976.

Jackson AA: Amino acids: Essential and non-essential? Lancet 1:1034, 1983.

Karplus M and McCamon JA: The dynamics of proteins. Sci Am 254:42, 1986.

Kendler BD: Taurine: An overview of its role in preventive medicine. Prev Med 18:79, 1989.

Kopple JD and Swendseid ME: Evidence that histidine is an essential amino acid in normal and chronically uremic men. J Clin Invest 55:881, 1975.

McLaren DS: The great protein fiasco. Lancet 2:93, 1974.

Rao KS: Evolution of kwashiorkor and marasmus. Lancet 1:709, 1974.

Rose WC et al: The amino acid requirements of man. J Biol Chem 217:987, 1955.

Rossouw JE: Kwashiorkor in North America. Am J Clin Nutr 49:588, 1989.

Rudman D et al: Hypotyrosinemia, hypocystinemia and failure to retain nitrogen during total parenteral nutrition of cirrhotic patients. Gastroenterology 81:1025, 1981.

Snyderman SE: The protein and amino acid requirements of the premature infant. *In* Ionxix JHP et al(ed): Metabolic Processes in the Fetus and Newborn Infant. Leiden, HE Stenfert Kroesse, 1971.

CHAPTER 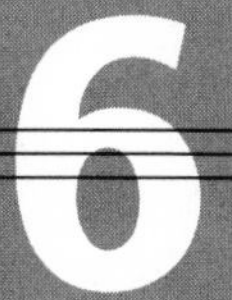

VITAMINS

CHAPTER OUTLINE

KEY TERMS

ANTIVITAMIN—a substance that interferes with the synthesis or metabolism of vitamins
ASCORBIC ACID—a hexose derivative; vitamin C
BERIBERI—thiamin deficiency disease
BIOTIN—a sulfur-containing vitamin that is synthesized by microorganisms in the lower gastrointestinal tract
CALCITRIOL—metabolically active form of vitamin D produced by the kidney and which functions as a hormone; 1,25-dihydroxycholecalciferol (1,25$(OH)_2D_3$)
CAROTENE—a yellow or red pigment found in carrots, sweet potatoes, leafy vegetables, milk fat, and egg yolk and which can be converted into vitamin A in the body
CHOLECALCIFEROL—vitamin D_3; 7-dehydrocholesterol that has been activated by ultraviolet irradiation
CHOLINE—a natural amine and precursor of acetylcholine; often classed with the B-complex vitamins but can be synthesized by humans
COBALAMIN—vitamin B_{12} in food
CYANOCOBALAMIN—commercially available form of vitamin B_{12}
7-DEHYDROCHOLESTEROL—a precursor of vitamin D found in the epidermal layer of the skin, which upon ultraviolet irradiation converts to vitamin D_3
ERGOCALCIFEROL—vitamin D_2; ergosterol that has been activated by ultraviolet irradiation
ERGOSTEROL—a precursor of vitamin D found in plants, which upon irradiation converts to vitamin D_2
FOLATE (FOLACIN)—a generic term for a group of compounds chemically and nutritionally similar to folic acid
FOLIC ACID—pteroylglutamic acid
MENADIONE—a fat-soluble, synthetic form of vitamin K
MENAQUINONE—vitamin K formed as the result of bacterial action in the intestinal tract; vitamin K as it occurs in animal tissue
NIACIN—generic term for nicotinamide (niacinamide) and nicotinic acid; vitamin B_3
NICOTINAMIDE—an amide of niacin without the vasodilating activity of niacin
PANTOTHENIC ACID—a B-complex vitamin
PELLAGRA—niacin deficiency disease
PYRIDOXINE—vitamin B_6
RETINOL—vitamin A
RETINOL EQUIVALENT—a measure of the vitamin A activity in foods
RIBOFLAVIN—vitamin B_2
RICKETS—a disease of abnormal ossification of the bone caused by a deficiency of vitamin D
SCURVY—vitamin C deficiency disease
THIAMIN—vitamin B_1
TOCOPHEROL—a molecule with a ring system and long saturated side chain, which has vitamin E biologic activity
TRYPTOPHAN—an amino acid; precursor of niacin
VITAMIN—an organic compound that is essential in small amounts for control of metabolic processes and that cannot be synthesized by the body
XEROPHTHALMIA (XEROSIS CONJUNCTIVAE)—dryness of the conjunctiva and cornea owing to vitamin A deficiency

Vitamins are organic compounds essential for specific metabolic reactions that cannot be synthesized by human tissue cells from simple metabolites. Many act as coenzymes or as parts of enzymes responsible for promoting essential chemical reactions. Vitamin A and niacin can be formed in the body if their precursors are supplied. Vitamin K, biotin, folacin, and vitamin B_{12} are produced by microorganisms in the intestinal tract. Vitamin D is synthesized from a cholesterol precursor in the skin upon exposure to sunlight.

The term *vitamine* was coined in 1912 by Casimir Funk to designate the accessory food factors necessary to life. The original theory that these substances were *vital amines* has been discredited, but the designation, minus the terminal "e," remains.

Because the existence of many vitamins was recognized before their chemical natures were identified, they were designated by letters and sometimes nomenclature descriptive of their function. Correct usage currently derives names from their chemical structure; however, the more familiar and frequently more convenient alphabetic terminology continues in wide use.

Vitamins are usually classified into two groups on the basis of solubility, which determines to some degree their stability, occurrence in foodstuffs, distribution in body fluids, and tissue storage capacity.

FAT-SOLUBLE VITAMINS

Each of the fat-soluble vitamins A, D, E, and K has a distinct and separate physiologic role. For the most part they are absorbed with other lipids, and efficient absorption requires the presence of bile and pancreatic juice. They are transported to the liver via the lymph as a part of lipoproteins and are stored in various body tissues, although not all in the same tissues or to the same extent. They are not normally excreted in the urine.

Vitamin A (Retinol)

The first fat-soluble vitamin to be recognized was vitamin A. Two groups of research workers, McCollum and Davis at the University of Wisconsin, and Osborne and Mendel at Yale University, made the discovery almost simultaneously in 1913.

Vitamin A is the generic term used to describe all retinoids having the biologic activity of all-trans retinol. Vitamin A, a light yellow crystalline alcohol, has been named retinol in reference to its specific function in the retina of the eye. Natural vitamin A usually occurs in the form of long-chain retinyl esters. Metabolically active forms of the vitamin include the corresponding aldehyde (retinal) and acid (retinoic acid).

The yellow-orange-red provitamin carotenoids, which are converted to vitamin A within the body with varying degrees of efficiency, are described in terms of beta-carotene, the most active. Of the several hundred naturally occurring carotenoids, only 50 have significant biologic activity.

Absorption, Transport, and Storage

Preformed vitamin A and carotenoids are released from proteins in the stomach. Retinyl esters are hydrolyzed in the small intestine to retinol, which is absorbed more efficiently than the esters. Beta-carotene is split in the cytoplasm of the intestinal mucosal cells into two molecules of retinaldehyde, which are reduced and esterified to form retinyl esters. The bioavailability of carotenoids is uncertain because of variability of absorption and conversion to retinol. Conversion of beta-carotene to vitamin A is regulated so that excess vitamin A is not absorbed from carotene sources. About 80 to 90% of retinyl esters but only 40 to 60% of carotenoids are absorbed. Dietary factors affecting carotenoid absorption include level and origin of dietary fat, amount of carotenoid, and digestibility of foods.

The retinyl esters are transported in the lymph to the blood and then to the liver as a part of chylomicrons and lipoproteins. At the time of mobilization from the liver, retinol is bound to *retinol-binding protein (RBP)* and travels to designated tissues in a complex with serum prealbumin. RBP transports vitamin A in the circulation and then may be removed from the circulation by the kidney (Fig. 6–1).

Approximately 90% of the vitamin A in the body is stored in the liver. The remainder is deposited in the fat depots, lungs, and kidneys. The liver gradually accumulates a reserve supply, which reaches its peak in adult life. This storage capacity allows for a temporarily reduced daily intake of vitamin A.

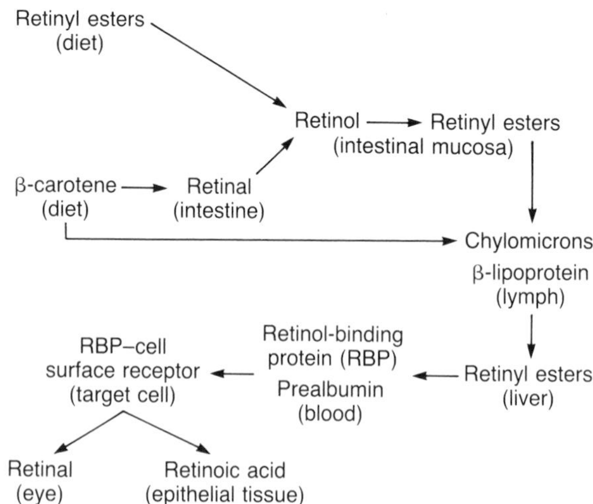

FIGURE 6–1. *The pathway by which dietary vitamin A reaches target cells of an organ.*

Functions

Vitamin A occupies essential roles in vision, growth, bone development, the development and maintenance of epithelial tissue, the immunity process, and normal reproduction.

The vitamin is a component of the visual pigments, and as such is essential to the integrity of photoreception in the rods and cones in the retina. The 11-cis isomer of vitamin A aldehyde *(retinal)* combines with the protein *opsin* to produce *rhodopsin* in the rods and *iodopsin* in the cones. Light changes the 11-cis configuration to the all-trans form of the retinaldehyde, causing visual excitation.

Vitamin A is necessary for growth and development of skeletal and soft tissues through its effect upon protein synthesis and bone cell differentiation. It is necessary for development of normal bone and of the enamel-forming epithelial cells in the development of teeth.

Vitamin A also has a role in the maintenance of normal epithelial structures. It is necessary in the differentiation of basal cells into mucous epithelial cells.

Nutrient Interactions

Although the exact role of vitamin A in iron metabolism is not clear, vitamin A deficiency ultimately results in anemia correctable by supplementation with vitamin A, iron, or both (Meija and Chew, 1988). This interrelationship may be important in areas where intakes of both nutrients are low. Hemoglobin concentration has been seen to increase in children receiving vitamin A-supplemented monosodium glutamate (MSG) (Muhilal et al, 1988a).

Measurement

Vitamin A was originally defined in terms of International Units (IU), which continue in wide use. However, the preferred measurement expresses vitamin A activity in chemical terms as micrograms (μg) of vitamin A alcohol *(retinol)*, beta-carotene, or other mixed carotenoids. Retinol equivalents (RE) are useful in calculating the vitamin A value of diets, as they permit summation of preformed vitamin A and carotenoids that occur in foods in different proportions and have different levels of biologic activity. These measurements are listed in Table 6-1.

TABLE 6-1. Retinol Equivalents (RE)

1 retinol equivalent = 1 μg retinol
= 6 μg β-carotene
= 12 μg other provitamin A carotenoids
= 3.33 IU vitamin A activity from retinol
= 10 IU vitamin A activity from β-carotene

Recommended Dietary Allowance

The RDA for vitamin A, expressed in μg of retinol, or *retinol equivalents* (RE), is listed in Table 6-2. The infant allowance is based on the amount of *retinol* in human milk. Adult allowances are based on levels that provide adequate blood levels and liver stores. Lower levels for women reflect smaller body size. Increased amounts in pregnancy and lactation provide for fetal storage and the vitamin A in breast milk.

Adequacy of vitamin A status is most often measured as serum vitamin A. Guidelines for interpretation of serum vitamin A values are given in Appendix 30.

The minimum requirement for adults to maintain adequate blood concentration and to prevent deficiency symptoms is 500 to 600 μg retinol or twice as much beta-carotene.

Sources

Some dietary sources of vitamin A are listed in Table 6-3. Preformed vitamin A occurs only in foods of animal origin, either in storage areas such as liver or asso-

TABLE 6-2. Recommended Dietary Allowances for Vitamin A in Retinol Equivalents*

Age (Years)	RDA† (in μg RE)
Infants	
0.0-0.5	375
0.5-1.0	375
Children	
1-3	400
4-6	500
7-10	700t
Males	
11-14	1,000
15-18	1,000
19-24	1,000
25-50	1,000
51+	1,000
Females	
11-14	800
15-18	800
19-24	800
25-50	800
51+	800
Pregnant	800
Lactating	
1st 6 months	1,300
2nd 6 months	1,200

* Food and Nutrition Board, National Research Council, NAS: Recommended Dietary Allowances, 10th ed. Washington, DC, National Academy Press, 1989.
† RDA = recommended dietary allowances; RE = retinol equivalents.

TABLE 6–3. Vitamin A Content of Selected Foods*

Food	RE†
Liver, beef, 3 oz.	9,011
Sweet potato, baked, 1 small	2,488
Carrots, raw, 1	2,025
Spinach, cooked, ½ cup	875
Squash, butternut, ½ cup	857
Cantaloupe, ¼ melon	516
Apricots, dried, 8 large halves	253
Milk, 2%, 1 cup	140
Broccoli, cooked, ½ cup	110
Egg yolk, 1	97
Cheese, cheddar, 1 oz	86
Margarine, fortified, 1 tsp	47
Peach, 1 medium	47
Halibut, baked, 3 oz	46
Butter, 1 tsp	38
Orange, 1 medium	27
Crab, 100 g	14
Apple, 1 medium	7

* From USDA: Composition of Foods. Handbook No. 8 Series. Washington, DC, ARS, USDA, 1976–1986.
† RE = retinol equivalents.

ciated with the fat of milk and eggs. Nonfat milk is fortified with retinol. The carotene forms are found in dark green, leafy, and yellow-orange vegetables and fruit; deeper colors are associated with higher levels of the provitamin. Vitamin A occurs at therapeutic levels in cod and halibut liver oils. About half of the total vitamin A activity in the usual foods available in the United States is in the form of retinol and half as provitamin A carotenoids.

Vitamin A is relatively stable to heat and light; however, it is destroyed by oxidation. Its bioavailability is enhanced by the presence of vitamin E and other antioxidants.

Cooking increases bioavailability of carotenoids; however, overcooking dramatically decreases them. Dehydration has also been shown to reduce the carotene in carrots, broccoli, and spinach.

Deficiency

An estimated 1 to 5 million people, mainly infants and preschool children, develop vitamin A deficiency. It is a major killer of children in developing countries, the increased mortality and morbidity resulting from increased rates of respiratory disease and diarrhea. This was shown effectively by the decrease in mortality and morbidity from measles produced by supplementation of marginally deficient children (Barclay et al, 1987). Infections cause an accelerated depletion of liver reserves of vitamin A (Campos et al, 1987). In children with low dietary intake, infections may precipitate marginal vitamin A deficiency (Sommer et al, 1987).

A deficiency of this vitamin is accompanied by keratinization of the mucous membranes that line the respiratory tract, the alimentary canal, and the urinary tract, and by keratinization of the body skin and epithelium of the eye, which lowers the barrier role played by these membranes in protection of the body against infections.

Prolonged deficiency of vitamin A may produce skin changes, night blindness, and corneal ulcerations. In extreme deficiency states, the mucous membranes of the respiratory, gastrointestinal, and genitourinary tracts are affected. Other symptoms of vitamin A deficiency are loss of appetite, inhibited growth, skeletal abnormalities, keratinization of taste buds, and loss of the sense of taste.

Primary deficiencies of vitamin A are the result of dietary inadequacies. Secondary deficiencies can result from liver disease, protein-energy malnutrition, abetalipoproteinemia, or malabsorption due to bile acid insufficiency.

NIGHT BLINDNESS (NYCTALOPIA). Impairment of dark adaptation—the ability to adapt from a bright light or glare to darkness, as encountered in night driving or upon entering a dark room from a brightly lighted one—is symptomatic of vitamin A deficiency. Night blindness is attributed to functional failure of the retina in the proper regeneration of rhodopsin. The ability to perceive details at low levels of illumination is related to tiny nerve endings (rods and cones) that are found in the retina. Cones are concerned primarily with day sight and the perception of color, and the rods control night vision. Individuals afflicted with night blindness cannot see in a dim light or at twilight.

XEROPHTHALMIA (XEROSIS CONJUNCTIVAE). Xerophthalmia, one of the serious eye conditions caused by vitamin A deficiency, occurs rarely in the United States where it is usually associated with malabsorption, chronic cachexia, and weight loss from a debilitating disease such as cancer. It is more commonly found in developing countries throughout much of the world. It is associated with atrophy of the periocular glands, hyperkeratosis of the conjunctiva and, finally, involvement of the cornea, leading to softening or keratomalacia and blindness. It proceeds more rapidly and is most severe in very young children.

INFECTION. Vitamin A deficiency increases host susceptibility to bacterial, viral, or parasitic infections through its role in maintaining the integrity of the mucous membranes. Without vitamin A, the "barrier" system against infection is gone. The number of circulating T lymphocytes as well as their response to mitogens is reduced in vitamin A deficiency.

CUTANEOUS CHANGES. Vitamin A deficiency produces characteristic changes in skin texture such as *follicular hyperkeratosis* (phrynoderma), in which blockage of the hair follicles with plugs of keratin causes the "goose flesh" or "toad skin" shown in Figure 6-2. The skin becomes dry, scaly, and rough. At first the forearms and thighs — but in advanced stages, the whole body — may be involved. The same condition may be caused by essential fatty acid deficiency, a vitamin B deficiency, exposure to sunlight, or lack of cleanliness.

Topical applications of retinoic acid have been used in the treatment of wrinkles, acne vulgaris, ichthyosis, psoriasis, keratosis, and other skin disorders. External use produces cytologic changes that lead to inflammation and an improvement in skin condition without systemic effects of toxicity.

PREVENTION AND TREATMENT OF AVITAMINOSIS A. Acute vitamin A deficiency is treated with large oral doses of vitamin A and correction of the usually concomitant protein-energy malnutrition. The symptoms of deficiency respond to diet and supplementation in about the same order as they appear. For example, night blindness responds very quickly, while the skin abnormalities may take several weeks to disappear.

Most corrective programs involve underdeveloped countries. Massive intermittent dosing with 200,000 IU (60,000 RE) of vitamin A can reduce mortality by 35 to 70% but is very costly. Fortification of MSG used in cooking with vitamin A has effectively increased serum and human milk concentrations, reduced mortality, and improved anthropometric status in those supplemented (Muhilal et al, 1988a and b). Encouraging use of natural sources high in the vitamin would seem to be appropriate, but cultural food practices often interfere with such an approach.

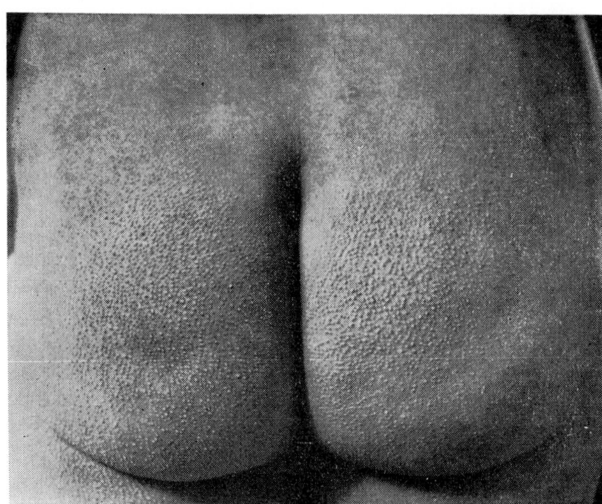

FIGURE 6-2. *Vitamin A deficiency showing early follicular hyperkeratosis resembling "goose flesh." (Reproduced by courtesy of Section of Dermatology and Syphilology, Mayo Clinic, Rochester, Minnesota.)*

Toxicity

Excess retinol causes changes in biologic membranes when the amount ingested exceeds the binding capacity of RBP.

Acute hypervitaminosis A can be induced by single doses of greater than 200 mg (660,000 IU) of retinol in adults or greater than 100 mg (330,000 IU) in children. Symptoms include nausea, vomiting, fatigue, weakness, headache, and anorexia (Table 6-4). A bulging fontanel may also be seen in infants. Dramatic stories in the literature describe reddening and exfoliation of the skin in Arctic explorers and fishermen who feasted on polar bear liver (10 million IU/lb) or halibut liver.

Chronic hypervitaminosis A, usually reflecting misuse of supplements, can follow the repeated intake of vitamin A in amounts at least 10 times the RDA: 4.2 mg of retinol (14,000 IU) for an infant or 10 mg of retinol (33,000 IU) for an adult (Olson, 1988). Response to chronic excess is highly variable among individuals (Bendich and Langseth, 1989; Carpenter et al, 1987; Krasinski et al, 1989). Symptoms disappear in weeks or months when the supplementation is discontinued (Olson, 1988).

Accutane, a drug closely related to vitamin A that was developed for the treatment of severe cystic acne, is a known teratogen. Failure to screen for pregnancy prior to use has resulted in infants with severe birth defects.

Toxicity studies in animals have shown that beta-carotene is not carcinogenic, mutagenic, or teratogenic. Foods such as carrot juice and tomato juice that are high in beta-carotene can be consumed in enormous amounts without harm except for the often alarming yellowing of the skin that follows deposition of carotene in the tissues. Unlike jaundice, in *hypercarotenodermia* the sclera (white) of the eye is clear. When excess intakes are discontinued, the skin clears normally in a short time.

TABLE 6-4. Signs of Vitamin A Toxicity

Serum vitamin A of 250-6,600 IU/100 ml
Bone pain and fragility
Hydrocephalus and vomiting (infants and children)
Dry, fissured skin
Brittle nails
Hair loss (alopecia)
Gingivitis
Cheilosis
Anorexia
Irritability
Fatigue
Hepatomegaly and abnormal liver function
Ascites and portal hypertension

Vitamin D (Calciferol)

Vitamin D has had an active history from the time when it was first recognized by McCollum as the component of cod liver oil that was capable of curing rickets to the discovery by DeLuca almost 50 years later that the metabolically active form requires synthesis in the kidney. The metabolism of this interesting vitamin continues to be clarified (Fig. 6–3).

The precursors of vitamin D are present in sterol fractions of both animal and plant tissues in the form of *7-dehydrocholesterol* and *ergosterol,* respectively. Both require ultraviolet irradiation to convert to the provitamin form (D_3 [cholecalciferol] and D_2, respectively), and both provitamins require conversion in the kidney to the metabolically active form (Table 6–5). The plant form is of interest primarily as a food additive.

The animal form of the precursor (7-dehydrocholesterol) is found in the epidermal layer of the skin, where it is very efficiently converted to the provitamin D_3, cholecalciferol, by ultraviolet irradiation. When described in these terms, vitamin D is more appropriately called a *prohormone* rather than a *vitamin* inasmuch as it does not need to be supplied from a source outside the body. The metabolically active forms, *calcitriol* and *ercalcitriol,* are produced by the kidney and function as a hormone, with the intestine and bone as target organs.

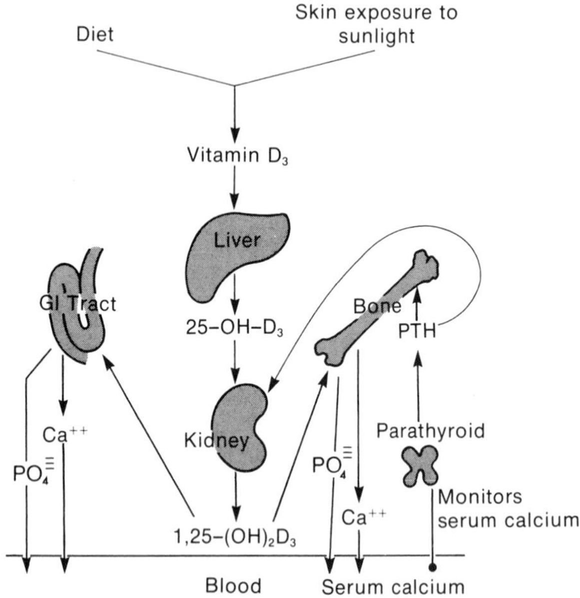

FIGURE 6–3. *The metabolism and functions of vitamin D. Vitamin D_3 (cholecalciferol) is changed to its biologically active forms, 25-OHD$_3$ and 1,25-(OH)$_2$D$_3$. 1,25-(OH)$_2$D$_3$ acts on the intestine to increase calcium and phosphate absorption and on the bones to increase calcium and phosphate resorption.*

TABLE 6–5. Vitamin D Terminology and Equivalents

Terminology	
7-Dehydrocholesterol (vitamin D_3 precursor) (Source: animal epidermis)	Ergosterol (vitamin D_2 precursor) (Source: plant tissue)
Vitamin D_3 25-hydroxycholecalciferol Cholecalciferol 25(OH)D_3 (Source: precursor irradiation)	Vitamin D_2 25-hydroxyergocalciferol Ergocalciferol 25(OH)D_2 (Source: precursor irradiation)
Vitamin D_3 (active form)* 1,25-dihydroxycholecalciferol Calcitriol 1,25(OH)$_2$$D_3$ (Source: kidney activation)	Vitamin D_2 (active form)* 1,25-dihydroxyergocalciferol Ercalcitriol 1,25(OH)$_2$$D_2$ (Source: kidney activation)
Equivalents	
1 International Unit (IU) = 0.025 μg of cholecalciferol (vitamin D_3)	
1 μg cholecalciferol (vitamin D_3) = 40 IU vitamin D	

* Vitamin D_3 usually used to denote both active forms.

Absorption, Transport, and Storage

Ingested vitamin D is absorbed from the intestine along with lipids with the aid of bile. Vitamin D from the skin or intestine is bound to vitamin D plasma-binding protein (DBP) for transport to storage sites in the liver, skin, brain, bones, and probably other tissues. Healthy elderly persons absorb vitamin D at the same rate as younger adults. However, older adults are less able to increase efficiency of calcium absorption when consuming a low-calcium diet, possibly as the result of a renal defect in vitamin D metabolism.

Metabolism

Vitamin D_3 *(cholecalciferol)* is formed in the skin by the action of ultraviolet (UV) rays in sunlight on 7-dehydrocholesterol. Sunlight can also convert provitamin D_3 to inert compounds. The relative amount of provitamin D_3 and inert compounds produced depends on intensity of UV radiation, which diminishes with increasing latitude. Other factors affecting the amount of provitamin D_3 synthesized by the skin are pigmentation, use of sunscreen, and length of time of exposure to sunlight (Webb and Holick, 1988).

Vitamin D_3 is converted in the liver to the biologically active metabolite, *25-hydroxycholecalciferol (25-OHD$_3$),* which is five times as potent as vitamin D_3. The blood level of 25-OHD$_3$, the predominant vitamin D sterol in the blood, is dependent on both intake and exposure to sunlight.

The most active form of vitamin D, *calcitriol,* or *1,25-dihydroxycholecalciferol (1,25-(OH)$_2$D$_3$),* with ten times the potency of vitamin D_3, is produced by the kidneys. It increases uptake of calcium and phosphate by acting on the intestine to increase their absorption and on the bone to increase their mobilization. Several other naturally occurring vitamin D metabolites have been identified, but their roles are not defined at present.

Calcitriol synthesis is regulated by the serum levels of calcium and phosphorus. *Parathyroid hormone (PTH),* which is released in response to low serum calcium, appears to be the mediator that stimulates the production of $1{,}25(OH)_2D_3$ by the kidney.

Thus it is proposed that a low dietary calcium intake is reflected in a lower serum calcium, which in turn affects PTH secretion and a subsequent increase in kidney synthesis of calcitriol. Dietary phosphate has a similar effect but does not require the intermediate action of PTH.

Functions

Calcitriol promotes the active, energy-requiring intestinal absorption of calcium through stimulation of the synthesis of calcium-binding protein in the brush border of the intestinal mucosa. Alkaline phosphatase, whose synthesis is also induced by calcitriol, may be involved as well. Vitamin D also stimulates the active phosphate transport system in the intestine. In conjunction with parathyroid hormone, it acts to mobilize calcium from bone and increases renal tubular reabsorption of calcium and phosphate.

Measurement

Although vitamin D continues to be discussed in terms of International Units, the preferred terminology is based on micrograms (μg) of vitamin D_3. Table 6–5 summarizes these relationships as well as the terminology for the various forms of vitamin D. Vitamins D_2 (ergocalciferol) and D_3 (cholecalciferol) have equal biologic activity and are usually both described in terms of vitamin D_3.

Recommended Dietary Allowance

Although 2.5 μg of vitamin D daily is sufficient to prevent rickets, higher levels are prescribed for infants and through the period of skeletal development on the basis of amounts that promote optimal growth (Table 6–6). Lower levels in adulthood provide for continued bone remodeling and adequate calcium and phosphorus homeostasis. Increased allowances for pregnancy and lactation reflect demands of fetal growth and calcium content of breast milk.

TABLE 6–6. Recommended Dietary Allowances for Vitamin D*

Age (Years)	RDA† (μg cholecalciferol)
Infants	
0.0–0.5	7.5
0.5–1.0	10
Children	
1–3	10
4–6	10
7–10	10
Males	
11–14	10
15–18	10
19–24	10
25–50	5
51+	5
Females	
11–14	10
15–18	10
19–24	10
25–50	5
51+	5
Pregnant	10
Lactating	
1st 6 months	10
2nd 6 months	10

* From Food and Nutrition Board, National Research Council, NAS: Recommended Dietary Allowances, 10th ed. Washington, DC, National Academy Press, 1989.

† RDA = recommended dietary allowance.

The normal adult is presumed to obtain sufficient vitamin D from exposure to sunlight and from the incidental ingestion of small amounts with foods. Exposure of the hands and face to summer sunlight for as little as 10 to 15 minutes per day will provide sufficient vitamin D to prevent rickets (DeLuca, 1988). The heavy pigment of dark-skinned people can prevent up to 95% of ultraviolet radiation from reaching the deeper layers of the skin where vitamin D is synthesized. However, pigmentation is only limiting if exposure periods are short. With longer exposure and higher intensity of irradiation, the same circulating concentrations of vitamin D_3 can be reached.

Supplemental vitamin D is unnecessary with the exception of those who are chronically shielded from sunlight, such as persons who are housebound, living in sunless areas with high atmospheric pollution, wearing clothes that completely cover the body, or working at night and staying indoors during the day. More exotic circumstances include long submarine voyages and living in the Antarctic. In these special cases, a small daily supplement of vitamin D is desirable.

Sources

Vitamin D occurs naturally in animal foods in the form of cholecalciferol. It is found in only small and highly variable amounts in butter, cream, egg yolk, and liver. The best food sources are the fish liver oils. Both human and cow's milk are poor sources of the vitamin, providing only 15 to 40 IU/l. However, approximately 98% of all fluid milk is fortified with vitamin D_2 (irradiated ergosterol), usually at the level of 400 IU/qt. Most dried whole milk and evaporated milk are fortified, as well as some margarines, butter, certain cereals, and infant formula products. The milk used to make cheese or yogurt is usually not vitamin D–fortified. Vitamin D is remarkably stable and does not deteriorate when foods are heated or stored for long periods. Vitamin D in both supplements and the preparations added to foods is in the form of vitamin D_2, which is prepared commercially by the irradiation of plant sterols, usually from yeast.

Table 6–7 gives the vitamin D content of selected foods.

Deficiency

Vitamin D deficiency is manifested as rickets in children and as osteomalacia in adults. Lack of the vitamin in adults may also contribute to the development of osteoporosis.

RICKETS. Vitamin D is specific for the prevention and cure of rickets, a disease associated with malformation of bones due to deficient mineralization of the organic matrix. Rachitic bones are not able to withstand ordinary stresses and strains, resulting in the appearance of bowlegs, knock-knees, pigeon breast, and frontal bossing of the skull. Rickets is rarely completely cured and the stature remains short.

TABLE 6–7. Vitamin D Content of Selected Foods*

Food	IU
Herring, fresh, raw, 1 oz	255
Salmon, 1 oz	142
Milk, cow's fortified, 1 cup	100
Sardines, canned, 1 oz	85
Liver, chicken, cooked, 3 oz	45
Shrimp, canned, 1 oz	30
Egg yolk	25
Milk, human, 1 cup	1–24
Liver, calf, cooked, 3 oz	12
Cream, light, 1 T	8
Cheese, cheddar, 1 oz	3
Oysters, 4	3
Butter, 1 tsp	1.4

* From USDA: Composition of Foods, Handbook No. 8 Series. Washington, DC, ARS, USDA, 1976–1986.

Skeletal and biochemical abnormalities seen in the disease may be the result of PTH activity. Failure to absorb calcium because of a vitamin D deficiency causes the renal threshold for phosphate to be lowered, with the result that larger amounts of phosphate are excreted in order to maintain a proper balance between calcium and phosphorus in the blood. Increased mobilization of phosphate from the bones to balance plasma calcium levels may account for skeletal and biochemical abnormalities seen in the disease.

Traditional victims of rickets are poor children in industrialized cities where exposure to sunlight is limited. In northern regions, 22% of the children under 7 years of age show signs of rickets. It is the second most common nutrition problem in China (Specker and Tsang, 1988). Dark-skinned children living in northern countries such as England or Scotland are particularly vulnerable. In the United States, black children are at greater risk for vitamin D deficiency than are white children because increased skin pigment (melanin) shields the precursor from irradiation.

Supplementation of foods with vitamin D has almost eliminated the disease as a pediatric problem in North America. However, some cases of active rickets persist despite the administration of conventional doses of vitamin D. Hypophosphatemic vitamin D refractory rickets of the simple type, resulting from renal tubular dysfunction, is the most common and may be classified as an inborn error of metabolism. However, not all examples of vitamin D refractory rickets have been related to an inherited background. This form of rickets may develop in infancy but not infrequently appears in late childhood and may not appear until adult life. Currently, oral administration of massive doses of vitamin D_2 (50,000 to 500,000 IU/day) is used, but the treatment of choice is use of one of the active metabolites of vitamin D_3 (25-D_3 or 1,25-D_3) or a synthetic analogue. Use of these forms will bypass the metabolic defect that is causing the vitamin D–deficient state. Synthetic analogues and available active metabolites of vitamin D_3 are discussed in Chapter 35.

Prolonged breast-feeding without vitamin D supplementation or omission of fortified formula can lead to rickets. It can also occur in children with malabsorption or in children who are receiving long-term anticonvulsant therapy for epilepsy (see Chapter 25).

Symptoms. The first visible symptoms of rickets are profuse sweating and restlessness; in addition, sleeping infants often move their heads from side to side and rub off their hair. Contrary to the usual deficiency disease symptoms, the patient does not become thin or emaciated and often parents will not recognize the symptoms of rickets until the child starts to walk. At that time the legs will bow because the bones are not strong enough to support the child's weight (Fig. 6–4). A pot belly and beading of the ribs (the rachitic rosary) as illustrated in Figure 6–5 may pass unobserved in a plump yet malnourished baby. If the deficiency appears during the third or fourth month of life when the skull is growing rapidly, the structure of the head will be larger than normal with a shape that is inclined to be square, with bulging on the sides and front. The softened and deformed bones cause other deformities, such as pigeon chest and enlarged wrists and ankles. Lesser defects sometimes ensue when the ailment is mild.

The severity of the condition may be identified chemically through studies of the calcium, 25-D_3, and phosphorus content of the blood, and clinically with roentgenograms of the bones. Radiologic evidence is a loss of metaphyseal definition. Increased serum levels of alkaline phosphatase, an enzyme released by the osteoblasts that is involved in bone formation, indicate failure of bone formation caused by a lack of calcium, which is secondary to a lack of vitamin D.

Prevention and Dietary Treatment. To prevent rickets in the newborn baby, it is important to start appropriate administration of vitamin D early and continue throughout the growth period. The vitamin D concentration of human milk varies depending upon the season and the mother's vitamin D supplementation (Ala-Houhala et al, 1988). A breast-fed baby can become vitamin D-deficient if not exposed regularly to sunlight (see Chapter 10).

Vitamin D concentrates of fish liver oil are often prescribed to prevent vitamin D deficiency. One teaspoon (4 ml) of cod liver oil contains 360 IU of vitamin D. Irradiated ergosterol is also an excellent source. However, mothers should be warned against the simultaneous use of several preparations, inasmuch as excesses are toxic.

OSTEOMALACIA. Vitamin D deficiency in adulthood results in *osteomalacia,* a condition characterized by pronounced softening of the bones, which leads to deformities, especially of the limbs, spine, thorax, and pelvis. Osteomalacia is frequently confused with osteoporosis, a disease having similar symptoms and with which it often occurs (see Chapter 22). Radiographic findings of translucent bands in the bones (Looser's zones) are diagnostic of osteomalacia.

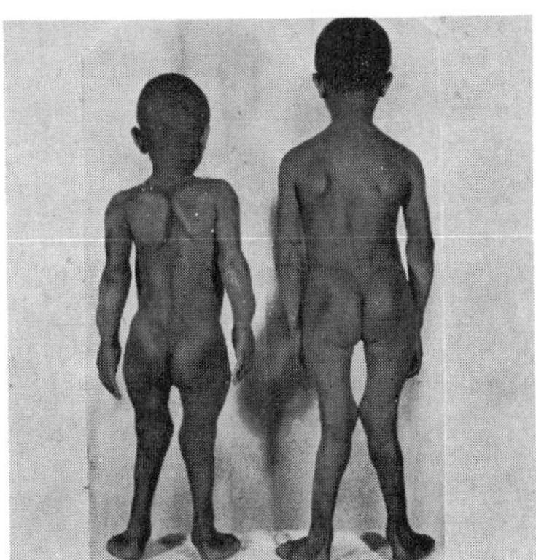

FIGURE 6–4. *Rachitic deformities. Note knock-knees and enlarged joints. (From Jolliffe N [ed]: Clinical Nutrition, 2nd ed. New York, Harper & Row, 1962.)*

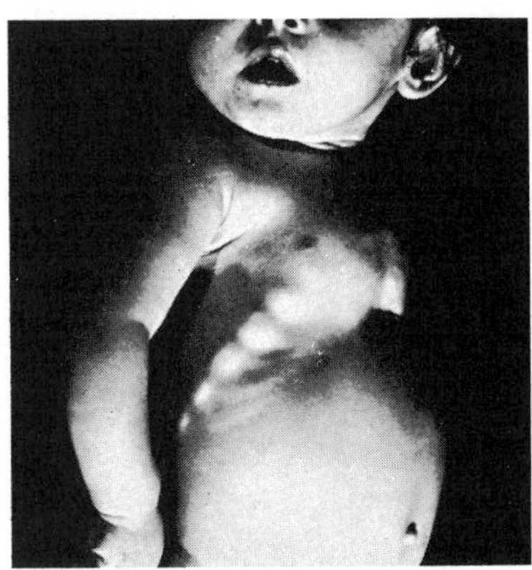

FIGURE 6–5. *Child suffering from rickets. Note rachitic rosary and pot belly. (From Jolliffe N [ed]: Clinical Nutrition, 2nd ed. New York, Harper & Row, 1962.)*

Typical symptoms are a rheumatic type of pain and general weakness. There may also be a waddling gait and tetany manifested by facial twitching. Although it is seen occasionally in men, it is most often observed in women of childbearing age who have become depleted of calcium because of multiple pregnancies and inadequate diet, or in women who are heavily clothed and have little exposure to the sun, such as Indian women who practice purdah. In the United States, osteomalacia is sometimes encountered among elderly persons living alone, consuming an inadequate diet, and getting inadequate sunshine or other source of vitamin D. It is seldom encountered among those who wear less clothing and who work outdoors in the sun, or among people who have an abundant diet. Constant hypocalcemia at a level that induces parathyroid activity can induce secondary hyperparathyroidism, characterized by lesions of osteitis fibrosa cystica in the bones.

Prevention and Treatment. Prevention of osteomalacia is usually possible through the adequate supply of vitamin D, calcium, and phosphorus in the diet. Vitamin D must be assured from either sunshine, UV lamp, natural food source, fortified food source, or a concentrated supplement. Adequate exposure must be qualified with time and place. For example, exposure of 10 to 15 minutes on a clear summer day, two to three times a week, should be sufficient for elderly whites in Boston (Webb and Holick, 1988).

If osteomalacia is already present, doses of 25 to 125 μg (1,000 to 5,000 IU) per day of vitamin D_3 are usually given unless there is evidence of malabsorption, in which case the dose should be 1250 μg (50,000 IU) daily. Calcium supplements may also be necessary. The

TABLE 6–8. Signs of Vitamin D Toxicity

Excessive calcification of bone
Kidney stones
Metastatic calcification of soft tissues (kidney and lung)
Hypercalcemia
Headache
Weakness
Nausea and vomiting
Constipation
Polyuria
Polydipsia

pain and weakness usually disappears within 1 to 2 months after treatment is started.

Toxicity

It is known that hypervitaminosis D can cause pathologic changes in the body when vitamin D is taken in excess. These changes, consequences of hypercalcemia, are excessive calcification of bone and calcification of soft tissues such as the kidney (including kidney stones), lungs, and even the tympanic membrane of the ear, which can result in deafness. Headache and nausea are often among the subjective findings (Table 6–8). Infants given excessive amounts of vitamin D may have gastrointestinal upsets, bone fragility, retarded growth, and mental retardation.

Vitamin D toxicity develops over time, and individuals vary in susceptibility. The toxic level has not been established for all ages, but infants and small children are most susceptible. Consumption of as little as 45 μg (1,800 IU) per day has been associated with hypervitaminosis in young children (American Academy of Pediatrics, 1963). Toxicity should always be monitored when large doses of vitamin D (25 μg or more) are given for an extended period.

Vitamin E (Tocopherol)

Vitamin E was first discovered in 1922, when it was found that reproductive abnormalities in rats reared on a basic diet were cured by a substance isolated from vegetable oils. A pure fraction was chemically identified in 1938 and named tocopherol after the Greek word *tokos,* which means *childbirth,* and *phero,* which means *to bring forth.*

Metabolism

Vitamin E activity in foods is contributed by the tocopherols — alpha, beta, gamma, and delta — and the tocotrienols. Their most important chemical characteristic is their antioxidant property.

Vitamin E is fairly stable to heat and acids and unstable to alkalis, ultraviolet light, and oxygen. It is destroyed when in contact with rancid fats, lead, and iron. Because the vitamin components are insoluble in water, there is no loss by extraction in cooking; however, freezing and deep-fat frying destroy most of the tocopherol present. Esters of tocopherol such as tocopherol acetate, the most common naturally occurring form, are not appreciably destroyed.

Absorption of vitamin E is relatively inefficient, ranging between 20 and 80%. It is stored in liver and to a larger extent in fatty tissues.

Functions

Vitamin E acts in foods to prevent the peroxidation of polyunsaturated fatty acids. At the gut level, it enhances the activity of vitamin A by preventing its oxidation in the intestinal tract.

At the cellular level, vitamin E appears to protect cellular and subcellular membranes from deterioration by scavenging free radicals that contain oxygen. In the absence of vitamin E, free radicals catalyze peroxidation of the polyunsaturated fatty acids (PUFAs) that constitute structural components of the membranes. The ensuing destruction leads to development of abnormal cellular structure and compromising of cellular function. The ability of vitamin E to circumvent such destruction has led to suggestions that it may eventually be useful in preventing conditions associated with free radical destruction, such as aging, effects of environmental toxins, and triggering of some forms of carcinogenesis. However, such relationships remain conjectural and controversial.

The long-recognized relationship between vitamin E and selenium appears to reflect the presence of other antioxidant systems, one of which contains a selenoenzyme, glutathione peroxidase.

Findings from animal research suggest other possibilities for the role of tocopherols in human nutrition. However, the many enthusiastic claims for the effectiveness of vitamin E in relieving or preventing ischemic heart disease, thrombophlebitis, fibrocystic breast disease, rheumatic fever, dystrophy, menstrual disorders, toxemias of pregnancy, spontaneous abortion, and sterility have not been substantiated.

Measurement

Although units of vitamin E continue to be expressed as IU in some circumstances, the RDA for this vitamin is listed, by international agreement, in the more appropriate usage of milligrams of RRR-alpha-tocopherol (formerly d-alpha-tocopherol) equivalents (alpha-TE). One milligram of synthetic all-rac-alpha-tocopherol (formerly dl-alpha tocopherol) equals 0.74 alpha-TE (Food and Nutrition Board, 1989). One milligram of the naturally occurring d-alpha-tocopherol is equivalent to 1.49 IU.

Because vitamin E occurs in foodstuffs in several forms with varying biologic activity, the expression of the dietary total as alpha-TEs requires calculation based on the quantity and relative biologic activity of each form. Multipliers of milligrams of alpha-tocopherol, beta-tocopherol, gamma-tocopherol, and alpha-tocotrienol are 1.0, 0.5, 0.1, and 0.3, respectively. When only information on alpha-tocopherol is available, the value in milligrams should be multiplied by 1.2 to derive a total of alpha-TEs that reflects the presence of other tocopherols in food (Food and Nutrition Board, 1989).

Recommended Dietary Allowance

The requirement for vitamin E depends upon the amount of PUFA consumed. Because this varies widely among individuals, it is not possible to establish a precise recommendation. Because there is no evidence to suggest that a deficiency of vitamin E occurs among persons in the United States, the RDAs are based on the amount consumed in the average diet. Increasing levels of PUFA that would require increased levels of the antioxidant are usually from vegetable oils, which are themselves among the richest sources of vitamin E. The amount required to balance the minimum requirement for the polyunsaturated essential fatty acids is not known but is estimated to be 3 to 4 mg alpha-TE (4.5 to 6.0 IU) per day.

The average daily intake of Americans has been estimated at 7.4 to 9.0 mg of alpha-TE and 21 g of PUFA. This is equivalent to an alpha-TE : PUFA ratio of approximately 0.4, which appears to be adequate (Food and Nutrition Board, 1989). Table 6–9 lists the vitamin E RDA for the various age-sex groups.

TABLE 6–9. Recommended Dietary Allowances for Vitamin E*

Age (Years)	RDA† (mg alpha-tocopherol equivalents)
Infants	
0.0–0.5	3
0.5–1.0	4
Children	
1–3	6
4–6	7
7–10	7
Males	
11–14	10
15–18	10
19–24	10
25–50	10
51+	10
Females	
11–14	8
15–18	8
19–24	8
25–50	8
51+	8
Pregnant	10
Lactating	
1st 6 months	12
2nd 6 months	11

* From Food and Nutrition Board, National Research Council, NAS: Recommended Dietary Allowances, 10th ed. Washington, DC, National Academy Press, 1989.

† RDA = recommended dietary allowance.

Sources

Vitamin E is widely available in common foodstuffs. Seed oils, particularly wheat germ oil, are the richest source, although lesser amounts also occur in fruits, vegetables, and animal fats. Peanut, olive, and coconut and fish oils are poor sources of the vitamin. Table 6–10 gives the total alpha-TE of selected foods. About 64% of the vitamin E in the customary American diet is supplied by salad oils, margarine, and shortening; about 11% by fruits and vegetables; and about 7% by grains and grain products. It is also produced synthetically.

TABLE 6–10. Vitamin E Content of Selected Foods*

Food	Total Vitamin E (mg)
Wheat germ oil, 1 T	34.6
Chocolate-covered almonds, ½ c	14.3
Corn oil, 1 T	11–14
Soybean oil, 1 T	8.8–14
Sunflower oil, 1 T	8.5–8.8
Milk, nonfat or whole, 1 c	7.6
Avocado, Florida, 1	4.0
Macaroni and cheese, 1 c	3.5
Peas, ckd from fresh, 1 c	3.4
Apricots, dried, 10	2.2
Olive oil, 1 T	1.8
Margarine, 1 T	1.6
Baked beans, canned with pork, 1 c	1.5
Chocolate milk, plain, 1 oz	1.4
Salmon, baked or broiled, 3 oz	1.3
Mayonnaise, 1 T	1.0
Chicken, roasted, 5 oz	0.8
Butter, 1 T	0.2

* Data from Hands ES: Food Finder. Salem, Oregon, ESHA Research, 1990.

Deficiency

Because of the widespread dietary availability of vitamin E, deficiencies are uncommon. When they do occur, they are usually associated with malabsorption or lipid transport abnormalities such as abetalipoproteinemia.

Newborn infants have low tissue concentrations of vitamin E because there is little transfer across the placenta. The amount of vitamin E in human milk is apparently sufficient to meet the infant's requirement. Serum vitamin E levels should be monitored in very low birthweight infants (less than 1.5 kg) to assure that supplementation is adequate. Premature infants may show signs of vitamin E deficiency because of inadequate tissue storage, malabsorption, or rapid growth rates that increase tissue requirements (see Chapter 11).

Vitamin E deficiency is associated with symptoms of peripheral neuropathy. Alpha-tocopherol is used to treat intermittent claudication (tension and pain in the legs when walking). Plasma levels of tocopherol may reflect abnormal lipoprotein levels.

Toxicity

Most individuals studied while taking large doses of vitamin E have not shown toxic effects. This is fortunate considering the large amounts (100 to 800 mg/day) with which many people medicate themselves. However, the known toxicity of fat-soluble vitamins A and K suggests caution with respect to long-term megadoses of this vitamin.

Vitamin K

In 1935 Dam in Copenhagen discovered a severe hemorrhagic disease in newly hatched chicks on a ration adequate in all then-known vitamins and dietary essentials. The antihemorrhagic factor was named vitamin K or *Koagulationsvitamin.* The vitamin was isolated and synthesized in 1939.

Chemical and Physical Properties

Vitamin K exists in at least three forms, all belonging to a group of chemical compounds known as quinones. The naturally occurring forms are vitamin K_1 *(phylloquinone),* which occurs in green plants, and vitamin K_2 *(menaquinone),* which is formed as the result of bacterial action in the intestinal tract. Water-soluble forms of vitamins K_1 and K_2 are also available. The fat-soluble synthetic compound, *menadione* (vitamin K_3), is about twice as potent biologically as the naturally occurring vitamins K_1 and K_2 on a weight basis because it lacks the long side chain of the natural vitamin. The body must add the side chain to the menadione before it can function as vitamin K. None of the forms of vitamin K are stored in appreciable amounts.

Vitamin K is fairly resistant to heat. The vitamin is not destroyed by ordinary cooking methods and, because vitamin K is fat soluble, there is no loss in cooking water. All vitamin K compounds tend to be unstable in the presence of alkali and light.

Absorption and Transport

The absorption of vitamin K requires bile and pancreatic juice. After absorption in the upper intestine, it is incorporated into chylomicrons and lipoproteins and carried to the liver. Elevated plasma levels of vitamin K are seen in hyperlipidemia, especially hypertriglyceridemia.

Functions

Vitamin K functions in the liver as an essential cofactor for carboxylase. This enzyme converts specific glutamic acid residues of precursor proteins to a new amino acid, *gamma-carboxyglutamic acid* (Gla). The proteins involved include the vitamin K–dependent blood clotting factor *prothrombin* (factor II) and factors VII, IX, and X. The presence of other Gla-containing proteins in tissues leads to the speculation that vitamin K may have functions in addition to its role in blood clotting. The calcium-binding action of Gla gives prothrombin its unique place in coagulation. Figure 6–6 outlines the complex clotting mechanism that involves vitamin K in several steps through its relationship to Gla.

The coumarin anticoagulant drugs *warfarin* and *dicumarol* act to prevent coagulation by antagonizing the action of vitamin K, but it is not completely clear how this is done.

Measurement

At present there is no standard unit to measure vitamin K activity, but it is usually expressed as μg of vitamin K.

Recommended Dietary Allowance

The RDA for vitamin K was established for the first time with the revision of 1989. Of the recommended level of 1 μg/kg body weight, it is assumed that half is supplied by intestinal synthesis and the remainder by the diet. In the United States, this amount is easily supplied by diet. Table 6–11 lists the RDA for all age-sex groups.

Sources

Vitamin K is found in large amounts in green leafy vegetables, especially broccoli, cabbage, turnip greens, and lettuce. Other vegetables, fruits, cereals, dairy products, eggs, and meat contain smaller amounts. Be-

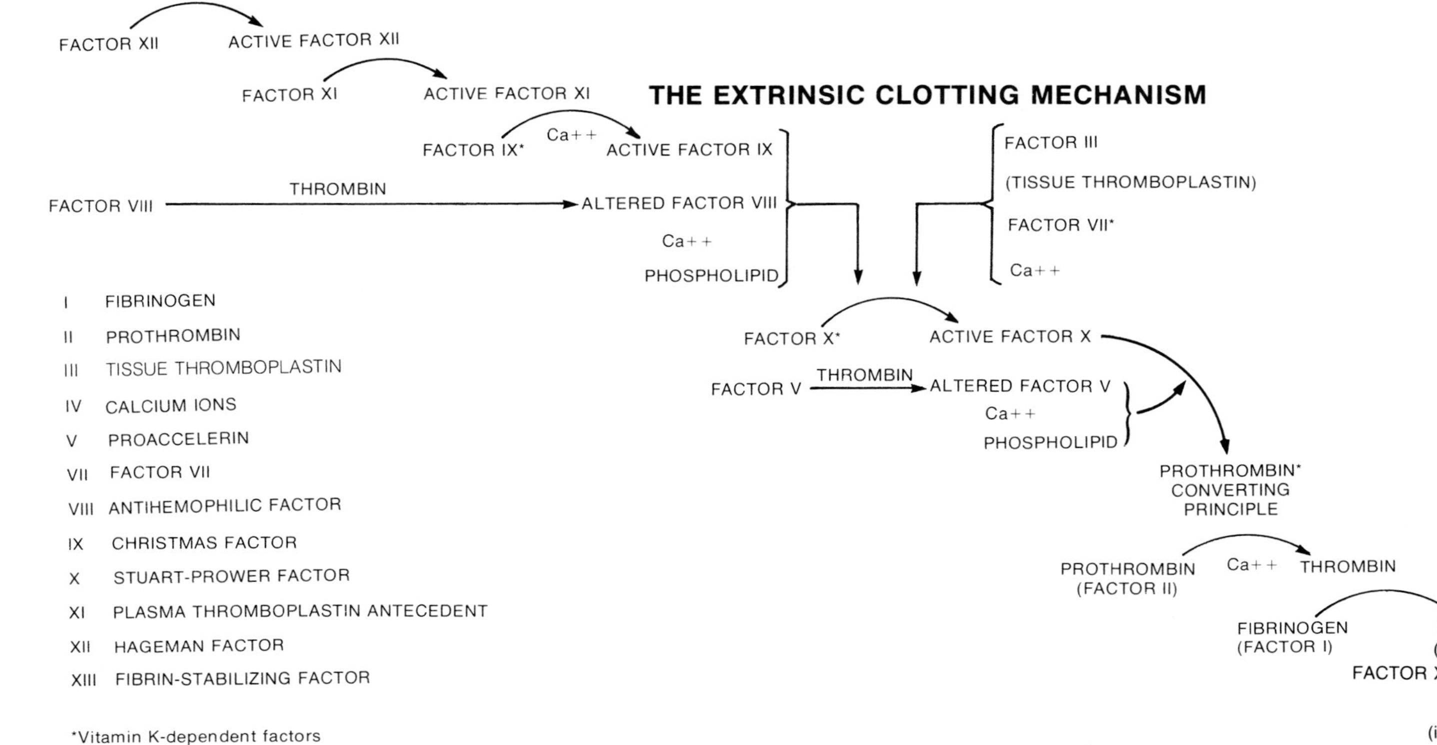

FIGURE 6–6. *Cascade theory of blood coagulation. (Adapted from Sauberlich HE, Skala JH, and Dowdy RP: Laboratory Tests for the Assessment of Nutritional Status. Cleveland, OH, CRC Press, 1974, p 85.)*

TABLE 6–11. Recommended Dietary Allowances for Vitamin K*

Age (Years)	RDA† (μg)
Infants	
0.0–0.5	5
0.5–1.0	10
Children	
1–3	15
4–6	20
7–10	30
Males	
11–14	45
15–18	65
19–24	70
25–50	80
51+	80
Females	
11–14	45
15–18	55
19–24	60
25–50	65
51+	65
Pregnant	65
Lactating	
1st 6 months	65
2nd 6 months	65

* From Food and Nutrition Board, National Research Council, NAS: Recommended Dietary Allowances, 10th ed. Washington, DC, National Academy Press, 1989.
† RDA = recommended dietary allowance.

cause vitamin K content cannot be determined with precision, values are not usually shown in food composition tables. Table 6–12 lists the average vitamin K content of a variety of foods. An average mixed diet provides about 300 to 500 μg/day of vitamin K (Olson, 1988). A significant amount is formed by the bacterial flora of the human lower intestinal tract.

Deficiency

Vitamin K deficiencies, when they rarely occur, are associated with lipid malabsorption or destruction of intestinal flora by continued antibiotic therapy. Liver disease that interferes with vitamin K utilization may produce a severe deficiency.

Newborn infants are susceptible to prothrombin deficiency during the first few days of life as the result of poor placental transfer of vitamin K and failure to establish vitamin K–producing intestinal flora. *Hemorrhagic disease of the newborn* is manifested by abnormal bleeding. It is therefore necessary to administer vitamin K intramuscularly upon delivery of some infants as a preventive measure. Premature infants and infants who are to be breast-fed are at higher risk of hemorrhagic disease. Breast milk contains less vitamin K than cow's milk, and because it is sterile, its consumption delays the development of intestinal flora.

The use of coumarin anticoagulants (e.g., dicumarol) affects vitamin K–dependent clotting factors, and excessive bleeding is mitigated by administration of the vitamin. Vitamin K is frequently given before surgery to prevent abnormal bleeding. Excessive use of aspirin can prevent normal clotting of blood by interfering with platelet aggregation and depressing the levels of vitamin K–dependent factors.

TABLE 6–12. Average Vitamin K Content of Selected Foods*

Food	μg/100 g	Food	μg/100 g	Food	μg/100 g	Food	μg/100 g
Milk and Milk Products		*Fats*		*Vegetables*		*Fruits*	
Butter	30	Beef fat	15	Asparagus	57	Applesauce	2
Cheese	35	Corn oil	0	Beans, green	40	Banana	2
Milk (cow's)	1	Safflower oil	10	Broccoli	175	Orange	1
Milk (human)	0.2	*Cereals and Grain Products*		Cabbage	125	Peach	8
Eggs		Bread	4	Kale	729	Raisin	6
Hens (whole)	11	Maize	5	Lettuce	129	Strawberry	10
Meat and Meat Products		Oats	10	Peas, green	29	*Beverages*	
Bacon	46	Rice	3	Potato	1	Coffee	38
Beef liver	92	Wheat flour	4	Pumpkin	2	Cola	2
Chicken liver	7	Whole wheat	17	Spinach	415	Tea, black	—
Ground beef	7			Tomato	10	Tea, green	712
Ham	15			Turnip greens	650	*Tobacco*	
Pork liver	25			Watercress	80	Cigarettes	5,000†
Pork tenderloin	11						

* From Olson RE: Vitamin K. *In* Shils ME and Young VR (eds): Modern Nutrition in Health and Disease, 7th ed. Philadelphia, Lea & Febiger, 1988, p 330.
† Only a small percentage is volatilized and absorbed by mucous membranes.

Toxicity

Excessive doses of synthetic vitamin K (menadione) have produced hemolytic anemia in the rat and kernicterus in the infant. The water-miscible forms of vitamin K have a much wider margin of safety.

WATER-SOLUBLE VITAMINS

Most of the water-soluble vitamins are components of essential enzyme systems. Many are involved in the reactions supporting energy metabolism. These vitamins are not normally stored in the body in appreciable amounts and are normally excreted in small quantities in the urine; thus, a daily supply is desirable to avoid depletion and interruption of normal physiologic functions.

The essential nature of vitamin B in the diet was first identified in 1897 by Eijkman, a Dutch physician in Java, who observed that adding rice bran to polished rice table scraps prevented beriberi in fowl. The significance of his findings was not recognized at the time, and it was not until 1911 that Funk and others described an essential food factor they designated as vitamin B. Later work demonstrated that the antiberiberi factor was only one of several parts, of which a total of 10 have now been identified. Their grouping under the term *B complex* is based upon their common source distribution, their close relationship in vegetable and animal tissues, and their intimate functional interrelationships.

Members of the B complex have an essential role in the metabolic processes of living cells, both plant and animal. They function as coenzymes or as prosthetic groups bound to apoenzymes. Four of these (thiamin, niacin, riboflavin, and pantothenic acid) are essential to the derivation of energy from glycolysis and the tricarboxylic acid cycle.

Because of the close interrelationships among the B vitamins, an inadequate intake of one may impair utilization of others. Discrete deficiencies of single B vitamins are rarely seen clinically.

Thiamin (Vitamin B_1)

Thiamin as either the *pyrophosphate (TPP)* or the *triphosphate (TTP)* has essential roles in energy transformation and membrane and nerve conduction and also in the synthesis of pentoses and the reduced coenzyme form of niacin.

History

An *antineuritic vitamin* was identified by Eijkman in 1897, but it was not until 1936 that Williams synthesized the vitamin and determined the chemical formula. The vitamin was named *thiamin* to designate the presence of sulfur and an amino group in the complex molecule.

Chemical Characteristics and Stability

Pure thiamin hydrochloride is a crystalline yellowish white powder with a salty, nutlike taste. The dry vitamin is fairly stable, but only acid solutions are heat stable. Cooking losses of thiamin are highly variable, depending on cooking time, pH, temperature, quantity of water used and discarded, and whether the water is chlorinated. Freezing has little or no effect on the thiamin content of foods. Thiaminase present in uncooked freshwater fish and shellfish destroys approximately 50% of the thiamin. Tea also contains an antithiamin factor. The thiamin decrease in microwave-cooked foods is comparable with that in conventionally cooked meals.

Absorption, Synthesis, and Storage

Thiamin is absorbed readily by active transport in the acid medium of the proximal duodenum and to some extent in the lower duodenum. Amounts in excess of 5 mg/day are partially absorbed by passive diffusion. Absorption may be inhibited by alcohol consumption, which interferes with active transport of the vitamin, and folate deficiency, which interferes with replication of enterocytes. Thiamin is phosphorylated in the mucosal cell to thiamin pyrophosphate, and in this form is carried to the liver by the portal circulation. It can be synthesized by microorganisms in human and animal intestinal tracts, but the amount available to the body is small.

Functions

In the pyrophosphate or diphosphate form, *TPP* functions as a coenzyme vital to tissue respiration. It is required for the oxidative decarboxylation of pyruvate to acetyl CoA, providing entry of oxidizable substrate into the Krebs cycle for the generation of energy. TPP is also required for the oxidative decarboxylation of other alpha-keto acids such as alpha-ketoglutaric acid and the 2-ketocarboxylates derived from the amino acids methionine, threonine, leucine, isoleucine, and valine. It is also the coenzyme for the transketolase reaction, which functions in the pentose phosphate shunt, an alternate pathway for glucose oxidation.

Although thiamin is needed for the metabolism of fats, proteins, and nucleic acids, it is most strongly linked with carbohydrate metabolism. The decarboxylation of pyruvate, which is concerned only with carbohydrate metabolism, is the first to suffer from a thiamin deficiency.

TABLE 6–13. Recommended Dietary Allowances for Thiamin*

Age (Years)	RDA† (mg)
Infants	
0.0–0.5	0.3
0.5–1.0	0.4
Children	
1–3	0.7
4–6	0.9
7–10	1.0
Males	
11–14	1.3
15–18	1.5
19–24	1.5
25–50	1.5
51+	1.2
Females	
11–14	1.1
15–18	1.1
19–24	1.1
25–50	1.1
51+	1.0
Pregnant	1.5
Lactating	
1st 6 months	1.6
2nd 6 months	1.6

* Reprinted with permission from *Recommended Dietary Allowances*, 10th edition, c. 1989 by the National Academy of Sciences. Published by National Academy Press, Washington, DC.

† RDA = recommended dietary allowance.

Recommended Dietary Allowance

Because of the close relationship of thiamin to energy metabolism, the RDA is based on units of energy intake. The allowance for children, adolescents, and adults is 0.5 mg/1,000 kcal with a minimum of 1 mg/day regardless of total intake. An additional 0.4 mg/day for pregnancy and 0.5 throughout lactation are recommended to allow for increased energy needs and the excretion of thiamin in milk. The RDA for infants is based on the level of thiamin in human milk (Food and Nutrition Board, 1989). The RDA for all age-sex levels are shown in Table 6–13.

Sources

Thiamin is found in a large variety of animal and vegetable materials. Lean pork and wheat germ are outstanding sources. All organ meats, lean meats and poultry, egg yolk, fish, legumes, whole grain and enriched breads, and cereals are also excellent sources. Milk and milk products, fruit, and vegetables are not rich in thiamin, but when consumed in sufficient quantities, they contribute significantly to the total intake. Table 6–14 gives the thiamin content of selected foods.

Average intakes for adults (1.75 mg or 0.68 mg/1,000 kcal for men and 1.05 mg or 0.69 mg/1,000 kcal for women) (USDA, 1986) and children (1.12 mg or 0.79 mg/1,000 kcal) (USDA, 1987) provide adequate amounts of dietary thiamin. Groups in which some people may have a thiamin:calorie ratio less than recommended include children, teenagers, elderly, adults in stress, alcoholics, and some Olympic-level athletes.

Deficiency

Thiamin deficiencies are no longer common in the United States and are seen most frequently in alcoholics. Alcohol-related thiamin deficiency, caused by inadequate intakes as well as impaired absorption and storage, is the third most common cause of dementia in the United States. Elsewhere deficiencies are seen where refined, unenriched cereal grains are major dietary staples, or where diets are high in raw fish containing microbial thiaminase.

Clinical signs of thiamin deficiency primarily involve the nervous and cardiovascular systems, eventually expressed in the deficiency disease of *beriberi.* Symptoms include mental confusion, muscular wasting (dry beriberi), edema (wet beriberi), peripheral paralysis, tachycardia, and enlarged heart. The "dry" form of the disease, associated with energy deprivation and inactivity, is characterized by peripheral neuropathy with loss of function or paralysis of the lower ex-

TABLE 6–14. Thiamin Content of Selected Foods*

Food	mg
Yeast, brewer's, 1 T	1.25
Sunflower seeds, shelled, ¼ cup	0.83
Pork chop, lean, 2 oz	0.75
Ham, lean, 3 oz	0.58
Malt-o-meal, 1 cup	0.48
Peanuts, roasted, shelled, ½ cup	0.48
Weat germ, raw, ¼ cup	0.47
Rice, white, enriched, cooked, 1 cup	0.44
Milk, soy, 1 cup	0.4
Beans, baked, 1 cup	0.34
Doughnut, years, 1	0.3
Pasta, cooked, 1 cup	0.30
Orange juice, 1 cup	0.28
Potato, baked, 1	0.24
Squash, acorn, baked, ½ cup	0.20
Salmon, baked, 2 oz	0.18
Bread, white, 1 slice	0.1
Milk, 2%, 1 cup	0.09
Chicken, breast, 3 oz	0.07
Tomato, 1	0.07
Halibut, baked, 3.5 oz	0.06
Lettuce, romaine, 1 cup	0.06
Hamberger, lean, 3 oz	0.05
Egg, 1	0.03

* From USDA: Composition of Foods. Handbook No. 8 Series. Washington, DC, ARS, USDA, 1976–1986.

TABLE 6-15. Clinical Features of Thiamin Deficiency

Deficiency Type	Features
Early stage of deficiency	Anorexia Indigestion Constipation Malaise Heaviness and weakness of legs Calf muscle tenderness "Pins and needles" and numbness in legs Anesthesia of skin, particularly at the tibia Increased pulse rate and palpitations
Wet beriberi	Edema of legs, face, trunk, and serous cavities Tense calf muscles Fast pulse Distended neck veins High blood pressure Decreased urine volume
Dry beriberi	Worsening of polyneuritis of early stage Difficulty walking Wernicke-Korsakoff syndrome: encephalopathy may occur — loss of immediate memory — disorientation — nystagmus (jerky movements of eyes) — ataxia (staggering gait)
Infantile beriberi (2-5 months of age)	Acute — decreased urine output — excessive crying; thin and plaintive whining — cardiac failure Chronic — constipation and vomiting — fretfulness — soft, toneless muscles — pallor of skin with cyanosis

tremities. The "wet" type, precipitated by a high carbohydrate intake along with strenuous physical exertion, is characterized by edema due to biventricular heart failure with pulmonary congestion (Table 6-15; Fig. 6-7). Without TPP, pyruvate cannot enter the Krebs (citric acid) cycle, and energy deprivation of the heart muscle results in heart failure. Administration of glucose in total parenteral nutrition (TPN) with less than the requirement of thiamin can result in the rapid development of wet beriberi (Beriberi. . ., 1987).

Infantile beriberi, although rare, has occurred in infants fed unusual formulas without thiamin supplements. Deterioration can be sudden and rapid, with cardiac failure and cyanosis.

Beriberi responds well to treatment with thiamin. Because most patients suffer from multiple deficiencies, a B-complex concentrate is frequently prescribed. If the damage to the nervous system is not too great, the response to treatment is usually good. In cases where acute heart failure has developed, the outlook is grave.

Toxicity

There are no known toxic effects from thiamin.

Riboflavin

Riboflavin functions primarily as a component of the coenzymes *flavin adenine dinucleotide (FAD)* and *flavin adenine mononucleotide (FMN).* FAD, the predominant form, is an essential component of energy production via the respiratory chain.

History

The biologic significance of a yellow-green fluorescent pigment in milk, first recognized in 1879, was first understood in 1932. The vitamin was synthesized and named *riboflavin* in 1935.

Chemical Characteristics and Stability

Riboflavin is a flavin in which the flavin ring is attached to an alcohol related to ribose. In pure state it appears as yellow crystals. It is stable to heat, oxidation, and acid, is sparingly soluble in water but disintegrates in the presence of alkali or light, especially ultraviolet. Very little is lost in the cooking and processing of foods; however, because it is sensitive to alkali, the common practice of adding baking soda to soften dried peas or beans destroys much of their riboflavin content. Milk in wax-lined paper containers is protected against loss through exposure to sunlight.

Absorption, Transport, and Excretion

Riboflavin is actively absorbed from the proximal small intestine by a saturable transport system. The absorp-

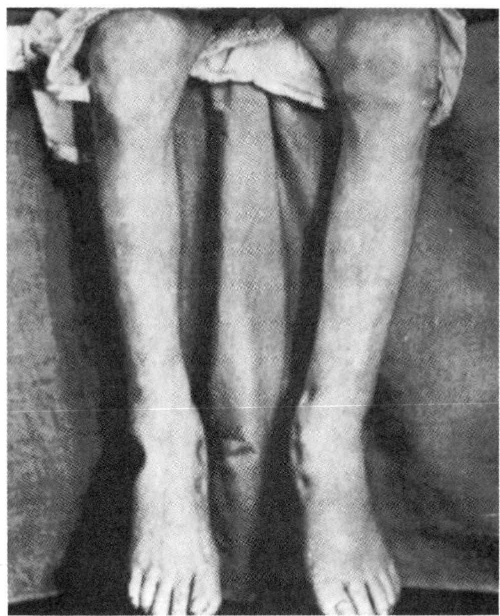

FIGURE 6-7. *Swelling of the legs and pitting edema in ankles typical of "wet" beriberi as a result of vitamin B_1 deficiency. (From Spies TD: Rehabilitation Through Better Nutrition. Philadelphia, WB Saunders, 1947.)*

tion of riboflavin is increased by the presence of food in the gastrointestinal tract.

Although small amounts of riboflavin are found in the liver and kidney, it is not stored to any great degree in the body and must therefore be supplied in the diet regularly. It is excreted in the urine in amounts depending on the intake and relative need of the tissues.

Functions

Riboflavin combines with phosphoric acid to become part of the structure of the two flavin coenzymes, FMN and FAD. These coenzymes constitute the prosthetic group of the flavoprotein enzymes, which catalyze oxidation-reduction reactions in the cells and function as hydrogen carriers in the mitochondrial electron transport system. They are also coenzymes of the dehydrogenases, which catalyze the first step in oxidation of several intermediates in glucose metabolism and of fatty acids. FMN is required for the conversion of phosphorylated pyridoxine (vitamin B_6) to its functional coenzyme and FAD for the conversion of tryptophan to niacin.

TABLE 6–16. Recommended Dietary Allowances for Riboflavin*

Age (Years)	RDA† (mg)
Infants	
0.0–0.5	0.4
0.5–1.0	0.5
Children	
1–3	0.8
4–6	1.1
7–10	1.2
Males	
11–14	1.5
15–18	1.8
19–24	1.7
25–50	1.7
51+	1.4
Females	
11–14	1.3
15–18	1.3
19–24	1.3
25–50	1.3
51+	1.2
Pregnant	1.6
Lactating	
1st 6 months	1.8
2nd 6 months	1.7

* Reprinted with permission from *Recommended Dietary Allowances*, 10th edition, c. 1989 by the National Academy of Sciences. Published by National Academy Press, Washington, DC.

† RDA = recommended dietary allowance.

Flavokinase, the enzyme that catalyzes the phosphorylation necessary for conversion of riboflavin to the coenzyme form, is regulated by thyroxine. Adults with hypothyroidism have biochemical evidence of riboflavin deficiency (Cimino et al, 1987). Adrenocorticotropic hormone (ACTH) and aldosterone also accelerate the activity of flavokinase.

Recommended Dietary Allowance

Riboflavin requirements are based on the amount calculated to maintain tissue reserves on the basis of urinary excretion, red cell riboflavin, and erythrocyte glutathione reductase (EGR) activity. On the basis of long-term studies indicating a need of 0.6 mg/day for healthy people, the RDA for adults has been established at a minimum of 1.2 mg/day. Requirements are increased during pregnancy and lactation to meet the needs of increased tissue synthesis and the riboflavin secreted in milk. Table 6–16 lists riboflavin RDA for all age-sex groups.

USDA surveys indicate that in 1985, adult men consumed an average of 2.08 mg of riboflavin per day while women and children 1 to 5 years old consumed 1.35 mg and 1.57 mg/day, respectively (USDA, 1986 and 1987).

Although it has been generally held that riboflavin differs from thiamin in that requirements are not increased by exercise, some evidence suggests a higher need with increased physical activity (van der Beek et al, 1988).

Sources

Riboflavin in small amounts is widely distributed in foods. The best daily sources are milk (fresh, canned, or dried), cheddar cheese, and cottage cheese. Organ meats contain appreciable amounts, and other lean meats, eggs, and green leafy vegetables are important sources. Sixty per cent of the vitamin is lost when flour is milled; however, breads and cereals enriched with riboflavin contribute appreciably to the total daily intake. Some synthesis of riboflavin by gut microorganisms occurs but the amounts are not appreciable.

Table 6–17 gives the riboflavin content of selected foods.

Deficiency

Deficiencies of riboflavin, when they occur, are usually in combination with deficiency of other water-soluble vitamins. Symptoms of deficiency may be secondary to the results of other nutrient deficiencies, or may follow extended periods of food deprivation or consumption of marginal diets lacking in animal protein and leafy veg-

TABLE 6–17. Riboflavin Content of Selected Foods*

Food	mg
Liver, beef, 3 oz	3.52
Ice milk, soft serve, 1 cup	0.54
Milk, 2% fat, 1 cup	0.40
Yogurt, fruit flavored, low fat, 1 cup	0.40
Yeast, brewer's, 1 T	0.34
Egg, 1	0.26
Custard, bkd, ½ cup	0.25
Pork, roast loin, 3 oz	0.24
Cheese, feta, 1 oz	0.23
Hamburger, lean, 3 oz	0.22
Spinach, fresh, ckd, ½ cup	0.22
Cheese, cottage, 2% fat, ½ cup	0.21
Bagel, plain, 1	0.20
Trout, bkd, 3 oz	0.19
Chicken, dark meat, 3 oz	0.19
Clams, canned, ¼ cup	0.17
Wheat germ, raw, ¼ cup	0.13
Cheese, colby, 1 oz	0.10
Milk, human, 1 cup	0.09
Rice, brown, cooked, 1 cup	0.05
Orange, 1	0.05
Rye Krisp, 2	0.03
Apple, 1	0.02

* From USDA: Composition of Foods. Handbook No. 8 series. Washington, DC, ARS, USDA, 1976–1986.

etables. The intake of riboflavin must be low for several months for signs of deficiency to develop.

Early deficiency symptoms include photophobia, lacrimation, burning and itching of the eyes, loss of visual acuity, and soreness and burning of lips, mouth, and tongue. *Ariboflavinosis* is characterized by the development of cheilosis (fissuring of the lips); angular stomatitis (cracks in the skin at the corners of the mouth); a greasy eruption of the skin in the nasolabial folds, scrotum, or vulva; a purple swollen tongue; and capillary overgrowth around the cornea of the eye. Table 6–18 summarizes signs of possible riboflavin deficiency.

Toxicity

There is no known toxicity level for riboflavin.

Niacin

Niacin is the generic term for nicotinamide (niacinamide) and nicotinic acid. Niacin functions as a component of the coenzymes *nicotinamide adenine dinucleotide (NAD)* and *nicotinamide adenine dinucleotide phosphate (NADP),* which are present in all cells.

History

The identification of niacin is closely related to the search for the cause and cure of pellagra, a disease common in Spain and Italy in the 18th century. The problem had reached sufficient proportions in the United States in the early 1900s to encourage the Public Health Service to dispatch Goldberger to investigate pellagra that was rampant in the southern states (Goldberger et al, 1918), where diets were based on cornmeal. He established that a nutrient deficiency was the cause of the disease and that it could be cured by a diet featuring high-quality protein. Recognition of pellagra as a niacin deficiency disease followed the discovery in 1937 by Elvehjem that the pellagrous disease of black tongue in dogs was caused by lack of niacin. It has been established since then that tryptophan is a precursor of niacin and that tryptophan deficiency is also involved in pellagra.

Chemical Characteristics and Stability

Niacin, or nicotinic acid, is a whitish crystalline material. When dry it is much more stable than thiamin and riboflavin, and is remarkably resistant to heat, light, air, acids, and alkalis, although small amounts may be lost in discarded cooking water. It is easily converted to the active form of nicotinamide and is frequently administered therapeutically in that form to avoid the vasodilating effect of nicotinic acid.

Absorption and Storage

Absorption takes place in the intestine. Little storage occurs in the body, and any excess is eliminated through the urine.

Functions

Nicotinamide functions in the body as a component of the coenzymes NAD and NADP (NADH and NADPH in their reduced forms). These coenzymes are essential

TABLE 6–18. Signs of Possible Riboflavin Deficiency*

Soreness and burning of lips, mouth, and tongue†
Cheilosis†
Angular stomatitis†
Glossitis†
Seborrheic dermatitis of nasolabial folds, vestibule of nose, and sometimes the ears and eyelids, scrotum, and vulva
Ocular pathology (sometimes)
— inflammation of conjunctiva
— superficial vascularization of cornea
— ulcerations of cornea
— photophobia
Anemia — normocytic and normochromic
Neuropathy
Purplish or magenta tongue†
Hypertrophy or atrophy of tongue papillae†

* Adapted from Goldsmith GA: Riboflavin deficiency. *In* Rivlin RS (ed): Riboflavin. New York, Plenum Press, 1975.

† Tongue and mouth changes are difficult to differentiate from those in niacin, folic acid, thiamin, vitamin B_6 or vitamin B_{12} deficiency.

in the oxidation-reduction reactions involved in the release of energy from carbohydrates, fats, and proteins, where they serve as hydrogen acceptors capable of accepting and releasing hydrogen atoms as they are removed by the dehydrogenase enzymes. NAD is also used in glycogen synthesis.

Clinical Uses

Niacin, but not nicotinamide, in pharmacologic doses of 3 g/day or more lowers serum cholesterol in some people. However, this use should be considered only after diet and the bile acid sequestrants have proved ineffective. Side effects include flushing as a result of vascular dilation.

Recommended Dietary Allowance

The RDA for niacin is expressed in terms of *niacin equivalents (NE)* in recognition of the tryptophan contribution to the total. Sixty milligrams of tryptophan is considered to be equivalent to 1 mg of niacin. Either one is expressed as an NE. Current recommendations for adults and children over 6 months of age are 6.6 NE/1,000 kcal with a minimum of 13 NE. Recommendations are increased in pregnancy (by 2 NE/day) and in lactation (by 5 NE/day). The RDA is given in Table 6–19.

TABLE 6–19. Recommended Dietary Allowances for Niacin*

Age (Years)	RDA (mg NE)†
Infants	
0.0–0.5	5
0.5–1.0	6
Children	
1–3	9
4–6	12
7–10	13
Males	
11–14	17
15–18	20
19–24	19
25–50	19
51+	15
Females	
11–14	15
15–18	15
19–24	15
25–50	15
51+	13
Pregnant	17
Lactating	
1st 6 months	20
2nd 6 months	20

* Reprinted with permission from *Recommended Dietary Allowances*, 10th edition, c. 1989 by the National Academy of Sciences. Published by National Academy Press, Washington, DC.

† RDA = recommended dietary allowance; NE = niacin equivalents.

TABLE 6–20. Niacin Equivalents in Selected Foods*

Food	Niacin (mg/1,000 kcal)	Tryptophan (mg/1,000 kcal)	Niacin Equivalents (per 1,000 kcal)
Cow's milk	1.2	673	12.4
Human milk	2.5	443	9.9
Beef, round	24.7	1,280	46.0
Whole eggs	0.6	1,150	19.8
Salt pork	1.2	61	2.2
Wheat flour, white	2.5	297	7.4
Corn grits	1.8	70	3.0
Corn	5.0	106	6.7

* From Horwitt MK, Harper AE, and Henderson LM: Niacin-tryptophan relationships for evaluating niacin equivalents. Am J Clin Nutr 34:423, 1981. Originally printed in Horwitt MK et al: Tryptophan-niacin relationships in man. Studies with diets deficient in riboflavin and niacin, together with observations on excretion of nitrogen and niacin metabolites. J Nutr 60 (Suppl 1):1, 1956.

Calculated intakes of total NEs are 27 mg for women and 41 mg for men (USDA, 1986 and 1987).

Sources

Both niacin and tryptophan are included in determining the niacin content of foods. However, most tables of nutrition composition give only the amount of preformed niacin in food, thus underestimating the total NE of the diet. Table 6–20 shows the niacin equivalents of selected foods.

Most diets consumed in the United States average 500 to 1,000 mg or more of tryptophan daily and 8 to 17 mg of preformed niacin, for a total of 16 to 34 NE. Lean meats, poultry, fish, and peanuts are rich daily sources of both. Organ meats, brewers' yeast, peanuts, and peanut butter are the richest sources of niacin. Vegetables and fruits are poor sources. Milk and eggs contain small amounts of niacin but are excellent sources of tryptophan. To a lesser extent, beans, peas, other legumes, most nuts, and whole grains or enriched cereals also contain niacin and tryptophan.

Most foods rich in animal protein are also rich in tryptophan. A dietary intake of 60 grams of predominantly complete protein provides 0.5 grams of tryptophan. A simple approximation of tryptophan intake can be made by assuming that dietary protein contains 1% tryptophan. If more precision is required, the following approximations can be used: corn products, 0.6%; other grains, fruits, and vegetables, 1%; meats, 1.1%; milk, 1.4%; and eggs, 1.5%.

Some niacin may be synthesized by intestinal bacteria.

Deficiency

Symptoms of niacin deficiency in the early stages include muscular weakness, anorexia, indigestion, and skin eruptions. Severe deficiency of niacin leads to pellagra, which is characterized by dermatitis, dementia, and diarrhea (the "3 Ds" of pellagra); tremors; and sore tongue ("beef tongue") (Fig. 6–8). The skin develops a cracked, pigmented, scaly dermatitis in the areas exposed to sunlight. Lesions in the central nervous system (CNS) lead to confusion, disorientation, and neuritis. Digestive abnormalities cause irritation and inflammation of the mucous membranes of the mouth and the gastrointestinal tract. Clinical symptoms of severe riboflavin deficiency appear, accenting the close interrelationships of riboflavin and niacin in cell metabolism.

Frequently those people who suffer from pellagra are on highly inadequate diets in which corn is a mainstay. There is very little niacin in the diet, and the tryptophan in the corn is unavailable for absorption from the intestine.

Niacin occurs in immature seeds as part of the biologically available coenzyme necessary for seed metabolism. In the mature seed, it is bound to carbohydrate, impairing its availability to humans and to animals (Wall and Carpenter, 1988). Hot alkali treatment makes niacin available. Hopi Indians boil immature sweet corn, but cook mature corn in alkaline wood ash, thus releasing the niacin. Unlike others with high-grain diets, the Hopi do not have pellagra.

In severe cases of pellagra, oral administration of 150 to 600 mg of nicotinic acid or nicotinamide per day in several doses is effective. Nicotinamide is preferred because it does not cause the unpleasant flushing and burning sensations that accompany nicotinic acid therapy. Within 24 hours there is a response to nicotinamide, with cessation of diarrhea and less redness of the tongue. Unfortunately, some of the mental problems do not ever respond, probably because of the previous prolonged state of malnutrition.

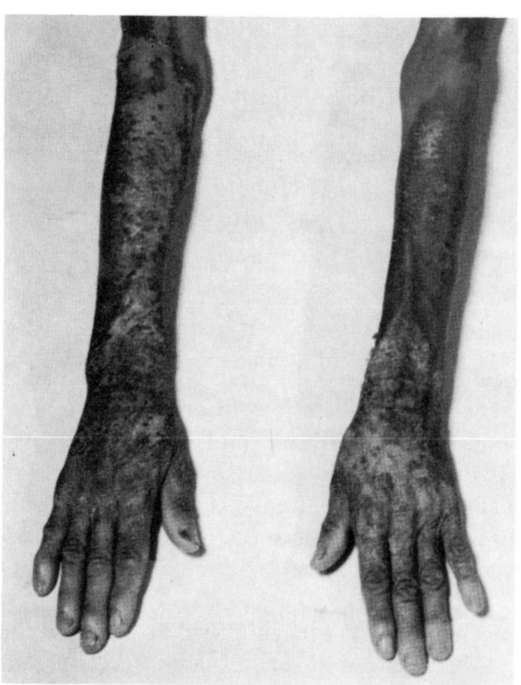

FIGURE 6–8. *Pellagra caused by niacin deficiency. (From Jarvis C: Physical Examination and Health Assessment. Philadelphia, WB Saunders [in press].*

Toxicity

Large doses of niacin have been used in an attempt to lower blood cholesterol concentration. Usually 1 to 2 g of niacin three times a day are given under medical supervision. The histamine release that causes the flushing may be injurious to persons with asthma or peptic ulcer disease.

Vitamin B_6 (Pyridoxine, Pyridoxal, and Pyridoxamine)

Vitamin B_6 (pyridoxine) exists in three interchangeable forms. The phosphorylated forms *pyridoxal phosphate (PLP)* and *pyridoxamine phosphate (PMP)* are coenzymes in transamination reactions. PLP is critical to many other reactions.

History

Pyridoxine was identified as another fraction of the vitamin B complex in 1938 and synthesized in 1939. Later it was found that *pyridoxamine (PM)* and *pyridoxal (PL),* both derivatives of pyridoxine, were also metabolically and functionally related. *Vitamin B_6* or *pyridoxine* designates this entire complex of closely related chemical compounds.

Chemical Properties

Pyridoxine, a white, crystalline, odorless compound, is soluble in water and alcohol. It is stable to heat in an acid medium, relatively unstable in alkaline solutions, and very unstable to light. Losses during freezing range from 36 to 55% (Sauberlich, 1987).

Absorption, Transport, and Excretion

All three forms of the vitamin are absorbed into the mucosal cells of the upper small intestine where they are phosphorylated to form PLP and PMP. PLP can be oxidized further to pyridoxic acid and other metabolites that are excreted in the urine. PLP is transported bound to albumin. Total excretion does not account completely for intake, suggesting some retention. Muscle, with 50% of the total body content of vitamin B_6, appears to be the prime reservoir in humans.

Functions

PLP and PMP are coenzymes that function primarily in transamination and other reactions related to protein metabolism. In addition, pyridoxal phosphate is necessary for the formation of alpha-aminolevulinic acid, a precursor of heme in hemoglobin. Vitamin B_6 is essential for the metabolism of tryptophan and for the conversion of tryptophan to niacin. As a coenzyme for phosphorylase, pyridoxine facilitates the release of glycogen from the liver and muscle as glucose-1-phosphate. It is also involved in the conversion of linoleic acid to the biologically important arachidonic acid. The formation of sphingolipids involved in the development of the myelin sheath surrounding nerve cells is also vitamin B_6-dependent. PLP regulates the synthesis of gamma-aminobutyric acid (GABA), a neurotransmitter. High levels of pyridoxine are maintained in the brain even at low plasma concentrations. Certain brain abnormalities such as dementia may result from inadequate cerebral uptake of certain vitamins, particularly vitamin B_6 (Spector et al, 1979).

Recommended Dietary Allowance

The requirement for vitamin B_6 increases as the intake of protein increases. Adequate vitamin B_6 status appears to be maintained when it is consumed in a ratio of 0.016 mg/g of protein. The RDA was established at the upper level of intake that is acceptable with a protein intake two times as large as the RDA. Extra protein allowances for pregnancy and lactation are paralleled by increases in the vitamin B_6 RDAs (Table 6–21). The vitamin B_6 concentration of human milk reflects the adequacy of the maternal diet. Infants who are breastfed by women whose intakes are less than 2 mg/day show some evidence of vitamin B_6 deficiency. Recommendations are 0.3 mg/day for the first 6 months of infancy and 0.6 mg/day for older infants. RDAs for children and adolescents are based on average protein intakes.

Separate RDA have not been established for the elderly, although numerous studies have shown a substantial number of individuals among elderly populations with biochemical evidence of deficiency (Suter and Russell, 1987). This may be due to low intake, a higher requirement, the presence of health problems that alter vitamin B_6 status, or a combination of these factors. Low-income, elderly persons with multiple health problems are particularly at risk (Manore et al, 1989; Löwik et al, 1989).

Sources

The best sources of pyridoxine are yeast, wheat germ, pork, glandular meats (especially liver), whole-grain cereals, legumes, potatoes, bananas, and oatmeal. Milk, eggs, vegetables, and fruit contain small amounts. Table 6–22 lists the pyridoxine content of selected foods.

TABLE 6–21. Recommended Dietary Allowances for Vitamin B_6*

Age (Years)	RDA† (mg)
Infants	
0.0–0.5	0.3
0.5–1.0	0.6
Children	
1–3	1.0
4–6	1.1
7–10	1.4
Males	
11–14	1.7
15–18	2.0
19–24	2.0
25–50	2.0
51+	2.0
Females	
11–14	1.4
15–18	1.5
19–24	1.6
25–50	1.6
51+	1.6
Pregnant	2.2
Lactating	
1st 6 months	2.1
2nd 6 months	2.1

* From Food and Nutrition Board, National Research Council, NAS: Recommended Dietary Allowances, 10th ed. Washington, DC, National Academy Press, 1989.

† RDA = recommended dietary allowance.

The presence in vegetables of a conjugated form of pyridoxine, a beta-glucoside that is absorbed but not well utilized, may account for the difference in bioavailability of this vitamin in vegetable and animal foods (Leklem, 1988). Vegetables such as potatoes, spinach, beans, and other legumes are high in the beta-glucoside. Intestinal microflora contribute little to vitamin B_6 nutriture according to studies using germ-free animals.

Deficiency

Dietary deficiencies of vitamin B_6 are relatively rare. However, many medications interfere with vitamin B_6 metabolism or performance. Isoniazid (isonicotinic acid hydrazide [INH]) used as a chemotherapeutic agent for tubercular patients, is a potent antagonist of vitamin B_6. Patients develop peripheral neuritis and many of the symptoms of pyridoxine deficiency (see Chapter 25).

Fifteen to 20% of women taking oral steroid contraceptives have been shown to have increased urinary excretion of tryptophan metabolites, suggestive of vitamin B_6 deficiency. This and the accompanying states

TABLE 6–22. Pyridoxine (Vitamin B_6) Content of Selected Foods*

Food	mg	Food	mg
Liver, beef, 3 oz	1.22	Rice, white, 1 cup	0.19
Oatmeal, ¾ cup	0.74	Brussels sprouts, cooked, ½ cup	0.16
Banana, 1	0.66	Cauliflower, cooked, ½ cup	0.13
Chicken, light meat, 3 oz	0.51	Orange juice, 1 cup	0.13
Potatoes, mashed, 1 cup	0.49	Peanut butter, 2 T	0.12
Avocado, California, 1	0.48	Milk, 2%, 1 cup	0.11
Sunflower seeds, kernels, ¼ cup	0.45	Yogurt, low fat, plain, 1 cup	0.11
Yeast, brewer's, 1 T	0.40	Tomato, raw	0.10
Halibut, baked, 3.5 oz	0.34	Frankfurter, 1	0.08
Chicken, dark meat, 3 oz	0.30	Apple, 1	0.07
Pork chop, baked, 3 oz	0.30	Apricots, dried halves, 10	0.06
Wheat germ, tasted, ¼ cup	0.30	Egg, large, 1	0.06
Rice, brown, cooked, 1 cup	0.28	Bread, whole wheat, 1 slice	0.05
Corn, canned, ½ cup	0.26	Milk, human, 1 cup	0.03
Beef, hamburger, 3 oz.	0.23	Cheese, cheddar, 1 oz	0.02
Prunes, dried, 10	0.22	Bread, white, 1 slice	0.01

* From USDA: Composition of Foods. Handbook No. 8 series. Washington, DC, ARS, USDA, 1976–1986.

of malaise, depression, and glucose intolerance are relieved by 10 to 15 mg/day of vitamin B_6. However, it is not clear that these effects represent a true vitamin B_6 deficiency.

Vitamin B_6 deficiency may accompany alcoholism, because alcohol and alcoholic liver disease can interfere with normal vitamin B_6 metabolism.

Extreme pyridoxine deficiency leads to CNS abnormalities. Infants fed a liquid milk formula in which much of the vitamin was unknowingly destroyed in processing developed irritability and convulsions but recovered rapidly after an injection of the vitamin. A deficiency syndrome has been identified in mentally retarded children with uncontrollable convulsions from birth due to an inborn error of vitamin B_6 metabolism. It is thought that these children are unable to synthesize GABA. Correction of the convulsions requires daily ingestion of large amounts of the vitamin and must be started in the neonatal period in order to prevent the development of irreversible mental retardation.

Studies of the relationship of vitamin B_6 and *premenstrual syndrome (PMS)* have produced conflicting results (see Further Reading 9–1, p. 159.). Few controlled trials have yielded significant effects; however, one study reported that 434 of 617 women showed improvement in seven of nine symptoms when given pyridoxine therapy (Williams et al, 1985). Part of the confusion may arise from differences in vitamin B_6 status of the women in a particular study.

Toxicity

Although acute toxicity from large doses of pyridoxine is low, prolonged ingestion of high dosages has resulted in ataxia and severe sensory neuropathy (Schaumberg et al, 1983). However, discontinuation of supplements has resulted in complete recovery within 6 months (Dalton and Dalton, 1987).

Folate (Folic Acid, Folacin, or Pteroylmonoglutamate)

Folacin and folate are generic descriptors for a group of compounds chemically and nutritionally similar to folic acid. They function as coenzymes in transport of single-carbon fragments in amino acid metabolism and nucleic acid synthesis.

History

Folate was known under several names in the study of unidentified growth factors in bacteria and experimental animals and in the study and treatment of anemias. It was synthesized and established as a dietary essential in 1946.

Chemical and Physical Properties

Folic acid, also known as *folacin* and *pteroylglutamic acid,* is a yellow, crystalline substance that belongs to a group of compounds known as *pterins* (found in the pigment of butterfly wings and named for the Greek *wing*). As the free acid, it is insoluble in cold water, but the disodium salt is more soluble.

Folate occurs in 150 different forms. The majority is present in foods in reduced forms and is labile and easily oxidized. Fifty to 95% is lost during home preparation and food processing.

Pteroylglutamic acid is formed by the linkage of pteridine and para-aminobenzoic acid (PABA) conjugated with 1 to 7 and sometimes up to 11 molecules of glutamic acid. Some of the glutamic acid molecules must be split off to form an unconjugated folic acid molecule, *pteroylmonoglutamic acid (PGA),* which is the active form. Vitamin B_{12} is involved in the reaction.

The various forms of folacin are highly variable in their response to heat and acid. Considerable loss of folic acid occurs during storage of vegetables at room temperature, and additional loss can occur during processing at high temperatures.

Absorption, Metabolism, and Storage

Only monoglutamates are absorbed from the small intestine. Folate, usually present in the polyglutamate form in food, is broken down to the monoglutamate form by folyl conjugase from the pancreas and mucosal conjugase from the intestinal wall. Most is then absorbed by carrier-mediated active transport. A small percentage is absorbed by a pH-sensitive passive diffusion. Bioavailability of folate in a typical diet is about one half that of crystalline folic acid (Sauberlich, 1987).

During or after absorption, monoglutamic acid is changed to methyltetrahydrofolic acid and stored. The exact amount of food folate that is absorbed is not clear, but it is assumed that all of the free folic acid and a good portion of the polyglutamates are absorbed. Folic acid in the presence of NAD is reduced to tetrahydrofolic acid (THFA). THFA unites with a single carbon unit to form *formyltetrahydrofolic acid* or *citrovorum factor,* which is much more stable.

Functions

Tetrahydrofolic acid is a carrier for the single-carbon formyl, hydroxymethyl, or methyl groups. It plays an important role in the synthesis of the purines guanine and adenine and of the pyrimidine thymine, compounds that are utilized for the formation of nucleoproteins deoxyribonucleic acid (DNA) and ribonucleic acid (RNA), which are essential to cell division.

THFA participates in the interconversion of serine and glycine, the oxidation of glycine, methylation of homocysteine to methionine with vitamin B_{12} as cofactor, and the methylation of the precursor ethanolamine to the vitamin choline. The conversion of nicotinamide to *N*-methyl nicotinamide by addition of a single methyl group and the oxidation of phenylalanine to tyrosine require folacin.

Folate is required for one step in the conversion of histidine to glutamic acid. An impaired metabolism of histidine results in accumulation of the intermediary product, *formiminoglutamic acid (FIGLU),* which is excreted in the urine.

Folate is essential for the formation of both red and white blood cells in the bone marrow and for their maturation. It serves as a single carbon carrier in the formation of heme. Folate supplementation produces marked alleviation of pernicious anemia; however, the gastrointestinal symptoms and neurologic lesions of the anemia continue to progress. This "masking effect" is described in Chapter 32.

Recommended Dietary Allowance

RDAs for folate have been established at 3 μg/kg of body weight, which is equivalent to the average intake of the populations of the United States and Canada. Although low folate stores are found in approximately 10% of the population, these are not accompanied by signs of deficiency and it is assumed that the RDA is sufficient to provide for storage and daily needs. Additional intakes recommended for pregnancy and lactation, based on a 50% absorption from food, can be met from an ordinary diet without added supplementation. Specific values for the various age-sex levels are listed in Table 6–23.

TABLE 6–23. Recommended Dietary Allowances for Folate*

Age (Years)	RDA† (μg)
Infants	
0.0–0.5	25
0.5–1.0	35
Children	
1–3	50
4–6	75
7–10	100
Males	
11–14	150
15–18	200
19–24	200
25–50	200
51+	200
Females	
11–14	150
15–18	180
19–24	180
25–50	180
51+	180
Pregnant	400
Lactating	
1st 6 months	280
2nd 6 months	260

* From Food and Nutrition Board, National Research Council, NAS: Recommended Dietary Allowances, 10th ed. Washington, DC, National Academy Press, 1989.

† RDA = recommended dietary allowance.

TABLE 6–24. Folic Acid Content of Selected Foods*

Food	μg
Yeast	
brewer's, 1 T	313
active, dry	285
Liver, beef, fried, 3 oz	187
Spinach (cooked), ½ cup	131
Beans, white, baked, ½ cup	122
Broccoli (cooked), 1 cup	78
Romaine lettuce, 1 cup	76
Wheat germ, raw, ¼ cup	70
Fresh orange juice, ½ cup	55
Cabbage, raw, 1 cup	40
Banana, 1	24
Egg, yolk, 1	23
Almonds, raw, ¼ cup	21
Whole wheat bread, 1 slice	16
Milk, 2%, 1 cup	12
Wheat bran, ¼ cup	12
White bread, 1 slice	10

* From USDA: Composition of Foods. Handbook No. 8 series. Washington, DC, ARS, USDA, 1976–1986.

Sources

Folate occurs widely in foods, usually in the polyglutamate form, and an adequate supply is easily obtained. The best sources are liver, kidney beans, lima beans, and fresh dark green leafy vegetables, especially spinach, asparagus, and broccoli. Good sources are lean beef, potatoes, whole-wheat bread, and dried beans. Poor sources include most meats, milk, eggs, most fruits except oranges, and root vegetables. The folic acid content of various foods is listed in Table 6–24.

The availability of measurable folate varies depending upon the presence of conjugase inhibitors, binders, or other unknown factors. Probably 25 to 50% of dietary folate is nutritionally available. As much as 50% of the folate in foods can be destroyed in preparation, either commercial or household. Intestinal bacteria synthesize large amounts of folate, which add to the daily balance.

Mean daily intakes of American adults between ages 19 and 74 in the National Health and Nutrition Examination Survey (NHANES) II were 242 μg for all adults, 281 μg for men, and 207 μg for women. In a 10% sample of this population aged 20 to 74 years, 12% had low serum folate and 8% had low red blood cell folate (Subar et al, 1989).

Methods for analyzing the concentration of folate in foods are difficult, and values in tables of food composition may be too low. Orange juice, white breads, dried beans, green salad, and ready-to-eat cereals are the major food sources of folate, contributing 37% of the total intake (Subar et al, 1989).

Deficiency

The main metabolic consequence of folic acid deficiency is alteration of DNA metabolism. This results in changes in cellular nuclear morphology, especially in those cells with the most rapid rates of multiplication — red blood cells, leukocytes, and epithelial cells of the stomach, intestine, vagina, and uterine cervix.

Folate deficiency may be the most common hypovitaminosis of humans, affecting mainly the indigent of the world. Deficiency of folate results in poor growth, megaloblastic anemia and other blood disorders, glossitis, and gastrointestinal (GI) tract disturbances (Fig. 6–9). Utilization and function of folate may be impaired in protein malnutrition and by conditions that enhance demands, such as pregnancy, hemolytic anemia, leukemia, Hodgkin's disease, and the use of certain drugs. Alcoholism interferes with folate absorption or increases excretion.

Despite an apparently low intake of folate, most elderly persons have normal whole blood folate concentrations. Age has not been shown to influence either the activity of mucosal folate conjugase or intestinal absorption. Folate status may be more related to health and socioeconomic status or institutionalization in the elderly. Drugs such as sulfasalazine, diphenylhydantoin, and barbiturate may impair folate absorption.

Toxicity

No toxicity from folate has been reported in adults with daily doses as high as 15 mg (Butterworth and Tamura, 1989).

Pregnant women in one study who took folate supplements had intakes as high as 15 times the 1989 RDA.

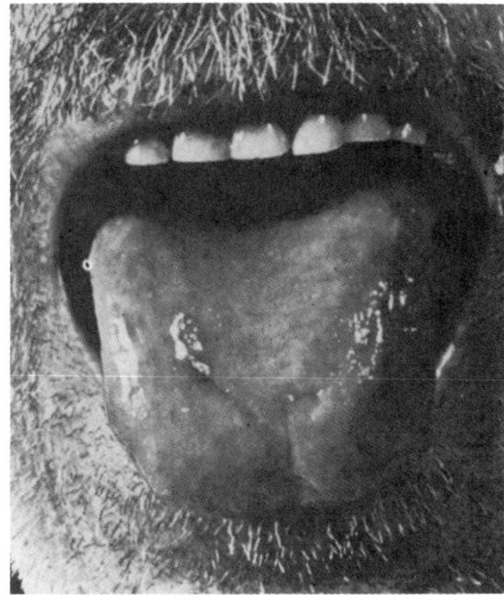

FIGURE 6–9. *Folic acid deficiency glossitis. (From Nizel AE: Nutrition in Preventive Dentistry, 2nd ed. Philadelphia, WB Saunders, 1981, p 145.)*

The mean intake of those who were consuming twice the RDA or more was 1,121 μg/day; approximately 70% of the 566 women in the study were in this category. Although not toxic to adults at these levels, the effect on the fetus is unknown as are possible subtle effects on maternal metabolism. Although the evidence for a zinc-folate interaction is still inconclusive, it has been stated in a review of folate safety that doses of 5 to 10 mg of folate are "without toxicity in normal, non-pregnant subjects" (Butterworth, 1989). The safest course during pregnancy would be to avoid intakes greater than 2½ times the RDA.

Vitamin B_{12} (Cobalamin)

Vitamin B_{12} (cobalamin) was isolated from liver extract in 1948 and identified as the extrinsic factor of food that is effective in the treatment of pernicious anemia. Of the several different cobalamin compounds that exhibit vitamin B_{12} activity, cyanocobalamin and hydroxycobalamin are the most active forms.

Chemical Characteristics and Stability

Vitamin B_{12} is a red crystalline substance that is water soluble. The red color is due to the presence of the heavy metal cobalt, which is chelated in a large tetrapyrrole ring very similar to the porphyrin ring of heme. Vitamin B_{12} is slowly destroyed by dilute acid, alkali, light, and oxidizing or reducing agents. Approximately 70% of the vitamin activity is retained during cooking.

Cyanocobalamin is the most stable form and therefore the form in which the vitamin is produced commercially from bacterial fermentation.

Absorption, Transport, and Storage

Cobalamin is released from its peptide bonds by hydrochloric acid in the stomach. However, it is poorly absorbed from the intestinal tract unless the *intrinsic factor* (a mucoprotein enzyme called "Castle's intrinsic factor") is present in the gastric secretion. The intrinsic factor combines with cobalamin and in the bound form is adsorbed to a receptor in the membranes of the ileum, through which it is transported into the cells in pinocytic vesicles. Calcium is necessary for the transfer.

After absorption, cobalamin is circulated to the various tissues bound to serum proteins *transcobalamin I and II* (II being more important). The highest concentration is found in the liver and to some extent in the kidney, from where it is released as needed to the bone marrow and other tissues.

The body store of the vitamin (~2,000 μg) is substantial. In addition, an enterohepatic circulation recycles it from bile and other intestinal secretions, thus reducing the necessary dietary intake to very small amounts. Thus it may take 5 or 6 years for deficiency symptoms to appear after restriction of the vitamin from natural sources. Any excess intake is excreted in the urine.

Functions

Cobalamin is essential for normal function in the metabolism of all cells, especially for those of the gastrointestinal tract, bone marrow, and nervous tissue. With folic acid, choline, and methionine, it participates in the transfer of methyl groups in the synthesis of nucleic acids, purines, and pyrimidine intermediates. It is necessary for removal of a methyl group from methylfolate and for generation of tetrahydrofolate necessary for DNA synthesis. Vitamin B_{12} affects myelin formation.

Recommended Dietary Allowance

The adult RDA of 2 μg provides for substantial body stores in view of the increasing prevalence of achlorhydria and pernicious anemia in persons over 60 years of

TABLE 6–25. Recommended Dietary Allowances for Vitamin B_{12}*

Age (Years)	RDA† (μg)
Infants	
0.0–0.5	0.3
0.5–1.0	0.5
Children	
1–3	0.7
4–6	1.0
7–10	1.4
Males	
11–14	2.0
15–18	2.0
19–24	2.0
25–50	2.0
51+	2.0
Females	
11–14	2.0
15–18	2.0
19–24	2.0
25–50	2.0
51+	2.0
Pregnant	2.2
Lactating	
1st 6 months	2.6
2nd 6 months	2.6

* From Food and Nutrition Board, National Research Council, NAS: Recommended Dietary Allowances, 10th ed. Washington, DC, National Academy Press, 1989.

† RDA = recommended dietary allowance.

age. Serum vitamin B_{12} concentrations have been reported to decline in the elderly, although they remain within the range of normal. The clinical significance of subclinical deficiencies, particularly in the elderly, has yet to be determined.

Additional allowances are recommended for pregnancy and lactation. The RDA for young infants is 0.3 μg/day; for older infants and children, it is based on progressive increases until the RDA for adults is reached (Table 6–25).

Sources

Vitamin B_{12} is present in animal protein foods, including those listed in Table 6–26. The richest sources are liver and kidney, followed by milk, eggs, fish, cheese, and muscle meats. Forty to 90% of the vitamin is lost when milk is pasteurized or evaporated. Foods of vegetable origin contain cobalamin only through contamination or bacterial synthesis. The vitamin B_{12} from the limited bacterial synthesis that occurs in humans is not absorbed because it takes place in the colon beyond the terminal ileum.

Many people believe that fermented foods contain sufficient vitamin B_{12} to meet their needs; however, this theory is not supported by analysis (Specker et al, 1988). Six samples of tempeh (a fermented soybean product) were analyzed and the vitamin B_{12} concentrations were negligible. In contrast, some cooked sea vegetables contained vitamin B_{12} in the same range as beef liver.

Deficiency

Cobalamin deficiency produces two clinical syndromes. Impaired DNA synthesis results in defective proliferation of rapidly dividing cells and is manifested by *megaloblastic anemia,* glossitis, and hypospermia. Distortion of intestinal architecture results in GI disorders.

A second neurologic syndrome is more difficult to understand because of the vagueness of initial symptoms. Megaloblastic anemia precedes neurologic change in the majority of patients (Carmel, 1988; Lindenbaum et al, 1988). Treatment may reverse neuropsychiatric abnormalities, but this may not occur, particularly when symptoms have been present for a long time.

A lack of vitamin B_{12} results in subacute degeneration of cerebral white matter, optic nerves, spinal cord, and peripheral nerves. Symptoms include numbness, tingling, and burning of the feet as well as stiffness and generalized weakness of the legs.

Many believe vitamin B_{12} deficiency to be a common disorder in the elderly (Carethers, 1988). It often presents with (1) a lemon-yellow tint resulting from concurrent anemia and jaundice from ineffective erythropoeisis; (2) a smooth, beefy red tongue and; (3) neurologic disorders. Psychiatric manifestations such as impaired mentation and depression may be present.

USDA survey data place the average dietary intake of American men, women, and children at 7.8, 4.8, and 3.8 μg/day, respectively (USDA, 1986 and 1987). While average figures suggest intake is more than adequate, intake of subsets of the population such as the elderly might be substantially less.

Breast-fed infants of vegetarian mothers may also be at risk (Specker et al, 1988).

TABLE 6–26. Vitamin B_{12} Content of Selected Foods*

Food	μg
Liver, beef, 3 oz	95
Clams, canned, ½ cup	80
Oysters, raw, Pacific, ½ cup	20
Crab, Dungeness, ¾ cup	10
Tuna, canned, 3 oz	2.8
Beef, hamburger, 3 oz	1.77
Halibut, baked, 3.5 oz	1.2
Milk, 2%, 1 cup	0.89
Frankfurters, 1	0.74
Yogurt, low fat, plain, ½ cup	0.64
Egg, 1	0.59
Pork chop, baked, 3 oz	0.50
Cheese, Edam, 1 oz	0.44
Ice cream, ½ cup	0.31
Chicken, white meat, 3 oz	0.29

* From USDA: Composition of Foods. Handbook No. 8 series. Washington, DC, ARS, USDA, 1976–1986.

Toxicity

No toxic effects are known. Self-prescribed intakes up to 100 μg appear to be without harm, but do not have any prophylactic benefit.

Pantothenic Acid

Pantothenic acid was synthesized in 1940. It is a white, crystalline compound that is bitter to the taste, more stable in solution than in dry form, and easily decomposed by acid, alkali, and dry heat. It is water soluble and stable in moist heat in neutral solution.

Functions

The primary role of pantothenic acid is as a constituent of coenzyme A and as such it is essential to many areas of cellular metabolism. As a part of acetyl CoA, it is involved in the release of energy from carbohydrate and in the degradation and metabolism of fatty acids. Besides functioning in the citric acid cycle, CoA is involved as an acceptor acetate group for amino acids, vitamins, and sulfonamides. It is involved in the synthesis of cholesterol, phospholipids, steroid hormones, and porphyrin for hemoglobin.

Estimated Safe and Adequate Daily Dietary Intake

A daily intake of 4 to 7 mg of pantothenic acid is probably adequate for adults, and a higher intake may be needed during pregnancy and lactation. However, there is insufficient evidence to define a recommended allowance.

Usual intake of pantothenic acid in the American diet is about 7 mg/day with a range of 5 to 20 mg. Estimated safe and adequate intakes are listed in Table 6–27.

Sources

Pantothenic acid is present in all plant and animal tissue, hence its name meaning *widespread.* Excellent sources include egg yolk, kidney, liver, and yeast; fair sources are broccoli, lean beef, skimmed milk, sweet potatoes, and molasses. Much of the pantothenate in meat is lost during thawing, and approximately 33% is lost in cooking. About 50% is lost in the milling of flour. Table 6–28 presents the pantothenate content of some foods.

Deficiency and Toxicity

Because panthothenic acid is so widely distributed in foods, no deficiency disease due to lack of the vitamin has been observed in humans.

No serious toxic effects of this substance are known; however, ingestion of large amounts may cause diarrhea.

TABLE 6–27. Estimated Safe and Adequate Daily Dietary Intakes for Pantothenic Acid*

Age (Years)	Intake (mg)
Infants	
0.0–0.5	2
0.5–1.0	3
Children	
1–3	3
4–6	3–4
7–10	4–5
11+	4–7
Adults	
Male and female, all ages	4–7

* From Food and Nutrition Board, National Research Council, NAS: Recommended Dietary Allowances, 10th ed. Washington, DC, National Academy Press, 1989.

TABLE 6–28. Panthothenic Acid Content of Selected Foods*

Food	mg
Liver, beef, 3 oz	5.03
Yogurt, low fat, w/fruit, 1 cup	1.11
Ice milk, soft serve, 1 cup	1.03
Liverwurst, 1 oz	1.0
Salmon, baked, 3 oz	0.94
Chicken, white meat, baked, 3 oz	0.83
Milk, 2% fat, 1 cup	0.78
Corn, cooked, ½ cup	0.72
Dates, 10	0.65
Wheat germ, raw, ¼ cup	0.56
Peanuts, roasted, shelled, ¼ cup	0.5
Cheese, blue, 1 oz	0.49
Oatmeal, regular, cooked, 1 cup	0.47
Papaya, ½	0.33
Cheese, cottage, 2% fat, ½ cup	0.27
Bread, whole wheat, 1 slice	0.26
Strawberries, ½ cup	0.25
Orange juice, ½ cup	0.24

* From USDA: Composition of Foods. Handbook No. 8 series. Washington, DC, ARS, USDA, 1976–1986.

Biotin

Biotin functions in metabolism via biotin-dependent enzymes that are involved in gluconeogenesis, synthesis and oxidation of fatty acids, degradation of some amino acids, and purine synthesis.

History

Biotin was first isolated in 1936 and synthesized in 1943. It had been previously observed that chicks and rats fed large amounts of raw egg whites developed eczema accompanied by alopecia around the eyes. The syndrome was cured by adding egg yolks to the diet of the affected animals, and the corrective factor in the yolk was named vitamin H. This proved to be the same as a potent growth factor in yeast called coenzyme R, and the factor was renamed *biotin.*

Chemistry and Stability

Biotin is a monocarboxylic acid, stable to heat, soluble in water and alcohol, and susceptible to oxidation.

Functions

Biotin functions as the coenzyme for reactions involving the addition or removal of carbon dioxide to or from active compounds. The synthesis and oxidation of fatty acids requires biotin as a coenzyme. It functions in deamination in the removal of NH_2 from certain amino acids, notably aspartic acid, threonine, and serine. Biotin is closely related metabolically to folic acid, pantothenic acid, and vitamin B_{12}.

Absorption, Transport, and Excretion

Biotin and *biocytin* (a large natural fragment released by the degradation of biotinyl enzymes) are readily absorbed. Biocytin is hydrolyzed in the plasma to release biotin, which is taken up by liver, muscle, and kidney. Biotin synthesized by microflora contributes substantially to tissue requirements. Fecal and urinary excretion considerably higher than dietary intake reflects the magnitude of microfloral synthesis. A vegetarian diet may alter the enteric flora to enhance synthesis of biotin or promote absorption, or both (Lombard and Mock, 1989).

Estimated Safe and Adequate Daily Dietary Intake

Definitive studies on biotin requirements have not been performed because of the lack of knowledge of bioavailability of biotin in foods and the uncertain contribution of microbial synthesis. The 1989 RDA is based on the probable daily intake of Americans, which appears to meet the needs of most healthy adults. Estimated safe and adequate intakes are listed in Table 6–29.

Sources

Biotin is found in a great many foods, and a considerable amount is synthesized by intestinal bacteria and absorbed by the body. Good sources are kidney, liver, egg yolk, some vegetables (mushrooms), a number of fruits (bananas, grapefruit, watermelon, strawberries), peanuts, and yeast. Moderate sources are eggs, human milk, fish, nuts, and oatmeal. Poor sources are meat, some fruits, and cow's milk. Biotin is frequently added to multiple vitamin preparations even though its need has not been definitely established. Table 6–30 presents the biotin content of some foods.

TABLE 6–29. Estimated Safe and Adequate Daily Dietary Intakes for Biotin*

Age (Years)	Intake (μg)
Infants	
0.0–0.5	10
0.5–1.0	15
Children	
1–3	20
4–6	25
7–10	30
11+	30–100
Adults	
Male and female, all ages	30–100

* From Food and Nutrition Board, National Research Council, NAS: Recommended Dietary Allowances, 10th ed. Washington, DC, National Academy Press, 1989.

Deficiency

Biotin deficiency has been described in patients receiving TPN for several years. Deficiency symptoms in adults include a dry, scaly dermatitis; pallor; nausea; vomiting; and anorexia. In infants under 6 months of age, the symptoms are seborrheic dermatitis and alopecia.

Avidin, a substance in raw egg white, combines with biotin in the intestine and prevents its absorption. Deficiency symptoms induced by feeding raw egg whites (the equivalent of 24/day) are alleviated by a concentrate of the vitamin. An occasional raw egg white does not precipitate a deficiency of biotin. Avidin is denatured by cooking.

Carbamazepine and primidone (anticonvulsant drugs) inhibit biotin transport in the human intestine (Said et al, 1989). This may be one of the causes of impairment of biotin status observed in patients on long-term anticonvulsant therapy (Krause, 1985). Diets low in fat and cholesterol are also low in biotin.

Toxicity

There are no known toxic effects from biotin.

Ascorbic Acid

History

Vitamin C is the antiscorbutic vitamin. Although scurvy was first described during the Crusades and commonly plagued early explorers and voyagers, the specific relationship between scurvy, citrus foods, and ascorbic acid was not established until the 20th century. English sailors have been nicknamed "limeys" since the days when ships were required to carry citrus fruits (actually lemons) as a scurvy preventive.

The antiscorbutic factor was isolated in 1928 by Szent-Gyorgyi, who found it in adrenal tissue, orange, and cabbage, and named it hexuronic acid. In 1932 both he and C. Glenn King demonstrated that hexuronic acid was vitamin C.

Chemical Characteristics

Ascorbic acid is a white, water-soluble crystalline material that is stable in dry form. It is easily oxidized in solution, especially on exposure to heat. Oxidation can

TABLE 6–30. Biotin Content of Selected Foods*

Food	Range (μg/100 g)	Food	Range (μg/100 g)
Cereals		***Poultry***	10–11.3
Wheat germ	22–38	***Fish and Shellfish***	3–24
Oatmeal	22–31		
Wheat bran	22.4–25.5	***Vegetables***	0.2–4.1
Oatmeal; rolled oats	15.3–24.6	***Fruit***	0.2–2
Wheat bran	22.4–33.4		
Milk and Milk Products		***Nuts***	
Fresh whole; dried	2–16	Almonds, raw	18
Whole	1.6–2.4	Peanuts, roasted	34
Instant	16–24	Pecans	27
		Walnuts, peanut butter	37–39
Eggs		***Miscellaneous***	
Whole, cooked	20–25	Chocolate	32
Yolk, raw	60	Molasses	9
Yolk, raw	51.5–58	Yeast, brewer's	200
Meat and Meat Products		Yeast, *Torula*	100
Beef, liver	96	***Human Milk***	18–22
Beef, other	2.6–3.4		
Chicken, liver	170–210		

* From Marshall MW: The nutritional importance of biotin—An update. Nutrition Today 22:26, 1987.

be accelerated by the presence of copper or iron and by alkaline pH.

Ascorbic acid is a hexose derivative and classified as a carbohydrate closely related to the monosaccharides. Plants and many mammals are able to synthesize it from glucose and galactose. The reduced form of ascorbic acid, which is the most active, is readily oxidized to dehydroascorbic acid; both forms are antiscorbutic. Further oxidation of dehydroascorbic acid produces diketogulonic acid, which has no antiscorbutic acid properties and cannot be reduced to an active form.

Absorption and Storage

Ascorbic acid is easily absorbed from the small intestine into the blood by an active mechanism and probably also by diffusion. Average absorption is 90% (Sauberlich, 1985) for intakes between 20 and 120 mg; however, at very high intakes such as 12 grams, which are often self-medicated, absorption is only 16%. Diets high in zinc or pectin may decrease absorption, whereas absorption may be increased by substances in natural citrus extract (Vinson and Bose, 1988).

Ascorbic acid readily passes into tissues of the adrenals, kidney, liver, and spleen, most of which appear to be in equilibrium with serum levels. Excess amounts ingested over the saturation level of various tissues are excreted in the urine as oxalic acid, although at intakes greater than 100 g/day, excesses are excreted as ascorbic acid or are exhaled as carbon dioxide.

Functions

Ascorbic acid has multiple functions either as a coenzyme or cofactor. Its ability to lose and take on hydrogen gives it an essential role in metabolism. Its role in enhancing absorption of iron is well recognized (see Chapters 7 and 32). In addition, ascorbic acid blocks the degradation of ferritin to hemosiderin, from which iron is poorly mobilized, thus assuring a more available supply in the form of ferritin (Bridges, 1987).

Vitamin C is involved in the hydroxylation of proline to form hydroxyproline in the synthesis of *collagen,* a protein substance upon which the integrity of cellular structure in all fibrous tissues depends. These include connective tissue, cartilage, bone matrix, tooth dentin, skin, and tendon. It is thus involved in healing of wounds, fractures, bruises, pinpoint hemorrhages, and bleeding gums. It also reduces liability to infections.

Vitamin C is essential for the oxidation of phenylalanine and tyrosine, for the conversion of folacin to tetrahydrofolic acid, for the conversion of tryptophan to 5-hydroxytryptophan and the neurotransmitter serotonin, and in the formation of norepinephrine from dopamine. It also reduces ferric to ferrous iron in the intestinal tract to facilitate absorption and is involved in the transfer of iron from plasma transferrin to liver ferritin.

Ascorbic acid participates in the hydroxylation of certain steroids synthesized in adrenal tissue. Concentration is decreased under stress when adrenal cortical hormone activity is high. Injection of ACTH causes considerable loss of ascorbic acid from the adrenal cortex. During periods of emotional, psychologic, or physiologic stress, the urinary excretion of ascorbic acid is increased.

Vitamin C promotes resistance to infection through the immunologic activity of leukocytes, the production of interferon, the process of inflammatory reaction, or the integrity of the mucous membranes. The value of large amounts of ascorbic acid to prevent and cure the common cold has been reported but these findings are controversial. If there is an effect, it is a small one, and routine large intakes of vitamin C are not recommended (Clinical Insight, see below).

The relationship of vitamin C to cancer is discussed in Chapter 36.

Recommended Dietary Allowance

The minimal daily intake of vitamin C needed to prevent scurvy is approximately 10 mg; however, this does not provide acceptable reserves of the vitamin. The RDA of 60 mg for adults has been established on the basis of the amount needed to prevent the onset of scorbutic symptoms for 4 weeks and provide a margin of safety. Several hundred absorption studies in humans have led to the suggestion that each main meal should contain at least 25 to 50 mg of ascorbate because of its key physiologic role in iron absorption (Hallberg et al, 1987). Table 6–31 presents the RDA for vitamin C.

Increased intakes of vitamin C are required to maintain normal plasma levels under acute emotional or environmental stress such as trauma, fever, infection, or elevated environmental temperatures. Because of the lower concentrations of ascorbic acid in the serum of cigarette smokers, it is recommended that smokers increase their intake to at least 100 mg/day (Food and Nutrition Board, 1989) (see Research Trends, p. 588).

Sources

Ascorbic acid is easily destroyed by oxidation, particularly in the presence of heat and alkalinity, and because it is highly soluble in water, it is often discarded in cooking water. Although the vitamin occurs in small amounts in animal tissues, it is usually destroyed either

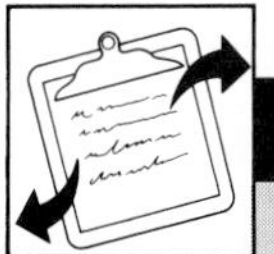

CLINICAL INSIGHT: Vitamin C and the Common Cold

Interest in the use of vitamin C for treatment of the common cold dates from the 1940s, but the theory did not become popular until Linus Pauling wrote a book claiming that vitamin C in massive doses would protect against and cure the common cold. Sales of the vitamin skyrocketed despite considerable skepticism from the nutrition community. In subsequent years, several studies have modified or even discredited the original hypothesis.

1. Anderson and colleagues conducted a double-blind trial with 818 individuals in which a placebo group was compared with a treatment group that took 1 g/day of vitamin C and 4 g/day during the first 3 days of a cold. Although the vitamin C group experienced less illness, the differences were statistically insignificant. However, when those taking vitamin C did contract a cold it was less severe and resulted in 30% fewer days of disability (Anderson, 1972 and 1975).
2. In a study involving 641 children taking a placebo or 1 to 2 grams of vitamin C, Coulehan and colleagues found that although taking the vitamin did not prevent colds, those children who were taking vitamin C had 24 to 28% fewer days of sickness as compared with a placebo group. However, a later study by the same investigator could not confirm the effectiveness of 1 g/day doses in reducing the severity of cold symptoms (Coulehan, 1974 and 1976).
3. Wilson and colleagues found that prophylactic doses of 200 to 500 mg/day reduced cold symptoms in girls but had no effect in boys (Wilson, 1973).
4. Miller and coworkers conducted a double-blind study on co-twins ranging in age from 6 to 15 years in which subjects received either a placebo or 500 to 1,000 mg of vitamin C per day depending on their size. They observed a 28% reduction in incidence of cold symptoms, a 17% reduction in total severity, and a 21% variation in total duration. The effect of the vitamin was more pronounced in younger girls. The authors concluded that even though large doses of vitamin C may have a detectable prophylactic effect in some age and sex groups, the genetic, environmental, or subjective factors would appear to account for a substantially greater fraction of the total morbidity (Miller, 1977).
5. Carr and colleagues studied a series of pairs of monozygotic twins aged 14 to 64 years who received either 1 g/day of vitamin C or placebo for 100 days. The perception of treatment was important, as those who thought they were on a "high dose" reported markedly fewer, shorter, and less severe colds than their co-twins who thought they were on a "low dose." In addition, there were significant correlations between cold symptoms reported and the personality trait of neuroticism (Carr, 1981).
6. One investigator concluded that ascorbic acid had an antihistaminic effect (Bouhuys, 1974). Other work has shown that persons with low plasma ascorbic acid levels have elevated blood histamine levels, which are lowered by supplementation with the vitamin.

It has been concluded that benefits from ascorbic acid in fighting the common cold are not great enough to recommend routine large intakes. If there are benefits, they appear to be in reducing the severity of symptoms rather than in preventing the cold.

TABLE 6–31. Recommended Dietary Allowances for Vitamin C*

Age (Years)	RDA† (mg)
Infants	
0.0–0.5	30
0.5–1.0	35
Children	
1–3	40
4–6	45
7–10	45
Males	
11–14	50
15–18	60
19–24	60
25–50	60
51+	60
Females	
11–14	50
15–18	60
19–24	60
25–50	60
51+	60
Pregnant	70
Lactating	
1st 6 months	95
2nd 6 months	90

* From Food and Nutrition Board, National Research Council, NAS: Recommended Dietary Allowances, 10th ed. Washington, DC, National Academy Press, 1989.

† RDA = recommended dietary allowance.

by exposure to air or by processing before it reaches the table. Therefore the best sources are fruits and vegetables, preferably acidic, fresh, and when necessary, cooked rapidly in very little water and served immediately. Adding sodium bicarbonate to preserve and improve the color of cooked vegetables is highly destructive of vitamin C.

Cumulative losses when vegetables are prepared and held for 24 hours in a refrigerator can be as high as 45% for fresh products and 52% for frozen products. As consumers eat out more frequently and as more foods are supplied to restaurants or institutions partially prepared (e.g., shredded lettuce, peeled and diced vegetables) this loss must be considered when evaluating dietary intake (Carlson and Tabacchi, 1988).

The ascorbic acid content of fruits and vegetables varies with the conditions under which they are grown and the degree of ripeness when harvested. Refrigeration and quick freezing help retain the vitamin. Most commercially frozen foods are processed so close to the source of supply that their ascorbic acid content is often higher than that of fresh foods that have been shipped across the country and spent time in storage and on supermarket shelves.

Ascorbic acid is widely found in citrus fruits, raw leafy vegetables, and tomatoes. Strawberries, cantaloupe, cabbage, and green peppers are good sources. When properly prepared, potatoes are a good source because of the quantity eaten. Table 6–32 lists the vitamin C content of selected fruits and vegetables (Fig. 6–10); Table 6–33 summarizes selected information for vitamin C as well as other vitamins.

TABLE 6–32. Vitamin C Content of Selected Foods*

Food	Amount	mg
Kiwi	1	74
Broccoli		
fresh	1 spear	141
frozen, chopped	½ cup	37
Brussels sprouts, frozen	½ cup	36
Cantaloupe	½ melon (5″ diameter)	113
Collards (cooked)	½ cup	72
Peppers		
sweet	1	95
hot chili, raw	½ cup	109
Orange	1 (2½″ diameter)	70
Orange juice		
fresh	½ cup	62
frozen, diluted	½ cup	49
canned	½ cup	36
Kale, from raw, cooked	½ cup	27
Turnip greens, from raw, cooked	½ cup	20
Strawberries	½ cup	42
Grapefruit juice		
canned, unsweetened	½ cup	36
Tomatoes		
fresh	1 (3″ diameter)	22†
canned	½ cup	18
juice	½ cup	22
Mango	1	57
Papaya	½ cup (½″ cubes)	46
Lemon	1 (2½″ diameter)	31
Grapefruit	½	41
Honeydew melon	¹⁄₁₀ melon (6¼″ diameter)	32
Cauliflower, from raw, cooked	½ cup	35
Mustard greens, cooked	½ cup	18
Potato		
baked, then peeled	1 medium	26
boiled, then peeled	1 medium	18
peeled, then boiled	1 medium	10
mashed	½ cup	7
French fries	10	5
chips	10	8
Watermelon	1 slice (4″ × 8″ wedge)	46
Sweet potato, baked	1 medium	28
Spinach		
fresh	½ cup	8
frozen	½ cup	16
canned	½ cup	3
Cabbage		
cooked	½ cup	18
raw	½ cup	17
Tangerine	1 (2¼″ diameter)	26
Okra, cooked	8 3″ pods	14
Cranberry juice cocktail (vitamin C added)	½ cup	54

* From USDA, HNIS: Nutrition Value of Foods. Home and Garden Bulletin No. 72, 1986.

† Vitamin C content depends on type of cultivation and harvest and time of year.

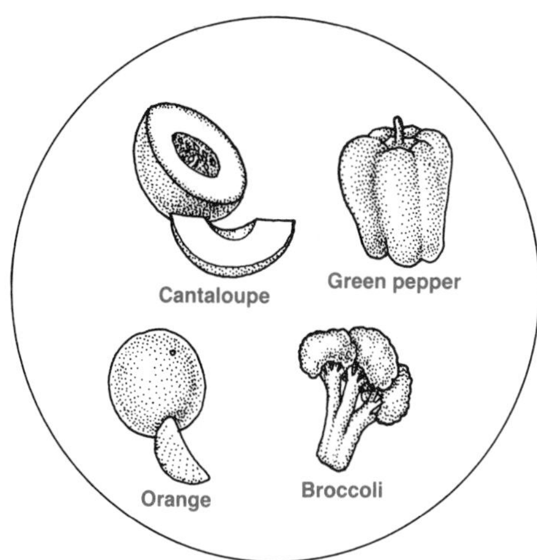

FIGURE 6–10. *Foods high in vitamin C.*

Deficiency

Although occurrence of frank scurvy is rare, marginal deficiencies of ascorbic acid may occur in people who consume a diet devoid of fruits and vegetables, alcoholics, aged people on very limited diets, severely ill people under chronic stress, and infants nourished exclusively on cow's milk.

Severe deficiency of ascorbic acid causes scurvy. Symptoms appear when the serum level falls below 0.2 mg/dl. Classic symptoms include follicular hyperkeratosis, swollen and inflamed gums, loosening of teeth, dryness of the mouth and eyes, loss of hair, and dry itchy skin (Fig. 6–11). Because of defects in collagen synthesis, wounds fail to heal and scars of previous wounds break down. Secondary infections develop easily in the bleeding areas. Neurotic disturbances consisting of hypochondriasis, hysteria, and depression followed by decreased psychomotor performance are common.

Toxicity

Hemolytic anemia has been linked to administration of a multivitamin preparation to a premature infant (Ballin et al, 1988). The erythrocytes of premature infants may be at greater risk for oxidative damage from vitamin C because lower glomerular filtration rates decrease the rate of excretion and permit circulating levels of ascorbic acid to remain high for longer periods.

Excess ascorbic acid excreted in the urine gives a false positive test for sugar. It has been implicated in the formation of urate and oxalate stones, but recent evidence shows that massive vitamin C ingestion (90 g/day) produces only a small increase in urinary oxalate concentration and no change in urate or inorganic phosphate.

It has also been reported that those on massive intakes of vitamin C have a "rebound scurvy" when the dosage is discontinued. Thus supplements should be decreased gradually (Omaye et al, 1988).

FACTORS NOT PROVED TO BE VITAMINS

A number of food factors have vitamin characteristics but for various reasons are not classified as vitamins. Some have been observed only in animals other than humans. Others can be synthesized to some extent in the body but require dietary supplementation in periods of stress. Some are simply substances that are known to occur in human tissues for which no purpose has yet been identified.

Choline

Choline is an essential component of animal tissues and has been classified as having vitamin-like activity in experimental animals. Humans, however, can synthesize choline from ethanolamine and methyl groups derived from methionine, but most of the time, choline probably comes from dietary phosphatides.

Functions

The only function of choline is as a component of larger molecules. Lecithin (phosphatidylcholine) is a structural component of cell membranes and plasma lipoproteins, and functions as a pulmonary surfactant. Sphingomyelin is also a structural component. Acetylcholine functions as a neurotransmitter.

Dietary Intake

The need for choline is high during growth and development and may exceed the synthetic capacity of the

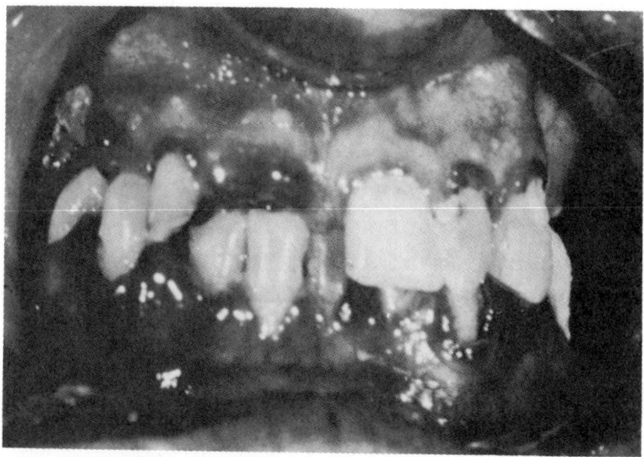

FIGURE 6–11. *Gingival enlargement due to vitamin C deficiency. (From Nizel AE: Nutrition in Preventive Dentistry, 2nd ed. Philadelphia, WB Saunders, 1981, p 166.)*

newborn. Therefore, the American Academy of Pediatrics (1985) recommended that infant formulas contain 7 mg/100 kcal of choline, the amount found in human milk. Human milk also contains phosphatidylcholine and sphingomyelin.

Daily requirements are not known, and no toxic effects have been observed. The amount required is influenced by the amount and type of fat, total energy, type of carbohydrate, amount of protein, and amount of cholesterol in the diet. The average diet has been estimated to contain 400 to 900 mg/day of choline. This amount is apparently adequate for health but should not be equated with the dietary requirement.

Sources

Free choline is present in liver, oatmeal, soybeans, cauliflower, kale, and cabbage. Eggs, liver, soybeans, and peanuts are rich in phosphatidylcholine.

Deficiency

Deficiency in animals is associated with fatty deposition in the liver and hemorrhagic kidney disease. Choline deficiency in humans has not been demonstrated.

Administration of pharmacologic doses of choline seems to alleviate symptoms of tardive dyskinesia and Huntington's disease in humans, but the dosage required to achieve this effect, up to 20 g/day, appears to be beyond the specific dietary needs for choline.

Myo-Inositol

Inositol is found in fruits, grains, vegetables, nuts, legumes, and organ meats such as liver and heart. It occurs abundantly in the average diet, usually as inositol phospholipids and as *phytic acid* (inositol hexaphosphate). Phytic acid interferes with the absorption of calcium, iron, and zinc. It is estimated that a mixed North American diet provides the adult with 300 to 1,000 mg/day.

Functions

Myo-inositol is the only one of the nine isomers of inositol that has metabolic importance. It is a cyclic six-carbon compound with six hydroxyl groups and a structure resembling glucose. It occurs in animal tissues as a component of phospholipids. It is concentrated in the brain and cerebrospinal fluid but occurs in skeletal and heart muscles and other tissues. The level of free inositol is especially high in all of the organs of the male reproductive tract, particularly in semen.

The physiologic role of inositol is related to its presence in phosphatidylinositol and thus to the function of phospholipids in cell membranes. Its functions include the mediation of cellular responses to external stimuli, nerve transmissions, and regulation of enzyme activity. Through its role in phospholipid synthesis, which affects the function of the lipoproteins, it exerts lipotropic activity.

Inositol metabolism is affected by dietary choline content, the amount and degree of saturation of dietary fat, and the specific fatty acid composition.

Deficiency

Because diabetic patients show high *myo*-inositol metabolism levels in urine and lowered levels in nerve membranes, attempts have been made to explain diabetic peripheral neuropathies on the basis of change in *myo*-inositol metabolism. However, findings have not been consistent.

Inositol deficiency in animals produces an accumulation of triglyceride in liver, intestinal lipodystrophy, and other abnormalities. Signs of inositol deficiency have not been found in humans and a deficiency is not likely, considering the widespread occurrence in food. However, because it could possibly occur in infants on non–cow's milk formulas, the American Academy of Pediatrics has recommended that it should be added to formulas based on non–cow's milk protein as a preventive measure.

Toxicity

No toxic effects have been reported. Patients with chronic renal failure show elevated serum inositol levels.

ANTIVITAMINS (VITAMIN ANTAGONISTS OR ANTIMETABOLITES)

An antivitamin or antagonist is a substance that interferes with the synthesis or metabolism of vitamins. Many vitamin antagonists are compounds similar in structure to the active molecule. By taking the place of the vitamin, they render the coenzyme inactive. Isonicotinic acid hydrazide (INH), a chemotherapeutic agent in the treatment of tuberculosis, is an antagonist for pyridoxine. Aminopterin, a drug used in the treatment of leukemia, is an antagonist of folacin. Dicumarol, an anticoagulant, acts as an antagonist to vitamin K.

Another type of antivitamin is avidin, found in raw egg white, which combines with biotin and forms a compound that cannot be absorbed from the intestinal tract.

TABLE 6–33. Summary of Information on Vitamins

Name	RDA for Adults*	Sources	Stability	Comments
		Fat-Soluble Vitamins		
Vitamin A (retinol; α-, β-, γ-carotene)	M: 1,000 RE F: 800 RE	Liver, kidney, milk fat, fortified margarine, egg yolk, yellow and dark green leafy vegetables, apricots, cantaloupe, peaches.	Stable to light, heat, and usual cooking methods. Destroyed by oxidation, drying, very high temperature, ultraviolet light.	Essential for normal growth, development and maintenance of epithelial tissue. Essential to the integrity of night vision. Helps provide for normal bone development and influences normal tooth formation. Toxic in large quantities.
Vitamin D (calciferol)	M: 5 μg F: 5 μg	Vitamin D milk, irradiated foods, some in milk fat, liver, egg yolk, salmon, tuna fish, sardines. Sunlight converts 7-dehydrocholesterol to cholecalciferol.	Stable to heat and oxidation.	Really a prohormone. Essential for normal growth and development; important for formation of normal bones and teeth. Influences absorption and metabolism of phosphorus and calcium. Toxic in large quantities.
Vitamin E (tocopherols and tocotrienols)	M: 10 α-TE F: 8 α-TE	Wheat germ, vegetable oils, green leafy vegetables, milk fat, egg yolk, nuts.	Stable to heat and acids. Destroyed by rancid fats, alkali, oxygen, lead, iron salts, and ultraviolet irradiation.	Is a strong antioxidant. May help prevent oxidation of unsaturated fatty acids and vitamin A in intestinal tract and body tissues. Protects red blood cells from hemolysis. Role in reproduction (in animals). Role in epithelial tissue maintenance and prostaglandin synthesis.
Vitamin K (phylloquinone and menaquinone)	M: 80 μg F: 65 μg	Liver, soybean oil, other vegetable oils, green leafy vegetables, wheat bran. Synthesized in intestinal tract.	Resistant to heat, oxygen, and moisture. Destroyed by alkali and ultraviolet light.	Aids in production of prothrombin, a compound required for normal clotting of blood. Toxic in large amounts.
		Water-Soluble Vitamins		
Thiamin	M: 1.5 mg F: 1.1 mg	Pork, liver, organ meats, legumes, whole-grain and enriched cereals and breads, wheat germ, potatoes. Synthesized in intestinal tract.	Unstable in presence of heat, alkali, or oxygen. Heat stable in acid solution.	As part of cocarboxylase, aids in removal of CO_2 from alpha-keto acids during oxidation of carbohydrates. Essential for growth, normal appetite, digestion, and healthy nerves.
Riboflavin	M: 1.7 mg F: 1.3 mg	Milk and dairy foods, organ meats, green leafy vegetables, enriched cereals and breads, eggs.	Stable to heat, oxygen, and acid. Unstable to light (especially ultraviolet) or alkali.	Essential for growth. Plays enzymatic role in tissue respiration and acts as a transporter of hydrogen ions. Coenzyme forms FMN and FAD.
Niacin (nicotinic acid and nicotinamide)	M: 19 mg NE F: 15 mg NE	Fish, liver, meat, poultry, many grains, eggs, peanuts, milk, legumes, enriched grains. Synthesized by intestinal bacteria.	Stable to heat, light, oxidation, acid and alkali.	As part of enzyme system, aids in transfer of hydrogen and acts in metabolism of carbohydrates and amino acids. Involved in glycolysis, fat synthesis, and tissue respiration.
Vitamin B_6 (pyridoxine, pyridoxal, and pyridoxamine)	M: 2.0 mg F: 1.6 mg	Pork, glandular meats, cereal bran and germ, milk, egg yolk, oatmeal, and legumes. Synthesized by intestinal bacteria.	Stable to heat, light, and oxidation.	As a coenzyme, aids in the synthesis and breakdown of amino acids and in the synthesis of unsaturated fatty acids from essential fatty acids. Essential for conversion of tryptophan to niacin. Essential for normal growth.

Table continued on following page

TABLE 6–33. Summary of Information on Vitamins *Continued*

		Sources	Stability	Comments
Folate	M: 200 μg F: 180 μg	Green leafy vegetables, organ meats (liver), lean beef, wheat, eggs, fish, dry beans, lentils, cowpeas, asparagus, broccoli, collards, yeast. Synthesized in intestinal tract.	Stable to sunlight when in solution; unstable to heat in acid media.	Appears essential for biosynthesis of nucleic acids. Essential for normal maturation of red blood cells. Functions as a coenzyme: tetrahydrofolic acid.
Vitamin B_{12}	2 μg	Liver, kidney, milk and dairy foods, meat, eggs. Vegans require supplement.	Slowly destroyed by acid, alkali, light, and oxidation.	Involved in the metabolism of single-carbon fragments. Essential for biosynthesis of nucleic acids and nucleoproteins. Role in metabolism of nervous tissue. Involved with folate metabolism. Related to growth.
Pantothenic acid	Level not yet determined but 4–7 mg believed safe and adequate.	Present in all plant and animal foods. Eggs, kidney, liver, salmon, and yeast are best sources. Possibly synthesized by intestinal bacteria.	Unstable to acid, alkali, heat, and certain salts.	As part of coenzyme A, functions in the synthesis and breakdown of many vital body compounds. Essential in the intermediary metabolism of carbohydrate, fat, and protein.
Biotin	Not known but 30–100 μg believed safe and adequate.	Liver, mushrooms, peanuts, yeast, milk, meat, egg yolk, most vegetables, banana, grapefruit, tomato, watermelon, and strawberries. Synthesized in intestinal tract.	Stable.	Essential component of enzymes. Involved in synthesis and breakdown of fatty acids and amino acids through aiding the addition and removal of CO_2 to or from active compounds, and the removal of NH_2 from amino acids.
Vitamin C (ascorbic acid)	60 mg	Acerola (West Indian cherry-like fruit), citrus fruit, tomato, melon, peppers, greens, raw cabbage, guava, strawberries, pineapple, potato.	Unstable to heat, alkali, and oxidation, except in acids. Destroyed by storage.	Maintains intracellular cement substance with preservation of capillary integrity. Cosubstrate in hydroxylations requiring molecular oxygen. Important in immune responses, wound healing, and allergic reactions. Increases absorption of nonheme iron.

* M = male; F = female; RE = retinol equivalents; α-TE = alpha-tocopherol equivalents; NE = niacin equivalents.

CITED REFERENCES

Ala-Houhala M et al: 25-hydroxyvitamin D and vitamin D in human milk: Effects of supplementation and season. Am J Clin Nutr 48:1057, 1988.

American Academy of Pediatrics: Pediatric Nutrition Handbook, 2nd ed. Elk Grove Village, Ill, American Academy of Pediatrics, 1985.

American Academy of Pediatrics: The prophylactic requirement and toxicity of vitamin D. Pediatrics 31:512, 1963.

Anderson TW, et al: Vitamin C and the common cold: A double-blind trial. Can Med Assoc J 107:503, 1972.

Anderson TW: Large scale trials of vitamin C. Ann NY Acad Sci 258:498, 1975.

Ballin A et al: Vitamin C induced erythrocyte damage in premature infants. J Pediatr 113:114, 1988.

Barclay AJG et al: Vitamin A supplements and mortality related to measles: A randomized clinical trial. Br Med J 294:294, 1987.

Bendich A and Langseth L: Safety of vitamin A. Am J Clin Nutr 49:358, 1989.

Beriberi can complicate TPN. Nutr Rev 45:239, 1987.

Bouhuys A: Colds and antihistamine effects of vitamin C. N Engl J Med 290:633, 1974.

Bridges KR: Ascorbic acid inhibits lysosomal autophagy of ferritin. J Biol Chem 262:1473, 1987.

Butterworth CE and Tamura T: Folic acid safety and toxicity: A brief review. Am J Clin Nutr 50:353, 1989.

Campos FACS et al: Effect of an infection on vitamin A status of children as measured by the relative dose response (RDR). Am J Clin Nutr 46:91, 1987.

Carethers M: Diagnosing vitamin B_{12} deficiency, a common geriatric disorder. Geriatrics 43:89, 1988.

Carlson BL and Tabacchi MH: Loss of vitamin C in vegetables during the food service cycle. J Am Diet Assoc 88:65, 1988.
Carmel R: Pernicious anemia: The expected findings of very low cobalamin levels, anemia and macrocytosis are often lacking. Arch Intern Med 148:1712, 1988.
Carpenter TO et al: Severe hypervitaminosis A in siblings: Evidence of variable tolerance to retinol intake. J Pediatr 111:507, 1987.
Carr AB et al: Vitamin C and the common cold: A second MZ cotwin control study. Acta Genet Med Gemellol 30:249, 1981.
Cimino JA et al: Riboflavin metabolism in the hypothyroid human adult. Proc Soc Exp Biol Med 184:151, 1987.
Coulehan JL et al: Vitamin C and acute illness in Navaho children. N Engl J Med 295:973, 1976.
Coulehan JL et al: Vitamin C prophylaxis in a boarding school. N Engl J Med 290:6, 1974.
Dalton K and Dalton MJT: Characteristics of pyridoxine overdose neuropathy syndrome. Acta Neurol Scand 76:8, 1987.
DeLuca H: Vitamin D and its metabolites. *In* Shils ME and Young VR (eds): Modern Nutrition in Health and Disease, 7th ed. Philadelphia, Lea and Febiger, 1988.
Food and Nutrition Board (FNB), National Research Council, NAS: Recommended Dietary Allowances, 10th ed. Washington, DC, National Academy Press, 1989.
Goldberger J et al: A study of the diet of nonpellagrous and pellagrous households. JAMA 71:944, 1918.
Hallberg L et al: Is there a physiological role of vitamin C in iron absorption? *In* Burns JJ, Rivers JM, and Machlin LJ (eds): Third Conference on Vitamin C. Ann NY Acad Sci 498:324, 1987.
Krasinski SD et al: Relationship of vitamin A and vitamin E intake to fasting plasma retinol, retinol-binding protein, retinyl esters, carotene, alpha-tocopherol and cholesterol among elderly people and young adults: Increased plasma retinyl esters among vitamin A-supplement users. Am J Clin Nutr 49:112, 1989.
Krause KH et al: Biotin status of epileptics. Ann NY Acad Sci 447:297, 1985.
Leklem JE: Vitamin B_6 bioavailability and its applications to human nutrition. Food Technology 42:195, 1988.
Lindenbaum J et al: Neuropsychiatric disorders caused by cobalamin deficiency in the absence of anemia or macrocytosis. N Engl J Med 318:1720, 1988.
Lombard KA and Mock DM: Biotin nutritional status of vegans, lactoovovegetarians and nonvegetarians. Am J Clin Nutr 50:486, 1989.
Löwik MRH et al: Dose-response relationships regarding vitamin B_6 in elderly people: A nationwide nutritional survey (Dutch Nutritional Surveillance System). Am J Clin Nutr 50:391, 1989.
Manore MM et al: Plasma pyridoxal 5′-phosphate concentration and dietary vitamin B_6 intake of free-living, low-income elderly people. Am J Clin Nutr 50:339, 1989.
Meija LA and Chew F: Hematological effect of supplementing anemic children with vitamin A alone or in combination with iron. Am J Clin Nutr 48:595, 1988.
Miller JZ et al: Therapeutic effect of vitamin C. A co-twin control study. JAMA 237:248, 1977.
Muhilal et al: Vitamin A-fortified monosodium glutamate and health, growth and survival of children: A controlled field trial. Am J Clin Nutr 48:1271, 1988a.
Muhilal et al: Vitamin A-fortified monosodium glutamate and vitamin A status: A controlled field trial. Am J Clin Nutr 48:1265, 1988b.
Olson RE: Vitamin K. *In* Shils ME and Young VR (eds): Modern Nutrition in Health and Disease, 7th ed. Philadelphia, Lea and Febiger, 1988.
Omaye ST et al: Rebound effect with ascorbic acid in adult males (Letter). Am J Clin Nutr 48:379, 1988.
Said HM et al: Biotin transport in the human intestine: Inhibition by anticonvulsant drugs. Am J Clin Nutr 49:127, 1989.
Sauberlich HE: Bioavailability of vitamins. Prog Food Nutr Sci 4:1, 1985.
Sauberlich HE: Vitamins—How much is for keeps? Nutrition Today 22:20, 1987.
Schaumberg HJ et al: Sensory neuropathy from pyridoxine abuse. N Engl J Med 309:445, 1983.
Sommer A et al: Increased risk of xerophthalmia following diarrhea and respiratory disease. Am J Clin Nutr 45:977, 1987.
Specker BL and Tsang RC: Vitamin D in infancy. Cereal Foods World 33:788, 1988.
Specker BL et al: Increased urinary methylmalonic acid excretion in breast-fed infants of vegetarian mothers and identification of an acceptable dietary source of vitamin B_{12}. Am J Clin Nutr 47:89, 1988.
Spector R et al: Idiopathic dementia a regional vitamin deficiency state? Med Hypotheses 5:763, 1979.
Subar AR et al: Folate intake and food sources in the U.S. population. Am J Clin Nutr 50:508, 1989.
Suter PM and Russell RM: Vitamin requirements of the elderly. Am J Clin Nutr 45:501, 1987.
USDA: Nationwide Food Consumption Survey. Continuing Survey of Food Intakes by Individuals: Men 19–50 years, 1 day, 1985. Report No 85-3, Nutrition Monitoring Division, Human Nutrition Information Service. Hyattsville, MD, USDA, 1986.
USDA: Nationwide Food Consumption Survey. Continuing Survey of Food Intakes by Individuals: Women 19–50 years and Their children 1–5 years, 4 days, 1985. Report No 85-4, Nutrition Monitoring Division, Human Nutrition Information Service. Hyattsville, MD, USDA, 1987.
Van der Beek EJ et al: Thiamin, riboflavin and vitamins B_6 and C: Impact of combined restricted intake on functional performance in man. Am J Clin Nutr 48:1451, 1988.
Vinson JA and Bose P: Comparative bioavailability to humans of ascorbic acid alone or in a citrus extract. Am J Clin Nutr 48:601, 1988.
Wall JS and Carpenter KJ: Variation in availability of niacin in grain products. Food Technology 42:198, 1988.
Webb AR and Holick MF: The role of sunlight in the cutaneous production of vitamin D_3. Annu Rev Nutr 8:375, 1988.
Williams MJ et al: Controlled trial of pyridoxine in the premenstrual syndrome. J Int Med Res 13:174, 1985.
Wilson CW and Loh HS: Common cold and vitamin C. Lancet 1:638, 1973.

ADDITIONAL REFERENCES

Vitamin A

Bendich A: The safety of β-carotene. Nutr Cancer 11:207, 1988.
Beta-carotene supplements. Nutr MD 18(4):4, 1989.
De Vet HCW: The puzzling role of vitamin A in cancer prevention. Anticancer Res 9:145, 1989.
Goldberg J: Vitamin A and eyesight. Am J Epidemiol 128:700, 1988.
Hathcock JN et al: Evaluation of vitamin A toxicity. Am J Clin Nutr 52:183, 1990.
Majewski S et al: Decreased levels of vitamin A in serum of patients with psoriasis. Arch Dermatol Res 280:499, 1989.
Mathews-Roth MM: Photoprotection by carotenoids. Fed Proc 46:1890, 1987.
Micozzi MS et al: Carotenodermia in men with elevated carotenoid intake from foods and beta-carotene supplements. Am J Clin Nutr 48:1061, 1988.
Vitamin A and iron deficiency. Nutr Rev 47:119, 1989.

Vitamin D

De Luca HF: The vitamin D story: A collaborative effort of basic science and clinical medicine. FASEB J 2:224, 1988.
Quesada JM et al: Immunologic effects of vitamin D. N Engl J Med 321:833, 1989.
Season, latitude, and ability of sunlight to promote synthesis of vitamin D_3 in skin. Nutr Rev 47:252, 1989.
Vitamin D and psoriasis. Nutr MD 18(4):3, 1989.

Vitamin E

Halliwell B: Oxidants and human disease: Some new concepts. FASEB J 1:358, 1987.
Lloyd JK: The importance of vitamin E in human nutrition. Acta Paediatr Scand 79:6, 1990.
Murphy SP et al: Vitamin E intakes and sources in the United States. Am J Clin Nutr 52:361, 1990.
The effect of vitamin E on immune responses. Nutr Rev 45:27, 1987.
Traber MG et al: Lack of tocopherol in peripheral nerves of vitamin

E-deficient patients with peripheral neuropathy. N Engl J Med 317:262, 1987.

Vitamin K

Suttie JW et al: Vitamin K deficiency from dietary vitamin K restriction in humans. Am J Clin Nutr 47:475, 1988.

Thiamin

Haas RH: Thiamin and the brain. Annu Rev Nutr 8:483, 1988.

Riboflavin

Bunce GE and Hess JL: Cataract—What is the role of nutrition in lens health? Nutrition Today 23(6):6, 1988.

Vitamin B_6

Bender DA: Vitamin B_6 requirements and recommendations. Eur J Clin Nutr 43:289, 1989.
Merrill AH and Henderson JM: Diseases associated with defects in vitamin B_6 metabolism or utilization. Annu Rev Nutr 7:137, 1987.
Pyridoxine and autism. Nutr MD 15(3):4, 1989.
Talbott MC et al: Pyridoxine supplementation: Effect on lymphocyte responses in elderly persons. Am J Clin Nutr 46:659, 1987.

Folic Acid

Butterworth CE and Tamura T: Folic acid safety and toxicity: A brief review. Am J Clin Nutr 50:353, 1989.
Herbert V: The 1986 Herman Award Lecture. Nutrition science as a continually unfolding story: The folate and vitamin B_{12} paradigm. Am J Clin Nutr 46:387, 1987.
Rosenberg IH: Folate absorption: Clinical questions and metabolic answers. Am J Clin Nutr 51:531, 1990.

Vitamin B_{12}

Clementz GL: The spectrum of vitamin B_{12} deficiency. Am Fam Physician 41(1):150, 1990.
Unrecognized cobalamin-responsive neuropsychiatric disorders. Nutr Rev 47:208, 1989.

Biotin

A role for biotin in bone growth. Nutr Rev 47:157, 1989.
Marshall MW: The nutritional importance of biotin—An update. Nutrition Today 22(6):26, 1987.

Vitamin C

Jacob R, et al: Vitamin C and B_{12}. Am J Clin Nutr 48:1436, 1989.
Lee W et al: Ascorbic acid status: Biochemical and clinical considerations. Am J Clin Nutr 48:286, 1988.
Machlin LJ and Bendich A: Free radical tissue damage: Protective role of antioxidant nutrients. FASEB J 1:441, 1988.
Vitamin C and cervical dysplasia. Nutr MD 18(4):2, 1989.

Choline

McMahon KE: Choline, an essential nutrient? Nutrition Today 22(2):18, 1987.

CHAPTER 7

MINERALS

Dorice M. Czajka-Narins, Ph.D.

CHAPTER OUTLINE

KEY TERMS

CERULOPLASMIN—a plasma glycoprotein in which copper is transported

CRETINISM—congenital condition often caused by severe iodine deficiency during gestation, which is characterized by arrested physical and mental development

FERRITIN—an iron-apoferritin complex that is a major storage form of iron

GLUCOSE TOLERANCE FACTOR—a biologically active chromium complex consisting of chromium, nicotinic acid, and glutathione

GLUTATHIONE PEROXIDASE—a selenium-containing enzyme that is the major active form of selenium in tissues

GOITER—a chronic enlargement of the thyroid gland, visible as a swelling at the front of the neck, which is usually associated with iodine deficiency

GOITROGEN—a compound that blocks the absorption and utilization of iodine

HEME—the nonprotein, insoluble iron protoporphyrin constituent of hemoglobin

HEMOGLOBIN—a conjugated protein containing four heme groups and globin with the property of reversible oxygenation

HEMOSIDERIN—an insoluble form of storage iron

HYDROXYAPATITE—a crystalline structure in bone, consisting of calcium phosphate and calcium carbonate

MACROMINERAL—a naturally occurring, homogeneous, inorganic substance required by humans in amounts of 100 mg/day or more

METALLOTHIONEIN—an abundant nonenzymatic zinc-containing protein

MICROMINERAL (TRACE ELEMENT)—a naturally occurring, homogeneous, inorganic substance required by humans in amounts of less than 100 mg/day

MYOGLOBIN—a ferrous protoporphyrin globin complex present in muscle that stores oxygen

NONHEME IRON—the form of iron found in plants, which is less well absorbed than heme iron

OXALIC ACID—an organic acid found in certain leafy vegetables that binds with calcium and inhibits its absorption from these foods

PHYTIC ACID (PHYTATE)—a phosphorus-containing compound found in the outer husks of cereal grains that binds with calcium and inhibits its absorption

TETANY—muscle twitchings, spasms, and eventually convulsions caused by low levels of blood calcium or magnesium

THYROXINE (T_4)—an iodine-containing hormone secreted by the thyroid gland to regulate the rate of cell metabolism

TRANSFERRIN—a protein synthesized in the liver that transports iron in the blood to the erythroblasts for use in heme synthesis

TRIIODOTHYRONINE (T_3)—an iodine-containing thyroid hormone with several times the biologic activity of thyroxine

Analysis of the human body reveals the presence of a wide variety of minerals. However, the function and requirements of only a few are well enough defined, whereas others whose purpose is well established remain to be identified with respect to specific requirements. The relatively recent development of more sophisticated measuring techniques has increased the amount of knowledge about minerals, particularly those occurring in minute amounts. Others that remain unexplained may in fact be essential or may occur only in human flesh and in fluids as contaminants.

Minerals such as calcium and phosphorus, which are required in amounts of 100 mg/day or more, have been designated arbitrarily as *macrominerals*. The *microminerals* that are present or required in small amounts are also called *trace* or *ultratrace* elements.

Minerals occur in the body and in food chiefly in their ionic form. Metals such as sodium, potassium, and calcium form positive ions (cations); nonmetals form negative ions (anions). The latter include chlorine, sulfur (as sulfate), and phosphorus (as phosphate). Salts such as sodium chloride and calcium phosphate dissociate in solution and thus are found in the body fluids as Na^+, Cl^-, Ca^{2+}, and $H_2PO_4^{2-}$. The minerals also occur as components of organic compounds, such as phosphoproteins, phospholipids, metalloenzymes, and hemoglobin.

STRUCTURE AND FUNCTION

Mineral Composition of the Body

Collectively, minerals represent about 4 to 5% of body weight or 2.8 kg in a 70-kg man. About half of this body weight is calcium, and another quarter is phosphorus. The five other macrominerals (magnesium, sodium, chloride, potassium, and sulfur) and the 14 microminerals (iron, zinc, copper, iodide, manganese, fluoride, molybdenum, cobalt, selenium, chromium, tin, nickel, vanadium, and silicon) constitute the remaining 25%.

Function of Minerals

Mineral elements have many essential roles, both as dissolved ions in body fluids and as constituents of essential compounds. The balance of mineral ions in body fluids regulates the activity of many enzymes, maintains acid-base balance and osmotic pressure, facilitates membrane transfer of essential compounds, and maintains nerve and muscular irritability. In some cases, mineral ions are structural constituents of body tissues. Many minerals are involved indirectly in the growth process as well.

It is important to recognize the interrelationship of nutrients with respect to absorption, transport, utilization, and requirement.

For example, the absorption of zinc can be reduced by iron supplementation, whereas excessive intake of zinc can reduce the absorption of copper. The level of zinc transport depends not only on the availability of zinc but also of albumin, the transport protein.

MACROMINERALS

Minerals essential at levels of 100 mg/day or more for adult humans include calcium, phosphorus, magnesium, sulfur, sodium, chloride, and potassium.

Calcium

Calcium is the most abundant mineral in the body. It makes up about 1.5 to 2% of the body weight and 39% of the total body minerals. Ninety-nine per cent of the calcium is in the bones and teeth. The remaining 1% is in the blood and extracellular fluids and within the cells of soft tissues where it regulates many important metabolic functions.

Skeletal Calcium

Skeletal calcium is distributed between a relatively *nonexchangeable* pool, which is stable and not available for short-term regulation of calcium homeostasis, and a rapidly *exchangeable* pool (about 1% of skeletal calcium), which is involved in metabolic activities. The exchangeable component may be considered a reserve that is accumulated when the diet provides an adequate intake of calcium. It is stored primarily in the ends of the long bones in crystalline structures known as *trabeculae* and may be mobilized to meet increased needs of growth, pregnancy, and lactation. In the absence of such a reserve, calcium must be drawn from the more stable bone substance itself. Prolonged, inadequate intake of calcium results in deficient bone structure.

Bone is constantly being synthesized and resorbed. The question of which aspect of the process is predominant depends on the age and physiologic state of the individual. Bone synthesis predominates in children; in the normal adult, these processes are in balance, with approximately 600 to 700 mg of calcium exchanged every day. Aging bone is gradually diminished when resorption dominates. Adult bone loss begins during the fifth decade in both sexes but progresses more rapidly in the female (see Chapter 22).

Calcium occurs in the bones in the form of *hydroxyapatite,* a crystalline structure that consists of calcium phosphate and is arranged around an organic matrix of collagenous protein to provide strength and rigidity. Many other ions are also present, including fluoride, magnesium, zinc, and sodium. Blood and lymph vessels, nerves, and bone marrow pass through the matrix and between the crystal structures. The mineral ions diffuse into the extracellular fluid, bathing the crystals and permitting deposition of new mineral or its resorption from bones.

The same types of crystals are present in the enamel and dentin of teeth, although the crystals are slightly larger. In contrast to bone, there is little turnover of minerals in teeth, and calcium is not readily available from this source during periods of deprivation.

Serum Calcium

Total serum calcium consists of three distinct fractions: free or ionized calcium (50%); anion-complexed calcium bound with phosphate, bicarbonate, or citrate (5%); and protein-bound calcium bound with albumin (primarily) or globulin (45%). Total serum calcium is maintained within a narrow range of 8.8 to 10.8 mg/dl, of which the ionized calcium concentrations range from 4.4 to 5.2 mg/dl.

Many factors affect the relative distribution of calcium. One of these is pH; the ionized fraction is increased in acidosis and decreased in alkalosis. Total calcium changes along with changes in plasma protein levels; however, the ionized fraction usually remains within normal limits. The strict regulation of ionized calcium makes it a useful diagnostic tool in assessing parathyroid gland function, monitoring kidney disease or sick neonates for whom hypocalcemia could be life-threatening, and during situations in which many transfusions are given.

Functions

In addition to its major function in building and maintaining bones and teeth, calcium also has a number of metabolic roles.

It affects the transport function of cell membranes, possibly acting as a membrane stabilizer. It also influences the transmission of ions across membranes of cell organelles, the release of neurotransmitters at synaptic junctions, the function of protein hormones, and the release or activation of intracellular and extracellular enzymes.

Calcium is required in nerve transmission and regulation of heart beat. The proper balance of calcium, sodium, potassium, and magnesium ions maintains muscle tone and controls nerve irritability. A significant increase in serum calcium can cause cardiac or respiratory failure; a decrease results in tetany.

Ionized calcium initiates the formation of a blood clot by stimulating the release of thromboplastin from the blood platelets. It is also a necessary co-factor in the conversion of prothrombin to thrombin, which aids in the polymerization of fibrinogen to fibrin.

Absorption and Utilization

Calcium is absorbed mainly in the part of the duodenum where an acid medium prevails; consequently, absorption is greatly reduced in the lower part of the intestinal tract where the contents become alkaline. Usually only 20 to 30% of ingested calcium, and sometimes as little as 10%, is absorbed.

Absorption of calcium in the duodenum is primarily controlled through the action of $1,25(OH)_2D_3$ (vitamin D). This hormone increases calcium uptake at the brush border of the intestinal mucosal cell by stimulating production of a calcium-binding protein. Vitamin D also stimulates the activity of enzymes, such as intestinal alkaline phosphatase. A second transport mechanism, passive diffusion, occurs along the length of the intestine.

Calcium is absorbed only if it is present in a water-soluble form and is not precipitated by another dietary constituent, such as oxalate. Unabsorbed calcium is excreted in the feces.

FACTORS THAT INCREASE CALCIUM ABSORPTION. A number of factors favorably influence the absorption of calcium. In general, the greater the need and the smaller the dietary supply, the more efficient will be the absorption. *Increased needs* encountered in growth, pregnancy, lactation, calcium deficiency, and levels of exercise resulting in high bone density will enhance calcium absorption.

Vitamin D in its active form ($1,25(OH)_2D_3$) stimulates intestinal absorption through a complex series of steps, including transfer across the mucosal brush border. Calcium is best absorbed in an *acid medium;* thus, the hydrochloric acid secreted in the stomach favors calcium absorption by lowering the pH in the proximal duodenum. *Lactose* enhances calcium absorption in humans with a normal lactase supply; however, in the presence of a lactase deficiency, lactose inhibits calcium absorption. Moderate amounts of *fat* increase transit time through the digestive tract, allowing more time for mineral absorption. Certain *amino acids* exert a favorable effect on intestinal pH. Taking calcium with a meal improves absorption (Heaney et al, 1989).

FACTORS THAT DECREASE CALCIUM ABSORPTION. Lack of or an insufficient amount of *vitamin D* in its active form inhibits the absorption of calcium. *Oxalic acid* in rhubarb, spinach, chard, and beet greens forms insoluble calcium oxalate in the digestive tract. For example, only 5% of the calcium in spinach is absorbed (Heaney et al, 1988). Cocoa is also high in oxalates; however, the amount of cocoa in chocolate milk is not large enough to interfere significantly with calcium absorption (Heaney and Weaver, 1989). *Phytic acid,* a phosphorus-containing compound found principally in the outer husks of cereal grains, combines with calcium to form calcium phytate, which is also insoluble and cannot be absorbed. *Fiber* may decrease calcium absorption. In an *alkaline medium,* calcium with phosphorus forms insoluble calcium phosphate. Excessive *gastrointestinal motility* decreases the opportunity for calcium absorption. *Mental* or *physical stress* tends to decrease absorption and increase excretion. *Medications* can affect bioavailability or increase calcium excretion, either of which can contribute to bone loss. *Aging* is characterized by a decreased efficiency of absorption and by a blunted adaptive response to decreased intake.

Maintenance of Serum Calcium Level

Calcium in the bones is in equilibrium with calcium in the blood. *Parathormone,* the hormone secreted by the parathyroid gland, and *thyrocalcitonin,* secreted by the thyroid gland, maintain serum calcium at a normal concentration of about 10 mg/100 ml of blood serum (2.5 mmol/l). When it falls below this level, parathormone promotes transfer of exchangeable calcium from the bone into the blood. At the same time the parathyroid causes the kidney to reabsorb calcium that normally might be excreted in the urine and stimulates increased absorption of calcium from the intestines. When the blood calcium level is above normal, calcitonin acts to lower it by inhibiting further bone resorption, and because the processes of renal excretion and endogenous fecal secretion continue, the net effect is to lower serum calcium.

Calcium : Phosphorus Ratio

It is frequently suggested that a high level of phosphorus in the diet will combine with the available calcium to form insoluble compounds. A relationship between a high phosphorus to calcium ratio has been postulated in the development of osteoporosis; however, adequate data are not available to support this theory. Calcium : phosphorus ratios between 1 : 1 and 2 : 1 are generally recommended. The ratio of current intake in the United States and Canada is 1 : 1.6.

Excretion

Normally, most of the ingested calcium (65 to 70%) is excreted in the feces and urine. Fecal calcium correlates with intake. Although a high urinary calcium excretion has been reported to accompany a high-protein diet, this effect appears to occur only in the presence of low intakes of calcium and phosphorus. The presence of phosphorus decreases calcium excretion. Therefore, when high intakes of calcium and phosphorus accompany the high-protein diet common in the United States, calcium balance is adequate (Schuette and Linkswiler, 1984). Caffeine and theophylline intakes are also related to calcium excretion in the short term and to decreased bone mineralization in the long term (Whitney and Whitney, 1987).

Dermal losses occur in the form of sweat and exfoliation of the skin. The loss of calcium in sweat is about 15 mg/day. Strenuous physical activity with sweating will increase loss, even in persons on a low intake.

Immobility, occurring in prolonged bed rest or in periods of weightlessness during space travel, promotes calcium loss in response to a lack of tension on the bones.

Recommended Dietary Allowance

The recommended dietary allowance (RDA) for adults is based on estimates of obligatory loss (200 to 250 mg/day) and an absorption rate of 30 to 40% (Food and Nutrition Board, 1989). Higher levels are recommended for adolescents to ensure adequate bone formation until 24 years of age, when peak bone mass is attained. Additional amounts are recommended to

TABLE 7–1. Recommended Dietary Allowances for Calcium*

Age (Years)	RDA† (mg)
Infants	
0.0–0.5	400
0.5–1.0	600
Children	
1–3	800
4–6	800
7–10	800
Males	
11–14	1,200
15–18	1,200
19–24	1,200
25–50	800
51+	800
Females	
11–14	1,200
15–18	1,200
19–24	1,200
25–50	800
51+	800
Pregnant	1,200
Lactating	
1st 6 mo	1,200
2nd 6 mo	1,200

* Reprinted with permission from *Recommended Dietary Allowances,* 10th ed., c. 1989 by the National Academy of Sciences. Published by National Academy Press, Washington, DC.

† RDA = recommended dietary allowance.

meet the needs of pregnancy and lactation. Calcium requirements in pregnancy, infancy, childhood, and adolescence are discussed in detail in Chapters 9 to 13. Table 7–1 lists the RDA for all age/sex groups.

The median daily calcium intake for males in the United States approaches the RDA for all age groups except those over 55 years. However, beginning about 14 years of age the median intake of women drops substantially below the recommended level, perhaps reflecting the concern for preventing weight gain by maintaining a low-energy intake. The average woman in the United States obtains approximately 500 mg/day of calcium (Pennington et al, 1986) (Fig. 7–1).

Sources and Intakes

It is difficult to meet the RDA for calcium without milk or milk products; 8 oz of milk (whole or nonfat) supply 288 to 298 mg. Dark green leafy vegetables, such as kale, collards, turnip greens, mustard greens, and broccoli, and sardines, clams, oysters, and canned salmon are good sources of calcium. Oxalic acid limits the availability of calcium in rhubarb, spinach, chard, and beet greens. Table 7–2 shows the calcium content of selected foods (Fig. 7–2).

Daily Calcium Intake (mg) for Females
U.S. Population, 1976-1980

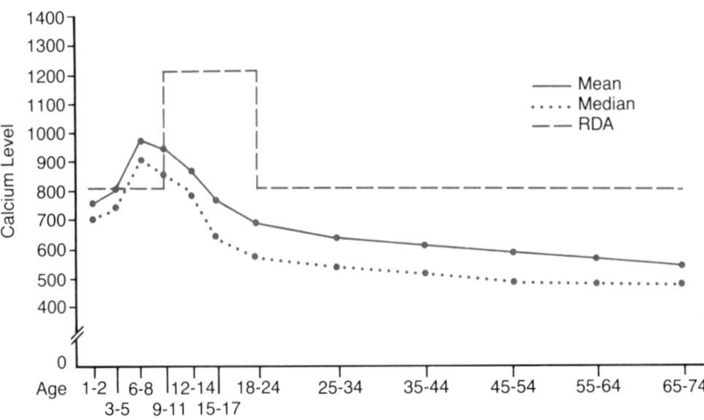

Daily Calcium Intake (mg) for Males
U.S. Population, 1976-1980

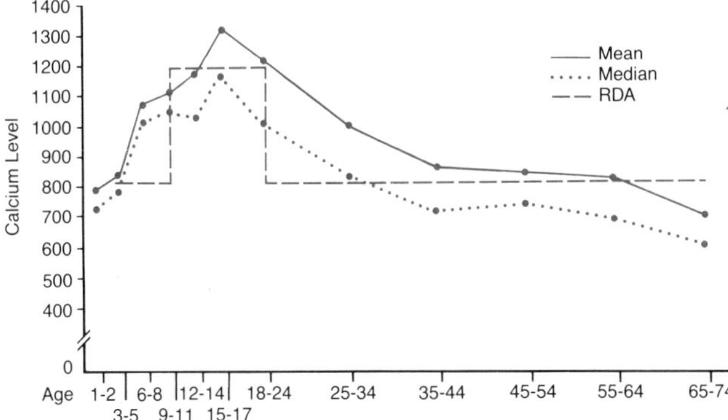

FIGURE 7–1. *Daily calcium intake for males and females in the United States. (Courtesy of the National Dairy Council.)*

TABLE 7–2. Calcium Content of Selected Foods*

Food	mg
Yogurt, low-fat, w/fruit, 1 cup	345
Milk, skim, 1 cup	302
Milk, 2%, 1 cup	297
Cheese, Gruyere, 1 oz	287
Ice milk, soft-serve, 1 cup	274
Tofu, firm, ½ cup	258
Yogurt, frozen, 1 cup	240
Cheese, mozarella, part-skim, 1 oz	207
Cheese, cheddar, 1 oz	204
Salmon, canned, w/bones, 3½ oz	185
Ice cream, vanilla, 1 cup	176
Cheese, American, 1 oz	174
Rhubarb, cooked, ½ cup	174
Cheese, ricotta, part-skim, ¼ cup	167
Oatmeal, fortified, instant, ¾ cup	163
Cheese, cottage, 2% fat, 1 cup	155
Waffle, homemade, 7″ diameter, 1	154
Spinach, frozen, cooked, ½ cup	138
Molasses, blackstrap, 1 T	137
Tofu, regular, ½ cup	130
Milk, dry, instant, nonfat, 2 T	104
Almonds, ¼ cup	92
Taco, chicken, 1	87
Baked beans, white, ½ cup	64
Frankfurter, turkey, 1	58
Mustard greens, cooked from fresh, ½ cup	52
Orange, 1 medium	52
Halibut, baked, 3 oz	51
Kale, fresh, cooked, ½ cup	47
Cookie, fig bar, 4	40
Broccoli, cooked from fresh, ½ cup	36
Bread, whole wheat, 1 slice	32
Waffle, frozen, 4″ diameter, 1	29
Cheese, cream, 2 T	23
Oatmeal, cooked, 1 cup	19
Cream, half and half, 1 T	16
Chicken, breast, baked, 3 oz	13
Apple, 1 medium	10
Pasta, cooked, 1 cup	10
Banana, 1 medium	7
Ground beef, lean, 3 oz	4

* From USDA: Composition of Foods. Handbook No. 8 series. Washington, DC, ARS, USDA, 1976–1986.

Deficiency

Bone Deformities. Abnormalities in bone structure due to calcium deficiency occur in osteoporosis, osteomalacia, and rickets. *Osteoporosis* is a metabolic disorder in which the amount of bone is reduced without change in composition. Skeletal strength cannot be maintained, and fractures occur with minimal stress. Whether deficient calcium intake is a factor is not clear. (Osteoporosis is discussed in depth in Chapter 22.) *Osteomalacia,* sometimes referred to as "adult rickets," is usually associated with a concurrent lack of vitamin D and an imbalance in the calcium : phosphorus intake. It is characterized by a failure to mineralize the bone matrix, resulting in a reduc-

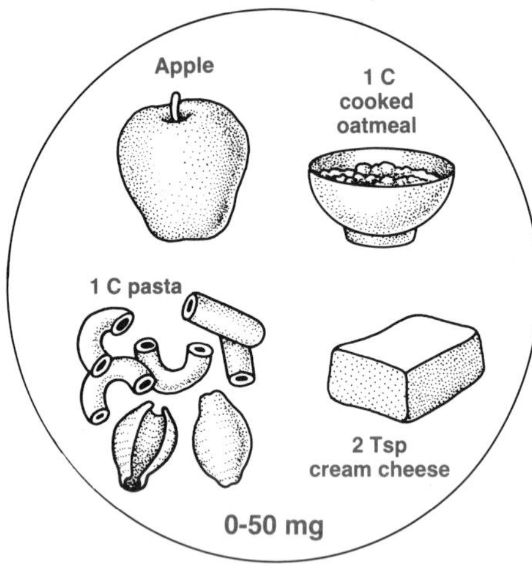

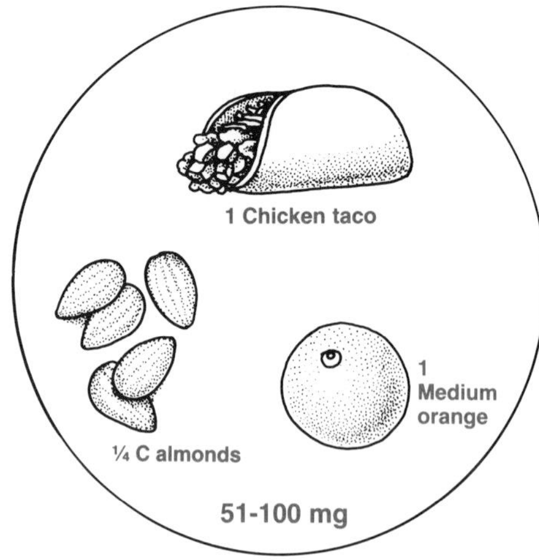

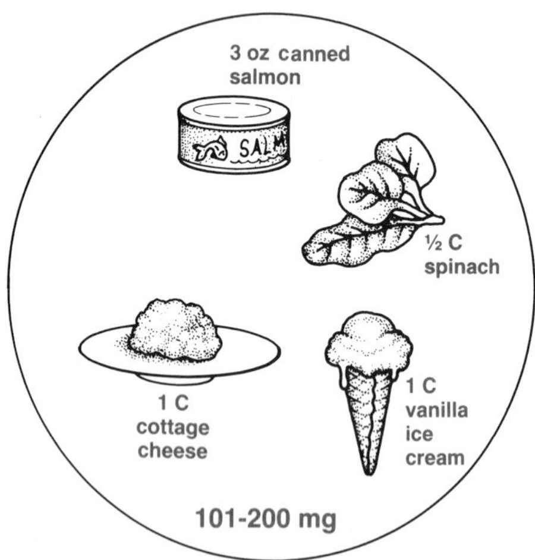

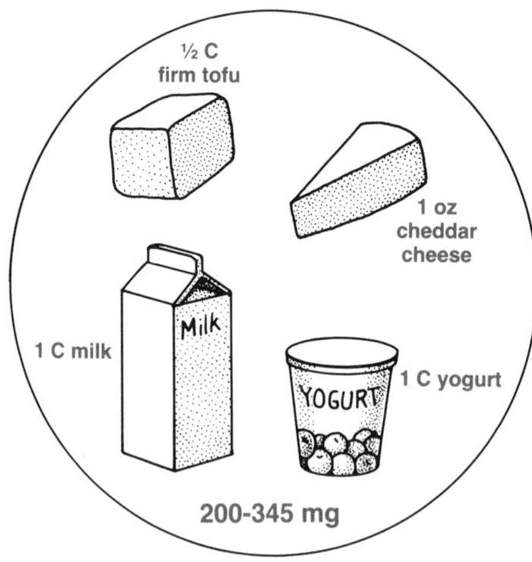

FIGURE 7–2. *Calcium content of some foods.*

tion in the mineral content of the bone. Calcium deficiency can also lead to a form of *rickets,* which exists in the presence of adequate vitamin D (Marie et al, 1982). Rickets due to vitamin D deficiency is discussed in Chapter 6.

TETANY. Extremely low levels of calcium in the blood may increase the irritability of nerve fibers and nerve centers, resulting in muscle spasms such as leg cramps, a condition that is known as *tetany.* It sometimes occurs during pregnancy in women who have consumed too little calcium or too much phosphorus. A rise in serum phosphorus leads to a compensatory decrease in serum calcium (see Chapter 9). Tetany sometimes occurs in newborn infants fed undiluted cow's milk that has a low calcium : phosphorus ratio (see Chapter 10).

HYPERTENSION. Abnormalities of calcium metabolism have been identified in both humans and animals with hypertension. Epidemiologic studies indicate an inverse correlation between the calcium content of the drinking water and the mean arterial pressure.

Oral calcium supplementation has been reported to lower blood pressure in hypertensive and normotensive patients (McCarron and Morris, 1987). However, because of inconsistent results, the role of calcium in hypertension remains controversial (see Chapter 21).

Toxicity

A very high intake of calcium and the presence of a high intake of vitamin D, which may occur in children receiving supplements, is a potential source of hypercalcemia. This may lead to excessive calcification in bone and in the soft tissues. Excessive urinary excretion of calcium may result in the formation of calcium-containing renal calculi.

Phosphorus

Phosphorus, one of the most essential elements, ranks second to calcium in abundance in human tissues. About 80% is present as calcium phosphate crystals in bones and teeth. The remainder is very active metabolically and is distributed in every cell in the body and in the extracellular fluid. The serum inorganic phosphorus is closely maintained by parathyroid activity at levels of 3 to 4 mg/100 ml in adults. Levels in infants are somewhat higher.

Functions

Phosphorus has numerous functions in addition to its structural role in the teeth and bony skeleton. It is an essential component of nucleic acids, and phospholipids are key components in the structure of cell membranes. Phosphorus participates in the energy cycle with the phosphorylation of glucose. High-energy phosphate compounds play a central role in many reactions, as does cyclic adenosine monophosphate (cyclic AMP). Phosphorus is part of some conjugated proteins, such as casein in human milk. The phosphate buffer system is particularly important in intracellular fluid and in the tubular fluids of the kidney.

TABLE 7–3. Recommended Dietary Allowances for Phosphorus*

Age (Years)	RDA (mg)
Infants	
0.0–0.5	300
0.5–1.0	500
Children	
1–3	800
4–6	800
7–10	800
Males	
11–14	1,200
15–18	1,200
19–24	1,200
25–50	800
51+	800
Females	
11–14	1,200
15–18	1,200
19–24	1,200
25–50	800
51+	800
Pregnant	1,200
Lactating	
1st 6 mo	1,200
2nd 6 mo	1,200

* Reprinted with permission from *Recommended Dietary Allowances,* 10th ed., c. 1989 by the National Academy of Sciences. Published by National Academy Press, Washington, DC.

Absorption

The factors that aid or deter the absorption of calcium act essentially in the same manner with regard to the absorption of phosphate. The most favorable absorption of inorganic phosphate takes place when calcium and phosphorus are ingested in approximately equal amounts, as they occur in milk. As with calcium, the presence of vitamin D also favors phosphate absorption.

In older children and adults, absorption from mixed diets varies between 50 and 70%. Infants absorb more than 85% of phosphorus from human milk and 65 to 75% from cow's milk.

Recommended Dietary Allowance

The Food and Nutrition Board recommends a daily intake of phosphorus approximately equal to that of calcium for all age groups (Table 7–3).

The average adult intake of phosphorus in the United States is approximately 1,500 to 1,600 mg/day. Food additives may contribute 20 to 30% of this amount; however, some forms are not hydrolyzed in the human gut and therefore may differ in their biologic effect.

Depending on the level of consumption, carbonated beverages may contribute amounts of phosphorus sufficient to adversely affect the calcium:phosphorus ratio. The average calcium:phosphorus ratio for adults is 1:1.6.

Sources

In general, good sources of protein are also good sources of phosphorus. Meat, poultry, fish, and eggs rank as excellent sources. Milk and milk products are good sources, as are nuts and legumes, cereals, and grains. However, in the outer coating of cereal grains, particularly wheat, phosphorus occurs in the form of phytic acid, which can complex with some minerals to form insoluble compounds. In conventional breads, phytic acid is converted to the soluble form of orthophosphate during the leavening process. However, in the unleavened breads that are commonly eaten in the Middle East, the availability of calcium, iron, and zinc is questionable. Table 7–4 lists the phosphorus content of various foods.

Deficiency

The widespread, severe, and ultimately fatal consequences of phosphorus depletion reflect its ubiquitous function and primarily result from decreased synthesis of adenosine triphosphate (ATP) and other organic

TABLE 7–4. Phosphorus Content of Selected Foods*

Food	mg
Grilled cheese sandwich, 1	531
Macaroni and cheese, 1 cup	322
Milkshake, vanilla, 10 oz	289
Sole, baked, 3 oz	248
Tostada with beans and beef, 1	247
Tofu, firm, ½ cup	239
Milk, 2% fat, 1 cup	232
Pizza, ⅛ of 15" diameter	216
Cheese, Swiss, processed, 1 oz	216
Split pea soup, 1 cup	213
Cheese, American, 1 oz	211
Ham, 3 oz	210
Ice milk, soft-serve, 1 cup	202
Almonds, ¼ cup	184
Oatmeal, 1 cup	178
Lentils, cooked, ½ cup	178
Cheese, cottage, 2% fat, ½ cup	170
Cheese, cheddar, 1 oz	146
Yeast, brewer's, 1 T	140
Cashews, ¼ cup	138
Shrimp, boiled, 2 large	137
Baked beans (white), ½ cup	137
Ground beef, 3 oz	135
Tofu, regular, ½ cup	120
Potato, baked, with skin, 1	115
Cheese sauce, ¼ cup	109
Garbanzo beans, canned, ½ cup	108
Egg, 1	86
Milk, dry, nonfat, instant, 2 T	84
Bread, whole wheat, 1 slice	74
Peas, frozen, cooked, ½ cup	72
Cola beverage, 1 can (12 oz)	46
Baking powder, 1 tsp	45
Potato chips, 14	43
Chocolate, dark, 1 oz	41
Cocoa powder, 1 T	38
Bread, white, 1 slice	30
Lettuce, romaine, 1 cup	25
Cauliflower, fresh, ½ cup	23
Orange, 1	18

* From USDA: Composition of Foods. Handbook No. 8 Series. Washington, DC, ARS, USDA, 1976–1986.

phosphate compounds. Neuromuscular, skeletal, hematologic, and renal abnormalities occur.

Because phosphorus is distributed so liberally in foods, there is little possibility of a dietary inadequacy, particularly if the food intake contains sufficient protein and calcium. Clinical phosphate depletion and hypophosphatemia result from long-term administration of glucose or total parenteral nutrition without sufficient phosphate, excessive use of phosphate-binding antacids, hyperparathyroidism, the treatment of diabetic acidosis, and alcoholism in patients with or without decompensated liver disease. Premature infants who are fed unfortified human milk can also develop hypophosphatemia.

Magnesium

Magnesium ranks second in quantity to potassium as an intracellular cation. The adult human body contains approximately 20 to 28 grams, of which approximately 60% is found in bone, 26% occurs in muscle, and the remainder occurs in soft tissues and body fluids. Normal serum levels are usually in the range of 1.5 to 2.1 mEq/l (0.75 to 1.1 mmol/l). About half the magnesium in blood is free, and approximately one third is bound to albumin; the remainder, including most in bone, is not exchangeable.

Functions

Magnesium is involved in a wide variety of biochemical and physiologic processes, including muscle contractility and nerve excitability. It is a normal constituent of bone.

Magnesium and calcium, with similar functions, are somewhat antagonistic. Excess magnesium inhibits bone calcification. In normal muscle contraction, calcium acts as a stimulator and magnesium acts as a relaxer. Excessive calcium may induce signs typical of magnesium deficiency.

Magnesium has been implicated in clinical problems, which share an underlying pathophysiology of vasospasm and increased coagulation. Low magnesium intakes have been shown experimentally to affect the ratio of prostacyclin and thromboxane in pregnancy-induced hypertension. The use of magnesium to inhibit atherogenesis or to prevent ischemic heart disease is the subject of continuing study.

Absorption and Excretion

The rate of absorption of magnesium varies widely from 24 to 85%. Many of the factors that govern calcium absorption from the upper intestine also influence the bioavailability of magnesium; however, vitamin D has no effect. As dietary calcium is decreased, magnesium absorption is increased.

The kidney conserves magnesium efficiently, particularly when intake is low. Renal reabsorption tends to vary inversely with that of calcium. Large losses of magnesium during vomiting reflect the high levels of this mineral in gastric juice.

Recommended Dietary Allowance

The average intake of magnesium by healthy adults in the United States and Western Europe ranges widely between 143 and 266 mg/day (Marier, 1986). In 1985 the average magnesium intake for adult American men was 329 mg/day and for adult women the intake was 207 mg/day (USDA, 1985 and 1986).

High intakes of calcium, protein, vitamin D, and alcohol all function to increase the requirement; physical or psychologic stress can also increase magnesium needs (Table 7–5).

TABLE 7-5. Recommended Dietary Allowances for Magnesium*

Age (Years)	RDA (mg)
Infants	
0.0-0.5	40
0.5-1.0	60
Children	
1-3	80
4-6	120
7-10	170
Males	
11-14	270
15-18	400
19-24	350
25-50	350
51+	350
Females	
11-14	280
15-18	300
19-24	280
25-50	280
51+	280
Pregnant	300
Lactating	
1st 6 mo	355
2nd 6 mo	340

* Reprinted with permission from *Recommended Dietary Allowances,* 10th ed., c. 1989 by the National Academy of Sciences. Published by National Academy Press, Washington, DC.

Sources and Intakes

Magnesium occurs abundantly in foods, and the ordinary diet is generally believed to provide adequate amounts. Good sources include seeds, nuts, legumes, and unmilled cereal grains, as well as dark green vegetables in which magnesium is an essential constituent of chlorophyll. Fish, meat, milk, and most commonly eaten fruits are poor sources of magnesium. Diets high in refined foods, meat, and dairy products are usually lower in magnesium than diets rich in vegetables and unrefined grains (Table 7-6). The mineral is lost during the refining and processing of foods such as flour, rice, and sugar.

Deficiency

Magnesium deficiency is manifested clinically by anorexia and by growth failure as well as cardiac and neuromuscular changes, such as muscle weakness, irritability, and mental derangement. Hypomagnesmic tetany is similar to hypocalcemic tetany.

A deficiency may be precipitated by any condition in which there is decreased intake or increased loss or a shift in electrolyte balance. Conditions in which acute deficiencies may develop are renal disease, diuretic therapy, malabsorption, hyperthyroidism, pancreatitis, kwashiorkor, diabetes, parathyroid gland disorders, postsurgical stress, and vitamin D-resistant rickets.

Sulfur

Sulfur occurs principally as a constituent of the amino acids cystine, cysteine, and methionine. It is present in all proteins but is most prevalent in insulin and in the keratin of skin, hair, and nails. Glutathione, a tripeptide containing cysteine, is important in cellular reactions involving the sulfur amino acids in protein.

Sulfur occurs also in carbohydrates, for example as a component of heparin, an anticoagulant found in liver and some other tissues, and of chondroitin sulfate, found in bone and cartilage. Thiamin, biotin, and pantothenic acid also contain sulfur.

Sulfur exists in the reduced form (-SH) in cysteine and in an oxidized form (-S-S-) in the double molecule, cystine. This is important in the specific configuration of some proteins and in the activity of some enzymes. For example, the poisonous effects of arsenic are due to its ability to combine with sulfhydryl groups.

Excess inorganic sulfur is excreted in the urine.

Sodium, Chloride, and Potassium

These three indispensable dietary constituents are so intimately related in the body that they are conveniently discussed together. Sodium constitutes 2%, potassium 5%, and chloride 3% of the total mineral content of the body. They are distributed ubiquitously throughout all body fluids and tissues, but sodium and chloride are primarily extracellular elements, whereas potassium is mainly an intracellular element. Sodium, potassium, and chloride are involved in maintaining at least four important physiologic functions of the body:

TABLE 7-6. Magnesium Content of Selected Foods*

Food	mg
Tofu, firm, ½ cup	118
Chili with beans, 1 cup	115
Wheat germ, toasted, ¼ cup	90
Cashews, roasted, ¼ cup	89
Halibut, baked, 3 oz	78
Swiss chard, cooked, ½ cup	75
Peanuts, roasted, ¼ cup	67
Chocolate chips, semisweet, ¼ cup	58
Baked potato with skin, 1	55
Cocoa powder, 2 T	52
Molasses, blackstrap, 1 T	52
Cereal, raisin bran, 1 oz	48
Spinach, fresh, 1 cup	44
Cheerios, 1 oz	39
Milk, 2% fat, 1 cup	33
Bread, whole wheat, 1 slice	26
Chicken, breast, 3 oz	25
Green peas, frozen, cooked, ½ cup	23
Ground beef, lean, 3 oz.	16
Bread, white, 1 slice	13
Fruits	10-25
Egg, 1	5

* From USDA: Composition of Foods. USDA Handbook No. 8 Series. Washington, DC, ARS, USDA, 1976-1986.

water balance and distribution, osmotic equilibrium, acid-base balance, and normal muscular irritability. The Na/K/Ca/ATPase "pump" system is important in volume regulation, maintenance of membrane potential, glucose transport, and transport of some amino acids, including alanine, proline, tyrosine, and tryptophan.

All three elements are readily absorbed through the intestinal tract and are excreted via the urine, feces, and sweat. Because these minerals are widely found in nature and in the ordinary diet, there is little chance of a deficiency in a healthy person. However, excesses do occur, particularly of sodium.

Estimated minimum requirements for these electrolytes were included with the 1989 RDA (see Table 8–16), since data are not yet available to support specific allowances. The electrolytes are discussed in more detail in Chapter 8.

TRACE ELEMENTS

A number of elements present in minute amounts in the tissues are essential to optimal growth and development. "Essential" trace elements are defined as those demonstrated through appropriately designed and corroborated experiments to be required for optimal performance of a particular function. Each element exhibits a spectrum of action that depends on the dosage and nutritional state of the recipient with respect to the element. Increasing amounts evoke an increasing biologic response until a plateau is reached beyond which larger intakes may produce pharmacologic effects and eventually toxicity.

Ranges for "safe and adequate" intakes for trace elements copper, manganese, fluoride, chromium, and molybdenum are given in Table 7–23. RDA are established for iron, iodine, selenium, and zinc. Appropriate ranges for the remaining trace minerals cannot be established on the basis of present knowledge.

General Characteristics

Functions

Many enzymes require small amounts of one or more trace metals for full activity. Metals function in enzyme systems by (1) direct participation in catalysis, (2) combination with substrate to form a complex on which the enzyme acts, (3) formation of a metalloenzyme that binds substrates, (4) combination with a reaction end-product, or (5) maintenance of quaternary structure.

Minute concentrations of trace minerals are able to affect the whole body through interaction with the enzymes or hormones that regulate masses of substrate. This ability is amplified if, in turn, the substrate has some regulatory function.

Sources

Foods of animal origin are generally superior sources of trace elements, because concentrations tend to be higher and the metals are available for absorption. Seafoods are usually rich in many micronutrients. One exception to the rule is manganese, which is readily available from plant sources. Trace elements are not distributed evenly in the wheat grain. The germ and outer layers that contain the most minerals are removed to a large extent by the milling process. However, the minerals that remain in white flour are more readily available than some of those in whole-wheat flour, which are firmly complexed by phytate and fiber.

Iron

Iron was first recognized as an essential nutrient for animals in the 1860s. Interest in iron and iron deficiency anemia has continued unabated to the present time. Although more information is available on iron than on any of the other trace minerals, many unresolved questions and problems remain.

The adult human body contains from 3 to 5 grams of iron, 30 to 40% of which is in storage form. Iron is well conserved by the body; approximately 90% is recovered and reused extensively.

Functions

Iron has a role in respiratory transport of oxygen and carbon dioxide and is involved as an active part of enzymes involved in the process of cellular respiration. Figure 7–3 presents a schematic outline of iron metabolism in adults. Iron also appears to be involved in the function of the immune system and in cognitive performance. Although these relationships have not been clearly identified, they reinforce the imperative of preventing iron-deficiency anemia in the world population. Table 7–7 lists the known iron compounds in the body and their functions.

Hemoglobin is present in red blood cells. The iron-containing protein *heme* combines with oxygen in the lungs and with carbon dioxide in the tissues. *Myoglobin,* also a heme protein, serves as an oxygen reservoir within muscle.

Oxidative production of ATP within the mitochondria involves many iron-containing enzymes, both heme and nonheme. The *cytochromes,* present in cells, function in the respiratory chain in the transfer of electrons and storage of energy through alternate oxidation and reduction of iron ($Fe^{2+} \leftrightarrows Fe^{3+}$). A number of water-insoluble drugs and endogenous materials are

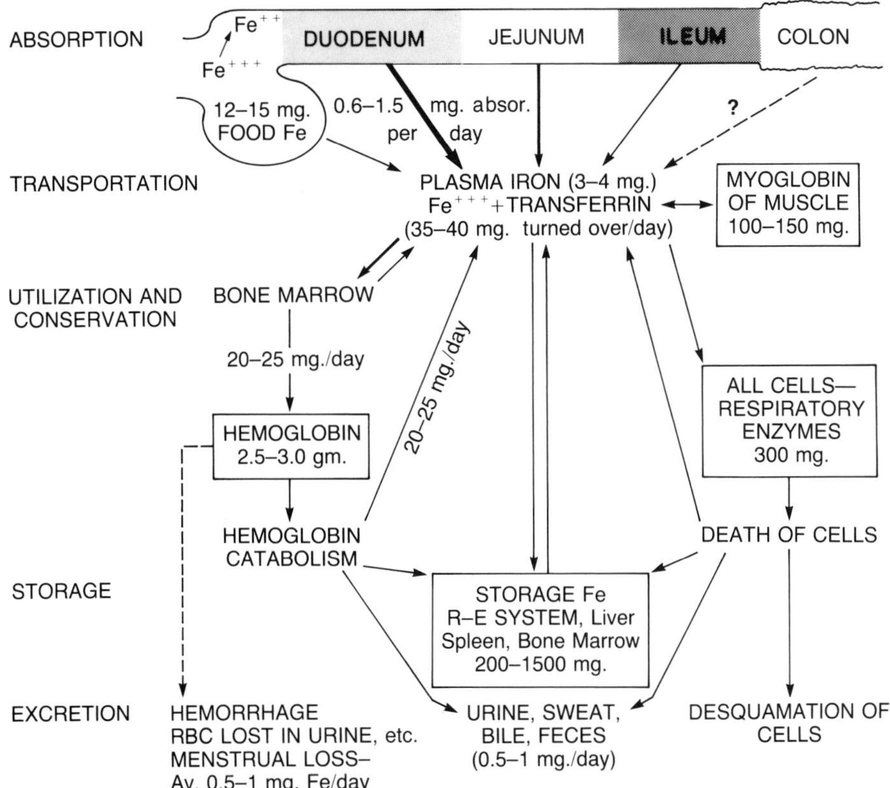

FIGURE 7–3. *Schematic outline of iron metabolism in adults. The majority of iron is absorbed from the duodenum and jejunum, after which it is transported as plasma iron or bound to transferrin.*

transformed by the *cytochrome P-450 system* to water-soluble compounds that can be excreted. Although these vital enzymes represent only a small part of the total iron, a drop in their cellular concentration can have a long-range effect.

Iron is clearly associated with the immune system, but the mechanisms by which it functions are not well defined. *Neutrophils,* white blood cells that engulf and destroy bacteria, are less effective in iron deficiency because their action involves several iron-dependent steps. Two iron-binding proteins, *transferrin* and *lactoferrin,* appear to protect against infection by withholding iron from microorganisms that need it for proliferation.

The role of iron in cognitive performance is also interesting. Differences have been found between the scholastic performance, sensorimotor competence, attention, learning, and memory of anemic children and control subjects (Pollitt et al, 1976). Iron supplementation of children with iron deficiency anemia benefited their learning processes as measured by the school achievement test scores (Soemantri et al, 1985).

TABLE 7–7. Iron Compounds in the Body

Metabolic Proteins	
Heme Proteins	
Hemoglobin	Oxygen transport from lungs to tissues
Myoglobin	Transports and stores oxygen in muscle
Enzymes—Heme	
Cytochromes	Electron transport
Cytochrome P-450	Oxidative degradation of drugs
Catalase	Converts hydrogen peroxide to oxygen and water
Enzymes—Nonheme	
Iron-sulfur and metalloproteins	Oxidative metabolism
Enzymes—Iron Dependent	
Tryptophan pyrrolase	Oxidation of tryptophan
Transport and Storage Proteins	
Transferrin	Transport of iron and other minerals
Ferritin	Storage
Hemosiderin	Storage

Absorption and Transport

Transport across the mucosal cells and in the blood relies on a specific protein carrier mechanism. *Transferrin,* a protein synthesized in the liver, transports iron in the blood to the erythroblasts for use in heme synthesis. *Mucosal transferrin* carries iron from the intestinal lumen into the mucosal cell. Two ferric ions are bound to transferrin for transport to the tissues. Current theory suggests that the number of transferrin receptors on a cell membrane can be adjusted to the needs of the individual cell. Deficiencies in dietary iron are reflected first in the saturation of circulating transferrin.

Dietary iron exists as *heme iron,* as found in hemoglobin and myoglobin, and *nonheme iron.* Heme iron is absorbed into the mucosal cells as the intact porphyrin complex. Absorption is affected only minimally by the composition of the meal and gastrointestinal secretions. Heme iron represents only 5 to 10% of dietary iron, but absorption may be 25% compared with 5% for nonheme iron.

Nonheme iron must be present in the duodenum and upper jejunum in a soluble form if it is to be absorbed. It is ionized by the acid gastric juice, reduced to the ferrous state, and chelated with solubilizing substances such as ascorbic acid, sugars, and the sulfur-containing amino acids. As the chyme passes from the stomach to the duodenum, the addition of duodenal secretions increases the pH to 7, at which point most ferric iron is precipitated unless it has been chelated. Ferrous iron is significantly more soluble at pH 7 and is therefore still available for absorption.

The rate of iron absorption appears to be under the control of the intestinal mucosa, which accepts amounts dictated by the body's needs. Mucosal transferrin excreted in the bile acts as a shuttle protein in facilitating iron absorption. It picks up iron in the intestinal lumen and takes it to the surface of the intestinal cell where it binds to the transferrin receptor, releases the iron into the cell, and returns to the lumen for more iron. Within the mucosal cell the iron may combine with *apoferritin* to form *ferritin* for temporary storage within the cell. Once in the mucosal cell, both apoferritin and ferritin form a common pool.

Transfer from mucosal cells to the body is slower than uptake and is affected by the size of the body stores and the quantity of iron in the diet. The rate at which the iron is released from the mucosal cells into general circulation may be regulated by the amount and saturation of transferrin. Transferrin is usually saturated to about one third of its *total iron-binding capacity (TIBC).* If iron is not needed, transferrin remains saturated and less is absorbed from the mucosal cells, and the transferrin remaining in the cells is sloughed with the cells at the end of their 2- to 3-day life. If iron is needed, the transferrin is less saturated when it reaches the intestinal mucosal cells, and more iron passes from the mucosal cell to the transferrin.

EFFICIENCY OF ABSORPTION. It is estimated that only 5 to 15% of the iron in food is absorbed by adults with normal hemoglobin values, although absorption can be as high as 50% in the presence of an iron deficiency. From 2 to 10% of iron in vegetables is absorbed, and from 10 to 30% of iron in animal protein can be absorbed.

FACTORS AFFECTING ABSORPTION. The efficiency of iron absorption is determined to some extent by the foods in which it occurs. These foods may contain enhancing substances, such as ascorbic acid and the meat, fish, and poultry (MFP) factor (see later), or they may contain complexing agents such as phytates that inhibit absorption. *Ascorbic acid,* the most potent enhancer of iron absorption, forms a chelate with iron that remains soluble at the higher pH of the small intestine. This effect is so well accepted that correction of total iron intake is now recommended to allow for the presence of ascorbic acid as well as for the intake of heme iron sources in meat, fish, and poultry (Clinical Insight, p. 562).

Cellular *animal proteins* from beef, pork, veal, lamb, liver, fish, and chicken enhance absorption; proteins from cow's milk, cheese, and eggs do not. The substance responsible for the enhancement of absorption, referred to as the MFP factor, is unknown.

Infants retain more iron from *human milk* than from cow's milk or infant formulas. Whether the increased retention results from the form in which the iron is present or other factors is not known.

The degree of *gastric acidity* enhances solubility and thus availability of iron in food. The lack of hydrochloric acid in the stomach or the administration of alkaline substances such as antacids interferes with iron absorption. Gastric secretions also include *intrinsic factor* which, because of the structural similarity of heme and vitamin B_{12}, increases absorption of heme iron.

Physiologic states such as pregnancy and growth that demand increased blood formation also stimulate iron absorption. More iron is absorbed in the presence of *deficiency.*

Foods with high *phytate* content have low iron bioavailability, but whether or not phytate is the cause is not clear (Monsen, 1988). *Tannins* in tea also reduce nonheme iron absorption. The presence of an adequate amount of *calcium* helps to remove phosphate, oxalate, and phytate that would combine with iron and inhibit its absorption.

The availability of iron from various compounds used for enrichment or supplementation varies widely according to their *chemical composition.* Although iron in the ferrous form is most readily absorbed, all ferrous compounds are not equally available. Ferrous pyrophosphate is used frequently in products such as breakfast cereals because it does not add a gray color to the food. However, this compound, as well as ferrous citrate and ferrous tartrate, is poorly absorbed. Iron is usually added to baby foods in an elemental form, whose absorbability depends on particle size.

Increased *intestinal motility* decreases iron absorption by decreasing contact time and also by rapidly removing the chyme from the area of highest intestinal acidity. Poor fat digestion leading to *steatorrhea* also decreases absorption.

Storage

About 200 to 1,500 mg of iron are stored in the body as *ferritin* and *hemosiderin;* 30% is in the liver, 30% occurs in the bone marrow, and the rest is found in the spleen and muscles. Up to 50 mg/day can be mobilized from storage iron, 20 mg of which is used in hemoglobin synthesis (see Fig. 7–3). Minute amounts of circulating ferritin, detectable by using sensitive immunoassay techniques, are correlated closely with body iron stores. Measurement of serum ferritin has been an invaluable tool for evaluating iron status clinically, as discussed in Chapters 17 and 32.

Long-term, high-level ingestion of iron or frequent blood transfusions can lead to abnormal accumulation of iron in the liver. Saturation of the apoferritin supply is followed by the appearance of hemosiderin, which is similar to ferritin but contains more iron and is very insoluble. *Hemosiderosis* is an iron storage condition developed by individuals who consume abnormally large amounts of iron or by those with a genetic defect resulting in excessive iron absorption. If the hemosiderosis is associated with tissue damage, it is called *hemochromatosis,* which is discussed further in Chapter 32.

Excretion

Iron is lost from the body only through bleeding and in very small amounts excreted via the feces, in the sweat, and in the normal exfoliation of hair and skin. Most of the iron lost in the feces consists of that not absorbed from food intake. The remainder comes from bile and from the cells exfoliated from the gastrointestinal epithelium. Almost no iron is excreted in the urine.

Daily iron loss amounts to approximately 1 mg in the adult male and slightly less in the nonmenstruating female. The loss of iron accompanying menstruation averages about 0.5 mg/day. Wide variations exist among individuals, however, and menstrual losses of more than 1.4 mg/day of iron have been reported in about 5% of normal women.

Recommended Dietary Allowance

The Food and Nutrition Board has recommended a daily intake of 10 mg of iron for men and postmenopausal women. An intake of 15 mg/day is recommended for women during child-bearing years to replace the losses of menstruation and to provide for iron stores sufficient to support a pregnancy. Female adolescent requirements are also set at 15 mg to provide for the needs of rapid growth. Teenage males have an RDA of 12 mg/day (Table 7–8).

An otherwise adequate diet frequently contains no more than 6 mg/1,000 kcal of iron. The average female consuming 1,800 kcal therefore consumes 10.8 mg of iron, or approximately 73% of the RDA. This appears to meet the needs of 86% of menstruating women. However, setting the RDA higher at 15 mg/day should meet the needs of all except 5% of menstruating women. Women with high losses appear to compensate with an increased rate of absorption.

Sources and Intake

By far the best source of dietary iron is liver, with oysters, shellfish, kidney, heart, lean meat, poultry, and fish as second choices. Dried beans and vegetables are the best plant sources. Some other foods that add iron are egg yolks, dried fruits, dark molasses, whole-grain and enriched breads, wines, and cereals. Milk and milk products are practically devoid of iron. However, the availability of food iron is important in the consideration of dietary sources. For example, only half or less of

TABLE 7–8. Recommended Dietary Allowances for Iron*

Age (Years)	RDA (mg)
Infants	
0.0–0.5	6
0.5–1.0	10
Children	
1–3	10
4–6	10
7–10	10
Males	
11–14	12
15–18	12
19–24	10
25–50	10
51+	10
Females	
11–14	15
15–18	15
19–24	15
25–50	15
51+	10
Pregnant	30
Lactating	
1st 6 mo	15
2nd 6 mo	15

* Reprinted with permission from *Recommended Dietary Allowances,* 10th ed., c. 1989 by the National Academy of Sciences. Published by National Academy Press, Washington, DC.

the iron in whole-grain cereals and some green leaves is available in utilizable form. Appendix 1 lists the iron content of foods. Table 7-9 gives the iron content of selected foods.

Iron fortification of cereals, flours, and bread has added significantly to the total iron intake. Fortified infant cereal is a substantial source of iron for children up to 12 months of age.

The infant is born with a reserve supply of iron and is apparently unable to utilize additional iron beyond this amount. The RDA for a normal term infant is based on an average need of 1.5 mg/kg/day of weight during the first year of life (Taylor et al, 1988). Therefore, the RDA is set at 10 mg/day and continues at that level until adolescence. Premature infants have limited iron stores because most of the iron and other trace minerals are transferred during the last trimester of pregnancy. The need for iron to support rapid growth in premature infants becomes apparent at approximately 2 to 3 months of age (see Chapter 12).

TABLE 7-9. Iron Content of Selected Foods*

Food	mg
Cereal, ready to eat, fortified, 1 cup	1-16
Clams, canned, ¼ cup	11.2
Malt-o-meal, fortified, 1 cup	9.6
Beef liver, fried, 3 oz	5.3
Braunschweiger, 2 oz	5.3
Baked beans, 1 cup	5.0
Molasses, blackstrap, 1 T	5.0
Oysters, cooked, 1 oz	3.8
Venison, roasted, 3 oz	3.8
Baked potato w/skin, 1	2.8
Soup, lentil and ham, 1 cup	2.6
Wheat germ, toasted, ¼ cup	2.5
Burrito, bean, 1	2.5
Soup, beef noodle, 1 cup	2.4
Rice, white, enriched, 1 cup	2.3
Spaghetti w/tomato sauce, 1 cup	2.3
Poptart, fortified, 1	2.2
Ground beef, lean, 3 oz	1.8
Apricots, dried halves, 10	1.7
Pumpkin, canned, ½ cup	1.7
Oatmeal, unfortified, 1 cup	1.6
Spinach, fresh, 1 cup	1.5
Spinach, frozen, cooked, ½ cup	1.5
Cocoa powder, 2 T	1.5
Almonds, dry roasted, ¼ cup	1.3
Peas, frozen, cooked, ½ cup	1.3
Bread, whole wheat, 1 slice	1.2
Chicken, breast, roasted, 1	0.9
Peanuts, dry roasted, ¼ cup	0.8
Pork chop, broiled, 1	0.7
Broccoli, fresh, cooked, ½ cup	0.7
Egg, 1	0.7
Asparagus, fresh, cooked, ½ cup	0.6
Blueberries, frozen, ½ cup	0.5
Wine, red, ½ cup	0.5
Raspberries, fresh, ½ cup	0.4
Kiwi fruit, 1	0.3
Cheese, cheddar, 1 oz	0.2
Milk, 2% fat, 1 cup	0.1

* From USDA: Composition of Foods. USDA Handbook No. 8 Series. Washington, DC, ARS, USDA, 1976-1986.

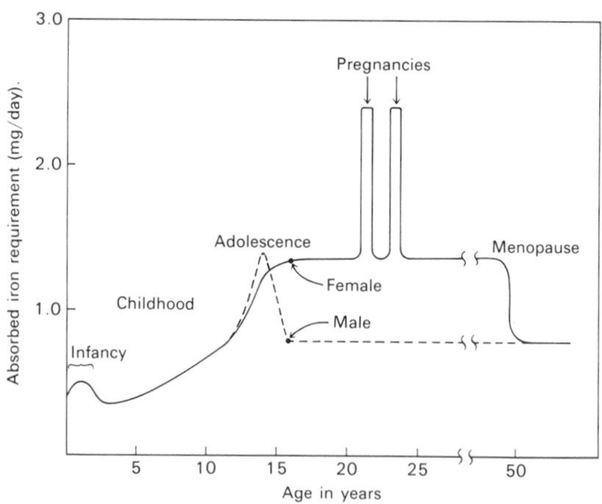

FIGURE 7-4. *The absorbed iron requirement in males and females of various ages. The greatest requirements in relation to food intake occur during infancy. During childhood, requirements are the same for both sexes. During the adolescent growth spurt there is an increase in iron needs—more in the male than in the female. Because of menstruation, the female's requirement remains high, while the requirement for the male decreases after adolescence. (From Wintrobe MS et al: Clinical Hematology, 7th ed. Philadelphia, Lea & Febiger, 1974.)*

Figure 7-4 shows the absorbed requirement in relation to age. Requirements are highest during infancy and adolescence. Male needs decrease after the adolescent growth spurt, whereas female needs continue to be high until after the menopause, with increases during pregnancies.

Deficiency

Iron deficiency is the most common of all deficiency diseases in humans in both developing and developed countries. Groups considered most frequently at risk are infants under 2 years of age, teenage girls, pregnant women, and the elderly. Pregnant teenagers are frequently at very high risk.

Iron deficiency manifests itself ultimately by the development of an anemia (hypochromic microcytic anemia), which is corrected by giving diets rich in absorbable iron and by providing iron supplements in the form of ferrous sulfate or ferrous gluconate. Iron deficiency can be caused by injury, hemorrhage, or illness (e.g., blood loss due to hookworms or gastrointestinal diseases that interfere with iron absorption). Deficiency can also be aggravated by a poorly balanced diet containing insufficient iron, protein, folate, and vitamins B_{12}, B_6, and C. Anemia may develop on a purely nutritional basis as a result of an inadequate diet or faulty iron absorption. Iron-deficiency anemia is discussed in detail in Chapter 32.

Zinc

Zinc has long been known to be essential for microorganisms, but human deficiency was demonstrated relatively recently (Halsted et al, 1972; Prasad et al, 1963). Zinc deficiency disease has been identified not only in malnourished populations but also in a marginal form that may be widespread in the United States (Clinical Insight, p. 124).

Zinc is distributed throughout the plant and animal kingdoms in abundance second only to iron. Two to 3 grams occur in the body of an adult, and the highest concentrations occur in the liver, pancreas, kidney, bone, and voluntary muscles. Other tissues with high concentrations include various parts of the eye, prostate gland, spermatozoa, skin, hair, fingernails, and toenails.

Functions

Many questions regarding the biologic role of zinc in humans remain unanswered. Zinc is known to participate in reactions involving either synthesis or degradation of major metabolites, such as carbohydrates, lipids, proteins, and nucleic acids. More than 200 zinc enzymes have been isolated from various species. Zinc is also involved in the stabilization of protein and nucleic acid structure and the integrity of subcellular organelles, as well as in transport processes, immune function, and expression of genetic information.

Metallothionein is the most abundant, nonenzymatic zinc-containing protein known at present. This low molecular weight protein is rich in cysteine and is exceptionally high in metals, among which are zinc and lesser amounts of copper, iron, cadmium, and mercury. The biologic role of metallothionein has not been defined conclusively. It may have a role in the detoxification of metals or, by inhibiting function of the metal-free thionein, it may influence metabolism of sulfur-containing amino acids (Vallee, 1988).

Zinc is abundant in the *nucleus,* where it stabilizes ribonucleic acid (RNA) and deoxyribonucleic acid (DNA) structure and is required for the activity of RNA polymerases important in cell division. Zinc also functions in chromatin proteins involved in transcription and replication.

Zinc appears in the crystalline structure of bone, in bone enzymes, and at the zone of demarcation. It is thought to be needed for adequate osteoblastic activity; formation of bone enzymes, such as alkaline phosphatase; and calcification. Unless bone resorption is occurring, the zinc in bone is not available.

Absorption

Zinc balance is maintained by the rate of absorption from and the rate of excretion into the intestine. Absorption occurs by a carrier-mediated process and by diffusion (Fig. 7–5). It is under homeostatic control and is affected by the level of zinc in the diet and the presence of interfering substances. With consumption of zinc in a meal, serum zinc rises and then falls in a pattern that is dose-responsive. A protein-rich diet promotes zinc absorption by forming zinc-amino acid chelates that present zinc in a more absorbable form. Absorbed zinc is taken up initially by the liver before redistribution to other tissues. Impaired absorption is associated with a variety of intestinal diseases, such as Crohn's disease or pancreatic insufficiency.

Albumin is the major plasma carrier, although some zinc is transported by transferrin and by alpha-2 macroglobulin. Most of the zinc in blood is localized in erythrocytes and leukocytes. Plasma zinc is metabolically active and fluctuates in response to low dietary intake as well as to physiologic factors, such as injury or inflammation. Plasma zinc levels drop by 50% in the acute phase response to injury, probably owing to the sequestering of zinc by the liver (Solomons, 1988).

When zinc is given intravenously, about 10% of the

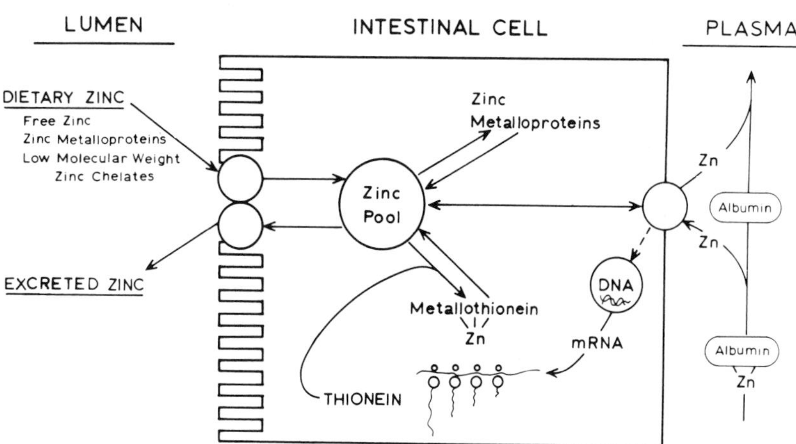

FIGURE 7–5. *Dietary zinc absorption. (Adapted from Cousins RJ: Regulatory aspects of zinc metabolism in liver and intestine. Nutr Rev 37:98, 1979.)*

CLINICAL INSIGHT: Zinc in Children's Growth

The first studies linking zinc and growth were done in Iran and Egypt almost 3 decades ago. "Nutritionally dwarfed" boys characterized by short stature, iron deficiency anemia, and delayed sexual maturity showed remarkable improvement with zinc supplementation. Some grew as much as 5 in. in 1 year along with a progression in gonadal development. The primary cause of zinc deficiency in these boys was identified as an impoverished diet consisting mainly of fibrous unleavened bread. Although the whole grains used to make the bread are relatively high in zinc, they also contain phytates that form insoluble complexes with both zinc and iron (Prasad, 1988).

At the time, it was believed that circumstances leading to growth impairment from zinc deficiency were unique to less developed countries. However, studies of preschool children from apparently well-nourished families in Denver demonstrated a correlation between short stature and low hair zinc levels (Hambidge et al, 1976). Other studies have supported these findings.

A more recent Canadian study found a significant negative correlation between hair zinc levels and height-for-age in boys but not in girls. Boys of shorter stature in the study group had lower intakes of meat, fish, and poultry and higher intakes of milk than boys of normal height (Smit Vanderkooy and Gibson, 1987).

The most readily available form of zinc occurs in animal flesh, particularly red meats and poultry. Meats are frequently low in diets of preschoolers because of personal preferences, possibly for socioeconomic reasons, but usually because meats are displaced by high intakes of the cereal foods, milk, and milk products that children tend to prefer. For example, some of the children in Hambidge's study were eating as little as 1 oz of meat daily. Milk is a good source of zinc, but high intakes of calcium can interfere with the absorption of both iron and zinc. Although the phytates in whole grains seriously limit zinc absorption in middle-Eastern diets, this is less likely to be a problem when breads, breakfast foods, and other cereal-based foods are made primarily from refined grains.

Diet assessment may suggest the presence of a mild zinc deficiency in young children with suboptimal stature. However, a positive response to zinc supplementation would be required to confirm such a diagnosis (Smit Vanderkooy and Gibson, 1987).

dose appears in the intestine in 30 minutes. Serum concentration falls after a zinc-free meal, possibly because the pancreas removes zinc from circulation to produce the metalloenzymes needed for digestion and absorption (Dinsmore et al, 1985).

INHIBITING FACTORS. *Fiber* or *phytate* decrease zinc absorption, but other complexing agents (e.g., tannins) do not. Higher than physiologic doses of *copper* inhibit zinc absorption. *Iron* competes with zinc for absorption; ratios of iron to zinc of 2:1 or 3:1 result in a significant reduction in zinc uptake (Solomons, 1988). Iron : zinc ratios greater than 3 : 1 are common to many vitamin-mineral supplements. On the other hand, high doses of zinc can impair absorption of iron from ferrous sulfate, the form found usually in vitamin/mineral supplements (Crofton et al, 1989).

ENHANCING FACTORS. Zinc absorption in animals is enhanced by either *glucose* or *lactose* and by *soy protein* fed alone or mixed with beef. Red table *wine* also increases zinc absorption, probably owing to the congeners present; white wine has not been studied. Zinc is better absorbed from *human milk* than from cow's milk.

Excretion

Excretion of zinc in normal individuals is almost entirely via the feces. Increased urinary excretion has been reported in starvation and in patients with nephrosis, diabetes, alcoholism, hepatic cirrhosis, and porphyria. Plasma and urine concentrations of amino acids, specifically cysteine and histidine, and other metabolites may have a role in determining zinc losses in these patients.

Recommended Dietary Allowance

Metabolic studies of healthy adults indicate that positive zinc balance is attained with intakes of 112.5 mg/day from a mixed diet, based on an efficiency of absorption of 20%. The 1989 RDA established 15 mg/day as the appropriate intake for male adolescents and adults. Because of the lower body weight of adolescent and adult women, their RDA is 12 mg/day. The requirement for preadolescents is estimated at 6 mg/day, but because of greater dermal losses and more variation, the RDA has been set at 10 mg. The RDA for infants is 5 mg/day during the first year of life (Table 7–10).

Oral contraceptive therapy may alter zinc distribution; however, no evidence is available showing that these changes alter the dietary requirement (King, 1986).

Sources and Intakes

Meat, fish, poultry, and milk and milk products provide 80% of the total dietary zinc (Moser-Veillon, 1990). Oysters, other shellfish, meat, liver, cheese, whole grain

TABLE 7–10. Recommended Dietary Allowances for Zinc*

Age (Years)	RDA (mg)
Infants	
0.0–0.5	5
0.5–1.0	5
Children	
1–3	10
4–6	10
7–10	10
Males	
11–14	15
15–18	15
19–24	15
25–50	15
51+	15
Females	
11–14	12
15–18	12
19–24	12
25–50	12
51+	12
Pregnant	15
Lactating	
1st 6 mo	19
2nd 6 mo	16

* Reprinted with permission from *Recommended Dietary Allowances,* 10th ed., c. 1989 by the National Academy of Sciences. Published by National Academy Press, Washington, DC.

cereal, dry beans, and nuts are sources of zinc (Table 7–11).

The zinc content of typical mixed diets of Canadian and American adults is between 10 and 15 mg/day (Food and Nutrition Board, 1989). Based on the 1985 Nationwide Food Consumption Survey, the mean zinc intake for women aged 19 to 50 was 8.7 to 9.2 mg/day and for men 14.1 mg/day (Moser-Veillon, 1990). The difference could be related to the difference in energy intake and not to the density of zinc in the diets of men and women. The zinc density of the American adult diet appears to be 5.6 to 5.7 mg/1,000 kcal.

Deficiency

The clinical entity of zinc deficiency in humans was first described in young males in Iran and Egypt and was characterized by short stature, hypogonadism, mild anemia, and low plasma zinc levels (Prasad et al, 1963) (Fig. 7–6). This deficiency is caused by a diet high in unrefined cereal and unleavened bread. These contain a high level of fiber and phytate, both of which chelate with zinc in the intestine and prevent absorption. The anemia seen in the young men may have reflected a coexisting iron deficiency from the same cause. Additional symptoms of zinc deficiency include hypogeusia (decreased taste acuity), delayed wound healing, alopecia, and diverse forms of skin lesions. A zinc-responsive night blindness has also been documented (Solomons, 1988). Acquired zinc deficiency may accrue as the result of malabsorption or increased loss via urinary, pancreatic, or other exocrine secretions.

Acrodermatitis enteropathica, an autosomal recessive disease characterized by zinc malabsorption, results in eczematoid skin lesions, alopecia, diarrhea, intercurrent bacterial and yeast infections, and eventually death if left untreated. Symptoms are generally first observed at weaning from human milk to cow's milk.

Zinc deficiency results in a variety of immunologic defects. Severe deficiency is accompanied by thymic atrophy, lymphopenia, reduced lymphocyte proliferative response to mitogens, a selective decrease in T4 helper cells, decreased natural killer (NK) cell activity, anergy, and deficient thymic hormone activity. Moderate zinc deficiency is associated with anergy and diminished NK activity but not with thymic atrophy or lymphopenia. Mild zinc deficiency is associated with impaired interleukin-2 production. Table 7–12 summarizes the clinical manifestations of zinc deficiency.

Similarities between patients with sickle cell anemia and zinc deficiency suggest the possibility of a secondary zinc deficiency in that disease (see Chapter 32).

TABLE 7–11. Zinc Content of Selected Foods*

Food	mg
Oysters, Eastern, ½ cup	113.0
Oysters, Pacific, ½ cup	21.0
Wheat germ, toasted, ¼ cup	4.7
Ground beef, lean, 3 oz	4.6
Liver, beef, fried, 3 oz	4.6
Turkey, dark meat, baked, 3 oz	3.8
Instant breakfast, 1 envelope	3.0
Beef enchilada, 1	2.3
Baked beans, with pork, ½ cup	1.9
Cheese, ricotta, part-skim, ½ cup	1.7
Pecans, ¼ cup	1.6
Tahini (sesame butter), 1 T	1.6
Peanuts, dry roasted, ¼ cup	1.4
Crab, canned, ¼ cup	1.3
Wild rice, cooked, ½ cup	1.1
Clams, canned, ¼ cup	1.1
Lobster, cooked, ½ cup	1.1
Cheese, Edam, 1 oz	1.1
Milk, 2% fat, 1 cup	1.0
Chicken, breast, baked, 1	1.0
Walnuts, English, ¼ cup	0.8
Bagel, 1	0.6
Gingerbread, 1 piece	0.6
Egg, 1	0.6
Salmon, baked, 3 oz	0.4

* From USDA: Composition of Foods. USDA Handbook Series No. 8. Washington, DC, ARS, USDA, 1976–1986.

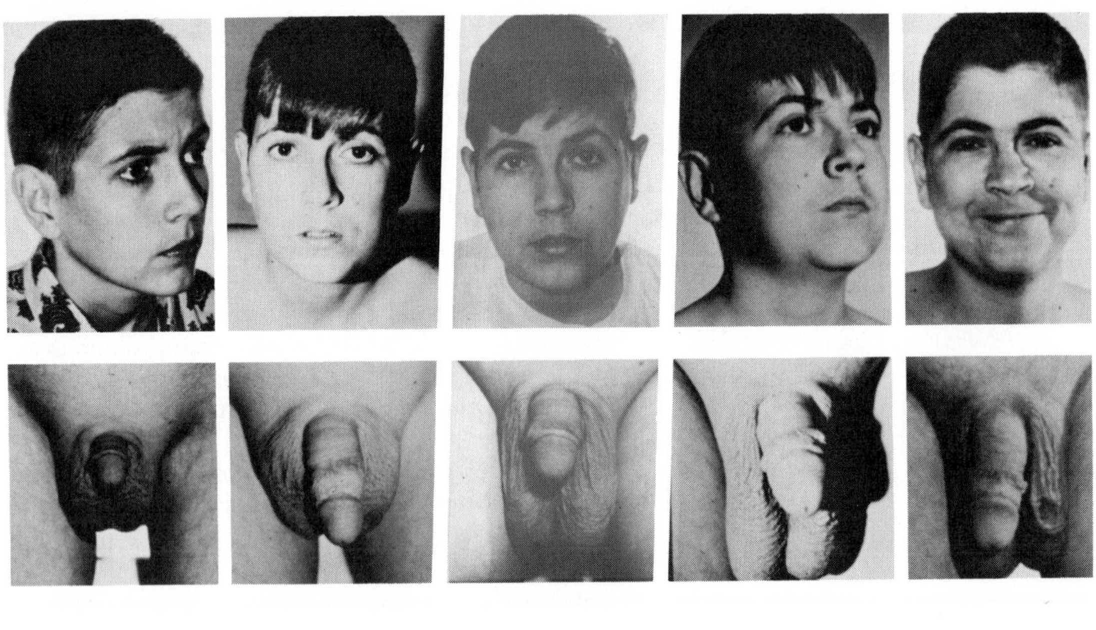

FIGURE 7–6. *Zinc deficiency from malabsorption and after treatment with zinc sulfate. Note the physical maturation and growth that result from zinc supplementation. (From Sandstead HH: Zinc as an unrecognized limiting nutrient. © Am J Clin Nutr 26:790, 1973. American Society for Clinical Nutrition.)*

Toxicity

Excess oral ingestion of zinc to the point of toxicity (100 to 300 mg/day) is rare. However, continued supplementation with zinc in excess of the RDA will interfere with copper absorption (Fosmire, 1990). Zinc supplementation of 50 mg/day has been found to cause a decrease in HDL-cholesterol in adult males (Black et al, 1988). Zinc sulfate in amounts of 2 g/day or more can cause gastrointestinal irritation and vomiting. Inhalation of zinc fumes during welding can be toxic but can be prevented with proper precautions.

The major type of zinc toxicity is seen in patients with renal failure on hemodialysis. Contamination of dialysis fluids from adhesive plastic used on the dialysis coils or from galvanized pipes has been reported. The toxic syndrome in this case is characterized by anemia, fever, and central nervous system disturbances.

TABLE 7–12. Clinical Manifestations of Human Zinc Deficiency*

Growth retardation
Delayed sexual maturation
Hypogonadism and hypospermia
Alopecia
Skin lesions
Impaired wound healing
Immune deficiencies
Behavioral disturbances
Night blindness
Impaired taste (hypogeusia)

* Adapted from Solomons NW: Zinc and copper. *In* Shils ME and Young VR (eds): Modern Nutrition in Health and Disease, 7th ed. Philadelphia, Lea & Febiger, 1988.

Copper

Copper, recognized around 1875 as a normal constituent of blood, has enjoyed increased nutritional interest along with other trace elements. Concentrations of copper are highest in liver, brain, heart, and kidney. Muscle has a lower concentration, but because of its large mass contains approximately 40% of all copper in the body. Approximately 90% of the copper in plasma is incorporated into *ceruloplasmin;* the rest is bound loosely to albumin, transcuprein, and amino acids.

Functions

Copper is a component of many enzymes, and clinical manifestations of copper deficiency are explicable mainly in terms of enzyme failure. Copper has a well-documented role in the oxidation of iron prior to transport in the plasma and in the cross-linking of collagen necessary for its tensile strength. Through the involvement of copper-containing enzymes, it also has roles in mitochondrial energy production, protection from oxidants, and synthesis of melanine and catecholamines.

Other functions have been suggested but as yet are not completely defined (Turnlund, 1988).

Absorption, Transport, and Excretion

Some copper is absorbed from the stomach, but absorption is maximal in the small intestine, both by active and passive transport. Reported absorption varies from 25 to 60%. Some of the variability may be the result of differing experimental conditions and of the short half-life of the radioisotopes used. The percentage of absorption decreases with increased intake (Turnlund, 1988).

Metabolism

Some evidence suggests that the amount of copper absorbed is regulated by the amount of metallothionein in the mucosal cells. For short-term transport to the liver, copper is carried primarily by albumin as well as by transcuprein and possibly by histidine. Copper-albumin may serve as a temporary storage site for copper. In the liver, copper is stored as metallothionein or incorporated into ceruloplasmin and secreted back into the plasma for long-term transport to the cells. Copper is also secreted from the liver as a component of bile. Once in the gastrointestinal tract, it becomes part of the pool and may be reabsorbed or excreted, depending on the body's need for copper. Biliary excretion increases substantially in response to copper overload.

Small amounts of copper are present in urine, sweat, and menstrual blood. Copper can be conserved by the kidney if necessary when substantial amounts are filtered through the glomerulus and are reabsorbed in the tubules. Unabsorbed copper is found in the feces.

The interaction of copper with other nutrients is an example of the inadvisability of supplementing with vitamins and minerals above levels established by the RDA. In amounts of 150 mg/day, zinc has induced copper deficiency by stimulating intestinal cells to produce more metallothionein (Copper . . . , 1985). Because metallothionein binds copper more avidly than zinc, more copper is lost with exfoliated intestinal cells. Ascorbic acid in excessive amounts reduces the oxidative activity and thus the functional properties of ceruloplasmin (Turnlund, 1988).

Fiber and phytate, known to affect bioavailability of some minerals, do not appear to have an adverse effect on copper absorption (Turnlund, 1988).

Estimated Safe and Adequate Daily Dietary Intake

Although sufficient data are not available to establish an RDA, the 1989 revision recommends an "estimated safe and adequate daily dietary intake" (ESADDI) for copper of 1.5 to 3 mg/day for adolescents and adults. The ESADDI for children is 0.7 to 2 mg/day, and for infants the ESADDI is 0.4 to 0.6 mg during the first 6 months and 0.6 to 0.7 mg/day during the second 6 months (Table 7–13). Premature infants, always born with low copper reserves, may require more. Copper concentration is greatest in the newborn and decreases during the first year of life.

Copper intakes of individuals in several age categories in the United States have been consistently below recommended amounts, with adolescent girls consuming about 50% of the ESADDI. The average intake for adults based on the 1986 Nationwide Food Consumption Survey was about 0.9 mg for women and 1.2 mg for men (Pennington et al, 1989). However, this analysis did not take drinking water into account, the copper content of which is directly related to the leaching of this mineral from copper water pipes.

Sources and Intakes

Copper is distributed widely in foods, and most diets provide about 2 mg/day. Foods high in copper are oysters, liver, kidney, chocolate, nuts, dried legumes, cereals, dried fruits, poultry, and shellfish (Table 7–14). Cow's milk, which is as poor a source of copper as it is of iron, contains 0.015 to 0.18 mg/l. The copper content of human milk, which ranges from 0.15 to 1.05 mg/l, is well absorbed.

Deficiency

Copper deficiency is signaled by a decrease in serum copper and ceruloplasmin levels, followed by failure of iron absorption, leading to a microcytic hemochromic anemia. Neutropenia, leukopenia, and bone demineralization follow, with subperiosteal hemorrhages, hair and skin depigmentation, defective elastin formation, and bone demineralization. Failure of erythropoiesis as well as cerebral and cerebellar degeneration finally lead to death. Neutropenia and leukopenia are the best early

TABLE 7–13. Estimated Safe and Adequate Daily Dietary Intakes for Copper*

	Age (Years)	ESADDI (mg)
Infants	0–0.5	0.4–0.6
	0.5–1	0.6–0.7
Children and Adolescents	1–3	0.7–1.0
	4–6	1.0–1.5
	7–10	1.0–2.0
	11+	1.5–2.5
Adults		1.5–3.0

* Reprinted with permission from *Recommended Dietary Allowances*, 10th ed., c. 1989 by the National Academy of Sciences. Published by National Academy Press, Washington, DC.

TABLE 7–14. Copper Content of Selected Foods*

Food	mg
Beef liver, fried, 3 oz	2.4
Cashews, dry roasted, ¼ cup	0.8
Black-eyed peas, dried, cooked, ½ cup	0.7
Molasses, blackstrap, 2 T	0.6
Sunflower seeds, ¼ cup	0.6
Chocolate chips, semisweet, ¼ cup	0.5
V-8 juice, 1 cup	0.5
Tofu, firm, ½ cup	0.5
Beans, refried, ½ cup	0.5
Instant breakfast, fortified, 1 envelope	0.5
Cocoa powder, 2 T	0.4
Prunes, dried, 10	0.4
Salmon, baked, 3 oz	0.3
Tahini (sesame butter), 1 T	0.2
Pizza, cheese, ⅛ of 15″	0.2
Bread, whole wheat, 1 slice	0.1
Milk chocolate, 1 oz	0.1
Milk, 2% fat, 1 cup	0.1

* From USDA: Composition of Foods. USDA Handbook No. 8 Series. Washington, DC, ARS, USDA, 1976–1986.

indications of copper deficiency in children. Copper deficiency anemia is discussed in Chapter 32.

Copper is stored in the liver, and therefore a deficiency develops slowly. Deficiencies have not been reported in otherwise healthy humans consuming a varied diet. Low serum copper, cerulopolasmin, and superoxide dismutase provide supportive evidence of copper deficiency but are not sensitive to marginal status. Bone changes including osteoporosis, metaphyseal spur formation, and soft-tissue calcification seen in infants receiving prolonged total parenteral nutrition (TPN) have improved with copper supplementation. The only signs of copper deficiency found in adults are neutropenia and microcytic anemia.

Menkes' disease is a sex-linked recessive defect that results in copper malabsorption, increased urinary loss, and abnormal intracellular copper transport, all of which cause an abnormal distribution of copper between organs and within cells. Affected infants have retarded growth, defective keratinization and pigmentation of the hair, hypothermia, degenerative changes in aortic elastin, abnormalities of the metaphyses of long bones, and progressive mental deterioration. Many of the features are due to interference with cross-linking of collagen and elastin. Brain tissue is practically devoid of cytochrome C oxidase and there is a marked accumulation of copper in the intestinal mucosa, although serum copper and ceruloplasmin are very low. Parenteral administration of copper results in transient improvement. Ataxia, mild learning difficulty, and connective tissue abnormalities are seen in patients with mild Menkes' disease (Procopis et al, 1981).

Decreased plasma copper is seen in patients with malabsorption diseases, such as celiac sprue, tropical sprue, protein-losing enteropathies, and nephrotic syndrome.

Toxicity

Ceruloplasmin concentrations increase during pregnancy and in women taking oral contraceptives. Serum copper concentrations in pregnant women are approximately twice the values of nonpregnant women. Serum copper concentration is increased in patients with acute and chronic infections, patients with liver disease, and patients with pellagra. The physiologic significance of these elevations is not known.

Bile contains substantial amounts of copper; therefore, copper retention is a possibility in any form of chronic liver disease that interferes with the excretion of bile. Primary biliary cirrhosis as well as mechanical obstruction of the bile ducts causes a progressive rise in liver copper.

Wilson's disease (hepatolenticular degeneration) is a disease characterized by accumulation of excessive copper in body tissue as the result of genetic deficiency in the liver synthesis of ceruloplasmin.

Iodine

The body normally contains 20 to 30 mg of iodine, with more than 75% in the thyroid gland and the rest distributed throughout the body, particularly in the lactating mammary gland, gastric mucosa, and blood. The only known function of iodine is related to its role as an integral part of the thyroid hormones.

Absorption and Excretion

Iodine is absorbed easily in the form of iodide. In circulation it occurs both as free and protein-bound iodine. Iodine is stored in the thyroid, where it is used for synthesis of triiodotyrosine (T_3) and thyroxine (T_4) when needed. The hormone is degraded in target cells and in the liver, and the iodine is conserved if needed. Excretion is primarily via urine; the small amounts in the feces come from the bile.

Recommended Dietary Allowance

An intake of 150 μg/day of iodine has been suggested as sufficient for all adults and adolescents. The RDA for pregnant and lactating women is increased 25 μg and 50 μg, respectively. The RDA for infants is 40 μg and 50 μg for older infants. The RDA for children is between 70 and 120 μg, depending on the age of the child (Table 7–15).

TABLE 7–15. Recommended Dietary Allowances for Iodine*

Age (Years)	RDA (μg)
Infants	
0.0–0.5	40
0.5–1.0	50
Children	
1–3	70
4–6	90
7–10	120
Males	
11–14	150
15–18	150
19–24	150
25–50	150
51+	150
Females	
11–14	150
15–18	150
19–24	150
25–50	150
51+	150
Pregnant	175
Lactating	
1st 6 mo	200
2nd 6 mo	200

* Reprinted with permission from *Recommended Dietary Allowances,* 10th ed., c. 1989 by the National Academy of Sciences. Published by National Academy Press, Washington, DC.

Dietary Sources

Iodine occurs in extremely variable amounts in food and drinking water. Seafoods such as clams, lobsters, oysters, sardines, and other saltwater fish are rich sources of iodine. Saltwater fish contain 300 to 3,000 μg/kg of flesh; freshwater fish contain 20 to 40 μg/kg and are potent sources of this mineral. The iodine content of cow's milk and eggs is determined by the iodides available in the diet of the animal, and the iodides in vegetables vary according to the amount in the soil in which they are grown. Bovine milk in the United States and Australia contains five to ten times as much iodine as found in many European countries (Aumont, 1987).

Iodine also enters the food chain through the use of iodophors as disinfectants, coloring agents, and dough conditioners. These sources add significant iodine to the food supply. (See Table 7–16 for ranges of iodine content of foods.)

The importance of iodized salt should still be emphasized in certain areas to prevent goiter. The best way to obtain an adequate intake of iodine is to use iodized salt (76 μg iodine per gram of salt for both United States and Canada) in the preparation of food. Over half of the amount of table salt sold in the United States is iodized; however, iodized salt is not used in processed foods. Mandatory iodization has been adopted by many nations, including Canada, but is not a policy in the United States, where iodine deficiency is not prevalent. Other methods of increasing iodine intake (adding iodine to water supplies and use of iodide tablets) have been tried in iodine-deficient areas of the world and have been impractical. Injections of iodized oil successfully provide protection for 2 to 4 years.

TABLE 7–16. Iodine Content of Selected Foods*

Food	μg
Salt, iodized, 1 tsp	400
Bread, made with iodate dough conditioner and continuous mix process, 1 slice	142
Haddock, 3 oz	104–145
Bread, made with regular process, 1 slice	35
Cheese, cottage, 2% fat, ½ cup	26–71
Shrimp, 3 oz	21–37
Egg, 1	18–26
Cheese, cheddar, 1 oz	5–23
Ground beef, 3 oz	8

* From USDA: Composition of Foods. Handbook No. 8 series. Washington, DC, ARS, USDA, 1976–1986.

The Total Diet Study of the FDA showed that the adult iodine intake in 1986 was 150 to 250 μg/day. The intake for teenagers was even higher, with that of adolescent males averaging 320 μg/day, over twice the RDA of 150 μg (Pennington et al, 1989).

Deficiency

Lack of iodine intake is associated with the development of endemic or simple *goiter,* which is an enlargement of the thyroid gland (Fig. 7–7). The deficiency may be absolute, especially in areas of subnormal iodine intake, or relative subsequent to increased need for thyroid hormones, such as in the female during adolescence, pregnancy, and lactation.

The World Health Organization has estimated that

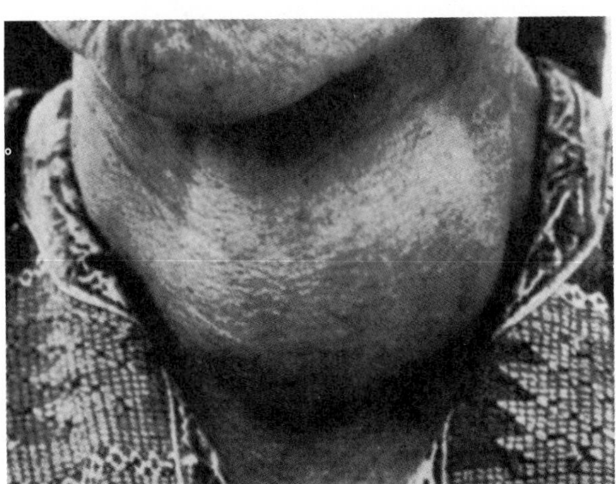

FIGURE 7–7. *Goiter caused by iodine deficiency. (From Nizel AE: Nutrition in Preventive Dentistry, 2nd ed. Philadelphia, WB Saunders, 1981, p 248.)*

the world incidence of goiter is approximately 200 million. In some countries, goiter is so common that it is regarded as a normal physical feature. According to one report, endemic goiter exists in at least 12 European countries, including some countries where iodine prophylaxis is mandatory (Subcommittee. . . , 1985). In the United States, the rate of goiter for all age groups is 1.9/1,000 persons. The rate is higher in women than in men and is higher for older age groups.

Goitrogens, substances occurring naturally in foods, can also cause goiter by blocking absorption or utilization of iodine. Some foods containing goitrogens are cabbage, turnips, rapeseeds, peanuts, cassava, and soybeans. These substances are inactivated by cooking. Other studies suggest that local water may contain goitrogenic substances from geologic origin or possibly from *Escherichia coli* in the water. This may explain the prevalence of goiter in some areas where it does not seem to be dependent on a deficient intake of iodine.

Severe iodine deficiency during gestation and early postnatal growth results in *cretinism,* a syndrome characterized by mental deficiency, spastic diplegia or quadriplegia, deaf mutism, dysarthria, a characteristic shuffling gait, shortened stature, and hypothyroidism (Fig. 7–8). Less severe variations of this syndrome may also exist, manifesting as deaf mutism alone or moderate retardation in intellectual or neuromotor maturation (Stanbury, 1988).

Toxicity

Iodine intake has a rather wide margin of safety. However, in some cases goiter is seen as a possible consequence of long-term iodine intakes well in excess of physiologic need. The significance of this relationship is not clear. At present, iodine in foods is not considered to be a significant public health problem in the United States and Canada. However, a study of iodine in a representative Canadian diet revealed consumption of this mineral at a level that was more than six times the recommendation for adults (Discher and Girous, 1987). Similar findings exist for the American diet. In every age group studied in one survey, the mean intake was at least equal to the RDA, and in the group of infants 6 to 11 months of age the iodine intake was almost three times that of the RDA (Pennington et al, 1986). This was less than in previous studies because of the decreased use of iodine-containing compounds in cereals. Adverse reactions are difficult to identify, but both intake and incidence of thyroid enlargement should continue to be monitored.

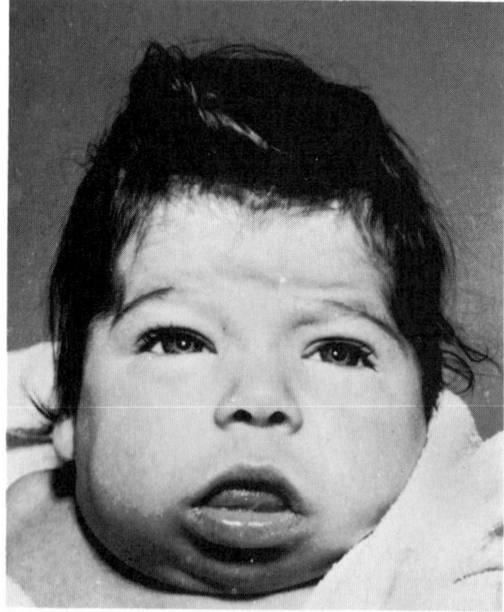

FIGURE 7–8. *Cretinism in a 6-month-old infant, caused by iodine deficiency. (From Di George AM: The Endocrine system.* In: *Behrman RE and Kliegman RM [eds]: Nelson Textbook of Pediatrics, 14th ed. Philadelphia, WB Saunders, 1991, p 123.)*

Fluoride

Fluoride is important for the health of bones and teeth. The average skeleton contains 2.5 mg of fluoride.

Functions

Fluoride is considered to be essential because of its beneficial effect on tooth enamel, conferring maximal resistance to dental caries. The prevalence of dental caries has decreased by 50% in the last 15 to 20 years, owing mainly to the fluoridation of drinking water. The prevalence of dental caries has also declined in communities without fluoridated water. The cause is unknown but probably includes the use of fluoridated toothpaste, topical application, and increased use of fluorides in the food chain, especially from the use of fluoridated water in food processing. The American Academy of Pediatrics recommends supplementation for infants and children if the fluoride concentration in the water supply is below 0.7 ppm (see Chapter 23).

Fluoride replaces the hydroxyl group in the calcium phosphorus salts of the bones and teeth to form fluoroapatite, which is less readily absorbed than hydroxyapatite. Some early studies suggested that this protected the bone against osteoporosis. However, larger and more complete studies have failed to find support for this hypothesis (Sowers et al, 1986).

Estimated Safe and Adequate Daily Dietary Intake

The estimated safe and adequate intake of fluoride for adults is 1.5 to 4 mg/day. Depending on the age, it is 0.5 to 2.5 mg/day for children and adolescents and 0.1 to 1 mg/day for infants (Table 7–17). An 8-oz glass of fluoridated water (1 part per million or 1 mg/l) provides about 0.2 mg of fluoride.

TABLE 7-17. Estimated Safe and Adequate Daily Dietary Intakes for Fluoride*

	Age (Years)	ESADDI (mg)
Infants	0-0.5	0.1-0.5
	0.5-1	0.2-1.0
Children and Adolescents	1-3	0.5-1.5
	4-6	1.0-2.5
	7-10	1.5-2.5
	11+	1.5-2.5
Adults		1.5-4.0

* Reprinted with permission from *Recommended Dietary Allowances*, 10th ed., c. 1989 by the National Academy of Sciences. Published by National Academy Press, Washington, DC.

Sources and Intakes

The major dietary sources of fluoride are drinking water and processed foods that have been prepared or reconstituted with fluoridated water. The reported difference in intake is 0.9 mg/day in an area with unfluoridated water to 1.7 mg/day in a fluoridated area (Singer et al, 1980). Although fluorides are widespread in fruits and vegetables, the amounts are not significant. However, the amount in tea leaves can be important, depending on the brewing strength and on the extent of tea consumption. One cup of tea can contain as much as 0.1 mg of fluoride (Sweeney and Shaw, 1988). Soups and stews made with fish and meat bones also provide fluoride in societies that depend extensively on such foods. Mechanically deboned meat and fowl, as well as seafood and beef liver, are high in fluoride. Cooking foods in Teflon pans (a fluoride-containing polymer) increases fluoride content of the food cooked in it.

Toxicity

A mild fluorosis can appear at doses of 0.1 mg/kg/day (see Chapter 23). This type of mottling is not usually visible and has no negative effect. However, the fact that it is increasing has generated concern that proliferating sources of fluorides may be leading to excessive intakes by toddlers in some cases (Leverett, 1982). In a study of cities where drinking water contains more than 0.7 ppm of fluoride, the mean dietary fluoride intake of 6-month-old infants was 0.418 mg/day and 0.621 mg/day for 1-year-old toddlers. When drinking water contained less fluoride, the average intake was less. Even the highest values did not exceed the recommendation of 0.08 mg/kg/day (Ophaug et al, 1985).

Chromium

The essentiality of chromium has been recognized, but its biologic function has not been well defined. The low levels of chromium in food, body tissues, and body fluids pose severe analytic problems. Because of the universal presence of chromium in the environment and unrecognized contamination of samples, the reliability of values for concentrations in urine, plasma, hair, and food must be evaluated carefully.

Functions

Chromium is required for normal lipid and carbohydrate metabolism and appears to be involved in the function of insulin. Inorganic chromium must be converted to the trivalent form in order to function physiologically.

The biologically active chromium complex called the "glucose tolerance factor" has been the subject of much research and is thought to consist of chromium, nicotinic acid, and glutathione. Its role in carbohydrate and lipid metabolism is discussed further in Chapter 31. Supplementation with chromium has also been shown to raise high-density lipoprotein cholesterol levels (Riales and Albrink, 1981).

Absorption and Excretion

The absorption of chromium in its trivalent form is about 10 to 25%; absorption of inorganic chromium is only 1%. The mechanism is not known, but it does not appear to be simple diffusion. Absorption is facilitated by amino acids that prevent chromium from precipitating in the alkaline medium of the small intestine. The amount absorbed remains constant at dietary intakes above 40 μg, at which point urinary excretion increases proportionally to intake (Anderson, 1986). Increased intake of simple sugar, strenuous exercise, or physical trauma also elevate urinary excretion.

Both chromium and iron are carried by transferrin; however, albumin is also capable of assuming this role in the presence of high iron transferrin saturation. A limited number of balance studies have identified serum chromium concentrations of 0.1 to 0.2 mg/ml (Anderson and Kozlovsky, 1985; Offenbacher et al, 1986).

Estimated Safe and Adequate Daily Dietary Intake

The ESADDI for chromium is 50 to 200 mcg/day for persons 7 years of age and older and, depending on the age of the child, 10 to 120 μg/day for younger children and infants (Table 7-18).

Sources and Intakes

Precise assessment of chromium in foods is difficult; biologically available chromium and inorganic chromium cannot be distinguished from each other. Brewer's yeast, oysters, liver, and potatoes have a high

TABLE 7–18. Estimated Safe and Adequate Daily Dietary Intakes for Chromium*

	Age (Years)	ESADDI (μg)
Infants	0–0.5	10–40
	0.5–1	20–60
Children and Adolescents	1–3	20–80
	4–6	30–120
	7–10	50–200
	11+	50–200
Adults		50–200

* Reprinted with permission from *Recommended Dietary Allowances,* 10th ed., c. 1989 by the National Academy of Sciences. Published by National Academy Press, Washington, DC.

chromium concentration; seafoods, whole grains, cheeses, chicken, meats, bran, fresh fruits, and vegetables are intermediate in content. Refining of wheat removes chromium along with the germ and the bran; refining sugar fractionates the chromium into the molasses portion.

A study of usual intake of chromium showed an average intake of 33 μg/day in self-selected diets containing 2,300 kcal and 25 μg/day in 1,600 kcal diets (Anderson and Kozlovsky, 1985).

Deficiency

Documenting moderate chromium deficiency is very difficult because of the lack of an indicator of chromium status. Even reliable measures of serum or plasma chromium may not accurately reflect tissue concentrations or body stores. Supplementation trials with high-risk groups (e.g., malnourished children, elderly subjects, or patients with noninsulin dependent diabetes) have yielded mixed results with respect to both glucose and lipid metabolism.

A chromium deficiency leads to signs of altered carbohydrate metabolism, such as impaired glucose tolerance, glycosuria, fasting hyperglycemia, elevated serum insulin levels, and decreased insulin binding. Impaired growth, peripheral neuropathy, and negative nitrogen balance are also seen. Stress appears to alter metabolism in the direction of increased chromium losses; however, supplemental chromium did not result in measurable improvement of glucose metabolism in traumatized patients receiving TPN (Anderson et al, 1988).

Hyperglycemia and weight loss seen in the three reported cases of chromium deficiency in patients receiving TPN were reversed with intravenous supplementation with inorganic chromium (Brown et al, 1986; Freund et al, 1979; Jeejeebhoy et al, 1977).

Cobalt

Most of the cobalt in the body appears with the vitamin B_{12} stores in the liver. Blood plasma contains approximately 1 μg/100 ml.

Functions

The only known biologic function of cobalt at present is as a component of vitamin B_{12} (cobalamin). This vitamin is essential for the maturation of red blood cells and normal functioning of all cells (see Chapter 6).

Absorption and Excretion

Cobalt may share at least part of the same intestinal transport mechanism with iron. Absorption is increased in patients with deficient iron intake, portal cirrhosis with iron overload, and idiopathic hemochromatosis. The major route of cobalt excretion is the urine, and small amounts are excreted with feces, sweat, and hair.

Recommended Intakes

The dietary requirement for cobalt for people 7 years of age and older is expressed in terms of vitamin B_{12}, of which 1.4 to 2 μg are needed daily (see Chapter 6).

Sources and Intakes

Cobalt occurs in foods; however, only microorganisms are able to synthesize vitamin B_{12}. Ruminant animals obtain cobalamin as the result of a symbiotic relationship with the microorganisms of their gastrointestinal tract. The microorganisms of monogastric species such as humans have an extremely limited capacity for synthesis in areas where the vitamin can be absorbed; therefore, humans must obtain their vitamin B_{12}, and thus cobalt, from animal foods such as organ and muscle meats. In some circumstances ordinary bacterial contamination of foods of vegetable origin may supply the minute amounts of this vitamin required for normal function. The 1984 Total Diet Survey showed cobalt intakes of the American population in the range of 6.3 to 10.8 μg/day for adults and 7.6 to 11.6 μg/day for 14- to 16-year-olds (Pennington and Jones, 1987).

Strict vegetarians who avoid all animal products may become deficient in vitamin B_{12}; however, the deficiency may only develop during a period of 3 to 6 years and sometimes never.

The dietary requirement for cobalt for people 7 years and older is expressed as 3 μg/day of vitamin B_{12} (see Chapter 6).

Deficiency

A deficiency of cobalt occurs only as it is related to a vitamin B_{12} deficiency. Insufficient vitamin B_{12} causes a macrocytic anemia. A genetic defect limiting vitamin B_{12} absorption results in pernicious anemia, which is treated appropriately with massive doses of the vitamin. These forms of anemia are discussed in detail in Chapter 32.

Toxicity

A high intake of inorganic cobalt in animal diets has been shown to produce polycythemia (overproduction of red blood cells), hyperplasia of bone marrow, reticulocytosis, and increased blood volume.

Selenium

Interest in selenium was concerned initially with its toxicity, because selenium poisoning was identified in animals grazing on land with high levels of this element. Later, a positive role was identified when selenium was shown to protect vitamin E–deficient rats against liver necrosis. In 1973, *glutathione peroxidase* was discovered to be a selenoenzyme and the major active form of selenium in tissues.

Selenium is metabolized in anionic form. Tissue levels are influenced by dietary intake and are reflective of the geochemical environment. Regions of North America deficient in selenium are northeastern, Pacific, southwestern, and extreme southeastern United States and north central and eastern Canada. Low selenium areas of the world include parts of China, Finland, and New Zealand.

Functions

Most of the pathologic changes observed in selenium deficiency can be explained on the basis of glutathione peroxidase, which acts together with other antioxidants and free-radical scavengers to reduce cellular peroxides to water and corresponding alcohols.

The antioxidant effects of selenium and vitamin E may reinforce each other by overlap of remedial action. Selenium functions with tocopherol to protect cell and organelle membranes from oxidative damage, to facilitate union between oxygen and hydrogen at the end of the metabolic chain, to transfer ions across cell membranes, and to aid in immunoglobulin and ubiquinone synthesis.

Glutathione peroxidase acts in the cytosol and mitochondrial matrix, whereas vitamin E is present in cell membranes. Other selenium-dependent enzymes, such as glycine reductase, have been identified in bacterial systems. In addition, selenium is incorporated in the amino acid portion of transfer RNA in microorganisms.

Absorption and Excretion

Absorption of selenium, which occurs in the upper segment of the small intestine, is more efficient when the animal is deficient. Selenium is transported initially by albumin and subsequently by alpha-2 globulin. Increased intake frequently results in increased excretion in the urine.

Selenium status is assessed by measuring selenium or glutathione peroxidase in plasma, platelets, and erythrocytes, or selenium in whole blood or urine. Erythrocyte selenium is an indicator of long-term status.

Recommended Dietary Allowance

A recommended allowance for selenium was defined for the first time in the 1989 RDA as 55 to 70 μg for adult women and men, respectively, and 40 to 50 μg/day for adolescents. The RDA for children is 20 to 30 μg/day, and the RDA for infants is 10 to 15 μg/day. Pregnancy increases the RDA by 10 μg, and lactation increases it still further (Table 7–19). Requirements may increase with the unsaturated fatty acid content of the diet.

TABLE 7–19. Recommended Dietary Allowances for Selenium*

Age (Years)	RDA (μg)
Infants	
0.0–0.5	10
0.5–1.0	15
Children	
1–3	20
4–6	20
7–10	30
Males	
11–14	40
15–18	50
19–24	70
25–50	70
51+	70
Females	
11–14	45
15–18	50
19–24	55
25–50	55
51+	55
Pregnant	65
Lactating	
1st 6 mo	75
2nd 6 mo	75

* Reprinted with permission from *Recommended Dietary Allowances*, 10th ed., c. 1989 by the National Academy of Sciences. Published by National Academy Press, Washington, DC.

Sources and Intakes

As yet there is no comprehensive table of the selenium composition of foods. Concentration in foods depends on the selenium content of soil and water where the food was grown. A further complication, common to other trace elements, is the continuing improvement of analysis techniques, which tends to cast doubt on early values. Table 7–20 lists the selenium concentrations of some foods.

Foods recognized as major sources of selenium are brazil nuts, seafoods, kidney, liver, meat, and poultry, whereas fruits and vegetables are low in selenium content. Grains vary depending on where they were grown.

Selenium content and glutathione peroxidase activity in human milk are influenced directly by maternal selenium nutrition (Mannan and Picciano, 1987). Blood concentration reflects the average dietary intake, and status of the human population in some regions tends to follow the pattern of selenium status of the livestock in the region.

Data from the 1986 Total Diet Study showed that the average selenium intake was 70 to 120 μg/day for adults and up to 110 μg/day for children. These are all higher than the RDA (Pennington et al, 1989). Mean intakes of 19 and 13 μg/day in men and women, respectively, have been described in a low selenium area where Keshan disease is present (Yang et al, 1988).

Deficiency

Despite a wide range of intake, selenium deficiency is rare in humans. Selenium status of humans can be categorized, ranging from deficiency to toxicity, as (1) overt clinical deficiency (blood levels less than 10 to 15 mg/ml); (2) no recognized human problems, but livestock requires selenium supplementation (blood levels in humans 40 to 75 μg/ml; intake 20 to 50 μg/day); (3) selenium adequate areas (blood levels 80 to 250 μg/ml; livestock have problems); and (4) high selenium areas (blood levels greater than 300 μg/ml; toxicity occurs in animals).

Two human diseases occur in areas where the soil is low in selenium. *Keshan disease* is a cardiomyopathy that mainly affects children and was first observed in the Keshan province of China. It can be prevented by supplementation of individuals at risk; however, if the disease is established, it does not respond to supplementation, probably because other causes contribute to the myopathy. *Kashin-Beck disease* in preadolescent and adolescent children initially involves symmetric stiffness, swelling, and often pain in the interphalangeal joints of the fingers, followed by a generalized osteoarthritis in which elbows, knees, and ankles are also involved (Sokoloff, 1988).

Selenium deficiency has occasionally been reported in malnourished patients maintained on long-term TPN (Brown et al, 1986.) Low blood levels have also been seen in some patients receiving long-term enteral nutrition, suggesting that long-term selenium status of these patients should be monitored (Feler et al, 1987). Selenium deficiency in patients with cystic fibrosis suggests that supplementation should be considered after assessment of underlying malnutrition (Dworkin et al, 1987) (see Chapter 34).

Selenium intake may be related to cancer mortality. Patients with cancer have lowered plasma selenium levels. Statistical analysis of data has shown lower cancer mortality in states with higher levels of selenium in forage crops and grains.

Although it has been suggested that human heart disease is due in part to dietary inadequacy of selenium and vitamin E, no clear relationships have been found between the risk of cardiovascular disease and low selenium and vitamin levels (Kok et al, 1987).

TABLE 7–20. Selenium Content of Selected Foods*

Food	μg
Brazil nuts, ¼ cup	380
Snapper, baked, 3 oz	148
Halibut, baked, 3 oz	113
Salmon, baked, 3 oz	70
Scallops, steamed, 3 oz	70
Clams, steamed, 20	52
Oysters, raw, ¼ cup	35
Lasagna, with meat, 1 piece	34
Wheat germ, toasted, ¼ cup	28
Molasses, blackstrap, 2 T	25
Sunflower seeds, ¼ cup	25
Granola, 1 cup	23
Ground beef, 3 oz	22
Chicken, breast, baked, 3 oz	17
Bread, whole wheat, 1 slice	16
Egg, 1	12
Milk, 2% fat, 1 cup	6
Cheese, cheddar, 1 oz	4

* From Hands ES: Food Finder: Food Sources of Vitamins and Minerals, 2nd ed. Salem, OR, ESHA Research, 1990.

Toxicity

Indicators of selenium toxicity and the level of dietary intake at which toxicity occurs are not known.

Manganese

Until 1972 when the first report of manganese deficiency in humans appeared it was doubted that such a deficiency could occur in humans (Doisy, 1973). Symptoms were weight loss, transient dermatitis, occasional nausea and vomiting, changes in color, and slow growth of hair and beard. Manganese deficiency in animals has been shown to affect reproductive capacity, pancreatic function, and several aspects of carbohydrate metabolism.

Functions

Concentration of the 10 to 20 mg of manganese in the adult human body tends to be high in tissues rich in mitochondria. Manganese is a component of several enzymes, including glutamine synthetase, pyruvate carboxylase, and mitochondrial superoxide dismutase. It is associated with the formation of connective and bony tissues, growth and reproduction, and carbohydrate and lipid metabolism.

Absorption and Excretion

Manganese is carried by *transmanganin,* a plasma protein, but the mechanism of absorption is unknown. Absorbed manganese appears rapidly in the bile and is excreted in the feces. Tissue levels seem to be regulated by selective excretion via bile. Concentration in the liver increases in patients with liver disease.

Estimated Safe and Adequate Daily Dietary Intake

In 1989 an ESADDI for manganese for adults and children 11 years and older in the range of 2 to 5 mg/day was established. One to 3 mg/day is suggested for children, depending on the age of the child (Table 7–21).

Sources and Intakes

The manganese content of foods varies greatly. The richest sources are whole grains, legumes, nuts, and tea. Fruits and vegetables are moderate sources. Animal tissues, seafood and dairy products are poor sources. Relatively high amounts occur in instant coffee and tea. Human milk is relatively low in manganese.

The Total Diet Study of 1986 indicated that the average manganese intake of adult males was 2.67 to 2.9 mg/day and was 2.2 to 2.3 mg/day for women, within the range of the ESADDI. In teenagers, the intake was 1.8 to 2.8 mg/day and 1.1 to 1.5 mg/day for older infants and 2-year-olds, respectively (Pennington et al, 1989). Based on the apparent lack of manganese deficiency in the population, these intakes appear to be sufficient (Food and Nutrition Board, 1989).

TABLE 7–21. Estimated Safe and Adequate Daily Dietary Intakes for Manganese*

	Age (Years)	ESADDI (mg)
Infants	0–0.5	0.3–0.6
	0.5–1	0.6–1.0
Children and Adolescents	1–3	1.0–1.5
	4–6	1.5–2.0
	7–10	2.0–3.0
	11+	2.0–5.0
Adults		2.0–5.0

* Reprinted with permission from *Recommended Dietary Allowances,* 10th ed., c. 1989 by the National Academy of Sciences. Published by National Academy Press, Washington, DC.

Deficiency

Data on physiologic effects resulting from manganese deficiency are confined to the results of animal studies. These have established the essentiality of manganese for reproduction. Sterility occurs in both sexes; striking skeletal abnormalities and ataxia characterize the offspring of deficient mothers.

Toxicity

Manganese toxicity has occurred in miners as a result of absorption of manganese through the respiratory tract. The excess, which accumulates in the liver and central nervous system, produces Parkinson-like symptoms.

Molybdenum

An interrelationship among molybdenum, copper, and sulfate absorption has been demonstrated in livestock and between molydenum intake and copper excretion in both humans and animals. Individuals on long-term TPN have displayed symptoms of molybdenum deficiency, including mental changes and abnormalities of sulfur and purine metabolism.

Xanthine oxidase, aldehyde oxidase, and sulfite oxidase, all enzymes that catalyze oxidation-reduction reactions, require a prosthetic group containing molybdenum. Sulfite oxidase is important to the degradation of cysteine and methionine and catalyzes the formation of sulfate from sulfite. Genetic sulfite oxidase deficiency is a fatal disorder resulting in a drastic reduction in brain size (Rajagopalan, 1987). Whether molybdenum is involved in the response of some asthmatics to sulfites is not known.

Molybdenum is found in minute amounts in the body, is readily absorbed from the gastrointestinal tract, and is excreted mainly in the urine.

Estimated Safe and Adequate Daily Dietary Intake

The daily requirement of molybdenum is not known; however, the 1989 ESADDI is 75 to 250 μg/day for adolescents and adults. Depending on the age of the child, the estimated safe intake is 25 to 150 μg/day (Table 7–22).

An excessive intake of 10 to 15 μg/day is associated with incidence of a gout-like syndrome (Nielsen, 1988).

TABLE 7–22. Estimated Safe and Adequate Daily Dietary Intakes for Molybdenum*

	Age (Years)	ESADDI (μg)
Infants	0–0.5	15–30
	0.5–1	20–40
Children and Adolescents	1–3	25–50
	4–6	30–75
	7–10	50–150
	11+	75–250
Adults		75–250

* Reprinted with permission from *Recommended Dietary Allowances*, 10th ed., c. 1989 by the National Academy of Sciences. Published by National Academy Press, Washington, DC.

Sources and Intakes

Molybdenum is distributed widely in commonly used foods, such as legumes, whole-grain cereals, milk and milk products, and dark green leafy vegetables. Intakes range from 50 μg/day in infants to peaks of 80 and 126 μg/day for 14- to 16-year-old females and males, respectively. Intakes decrease slowly to 74 and 101 μg/day for 60- to 65-year-old females and males, respectively (Pennington and Jones, 1987).

Summary Table

Information on the minerals known to be required by humans is summarized in Table 7–23.

TRACE ELEMENTS: REQUIREMENTS UNDEFINED

Silicon

Silicon has been recognized as an essential trace element only within the last 2 decades. The highest concentrations are in the epidermis and connective tissue. Silicon plays a role in initiating calcification of bone and promotes the synthesis of collagen.

Silicon is absorbed readily in the form of silicic acid and is excreted in the urine. Age, sex, and some hormones affect the concentration in tissues and blood. The concentration in plasma averages 0.5 mg/l.

With the exception of chicken skin, animal foods are poor sources of silicon. Plant foods, particularly unrefined grains, contain large amounts. The most concentrated source of silicon is beer.

Vanadium

Vanadium, named after the Scandinavian goddess of beauty, youth, and luster, was established as essential based on data from four laboratories on two different species.

Vanadium *in vitro* inhibits $Na^{+}K^{+}Ca^{2+}$ATPase and other phosphoryl transfer enzymes, but whether it performs a regulatory function under normal physiologic conditions is not clear. To date, no mammalian metalloproteins containing vanadium have been identified. Intakes range from 3 μg/day for infants 6 to 11 months of age to about 11 μg/day for adolescents and young adult males (Pennington and Jones, 1987).

Good sources of vanadium are grains and grain products and cereals. Meat, fish, and poultry contain moderate amounts.

Tin

The presence of tin in tissues was attributed originally to environmental contamination; however, careful work has met the standards of essentiality by demonstrating that tin produces growth acceleration in rats.

Tin tends to form covalent linkages and is similar to carbon in this respect. Tin has been shown to exert a potent induction effect on heme oxygenase, enhancing heme breakdown in the kidney and impairing heme-dependent cellular functions such as drug biotransformations mediated by cytochrome P-450.

A large proportion of tin is found in the lipid-extractable portion of commercial fats.

Nickel

Nickel was found in 1974 to be essential for chicks, rats, miniature pigs, and goats. The significance of alterations in blood nickel concentrations seen in a variety of pathologic conditions is not known.

Nickel is consistently present in RNA and DNA. It may stabilize the tertiary structure of nucleic acids and proteins or function as a co-factor or structural component of enzymes. It is important in iron absorption, in which it enhances the absorption of relatively unavailable ferric iron.

Nuts, some grains and grain products, and some legumes are good sources of dietary nickel. Relatively little occurs in foods of animal origin. Estimated intake of nickel in the FDA Total Diet Study ranged from about 70 μg/day for 6- to 11-month-old infants to slightly more than twice that amount (163 μg/day) for teenage males (Pennington and Jones, 1987).

Additional Trace Elements

Arsenic was thought to be an essential trace element, but this has not been confirmed. *Boron* was thought to have no function until recently, when studies with rats and chicks showed that boron affects metabolism of major minerals. In a study of postmenopausal women, boron supplementation produced changes that were consistent with the prevention of calcium loss and bone demineralization (Nielsen et al, 1987) (see Chapter 23).

TABLE 7–23. Minerals in Human Nutrition

Mineral	Location in Body and Some Biologic Functions	RDA* or ESADDI† for Adults	Food Sources	Comments on Likelihood of a Deficiency
I. Macronutrients essential at levels of 100 mg/day or more				
Calcium	99% in bones and teeth. Ionic calcium in body fluids essential for ion transport across cell membranes. Calcium is also bound to protein, citrate, or inorganic acids.	800 mg 1,200 mg for women 19–24 yr	Milk and milk products, sardines, clams, oysters, kale, turnip greens, mustard greens, tofu.	Dietary surveys indicate that many diets do not meet recommended dietary allowances for calcium. Since bone serves as a homeostatic mechanism to maintain calcium level in blood, many essential functions are maintained, regardless of diet. Long-term dietary deficiency is probably one of the factors responsible for development of osteoporosis in later life.
Phosphorus	About 80% in inorganic portion of bones and teeth. Phosphorus is a component of every cell and of highly important metabolites, including DNA, RNA, ATP (high energy compound), and phospholipids. Important to pH regulation.	800 mg 1,200 mg for women 19–24 yr	Cheese, egg yolk, milk, meat, fish, poultry, whole-grain cereals, legumes, nuts.	Dietary inadequacy not likely to occur if protein and calcium intake are adequate.
Magnesium	About 50% in bone. Remaining 50% is almost entirely inside body cells with only about 1% in extracellular fluid. Ionic Mg functions as an activator of many enzymes and thus influences almost all processes.	350 mg for male, 280 mg for female	Whole-grain cereals, tofu, nuts, meat, milk, green vegetables, legumes, chocolate.	Dietary inadequacy considered unlikely, but conditioned deficiency is often seen in clinical medicine, associated with surgery, alcoholism, malabsorption, loss of body fluids, certain hormonal and renal diseases.
Sodium	30 to 45% in bone. Major cation of extracellular fluid and only a small amount is inside cell. Regulates body fluid osmolarity, pH, and body fluid volume.	500–3,000 mg	Common table salt, seafoods, animal foods, milk, eggs. Abundant in most foods except fruit.	Dietary inadequacy probably never occurs, although low blood sodium requires treatment in certain clinical disorders. Sodium restriction necessary practice in certain cardiovascular disorders.
Chloride	Major anion of extracellular fluid, functioning in combination with sodium. Serves as a buffer, enzyme activator; component of gastric hydrochloric acid. Mostly present in extracellular fluid; less than 15% inside cells.	750–3,000 mg	Common table salt, seafoods, milk, meat, eggs.	In most cases dietary intake has little significance except in the presence of vomiting, diarrhea, or profuse sweating, when a deficiency may develop.
Potassium	Major cation of intracellular fluid, with only small amounts in extracellular fluid. Functions in regulating pH and osmolarity, and cell membrane transfer. Ion is necessary for carbohydrate and protein metabolism.	2,000 mg	Fruits, milk, meat, cereals, vegetables, legumes.	Dietary inadequacy unlikely, but conditioned deficiency may be found in kidney disease, diabetic acidosis, excessive vomiting, diarrhea, or sweating. Potassium excess may be a problem in renal failure and severe acidosis.
Sulfur	Bulk of dietary sulfur is present in sulfur-containing amino acids needed for synthesis of essential metabolites. Functions in oxidation-reduction reactions. Sulfur also functions in thiamin and biotin, and as inorganic sulfur.	Need for sulfur is satisfied by essential sulfur-containing amino acids.	Protein foods such as meat, fish, poultry, eggs, milk, cheese, legumes, nuts.	Dietary intake is chiefly from sulfur-containing amino acids and adequacy is related to protein intake.
II. Micronutrients essential at levels of a few milligrams				
Iron	About 70% is in hemoglobin; about 26% stored in liver, spleen and bone. Iron is a component of hemoglobin and myoglobin, important in oxygen transfer; also present in serum transferrin and certain enzymes. Almost none in ionic form.	10 mg for male, 15 mg for female	Liver, meat, egg yolk, legumes, whole or enriched grains, dark green vegetables, dark molasses, shrimp, oysters.	Iron-deficiency anemia occurs in women in reproductive years and in infants and preschool children. May be associated in some cases with unusual blood loss, parasites, and malabsorption. Anemia is last effect of deficient state.
Zinc	Present in most tissues, with higher amounts in liver, voluntary muscle and bone. Constituent of many enzymes and insulin; of importance in nucleic acid metabolism.	15 mg for male, 12 mg for female	Oysters, shellfish, herring, liver, legumes, milk, wheat bran.	Extent of dietary inadequacy in this country not known. Conditioned deficiency may be seen in systemic childhood illnesses and in patients who are nutritionally depleted or have been subjected to severe stress, such as surgery.

Table continued on the following page

TABLE 7–23. Minerals in Human Nutrition (*Continued*)

Mineral	Location in Body and Some Biologic Functions	RDA* or ESADDI† for Adults	Food Sources	Comments on Likelihood of a Deficiency
Copper	Found in all body tissues; larger amounts in liver, brain, heart, and kidney. Constituent of enzymes and of ceruloplasmin and erythrocuprein in blood. May be integral part of DNA or RNA molecule.	1.5–3 mg	Liver, shellfish, whole grains, cherries, legumes, kidney, poultry, oysters, chocolate, nuts.	No evidence that specific deficiencies of copper occur in the human. Menkes' disease is genetic disorder resulting in copper deficiency.
Iodine	Constituent of thyroxine and related compounds synthesized by thyroid gland. Thyroxine functions in control of reactions involving cellular energy.	150 μg	Iodized table salt, seafoods, water and vegetables in nongoitrous regions.	Iodization of table salt is recommended especially in areas where food is low in iodine.
Manganese	Highest concentration is in bone; also relatively high concentrations in pituitary, liver, pancreas and gastrointestinal tissue. Constituent of essential enzyme systems; rich in mitochondria of liver cells.	2.5–5.0 mg	Beet greens, blueberries, whole grains, nuts, legumes, fruit, tea.	Unlikely that deficiency occurs in humans.
Fluoride	Present in bone and teeth. In optimal amounts in water and diet, reduces dental caries and may minimize bone loss.	1.5–4.0 mg	Drinking water (1 ppm), tea, coffee, rice, soybeans, spinach, gelatin, onions, lettuce.	In areas where fluoride content of water is low, fluoridation of water (1 ppm) has been found beneficial in reducing incidence of dental caries.
Molybdenum	Constituent of an essential enzyme xanthine oxidase and of flavoproteins.	75–250 μg	Legumes, cereal grains, dark green leafy vegetables, organs.	No information.
Cobalt	Constituent of cyanocobalamin (vitamin B_{12}), occurring bound to protein in foods of animal origin. Essential to normal function of all cells, particularly cells of bone marrow, nervous system, and gastrointestinal system.	2.0 μg of vitamin B_{12}	Liver, kidney, oysters, clams, poultry, milk.	Primary dietary inadequacy is rare except when no animal products are consumed. Deficiency may be found in such conditions as lack of gastric intrinsic factor, gastrectomy, and malabsorption syndromes.
Selenium	Associated with fat metabolism, vitamin E, and antioxidant functions.	70 μg—male 55 μg—female	Grains, onions, meats, milk, vegetables variable—depends on selenium content of soil.	Keshan disease is a selenium deficient state. Deficiency has occurred in patients receiving long-term TPN without selenium.
Chromium	Associated with glucose metabolism.	0.05–0.2 mg	Corn oil, clams, wholegrain cereals, meats, drinking water variable.	Deficiency found in severe malnutrition, may be factor in diabetes in the elderly and cardiovascular diseases.
Tin Nickel Vanadium Silicon	Now known to be essential but no RDA or ESADDI established.			

* RDA = recommended dietary allowance.
† ESADDI = estimated safe and adequate daily dietary intake.

CITED REFERENCES

Anderson RA: Chromium metabolism and its role in disease processes in man. Clin Physiol Biochem 4:31, 1986.

Anderson RA and Kozlovsky AS: Chromium intake, absorption, and excretion of subjects consuming self-selected diets. Am J Clin Nutr 41:1177, 1985.

Anderson RA et al: Chromium intake and excretion of patients receiving total parenteral nutrition: Effects of supplemental chromium. J Trace Elem Exper Med 1:9, 1988.

Aumont G et al: Iodine content of dairy milk in France in 1983 and 1984. J Food Protection 50:490, 1987.

Black MR et al: Zinc supplements and serum lipids in young adult white males. Am J Clin Nutr 47:970, 1988.

Brown MR et al: Proximal muscle weakness and selenium deficiency associated with long-term parenteral nutrition. Am J Clin Nutr 43:549, 1986.

Copper deficiency induced by megadoses of zinc. Nutr Rev 43:148, 1985.

Cordano A and Graham GG: Copper deficiency complicating severe chronic intestinal malabsorption. Pediatrics 38:596, 1966.

Crofton RW et al: Inorganic zinc and the intestinal absorption of ferrous iron. Am J Clin Nutr 50:141, 1989.

Dinsmore WW et al: The absorption of Zn from a standardized meal in alcoholics and in normal volunteers. Am J Clin Nutr 42:688, 1985.

Discher PWF and Girous A: Iodine content of a representative Canadian diet. J Can Diet Assoc 48:24, 1987.

Doisy EA Jr: Micronutrient controls on biosynthesis of clotting proteins and cholesterol. *In* Hemphill DD (ed): Trace Substances in Environmental Health, Vol VI. Columbia, MO, University of Missouri, 1973, pp 193–199.

Dworkin B et al: Low blood selenium levels in patients with cystic fibrosis compared to controls and healthy adults. JPEN 11:38, 1987.

Feler AG et al: Subnormal concentrations of serum selenium and plasma carnitine in chronically tube-fed patients. Am J Clin Nutr 45:476, 1987.

Food and Nutrition Board, National Research Council, National Academy of Sciences: Recommended Dietary Allowances, 10th ed. Washington, DC, National Academy Press, 1989.

Fosmire GJ: Zinc toxicity. Am J Clin Nutr 51:225, 1990.

Freund H, Alamian S, and Fischer JE: Chromium deficiency during total parenteral nutrition. JAMA 241:496, 1979.

Halsted JA et al: Zinc deficiency in man—the Shivaz experiment. Am J Med 43:277, 1972.

Hambidge KM et al: Zinc nutrition of preschool children in the Denver Head Start program. Am J Clin Nutr 29:734, 1976.

Heaney RP and Weaver CM: Oxalate: Effect on calcium absorbability. Am J Clin Nutr 50:830, 1989.

Heaney RP, Weaver CM, and Recker RR: Calcium absorbability from spinach. Am J Clin Nutr 47:707, 1988.

Heaney RP et al: Meal effects on calcium absorption. Am J Clin Nutr 49:372, 1989.

Jeejeebhoy KN et al: Chromium deficiency, glucose intolerance and neuropathy reversed by chromium supplementation in a patient receiving long-term total parenteral nutrition. Am J Clin Nutr 30:531, 1977.

Jensen R, Closson W, and Rothenberg R: Selenium intoxication—New York. MMWR 33:157, 1984.

King JC: Do women using oral contraceptive agents require extra zinc? J Nutr 117:217, 1986.

Kok FJ et al: Serum selenium, vitamin antioxidants and cardiovascular mortality: A 9-year follow up study in the Netherlands. Am J Clin Nutr 45:462, 1987.

Leverett DH: Fluorides and the changing prevalence of dental caries. Science 217:26, 1982.

Mannan S and Picciano MF: Influence of maternal selenium status on human milk selenium concentration and glutathione peroxidase activity. Am J Clin Nutr 46:95, 1987.

Marie PJ et al: Histological osteomalacia due to dietary calcium deficiency in children, N Engl J Med 307:584, 1982.

Marier JR: Magnesium content of the food supply in the modern-day world. Magnesium 5:1, 1986.

McCarron DA and Morris CD: The calcium deficiency hypothesis of hypertension. Ann Int Med 107:919, 1987.

Monsen ER: Iron nutrition and absorption: Dietary factors which impact iron bioavailability. J Am Diet Assoc 88:786, 1988.

Moser-Veillon PB: Zinc: Consumption patterns and dietary recommendations. J Am Diet Assoc 90:1089, 1990.

Nielsen FH et al: Effect of dietary boron on mineral, estrogen and testosterone metabolism in postmenopausal women. FASEB J 1:394, 1987.

Nielsen FH: Ultratrace minerals. *In* Shils ME and Young VR (eds): Modern Nutrition in Health and Disease, 7th ed. Philadelphia, Lea & Febiger, 1988.

Offenbacher EG et al: Metabolic chromium balances in men. Am J Clin Nutr 44:77, 1986.

Ophaug RH, Singer L, and Harland BF: Dietary fluoride intake of 6-month and 2-year-old children in four dietary regions of the United States. Am J Clin Nutr 42:701, 1985.

Pennington JAT and Jones JW: Molybdenum, nickel, cobalt, vanadium, and strontium in total diets. J Am Diet Assoc 87:1644, 1987.

Pennington JAT, Young BE, and Wilson DB: Nutritional elements in U.S. diets: Results from the Total Diet Study, 1982 to 1986. J Am Diet Assoc 89:659, 1989.

Pennington JAT et al: Mineral content of foods and total diets: The Selected Minerals in Foods Survey, 1982–1984. J Am Diet Assoc 86:876, 1986.

Pollitt E, Greenfield D, and Leibel RL: Behavioral effects of iron deficiency among preschool children in Cambridge, MA. Fed Proc 37:487, 1976.

Prasad AS: Zinc and growth and development and spectrum of human zinc deficiency. J Am Coll Nutr 7:377, 1988.

Prasad AS et al: Zinc metabolism in patients with the syndrome of iron deficiency anemia, hepatosplenomegaly, dwarfism and hypogonadism. J Lab Clin Med 61:537, 1963.

Procopis P, Camakaris J, and Danks DM: A milk form of Menkes' syndrome. J Pediatr 98:97, 1981.

Rajagopalan KV: Molybdenum—an essential trace element. Nutr Rev 45:321, 1987.

Riales B and Albrink MJ: Effect of chromium chloride supplementation on glucose tolerance and serum lipids including high density lipoprotein of adult men. Am J Clin Nutr 34:2670, 1981.

Schuette SA and Linkswiler HM: Calcium. *In* Olson RE (ed): Nutrition Review's Present Knowledge in Nutrition. Washington, DC, The Nutrition Foundation, Inc, 1984.

Singer L, Ophaug RH, and Harland BF: Fluoride intake of young male adults in the United States. Am J Clin Nutr 33:328, 1980.

Smit Vanderkooy, PD and Gibson RS: Food consumption patterns of Canadian preschool children in relation to zinc and growth status. Am J Clin Nutr 45:609, 1987.

Soemantri AG, Pollitt E, and Kim I: Iron deficiency anemia and educational achievement. Am J Clin Nutr 42:1221, 1985.

Sokoloff L: Kashin-Beck disease: Current status. Nutr Rev 46:113, 1988.

Solomons NW: Zinc and copper. *In* Shils ME and Young VR (eds): Modern Nutrition in Health and Disease, 7th ed. Philadelphia, Lea & Febiger, 1988.

Sowers MR, Wallace RB, and Lemke JH: The relationship of bone mass and fracture history to fluoride and calcium intake: A study of three communities. Am J Clin Nutr 44:889, 1986.

Stanbury JB: Iodine. *In* Shils ME and Young VR (eds): Modern Nutrition in Health and Disease, 7th ed. Philadelphia, Lea & Febiger, 1988.

Subcommittee for the Study of Endemic Goiter and Iodine Deficiency of the European Thyroid Association: Goitre and iodine deficiency in Europe. Lancet 2:1289, 1985.

Sweeney EA and Shaw JH: Nutrition in relation to dental medicine. *In* Shils ME and Young VR (eds): Modern Nutrition in Health and Disease, 7th ed. Philadelphia, Lea & Febiger, 1988.

Taylor PG et al: Daily physiological iron requirements in children. J Am Diet Assoc 88:454, 1988.

Turnlund JR: Copper nutriture, bioavailability, and the influence of dietary factors. J Am Diet Assoc 88:303, 1988.

USDA: Nationwide Food Consumption Survey: Continuing Survey of Food Intakes by Individuals: Women 19–50 years and Their Children 1–5 years, 1 Day, 1985. Report No. 85-1, Nutrition Monitoring Division, Human Nutrition Information Service, Hyattsville, MD, USDA, 1985.

USDA: Nationwide Food Consumption Survey: Continuing Survey of Food Intakes by Individuals: Men 19–50 Years, 1 Day, 1985. Report No. 85-3, Nutrition Monitoring Division, Human Nutrition Information Service, Hyattsville, MD, USDA, 1986.

Vallee BL: Zinc: Biochemistry, physiology, toxicology and clinical pathology. BioFactors 1:31, 1988.

Whitney SJ and Whitney HL: Effect of dietary caffeine and theophylline on urinary calcium excretion in the adult rat. J Nutr 117:1224, 1987.

Yang G et al: Selenium-related endemic diseases and the daily selenium requirement of humans. World Rev Nutr Diet 55:98, 1988.

ADDITIONAL REFERENCES

General

Murphy SP and Calloway DH: Nutrient intakes of women in NHANES II emphasizing trace minerals, fiber and phytate. J Am Diet Assoc 86:1366, 1986.

Nielsen FH: Nutritional significance of the ultratrace elements. Nutr Rev 46:337, 1988.

Sandstead HH: A brief history of the influence of trace elements on brain function. Am J Clin Nutr 43:293, 1986.

Symposium on trace elements and human health. Proc Nutr Soc 47:21, 1988.

USDA: Nationwide Food Consumption Survey: Continuing Survey of Food Intakes by Individuals: Women 19–50 Years and Their Children 1–5 years, 1 Day, 1986. Report No. 86-1, Nutrition Monitoring Division, Human Nutrition Information Service, Hyattsville, MD, USDA, 1987.

USDA: Nationwide Food Consumption Survey: Continuing Survey of Food Intakes by Individuals: Women 19–50 Years and Their Children 1–5 years, 4 Days, 1986. Report No. 86-3, Nutrition

Monitoring Division, Human Nutrition Information Service, Hyattsville, MD, USDA, 1988.

Calcium and Phosphorus

Bronner F: Intestinal calcium absorption: Mechanisms and applications. J Nutr 117:1347, 1987.
Calcium absorption from chocolate milk. Nutr MD 14(9):5, 1988.
Calcium supplement absorption. Nutr MD 14(5):2, 1988.
Dawson-Hughes B et al: Effect of lowering dietary calcium intake on fractional whole body calcium retention. J Clin Endocrin Metab 67:62, 1988.
Dietary caffeine and calcium excretion. Nutr Rev 46:232, 1988.
Enhancing calcium absorption. Nutr MD 15(10):8, 1989.
Heaney RP and Recker RR: Distribution of calcium absorption in middle-aged women. Am J Clin Nutr 43:299, 1986.
Heaney RP, Recker RR, and Hinders SM: Variability of calcium absorption. Am J Clin Nutr 47:262, 1988.
Mickelsen O and Marsh AG: Calcium requirement and diet. Nutr Today 24:28, 1989.
Miller JZ et al: Calcium absorption from calcium carbonate and a new form of calcium (CCM) in healthy male and female adolescents. Am J Clin Nutr 48:1291, 1988.
Mistry AN, Brittin HC, and Stoecker BJ: Availability of iron from food cooked in an iron utensil determined by an in vitro method. J Food Sci 53:1546, 1988.
Not all calcium pills provide calcium. Tufts Univ Diet and Nutrition Letter 6(2):1, 1988.
Resnick LM: Dietary calcium and hypertension. J Nutr 117:1806, 1987.
Sheikh MS et al: Role of vitamin D-dependent and vitamin D-independent mechanisms in absorption of food calcium. J Clin Invest 81:126, 1988.
Spencer H, Kramer L, and Osis D: Do protein and phosphorus cause calcium loss? J Nutr 118:657, 1988.

Magnesium

Brady H, Ryan M, and Horgan J: Magnesium: the forgotten cation. Irish Med J 80:250, 1987.
Franz KB: Magnesium in human nutrition. Nutr MD 14(11):1, 1988.
Magnesium and blood pressure. Nutr MD 14(5):1, 1988.

Iron

Hallberg L, Brune M, and Rossander L: Iron absorption in man: ascorbic acid and dose-dependent inhibition by phytate. Am J Clin Nutr 49:140, 1989.
Hershko C, Peto TEA, and Weatherall DJ: Iron and infection. Br Med J 296:660, 1988.
Iron deficiency and brain proteins. Nutr Rev 45:317, 1987.
Kuvibidila S: Iron deficiency, cell-mediated immunity and resistance against infections: Present knowledge and controversies. Nutr Res 7:989, 1987.
Macfarlane BJ et al: Inhibitory effect of nuts on iron absorption. Am J Clin Nutr 47:270, 1988.
Stevens R et al: Iron and cancer. N Engl J Med 319:1047, 1988.
Woods S et al: Iron metabolism. Am J Gastroenterology 85:1, 1990.

Zinc

Calesnick B and Dinan A: Zinc deficiency and zinc toxicity. Am Fam Phys 37:267, 1988.
Prasad AS: Zinc in growth and development and spectrum of human zinc deficiency. J Am Coll Nutr 7:377, 1988.
Yedrick MK, Kenney MA, and Winterfeldt EA: Iron, copper and zinc status: Response to supplementation with zinc or zinc and iron in adult females. Am J Clin Nutr 49:145, 1989.
Zinc in the elderly. Nutr MD 14(5):2, 1988.

Copper

A unified hypothesis of copper transport and uptake. Nutr Rev 46:332, 1988.
Copper, for where the heart is. Tufts Univ Diet and Nutrition Letter 6(3):1, 1988.
Johnson MA and Kays SE: Copper: Its role in human nutrition. Nutr Today 25:6, 1990.

Iodine

Hershman JM: Iodine intake—Deficiency, excess, and hypersensitivity. Nutr MD 14(5):1, 1988.

Chromium

Anderson RA: Chromium in human health and disease. Nutr MD 14(3):1, 1988.
Offenbacher EG and Pi-Sunyer FX: Chromium in human nutrition. Annu Rev Nutr 8:543, 1988.

Selenium

Burk RF: Newer roles of selenium. J Nutr 119:1051, 1989.
Levander OA: A global view of human selenium nutrition. Annu Rev Nutr 7:227, 1987.
Newly recognized signs of selenium deficiency in humans. Nutr Rev 47:117, 1989.
Schubert A, Holden JM, and Wolf WR: Selenium content of a core group of foods based on a critical evaluation of published data. J Am Diet Assoc 87:285, 1987.
Thomson CD et al: Selenium and vitamin E supplementation: Activities of glutathione peroxidase in human tissues. Am J Clin Nutr 48:316, 1988.

Manganese

Freeland-Graves JH: Manganese: An essential nutrient for humans. Nutr Today 23(6):13, 1988.

Boron

Nielsen FH: Boron—an overlooked element of potential nutritional importance. Nutr Today 23(1):4, 1988.

Aluminum

Caster WO and Wang M: Dietary aluminum and Alzheimer's disease: A review. Sci Total Environ 17:31, 1981.
Pennington JAT: Aluminum content of foods and diets. Food Additives Contamin 5:161, 1988.

CHAPTER 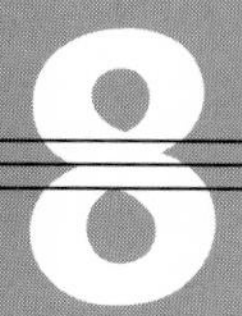

WATER, ELECTROLYTES, AND ACID-BASE BALANCE

Dorice M. Czajka-Narins, Ph.D.

CHAPTER OUTLINE

KEY TERMS

ACID-BASE BALANCE—dynamic state of equilibrium with regard to hydrogen ion concentration in the body

ACIDOSIS—the excessive accumulation of acid or hydrogen ions, or the loss of base from the body

ALKALOSIS—excessive accumulation of base or the loss of hydrogen ions or acid from the body

BUFFER—a proton donor and acceptor system that helps to preserve homeostasis of the hydrogen ion concentration

DEHYDRATION—excessive loss of body water

EDEMA—the abnormal accumulation of fluid in the intercellular tissue spaces or body cavities

ELECTROLYTE—a substance that dissociates into positively and negatively charged ions when dissolved in water

EXTRACELLULAR WATER—the water in the plasma, lymph, spinal fluid, and secretions

HYPERTONIC—describing a solution that, when bathing body cells, causes a net flow of water across the semipermeable cell membrane out of the cell

HYPOTONIC—describing a solution that, when bathing body cells, causes a net flow of water across the semipermeable cell membrane into the cell

INTERCELLULAR (INTERSTITIAL) WATER—the water between and around the cells

INSENSIBLE WATER LOSS—water lost with air expired from the lungs or sweat evaporated from the skin

INTRACELLULAR WATER—water contained within the cell

METABOLIC ALKALOSIS—a disturbance in which the acid-base status of the body shifts toward the alkaline side because of retention of base or loss of noncarbonic acid that is usually due to renal changes or failure

METABOLIC WATER—water derived from the metabolism of carbohydrate, protein, or fat

ONCOTIC PRESSURE (COLLOID OSMOTIC PRESSURE)—the pressure at the capillary membrane due to dissolved proteins in the plasma and interstitial fluids

OSMOLALITY—a measure of the osmotically active particles per kilogram of solvent in which the particles are dispersed

OSMOLARITY—a measure of the osmotically active particles per liter of the entire solution

OSMOTIC PRESSURE—the pressure of a solution directly related to its solute osmolar concentration

RESPIRATORY ALKALOSIS—a disturbance in which the acid-base status of the body shifts toward the alkaline side because of excessive expiration of carbon dioxide

SENSIBLE WATER LOSS—water lost with urine and feces

WATER INTOXICATION—excess water increasing intercellular volume and dilution of body fluids

Water is closer to being a universal solvent than any other material. Water is, however, more than a passive solvent; it also participates actively in reactions and provides form and structure to the cells through the turgor it provides. It also provides a means of stabilizing body temperature.

Electrolytes are substances or compounds that, when dissolved in water, dissociate into positively and negatively charged ions. Electrolytes can be simple inorganic salts of sodium, potassium, or magnesium or complex organic molecules.

Acid-base balance is the dynamic state of equilibrium with regard to hydrogen ion concentration. Marked alterations in rates of chemical reactions can occur with only slight changes in hydrogen ion concentration. Protein-energy malnutrition, illness, trauma, or surgery can cause an alteration in the amount and composition of tissue fluids which, if not corrected, can result in dehydration, shock, and death (Table 8–1).

BODY WATER

Water is the largest single component of the body. Metabolically active cells of the muscle and viscera have the highest concentration, and calcified tissue cells have the lowest concentration. As a percentage of body weight, water varies among individuals, depending on the proportion of muscle to adipose tissue. Total body water decreases significantly with age and is higher in athletes than in nonathletes (Fig. 8–1).

Functions of Water

Water is an essential component of all body tissues. It is the solvent in which many solutes available for cell function are dissolved and is the medium for all reactions. It also participates as a substrate in metabolic reactions and as a structural material in providing form to the cells. Water is essential to the physiologic processes of digestion and absorption and excretion of metabolic and indigestible wastes, as well as to the structure and function of the circulatory system. It acts as a transport medium for nutrients and all body substances. It maintains the physical and chemical constancy of intracellular and extracellular fluids and has a direct role in the maintenance of body temperature. Evaporation of perspiration during warm weather cools the body; 600 kcal of body heat are removed during the evaporation of 1 liter of perspired water.

Loss of 20% of body water may cause death, and a loss of only 10% causes severe disorders (Fig. 8–2). In moderate weather adults can live up to 10 days without water; children can live up to 5 days. In contrast, it is possible to survive without food for several weeks.

Distribution of Body Water

Intracellular water (ICW) consists of the water contained within cells. *Extracellular water* (ECW), commonly estimated to be 20% of body weight, includes the water in plasma, lymph, spinal fluid, and secretions, as well as the *intercellular (interstitial) water* that occurs between and around the cells. Most interstitial water is held in a gel in the intercellular spaces and communicates continually with the plasma through pores in the capillaries. The abnormal accumulation of fluid in the intercellular tissue spaces or body cavities is called *edema*.

The distribution of body water can vary under different circumstances, but the total amount in the body remains relatively constant. Our understanding of body water in health and disease is improving through the use of bioelectrical impedance, a measurement of

TABLE 8–1. Classification of the Four Major Hydrogen Ion Imbalances and Some of the Conditions Leading to These Imbalances

	Pulmonary		Renal	
	Respiratory acidosis	Respiratory alkalosis	Metabolic acidosis	Metabolic alkalosis
Nature of failure Imbalance	↑ H_2CO_3 due to retention of CO_2	↓ H_2CO_3 due to excessive expiration of CO_2 and H_2O	↑ H^+ concentration due to ↑ production or ↑ retention	↓ H^+ concentration due to losses
			OR	OR
			↓ HCO_3^- due to excretion of large amounts of base from ECF	↑ HCO_3^- due to abnormal retention of alkali in ECF
Diseases that may cause	Conditions of ↓ lung surface area, such as emphysema	Aftermath of severe exercise Anxiety reaction	Diarrhea Vomiting Uremia Uncontrolled diabetes mellitus Starvation Drugs High-fat or low-CHO diet	Diuretics ↑ Ingestion of alkali Loss of chloride

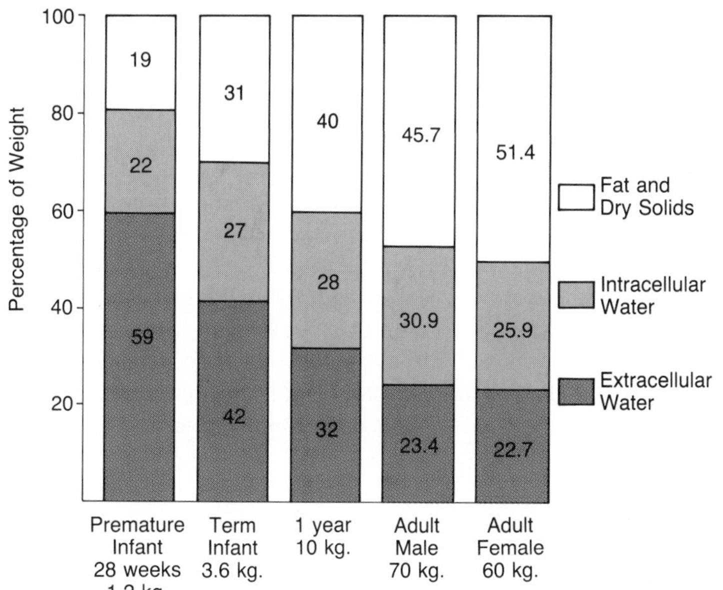

FIGURE 8–1. *Distribution of body water as percentage of body weight. (Data from Foman SJ et al: Body composition of reference children, birth to age ten years. Am J Clin Nutr 35:1169, 1982; and Moore FD et al: Body Cell Mass and Its Supporting Environment. Philadelphia, WB Saunders, 1963.)*

electrical conduction, to estimate body water (Kushner and Schoeller, 1986).

Water Balance

The water content of the fat-free body weight remains fairly constant by homeostatic regulation resulting from interactions among antidiuretic hormone (ADH), the gastrointestinal tract, the kidneys, and the brain. The amount of water taken in daily is approximately equivalent to the amount of water lost (Table 8–2).

Water Intake

In healthy individuals, water intake is controlled mainly by thirst. The thirst control centers are located in the ventromedial and anterior hypothalamus, in close relationship to the centers that regulate ADH. Thirst is stimulated when osmolality increases with a change in volume or when extracellular volume decreases. The sensation of thirst serves as a signal to seek fluids.

Water is ingested as such and also as part of ingested food. The oxidation of these foods in the body also produces *metabolic water* as an end-product. The oxidation of 100 grams of fat, carbohydrate, or protein yields 107, 55, and 41 grams of water, respectively, for a total of approximately 200 to 300 ml/day.

Water is absorbed rapidly because it moves freely by diffusion through membranes. This movement is controlled mainly by osmotic forces generated by the inor-

% Body Weight Lost	*Effect*
0	
	Thirst
1	
2	Stronger thirst, vague discomfort, loss of appetite
3	Decreasing blood volume, impaired physical performance
4	Increased effort for physical work, nausea
5	Difficulty in concentrating
6	Failure to regulate excess temperature
7	
8	Dizziness, labored breathing with exercise; increasing weakness
9	
10	Muscle spasms, delirium, and wakefulness
11	Inability of decreased blood volume to circulate normally; failing renal function

FIGURE 8–2. *Adverse effects of dehydration. (Adapted from Greenleaf JE: The body's need for fluids.* In *Haskell W, Scala J, and Whitten J [eds]: Nutrition and Athletic Performance. Palo Alto, CA, Bull Publishing Co, 1982.)*

TABLE 8–2. Water Balance*
(Average Figures in Milliliters)

			Water Intake
Fluids			1,400
Water in food			700
Water from cellular oxidation of food			200
Total			2,300
		Water Output	
	Normal Temperature	***Hot Weather***	***Prolonged Exercise***
Urine	1,400	1,200	500
Water in feces	100	100	100
Skin (perspiration)	100	1,400	5,000
Insensible Loss			
Skin	350	350	350
Respiratory tract	350	250	650
Total	2,300	3,300	6,600

* From Guyton AC: Textbook of Medical Physiology, 6th ed. Philadelphia, WB Saunders, 1981, p. 392.

ganic ions found in solution in the body (Clinical Insight, below).

When water cannot be taken orally, it may be given intravenously in the form of salt (saline) solutions that resemble closely the fluids of the body, as glucose solutions, or as blood, plasma, or protein hydrolysate mixtures.

Water Elimination

Water loss is normally through the kidneys as urine and as a part of feces (*sensible*, or measurable water), or with air expired from the lungs or sweat evaporated from the skin *(insensible)* (see Table 8–2). The kidney is the main regulator of water loss. Insensible water loss is continuous and usually occurs unconsciously. Perspiration losses vary greatly. Athletes can lose 3 to 4 lb during practice at 80° F and low humidity and even more at higher temperatures and humidity (see Chapter 19).

Under normal conditions, the water component of the 7 to 9 liters of digestive juices and other extracellular fluids secreted daily into the gastrointestinal tract is almost entirely reabsorbed in the ileum and colon, except for about 100 ml that is excreted in the feces. Because this volume of reabsorbed fluid is about twice that of the blood plasma, the loss of large amounts from the gastrointestinal tract in diarrhea may have serious

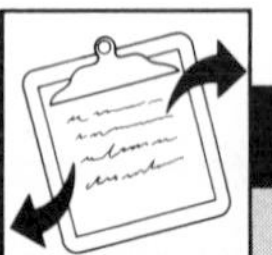

CLINICAL INSIGHT: Osmotic Forces

OSMOTIC PRESSURE

Osmotic pressure is directly proportional to the number of particles in solution and usually refers to pressure at the *cell membrane.*

It is convenient (although not entirely accurate) to consider the osmotic pressure of the intracellular fluid as a function of its content of potassium, which is the predominant cation in the intracellular fluid, whereas the osmotic pressure of the extracellular fluid may be conveniently considered to relate to its content of sodium, the major cation present in extracellular fluid. Although variations in the distribution of sodium and potassium ions are the principal cause of shifts of water between the various fluid compartments, chloride and phosphate can also influence water balance.

Proteins, nondiffusible because of their size, also have an important part in maintaining osmotic equilibrium.

ONCOTIC PRESSURE

Oncotic pressure or *colloid osmotic pressure* is the pressure at the *capillary membrane* due to dissolved proteins in the plasma and interstitial fluids.

The oncotic pressure helps to retain water within the blood vessel, thus preventing the leakage of water from plasma into the interstitial fluid. In disease states such as protein-energy malnutrition, where the protein content of plasma is exceptionally low, water does leak into the interstitial fluids and causes edema.

OSMOLE AND MILLIOSMOLE

Electrolyte concentrations of individual ionic constituents of extracellular or intracellular fluids are expressed in terms of *milliosmoles* per liter.

1 mol (M) = 1 gram-molecular weight of a substance. Dissolved in 1 liter of water, it becomes 1 osmole. 1 milliosmole (mOsm or mO) is 1/1,000th of an osmole.

1 millimol
= 1 milliosmol (mOsm) for a nonelectrolyte (e.g., glucose)
= 2 milliosmols for an electrolyte ($Na^+ + Cl^-$)

One milliosmole dissolved in 1 liter of water has an osmotic pressure of 17 mm Hg.

OSMOLALITY AND OSMOLARITY

Osmolality is a measure of the osmotically active particles per kilogram of the solvent in which the particles are dispersed. It is expressed as milliosmoles of solute per kilogram of solvent or mOsm/kg. *Osmolarity* was formerly the term used to describe concentration in mOsm per liter of the entire solution; however, osmolality is now designated in mOsm/l for most clinical work. In some disease states, such as hyperlipidemia, it makes a difference whether it is stated as mOsm/kg of solvent or per liter of solution.

SERUM OSMOLALITY

Osmolality can be calculated for serum and extracellular fluids as follows:

$$\text{Osmolality} = (\text{serum Na (mEq/l)} \times 2) + \frac{\text{glucose (mg/dl)}}{18} + \frac{\text{BUN (mg/dl)}}{2.8}$$

The average sum of the concentration of all the cations in serum is about 150 mEq/l. This is balanced by 150 mEq/l of anions to make a total serum osmolarity of about 300 mEq/l.

Osmolar imbalance is caused by a gain or loss of water relative to a solute or by a gain or loss of solute relative to water. An osmolality of less than 285 mOsm/l indicates water excess; an osmolality of greater than 295 mOsm/l indicates water deficit.

consequences, particularly for the very young and the very old.

Fluid loss secondary to diarrhea has been responsible for thousands of deaths of children in developing countries. Oral rehydration therapy, a simple mixture of water, sugar, and salts, has been highly effective in reducing the number of deaths (see Chapter 27). Other abnormal losses occur through vomiting, hemorrhage, draining fistulas, exuding of burns, draining of nasogastric and surgical tubes, and the ingestion of diuretics.

When water intake is insufficient or water loss occurs, the kidney compensates by conserving water and excreting a more concentrated urine. Renal tubules increase the reabsorption of water in response to hormonal action of ADH. During dehydration, the specific gravity of urine increases above normal levels of 1.008 to 1.030.

Water balance is related directly to the homeostatic functioning of the internal environment. When excess water is lost, changes in electrolyte balance occur. Dehydration by excess sweating or fluid restriction has frequently been used by young wrestlers trying to "make weight," a harmful practice that can adversely affect performance. Diets such as the Zen macrobiotic diet, which recommends severely restricted intakes of water and other fluids, can be extremely dangerous.

Water intoxication exists when there is an excess of water and intracellular fluid (ICF) volume and osmolar dilution. If an excess of water is given after surgery, trauma, or any condition resulting in a loss of salt and water, and ADH and the kidney are unable to respond, water intoxication can result. The increased volume of ICF causes the cells, particularly the brain cells, to swell, leading to the symptoms of headache, nausea, vomiting, muscle twitching, convulsion with intervening stupor, and death. Papilledema, blurring of vision, and eventual blindness may also result.

Requirement for Water

There is no provision for water storage in the body; therefore, the amount lost every 24 hours must be replaced to maintain health and efficiency. Under ordinary circumstances, a reasonable allowance based on recommended caloric intake is 1 ml/kcal for adults and 1.5 ml/kcal for infants. This translates into 35 ml/kg of usual body weight in adults, 50 to 60 ml/kg for children, and 150 ml/kg for infants. A suitable daily allowance for adults in most cases is 2.5 liters or approximately 2.5 to 3 quarts. Infants have a greater need for water because of the limited capacity of their kidneys for handling the renal solute load, their higher percentage of body water, and their large surface area per unit of body weight.

Thirst is usually an adequate guide for water intake, except in infants, the sick, and sometimes the elderly, in whom the thirst sensation is diminished. Anyone sick enough to be hospitalized, regardless of diagnosis, is at risk of water and electrolyte imbalance. In cases of extreme heat or excessive sweating, thirst may not keep pace with the actual water requirement (see Chapter 19).

During lactation the need for water is increased because of the high amounts required for milk production, theoretically an additional 600 to 700 ml/day (Food and Nutrition Board, 1989). Many successfully lactating women do not consume enough water to satisfy theoretical recommendations and evidently meet their needs with water from foods (Stumbo et al, 1985) (Table 8-3).

The 1985 Nationwide Food Consumption Survey showed that respondents' intake of fluid as nonalcoholic beverages, excluding milk, averaged about 3.5 cups/day (USDA, 1983).

ELECTROLYTES

Electrolytes are substances or compounds that, when dissolved in water, dissociate into positively and negatively charged ions (cations and anions). Electrolytes can be simple inorganic salts of sodium, potassium, or magnesium or complex organic molecules (Table 8-4).

TABLE 8-3. Percentage Water of Some Common Foods*

Food	%
Collards	96
Lettuce (iceberg)	96
Radishes	95
Celery	95
Cabbage (raw)	93
Watermelon	92
Broccoli, beets	91
Snapbeans	89
Milk	88
Carrots	87
Orange	87
Cereals (cooked)	85
Apples	84
Fish (baked flounder)	78
Potatoes (boiled)	77
Eggs	75
Bananas	74
Corn	70
Prunes (cooked)	70
Chicken (roast)	67
Beef (lean), sirloin	59
Cheese, Swiss	42
Bread, white	37
Cake (Devil's food)	24
Butter	16
Almonds	4
Soda crackers	4
Sugar (white)	1
Oils	0

* From Nutritive Value of Foods, US Department of Agriculture. Home Garden Bull No. 72, revised 1985.

TABLE 8–4. Normal Electrolyte Concentration of Serum

Electrolytes	Range of Normal
Cations	
Sodium	136–145 mEq/l
Potassium	3.5–5 mEq/l
Calcium	4.5–5.5 mEq/l (9.0–11 mg/dl)
Magnesium	1.5–2.5 mEq/l (1.8–3 mg/dl)
Anions	
Chloride	96–106 mEq/l
CO_2 (content) TCO_2	24–28.8 mEq/l
Phosphorus (inorganic)	3–4.5 mg/dl (1.9–2.85 mEq/l as HPO_4^{-2})
Sulfate (as S)	0.8–1.2 mg/dl (0.5–0.75 mEq/L as SO_2^{-2})
Lactate	0.7–1.8 mEq/l (6–16 mg/dl)
Protein	6–7.6 g/dl (14–18 mEq/l) Depends on albumin

Sodium

Sodium is the major cation of extracellular fluid. Various intestinal secretions, such as bile and pancreatic juice, contain substantial amounts of sodium. Thirty-five to 40% of the sodium is in the skeleton; however, most of this sodium is unexchangeable or only slowly exchangeable with that in body fluids.

Functions

As the dominant ion of extracellular fluid, sodium regulates the size of this compartment as well as plasma volume. Sodium also aids in the conduction of nerve impulses and the control of muscle contraction.

Absorption and Excretion

Sodium is readily absorbed from the intestine and is carried to the kidneys, where it is filtered out and returned to the blood in amounts needed to maintain appropriate levels. The amount absorbed is proportional to the intake.

About 90 to 95% of normal body sodium loss is via the urine, and the rest is lost in feces and sweat. Normally, the quantity of sodium excreted daily is equal to the amount ingested. Sodium excretion is maintained by a mechanism involving glomerular filtration rate, the cells of the juxtaglomerular apparatus of the kidneys, the renin-aldosterone system, the sympathetic nervous system, circulating catecholamines, and blood pressure.

Regulation of sodium balance is controlled by *aldosterone,* a mineralocorticoid secreted by the adrenal cortex. When blood sodium levels rise, the thirst receptors in the hypothalamus stimulate the thirst sensation. When blood levels are low, the excretion of sodium through the urine decreases.

Estrogen, with its slight resemblance to aldosterone, causes sodium and water retention. Changes in water and sodium balance during the menstrual cycle and pregnancy and with oral contraceptive use are due in part to changes in progesterone and estrogen levels.

Recommended Intake

Daily requirements for sodium are not known. Estimates of human requirements are as low as 200 mg/day. The estimated minimum requirements for all ages as recommended in the 1989 recommended daily allowance (RDA) are shown in Table 8–5. Discussion of the low-salt syndrome appears in Chapter 33.

Acutely excessive intake of sodium leads to edema and hypertension; however, the kidney is usually able to excrete the excess sodium (Fig. 8–3). Of more concern is chronic excessive intake. Recently, an upper limit of 6 g/day of sodium chloride has been recommended, based on the potential role of sodium in the development of hypertension (see Chapter 21) (Food and Nutrition Board, 1989).

Sources

The major source of sodium is sodium chloride, or common table salt, of which sodium constitutes 40%. The mean daily salt intake is about 10 to 12 grams (4 grams of sodium) per capita in Western societies. Approximately 3 grams of the daily intake of salt occurs naturally in foods; 3 grams is added during processing; and 4 grams is added by the individual. Protein foods generally contain more sodium than do vegetables and grains, whereas fruits contain little or none. See Chap-

TABLE 8–5. Estimated Sodium, Chloride, and Potassium Minimum Requirements of Healthy Persons*

Age	Weight (kg)	Sodium (mg)†‡	Chloride (mg)†‡	Potassium (mg)§
Months				
0–5	4.5	120	180	500
6–11	8.9	200	300	700
Years				
1	11.0	225	350	1,000
2–5	16.0	300	500	1,400
6–9	25.0	400	600	1,600
10–18	50.0	500	750	2,000
>18‖	70.0	500	750	2,000

* Reproduced with permission from *Recommended Dietary Allowances,* 10th ed., c. 1989 by the National Academy of Sciences. Published by National Academy Press.

† No allowance has been included for large, prolonged losses from the skin through sweat.

‡ There is no evidence that higher intakes confer any health benefit.

§ Desirable intakes of potassium may considerably exceed these values (~3,500 mg for adults).

‖ No allowance included for growth. Values for those below 18 years assume a growth rate at the 50th percentile reported by the National Center for Health Statistics and averaged for males and females. See Chapter 9 for information on pregnancy and lactation.

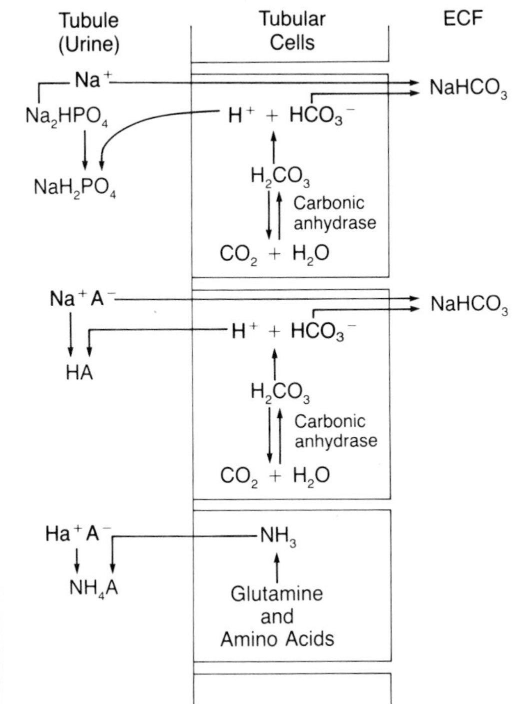

FIGURE 8–3. *Generation of $NaHCO_3$ and clearance of H^+ by the three buffer systems that function in the kidney. (ECF = extracellular fluid; HA = any acid in the body.)*

ter 33 and Appendix Table 1 for further discussion of the sodium content of foods.

Chloride

Functions

Chloride is widely distributed throughout the body as the principal anion of the extracellular fluids. Together with sodium, it helps to maintain water balance and osmotic pressure. The highest concentration is in the cerebrospinal fluid and in the gastric and pancreatic juices. Along with phosphate and sulfate, chloride helps to maintain acid-base balance in the body fluids. Chloride ions maintain osmotic equilibrium in the face of changing levels of bicarbonate in the plasma and red blood cells. It has been suggested that chloride is a regulator of the renin-angiotensin-aldosterone system (Koletsky et al, 1981).

Absorption and Excretion

Chloride is almost completely absorbed in the intestine and is excreted in urine and sweat. Chloride loss parallels sodium loss. Excessive sweat loss is minimized by the action of aldosterone, which acts directly on the sweat glands. Extra chloride is necessary to correct the metabolic alkalosis resulting from disease or from the use of diuretics.

Sources

Most of the chloride ingested in the diet occurs as sodium chloride, and the amount in food and added table salt provides approximately 3 to 9 g/day. Chloride in water contributes to the total, but it is a very small fraction of the 6 grams of chloride consumed in the diet.

Recommended Intake

The safe range of chloride intake for all ages as determined by the Food and Nutrition Board is shown in Table 8–5.

A syndrome of chloride deficiency has been described in infants receiving a chloride-deficient formula. The syndrome is characterized by loss of appetite, failure to thrive, muscle weakness, lethargy, and severe hypokalemic metabolic acidosis (Grossman et al, 1980). See Chapter 21 for the possible role of chloride in hypertension.

Potassium

Functions

Potassium is the major cation of the intracellular fluid and is present in small amounts in the extracellular fluid. Along with sodium, it is involved in the maintenance of normal water balance, osmotic equilibrium, and acid-base balance. Along with calcium it is important in the regulation of neuromuscular activity. Potassium also promotes cellular growth. Potassium level in muscle is related to muscle mass and glycogen storage; therefore, if muscle is being formed, an adequate supply of potassium is essential.

Absorption and Excretion

Potassium is readily absorbed from the small intestine. Eighty to 90% of ingested potassium is excreted in the urine; the remainder is lost in the feces. Normal serum levels are maintained by the kidney through its ability to filter, reabsorb, and excrete potassium under the influence of aldosterone. Ionized potassium is excreted in place of ionized sodium by means of the exchange mechanism in the renal tubules.

Sources

Dietary sources of potassium are given in Chapter 35 and in Appendix Table 1. In general, fruits, vegetables, and fresh meat are good sources of potassium. According to the 1985 Nationwide Food Consumption Survey, the mean potassium intake of women and men 19 to 50 years of age is 1.36 mg/day (USDA, 1987). This can vary widely depending on the intake of fruits and vegetables.

Recommended Intake

A potassium deficiency from inadequate intake is not likely in healthy individuals, because potassium is widely distributed in foods. The minimum requirement for adults is 1.6 to 2 grams (40 to 50 mEq) per day, but higher levels are recommended because of the possible protective effect of potassium against hypertension (Food and Nutrition Board, 1989; National Research Council, 1989). The safe range of recommended intakes for all ages is given in Table 8–4. The average intake is estimated to range from 0.8 to 1.5 grams of potassium per 1,000 kcal. An adequate intake of milk, meats, cereals, vegetables, and fruits will provide ample potassium.

CITED REFERENCES

Food and Nutrition Board, National Research Council: Recommended Dietary Allowances, 10th ed. Washington, DC, National Academy Press, 1989.

Grossman H et al: The dietary chloride deficiency syndrome. Pediatrics 66:366, 1980.

Koletsky RJ et al: Dietary chloride release in normal humans. Am J Physiol 241:F361, 1981.

Kushner RF and Schoeller DA: Estimation of total body water by bioelectrical impedance analysis. Am J Clin Nutr 4:417, 1986.

National Research Council: Diet and Health: Implications for Reducing Chronic Disease Risk. Washington, DC, National Academy Press, 1989.

Stumbo PJ et al: Water intakes of lactating women. Am J Clin Nutr 42:870, 1985.

USDA: Nationwide Food Consumption Survey 1977–78. Food Intakes: Individuals in 48 States, Year 1977–78. Report I-1, Consumer Nutrition Division, Human Nutrition Information Service. Hyattsville, MD, USDA, 1983.

USDA: Nationwide Food Consumption Survey. Continuing Survey of Food Intakes by Individuals. Women 19–50 Years and Their Children 1–5 Years, 4 Days, 1985, Report No. 85-4, Nutrition Monitoring Division, Human Nutrition Information Service. Hyattsville, MD, USDA, 1987.

ADDITIONAL REFERENCES

Askanazi J et al: Fluid and Electrolyte Management in Critical Care. Boston, Butterworths, 1986.

Groer ME: Physiology and Pathophysiology of Body Fluids. St Louis, CV Mosby, 1981.

Guyton AC: Textbook of Medical Physiology, 8th ed. Philadelphia, WB Saunders, 1991.

Kokko JP and Tannen RL: Fluid and Electrolytes. Philadelphia, WB Saunders, 1986.

Masiak MJ et al: Fluids and Electrolytes Through the Life Cycle. Norwalk, CT, Appleton-Century-Crofts, 1985.

Pestana C: Fluids and Electrolytes in the Surgical Patient, 3rd ed. Baltimore, Williams and Wilkins, 1985.

Pullman A et al: Water and Ions in Biological Systems. New York, Plenum Press, 1985.

Rosen RA et al: On the mechanism by which chloride corrects metabolic alkalosis in man. Am J Med 84:449, 1988.

Vanatta JC and Fogelman MJ: Moyer's Fluid Balance: A Clinical Manual, 4th ed. Chicago, Year Book Medical Publishers, Inc, 1988.

Vokes T: Water homeostasis. Annu Rev Nutr 7:383, 1987.

PART 2

NUTRITION IN THE LIFE CYCLE

The importance of nutrition throughout the life cycle seems fairly obvious. After all, we must eat to live. However, the significance of nutrition at specific times of growth, development, and aging is becoming increasingly appreciated.

The effect of proper nutrition during pregnancy on the health of the infant and of the mother in post-childbearing years has long been recognized. It now appears that maternal, and possibly even paternal, nutrition prior to conception affects the health of the newborn.

Establishing good food habits during childhood lessens the possibility of inappropriate eating behavior, which occurs with disturbing frequency during adolescence. Although the influence of proper nutrition on one's own morbidity and mortality usually remains unacknowledged until adulthood, it now appears even more obvious that prevention of the degenerative diseases that appear later in life should begin in childhood.

With the rapid growth in the elderly population has evolved a need to amplify the limited data currently available in that area. Although it is obvious that energy needs decrease with aging, little is known about whether requirements for specific nutrients are increased or decreased. The identification of unique differences in the stages of aging assumes increased significance as it becomes more common for old age to extend well into the ninth decade.

CHAPTER 9

NUTRITION DURING PREGNANCY AND LACTATION

Bonnie S. Worthington-Roberts, Ph.D.*

CHAPTER OUTLINE

KEY TERMS

AMYLOPHAGIA—a form of pica involving consumption of excessive amounts of starch such as laundry starch

COLOSTRUM—the thin, yellow, milky fluid secreted by the mammary gland a few days before and after birth, before the secretion of mature milk

CONGENITAL MALFORMATION—an abnormality present in the infant at birth

ECLAMPSIA—the late stage of pregnancy-induced hypertension characterized by proteinuria and often grand mal seizure occurring near the time of labor

FETAL ALCOHOL SYNDROME—a specific set of abnormal features resulting from exposure of the fetus to alcohol during gestation

GEOPHAGIA—a common pica of pregnancy involving the consumption of dirt or clay

GESTATIONAL DIABETES—diabetes that exists only during pregnancy

HYPEREMESIS GRAVIDARUM—prolonged persistent vomiting during pregnancy

INFANT MORTALITY—infant deaths in the first year of life

LACTATION—the period of secretion of milk

LET-DOWN—a distinct tingling sensation accompanying the movement of milk from the alveoli through the duct system and lactiferous sinuses to the nipple

OXYTOCIN—a hormone from the posterior pituitary that stimulates the movement of milk down to the nipple and the contraction of the uterine muscle

PERINATAL MORTALITY—the number of infant deaths occurring in the period from 28 weeks' gestation to 4 weeks after birth

PICA—compulsive ingestion of unsuitable substances having little or no nutritional value

PREECLAMPSIA—the early stage of pregnancy-induced hypertension

PREGNANCY-INDUCED HYPERTENSION—a syndrome sometimes occurring during pregnancy characterized by hypertension, proteinuria, and edema

PREMENSTRUAL SYNDROME—a syndrome occurring around menses that is characterized by anxiety, mood swings, breast pain, fatigue, and cramps

PROLACTIN—one of the hormones of the anterior pituitary gland that stimulates milk production by alveolar cells

* *Sections of these chapters are modified with permission from Worthington-Roberts BS and Williams SR: Nutrition in Pregnancy and Lactation, 4th ed. St Louis, CV Mosby, 1989.*

PREGNANCY

Numerous factors interact to determine the progress and outcome of pregnancy. Although much remains to be learned about the role of nutrition in modifying this process, it is well accepted that the nutritional status of the pregnant woman affects the outcome of her pregnancy. This is especially true with respect to the birthweight of her infant, a factor closely related to infant mortality.

Effect of Nutritional Status on Pregnancy Outcome

Historical Perspective

The effects of undernutrition and the accompanying stress on previously well-nourished populations have been explored as a consequence of World War II, when severe food deprivation occurred in many parts of Europe. Retrospective studies in Germany, the Netherlands, and Leningrad indicate that the incidence of amenorrhea increased significantly, a protective phenomenon that reflects the nutritional unpreparedness of such women for pregnancy. In the Netherlands, 50% of the female population stopped menstruating. The smallest decline in fertility was among those who lived in rural areas or had priority access to food rations. As living conditions improved, mean birthweight rose steadily, returning to normal by 1948. Miscarriages and abortions, stillbirths, neonatal deaths, and malformations all increased in infants conceived during famine. Surviving infants showed a significant reduction in mean birthweights and birth lengths (Hytton and Leitch, 1971).

Relation of Perinatal Mortality and Birthweight

Low birthweight (<2,500 grams) is a major factor in two thirds of all infant deaths (Institute of Medicine, 1985). Deaths of low-birthweight infants, whether because of intrauterine growth retardation or prematurity, are 30 times more frequent than deaths of newborns of normal weight. Because perinatal mortality seems to correlate better with birthweight than with length of gestation, it is widely believed that if birthweight distribution could be improved, there would be a substantial reduction in infant mortality.

Although many inherited problems or perinatal insults cannot be prevented, poor gestational nutrition and low maternal weight gain, both factors in low birthweight, can be modified. In addition, it appears that poor nutritional status and low prepregnant weight of the mother negatively influence infant birthweight (Kramer, 1987).

Two indicators of maternal nutritional status have shown consistent relationship to infant birthweight: maternal size (height and prepregnancy weight) and the amount of weight gained during pregnancy.

MATERNAL SIZE. Big mothers have big babies, and it is proposed that maternal size is a conditioning factor on the ultimate size of the placenta. The size of the placenta determines the amount of nutrition available to the fetus, and eventually the birthweight of the neonate. Mothers with low prepregnancy weights have much lighter weight placentas than heavier mothers (Naeye, 1979). There is a greater incidence of lower birthweight and prematurity in babies born to underweight mothers than in those born to normal weight mothers (Edwards et al, 1979). Adequate pregravid weight and satisfactory weight gain are particularly important for the offspring of short women (Luke et al, 1984). By reaching a higher prepregnancy weight or gaining extra weight during pregnancy, these women can improve their pregnancy outcome (Naeye, 1981).

MATERNAL WEIGHT GAIN DURING PREGNANCY. The normal composition of weight gain is illustrated in Figure 9-1. Less than half of the total weight gain resides in the fetus, placenta, and amniotic fluid; the remainder is

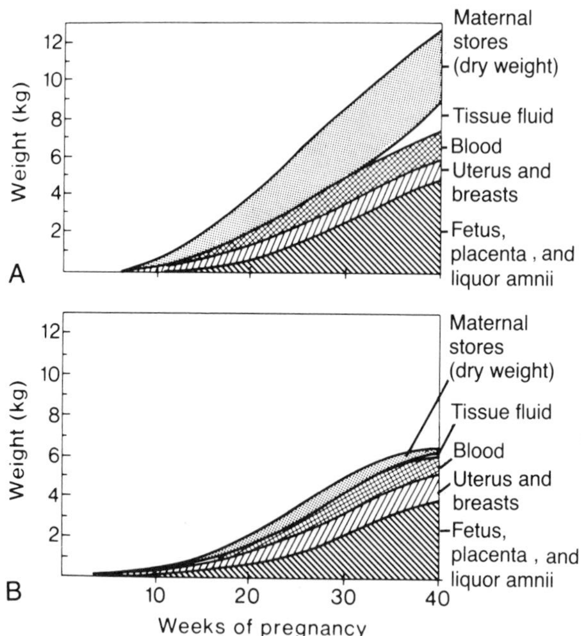

FIGURE 9-1. *Estimated composition of weight gain during pregnancy for a normal, healthy Northern European woman (A) and a poor, underfed woman from India (B). (Adapted from Hurley LS: Developmental Nutrition. Englewood Cliffs, NJ, Prentice-Hall, 1980. After Committee on Maternal Nutrition, National Research Council: Maternal Nutrition and the Course of Pregnancy. Washington, DC, National Academy of Sciences, 1970.)*

found in maternal reproductive tissues, fluid, blood, and "maternal stores," a component largely composed of body fat. A gradual increase in subcutaneous fat at the abdomen, back, and upper thigh serves as an energy reserve for pregnancy and lactation.

Over the years, attitudes about the amount of weight gained during pregnancy have changed dramatically. In the early 1900s, a popular view held that larger babies complicated the process of labor and delivery. Inasmuch as cesarean sections were rarely done and maternal mortality was high, restriction of fetal size seemed justifiable at the time. The philosophy of restricting maternal weight gain to this end prevailed into the 1960s and is still espoused by a minority of clinicians. In 1915, however, poor maternal nutritional status was reported to have a profound influence on birthweight and outcome of pregnancy (Smith, 1916). The majority of subsequent studies have corroborated the observation that an increase in weight gain during pregnancy is associated with a parallel increase in birthweight and a progressive decrease in the number of low-birthweight infants (National Center for Health Statistics, 1980) (Fig. 9–2). This relationship exists up to a weight gain of 26 to 35 lb, the range associated with optimal outcome; however, in very overweight mothers, increasing weight gain is usually not associated with substantial increments in birthweight (Abrams and Laros, 1986). The National Academy of Sciences (NAS) recommends a weight gain of 25 to 35 lb for women of normal weight, 28 to 40 lb for underweight women, and 15 to 25 lb for overweight women (The Latest . . . , 1990) (Table 9–1).

The trend is toward development of new weight-gain curves based on large groups of women in which a range of weight gains would reflect the prepregnancy weight, height, and age of the mother. Figure 9–3 presents curves of desirable weight gains during pregnancy as recommended by the Subcommittee on Nutritional Status and Weight Gain During Pregnancy (Subcommittee . . . , 1990).

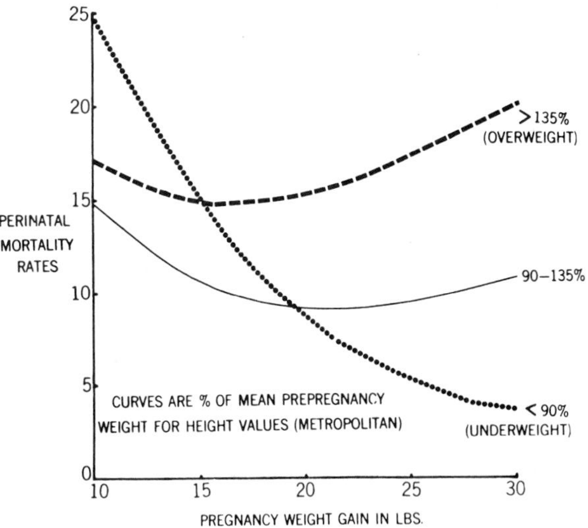

FIGURE 9–2. *Perinatal mortality rates related to weight gain of mother during pregnancy.* Dashed line *indicates overweight mothers, with prepregnancy weight greater than 135% of ideal weight;* solid line *indicates normal weight mothers, with prepregnancy weight 90 to 135% of ideal weight;* dotted line *indicates underweight mothers, with prepregnancy weight less than 90% of ideal weight. (From Naeye RL: Weight gain and the outcome of pregnancy. Am J Obstet Gynecol 135:3, 1979.)*

OBESITY. No ideal weight gain is known for obese women; these women tend to produce big babies at all levels of weight gain. However, gains of 15 to 25 lb have been recommended. Obese women have a higher incidence of obstetric complications including prolonged labor, pyelonephritis, diabetes, hypertension, and thromboembolism. For this group, the nutritional goal

TABLE 9–1. Recommended Weight Gain for Pregnant Women Based on Body Mass Index*

Weight Category Based on BMI†	Total Weight Gain‡		1st Trimester Gain		2nd and 3rd Trimester Weekly Gain	
	lb	*kg*	*lb*	*kg*	*lb*	*kg*
Underweight (BMI <19.8)	28–40	12.5–18	5	2.3	1.07	0.49
Normal weight (BMI = 19.8–26)	25–35	11.5–16	3.5	1.6	0.97	0.44
Overweight (BMI >26–29)	15–25	7–11.5	2	0.9	0.67	0.3
Obese (BMI >29)	at least 15	6				

* Data from Subcommittee on Nutritional Status and Weight Gain During Pregnancy and Subcommittee on Dietary Intake and Nutrient Supplements During Pregnancy, Food and Nutrition Board, National Academy of Sciences: Nutrition During Pregnancy, Parts I and II. Washington, DC, National Academy Press, 1990.

† BMI = body mass index; metric BMI = weight (kg)/height $(m)^2$

‡ Young adolescents and black women should strive for gains at the upper end of the recommended range. Short women (<62 in or <157 cm) should strive for gains at the lower end of the range.

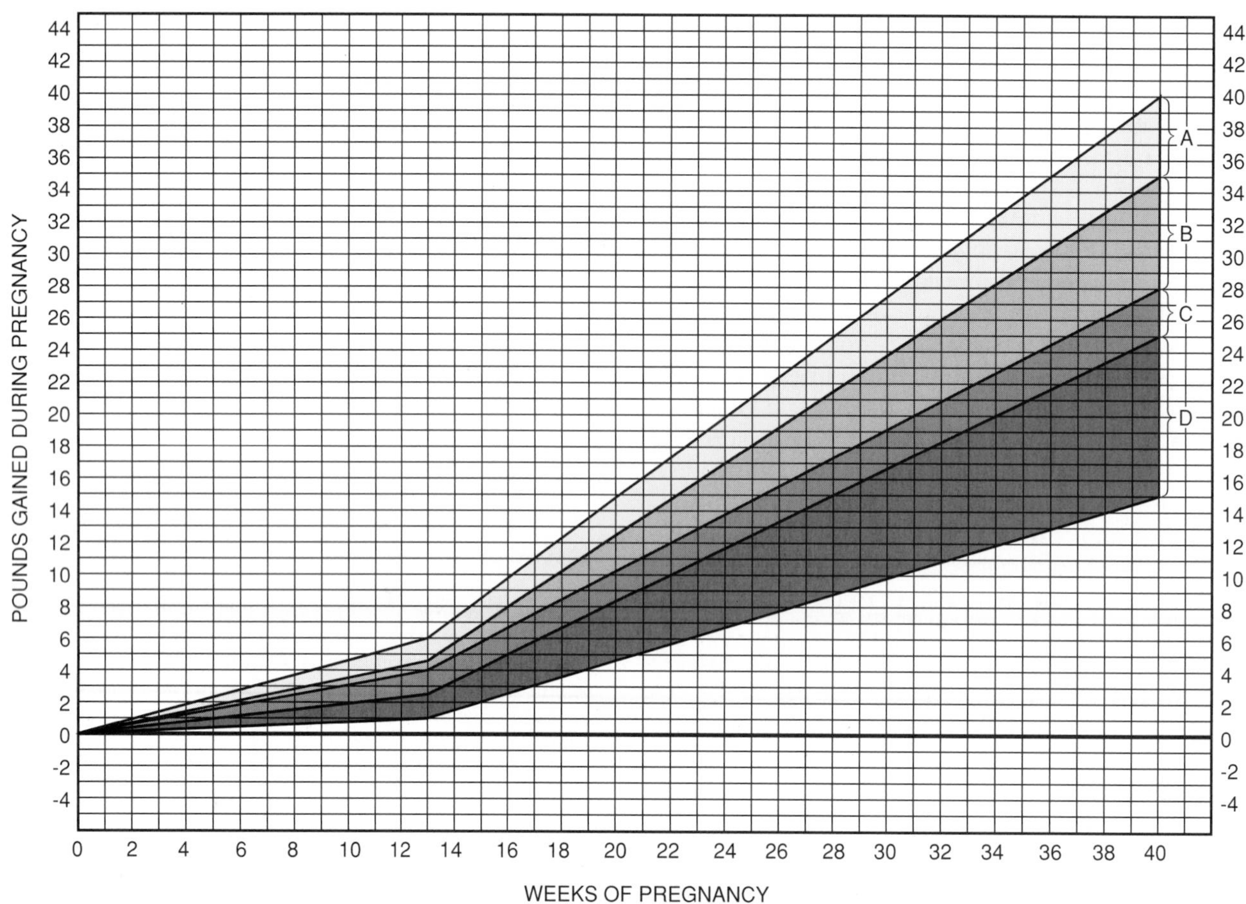

FIGURE 9–3. *The woman who is of normal weight prior to pregnancy should gain in the B-C range, 25 to 35 lb during the pregnancy. The underweight woman should gain in the A-B range, 28 to 40 lb. The woman who is overweight prior to pregancy should gain in the D range, 15 to 25 lb. (From the National Dairy Council: Great Beginnings: The Weighting Game Graph. Rosemont, IL, National Dairy Council, 1991; adapted from the National Academy of Sciences: Nutrition During Pregnancy. Washington, DC, National Academy Press, 1990.)*

would be emphasis on food choices of high nutritional quality and avoidance of unnecessary calorie-rich foods.

ADOLESCENCE. It is recommended that adolescents, as a group, gain 28 to 40 lb during pregnancy but obviously this should be individualized depending upon prepregnant weight and gynecologic age (years since menarche) (Loris et al, 1985) (see Chapter 13).

MULTIPLE BIRTHS. Women pregnant with twins or multiple fetuses should obviously gain more weight than those pregnant with singletons. Although there has been no study of large numbers of multiple births, one study showed that a mean weight gain in the group with optimal outcomes of pregnancy was 44 lb. The mean weight gain of those with less than optimal outcome (babies with birthweight of less than 2,500 grams, or with gestational age of 37 weeks or less, or Apgar scores at 5 minutes of less than 7) was 37 lb, and this group showed a slowing of weight gain during the last 10 weeks of pregnancy (Pederson, 1989).

Nutritional Supplementation During Pregnancy

The findings from the many studies of supplementation appear to suggest that the worse the nutritional condition of the mother entering pregnancy, the more valuable the improved prenatal diet or nutritional supplement, or both, will be in improving her pregnancy course and outcome.

A comprehensive study in Guatemala, in which women were supplemented with either calories or calories and protein during their pregnancies, showed that for full-term infants there was a consistent increase in birthweight as the total supplemental kilocalories of the mother increased (Lechtig et al, 1975a). On the average, the group with low maternal supplementation (<20,000 kcal total) through the pregnancy had placentas weighing 11% less than the group with high maternal supplementation (20,000 kcal or more total). Even more intriguing was the finding that there was no difference in placental weight, mean birthweight, or the percentage of low-birthweight babies associated with the presence of protein in the calorie supplements.

In a Canadian study of high-risk poor women who received supplements along with nutritional counseling, there was a direct relationship between maternal weight gains and birthweights, which were in turn related directly to the length of time that the women received service from the Montreal Diet Dispensary (Primrose and Higgins, 1971).

In this country, the major food program for pregnant women is the Special Supplemental Food Program for Women, Infants and Children, better known as WIC, which was originally authorized in 1972. An evaluation of the effectiveness of the program found the following:

1. A significant increase in mean birthweight of 23 grams.
2. A substantial, but not statistically significant, reduction in low birthweight among less educated whites and more educated blacks.
3. A significantly longer mean pregnancy duration (1.4 days).
4. A reduction in preterm delivery by 9 per 1,000 births.
5. A statistically significant reduction of 2.3 fetal deaths per 1,000 births.
6. A 20% reduction in low birthweight among WIC participants with less than 12 years' education.

The author concluded that WIC had a significant effect on duration of pregnancy, birthweight, head growth, fetal mortality, and perhaps neonatal mortality (Rush, 1986).

Whereas poor women in developing countries often suffer some degree of malnutrition before and during pregnancy, only a minority of women from low socioeconomic groups in developed countries are truly undernourished. Nutritional supplementation of the latter will clearly yield less dramatic improvements in outcome. In developed countries, nutrition intervention should focus on women whose prepregnancy status is inferior.

Physiologic Changes of Pregnancy

Blood Volume and Composition

Many physical and biochemical changes occur in normal pregnancy. Blood volume expands by 50%, resulting in a decrease in hemoglobin and in serum levels of albumin, other serum proteins, and water-soluble vitamins. The fall in serum albumin contributes to the tendency for extracellular water accumulation during pregnancy. The decrease in water-soluble vitamin concentrations makes determination of an inadequate intake or a deficient state for a nutrient difficult. On the other hand, serum concentrations of fat-soluble vitamins and other lipid fractions such as triglycerides, cholesterol, and free fatty acids increase.

Cardiovascular and Pulmonary

To provide for increased cardiac output there is slight cardiac hypertrophy and increased pulse rate. Blood pressure usually decreases and then returns to normal in the third trimester. Maternal oxygen requirements increase and there is a lowered threshold for CO_2, making the pregnant woman feel dyspneic with an increased need to breathe. Adding to this feeling of dyspnea is the fact that the growing uterus pushes the diaphragm upward, making breathing difficult. Fortunately there is also more efficient gas exchange in the lungs.

Gastrointestinal

The functioning of the gastrointestinal system changes in several ways that affect nutritional status. Early on, nausea and vomiting may occur, followed by a return of appetite that can be ravenous. Cravings for and aversions to foods may be accompanied by less ability to taste saltiness. This may be a physiologic mechanism for increasing salt intake (Brown and Toma, 1986). At the same time that an increased progesterone level relaxes the uterine muscle so that it can expand with fetal growth, it also causes diminished gastrointestinal motility so that constipation is often a problem. A relaxed lower esophageal sphincter can result in regurgitation and "heartburn." Intestinal secretions are reduced, but absorption is enhanced.

Renal

Because of increased blood volume, there is a high glomerular filtration rate. It appears that the kidney tubules are unable to adjust completely and a percentage of nutrients that would have been reabsorbed in the nonpregnant woman are excreted in the urine. Greater amounts of amino acids, glucose, and water-soluble vitamins may appear in the urine. The ability to excrete water is lowered, and edema in the legs and ankles is common and normal. This edema is not associated with perinatal mortality when the other symptoms of preeclampsia — hypertension and proteinuria — are absent. In fact, if it is not associated with other symptoms of preeclampsia, the presence of mild edema results in slightly larger babies and a lower rate of prematurity (Worthington-Roberts and Williams, 1989).

Placenta

Not only is the placenta the principal site of production for several hormones responsible for the regulation of maternal growth and development, but it is also the conduit for exchange of nutrients, oxygen, and waste products. Any damage to the placenta or inadequacy in the placenta compromises its ability to nourish the fetus regardless of how well nourished the mother is or how optimal her intake. The placental size and the number of placental cells are 15 to 20% below normal when infants experience intrauterine growth failure (Lechtig et al, 1975b). A small placenta has a smaller surface area of placental peripheral villi, which are responsible for the transfer of nutrients to the fetus. The small surface area may be the means by which maternal nutrition affects birthweight (Lechtig et al, 1975b).

Nutritional Requirements

Pregnancy is a time for growth and additional demand for nutrients. The choice of appropriate standards for assessing nutritional status and requirements during pregnancy is a difficult one. Increased plasma volume with consequently low serum values of some nutrients, as well as the tendency of the kidney to excrete nutrients in larger amounts, leads to values that would be judged deficient if seen in a nonpregnant woman. Whether this is considered a normal expression of the profound metabolic changes seen in pregnancy, or whether lowered serum values are viewed as indicators of increased risk, will determine the course of nutritional management to some extent. Normal values may not be reached without an inordinate increase in energy intake, which raises the question of whether particular nutrient supplements should be used to achieve that purpose.

Energy

Additional energy is required during pregnancy to support the metabolic demands of pregnancy and fetal growth.

RECOMMENDED INTAKE. It is difficult to specify precise energy requirements because these vary with prepregnancy weight, amount and composition of weight gain, and stage of pregnancy and activity level. Rather than establish a recommendation applicable to all women, it has been suggested that energy requirements should be evaluated in terms of rate of weight gain (Worthington-Roberts and Williams, 1989).

The theoretical energy demands of a pregnancy in which a well-nourished Northern European woman gains 12.5 kg have been estimated to total around 80,000 kcal. This value includes 36,000 kcal for increased basal metabolic rate (BMR) and 44,000 kcal for synthesis of new tissue (Hytton and Leitch, 1971). Recent observations of smaller women from developing countries suggest that their energy needs are much lower. The 1989 Recommended Dietary Allowance (RDA) is an additional 300 kcal/day, with the qualification that unless body reserves are depleted at the onset of pregnancy, the extra 300 kcal should be added only in the second and third trimesters (Food and Nutrition Board, 1989). However, it should be recognized that there is a wide range of energy intakes with good pregnancy outcomes (Durnin, 1986; Forsum et al, 1988; Van Raaij et al, 1989).

EXERCISE. Energy expended in voluntary physical activity is the largest variable in overall energy expenditure. Activities involving body movement require an increase in energy expenditure proportional to the increase in body weight. Most pregnant women compensate, however, by slowing their work pace as weight gain proceeds, so that total energy expenditure during a day may not be substantially greater than before.

Studies of pregnancy outcomes as related to physical activity are not conclusive with respect to effects of severity and timing of exercise programs. One study compared a sedentary group with women who engaged in vigorous endurance exercise such as running and aerobic dancing through either the first half or the entire pregnancy. Although incidence of complications was similar in all groups, increasing exertion either in vigorousness or duration of activity was associated with shorter gestational lengths and lower birthweights of infants (Clapp and Dickstein, 1984). Other studies have supported the recommendation that only moderate exercise should be continued through the third trimester. The American College of Obstetricians and Gynecologists provides exercise guidelines (American College of Obstetricians and Gynecologists, 1985).

Because individuals vary considerably in level and intensity of activity, it is best to advise women to eat enough to satisfy physiologic appetite and to support an appropriate rate of weight gain.

CONSEQUENCES OF ENERGY RESTRICTION. Optimal fetal growth occurs only when the mother is able to accumulate a critical amount of extra body stores during pregnancy. The effect of maternal malnutrition on the development of the fetus is a matter of concern not only with respect to nutritionally deprived populations but also to the deliberate practice of restricting food intake to lose weight or prevent weight gain.

A once-popular concept held that the fetus can protect itself by parasitizing the mother when nutritional status is less than optimal. However, evidence from famines experienced in Holland and Germany during World War II clearly contradict this assumption (Hytton and Leitch, 1971). The deprived mothers appeared to be proportionately less affected than their infants, an observation also consistent with animal data.

One recognized consequence of energy restriction is the increased production of ketone bodies and their ultimate spillage into the urine. Although it is known that the fetus can metabolize ketone bodies to some degree, the short- and long-term effects of maternal ketonemia are unclear. Both animal and human data indicate that ketone bodies are probably normally presented to the fetal brain at various times during pregnancy. After an overnight fast, maternal ketone body concentrations in the blood are greater in pregnant than in nonpregnant women and ketonuria will sometimes be seen. Extreme levels of ketonemia, however, may be indicators of maternal malnutrition, with maternal-fetal competition for nutrients and the associated increased risk of fetal or neonatal death (Naeye, 1981).

Protein

Although the need for additional protein to support the synthesis of maternal and fetal tissues is obvious, the magnitude of the extra need is uncertain. Efficiency of protein utilization in pregnant women appears to be about 70%, the same as that observed in infants. Needs are also variable, increasing as pregnancy proceeds, with greater demands occurring during the second and third trimesters. The current RDA of 60 grams for pregnant women includes an additional 10 to 16 g/day over nonpregnant requirements (Food and Nutrition Board, 1989).

Protein deficiency during pregnancy has adverse consequences, but limited intakes of protein and energy usually occur together, making it hard to separate effects of energy deficiency from protein deficiency. Studies have shown that providing extra energy to mothers has as much influence on pregnancy outcome as providing energy and protein together (Lechtig, 1975a; Zlatnick and Burmeister, 1983). Thus it appears that it is usually the energy deficit and not the protein deficit that determines unfavorable pregnancy outcome.

Vitamins

Maintenance of health during the course of pregnancy requires an adequate supply of vitamins and minerals, some of particular significance.

FOLACIN. Folacin needs increase during pregnancy in response to the demands of maternal erythropoiesis and fetal-placental growth. The 1989 RDA is for 400 μg, or over twice the amount recommended in the nonpregnant state. This level can usually be met by a well-selected diet, assuming that 50% of food folate is absorbed.

Folic acid deficiency is marked by a reduction in the rate of DNA synthesis and mitotic activity of individual cells. Megaloblastic anemia develops, usually during the third trimester; however, preliminary morphologic and biochemical signs of deficiency may precede this state.

The consequences of folic acid deficiency in the absence of anemia are controversial. Maternal folic acid deficiency in experimental animals is associated with increased incidence of problems related to pregnancy including congenital malformations in the offspring. Malformations have been described in offspring of women using drugs that are folate antagonists, such as methotrexate (Dansky, 1987). Limited evidence in humans also suggests that deficiency of this vitamin may be associated with spontaneous abortion and congenital malformations; however, these relationships are poorly documented and therefore highly controversial.

The role of folic acid deficiency (or deficiency of some other vitamin) in the etiology of neural tube defects is currently a subject of considerable research. Studies in Northern Europe have suggested that periconceptional multivitamin or folic acid supplementation of women with previous neural tube defect offspring is associated with significant reduction in recurrence of the problem. However, difficulties in obtaining randomized samples of adequate size have led to criticism of the results (Laurence et al, 1981; Sheppard et al, 1989; Smithells et al, 1980, 1981, and 1983).

Research in the United States has yielded conflicting results. A retrospective project using data from the Atlanta Birth Defects Case-Control Study reported an apparent protective effect of periconceptional multivitamin use (Mulinare et al, 1988). Another study, which examined the relation of multivitamin intake in general and folic acid in particular to the risk of neural tube defects, found that the prevalence of neural tube defect for women who used folic acid–containing multivitamins during the first 6 weeks of pregnancy was substantially lower than the prevalence among those who never used multivitamins before or after conception or who used multivitamins before conception only (Milunsky et al, 1989). However, a similar study involving women from Illinois and California did not find an association between periconceptional use of multivitamins or folate-containing supplements and a decreased risk of having an infant with a neural tube defect (Mills et al, 1989).

A randomized controlled supplementation trial currently under way in Northern Europe may clarify the role of vitamin deficiency in the etiology of neural tube defects (Wald, 1984). In the meantime, preconceptional nutrition counseling should include information about sources of vitamin-rich foods. At least one expert panel has recommended that women with previous neural tube defect outcome should be advised that folic acid supplementation may be protective (Expert Panel . . . , 1989).

VITAMIN B_6. The current RDA for vitamin B_6 during pregnancy is 2.2 mg/day. The additional 0.6 mg above the recommendation for adult women provides for increased needs associated with synthesis of nonessential amino acids in growth and vitamin B_6-dependent niacin synthesis from tryptophan.

Some evidence suggests that a significant number of pregnant women on presumably normal diets develop biochemical abnormalities suggestive of vitamin B_6 deficiency (Bapurao et al, 1982). Depression of pregnancy has been correlated negatively with serum vitamin B_6 concentrations (Pulkkinen et al, 1978). Administration of vitamin B_6 supplements corrects the biochemical deficit, and dosages amounting to 10 mg/day have been recommended by several investigators.

The apparent alterations in vitamin B_6 status are regarded as indicative of some poorly understood physiologic adjustment to pregnancy. However, some assessments of babies born to mothers with varying vitamin B_6 status have associated unsatisfactory Apgar scores with lower levels of the vitamin in both maternal and cord serum and breast milk (Roepke and Kirksey, 1981; Schuster et al, 1981).

Vitamin B_6 has also been administered in the management of severe nausea and vomiting of pregnancy. Although this vitamin is known to catalyze a number of reactions involving neurotransmitter production, it is not known whether this function is involved in the relief sometimes observed following its administration (Schuster et al, 1985).

Further Reading, p. 159, presents a discussion of vitamin B_6 and premenstrual syndrome.

ASCORBIC ACID. An extra 10 mg/day of vitamin C is recommended for the pregnant woman. The total recommendation of 70 mg/day is easily met by the American diet.

Ascorbic acid deficiency has not been shown to affect the course or outcome of pregnancy in humans. However, low plasma levels of vitamin C have been reported in association with preeclampsia as well as premature rupture of the membranes.

VITAMIN A. The RDA of 800 retinol equivalents (RE) for vitamin A is not increased for pregnancy in view of maternal stores that easily meet the fetal accretion rate. Vitamin A deficiency is teratogenic in lower animals, but confirmatory evidence of its teratogenicity in humans is lacking. However, excessive consumption of vitamin A does appear to be teratogenic. At least seven case reports of adverse pregnancy outcome have been associated with a daily ingestion of 25,000 IU or more (Rosa et al, 1986). In addition, epidemiologic evidence indicates that the drug isotretinoin, a vitamin A analogue used for treatment of cystic acne, causes major malformations involving craniofacial, central nervous system, cardiac, and thymic changes (Benke, 1984; Lammer et al, 1985). The Teratology Society (1987) urges that women in their reproductive years be informed that the excessive use of vitamin A shortly before and during pregnancy could be harmful to their babies. This group also suggests that manufacturers of vitamin A-containing supplements should lower the maximum amount of vitamin A per unit dosage to 5,000 to 8,000 IU and identify the source of the vitamin. They further support the practice of labeling products containing vitamin A to indicate that consumption of excessive amounts of vitamin A may be hazardous to the embryo or to the fetus when taken during pregnancy and that women of childbearing age should consult with their physicians before consuming these products. The NAS similarly advises pregnant women to avoid vitamin A-containing supplements during the first trimester unless a vitamin A deficiency has been diagnosed (The Latest . . . , 1990).

VITAMIN D. The RDA for vitamin D of 10 μg/day includes an additional increment of 5 μg (200 IU) above the amount recommended for nonpregnant women.

Vitamin D has long been appreciated for its positive effects on calcium balance during pregnancy. This vitamin and its metabolites cross the placenta and appear in fetal blood in the same concentration as found in maternal circulation.

Maternal deficiency of vitamin D and subsequent limitation in placental transport to the fetus has been associated with the appearance of neonatal hypocalcemia or enamel hypoplasia, or both. Vitamin D levels are often low in such infants. Excessive amounts of vitamin D may be harmful during gestation. Severe infantile hypercalcemia and associated problems have been reported in newborn animals and in human infants.

VITAMIN E. Vitamin E needs are believed to increase somewhat during pregnancy, but deficiency in humans rarely occurs and has not been linked with either damage to offspring or reduced fertility. However, the 1989 RDA of 10 mg alpha-tocopherol equivalents (alpha-TE) includes a daily increase of 2 mg of alpha-TE to compensate for the amount deposited in the fetus.

Vitamin E deficiency has long been associated with spontaneous abortion in experimental animals. However, studies have failed to support the use of this vitamin as an abortion preventive in humans.

VITAMIN K. An RDA for vitamin K during pregnancy has not been established because information is lacking; therefore, the recommendation of 65 μg for adult women aged 25 to 50 is continued. Usual diets provide adequate amounts of vitamin K.

FURTHER READING: Premenstrual Syndrome

Many women experience menses-related mood fluctuations and general discomfort. For about 10 to 20% of these women, the symptoms are sufficiently severe to create personal hardship. The most common symptoms include anxiety, depression, mood swings, fatigue, weight gain, swelling, breast pain, cramps, and backache. Although labeled *premenstrual syndrome* (PMS), multiple configurations of these symptoms have been found to occur. Because peak severity usually develops during menses, the term *perimenstrual symptoms* has been proposed to more accurately describe what most women experience.

Despite over 50 years of research on the etiology and treatment of PMS, the underlying mechanisms remain poorly understood and an operational definition does not exist. Methodologic problems have plagued studies, preventing consistency in results of similar treatments. The fact that different symptoms may have distinct etiologies may partially explain why single-focus treatment trials have failed to yield consistent results. Also significant is the unusually high placebo response to interventions, reportedly from 40 to 80%.

While there are many attractive theories and a multiplicity of nutritional, drug, and psychotherapeutic treatments, evidence of their effectiveness is weak. There is no proof that PMS is caused by a poor diet or vitamin/mineral deficiency, or that it can be prevented or cured by dietary therapy. Although limited evidence suggests that moderate doses (50 mg/day) of vitamin B_6 may reduce emotional symptoms (depression, irritability, tiredness), confirmation of this finding is required. In any case, megadoses of vitamin/mineral supplements should be avoided. The best advice for premenopausal women is to follow the Dietary Guidelines for Americans, participate in regular exercise, and enjoy daily periods of relaxation and stress reduction.

Minerals

CALCIUM. The pregnant woman routinely exhibits extensive adjustments in calcium metabolism, largely under the influence of hormonal factors. *Human chorionic somatomammotropin* from the placenta progressively increases the rate of bone turnover. *Estrogen,* also largely from the placenta, inhibits bone resorption, provoking a compensatory release of *parathyroid hormone,* which maintains the serum calcium level while enhancing intestinal absorption. The net effect of these changes, which predate fetal skeletal mineralization, is the promotion of progressive calcium retention to meet progressively increasing fetal skeletal demands for mineralization. Fetal hypercalcemia and subsequent endocrine adjustments ultimately stimulate the mineralization process.

Approximately 30 grams of calcium is accumulated during pregnancy, almost all of it in the fetal skeleton (25 grams). The remainder is stored in the maternal skeleton, presumably in reserve for the calcium demands of lactation. Most of the accretion occurs during the latter part of pregnancy, with an estimated average of 300 mg/day deposited during the last trimester.

The current RDA for calcium during pregnancy provides for an extra 400 mg above the 800 mg recommended for the adult woman. It can be argued that this allowance is excessive, inasmuch as successful pregnancies occur in many other cultures with substantially lower calcium intakes. However, with lower intakes there may be a greater leaching of calcium from the calcium reservoir in the maternal skeleton, of which the total requirement of pregnancy (30 grams) amounts to about 2.5%. Multiparous women with poor calcium intake can exhibit evidence of clinical osteomalacia, and neonatal bone density may relate to the adequacy of maternal calcium consumption during pregnancy. Diets typical of other cultures often are lower in phosphorus and protein, which would reduce urinary calcium losses (see Chapter 7).

PHOSPHORUS. The RDA for phosphorus of 1,200 mg/day during pregnancy is the same as that for calcium. Phosphorus is found in such a wide variety of foods that a deficiency is rare.

The common occurrence of leg cramps during pregnancy, manifested nocturnally in sudden contractions of the gastrocnemius muscle, has been related to a decline in serum calcium related to a calcium/phosphorus imbalance. Prevention or relief of these leg cramps has been reported through reduction in intake of milk (a high-phosphorus, high-calcium beverage) followed by supplementation with nonphosphate calcium salts, along with regular ingestion of aluminum hydroxide to promote formation of insoluble aluminum phosphate salts in the gut. Although several studies confirmed the benefit of these measures on the total serum calcium level in affected women, other controlled and double-blind studies have failed to indicate a correlation between leg cramps and either intake of dairy products or type of calcium supplement employed.

IRON. A marked increase in the maternal blood supply during pregnancy greatly increases the demand for iron. In accord with the availability of this mineral, either dietary or supplemental, total erythrocyte volume increases by 20 to 30%. An active bone marrow may utilize an extra 500 mg of elemental iron during pregnancy and the term fetus and placenta accumulate 250 to 300 mg of elemental iron. Overall, the pregnant woman must have between 700 and 800 mg of extra iron, the majority of which is needed during the last half of pregnancy when the heaviest maternal and fetal demands occur. Averaged over the entire pregnancy, this amounts to a daily increment of 15 mg of iron. Adding this amount to the 15 mg/day recommendation for the nonpregnant state brings the 1989 RDA for iron during pregnancy to a total of 30 mg/day.

It is only rarely that women enter pregnancy with iron stores sufficient to cover all needs without compromising maternal well-being. Iron supplementation, usually in the form of ferrous salts, is thus often acknowledged as a necessary means of preventing iron deficiency anemia.

Maternal anemia, defined by a hematocrit of less than 32% and hemoglobin level of less than 11 g/dl, develops in some pregnant women who do not use iron supplements. An anemic woman is clearly less able to tolerate hemorrhage with delivery and is more prone to develop puerperal infection; however, the fetal effects of maternal anemia are poorly understood. Some data suggest that they are relatively mild, but several reports suggest that pregnancy outcome may be compromised. It might be hypothesized that poor iron consumption leads to poor hemoglobin production, followed by compromised delivery of oxygen to the uterus, placenta, and developing fetus. If maternal cardiac output increases to accommodate the insufficiency in hemoglobin content, the added workload undertaken by the heart could unduly stress maternal systems.

The pregnant woman with iron deficiency anemia should be treated for a finite period with iron supplements at therapeutic doses of 60 to 120 mg/day in divided doses. In a large proportion of anemic women treated in this fashion, an upward shift in hematocrit can be achieved easily. The 15 or 20% of women who do not respond may represent a population in which expanded plasma volume is significantly greater than normal. This phenomenon is reportedly common in multiple pregnancies.

Elevated maternal hemoglobin levels (greater than 13.2 g/dl) have been associated with increased fetal risk as well as increased maternal hypertension, possibly reflecting a failure in plasma volume expansion or harmful effect of high hemoglobin levels on uteroplacental circulation (Murphy et al, 1986).

ZINC. The 1989 RDA for zinc includes an additional 3 mg above the RDA for the nongravid woman. Zinc stored in maternal bones appears to be somewhat unavailable, so that a zinc-deficient diet does not effectively lead to mobilization of zinc stores. As a result, a dietary deficiency is quickly reflected in the maternal mineral balance.

Zinc deficiency is highly teratogenic in rats and leads to the development of a variety of congenital malformations. Nonhuman primates also are affected, and abnormal brain development and behavior have been described in offspring of zinc-deficient monkeys. Evidence from human populations suggests that malformation rates and other poor pregnancy outcomes may be higher in populations where zinc deficiency is recognized (Soltan and Jenkins, 1982).

It may be that the maternal zinc status is related inversely to the level of prenatal iron supplementation (Breskin et al, 1983; Hambidge et al, 1987).

COPPER. The copper content of many diets of pregnant women is only marginal; however, it is currently unknown whether moderate dietary copper deficiency is of consequence to the developing human fetus. Inasmuch as copper deficiency has been found to be teratogenic in animals, it is also possible that copper deficiency may compromise pregnancy outcome in humans.

SODIUM. Sodium metabolism is altered during pregnancy under the stimulus of a modified hormonal milieu. Glomerular filtration of the increased maternal blood volume typically leads to the filtration of an additional sodium load of 5,000 to 10,000 mEq/day. Compensatory mechanisms maintain fluid and electrolyte balance.

Restriction of dietary sodium has been common in the past among pregnant women who have edema; however, moderate edema appears to be a normal consequence of pregnancy and is no longer combated with diuretics or low-sodium diets. In fact, the increased fluid retention that is normal during pregnancy actually increases the body's demand for sodium. Rigorous sodium restriction in pregnant animals stresses the renin-angiotensin-aldosterone system to the point of breakdown; such animals tend to develop water intoxication along with renal and adrenal tissue degeneration. Neonatal hyponatremia (low blood sodium) has been observed in offspring of women who unduly restricted sodium intake before delivery.

Although moderation in use of salt and other sodium-rich foods is appropriate for everyone, *aggressive restriction is unwarranted in pregnancy and daily consumption of sodium should not fall below 2 to 3 grams.*

MAGNESIUM. The RDA for magnesium in pregnancy of 320 mg includes an increase of 40 mg to meet the needs of fetal and maternal tissue growth. This allows for individual variation and an absorption rate of 50%.

The term fetus will accumulate 1 g of magnesium during gestation.

FLUORIDE. The role of fluoride in prenatal development is somewhat controversial. Development of the primary dentition begins at 10 to 12 weeks of pregnancy; from the sixth to the ninth month, the first four permanent molars and eight of the permanent incisor teeth begin formation. Thus 32 teeth are forming and developing during gestation. Questions involve the extent to which fluoride is transported across the placenta and its value in utero in the development of caries-resistant permanent teeth.

IODINE. An additional increment of 25 μg/day has been included in the RDA of 175 μg/day to cover the extra demands of the fetus for iodine.

Maternal iodine deficiency has long been recognized as a cause of cretinism in offspring. Data also suggest that suboptimal iodine nutrition of the mother may compromise development of her fetus even when cretinism does not occur (Connolly et al, 1979). Findings indicate that iodine deficiency may lead to a spectrum of subclinical deficits that place the children at a developmental disadvantage.

The RDA for pregnancy are summarized in Table 9–2.

Guide for Eating During Pregnancy

Recommended Food Intake

The increased requirements of pregnancy can be met by the adequate diet pattern discussed in Chapter 16, with a few important changes and additions as listed in Table 9–3.

Four cups of milk per day will provide more than the additional 10 to 16 grams of high-quality protein needed, increase the calcium intake to 1.2 grams, and provide an additional 320 kcal from skim milk or 640 kcal from whole milk. A number of choices are available: whole milk, low-fat milk, skim milk, nonfat powdered milk, buttermilk, acidophilus milk, evaporated milk, yogurt, and cheese. If preferred, the required amount can be used in soups, custards, puddings, ice cream, or flavored beverages. Nonfat milk powder can be added in the preparation of meat loaf, soups, scrambled eggs, mashed and scalloped potatoes, sandwich spreads, cooked cereals, homemade breads, cookies, or pastries. Approximately one-third cup of dried skim milk is equivalent to 1 cup of fluid milk. Milk can be made richer in calcium, protein, and calories by adding 2 tablespoons of dried nonfat milk to a glass of fluid milk. Three to four cups of milk fortified with vitamin D provide 7.5 to 10 μg of cholecalciferol (300 to 400 IU). If fluid milk is used in limited amounts, a vitamin D supplement may be desirable, especially if exposure to sunlight is limited.

TABLE 9–2. Recommended Dietary Allowances for Women*

	15–18 Yr	19–24 Yr	25–50 Yr	Pregnant	Lactating	
					1st 6 Months	*2nd 6 Months*
Energy (kcal)	2,200	2,200	2,200	+0 1st tri† +300 2nd tri +300 3rd tri	+500	+500
Protein (gm)	44	46	50	60	65	62
Vitamin A (μg RE)	800	800	800	800	1,300	1,200
Vitamin D (μg)	10	10	5	10	10	10
Vitamin E (mg α-TE)	8	8	8	10	12	11
Vitamin K (μg)	55	60	65	65	65	65
Vitamin C (mg)	60	60	60	70	95	90
Thiamin (mg)	1.1	1.1	1.1	1.5	1.6	1.6
Riboflavin (mg)	1.3	1.3	1.3	1.6	1.8	1.7
Niacin (mg NE)	15	15	15	17	20	20
Vitamin B_6 (mg)	1.5	1.6	1.6	2.2	2.1	2.1
Folate (μg)	180	180	180	400	280	260
Vitamin B_{12} (μg)	2	2	2	2.2	2.6	2.6
Calcium (mg)	1,200	1,200	800	1,200	1,200	1,200
Phosphorous (mg)	1,200	1,200	800	1,200	1,200	1,200
Magnesium (mg)	300	280	280	320	355	340
Iron (mg)	15	15	15	30	15	15
Zinc (mg)	12	12	12	15	19	16
Iodine (μg)	150	150	150	175	200	200
Selenium (μg)	50	55	55	65	75	75

* Reprinted with permission from *Recommended Dietary Allowances,* 10th ed., c. 1989 by the National Academy of Sciences. Published by National Academy Press.

† tri = trimester.

TABLE 9–3. Daily Food Pattern for Pregnancy

Food	Amount	Protein (g)
Milk, nonfat or low fat, yogurt, and cheese	3 to 4 cups	24–32
Meat (lean), poultry, fish, egg	2 servings (total of 4–6 oz)	28–42
Vegetables, cooked or raw dark green/deep yellow, starchy, including potatoes, dried peas, and beans; all others	3 to 5 servings, all types often	6–10
Whole-grain and enriched breads and cereals	7 or more servings	14+
Fats and sweets	In moderate amounts	Variable
	Total protein	72+
	Vegetarian Pattern	
Milk, nonfat or low fat, yogurt, and cheese	3 to 4 cups	24–32
Beans, tofu, soy protein meat substitutes	2 servings	14–18
Vegetables, cooked or raw dark green/deep yellow, starchy, including potatoes, dried peas, and beans; all others	3 to 5 servings, all types often	6–10
Whole grain and enriched breads and cereals	7 or more 1-oz servings	14+
Fats and sweets	In moderate amounts	Variable
	Total protein	58+

Many women, primarily from the non-Caucasian populations, are unable to digest the lactose in milk (see Chapter 27). They are often able to tolerate milk when it is taken in small amounts at a time. Commercial enzyme preparations such as Lactaid that can be added to fluid milk are readily available. Cheese or yogurt, which contain only small amounts of lactose, can be substituted. If necessary, preparations such as calcium lactate or calcium carbonate may have to be prescribed (see Chapter 7).

The daily consumption of whole-grain bread and cereals, leafy green and yellow vegetables, and fresh and dried fruits should be encouraged to provide additional minerals, vitamins, and fiber. Careful attention to the selection of foods that are good sources of iron and folic acid is important (see Appendix Tables 1 and 3). Table 9–4 gives an example of a menu that meets the needs of the normal pregnant woman.

Drinking of six to eight glasses of water daily is encouraged. Intestinal stasis is often encountered as a result of the necessary restrictions of activities and the pressure of the enlarging uterus. However, for most individuals, the bulky content of the protective diet plus the suggested amount of water will counteract any difficulty with constipation.

Pregnant women are usually highly motivated and very receptive to well-presented nutrition advice. Full discussion of individual needs with involvement of the mother and perhaps the father-to-be in planning the diet changes is usually an effective approach (Fig. 9–4).

Alcohol

Abundant evidence from both animal studies and human experience has associated heavy alcohol consumption with teratogenicity. A pattern of abnormalities has been identified in affected offspring and labeled the *fetal alcohol syndrome* (Streissguth et al, 1980). Features associated with this syndrome include prenatal and postnatal growth failure, developmental delay, microcephaly, eye changes including the epicanthal fold, facial abnormalities, and skeletal joint abnormalities (Fig. 9–5). Infants born to moderately heavy drinkers may display limited features of the syndrome *(fetal alcohol effects).* These mothers also experience a higher rate of spontaneous abortion, abruptio placentae, and low-birthweight delivery (Council, 1983). Some evidence suggests a relationship between paternal alcohol use and the size of the offspring (Little and Sing, 1986).

TABLE 9–4. Suggested Menu for a Pregnant Woman*

Breakfast

Orange juice, ½ cup
Oatmeal, ½ cup
Whole grain or enriched toast, 1 slice
Peanut butter, 2 tsp
Decaffeinated coffee or tea

Midmorning

Apple
High bran cereal, ¼ cup
Nonfat yogurt, ½ cup

Lunch

Turkey (2 oz) sandwich on rye or whole grain bread with lettuce and tomato and 1 tsp mayonnaise
Green salad
Salad dressing, 2 tsp
Fresh peach
Nonfat or low-fat milk, 1 cup

Midafternoon

Nonfat or low-fat milk, 1 cup
Graham crackers, 4 squares

Dinner

Baked chicken breast, 3 oz
Baked potato with 2 T sour half-and-half
Peas and carrots, ½ cup
Green salad
Salad dressing, 2 tsp
Fresh pear

Evening

Nonfat frozen yogurt, 1 cup
Fresh strawberries

* Quantities of food should be adjusted to meet individual energy needs to promote appropriate weight gain. The pregnant adolescent, very active woman, or underweight woman will require more.

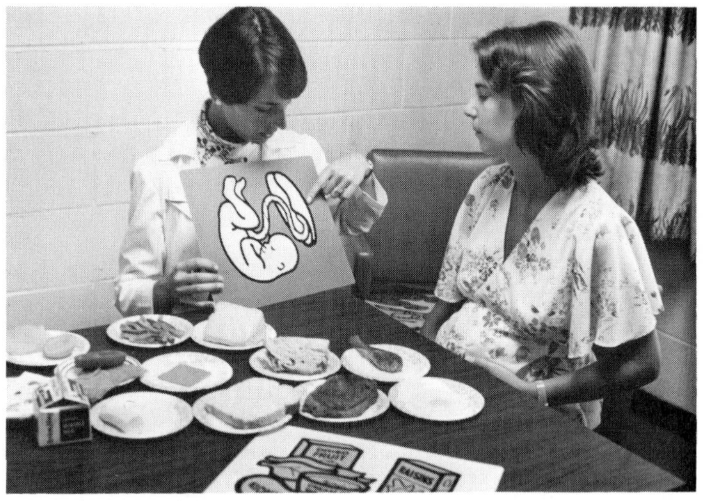

FIGURE 9–4. *A prospective mother learning about food in relation to her pregnancy. (Photograph courtesy of Nutrition Department, Lutheran General Hospital, Park Ridge, IL.)*

The impact of binge drinking has never been satisfactorily evaluated. Even the question of how much moderate drinking is safe during pregnancy has not been answered. It appears that moderate drinking (fewer than two drinks weekly) is not directly associated with any measurable adverse outcome of pregnancy (Halmesmaki et al, 1987).

The mechanisms by which alcohol affects the fetus are not completely understood. As alcohol crosses the placenta, it may accumulate to toxic levels that are particularly damaging during blastogenesis and cell differentiation (Figs. 9–6 and 9–7). Fetal damage may also be the result of deficiencies of folate, magnesium, and zinc that are common to alcoholics with poor diets.

There is evidence that the course and outcome of pregnancy can be significantly improved if problem drinkers change their habits even after conception has occurred (Rosett et al, 1983). However, those who reduce or eliminate alcohol consumption are usually the moderate drinkers, not the heavy drinkers (Streissguth et al, 1983).

Non-Nutritive Substances in Foods

CAFFEINE. Caffeine crosses the placenta and enters the fetus where it may affect fetal heart rate and breathing. Massive doses of caffeine are teratogenic in mice, but the effects of smaller quantities have not been satisfactorily examined. Human data are limited, but some surveys have suggested that heavy caffeine use is associated with increased reproductive loss and pregnancy complications (Scrisuphan and Bracken, 1986; Weathersbee et al, 1977). However, no studies to date show a definite link between caffeine consumption and birth defects in humans (Kurppa et al, 1982; Linn et al, 1982; Rosenberg et al, 1982). Because it has not been proved beyond a doubt that caffeine does not cause birth defects, the consumption of unnecessary caffeine during pregnancy is discouraged. It is recommended that pregnant and breast-feeding women consume no more caffeine than the amount in two 5-oz cups of coffee daily. Use of tea and caffeine-containing carbonated beverages should be moderate.

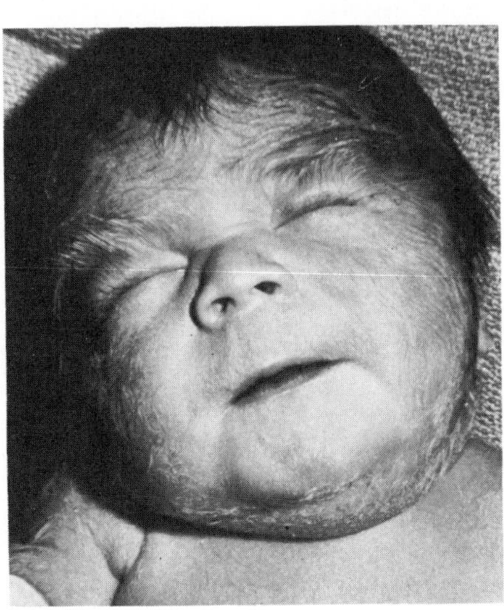

A

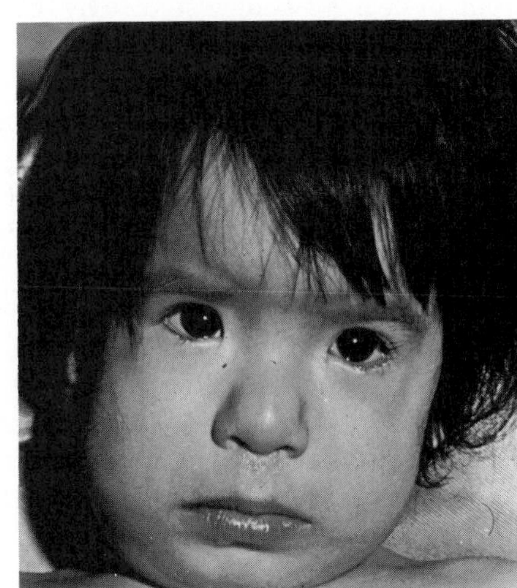

B

FIGURE 9–5. *Child with fetal alcohol syndrome at birth* (A) *and at one year* (B). *(From Moore KL: The Developing Human, 4th ed. Philadelphia, WB Saunders, 1989, p 146.)*

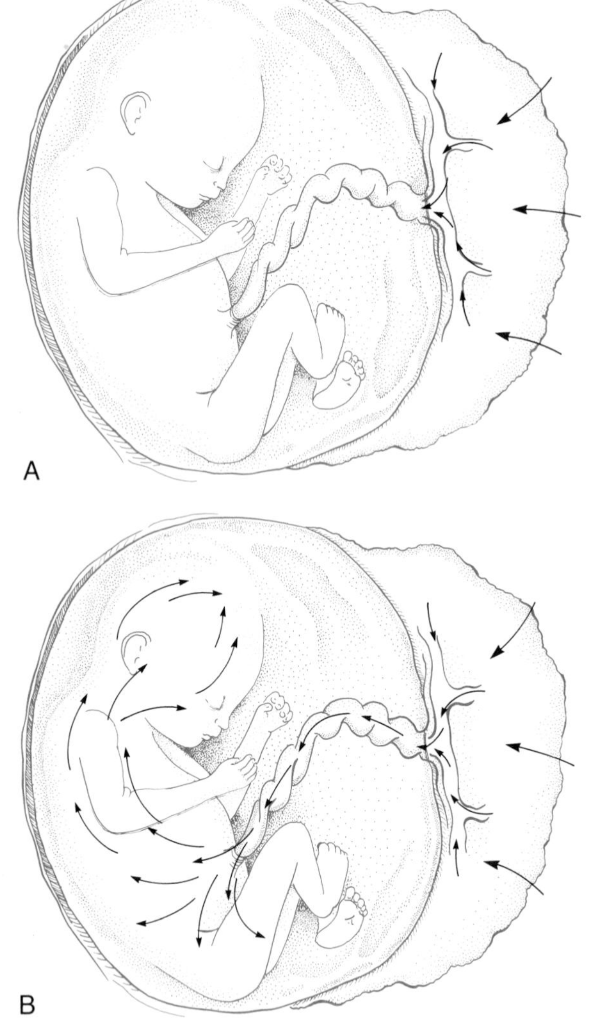

FIGURE 9–6. *Placental transfer of alcohol, tobacco smoke, caffeine, and drugs.*

Recently caffeine has been linked to infertility in a group of healthy women studied by the National Institute of Environmental Health Sciences. Women who consumed more caffeine per day than the amount in one cup of coffee (or three cans of caffeinated soda pop) were half as likely to conceive during a given menstrual cycle than women who drank less (Christianson et al, 1989). However, other research has not confirmed these findings (Joesoef et al, 1990).

ARTIFICIAL SWEETENERS. Saccharin has not been identified as a teratogen, but because it has been shown to be weakly carcinogenic in rats, moderation in its consumption seems appropriate.

Questions about the safety of aspartame use during pregnancy relate to the release of phenylalanine, an amino acid that is a product of its digestion. In most people, phenylalanine is rapidly broken down into a relatively harmless substance; however, persons with phenylketonuria (PKU) lack the enzyme necessary for its conversion and suffer brain damage as a consequence of the high levels of phenylalanine that accumulate in the blood (see Chapter 41). High circulating levels of this amino acid are known to damage the fetal brain; however, the amount of phenylalanine accumulating in the blood of a pregnant woman who does not suffer from PKU is extremely small. Consumption of the amount of aspartame necessary to raise serum phenylalanine to potentially dangerous levels has been calculated at one 12-oz can of diet soda every 8 minutes, 24 hours/day. In view of these practical considerations and the fact that no data suggest a danger, it seems unreasonable to counsel avoidance of this artificial sweetener during pregnancy (Sturtevant, 1985).

CONTAMINANTS. A number of contaminants are found in food, some of which may adversely affect the course and outcome of pregnancy if consumed in sufficient amounts. Most heavy metals are embryotoxic but only mercury, lead, cadmium, and possibly nickel and selenium have been implicated in this regard. Lead toxicity has been associated with abortion and menstrual disorders, but it is not clear that lead is a teratogen. Some authors report a correlation between atmospheric lead levels and congenital malformations, whereas others deny these associations.

Beliefs, Avoidances, Cravings, and Aversions

Most women change their diets during the course of pregnancy. Some changes are based on medical advice, others on folk medical beliefs or on changes in preferences and appetite that may be idiosyncratic or culturally patterned. Inasmuch as the latter will affect a woman's willingness to follow prescribed dietary regimes, the health care provider should be sensitized to their existence.

One important group of *beliefs* involves dietary means by which the mother can ensure an easier delivery. Most hazardous of these from the biomedical viewpoint are those that lead to elimination of animal proteins or to the avoidance of "excessive" weight gain. Low weight gain is deemed desirable because the smaller fetus is believed to be delivered more easily and the baby can "catch up" after birth.

Food avoidances reflect the mother's conscious choice not to consume certain foods during her pregnancy, usually for a reason she can articulate and that seems reasonable to her. The four most commonly avoided foods are sources of animal protein: milk, lean meats, pork, and liver.

Cravings and aversions are powerful urges toward or away from foods, including foods about which women experience no unusual attitudes outside of pregnancy. The most commonly reported craved foods are sweets

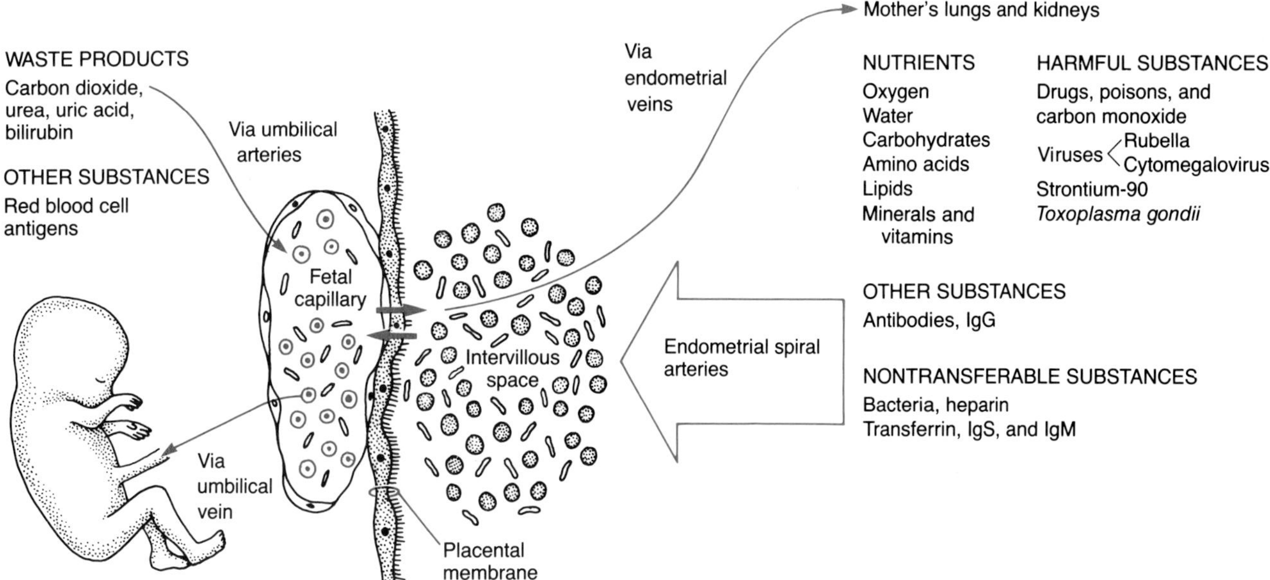

FIGURE 9–7. *Diagrammatic illustration of transfer across the placental membrane. (From Moore KL: The Developing Human, 4th ed. Philadelphia, WB Saunders, 1989, p 94.)*

and dairy products. The most common aversions reported are to alcohol, caffeinated drinks, and meats. However, cravings and aversions are not limited to any particular foods or food groups.

The significance of these behaviors is difficult to evaluate, inasmuch as information has often been collected in an anecdotal manner. The nutritional importance of such practices cannot be assessed without reference to the rest of the individual's diet. Cravings and aversions are not necessarily deleterious.

PICA. Pica refers to the compulsion for persistent ingestion of unsuitable substances having little or no nutritional value. Pica of pregnancy most often involves consumption of dirt or clay *(geophagia)* or starch *(amylophagia),* such as laundry starch. However, nonfood substances subject to compulsive consumption include a bizarre variety of such things as ice, paper, burnt matches, hair, stone or gravel, charcoal, soot, cigarette ashes, mothballs, antacid tablets, milk of magnesia, baking soda, coffee grounds, and tire inner tubes. The practice of pica is not limited to any one geographic area, race, sex, culture, or social status, nor is it limited to pregnancy. A familiar example of pica is the consumption of lead paint chips by young children.

Among the medical consequences of pica is malnutrition, as nonfood substances displace essential nutrients in the diet. Starch in the excessive amounts often seen can contribute to obesity. Some substances contain toxic compounds; others can interfere with the absorption of minerals, such as iron. Starch and clay in gross amounts can lead to intestinal obstruction.

The etiology of pica is poorly understood. One theory suggests that the ingestion of nonfood substances relieves nausea and vomiting. It has also been hypothesized that a deficiency of an essential nutrient such as calcium or iron results in the eating of nonfood substances that contain these nutrients. Much of this behavior appears to be based on fallacious superstitions, customs, and traditions that are often passed from mother to daughter.

Table 9–5 presents a summary of nutritional care for the pregnant woman.

Diet-Related Complications of Pregnancy

Nausea and Vomiting

Morning sickness or nausea is common during the early months of pregnancy, and the condition usually disappears as spontaneously as it appears. However, when early pregnancy is characterized by excessive vomiting, an acute protein and energy deficit and the loss of min-

TABLE 9–5. Summary of Nutritional Care for the Pregnant Woman

1. Energy to meet nutritional needs and allow for about a 0.4 kg (14 oz) gain per week during the last 30 weeks of pregnancy.
2. Protein to meet nutritional needs—about an additional 10–16 g/day.
3. Sodium should not be excessive, but should be no less than 2 g/day.
4. Minerals and vitamins to meet the RDA. For iron and folate, this may necessitate supplementation.
5. Alcohol should be omitted or at least restricted to very small amounts infrequently.
6. Caffeine should be reduced to less than 200 mg/day, the equivalent of 2 cups of coffee.

erals, vitamins, and electrolytes may result. Simple treatment generally improves food tolerance. Small frequent dry meals of easily digested carbohydrate foods are usually better tolerated. Liquids are best taken between meals.

Fats are often a problem. A low-fat diet should be followed until fats can be tolerated. Fats and fluids, as tolerated, are gradually added to the meals. Cooking odors may be problematic for some women.

The pregnant woman should be advised of the importance of eating during this period and be encouraged to eat as much as possible when she is not nauseated. Although anecdotal data indicate that vitamin B_6 has been sometimes used successfully in relieving nausea of pregnancy, this is not a routine recommendation.

Prolonged, persistent vomiting *(hyperemesis gravidarum)* develops in about 2% of pregnant women. Hospitalization is usually indicated, with intravenous fluid and electrolyte replacement required to prevent complications of dehydration. Parenteral nutritional support may be required in the rare persistent case.

Heartburn

Heartburn is a common complaint during the latter part of pregnancy. In most cases this is an effect of pressure of the enlarged uterus on the stomach in combination with the relaxed esophageal sphincter, resulting in occasional regurgitation of stomach contents into the esophagus. This can usually be relieved by limiting the amount of food consumed at one time. Attention to adequate chewing, eating slowly, and avoiding lying in a reclining position after meals may also help.

Constipation and Hemorrhoids

Pregnant women often develop constipation, most frequently during the latter stages of pregnancy. Causes of this problem include reduced gut motility, physical inactivity, and the pressure exerted on the bowel by the enlarged uterus. The weight of the fetus and downward pressure on the veins often leads to the development of hemorrhoids during this period. Increased consumption of fluid, fiber-rich foods, and dried fruits (especially prunes and figs) usually controls these problems, but some women may also require a bulking type of laxative (see Chapter 27).

Edema

Mild physiologic edema is usually present in the extremities in the third trimester (see page 155) and should not be confused with the pathologic generalized edema associated with pregnancy-induced hypertension. The swelling of the lower extremities may be caused by the pressure of the enlarging uterus on the veins returning fluid from the legs. Extravascular fluid is often mobilized in the evening when the woman is lying down, and this results in a tendency to urinate during the night. This normal edema requires no sodium restriction or other dietary change.

Diabetes Mellitus

Individualized, expert care is needed for the nutritional management of the pregnant diabetic. On the basis of nutritional history and assessment early in pregnancy and preferably prior to conception, an individually adapted dietary plan should be developed by a skilled nutritionist as part of the health care team (see Chapter 31).

The incidence of preeclampsia is high in the pregnant diabetic, and fetal morbidity and mortality are significantly greater than in normal pregnancy. It must be emphasized that unfavorable effects are in proportion to the care the mother receives. Early prenatal care from a team of professionals including a clinical nutritionist is an important factor. With good specialized care, the risk of complications in the pregnant diabetic woman can be reduced to the same level as that seen in nondiabetic pregnancies (Freinkel et al, 1985; Osbourne, 1988).

Infants born to diabetics are, as a rule, larger than those of nondiabetics. This is most likely caused by exposure of the infant in utero to supernormal levels of its own insulin, which in fact is a growth hormone. High fetal insulin levels reflect the hyperglycemia of the mother, which encourages high levels of glucose to cross the placenta. Infants of diabetic mothers also tend to become hypoglycemic shortly after birth, with the probability directly related to the maternal glucose intolerance.

Successful pregnancy depends on adequate dietary intake, frequent glucose monitoring, and insulin management to meet the growth needs of the fetus, maintain optimal blood glucose levels, and prevent ketosis and depletion of the mother's nutritional stores. The demands of pregnancy may impose a need for insulin in a diabetic gravid woman whose condition was adequately controlled by diet alone in the nonpregnant state. Insulin requirements decrease in the first half of pregnancy because of fetal use of glucose, and the mother may need only two thirds of her usual amount. In the second half of pregnancy, hormone changes induce an increase in insulin requirements of 70 to 100% over prepregnancy requirements. This increase occurs rather abruptly during the fifth month and may last through the ninth month. Frequent changes to the diet and the insulin dosage may be necessary.

Diabetes may exist only during the stress of pregnancy and resolve itself after delivery, a condition called *gestational diabetes.* The etiology of gestational diabetes is not understood, but it usually can be controlled by diet alone (see Chapter 31).

Pregnancy-Induced Hypertension (Preeclampsia and Eclampsia)

Pregnancy-induced hypertension (PIH) is a syndrome characterized by hypertension, proteinuria, and edema. Hypoalbuminemia, hypovolemia, and subsequent hemoconcentration also are present. It usually develops in the third trimester, affecting about 7 to 8% of the obstetric population, particularly those who are young, pregnant for the first time, or of low socioeconomic status. The terms *preeclampsia* and *eclampsia* refer to the nature and degree of the symptoms involved. Eclampsia is an extension of preeclampsia with grand mal seizure occurring near the time of labor.

PIH is usually defined by a systolic blood pressure of 140 mm Hg or a diastolic pressure of 90 mm Hg or both. However, because young women — the typical group to experience eclampsia — often have very low prepregnant blood pressures (90/60 to 120/80 mm Hg) it is more useful to look at blood pressure *change* during pregnancy. A rise of 20 to 30 mm Hg in systolic pressure or 10 to 15 mm Hg in diastolic pressure, or both, on two or more occasions 6 hours apart is a diagnostic tool.

The extent of proteinuria varies with the degree of PIH. Often it is fluctuating or transient, and may be minimal even in severe cases. The presence of 500 mg of protein in a 24-hour urine or 2+ protein on random collection defines the condition of preeclampsia. Eclampsia is defined by 5 g of protein/24 hr or 3 to 4+ protein on random collection.

When edema is generalized, it indicates that the kidneys are reabsorbing large amounts of sodium and the control of the extracellular fluid volume has been lost. With increased sensitivity to renin, some hypertension can be expected to develop. The edema of preeclampsia may also be associated with dizziness, headache, visual disturbances, facial edema, anorexia, nausea, and vomiting. In the severe state of eclampsia, convulsions occur near the time of labor.

The etiology of PIH is still unknown, but its development is associated with poverty, lack of prenatal care, and poor nutritional status. Most researchers agree that it is associated with a decreased uterine blood flow leading to a reduction in fetal nourishment. Of the proposed nutritional causes, protein deficiency has been the most popular idea. However, the link between protein intake and PIH is not clear, and evidence of the benefit of a high-protein diet in preventing the disorder is inconclusive.

An association has been proposed between calcium deficiency and PIH. The incidence of PIH seems to be higher in populations with low calcium intake, and supplementation of pregnant women with calcium has been associated with reduced blood pressure (Villar et al, 1987; Marya et al, 1987). A large randomized controlled, double-blind calcium supplementation trial may ultimately prove or disprove the protective effect of calcium. In the meantime, it seems reasonable to ensure that the pregnant woman consume at least the RDA for calcium.

In previous years, attempts to treat PIH have focused on sodium restriction and diuretics. Sodium restriction has failed to significantly alter blood pressure, weight gain, or proteinuria in gravid women and seems to have no place in treatment or prevention of PIH. The same can be said for diuretics; use of these drugs does not lower the incidence of PIH or aid in its management. In fact, it may be dangerous to recommend diuretics for the woman with PIH inasmuch as she is known to have a subnormal intravascular volume due to peripheral vasoconstriction. Diuretics would restrict intravascular volume even further through forced kidney diuresis of sodium and water. As with diuretics and sodium restriction, restricted energy intake has not been found to prevent preeclampsia in pregnant women with high weight gain.

LACTATION

Interest in breast-feeding has increased significantly since the beginning of the 1970s. Before that time, formulas were preferred and in many areas were considered the "modern" method of infant feeding. As information about the apparent superiority of human milk has accumulated, enthusiasm for breast-feeding has increased. Currently more than 50% of American mothers leave the hospital nursing and many plan to continue the practice well into the first year of their infants' lives. More than 15% of infants continue to breast-feed well beyond 6 months of age. Although the advantages of nursing vary among mother-infant pairs, those features of breast-feeding that are typically viewed as superior to formula feeding are defined in Table 9-6. The composition of human milk is discussed in Chapter 10.

TABLE 9-6. Advantages of Breast-Feeding

1. Breast milk is nutritionally superior to any alternative.
2. Breast milk is bacteriologically safe and always fresh.
3. Breast milk contains a variety of anti-infectious factors and immune cells.
4. Breast milk is the least allergenic of any infant food.
5. Breast-fed babies are least likely to be overfed.
6. Breast-feeding promotes good jaw and tooth development.
7. Breast-feeding generally costs less than the commercial infant formulas currently available.
8. Breast-feeding automatically promotes close mother-child contact.
9. Breast-feeding is generally more convenient once the process is established.

Physiology of Lactation

The mammary glands prepare for lactation through a series of developmental steps that occur during adolescence and pregnancy. Hormonal changes markedly increase breast, areola, and nipple size. The principal feature of mammary growth in pregnancy is a great increase in ducts and alveoli under the influence of many hormones. Late in pregnancy, the lobules of the alveolar system are maximally developed and small amounts of colostrum may be released for several months prior to delivery. Anatomic features of the human mammary gland are illustrated in Figure 9–8. Delivery of the infant is followed by a dramatic change in the hormonal pattern of the mother. A sudden drop in circulating levels of estrogen and progesterone accompanies a rapid rise in secretion of prolactin. These changes and others set the stage for the formal onset of lactation.

The typical stimulus for milk production and secretion is the suck of the infant at the mother's breast. Nerves beneath the skin of the areola send a message via the spinal cord to the hypothalamus, which in turn transmits a message to the pituitary gland, where both the anterior and posterior areas are stimulated to release their respective hormones. *Prolactin* from the anterior pituitary ultimately stimulates milk production by alveolar cells in the mammary tissue, as shown in Figure 9–9. *Oxytocin* from the posterior pituitary stimulates the myoepithelial cells of the mammary gland to contract, causing movement of milk through the duct system and lactiferous sinuses for ultimate arrival in the mouth of the infant. This latter process is referred to as *let-down* and is accompanied in the woman by a distinct sensation described as a "tingling feeling." Because oxytocin also stimulates the muscle cells of the uterus to contract, lactation immediately following delivery is considered useful in assisting in rapid shutdown of bleeding from this tissue.

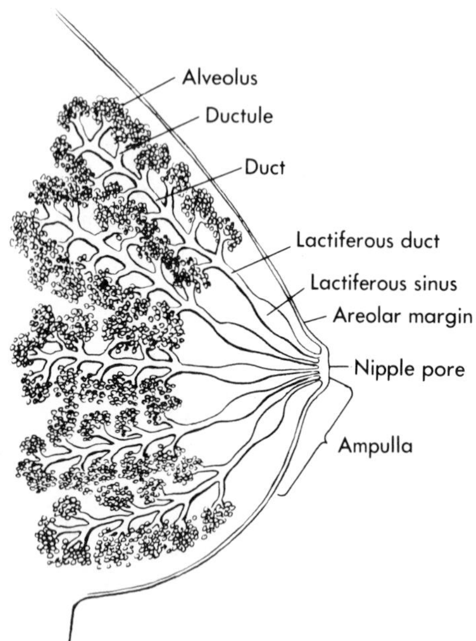

FIGURE 9–8. *Structural features of the human mammary gland showing the terminal glandular (alveolar) tissue of each lobule leading into the duct system, which enlarges eventually into the lactiferous duct and lactiferous sinus. The lactiferous sinuses rest beneath the areola and converge at the nipple pore. (From Worthington-Roberts BS and Williams SR: Nutrition in Pregnancy and Lactation, 4th ed. St Louis, CV Mosby, 1989.)*

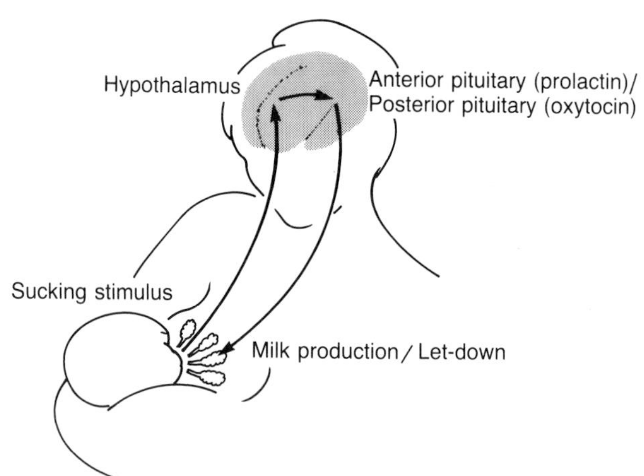

FIGURE 9–9. *Physiology of milk production and the let-down reflex.*

The process of let-down appears to be sensitive to small changes in circulating oxytocin levels; minor emotional disturbances or environmental stresses may influence the ease with which breast milk is provided to the infant. The attitude of the mother toward the process of breast-feeding is a powerful factor in determining her success at lactation. The support of the father, physician, nurse, extended family, and friends is also an important determinant of the degree of satisfaction and success derived from the breast-feeding experience.

Nutritional Requirements of Lactation

The process of lactation is nutritionally demanding, especially for the woman who fully nurses for a number of months. Increased intake of most nutrients is advised, as is indicated in Table 9–2.

The influence of maternal diet on the composition of human milk depends to some degree on the nutritional history of the mother. If her nutritional stores are substantial, consumption of a poor-quality diet for a period of time may have limited impact on the milk quality; nutrients will be drawn from her stores if her diet is suboptimal. However, this utilization of maternal stores has obvious limits, particularly with respect to the water-soluble vitamins, which typically are found in low levels in human milk when the maternal diet is low in these nutrients. Important antimicrobial proteins provided by human milk may also be secreted in reduced amounts if the mother is malnourished (Chang, 1990).

Energy

Milk is produced with about 80% efficiency; production of 100 ml of milk (about 67 kcal) requires an 85-kcal expenditure. Average milk secretion in the first 6 months is 750 ml/day and drops to 600 ml/day during the second 6 months.

The RDA for energy needs during lactation provides for an extra 500 kcal/day above the levels for nonpregnant women. Maternal fat stores accumulated during pregnancy provide about 100 to 150 kcal/day during the early months of lactation. When the reserve fat pad has been depleted, dietary energy support for lactation must be increased if the mother intends to provide all or most of her infant's nutrition through breast milk alone.

Lactation may be associated with increased efficiency of energy utilization. Lactating women may not need to increase energy intake to the extent suggested by current RDA.

The major effect on lactation of maternal undernutrition is the production of less milk each day. Such a consequence may be seen in the nursing mother who takes on a rigorous weight-reduction diet while attempting to breast-feed her infant. Suboptimal quantity of milk production may also result from inadequate fluid intake on the part of the mother. Breast-feeding mothers should be discouraged from dieting and encouraged to consume 3 to 4 quarts of fluid daily. They should also be advised that use of oral contraceptives may suppress lactation, especially in the first 6 to 10 weeks.

Once lactation is well established, modest reduction in energy intake to achieve an increased rate of fat utilization can usually be initiated without adverse impact on milk production. One investigation showed that lactating women who reduced their daily kcal intake from 2,300 to 1,600 for 1 week demonstrated no significant drop in daily milk output. However, inasmuch as studies exploring the impact on milk production of longer periods of dieting have not been reported, care should be taken when a woman attempts to combine lactation with weight-reduction strategies (Strode et al, 1986).

Protein

The RDA provides for an additional 15 grams of protein during the first 6 months of lactation and 12 grams during the second 6 months, when less milk is produced. The average protein requirement for lactation is estimated from milk composition data and the mean volume of 750 ml produced daily, assuming an efficiency of 70% in conversion of dietary protein to milk protein.

Lipids

The fat in breast milk directly reflects both the amount and saturation pattern of fat in the maternal diet. Severe restriction of energy intake results in mobilization of body fat, with the result that milk produced has a fatty acid composition resembling that of the mother's depot fat.

Human milk contains 10 to 20 mg/dl of cholesterol, resulting in an approximate daily consumption of 100 mg/day by the infant. The amount of cholesterol in milk does not seem to be influenced by the mother's diet; however, the cholesterol content of the milk is reduced as lactation progresses.

Vitamins and Minerals

Some mineral and vitamin concentrations in breast milk seem sensitive to maternal intake. Zinc supplementation of mothers may result in higher zinc concentrations in their milk. It appears that the selenium content of milk is strongly related to maternal selenium status (Mannan and Picciano, 1987). The vitamin D content of milk is related to the maternal vitamin D intake and the amount of sun exposure (Specker and Tsang, 1987). See Chapter 10 for further discussions of vitamin D intake in infancy.

Breast-Feeding an Infant

Preparation

Positive emphasis on the advantages of breast-feeding should be presented early in pregnancy if not before. Women should be encouraged to express their opinions and feelings so that they can be discussed and any misinformation can be corrected. During the last months of pregnancy, counseling on the process of lactation should be made available to women who have decided to breast-feed. Fathers should be encouraged to participate in counseling sessions, inasmuch as their encouragement and emotional support contribute to successful lactation. Many mothers have never seen a woman nursing an infant; they therefore find it especially helpful to have a woman who has successfully nursed an infant available to answer questions and provide positive reinforcement.

The Technique

The baby should be put to the breast as soon after birth as the mother feels ready. It is not essential that suckling occur immediately after delivery, but some mothers wish this experience and if possible their wishes should be accommodated. Milk may be expected to flow within 48 to 96 hours after delivery. Before this time, however, the thin yellow fluid called *colostrum* should appear; colostrum is higher in protein and lower in fat and carbohydrate than mature milk; it provides approximately 15 kcal/oz along with a rich source of antibodies. As it becomes replaced by transitional and mature milk, the breasts become enlarged and firm as they fill with milk.

For breast-feeding to be successful, it is important that both mother and infant get into a comfortable position, either sitting or lying down. The mother should hold the baby close, cradling the baby in her arm to support the head if she is sitting up. If the baby's cheek is touched, the baby will turn toward that side (the rooting reflex). The mother should hold her breast so that the areola and nipple are in the baby's mouth as much as possible. If the breast is very full, it helps to press the breast gently away from the baby's nose so that the infant can breathe more easily. Alternatively, it may be helpful for the mother to express a little milk before letting the baby nurse. The baby should be allowed to nurse from 5 to 10 minutes on each side initially, then longer if both wish.

The *let-down* reflex is detected by a tingling sensation, which is often accompanied by dripping from the opposite nipple and occasionally by uterine cramps. It may take some time for the let-down reflex to become fully functional and conditioned. Some women never feel the let-down, but swallowing by the baby is a definite sign that it has occurred. Rest or a hot shower before nursing may help the let-down reflex. If the woman has too much milk, the baby may need to nurse on only one side at a feeding for a while. This reduces overall stimulation and thus the milk supply. This could also be a good time to express milk from the other breast for storage for a future feeding when the mother needs to be away.

To remove the baby from the breast, a finger is placed in the corner of the baby's mouth until the suction is broken. The breast can then be comfortably removed. Most babies need to be burped before feeding from the second breast; the need for burping, however, is highly individual among babies.

Because breast milk is more easily digested than other infant feeds, breast-fed infants may wish to feed more often than formula-fed babies. If the baby wants to nurse, there is no reason not to let him or her do so; breast-fed babies consume what they need and no more. Breast-feeding whenever the baby is hungry is easy to do, because the milk is always ready. Some babies may be hungry as frequently as every hour or two on some days, whereas others may at times not become hungry until 4 hours after the previous feeding. The more often the baby nurses, the more milk the breasts produce; thus, whenever a woman's supply is low (e.g., during or after an illness, provided that there is no risk that the baby will contract the disease through breast-feeding), she should nurse more often.

Parents should realize that crying does not always mean that the baby is hungry. He or she may be physically uncomfortable or just want to be held, burped, or changed. Parents usually learn to distinguish the different needs of their infants.

Feeding time is perfectly suited for establishing and maintaining close mother-child interactions, as shown in Figure 9–11. The mother, however, need not be tied to her infant all of the time. On occasions when she wants or needs to be away from her infant at the usual time of feeding, a bottle can be given. The bottle might contain formula or breast milk that has been expressed earlier. It is best to avoid supplemental bottles other than water until the woman is satisfied that her milk supply is well established and regulated, usually around 6 weeks postpartum. She should consider taking the baby with her instead.

Duration of Breast-Feeding

The length of time a woman breast-feeds her infant will depend on her own feelings and situation. If she is working, she can continue to breast-feed by expressing milk and by instructing a caregiver to give it in a bottle. Milk will continue to be produced as long as there is demand for it and it is taken from the breast, although a breast may not be emptied at any given feeding.

Some mothers prefer to breast-feed until the baby can be weaned to a cup (thus avoiding bottles altogether); this can be accomplished when the baby is about 9 to 10 months of age. Some mothers choose to breast-feed much longer—for several years—letting the baby decide when to be weaned. There is a wide variability in ease of weaning, depending on the baby's overall interest in nursing, the relationship between mother and child, and the use of bottles. Babies who have had frequent supplemental bottles from birth are likely to wean themselves at an early age.

When a mother decides to wean her baby, it should be done gradually over a period of several weeks. At first, one feeding can be omitted for several days; two feedings may then be skipped until the baby is down to one feeding a day (usually the night or early morning feeding). Eventually this last feeding can be discontinued. Weaning in this gradual manner will be easier on the mother, avoiding engorgement of her breasts, and will make it easier for the baby to adjust to the new routine.

Common Problems

The inexperienced nursing mother is likely to encounter some problems in the course of adjustment to the breast-feeding experience. Some of the initial diffi-

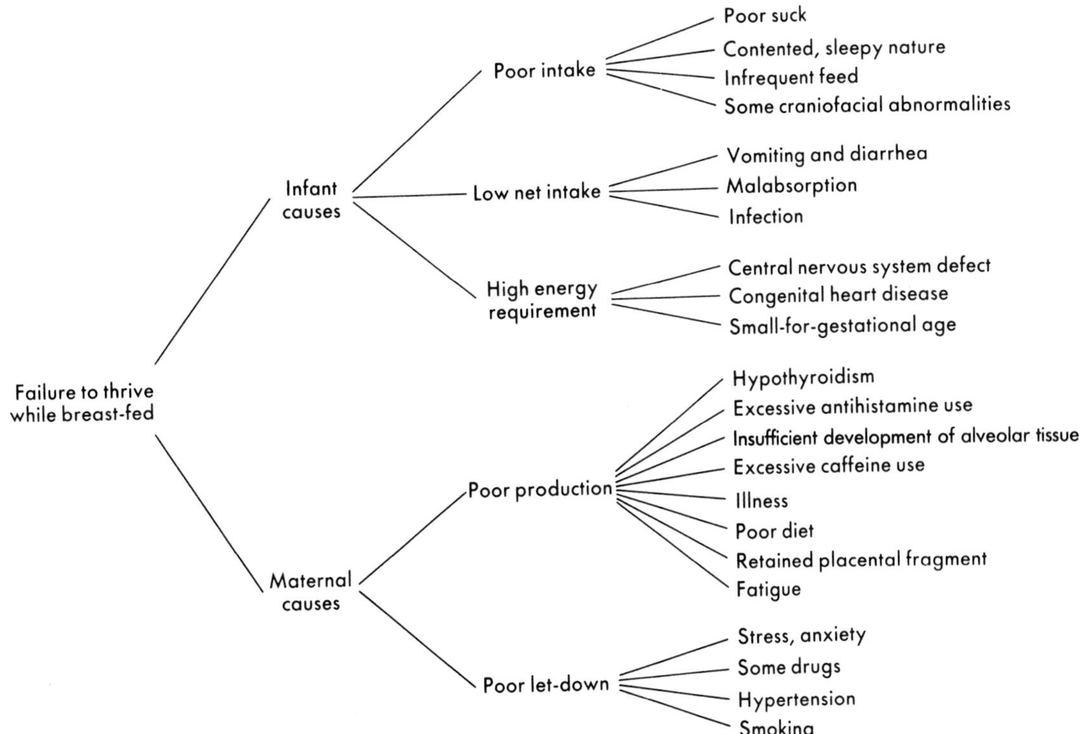

FIGURE 9–10. *Diagnostic flow chart for failure to thrive. (CNS = central nervous system problems; SGA = small for gestational age.) (Reproduced by permission from Worthington-Roberts BS and Williams SR: Nutrition in Pregnancy and Lactation, 2nd ed. St. Louis, Times Mirror/Mosby College Publishing. After Lawrence R: Breast-feeding: A Guide for the Medical Profession, 2nd ed. St Louis, CV Mosby, 1985.)*

culties are summarized in Table 9–7 along with comments about counseling strategies. Success or failure at the breast-feeding effort may depend mainly on the availability of help in the early weeks and on the support of a clinician or friend who provides useful tips.

TABLE 9–7. Management of Breast-Feeding Problems

Problem	Approaches to Management
Retracted nipple(s)	Before feeding the infant, roll the nipple gently between the fingers until erect.
Baby's mouth not open wide enough	Before feeding, depress the infant's lower jaw with one finger as the nipple is guided into the mouth.
Baby sucks poorly	Stimulate sucking motions by pressing upward under the baby's chin. Expression of colostrum often occurs and the taste may stimulate sucking.
Baby demonstrates rooting but does not grasp the nipple; eventually cries in frustration	Interrupt the feeding, comfort the infant; mother should take time to relax before trying again.
Baby falls asleep while nursing	If the infant falls asleep early in the feeding, mother should awaken the infant by holding him or her upright, rubbing his or her back, talking to him or her, or providing similar quiet stimuli; another effort can then be made. If the baby falls asleep again, the feeding should be postponed.

ENGORGED BREASTS. If nursing has been on demand since birth, painful engorgement of the breasts is not likely to occur. If the breasts become engorged, the discomfort can be relieved by applying wet cloths as hot as can be endured to the whole breast and, at the same time, by expressing milk from the nipple. This helps to relieve discomfort. As the wet cloth cools, it should be replaced with another hot one.

To express milk by hand, the thumb and forefinger are placed on opposite sides of the breast just outside the areola, pressed into the rib cage, and then squeezed together and downward; the nipple should not be pulled outward. The procedure is repeated, moving the thumb and forefinger around the nipple until as much milk as desired has been expressed. Sometimes it helps to do breast massage before expressing the milk; this is done by putting the thumbs together on top of the breast and the remaining fingers under the breast. Gentle traction is then exerted from around the breast toward the nipple. If the milk is to be used later, it should be expressed into a sterile bottle and refrigerated. Milk expression is not easy for some women at first, but persistence usually brings success if the mother takes the time.

SORE NIPPLES. The nipples may become sore at the beginning of breast-feeding. This problem may be minimized if the woman toughens the skin of the nipple and surrounding area by massage during the latter months of pregnancy. Nipple rolling is sometimes practiced, or alternatively frequent massage with a bath towel may be useful. During the early days of nursing, soreness may be limited by utilizing a correct nursing position, avoiding undue breast engorgement, and gradually increasing the length of time the baby is allowed to nurse. If soreness occurs, it is always temporary and occurs until the nipples become accustomed to the baby's sucking. One of the best ways to relieve the soreness is to expose the nipples to the air. This is done by removing the bra and wearing a loose cotton blouse or shirt. It is also helpful to briefly expose the bare nipples to a sunlamp or the sun. It may also help to apply a soothing ointment like lanolin. Persistence in breast-feeding is important because the soreness will be gone in several days. Until soreness subsides, nursing should be initiated on the side that feels the best. Limiting sucking leads to engorgement and increased soreness. However, nursing should be limited to 10 to 15 minutes at each side while the soreness persists.

INVERTED (RETRACTED) AND FLAT NIPPLES. Most nipples protrude a bit from the surrounding areola. Sometimes, however, they look flat, or even go inward partially or completely. These are called inverted or "turned in" nipples. Careful examination will determine whether these nipples are truly inverted or not.

Inverted nipples can cause serious difficulties, but they are rare. Most of these nipples are just flat and, with patience and care during pregnancy and the first part of breast-feeding, will become normal. If the nipple is pulled out (protracted) but slips away as if it is fastened to the tissues beneath the skin, it is potentially functional. If it is truly inverted, it may not be protracted at all. Usually, it is possible to pull the nipple out a short way, and such a nipple stretches when the baby sucks from it. Some flat-looking nipples protract very well.

A truly inverted (nonprotractible) nipple can be quite difficult to manage but must be treated if breast-feeding is to be attempted. The first step is to obtain plastic breast shields or something similar to wear inside the bra. The woman should wear these shells daily over her nipples from the seventh month of pregnancy until term. She must also do the "pulling exercise"—repeatedly pulling the nipple away from the areola. Also, during the early days of feeding she may wish to use a nipple shield. Some women with flat but protractible nipples may also use nipple shells and shields.

PLUGGED DUCTS. Occasionally a milk duct will become plugged, creating a tender spot on the breast that even appear lumpy and hot. This might result from inadequate emptying of the milk ducts or from wearing a bra that is too tight. Should a plugged duct develop, the following approaches might be taken:

1. Offer the sore breast first to the baby so that it will be emptied more completely.
2. Nurse longer and more often; if the breast gets too full, the plugged duct becomes worse and infection may develop.
3. Change positions at every feeding so that the pressure of the nursing will be applied to different places on the breast.
4. Apply warm compresses to the breasts between feedings to reduce the risk of infection.

INFECTION. If breast tenderness is accompanied by fever and a general flu-like feeling, a breast infection is probably present. Treatment involves bed rest, continued nursing (offering the sore breast first), application of heat with a hot water bottle or heating pad, supporting the breasts with a firm bra, and consulting a physician.

There is generally no danger from the baby becoming ill from nursing on the infected breast. The same bacteria as those responsible for the infection of the mother are usually already present in the baby's nose and throat. Breast infections are sometimes complicated by localized pus accumulation; this is referred to as a breast abscess and may require surgical opening and draining in addition to antibiotics. Women are advised not to nurse on the affected side until the abscess heals. During the interval when the woman is not nursing, the milk should be frequently expressed by hand from the affected breast.

LEAKING. Some mothers are bothered by leaking breasts either during or between feedings. Although this may help to relieve fullness in the early weeks of lactation, it soon becomes a nuisance. It can be stopped by simply pressing firmly with the palm of the hand against the leaking nipple. A less obvious way to stop both breasts from leaking is for the woman to cross her arms against her breasts and press firmly. Gauze pads with an outside plastic coat may be inserted inside the bra to catch any milk that may be released. If this is done, the pads should be changed frequently.

FAILURE TO THRIVE IN THE BREAST-FEEDING INFANT. Insufficient milk supply is rarely a problem for the well-fed mother. Because sucking stimulates the flow of milk, feeding on demand for adequate duration should supply ample amounts of milk. If the baby continues steadily to gain weight and length, has at least six wet diapers daily and normal stools, the milk supply is probably adequate.

Occasionally, however, an infant will fail to thrive while seemingly nursing properly. A variety of circumstances can be explored as likely bases for the unsatis-

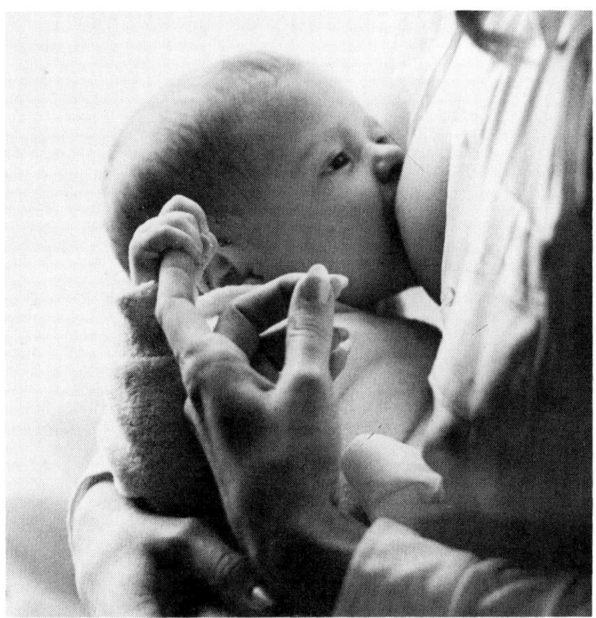

FIGURE 9–11. *A mother and her baby enjoying the close physical contact while nursing. (Photograph copyright of Kathryn Abbe, New York.)*

factory breast-feeding experience. Figure 9–10 illustrates diagrammatically potential problems in the mother or in the infant that should be investigated during the course of evaluation. If the cause of the problem cannot be identified or the defined problem cannot be corrected, it may be necessary to encourage the mother to turn to commercial infant formula for at least partial nutritional support of the infant.

Relactation and Induced Lactation

Occasionally a mother starts breast-feeding late or discontinues nursing but decides at a much later date that she would like to begin again. She can attempt "relactation" through providing the infant substantial opportunities to suck at the breast. With much sucking stimulus over several days' time, many patient and persistent women can initiate the lactation process late or once again. Their volume of milk production may be less than the infant demands, in which case a supplemental feeding following nursing may be necessary. Alternatively, some women find that the Lact-aid Nursing Trainer* nicely complements their own milk production. While the baby sucks at the breast, he or she also obtains milk via suction through a small tube leading to a bag of fresh formula that is clipped to the mother's bra. While sucking, the baby simultaneously builds up the mother's milk supply and receives adequate nutrition through the Lact-aid feeding device.

After adopting an infant, a minority of women decide to attempt lactation. Some of these women have never done so before, and others have breast-fed a previous baby of their own. With much sucking stimulus, lactation can often be induced, but only with great perseverance and in most cases only if a woman has once carried a pregnancy well into the second trimester. Because the mammary glands complete their development for lactation during the first 6 months of pregnancy, a woman who has never been pregnant or never carried a pregnancy beyond the first trimester is a poor candidate for successful induction of lactation.

Breast Pumping and Milk Storage

Mothers may wish to remove milk from their breasts for a number of reasons, for example, to save it for a later feeding, take it to their hospitalized neonate, or donate it to a milk bank. Under such circumstances, some women find it satisfactory to express milk by hand. For many women, however, a manual or electric breast pump provides a better stimulus for milk flow and a more efficient mode of milk collection. Instructions for use of these pumps accompany each apparatus, but individual counseling by a skilled clinician or experienced nursing mother can greatly simplify the process of learning to pump.

NUTRITION, FERTILITY, AND CONCEPTION

Although most American women have access to sufficient food sources of energy, protein, and micronutrients, individual circumstances sometimes prevent a woman from achieving nutritional well-being. The problem may be one of limited resources, but it is just as likely to be one of self-selected behaviors that lead to nutritional imbalances over time. Should poor dietary practices occur during childhood or adolescence, or both, growth and development can be temporarily or permanently limited. Stunted linear growth or incomplete development of the pelvic girdle might later interfere with normal fetal development due to restricted maternal space. Chronic dieting may lead to amenorrhea and the obvious consequence of reduced fertility. Deficiencies of specific nutrients may lead to eventual depletion of nutrient stores such that the functioning of many physiologic and biochemical processes may be adversely affected; resistance to disease may decrease and energy to perform daily activities may wane. Overeating associated with lack of exercise may lead to excessive deposition of body fat; massive obesity poses a serious risk to the well-being of both mother and child during and after pregnancy.

* Lact-aid Nursing Trainer is available from Resources in Human Nurturing International, 3885 Forest St, P.O. Box 6861, Denver, Colorado 80206.

The Dietary Guidelines for Americans provide an appropriate base for counseling women of reproductive age (see Chapter 16). Although the food industry is making an effort to assist consumers with dietary change, only small signs of recent dietary improvement have been recorded. Clearly there is need for continued focus on individualized nutrition counseling for women of reproductive age. Whether defined problems are due to lack of resources, lack of nutrition knowledge, self-imposed dietary manipulations, genetic idiosyncrasies, or a combination of the above, solutions to defined problems can often be found. Although the value of nutrition counseling may not be measurable immediately, the ultimate result may be improved preparation for reproduction and the accompanying responsibilities of parenting.

CITED REFERENCES

Abrams BF and Laros RK: Prepregnancy weight, weight gain and birth weight. Am J Obstet Gynecol 154:503, 1986.

American College of Obstetricians and Gynecologists: Exercise During Pregnancy and the Postnatal Period (ACOG Home Exercise Programs). Washington, DC, American College of Obstetricians and Gynecologists, 1985.

Bapurao S, Raman L, and Tulpule PG: Biochemical assessment of vitamin B_6 nutritional status in pregnant women with orolingual manifestations. Am J Clin Nutr 36:581, 1982.

Benke PJ: The isotretinoin teratogen syndrome. JAMA 251:3267, 1984.

Breskin MW et al: First trimester serum zinc concentrations in human pregnancy. Am J Clin Nutr 38:943, 1983.

Brown JE and Toma RB: Taste changes during pregnancy. Am J Clin Nutr 43:414, 1986.

Chang S-J: Antimicrobial proteins of maternal and cord sera and human milk in relation to maternal nutritional status. Am J Clin Nutr 51:183, 1990.

Christianson RE, Oechsli RLW, and van den Berg BJ: Caffeinated beverages and decreased fertility. Lancet 1:378, 1989.

Clapp JF and Dickstein S: Endurance exercise and pregnancy outcome. Med Sci Sports Exerc 16:556, 1984.

Connolly KJ, Pharoah POD, and Hetzel BS: Fetal iodine deficiency and motor performance during childhood. Lancet 2:1149, 1979.

Council on Scientific Affairs, American Medical Association: Fetal effects of maternal alcohol use. JAMA 249:2517, 1983.

Dansky LV: Anticonvulsants, folate levels and pregnancy outcome: A prospective study. Ann Neurol 21:176, 1987.

Durnin JVGA: Energy requirements of pregnancy: An integration of the longitudinal data from the 5-country study, Nestle Foundation Annual Report. Lausanne, Switzerland, Nestle Foundation, 1986, pp 147–154.

Edwards LE et al: Pregnancy in the underweight woman: Course, outcome and growth patterns of the infant. Am J Obstet Gynecol 135:297, 1979.

Expert Panel on the Content of Prenatal Care: Caring for Our Future: The Content of Prenatal Care. Washington, DC, DHHS, PHS, 1989.

Food and Nutrition Board, National Research Council, NAS: Recommended Dietary Allowances, 10th ed. Washington, DC, National Academy Press, 1989.

Forsum E, Sadurkis A, and Wagner J: Resting metabolic rate and body composition of healthy Swedish women during pregnancy. Am J Clin Nutr 47:942, 1988.

Freinkel N, Dooley SL, and Metzger BE: Care of the pregnant woman with insulin-dependent diabetes mellitus. N Engl J Med 313:96, 1985.

Halmesmaki E, Raivio KO, and Ylikorkala O: Patterns of alcohol consumption during pregnancy. Obstet Gynecol 69:594, 1987.

Hambidge KM et al: Acute effects of iron therapy on zinc status during pregnancy. Obstet Gynecol 70:593, 1987.

Hytton FE and Leitch I: The Physiology of Human Pregnancy, 2nd ed. Oxford, Blackwell Scientific Publications, 1971.

Institute of Medicine: Preventing Low Birthweight. National Academy Press, 1985.

Joesoef MR et al: Are caffeinated beverages risk factors for delayed conception? Lancet 335:136, 1990.

Kramer MS: Intrauterine growth and gestational duration determinants. Pediatrics 80:502, 1987.

Kurppa K et al: Coffee consumption during pregnancy. N Engl J Med 306:1548, 1982.

Lammer EJ et al: Retinoic acid embryopathy. N Engl J Med 313:837, 1985.

Laurence KM et al: Double-blind randomized controlled trial of folate treatment before conception to prevent recurrence of neural tube defects. Br Med J 282:1509, 1981.

Lechtig A et al: Effect of food supplementation during pregnancy on birth weight. Pediatrics 56:508, 1975a.

Lechtig A et al: Effect of moderate maternal malnutrition on the placenta. Am J Obstet Gynecol 123:191, 1975b.

Linn S et al: No association between coffee consumption and adverse outcomes of pregnancy. N Engl J Med 306:141, 1982.

Little RE and Sing CF: Association of father's drinking and infant's birth weight. N Engl J Med 314:1644, 1986.

Loris P, Dewey KG, and Poirier-Brode K: Weight gain and dietary intake of pregnant teenagers. J Am Diet Assoc 85:1296, 1985.

Luke B, Jonaitis MA, and Petrie RH: A consideration of height as a function of prepregnancy nutritional background and its potential influence on birth weight. J Am Diet Assoc 84:176, 1984.

Mannan S and Picciano MF: Influence of maternal selenium status on human milk selenium concentration and glutathione peroxidase activity. Am J Clin Nutr 46:95, 1987.

Marya RK, Rathee KLS, and Manrow M: Effect of calcium and vitamin D supplementation on toxaemia of pregnancy. Gynecol Obstet Invest 24:38, 1987.

Mills JL et al: National Institute of Child Health and Human Development Neural Tube Defects Study Group: The absence of a relation between the periconceptional use of vitamins and neural tube defects. N Engl J Med 321:430, 1989.

Milunsky A et al: Multivitamin/folic acid supplementation in early pregnancy reduces the prevalence of neural tube defects. JAMA 262:2847, 1989.

Mulinare J et al: Periconceptional use of multivitamins and the occurrence of neural tube defects. JAMA 260:3141, 1988.

Murphy JF et al: Relation of haemoglobin levels in first and second trimesters to outcome of pregnancy. Lancet 1:992, 1986.

Naeye RL: Teenaged and pre-teenaged pregnancies: Consequences of the fetal-maternal competition for nutrients. Pediatrics 67:146, 1981.

Naeye RL: Weight gain and the outcome of pregnancy. Am J Obstet Gynecol 135:3, 1979.

National Center for Health Statistics: Maternal weight gain and the outcome of pregnancy, 1980. DHHS, PHS, Series 21, No 44. Washington, DC, US Government Printing Office, 1986.

Osbourne J: Healthier pregnancies for women with diabetes. Diabetes Focus Spring 1988, p 15.

Pederson A et al: Weight gain patterns during twin gestation. J Am Diet Assoc 89:642, 1989.

Primrose T and Higgins A: A study of human antepartum nutrition. J Reprod Med 7:257, 1971.

Pulkkinen MO et al: Serum vitamin B_6 in pure pregnancy depression. Acta Obstet Scand 57:471, 1978.

Roepke JLB and Kirksey A: Effects of vitamin B_6 supplementation during pregnancy on the vitamin B_6 nutriture of previous long term oral contraceptive users and nonusers. Fed Proc 40:863, 1981.

Rosa FW et al: Vitamin A congeners. Teratology 33:355, 1986.

Rosenberg L et al: Selected birth defects in relation to caffeine-containing beverages. JAMA 247:1429, 1982.

Rosett HL et al: Treatment experience with pregnant problem drinkers. JAMA 249:2029, 1983.

Rush D: The National WIC Evaluation: An Evaluation of the Special Supplemental Food Program for Women, Infants and Children, vols I and II. New York, Research Triangle Institute and New York State Research Foundation for Mental Hygiene, 1986.

Schuster K, Bailey LB, and Mahan CS: Vitamin B_6 status of low income adolescent and adult pregnant women and the condition of their infants at birth. Am J Clin Nutr 34:1731, 1981.

Schuster K et al: Morning sickness and vitamin B_6 status of pregnant women. Human Nutr Clin Nutr 39C:75, 1985.

Scrisuphan W and Bracken MB: Caffeine consumption during pregnancy and association with late spontaneous abortion. Am J Obstet Gynecol 154:14, 1986.

Sheppard S et al: Neural tube defect recurrence after "partial" vitamin supplementation. J Med Genet 26:326, 1989.

Smith GFD: Effects of the state of nutrition of the mother during pregnancy and labour on the condition of the child at birth and for the first few days of life. Lancet 2:54, 1916.

Smithells RW et al: Apparent prevention of neural tube defects by periconceptional vitamin supplementation. Arch Dis Child 56:911, 1981.

Smithells RW et al: Further experience of vitamin supplementation for prevention of neural tube defect recurrences. Lancet 1:1027, 1983.

Smithells RW et al: Possible prevention of neural-tube defects by periconceptional vitamin supplementation. Lancet 1:339, 1980.

Soltan MH and Jenkins MH: Maternal and fetal plasma zinc concentration and fetal abnormality. Br J Obstet Gynaecol 89:56, 1982.

Specker BL and Tsang RC: Cyclical serum 25-hydroxyvitamin D concentrations paralleling sunshine exposure in exclusively breast-fed infants. J Pediatr 110:744, 1987.

Streissguth AP et al: Comparison of drinking and smoking patterns during pregnancy over a six-year interval. Am J Obstet Gynecol 145:716, 1983.

Streissguth AP et al: Teratogenic effects of alcohol in humans and laboratory animals. Science 209:353, 1980.

Strode MA et al: Effects of short-term caloric restriction on lactational performance of well-nourished women. Acta Paediatr Scand 75:222, 1986.

Sturtevant FM: Use of aspartame in pregnancy. Int J Fertil 30:85, 1985.

Subcommittee on Nutritional Status and Weight Gain During Pregnancy and Subcommittee on Dietary Intake and Nutrient Supplements During Pregnancy: Nutrition During Pregnancy, Parts I and II, Washington, DC, National Academy Press, 1990.

Teratology Society: Teratology Society position paper: Recommendations for vitamin A use during pregnancy. Teratology 35:269, 1987.

The latest on eating for two. Tufts University Dietetics and Nutrition Letter 8:7, 1990.

van Raaij JMA et al: Body fat mass and basal metabolic rate in Dutch women before, during, and after pregnancy: A reappraisal of energy cost of pregnancy. Am J Clin Nutr 49:765, 1989.

Villar J et al: Calcium supplementation reduces blood pressure during pregnancy: Results of a randomized controlled clinical trial. Obstet Gynecol 70:317, 1987.

Wald NJ: Neural tube defects and vitamins: The need for a randomized clinical trial. Br J Obstet Gynaecol 91:516, 1984.

Weathersbee PS, Olsen LK, and Lodge JR: Caffeine and pregnancy: A retrospective survey. Postgrad Med 62:64, 1977.

Worthington-Roberts BS and Williams SR: Nutrition in Pregnancy and Lactation, 4th ed. St Louis, CV Mosby, 1989.

Zlatnick FJ and Burmeister LF: Dietary protein in pregnancy: Effect on anthropometric indices of the newborn infant. Am J Obstet Gynecol 146:199, 1983.

ADDITIONAL REFERENCES

Belizan JM and Villar J: The relationship between calcium intake and edema-, proteinuria- and hypertension-gestosis: An hypothesis. Am J Clin Nutr 33:2202, 1980.

Glenn FB, Glenn WD, and Duncan RC: Fluoride tablet supplementation during pregnancy for caries immunity: A study of the offspring produced. Am J Obstet Gynecol 143:560, 1982.

Lauwers J and Woessner C: Counselling the Nursing Mother, 2nd ed. Garden City, NY, Avery Publishing Group, 1989.

Naeye RL: Causes of fetal and neonatal mortality by race in a selected U.S. population. Am J Public Health 69:857, 1979.

Rush D: Is WIC worthwhile? Am J Public Health 72:1101, 1982.

Subcommittee on Nutritional Status and Weight Gain During Pregnancy and Subcommittee on Dietary Intake and Nutrient Supplements During Pregnancy, National Academy of Sciences: Nutrition during pregnancy. Executive summary. Nutr Today 25:13, 1990.

Viegas OAC, Cole TJ, and Wharton BA: Impaired fat deposition in pregnancy: An indicator for nutritional intervention. Am J Clin Nutr 45:23, 1987.

CHAPTER 10

NUTRITION IN INFANCY

Peggy L. Pipes, M.A., M.P.H., R.D.

CHAPTER OUTLINE

KEY TERMS

CASEIN—the principal protein of cow's milk
CASEIN HYDROLYSATE—casein that has been split into smaller components by using acid, alkali, or enzyme
COLIC—severe abdominal pain in infants
ELECTROLYTICALLY REDUCED IRON—iron that has been fractionated into small particles for improved absorption; used in fortification of foods
LACTALBUMIN—an easy-to-digest protein found in milk
LAG DOWN—the phenomenon of growth in the first year of life when the rate of growth shifts downward to genetic potential
PALMAR GRASP—an immature way of holding an object, using the palm
PINCER GRASP—a more refined and mature way of holding an object, using the fingers
RENAL SOLUTE LOAD—the amount of nitrogenous waste and minerals that must be excreted by the kidney
WHEY PROTEINS—the proteins remaining in the watery fraction of milk after the curd and cream have been removed

The first 2 years of life, characterized by rapid physical and social growth and development, are years in which many changes that affect feeding and nutrient intake occur. Also, the adequacy of infants' nutrient intakes affects their interaction with their environment. Healthy, well-nourished infants have the energy to respond to and learn from the stimuli in their environment and to interact with their parents in a manner that encourages bonding and attachment.

PHYSIOLOGIC DEVELOPMENT

During the first few days of life infants lose weight, but birthweight is usually regained by the seventh to the tenth day of life. Thereafter growth proceeds at a rapid but decelerating rate. Infants usually double their birthweight by 4 to 6 months and triple it by 1 year of age. The number of pounds gained during the second year approximates the birthweight. Infants increase their length by 50% during the first year of life and double it by 4 years of age. Total body fat increases rapidly during the first 9 months, after which the rate of fat gain tapers off during the rest of childhood. Total body water decreases from 70% to 60% by 1 year of age.

The stomach capacity of infants increases from 10 to 20 ml at birth to 200 ml by 12 months, enabling infants to consume more food at a time and at less frequent intervals as they grow older. The rate of emptying depends on the size and composition of the meals. During the first weeks after birth gastric acidity decreases and remains lower than that of adults for the first few months.

Trypsin activity of duodenal fluids is less in infants than in older children. However, the enzymatic action is sufficient to digest the milk protein ingested by normal infants.

Newborns absorb 85 to 90% of human milk fat, but they sometimes absorb less than 70% of cow's milk fat. However, the fat in infant formulas is modified so that it is absorbed almost as well as that of human milk.

The bile acid pool of the infant per unit of body surface area is about one half that of the adult, so the absorption of fat does not begin to reach adult levels until 6 to 9 months of age.

The activity of the enzymes maltase, isomaltase, and sucrase reaches adult levels by 28 to 32 weeks of gestation. Lactase activity increases near term and reaches adult levels by birth, whereas pancreatic amylase, which digests starch, continues to remain low during the first 6 months after birth. If starch is fed before this time, there is usually compensation by an increased activity of salivary amylase and digestion in the colon.

The newborn has a functionally immature kidney. The concentrating capacity is limited to as little as 700 mOsm/l in some infants. Others have the concentrating capacity of adults—1,200 to 1,400 mOsm/l.

Development of Feeding Skills

Infants at birth coordinate sucking, breathing, and swallowing, and are prepared to suck or suckle liquids, but not foods with texture. During the first year, normal infants develop head control, the ability to move into and sustain a sitting posture, and the ability to grasp, first with a palmar grasp and then with a refined pincer grasp. They develop a mature suck and rotary chewing, and progress from being fed to finger feeding. In the second year, they learn to independently feed themselves with a spoon. They learn to walk and seek food for themselves.

MILK FOR INFANTS

Human milk is unquestionably the food of choice for the infant. Its composition is designed to provide the necessary energy and nutrients in appropriate amounts. It contains factors that provide protection against certain bacteriologic infections. Allergic reactions to human milk are minimal. The closeness of the mother and infant during feeding facilitates attachment and bonding.

Unmodified cow's milk is inappropriate for infants. The tough hard curd is difficult for young infants to digest, and the absorption of cow's milk fat is less than that of human milk. The much higher protein and ash content of cow's milk results in a higher *renal solute load,* which is the amount of nitrogenous waste and minerals that must be excreted by the kidney. Goat's milk contributes to an even higher renal solute load.

Commercial formulas made from heat-treated nonfat milk are designed to provide necessary nutrients in a well-absorbed form. Formulas prepared from a soy protein isolate or a casein hydrolysate and a variety of other formula and electrolyte replacement solutions are available for infants with special problems, as shown in Table 10-1.

Composition of Human and Cow's Milk

The composition of human milk is uniquely different from cow's milk; for this reason, cow's milk is not recommended for the human infant until at least 1 year of age (Ziegler, 1990). Both provide 20 kcal/oz; however, the nutrient source of the calories is different. Protein provides 6 to 7% of the calories in human milk and 20% of the calories in cow's milk. Whey proteins constitute 60% of the protein in human milk, whereas casein is the main protein in cow's milk, accounting for 80% of the total. Casein forms a tough, hard-to-digest curd in the infant's stomach; lactalbumin forms soft, flocculent, easy-to-digest curds. The amino acids taurine and cystine are present in higher concentrations in human milk than in cow's milk. These amino acids may be essential for premature infants.

Lactose provides 42% of calories in human milk and only 30% of the calories in cow's milk.

Lipids provide 50% of the calories in both human and cow's milk. Monounsaturated oleic acid is the predominant fatty acid in both milks. Linoleic acid, the essential fatty acid, provides 4% of calories in human milk and only 1% in cow's milk. The cholesterol content of human milk is 7 to 47 mg/dl and 10 to 35 mg/dl in cow's milk. An additional lipase in the nonfat fraction of human milk is stimulated by bile salts and contributes significantly to the hydrolysis of milk triglycerides.

All of the water-soluble vitamins in human milk reflect maternal intake. Cow's milk contains adequate quantities of the B complex vitamins but very little vitamin C. Both milks provide sufficient vitamin A. Human milk, providing 2 IU/l, is a richer source of vitamin E than cow's milk. Human milk contains five metabolites of vitamin D providing 40 to 50 IU/l of vitamin D activity; however, the need for additional vitamin D becomes progressively more important with age. Cow's milk is usually fortified with 400 IU/l.

The quantity of iron in human and cow's milk is small, 0.3 mg/l. Forty-nine per cent of iron in human milk but less than 1% of iron in cow's milk is absorbed. The bioavailability of zinc in human milk is higher. Cow's milk contains three times as much calcium and six times as much phosphorus, and the fluoride concentration is twice that of human milk. Because most of the fluoride in the water supply and in the mother's diet does not pass into her milk, the diet of the breast-fed infant needs to be supplemented.

The sodium and potassium concentrations of human milk are about one third that of cow's milk. The osmolality of human milk averages 286 mOsm/kg, whereas the osmolality of cow's milk is 400 mOsm/kg.

Anti-Infective Factors

Human milk and colostrum contain antibodies and anti-infective factors not present in cow's milk. Secretory IgA is the predominant immunoglobin in human milk and plays a role in protecting the infant's immature gut from infection. It appears that breast-feeding must be maintained until at least 3 months of age to offer this protection (Howie, 1990).

The iron-binding protein lactoferrin in human milk deprives bacteria of iron and thus slows their growth. Lysozymes, bacteriolytic enzymes found in human milk, destroy bacteria cell membranes after they have been inactivated by the peroxides and ascorbic acid also present in human milk. The growth of the bacterium *Lactobacillus bifidus* is enhanced by breast milk, and produces an acidic gastrointestinal environment, which interferes with the growth of certain pathogenic organisms. Because of these anti-infective factors, the incidence of infections is lower in breast-fed than in bottle-fed babies.

Formulas

Infants whose mothers are unwilling or unable to breast-feed will usually be fed a formula based on cow's milk or a soy-based product. Those who have special requirements will receive specially designed products.

Five formulas made from nonfat milk are available for normal infants and are designed to be as close as possible to the composition of human milk. Enfamil and SMA have been modified to provide a whey:casein protein ratio similar to that of human milk. Similac and Gerber Formula are subjected to heat treatment, which also reduces the curd tension. Good Start contains hydrolyzed reduced mineral whey. Vegetable oils are added so that fat absorption is similar to that from human milk. Vitamins and minerals are added to meet the recommended intake for infants. Advance and Follow-Up Formula are formulas for the older infant. Advance has fewer calories per ounce but is still fortified with all the necessary vitamins and minerals. Pediatricians feel there is no need for these "older infant" formulas (Committee on Nutrition, 1989c).

The declining prevalence of anemia in infants is credited to the use of the iron-fortified formula, and for this reason the American Academy of Pediatrics recommends that all infants should be using iron-fortified formulas. The impression that low-iron formulas are associated with fewer adverse gastrointestinal reactions is not supported by controlled comparisons (Committee on Nutrition, 1989b).

Formulas are available with and without additional iron. Table 10–1 shows the composition of various formulas and human milk.

A variety of products are available for infants who do not tolerate the milk in cow's milk–based formulas. Soy products designed to meet all the nutrient needs are recommended for: (1) children of vegetarian families; (2) the management of galactosemia, primary lactase deficiency, or recovery from secondary lactose intolerance; and (3) potentially allergic infants who have not shown clinical manifestations of allergy. It is not recommended for children known to have food allergies because many infants allergic to cow's milk also become or are allergic to soy milk (Committee on Nutrition, 1989a).

Infants intolerant of soy products may be fed formulas made from a casein hydrolysate (Nutramigen, Pregestimil, or Alimentum). Other formulas are available

TABLE 10–1. Composition of Infant Formulas per Liter

Milk or Formula	Kcal	Protein (g)	Fat (g)	Carbohydrate (g)	Calcium (mg)	Phosphorus (mg)	Sodium (mg)	Sodium (mEq)	Potassium (mg)	Potassium (mEq)	Iron (mg)	Protein Source	Fat Source	Carbohydrate Source	Comment
Human milk	750	11	45	70	340	140	161	7	570	15	0.2	Lactalbumin, casein	Human	Lactose	Protein readily digested; adequate in all nutrients except vitamin D and fluoride
Standard Formulas															
Similac	676	15	36.3	72.3	510	390	220	10	810	21	12/1.4^{+}	Casein	Soy, coconut, and corn oil	Lactose	Vitamins and minerals added
Enfamil	676	15	33	69	460	320	180	8	720	18	12/1.4^{+}	Reduced-mineral whey, casein	Coconut, and soy oils	Lactose	Whey predominant formula for normal infants; vitamins and minerals added
SMA	676	15	36	72	420	280	150	7	560	14	12/1.4^{+}	Casein, demineralized whey	Oleo, soybean, safflower, and coconut oils	Lactose	Whey predominant formula for normal infants; vitamins and minerals added
Advance	540	20	27	55	510	390	230	10	950	24	10	Casein, soy protein	Soy and corn oils	Corn syrup solids	Formula for infants over 6 months of age
Good Start	670	16	34	74	430	240		17				Hydrolyzed reduced-mineral whey	Palm, safflower, and coconut oils	Lactose, corn syrup	Whey-predominant formula for normal infants; vitamins and minerals added
Follow-Up Formula	670	21	27	85	900	600		24				Nonfat milk	Palm, safflower, and coconut oils	Lactose, corn syrup	Formula for infants over 6 months of age
Gerber Formula	670	15	36	71	500	380	232	10	760	19	trace	Casein	Soy and coconut oils	Lactose	Vitamins and minerals added

Cow's Milk															
Skim	360	36	1	51	1,210	950	520	23	1,450	37	trace	Casein	None	Lactose	Inappropriate for infants
2%	590	42	20	60	1,430	1,120	610	27	1,750	45	trace	Casein	Butterfat	Lactose	Inappropriate for infants
Whole	670	20	36	67	630	500	240	11	820	21	trace	Casein	Butterfat	Lactose	Inappropriate for infants less than 6 months of age
Special Formulas															
ProSobee	676	20	36	68	635	500	243	11	825	21	12.6	Soy protein	Soy oil	Corn syrup solids	Vitamins and minerals added; for infants allergic to cow's milk; lactose and sucrose-free
Isomil	676	18	37	68	710	509	318	14	946	24	12	Soy protein	Coconut and soy oils	Sucrose, corn syrup solids	Vitamins and minerals added; for infants allergic to cow's milk
Nutramigen	670	19	26	90	630	420	320	14	740	19	13	Casein hydrolysate	Corn oil	Modified tapioca, sucrose	Hydrolyzed casein; lactose-free; vitamins and minerals added; infants allergic to soy and cow's milk may tolerate
Similac PM 60/40	676	16	37.6	69	380	190	160	7	580	15	1.5	Casein, demineralized whey	Coconut and corn oils	Lactose	Vitamins and minerals added; protein easily digested
Pregestimil	670	19	27	90	630	420	320	14	740	17	13	Casein hydrolysate	MCT* oil, corn oil	Corn syrup solids, modified tapioca starch	Vitamins and minerals added; protein and fat easily digested; hydrolyzed casein; infants allergic to soy and cow's milk may tolerate; used in malabsorption
Alimentum	676	19	38	69	710	510	300	13	800	20	12.2	Casein hydrolysate	MCT, safflower, and soy oils	Sucrose, modified tapioca starch	Vitamins and minerals added; appropriate for infants allergic to cow's milk and soy formulas

* MCT = medium-chain triglyceride.
† Level depends on whether iron added or not.

for children with specific problems such as malabsorption or phenylketonuria.

Formula Preparation

Commercial formulas are available in ready-to-feed forms requiring no preparation, as concentrates prepared by mixing with equal parts of water, and in powder form made by mixing 2 oz of water with each level tablespoon of the powder.

In most households that maintain a reasonable level of sanitation, sterilization of formulas is seldom practiced. However, care should be taken in maintaining a very clean environment when formulas are made. All equipment, including bottles, nipples, mixers, and the top of the can of milk, should be thoroughly washed. The infant should be fed immediately after the formula is prepared, and any milk not consumed at that feeding should be discarded. Any open cans of formula should be covered and refrigerated.

FOODS FOR INFANTS

A variety of commercially prepared canned or freeze-dried foods are available for infants. These vary widely in nutrient value, as shown in Table 10–2.

Ready-to-serve dry infant cereals are fortified with electrolytically reduced iron. Three level tablespoons of cereal will provide about 5 mg of iron, or from one half to one third of what the infant requires. Therefore, cereal is usually the first food added to the infant's diet. Cereal and fruit mixtures in jars are fortified with ferrous sulfate to provide 7 to 9 mg of iron per 4.5-oz jar.

Strained and junior vegetables and fruits provide carbohydrate and variable amounts of vitamins A and C. Vitamin C is added to a number of fruits and all of the fruit juices. Several fruits, including apricots, have sugar added and are marketed as fruit desserts. Tapioca is added to a number of the fruits. Milk is added to creamed vegetables and wheat is incorporated into the mixed vegetables.

Strained and junior meats and egg yolk are prepared with only water, except for lamb, which has lemon juice added. Strained meats, which have the highest caloric density of any of the commercial baby foods, are an excellent source of high-quality protein and heme iron.

Water is the most abundant ingredient in vegetable and meat combinations and high-meat dinners. The introduction of these products should be delayed until it has been ascertained that an infant has no allergic reactions to any of the wide variety of ingredients they contain.

TABLE 10–2. Average Values of Selected Nutrients in Infant Food per 100 Grams*†

	Calories	Protein (g)	Iron (mg)	Vitamin A (μg RE)‡	Vitamin C (mg)
Infant Cereals, Dry (T)§					
Mixed	13.8	0.4	1.7	—	—
Oatmeal with banana	15	0.5	1.7	—	—
Strained cereal with applesauce and banana per 4.0-oz jar	89.3	1.4	6.8	—	15.7
Strained Fruits (per 100 g or jar [7T])					
Pears and pineapple	53	0.4	0.1	3	13.9
Prunes with tapioca	72	0.6	0.3	30	1.4
Strained Vegetables					
Green beans	31	1.4	0.5	32	1.4
Sweet potatoes	63	1.1	0.3	786	3.4
Strained Meat					
Beef	95	14.1	1.5	6	1.8
Chicken	138	14.4	0.9	1	2.4
Strained Egg Yolk	195	9.9	2.0	147	1.1
Strained Vegetables and Meat					
Vegetables and chicken	58	2.3	0.3	73	1.4
Macaroni and Cheese	67	3.0	0.3	6	0.8
Strained Desserts					
Fruit dessert	76	0.3	0.4	2	13.9
Vanilla custard pudding	85	1.7	0.2	14	0.6

* From Nutrient Values of Gerber Baby Foods. Fremont, MI, Gerber Products Company, 1991.
† Except where specified otherwise.
‡ RE = retinol equivalents.
§ 3.55 g = 1 tablespoon (T).

A number of dessert items are also available, including puddings and fruit desserts. The nutrient composition of these products varies, but all contain sugar and modified corn or tapioca starch.

Mothers who wish to make their own baby food can easily do so, as explained in Table 10–3. Home-prepared foods generally are more concentrated in nutrients than commercially prepared ones because less water is used. Salt should not be added to foods prepared for infants, and sugar should be added sparingly.

NUTRIENT NEEDS OF INFANTS

Nutrient needs of infants reflect rates of growth, energy expended in activity, basal metabolic needs, and the interaction of nutrients consumed. Balance studies have defined minimal acceptable levels of intakes for a few nutrients, but for most nutrients the suggested intakes have been extrapolated from intakes of normal thriving infants. The Recommended Dietary Allowances (RDA) for infants are shown in Table 10–4.

Energy

Normal infants who are breast-fed to satiety and infants fed a standard 20 kcal/oz formula whose mothers are sensitive to their cues of hunger and satiety will generally adjust their intake to meet their energy needs.

The best method to determine the adequacy of infants' energy intakes is to carefully monitor their gain in height and weight by plotting on the growth grids shown in Appendix Tables 7 and 11. It is important to recognize that during the first year *catch up* or *lag down* in growth may be seen. Infants who are genetically determined to be larger than indicated by their birth-weight will shift upward in channels of growth in the first 3 to 6 months of life (Fig. 10–1). Those whose genotypes are for smaller size tend to grow at their fetal rate or less and a growth "lag down" becomes evident. They may be 13 months old before their appropriate growth channel is evident (Smith et al, 1976).

Growth in height and weight should proceed at approximately the same rate. If an infant begins to reduce his or her rate of weight gain, does not gain weight, or loses weight, the energy and nutrient intake should be carefully monitored. If the rate of growth in height is reduced or ceases, the probability of malnutrition or undetected disease, or both, should be thoroughly investigated. If weight gain proceeds at a much more rapid rate than growth in height, the calorie concentration of the formula, quantity of formula consumed, and the amount and type of semisolids and table food offered should be investigated in an assessment of excess energy intake. Activity of the infant should also be explored.

Infants fed a calorically dilute milk such as nonfat milk, or formula to which more water has been added than instructions indicate will increase their intake of milk but not enough to provide for an adequate weight gain. If the formula is concentrated because insufficient water has been added to the powder concentrate, infants will become thirsty and cry. Parents may think that their infant is crying for food and offer more of the

TABLE 10–3. Directions for Home Preparation of Infant Foods

1. Select fresh, high-quality fruits, vegetables, or meats.
2. Be sure all utensils, including cutting boards, grinder, knives, etc, are thoroughly clean.
3. Wash hands before preparing the food.
4. Clean, wash, and trim the food in as little water as possible.
5. Cook the foods until tender in as little water as possible. Avoid overcooking, which may destroy heat-sensitive nutrients.
6. Do not add salt. Add sugar sparingly. Do not add honey or corn syrup to food for infants less than 1 year of age.*
7. Add enough water so that the food has a consistency that is easily puréed.
8. Strain or purée the food using an electric blender, a food mill, a baby food grinder, or a kitchen strainer.
9. Pour purée into ice cube tray and freeze.
10. When food is frozen hard, remove the cubes and store in freezer bags.
11. Defrost and heat in serving container the amount of food that will be consumed at a single feeding.

* Botulism spores have been reported in honey and corn syrup, and young infants do not have the immune capacity to resist this infection.

TABLE 10–4. Recommended Daily Allowances for Children, Birth to Age 3 Years*

Nutrient	Age (Years) 0.0–0.5	0.5–1.0	1–3
Energy needs (kcal)	kg × 108	kg × 98	kg × 102
Protein (g)	kg × 2.2	kg × 1.6	kg × 1.2
Vitamin A (μg RE)†	375	375	400
Vitamin D (μg)‡	7.5	10	10
Vitamin E (mg)§	3	4	6
Vitamin K (μg)	5	10	15
Vitamin C (mg)	30	35	40
Thiamine (mg)	0.3	0.4	0.7
Riboflavin (mg)	0.4	0.5	0.8
Niacin (mg NE)‖	5	6	9
Vitamin B_6 (mg)	0.3	0.6	1.0
Folacin (μg)	25	35	50
Vitamin B_{12} (μg)	0.3	0.5	0.7
Calcium (mg)	400	600	800
Phosphorus (mg)	300	500	800
Magnesium (mg)	40	60	80
Iron (mg)	6	10	10
Zinc (mg)	5	5	10
Iodine (μg)	40	50	70
Selenium (μg)	10	15	20

* Reprinted with permission from *Recommended Dietary Allowances*, 10th edition, c. 1989 by the National Academy of Sciences. Published by National Academy Press, Washington, DC.

† RE = retinol equivalents; 1 RE = 1 μg retinol or 6 μg β-carotene.

‡ As cholecalciferol; 10 μg cholecalciferol = 400 IU of vitamin D.

§ α-Tocopherol equivalents; 1 mg d,α-tocopherol = 1 α-TE.

‖ NE = niacin equivalent.

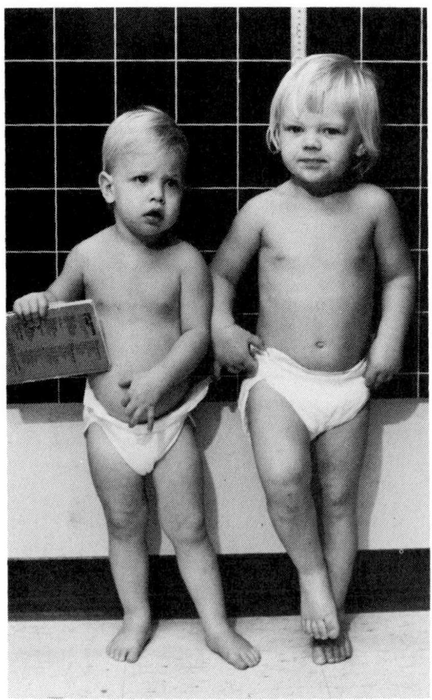

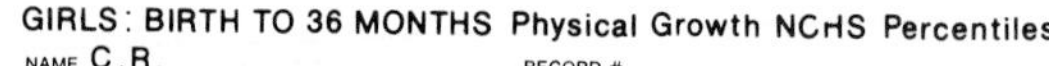

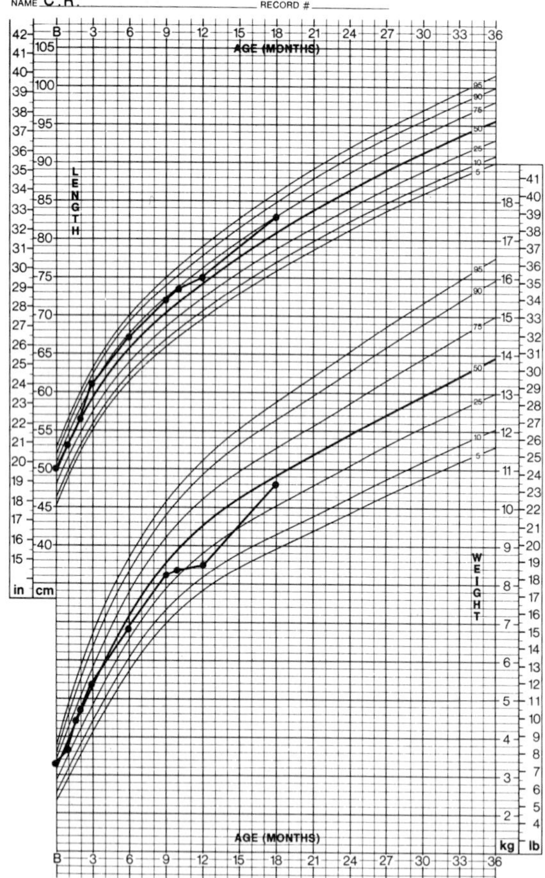

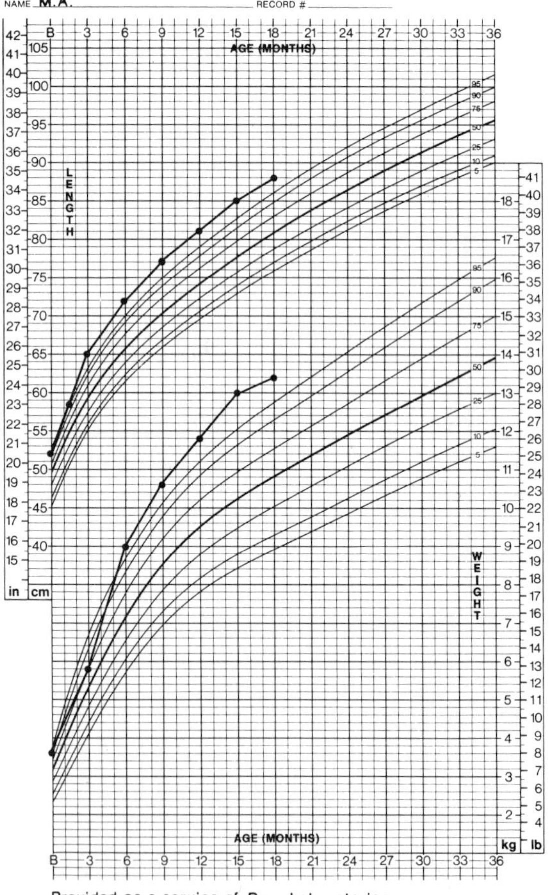

FIGURE 10–1. *These two little girls, born just 1 month apart with only a 1-lb difference in birthweight, show a marked difference in rates of growth and appearance. Note the early catch-up growth shown in the growth grid for M.A. to above the 95th percentile in height and weight prior to 3 months of age. Also note the effect of illness on both weight gain and linear growth in C.R. at age 12 months and the subsequent catch-up growth. The photograph shows the two girls at approximately 20 months of age. (Growth grids adapted from National Center for Health Statistics: NCHS Growth Charts, 1976. Monthly Vital Statistics Report. Vol. 25, No. 3, Suppl. (NRA) 76-1120. Health Resources Administration, Rockville, Maryland, June, 1976. Data from The Fels Research Institute, Yellow Springs, Ohio. Courtesy of Ross Laboratories, Columbus, Ohio.)*

concentrated formula. This will result in an inadequate intake of water and an excessive energy intake and weight gain.

Infants may not grow properly due to parental overconcern about the potential for obesity or eventual heart disease. Because of mistaken beliefs, or in imitation of their own diets, these parents limit the energy intakes of their infants by restricting sugar and fat, snacks, and fat-containing dairy products (Pugliese et al, 1987).

The type of feeding — breast or bottle — and the age at which semisolid foods are introduced do not appear to be etiologic factors in infantile obesity (Fomon et al, 1984). Important factors are the family attitudes toward feeding, parental recognition of cues of hunger and satiety, and the mother's confidence in her own parenting skills and bonding with the baby. Signs of satiety are listed in Table 10–5.

Protein

Protein requirements during the rapid growth of infancy are higher on a per kilogram basis than those of the adult or older child. Recommendations are based on the composition of human milk, assuming the efficiency of utilization of mother's milk to be 100%. Table 10–4 lists the RDA for protein in terms of g/kg body weight for children from birth to age 3 years. On the basis of g/kcal, advisable intakes are 1.9 g/100 kcal for infants 0 to 4 months of age, 1.7 g/100 kcal for infants 4 to 12 months of age, and 1.4 g/kg/day for infants 12 to 36 months of age (Fomon, 1973). These are about 15% lower for infants on breast milk because of the higher biologic value of human milk protein.

Histidine is an essential amino acid for the infant. The minimum requirement of 34 mg/kg/day is amply supplied by human or cow's milk as well as by the standard formulas. Tyrosine, cystine, and taurine may also be essential for the premature infant.

Human milk or formula provides the major portion of protein during the first year of life. Although considerably less than in formula, the amount of protein in human milk is perfectly adequate for the first 6 months. In the last 6 months of the first year, diets of breast-fed infants should be supplemented with additional sources of high-quality protein such as yogurt, strained meats, or cereal mixed with milk.

Inadequate intakes of protein may be the result of excessive dilution of formula, continuation of a regimen designed to treat diarrhea after an enteric illness, extreme vegetarian food patterns, multiple food allergies, or the deprivation associated with extreme poverty.

TABLE 10–5. Satiety Behaviors in Infants*

Age (Weeks)	Behavior
4–12	Draws head away from the nipple Falls asleep When nipple reinserted, closes lips tightly Bites nipple, purses lips, or smiles and lets go
16–24	Releases nipple and withdraws head Fusses or cries Obstructs mouth with hands Increased attention to surroundings Bites nipple
28–36	Changes posture Keeps mouth tightly closed Shakes head as if to say "no" Plays with utensils Hands become more active Throws utensils
40–52	Behaviors of above period Sputters with tongue and lips Hands bottle or cup to mother

* Adapted from Gesell A and Ilg FL: Feeding Behavior of Infants. Philadelphia, JB Lippincott, 1937. Reprinted with permission from Pipes PL: Health care professionals. *In* Garwood G and Fewell R (eds): Educating Handicapped Infants. Rockville, MD, Aspen Systems, 1982.

Lipid

It is recommended that infants consume a minimum of 3.8 g/100 kcal and a maximum of 6 g/100 kcal of fat (30 to 54% of calories). This quantity is present in human milk and all formulas prepared for infants. Significantly lower intakes, as in skim milk feedings, may result in an inadequate energy intake. The infant may try to correct the deficit by increasing the volume of milk, but usually cannot make up the entire amount. Increasing the intake of skim milk furnishes energy but the accompanying excess of protein, calcium, and phosphorus contributes to a high renal solute load and subsequent dehydration.

Linoleic acid, which is essential for growth and dermal integrity, should provide 3% of the total kilocalories. Five per cent of the kilocalories in human milk and 10% in most infant formulas are derived from linoleic acid.

Human milk is a relatively rich source of cholesterol, and it has been suggested that it may be essential in infancy to provide a cholesterol challenge to initiate a cholesterol degrading mechanism. However, infants who receive commercial formula that is very low in cholesterol have been found at the ages of 4 to 7 years to have cholesterol levels that reflect their current dietary intake.

Carbohydrate

Carbohydrate should supply 30 to 60% of the energy intake during infancy. Thirty-seven per cent of the calories in human milk and 40 to 50% of the calories in commercial formulas are derived from lactose or other carbohydrates. The rare infant who cannot tolerate lactose will require a special diet, as discussed in Chapters 27 and 41.

Botulism in infancy is caused by ingestion of the spores of *Clostridium botulinum,* which germinate and produce toxin in the lumen of the bowel. Honey and corn syrup, sometimes used in home-prepared foods, have been identified as the only food sources in infants' diets of these spores, which are extremely resistant to heat treatment and are not destroyed by present methods of processing. Honey and corn syrup should not be fed to infants less than 1 year of age because at this age they do not have the immunity to resist the botulism spore development (Kauter et al, 1982).

Water

The water requirement is determined by the amount lost from the skin and lungs and in the feces and urine plus a small amount needed for growth. The National Research Council recommends an intake of 1.5 ml/kcal/day. Water requirements per kilogram are shown in Table 10–6.

The renal concentrating capacity of the young infant may be less than that of older children and adults; therefore the infant is vulnerable to water imbalance. Human milk and properly prepared formula supply water in amounts adequate under ordinary conditions. When a formula is boiled, the water evaporates and solutes become concentrated; boiled milk or formulas are therefore inappropriate for infants. In very hot, humid environments, the infant may require additional water. When other than renal losses of water are high, as in cases of vomiting and diarrhea, infants should be carefully monitored for both fluid and electrolyte balance.

Water intoxication results in hyponatremia, restlessness, nausea, vomiting, diarrhea, and polyuria or oliguria. Convulsions can result. This may occur if water is fed as a replacement for milk or if the formula is excessively diluted.

TABLE 10–6. Water Requirements of Infants and Children

Age	Water Requirement (ml/kg/day)
10 days	125–150
3 months	140–160
6 months	130–155
1 year	120–135
2 years	115–125
6 years	90–100
10 years	70–85
14 years	50–60

* From Barness LA: Nutrition and nutritional disorders. *In* Behrman RE and Vaughan VC: Nelson Textbook of Pediatrics, 13th ed. Philadelphia, WB Saunders, 1987.

Minerals

Calcium

The RDA for calcium of 400 to 800 mg/day has been planned to meet the needs of infants fed cow's milk–based formula who retain approximately 25 to 30% of their intake. This amount is not applicable to breast-fed infants, who will retain approximately two thirds of their intake of calcium.

The calcium : phosphorus ratio in the infant's diet is no longer felt to be important (Food and Nutrition, 1989).

Iron

Normal infants have adequate stores of iron for growth up to a doubling of their birthweight. This occurs at approximately 4 months of age in full-term infants, and at a much earlier age in prematurely born infants. Recommended intakes of iron increase from 6 mg/day in the first 6 months to 10 mg/day until 3 years of age. Iron in human milk is highly bioavailable; however, both breast-fed and formula-fed infants should receive an additional source of iron by 4 to 6 months of age. Iron-fortified formula and cereals are the most commonly used food sources.

The commonly held belief that iron-fortified formula can cause constipation, loose stools, colic, and spitting up in some infants has not been found to be true in clinical studies (Nelson et al, 1988; Lack of adverse reactions . . . , 1989).

Fresh cow's milk has been shown to be associated with a small but chronic gastrointestinal blood loss that can lead to anemia. Therefore fresh cow's milk should not be used before the child is 1 yr of age.

Zinc

Normal newborns have no reserves of zinc and are therefore immediately dependent on a dietary source of this mineral. Human milk and infant formulas provide adequate zinc for the first year of life, and other foods should provide most of the zinc required during the second year. See Table 10–4 for the RDA for zinc.

Fluoride

The importance of fluoride in the prevention of dental caries has been well documented. Human milk contains little fluoride, and commercially prepared formulas are

TABLE 10–7. Supplemental Fluoride Dosage Schedule (mg/day)*†

Age	Concentration of Fluoride in Drinking Water (ppm)		
	<0.3	*0.3–0.7*	*>0.7*
2 weeks to 2 years	0.25	0	0
2 to 3 years	0.50	0.25	0
3 to 16 years	1.00	0.50	0

* Reproduced by permission of Pediatrics, Vol. 63, p. 150. © 1979.
† 2.2 mg of sodium fluoride contains 1 mg of fluoride.

made with nonfluoridated water. Therefore infants who are breast-fed, those who consume ready-to-feed formula, and those whose formulas are prepared with nonfluoridated water should receive supplemental fluoride. Suggested dosages are shown in Table 10–7.

Vitamins

Milk from an adequately fed lactating mother will supply all the vitamins that the term infant needs except for vitamin D. Breast-fed infants should receive a vitamin D supplement or be regularly exposed to sunlight. Exposure of 30 min/wk, with the infant wearing only a diaper, or 2 hr/wk fully clothed without a hat, is enough (Specker et al, 1985). Commercially prepared infant formulas are fortified with all necessary vitamins. Both evaporated and homogenized cow's milk are fortified with vitamin D but have very little vitamin C. Fresh goat's milk is deficient in vitamin D, vitamin C, and folate.

Vitamin deficiencies have been reported in infants fed formula products in which nutrients were destroyed or omitted during processing or in infants who were fed by a lactating mother whose diet was inadequate and who was not taking appropriate vitamin supplements. In the early 1950s, infants fed a formula in which vitamin B_6 was destroyed during processing were found to be pyridoxine-deficient (Coursin, 1954). A similar incident was reported again in the early 1980s when a manufacturer neglected to add vitamin B_6 during manufacturing of the formula. Fortunately there are very few such instances; however, when formula-fed infants are noted to have symptoms of vitamin deficiency, such errors must be considered.

Most infants can tolerate cow's milk or soy formulas. However, a small number with multiple food intolerances have been able to tolerate goat's milk as their only food for long periods in infancy. When their diets have not been supplemented with folate, these infants have failed to thrive.

The fact that human milk contains only 40 to 50 IU/l of vitamin D activity makes it important to expose these babies to sunlight or to supplement with this nutrient. Cases of rickets have often been diagnosed in breast-fed infants with dark skin and little exposure to sunlight (Bachrach et al, 1979).

Milk from lactating mothers who follow a strict vegan diet may be vitamin B_{12} deficient, especially if the mother has followed the regimen for a long time prior to and during the pregnancy. Also, vitamin B_{12} deficiency has been diagnosed in an infant breast-fed by a mother with pernicious anemia (Higgenbottom et al, 1978; Johnson and Roloff, 1982).

The vitamin K nutriture of the newborn requires special attention. A deficiency may develop and result in bleeding or *hemorrhagic disease of the newborn.* This is more common in breast-fed infants because breast milk contains only 15 μg/l of vitamin K, whereas cow's milk and cow's milk formulas contain approximately four times that amount. Breast-fed infants consume less milk during the first few days of life than do formula-fed infants, which also accounts for their low vitamin K intake. It is recommended that all formulas contain a minimum of 4 μg vitamin K per 100 kcal of formula. The suggested intake of 5 to 15 μg/day can be supplied by mature breast milk (15 μg/l), although perhaps not during the first few days to 1 week of life. Vitamin K supplementation may be necessary during that time. Many states require that infants should receive an injection of vitamin K as a prophylactic measure while they are in the nursery.

Vitamin and mineral supplements should be prescribed only after careful evaluation of the infant's intake and exposure to sunlight. Infants fed commercially prepared formula rarely need supplements. Breast-fed infants need additional vitamin D by 2 months of age. Infants fed homogenized milk or an evaporated milk formula need a food source or supplement of vitamin C, and those who receive goat's milk need a food source or supplement of vitamin C, folate, and vitamin D if it is fresh goat's milk. Evaporated goat's milk is fortified with vitamin D. Chapter 11 discusses the feeding of premature or high-risk infants and their special needs.

FEEDING THE INFANT

Early Feeding Patterns

Because milk from a mother who consumes an adequate diet is uniquely designed to meet the needs of the human infant, breast-feeding for the first 6 months is strongly recommended. Most chronic medical conditions do not contraindicate breast-feeding.

A mother should be encouraged to nurse her infant immediately after birth. Those who care for and counsel parents during the first postpartum days should acquaint themselves with ways in which they can be supportive. Ideally, counseling and preparation start in the last few months or weeks of pregnancy, as is discussed in Chapter 9.

During the first few days, the baby receives colostrum, a yellow transparent fluid that meets the infant's needs during the first week. It contains less fat and carbohydrate but more protein and greater concentrations of sodium, potassium, and chloride than mature milk.

Infants who are bottle-fed will most likely receive ready-to-feed formula in the hospital. At home, products such as concentrated formula that have been refrigerated should be mixed with warm water or heated to body temperature in a water bath. Refrigerated ready-to-feed formula also needs to be warmed.

Regardless of whether the infant is breast- or bottle-fed, the baby should be held and cuddled during feeding. Once a feeding rhythm is established, infants will become fussy or cry to indicate hunger; often they will smile and fall asleep when they are satiated. Infants, not adults, should establish their feeding schedules. Most will initially feed at intervals of 2 to 3 hours, and by 4 weeks of age, most infants have extended the intervals between feedings to 4 hours. By 2 to 4 months of age, sufficient maturation has occurred that most infants omit the night feeding.

Baby Bottle Tooth Decay

A pattern of tooth decay that involves the upper anterior and sometimes lower posterior teeth is common among infants and children who are given sugar-sweetened beverages or fruit juice in a bottle at bedtime (see Chapter 23 and Further Reading, p. 409). Infants should be fed, burped, and put to bed without food.

Whole Cow's Milk

Although it is generally recommended that infants receive human milk or iron-fortified formula for the first year, many parents make the transition from formula to fresh cow's milk when the infant is between 5 and 9 months of age. However, the Committee on Nutrition of the American Academy of Pediatrics has concluded that infants should not be fed whole cow's milk in the first year of life (Ziegler, 1990).

Low-fat (2%) and nonfat milk are also inappropriate feedings for infants during the first year of life. If there is concern about a very rapid weight gain, infants may be offered a formula prepared for the older infant that provides only 54 kcal/100 ml or about 16 kcal/oz, as shown in Table 10–1. Substitute or imitation milks are inappropriate and should not be fed to infants (Committee on Nutrition, 1984).

TABLE 10–8. Developmental Stages of Readiness to Progress in Feeding Behaviors During First Two Years of Life*

Developmental Landmarks	Change Indicated	Examples of Appropriate Foods
Tongue laterally transfers food in the mouth Voluntary and independent movements of the tongue and lips Sitting posture can be sustained Beginning of chewing movements (up and down movements of the jaw)	Introduction of soft, mashed table food	Tuna fish; mashed potatoes; well-cooked mashed vegetables; ground meats in gravy and sauces; soft diced fruit such as bananas, peaches, pears, etc.; liverwurst; flavored yogurt
Reaches for and grasps objects with scissor grasp Brings hand to mouth	Finger feeding (large pieces of food)	Oven-dried toast, teething biscuits, cheese sticks, peeled Vienna sausage (food should be soluble in the mouth to prevent choking)
Voluntary release (refined digital grasp)	Finger feeding (small pieces of food)	Bits of cottage cheese, dry cereal, peas, etc., small pieces of meat
Rotary chewing pattern	Introduction of more textured food from family menu	Well-cooked chopped meats and casseroles, cooked vegetables and canned fruit (not mashed), toast, potatoes, macaroni, spaghetti, peeled ripe fruit
Approximates lips to rim of the cup	Introduction of cup	
Understands relationship of container and contained	Beginning self-feeding (messiness should be expected)	Food that when scooped will adhere to the spoon, such as applesauce, cooked cereal, mashed potatoes, cottage cheese
Increased rotary movements of the jaw	More skilled at cup and spoon feeding	Chopped fibrous meats such as roast and steak
Ulnar deviation of wrist develops		Raw vegetables and fruit (introduce gradually)
Walks alone	May seek food and get food independently	Food of high nutrient value should be available
Names food, expresses preferences; prefers unmixed foods Goes on food jags Appetite appears to decrease		Balanced food intake should be offered and the child should be permitted to develop food preferences. Parents should not be concerned that these preferences will last forever

* Adapted from Pipes P: Nutrition in Infancy and Childhood, 4th ed. St Louis, CV Mosby, 1989.

Addition of Semisolid Foods

In the last decade developmental readiness and nutrient needs have been the criteria that determine appropriate times for the addition of various foods. Table 10–8 lists developmental landmarks and their indications for progression in semisolid and table food introduction. During the first 4 months the infant attains head and neck control and oral motor patterns change from a suck to a suckling to beginnings of a mature sucking pattern. If puréed foods are fed during this phase they are consumed in the same manner as liquids, with each suckle followed by a tongue thrust swallow.

Between 4 and 6 months of age, when the mature suck is refined and munching movements (up and down chopping motions) begin, the introduction of strained foods is appropriate. Infant cereal is usually introduced first. Thereafter, a variety of commercially or home-prepared foods may be offered. The sequence in which these foods are introduced is not important; however, it is important that only one food (e.g., peaches rather than peach cobbler with many ingredients) be introduced at a time. This helps parents to identify if the child has any allergies or intolerances to particular foods.

As oral-motor maturation proceeds, infants' rotary chewing develops, indicating a readiness for more textured foods such as well-cooked mashed vegetables, casseroles, and pasta from the family menu (Fig. 10–2). Learning to grasp, first with a palmar grasp, then an inferior and finally a refined pincer grasp, indicates a readiness for finger foods such as oven-dried toast, arrowroot biscuits, or cheese sticks. Table 10–9 gives recommendations for adding foods to the infant's diet. Hot dogs, grapes, and bread spread with peanut butter have been identified as causes of choking, and should not be offered at this age unless they are cut into small pieces (Harris et al, 1984).

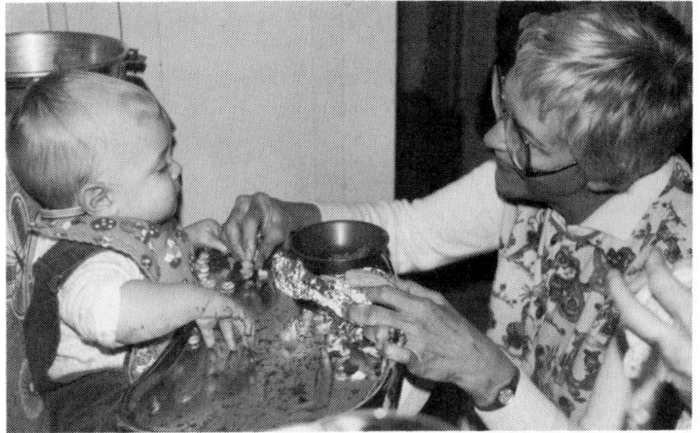

FIGURE 10–2. *Grandparents and relatives often enjoy feeding the infant.*

During the last quarter of the first year, babies can approximate their lips to the rim of the cup and can drink if the cup is held for them. During the second year they gain the ability to rotate their wrists and elevate their elbows, thus allowing them to hold the cup themselves. They feed very messily at first, but by 2 years of age, most normal children are skillful self-feeders (Fig. 10–3).

TABLE 10–9. Suggested Ages for the Introduction of Juice, Semisolid Foods, and Table Foods*

	Age (Months)		
Food	*4 to 6*	*6 to 8*	*9 to 12*
Iron-fortified cereals for infants	Add		
Vegetables		Add strained	Gradually delete strained foods, introduce table foods
Fruits		Add strained	Gradually delete strained foods, introduce chopped well-cooked or canned foods
Meats		Add strained or finely chopped table meats	Decrease the use of strained meats, increase the varieties of table meats
Finger foods such as arrowroot biscuits, oven-dried toast		Add those that can be secured with a palmar grasp	Increase the use of small-sized finger foods as the pincer grasp develops
Well-cooked mashed or chopped table foods, prepared without added salt or sugar			Add
Juice or formula by cup			Add

* From Pipes P: Nutrition in Infancy and Childhood, 4th ed. St Louis, CV Mosby, 1989.

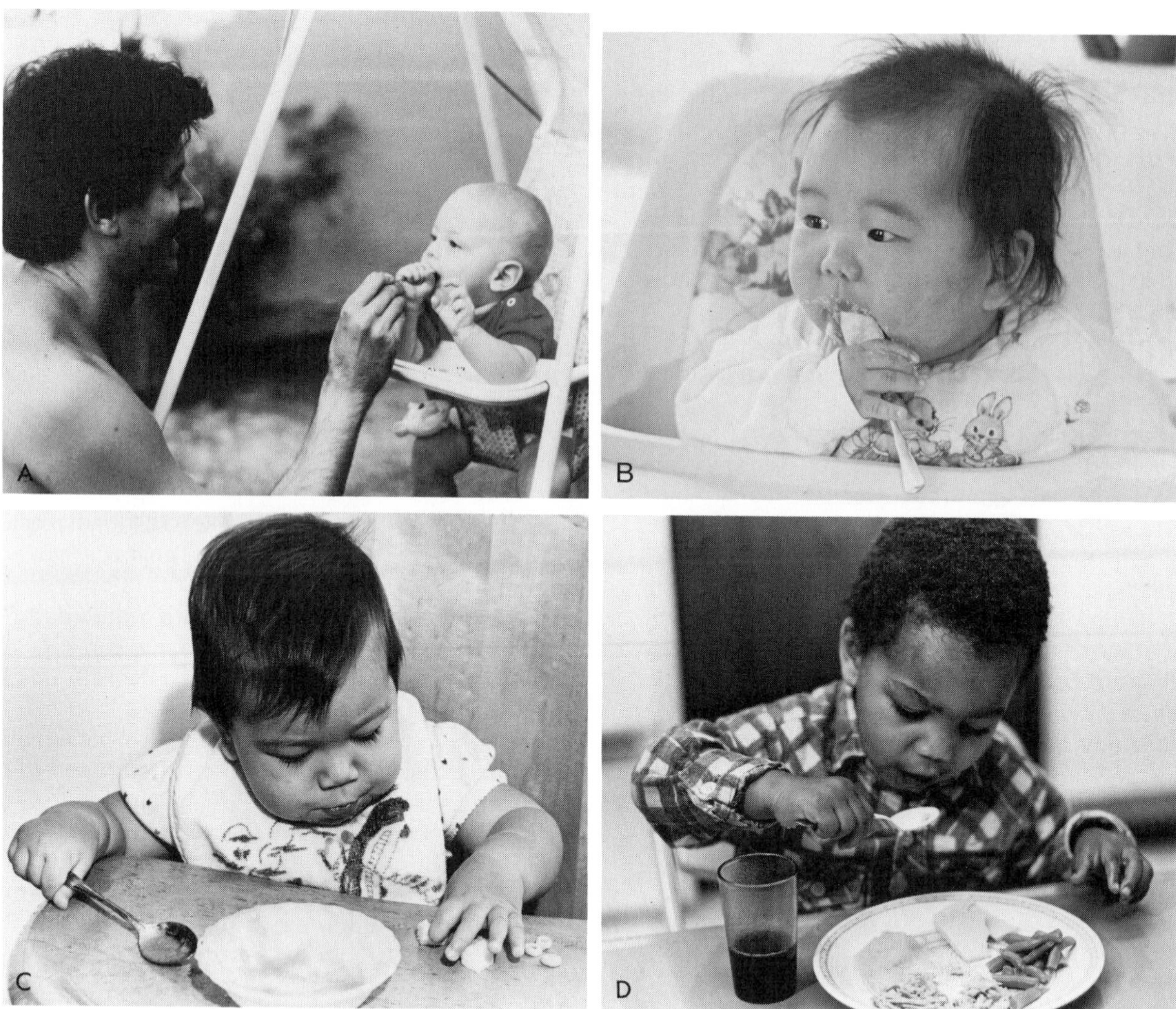

FIGURE 10–3. *Development of feeding skills in infants and toddlers.* A, *At 7 months this child shows beginning involvement with feeding and is reaching for the spoon.* B, *At 9 months this little boy is beginning to use his spoon independently, although he is not yet able to keep food on it.* C, *Here the 9-month-old shows a refined pincer grasp to pick up food.* D, *The 2-year-old is much more skillful at self-feeding, with the ability to both rotate the wrist and elevate the elbow to keep food on the spoon.*

Feeding the Older Infant

As maturation proceeds and the rate of growth slows down, infants' interest in and approach to food change. Between 9 and 18 months, most reduce their milk intake. They become finicky about what and how much they will eat and may go on food jags. However these are rarely dangerous and should not be major topics of concern. See Further Reading p. 191.

In the weaning stage, infants have to learn many manipulative skills, including chewing and swallowing solid food and the use of utensils. They learn to eat a variety of textures and flavors of food, to finger feed, and then to feed themselves. Very young children should be encouraged to feed themselves.

At the beginning of a meal, children are hungry and should be allowed to feed themselves; when they become tired, they can quietly be helped. Emphasis on table manners and the fine points of eating should be left until later when they have matured and developed enough to be ready for it.

The food should be in a form that is easy to handle and eat. Meat should be cut into bite-sized pieces. Potatoes and vegetables should be mashed so that a spoon can be used easily. Raw fruits and vegetables should be in sizes that can be picked up easily. In addition, the utensils should be small and manageable. The cup should be easy to hold, and dishes should be designed so that they do not tip over easily.

Size of Servings

The size of servings offered a child is very important. At 1 year, babies will eat one third to one half the amount

FURTHER READING: Self-Selected Diets of Infants and Young Children

Young children, if left to their own devices with a wide variety of wholesome foods at their disposal, will instinctively choose an adequate diet. This was shown as a result of studies conducted in the early 1920s by Davis, who was attempting to demonstrate that the prevailing practice of withholding solid foods until 1 year of age was not in the best interest of the child (Davis, 1928). Davis followed three children aged from 7 to 9 months at the onset of the study for 6 months to 1 year and later followed 12 more children for 6 months to 4½ years, during which time their diets were entirely self-selected. They were offered a variety of fresh, unprocessed, and unseasoned foods and allowed to eat as little or as much as they pleased of any or all items. A modern evaluation of their intakes indicates that the foods consumed equaled or exceeded the RDA for all nutrients except iron (Davis, 1939).

It would appear to be difficult for a child with a normal appetite to fail to obtain an adequate diet with choices limited to the following: beef, lamb, chicken, liver, kidney, brains, sweetbreads, haddock; whole wheat, oatmeal, barley, cornmeal, Ry-Krisp; bone marrow, bone jelly, eggs, raw milk, raw lactic milk; apples, oranges, bananas, peaches, pineapples; lettuce, cabbage, spinach, cauliflower, peas, beets, carrots, turnips, potatoes, tomatoes; and sea salt.

Items not included were any of the desserts or snacks common to the period and certainly none of the highly refined, energy-rich, and nutrient-dilute foods that are available today.

A preference for sweetness that is present at birth and persists throughout childhood would suggest that infants confronted with selections including desserts and sweetened snack foods would be unable to make the choices appropriate to a nutritious diet (Story and Brown, 1987).

However, it must also be noted that a similar study of children age 2½ to 4 years who were presented with wholesome food today also demonstrated an innate ability to select foods to meet their energy requirements. Unfortunately the nutrient adequacy of their selected diets was not determined (Birch, 1991).

an adult consumes. This proportion rises to one half or a little more by the time the child reaches 3 years of age and to about two thirds by 6 years of age. Little children should not be served a large plate full of food; the size of the plate and the amount should be kept in proportion to their age. A tablespoon (not heaping!) of each food offered for each year of age is a good guide to follow. Serving less than you think or hope will be eaten helps children to eat successfully and happily. They will ask for more food if their appetite is not satisfied.

Type of Food

In general, children prefer simple, uncomplicated foods (Lowenberg, 1989). Food from the family meal may be adapted for the child and served in child-sized portions. Children under 6 years of age usually prefer mild-flavored foods. Because the young child's stomach is small, a snack may be required between meals. Fruit, cheese, crackers, fruit juices, and milk contribute nutrients as well as energy. Children aged 2 to 6 years often prefer raw to cooked vegetables and fruits.

It is especially desirable that the baby receive foods varied in both texture and flavor. The infant who is accustomed to many kinds of foods is less likely to grow up with definite food dislikes. To add variety to the infant's diet, different vegetables and fruits may be added to cereal feedings. It is important to offer a variety of dishes and not to allow the youngster to continue on a diet consisting of one or two favorite foods. Older infants generally reject unfamiliar foods the first time they are offered. If the parent continues to offer small portions of these foods without comment, the infant will become familiar with the item and will often accept it.

Forced Feeding

Children should not be forced to eat; instead, the cause for the unwillingness to eat should be determined. A normal, healthy child will eat without coaxing. Refusal of food is sometimes due to a child's being too inactive to make him or her hungry or too active and overtired. Fatigue can be avoided by planning a short rest period for the child before meals or by providing a picture book for the child's quiet enjoyment. An overanxious parent can affect the appetite of the infant or the child. Emotions can retard the flow of gastric juice and inhibit digestion. Refusal to eat may also be the result of too much attention. Children enjoy the attention of their parents and soon learn that refusal to eat is one way to obtain it.

If a child refuses to eat, the family meal should be completed without comment and the plate should be removed. This procedure is usually harder on the parent than on the child. At the next mealtime, the child will be hungry enough to enjoy the food presented.

Where the Child Should Eat

Children should eat their meals at the family table. They then have an opportunity to learn table manners while enjoying meals with a family group. Sharing the family fare strengthens ties and makes mealtime a pleasant period. However, if the adult meal is delayed or if adult guests are present, the children should receive their meal at the usual time. When children eat with the family, everyone must be careful not to make unfavorable comments about any food. Children are great imitators of people they admire; thus, if the father or older siblings turn up their noses at squash, for example, they are likely to do the same.

CITED REFERENCES

Bachrach S, Fisher J, and Parks JS: An outbreak of vitamin D deficiency rickets in a susceptible population. Pediatrics 64:871, 1979.

Committee on Nutrition, American Academy of Pediatrics: Follow-up on weaning formulas. Pediatrics 83:1067, 1989c.

Committee on Nutrition, American Academy of Pediatrics: Hypoallergenic infant formulas. Pediatrics 83:1383, 1989a.

Committee on Nutrition, American Academy of Pediatrics: Imitation and substitute milks. Pediatrics 73:876, 1984.

Committee on Nutrition, American Academy of Pediatrics: Iron-fortified infant formulas. Pediatrics 84:1114, 1989b.

Committee on Nutrition, American Academy of Pediatrics: The use of whole cow's milk in infancy. Pediatrics 72:253, 1983.

Coursin DB: Convulsive seizures in infants with pyridoxine deficient diet. JAMA 154:406, 1954.

Davis CM: Results of the self-selection of diets by young children. Can Med Assoc J 41:257, 1939.

Davis CM: Self-selection of diet by newly weaned infants: An experimental study. Am J Dis Child 36:651, 1928.

Fomon SJ et al: Indices of fatness and cholesterol in relation to feeding and growth during early infancy. Pediatr Res 18:1233, 1984.

Fomon SJ et al: Requirements for protein and essential amino acids in early infancy. Acta Pediatr Scand 62:33, 1973.

Food and Nutrition Board, National Research Council, NAS: Recommended Dietary Allowances, 10th ed. Washington, DC, National Academy Press, 1989.

Harris CS et al: Childhood asphyxiation by food: A national analysis and overlook. JAMA 251:231, 1984.

Higgenbottom L, Sweetman L, and Nyhan WL: A syndrome of megaloblastic anemia and neurological abnormalities of a vitamin B_{12} deficient breast fed infant of a strict vegetarian. N Engl J Med 299:317, 1978.

Howie PW et al: Protective effect of breast feeding against infection. Br Med J 300:11, 1990.

Johnson PR and Roloff JS: Vitamin B_{12} deficiency in an infant strictly breast-fed by a mother with latent pernicious anemia. J Pediatr 100:917, 1982.

Kauter DA et al: Clostridium botulinum spores in infant foods: A survey. J Food Protection 45:1028, 1982.

Lack of adverse reactions to iron-fortified formula. Nutr Rev 47:41, 1989.

Lowenberg M: The development of food patterns in young children. *In* Pipes P: Nutrition in Infancy and Childhood, 4th ed. St Louis, CV Mosby, 1989.

Nelson SE et al: Lack of adverse reactions to iron-fortified formula. Pediatrics 81:360, 1988.

Pugliese MT et al: Parental health beliefs as a cause of nonorganic failure to thrive. Pediatrics 80:175, 1987.

Smith D et al: Shifting linear growth during infancy: illustration of genetic factors in growth from fetal life through infancy. J Pediatr 89:225, 1976.

Specker BL et al: Sunshine exposure and serum 25-hydroxyvitamin D concentrations in exclusively breast-fed infants. J Pediatr 107:372, 1985.

Ziegler EE: Milk and formulas for older infants. J Pediatr 117(Suppl):S76, 1990.

ADDITIONAL REFERENCES

Committee on Nutrition, American Academy of Pediatrics: Follow-up on weaning formulas. Pediatrics 83:1067, 1989.

Committee on Nutrition, American Academy of Pediatrics: On the feeding of supplemental foods to infants. Pediatrics 65:1178, 1980.

Committee on Nutrition, American Academy of Pediatrics: Soy-protein formulas: Recommendations for use in infant feeding. Pediatrics 72:359, 1983.

Complementary feedings for breast fed infants. Nutr MD 15(3):3, 1988.

Fomon SJ: Infant Nutrition. Philadelphia, WB Saunders, 1974.

Fomon SJ: Reflections on infant feeding in the 1970s and 1980s. Am J Clin Nutr 46:171, 1987.

Fomon SJ et al: Body composition of reference children from birth to age 10 years. Am J Clin Nutr 35:1169, 1982.

Fomon SJ and Heird WC (eds): Energy and Protein Needs During Infancy. San Diego, CA, Academic Press, 1986.

Lawless H: Sensory development in children: Research in taste and olfaction. J Am Diet Assoc 85:577, 1985.

McMillan JA, Landau SA, and Oski F: Iron sufficiency in breast-fed infants and the availability of iron from human milk. Pediatrics 58:686, 1976.

Moore DJ, Robb A, and Davidson GP: Breath hydrogen response to milk containing lactose in colicky and noncolicky infants. J Pediatr 113:979, 1988.

Parraga IM et al: Feeding patterns of urban black infants. J Am Diet Assoc 88:796, 1988.

Partridge JC et al: Water intoxication secondary to feeding mismanagement. Am J Dis Child 135:38, 1981.

Pipes P: Nutrition in Infancy and Childhood, 4th ed. St Louis, CV Mosby, 1989.

Reeve LE, Chesney RW, and DeLuca HF: Vitamin D of human milk: Identification of biologically active forms. Am J Clin Nutr 36:122, 1982.

Roche AR, Guo S, and Moore WM: Weight and recumbent length from 1 to 12 mo of age: Reference data for 1-mo increments. Am J Clin Nutr 49:599, 1989.

Sheard NF and Walker WA: The role of breast milk in the development of the gastrointestinal tract. Nutr Rev 46:1, 1988.

Sinatra FR and Merritt RJ: Iatrogenic kwashiorkor in infants. Am J Dis Child 135:21, 1981.

Stekel A et al: Absorption of fortification iron from milk formulas. Am J Clin Nutr 43:917, 1986.

Story M and Brown JE: Do young children instinctively know what to eat? N Engl J Med 316:103, 1987.

Tsang RC and Nichols BL: Nutrition During Infancy. Philadelphia, Hanley and Belfus, 1988.

Tunnessen WW and Oski FA: Consequences of starting whole cow milk at 6 months of age. J Pediatr 111:813, 1987.

Udall JN and Kilbourne KA: Selected aspects of infant feeding. Nutrition 4:409, 1988.

Weigley ES: Infant feeding practices — a century of transitions. Nutrition Today 23:20, 1988.

Willoughby A et al: Developmental outcome in children exposed to chloride deficient formulas. Pediatrics 79:851, 1987.

Wyatt DT, Noetzel MJ, and Hillman RE: Infantile beriberi presenting as subacute necrotizing encephalomyelopathy. J Pediatr 110:888, 1987.

Zlotkin, SH: Unconventional pediatric diets. Nutr MD 14(9):1, 1988.

CHAPTER 11

NUTRITIONAL CARE OF THE LOW-BIRTHWEIGHT INFANT*

Mary J. O'Leary, M.S., R.D.

CHAPTER OUTLINE

- Characteristics of Low-Birthweight Infants
- Parenteral Nutrition
- Transition from Parenteral to Enteral Nutrition
- Enteral Nutrition
- Growth and Nutritional Assessment
- Discharge Care
- Neurodevelopmental Outcome

KEY TERMS

APPROPRIATE FOR GESTATIONAL AGE—describing the infant who is between the 10th and 90th percentiles on the intrauterine growth grids for both height and weight

FULL-TERM INFANT—an infant born between the 37th and 42nd week of gestation

GASTRIC GAVAGE—a feeding method that involves inserting a soft feeding tube through the mouth or nose into the stomach for each feeding

GESTATIONAL AGE—the age of the infant at birth as determined by the length of the pregnancy—the number of weeks since the last menstrual period if known; also can be determined by clinical assessment

GLUCOSE LOAD—the amount of glucose received intravenously

HEMOLYTIC ANEMIA—anemia due to oxidative destruction of mature red blood cells; sometimes caused by vitamin E deficiency

HUMAN MILK FORTIFIER—a supplement of protein, carbohydrate, fat, calcium, and phosphorous that is added to human milk to make it more appropriate for the premature infant

INFANCY—birth to 1 year of age

INFANT MORTALITY RATE—number of infant deaths in the first year of life per 1,000 live births

LOW BIRTHWEIGHT (LBW)—referring to an infant who weighs less than 2,500 grams (5.5 lb) at birth

NEONATAL PERIOD—first 28 days of life

OSTEOPENIA OF PREMATURITY—reduced bone mass in the premature infant owing to a decrease in the rate of bone synthesis; often due to inadequate calcium and phosphorous intake

POSTNATAL PERIOD—from 28 days of age to the first birthday

PERINATAL—referring to the time period from 28 weeks of gestation to 4 weeks after birth

PREMATURE (PRE-TERM)—referring to an infant who is born before 37 weeks' gestation

SMALL FOR GESTATIONAL AGE (SGA)—referring to an infant who weighs less than the 10th percentile of the standard weight for gestational age

SURFACTANT—a mixture of lipoproteins secreted by alveolar cells into the alveoli and respiratory air passages that contributes to the elastic properties of pulmonary tissue

VERY LOW BIRTHWEIGHT (VLBW)—referring to an infant who weighs less than 1,500 grams (3½ lb) at birth

* *Sections of this chapter are modified from O'Leary MJ: Nourishing the premature and low-birthweight infant.* In *Pipes PL: Nutrition in Infancy and Childhood, 4th ed. St Louis CV Mosby, 1989 and from O'Leary MJ: Health-related concerns: Nutrition and feeding.* In *Johnson-Crowley N and Sumner GA: Nursing Systems Toward Effective Parenting: Preterm. Seattle, WA, NCAST Publications, 1989.*

The management of low birthweight (LBW) infants requiring intensive care has improved dramatically during the last 15 years. With new technologies, better understanding of pathophysiology, and cooperative interactions to regionalize the delivery of perinatal care, many immature infants are surviving (New Directions, see below). Studies indicate that the majority of these infants have the potential to have long and productive lives (Bennett, 1988).

Although there are many methods of providing nutrients to LBW infants, each has its benefits and limitations. Because of the complexities involved in the neonatal intensive care setting, a team including a skilled dietitian is necessary to promote optimal nutrition and to minimize undue delays and oversights of nutritional care. The dietitian may also function within a regionalized perinatal care system to provide consultation and guidance to community hospitals concerning the unique nutritional problems of premature infants.

CHARACTERISTICS OF LOW-BIRTHWEIGHT INFANTS

Gestational Age and Size

An infant who weighs less than 2,500 grams (5.5 lb) at birth is classified as being of *LBW,* whereas an infant

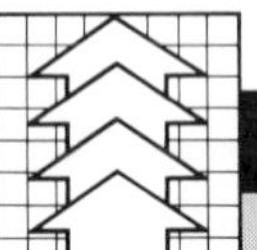

NEW DIRECTIONS: Some Demographics of Infant Mortality

The *infant mortality rate,* defined as the number of infant deaths in the first year of life per 1,000 live births, has declined 78% in the United States in the last 48 years. The decline in the white population during that period has been 80% as compared to 76% in the black population (Wegman, 1990).

In 1987, the American infant mortality rate was 8.6 for the white population, 15.4 for the nonwhite population (including blacks), and 17.9 for the black population only.

Prenatal care was started in the first trimester of pregnancy for 79% of white women and 61% of black women. Six per cent received essentially no prenatal care.

In 1988, 21 developed countries with populations greater than 2,500,000 had infant mortality rates lower than the United States (see the following Table). The range from the lowest to the highest represented a difference of 5 deaths per 1,000 live births.

In this ranking of the world's nations, Japan had the lowest infant mortality rate (4.4) and Guinea had the highest (176). The American rate was 10.0. (The provisional rate in the United States for 1990 was 9.3.)

Thirteen of the first 21 countries in the ranking have populations that are less than 10% of the American population. One half of the 21 countries, including Sweden and the other Scandinavian countries, are smaller than either New York City or Los Angeles. Japan has one half of the population of the United States.

Birth rate, or the number of births per 1,000 population, in the first 22 countries was lowest in Japan (10) and highest in Singapore (20). The American birth rate was 16.

In 1988, the United States had the highest *teenage pregnancy rate* among the developed countries (9.8% of females aged 15–19). Japan had the lowest rate (1%). Birth rate in the 15- to 17-year age group in the United States increased in 1988 by 6% to 33 compared with the overall birth rate of 16. Average age at menarche in the United States is 12½ to 13 years, and teenagers who become pregnant within 4 years after menarche are at high nutritional risk (Nutrition Management . . . , 1989).

Infant Mortality Rate, Birth Rate, and Population of Selected Countries*

Country†	Infant Mortality Rate (1988)‡	Birth Rate (1988)§	Population (Millions) (1990 est)	Population as % of the U.S. Population
Japan	4.8	10.1	123.8	50
Sweden	5.8	13.6	8.4	3
Finland	6.1	12.8	5.0	2
Taiwan	6.3	16	20.5	8
Switzerland	6.8	12.2	6.6	3
Singapore	7.0	20.0	2.7	1
Canada	7.2	14.5	26.5	11
Hong Kong	7.4	13.3	5.7	2
Netherlands	7.5	12.7	14.9	6
West Germany	7.5	10.9	61.0	24
Denmark	7.6	11.5	5.1	2
France	7.7	13.8	56.2	22
Austria	8.1	11.5	7.6	3
East Germany	8.1	12.0	16.6	7
Norway	8.4	14.0	4.2	2
United Kingdom	9.0	13.6	57.1	23
Belgium	9.1	11.9	9.9	4
Spain	9.2	11.2	39.6	16
Ireland	9.2	14.7	3.6	1
Australia	9.2	14.9	16.7	7
Italy	9.5	9.9	57.7	23
United States	**10.0‖**	**16.2**	**250.4**	**100**
USSR	25.2	18	290.9	116
China	33	23	1130.1	451
Mexico	42	30	83.3	33
India	91	31	850.1	340
Guinea	176	48	7.3	3

* Data from Wegman ME: Annual summary of vital statistics—1989. Pediatrics 86:835, 1990; The World Almanac and Book of Facts, 1991. New York, World Almanac, 1991.

† Countries with population greater than 2,500,000.

‡ Deaths per 1,000 live births.

§ Births per 1,000 population.

‖ 1989, 9.7; 1990 (provisional), 9.3.

weighing less than 1,500 grams (3½ lb) at birth is frequently referred to as having a *very low birthweight (VLBW)*. An infant may have an LBW owing to a shortened period of gestation, which means that he or she is premature, or because of a retarded rate of growth, which makes him or her *small for gestational age (SGA)*. The *full-term infant* is born between the 37th and 42nd week of gestation. A *premature infant* is one born before 37 weeks of gestation. Infants born before the 25th week rarely survive. Modern neonatal intensive care is not able to meet the metabolic and medical needs of most infants born before the third trimester of gestation.

The *gestational age* of the infant is determined primarily by clinical assessment. Clinical parameters fall into two groups: (1) a series of neurologic signs, dependent mainly on postures and tone, and (2) a series of external characteristics that reflect the physical maturity of the infant. Accurate assessment of gestational age is important in establishing nutritional goals for individual infants and in differentiating the premature infant from the SGA infant.

An SGA infant is defined as one who weighs less than the 10th percentile of the standard weight for that gestational age. This is usually a valid test, although an infant can sometimes be recognized as SGA only when compared with normal siblings who presumably have the same genetic potential. An SGA infant whose intrauterine weight gain is poor but whose linear and head growth are *appropriate for gestational age (AGA)* (i.e., between the 10th and 90th percentiles on the intrauterine growth grid), has experienced *asymmetric intrauterine growth retardation* (IUGR). An SGA infant whose length and occipital frontal circumference (OFC) are also below the 10th percentile of the standards is said to be *symmetrically growth retarded.* Symmetric *IUGR* usually reflects early and prolonged intrauterine deficit and is apparently more detrimental to later growth and development. The infant whose birthweight is above the 90th percentile on the intrauterine weight gain grid is referred to as *large for gestational age (LGA)*. Figure 11–1 shows the classification of newborns based on maturity and intrauterine growth.

Problems of Immaturity

The premature or LBW infant has not had the chance to develop fully *in utero* and is physiologically different from the full-term infant (Fig. 11–2). Because of this, LBW infants have a variety of clinical problems in the early postnatal period, depending on the intrauterine environment, degree of prematurity, birth-related trauma, and functioning of immature or stressed organ systems. Certain problems shown in Table 11–1 occur with such frequency as to be considered typical problems of prematurity.

Smaller Metabolic Reserves

Birth interrupts the influx of nutrients to the fetus, and thus premature infants enter the world with smaller metabolic reserves than full-term babies. Because most of the fetal glycogen is stored in the liver during the last 4 weeks of gestation, the glycogen reserve of the preterm infant is small and is rapidly depleted. Fat stores are also limited, because most fetal fat is deposited during the last 6 weeks of pregnancy. In the premature infant weighing 1,000 grams, fat contributes only 1% of total body weight; in contrast, the body of the full-term infant (3,500 grams) is about 16% fat.

In general, the smallest infants have the smallest energy reserves of glycogen and fat. Tiny newborns become rapidly dependent on exogenous energy intake to meet their metabolic needs and support basic life functions. The 1,000-gram AGA premature infant, for example, has a glycogen and fat reserve equivalent to about 110 kcal/kg of body weight. With basal metabolic needs of at least 50 kcal/kg/day, it is obvious that this baby will rapidly run out of fat and carbohydrate fuel

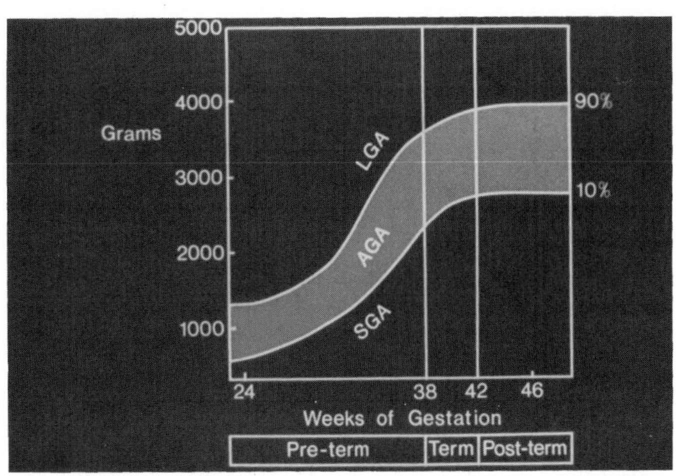

FIGURE 11–1. *Classification of newborns based on maturity and intrauterine growth. SGA = small for gestational age; AGA = appropriate for gestational age; LGA = large for gestational age.*

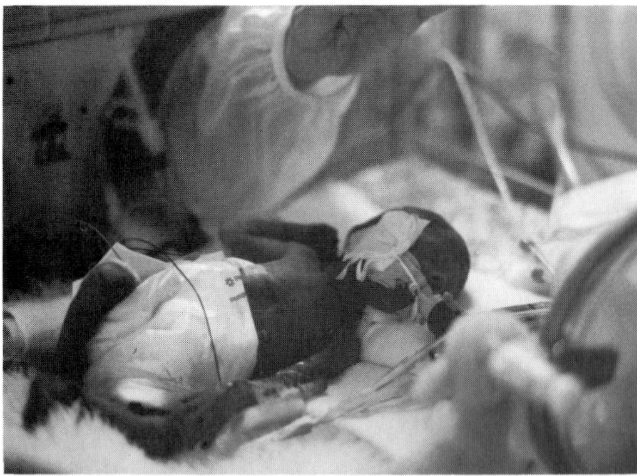

FIGURE 11–2. *A.R., born at 27 weeks' gestation weighing 870 g (1 lb 14 oz).*

unless adequate nutritional support is established. Depletion time varies between 2 and 4 days, depending on the volume and concentration of parenteral dextrose that can be tolerated. Obviously, depletion time will be even shorter for premature babies weighing less than 1,000 grams at birth. Nutrient reserves are depleted most quickly by tiny infants who have IUGR.

It is often difficult, however, to provide adequate nutritional intake during the first several days of life because of immaturity of the organ systems and severe medical problems. When adequate dietary intake cannot be achieved and fat and glycogen reserves have been exhausted, the infant begins to catabolize vital body protein tissue for energy. Theoretical estimates of survival time of starved and semistarved infants are shown in Table 11–2. These assume depletion of all glycogen and fat and about one third of body protein tissue, at a rate of 50 kcal/kg/day with fluids such as intravenous water (no exogenous calories) or 10% dextrose solution ($D_{10}W$). Even at the expense of protein tissue catabolism, the projected survival times are alarmingly short.

The small premature baby is particularly vulnerable to undernutrition; inadequate intake for even a few days may adversely affect the infant's clinical course. For example, immature infants with pulmonary disease may have weakening of respiratory muscles, depression of ventilatory drive, and increased difficulty in weaning from mechanical ventilation when protein-energy malnutrition complicates their clinical status (see Chapter 34). Furthermore, malnutrition in premature infants may increase the risk of infection, prolong chronic illness, and adversely affect brain growth and function.

TABLE 11–1. Examples of Problems Common to Premature or Low-Birthweight Infants in the Neonatal Period*

System	Problem
Respiratory	Hyaline membrane disease, also known as respiratory distress syndrome
Cardiovascular	Patent ductus arteriosus
Renal	Fluid or electrolyte imbalance
Neurologic	Intracranial hemorrhage
Metabolic	Hypoglycemia; hypocalcemia
Gastrointestinal	Hyperbilirubinemia; feeding intolerance; necrotizing enterocolitis
Hematologic	Anemia
Immunologic	Sepsis; pneumonia; meningitis

* From O'Leary MJ: Nourishing the premature and low-birthweight infant. *In* Pipes PL: Nutrition in Infancy and Childhood, 4th ed. St Louis, CV Mosby, 1989.

TABLE 11–2. Expected Duration of Survival of Infants in Starvation (H_2O Only) and Semistarvation ($D_{10}W$)*

	Estimated Survival Time (Days)	
Birthweight	*H_2O Only*	*$D_{10}W$*
1,000	4	11
2,000	12	30
3,500	32	80

* Data from Heird WC et al: Intravenous alimentation in pediatric patients. J Pediatr *80*:351, 1972.

PARENTERAL NUTRITION

Many critically ill LBW infants have difficulty working up to full enteral feedings in the first several days or even weeks of life. These sick premature babies are likely to develop protein-energy malnutrition unless adequate parenteral nutrition (PN) can be established.

A complete discussion of PN is given in Chapter 30, and only aspects particular to feeding the LBW infant are presented here. (Additional information about pediatric PN can be found in Kerner, 1983; Lebenthal, 1986; and American Academy of Pediatrics, 1983.)

Fluid

Parenteral fluid is required by LBW infants unable to tolerate an adequate enteral volume. Water requirements are estimated by the sum of the predicted losses. A major route of water loss in LBW infants is the evaporation of water through the skin and respiratory tract. This insensible water loss is highest in the smallest and least mature babies owing to their larger body surface area relative to body weight, increased permeability of the skin epidermis to water, and greater skin blood flow relative to metabolic rate. Insensible water loss is 10 to 60 ml/kg/day and is increased by radiant warmers and phototherapy lights and decreased by heat shields and thermal blankets. Excretion of urine is the other major route of water loss and varies between 60 and 125 ml/kg/day, depending on solute load presented to the kidneys and the ability of the kidneys to concentrate the urine that increases with maturity.

Fluid balance must be monitored carefully in the premature neonate. Inadequate intake can lead to dehydration, electrolyte imbalances, and hypotension. Excessive intake, on the other hand, can lead to edema, congestive heart failure, and possible opening of the ductus arteriosus. The premature infant has a greater percentage of body water (especially extracellular water) compared with the full-term infant, and reduction of this extracellular water in the first few days of life is especially important in the premature neonate. This reduction is accompanied by a normal loss of 10 to 15% of body weight and by an improvement in renal function. Failure of this transition in fluid dynamics and lack of diuresis may complicate the course of the respiratory disease in LBW infants.

Because of the many variables affecting fluid losses, most nurseries determine fluid needs on an individual basis. After initial fluid administration of 80 to 100 ml/kg/day, additional needs are determined by clinical parameters of urine output and specific gravity, serum electrolytes and blood urea nitrogen, blood pressure, peripheral circulatory status, mucous membrane moisture, skin turgor, and daily weights. Daily fluid administration is generally increased by 10 to 15 ml/kg/day, and most LBW infants receive 100 to 200 ml of fluid/kg/day by the second week of life. Fluid may need to be restricted in LBW infants with a patent ductus arteriosus (PDA), renin insufficiency, decreased cardiac output, and decreased urinary output and in conditions where cerebral edema may be present. Fluids may need to be increased in LBW infants under phototherapy lights or radiant warmers and when environmental or body temperature is elevated.

Energy

The energy needs of LBW infants fed parenterally are less than those of enterally fed infants because absorptive loss does not occur when nutritional intake bypasses the intestinal tract.

Enterally fed LBW infants usually require 120 to 130 kcal/kg/day to grow, whereas parenterally fed premature neonates can grow well on 70 to 90 kcal/kg/day. Minimal maintenance energy needs of about 60 kcal/kg/day and adequate protein should be provided as early as possible to prevent tissue catabolism. Energy intake should be increased as the infant's condition stabilizes and growth becomes the goal (Table 11–3).

Glucose

Glucose or dextrose is the principal energy source (3.4 kcal/g). However, glucose tolerance is limited in premature infants, especially VLBW infants. The reasons for this are inadequate insulin production or function and immature hepatic enzyme function. Glucose intolerance (hyperglycemia) is less likely when glucose is given with amino acids than when glucose is infused alone. Amino acids exert a stimulatory effect on insulin release. Avoidance of hyperglycemia is important because of its negative effects—diuresis and dehydration.

To avoid glucose intolerance in VLBW infants, glucose should be administered in small amounts. In order to accurately determine the amount of glucose an infant receives, it is necessary to calculate the glucose load. The *glucose load* is a function of both the concentration of the dextrose infusion and the rate at which it is administered. Glucose load should be calculated during the first 2 weeks of life for all VLBW infants, or whenever infants are at risk for glucose intolerance (Table 11–4).

To prevent hyperglycemia, infants weighing less than 1,000 grams should receive an initial glucose load of less than 6 mg/kg/min with daily increments of 1.5 to 2 mg/kg/day. For infants 1,001 to 1,500 grams a glucose load of 8 mg/kg/min is recommended with similar daily increments. Larger infants usually tolerate more rapid increments in glucose load (Kemer, 1983).

Hypoglycemia is not as common a problem as hyperglycemia. However, hypoglycemia may occur if the glucose infusion is abruptly decreased or interrupted.

TABLE 11–3. Comparison of Parenteral and Enteral Energy Needs of Low-Birthweight Infants

	Parenteral	Enteral
Maintenance		
Gradually increase to meet these needs by the end of the first week.	55–60 kcal/kg/day	60–80 kcal/kg/day
Growth		
Meet these needs as soon as infant is stable.	70–90 kcal/kg/day	120–130* kcal/kg/day
Use this formula to calculate caloric intake:		
Hydrated dextrose = 3.4 kcal/g/dl % dextrose = ___g/100 ml ___g/100 ml × 3.4 kcal/g = ___kcal/ml		

* May be higher, depending on factors described on page 201.

TABLE 11-4. Guidelines for Glucose Load in Low-Birthweight Infants

Birthweight (g)	Initial (mg/kg/min*)	Daily Increments (mg/kg/min)	Maximum (mg/kg/min)
<1,000	<6	1.5-2.0	As tolerated
1,001-1,500	<8	1.5-2.0	As tolerated
1,501-2,000	8	As tolerated	As tolerated

* Use this formula to calculate glucose load:

$$\frac{\frac{\text{g glucose}}{100\text{ ml}} \times \_\_\text{ml/kg/day} \times \frac{1{,}000\text{ mg}}{\text{g}}}{1{,}440\text{ min/day}} = \frac{\%\text{ dextrose} \times \_\_\text{ml/kg/day}}{144} = \text{mg/kg/min}$$

Amino Acids

Parenteral administration of 2 to 2.5 mg/kg/day of crystalline amino acids along with adequate energy intake results in nitrogen retention comparable with that observed in enterally fed infants. Protein in excess of these parenteral requirements should not be given to LBW infants, because additional protein offers no apparent advantage and increases the risk of metabolic problems. In practice, LBW infants are usually given a small amount of amino acids (0.5 to 1 g/kg/day within the first 2 to 5 days of life) and the amount is gradually increased to 2 to 2.5 g/kg/day as tolerated (Kerner, 1983).

Controversy surrounds the issue of the ideal amino acid mixture for LBW infants (Heird et al, 1988; Helms et al, 1987; Zlotkin, 1988). Two solutions have been designed for use in pediatrics: Trophamine (Kendell McGaw Laboratories), and Aminosyn PF (Abbott Laboratories), and Neopham (KabiVitrum). Compared with other solutions used with adults, the use of these pediatric solutions results in plasma amino acid profiles more like those of healthy infants fed with breast milk. Amino acid solutions such as Aminosyn (Abbott Laboratories), Freamine (McGaw Laboratories), and Travasol (Travenal Laboratories) were not designed to meet the particular needs of immature infants and may provoke imbalances in plasma amino acid levels. For example, cysteine, tyrosine, and taurine in these solutions are low relative to the needs of the LBW infant, but the methionine and glycine levels are relatively high. However, many LBW infants have received long-term parenteral nutrition with these amino acid mixtures without showing evidence of nutrient deficiency or excess. More research is needed to clarify which amino acid solutions are preferred for LBW infants.

In addition to plasma amino acid imbalances, other metabolic problems associated with amino acid infusions in LBW infants include metabolic acidosis, hyperammonemia, and azotemia. These problems can be minimized by gradual increases in protein load according to the guidelines in Table 11-5.

Lipid

Intravenous fat emulsions are used in LBW infants for two reasons: (1) to meet essential fatty acid (EFA) needs and (2) to provide a concentrated source of energy. EFA needs can be met by providing about 1 g/kg/day (Farrell et al, 1988). Biochemical evidence of EFA deficiency has been seen during the first week of life in VLBW infants fed parenterally without fat. Clinical consequences of EFA deficiency may include coagulation abnormalities, abnormal pulmonary surfactant, and adverse effects on lung metabolism (Lebenthal, 1986).

Lipid should be introduced slowly in LBW infants with regular monitoring of free fatty acid and plasma triglyceride levels. Infants with hyperbilirubinemia are at increased risk for developing kernicterus if free fatty acids displace bilirubin from albumin-binding sites and raise the level of free bilirubin in the blood. The free fatty acid to albumin ratio should be monitored and should be less than 6.0 to prevent this problem (Kerner, 1981). Hypertriglyceridemia should be avoided because of the possible pulmonary complications in VLBW infants with lung disease. Serum triglyceride levels should be less than 150 mg/dl in LBW infants and less than 100 mg/dl in VLBW infants with severe lung disease.

Initial lipid loads should not exceed EFA needs to avoid possible complications in LBW infants with hy-

TABLE 11-5. Guidelines for Parenteral Amino Acids for Low-Birthweight Infants

Birthweight (g)	Start (g/kg/day*)	Increments (g/kg/day)	Maximum (g/kg/day)
<1,000	0.5	0.5 every other day	2.0-2.5
1,001-1,500	0.5-1.0	0.5	2.0-2.5
1,501-2,500	0.5-1.0	0.5	2.0-2.5

* Use this formula to calculate protein load:

$$\%\text{ protein} = \_\_\text{g/100 ml}$$

$$\frac{\_\_\text{g} \times \_\_\text{ml/kg/day}}{100\text{ ml}} = \_\_\text{g/kg/day}$$

perbilirubinemia or lung disease. Once the infant is medically stable and there is need to provide additional energy for growth, lipid loads can be slowly increased. Lipid should be administered slowly for 24 hours, with increments of 0.25 to 0.5 g/kg/day each day or every other day to a maximum of 2 to 2.5 g/kg/day. Total lipid load should usually be less than—and should not exceed—40% of total calories (Table 11–6). The lipid emulsions presently in use are described in Chapter 30. In LBW infants, 10% solutions providing 1.1 kcal/g are usually preferred. Use of medium-chain triglycerides in neonatal PN is still experimental (Lima, 1989).

It has been suggested that the administration of heparin to infants receiving parenteral lipid may improve lipid clearance by stimulating the release of the enzymes lipoprotein lipase and hepatic lipase into the circulation and thus promoting the intravascular lipolysis of fat (Spear et al, 1988). However, more studies are needed before the routine use of heparin can be recommended.

Also under consideration is the supplemental use of *carnitine* in LBW babies receiving total parenteral nutrition (TPN). Carnitine facilitates the mechanism by which fatty acids are transported across the mitochondrial membrane so that they can be oxidized to provide energy. Enhanced lipid utilization in preterm neonates receiving parenteral nutrition supplemented with carnitine has been demonstrated (Helms et al, 1986). More studies are needed before this can be recommended.

Electrolytes

Sodium, potassium, and chloride are provided by the parenteral solutions. Actual requirements are variable depending on factors such as renal function, state of hydration, and the use of diuretics. Very immature infants may be limited in their ability to conserve sodium and sometimes require up to 8 to 9 mEq/kg/day to maintain a normal serum sodium concentration. Excess chloride intake is more common than inadequate intake; hyperchloremia is manifested as metabolic acidosis. The chloride in saline flushes may contribute to metabolic acidosis in LBW infants on TPN (Groh-Wargo et al, 1988). Serum electrolyte levels should be routinely monitored (Table 11–7).

TABLE 11–6. Guidelines for Parenteral Lipid

Birthweight (g)	Start (g/kg/day*)	Increments (g/kg/day)	Maximum (g/kg/day)
<1,000 g	0.5	0.25 every other day	2.0
1,001–1,500	0.5	0.25	2.0–2.5
1,501–2,500	0.5	0.25–0.5	2.0–2.5

* Use this formula to calculate lipid load:

10% lipid = 10 g/100 ml

$$\frac{10\text{ g} \times \underline{\quad}\text{ml/kg/day}}{100\text{ ml}} = \underline{\quad}\text{g/kg/day}$$

TABLE 11–7. Guidelines for Parenteral Electrolytes

Electrolytes	mEq/kg/day
Sodium	2–3
Chloride	2
Potassium	2

Minerals

Calcium and phosphorous are important components of the PN solution. Premature infants who receive TPN with low calcium and phosphorus concentrations are at risk for developing osteopenia of prematurity and eventually rickets (Kine et al, 1982). This poor bone mineralization is most likely to occur in VLBW infants on long-term PN. Calcium and phosphorus status should be monitored using serum calcium, serum phosphorus, alkaline phosphatase, and radiographic bone studies.

Preterm infants have higher calcium and phosphorus needs than full-term infants (Koo et al, 1988). However, it is difficult to add enough calcium and phosphorus to parenteral solutions to meet these higher requirements without causing precipitation of the minerals. Calcium and phosphorous should be provided simultaneously in TPN solutions. Alternate-day infusions are not recommended because calciuria occurs when phosphorus intake is low (Hoehn et al, 1987).

Recommendations for parenteral administration of increased amounts of calcium, phosphorus, and magnesium have been summarized by Greene and associates (1988). However, the intakes in Table 11–8 are

TABLE 11–8. Guidelines for Parenteral Minerals*

Minerals	mg/l†
Calcium	500–600
Phosphorus	400–450
Magnesium	50–70

* Data from Greene HL et al: Guidelines for the use of vitamins, trace elements, calcium, magnesium, and phosphorus in infants and children receiving total parenteral nutrition: Report of the Subcommittee on Pediatric Parenteral Nutrient Requirements from the Committee on Clinical Practice Issues of The American Society for Clinical Nutrition. Am J Clin Nutr 48:1324, 1988.

† Guidelines are given per liter to prevent administration of excessively high concentrations of calcium and phosphorus that may result if intakes are expressed per kilogram of body weight and/or if there is fluid restriction.

These recommendations assume an average fluid intake of 120–150 ml/kg/day with 2.5 g of amino acids per 100 ml. These dosages should *only* be given in central venous infusions.

described per liter to prevent administration of high concentrations of calcium and phosphorus that may result if intakes are expressed per kilogram of body weight or if there is fluid restriction.

Trace Elements

Zinc should be given to all LBW infants receiving PN. If enteral feedings cannot be started by 4 weeks of age, then additional trace elements should be added (Greene et al, 1988). However, the amounts of copper and manganese should be reduced in infants with hepatic dysfunction or cholestasis, and the amounts of selenium, chromium, and molybdenum should be reduced in infants with kidney dysfunction. Recommendations are not yet available for parenteral administration of iron or fluoride to LBW infants (Table 11–9).

Vitamins

The only intravenous multivitamin preparation currently approved for use in infants and children is MVI-Pediatric (Armour Pharmaceutical Co.). This preparation meets the 1979 recommendations of the Nutrition Advisory Group of the American Medical Association (1979). However, evidence suggests that LBW infants often receive too little retinol and too much riboflavin and other B vitamins (Greene et al, 1988). Until a newer, more appropriate product for LBW infants becomes available, the guidelines in Table 11–10 should be followed. The dosage of MVI-Pediatric should be adjusted according to body weight (MacDonald et al, 1987).

TRANSITION FROM PARENTERAL TO ENTERAL NUTRITION

It is desirable to begin enteral feedings in LBW infants as early as possible because feedings stimulate gastrointestinal enzymatic development and activity, promote bile flow, and increase small intestinal villous growth. Even small amounts of enteral feedings are beneficial and decrease the possibility that cholestatic jaundice will occur. Early introduction of small volume enteral feedings can improve subsequent feeding tolerance in VLBW infants (Slagle and Gross, 1988).

When making the transition from parenteral to enteral feeding, it is important to maintain parenteral feeding until enteral feeding is well established so that the net intake of fluid and nutrients remains adequate. Premature infants have poor motility as a result of motor immaturity of the gastrointestinal tract. Therefore, premature infants are more likely to tolerate initial feedings if small volumes are given. Initial feedings should simply be as small as possible. Depending on the infant's medical condition, feedings can be slowly advanced. The smallest, sickest infants are usually limited to increments of only 10 ml/kg/day. Larger, more stable LBW infants may tolerate increments of 20 ml/kg/day. See Chapter 30 for further discussion of transitional feeding.

TABLE 11–9. Guidelines for Parenteral Trace Elements*

Trace Elements	μg/kg/day
Zinc	400.0
Copper	20.0†
Manganese	1.0†
Selenium	2.0‡
Chromium	0.2‡
Molybdenum	0.25‡
Iodine	1.0

* Data from Greene HL et al: Guidelines for the use of vitamins, trace elements, calcium, magnesium, and phosphorus in infants and children receiving total parenteral nutrition: Report of the Subcommittee on Pediatric Parenteral Nutrient Requirements from the Committee on Clinical Practice Issues of The American Society for Clinical Nutrition. Am J Clin Nutr 48:1324, 1988.

† Reduce or omit in infants with cholestatic jaundice or hepatic dysfunction.

‡ Reduce or omit in infants with renal dysfunction.

TABLE 11–10. Guidelines for Parenteral Vitamins*

	<1,000 g	1,001–3,000 g	>3,000 g
% of one 5-ml vial of MVI-Pediatric	30%	65%	100%

* Data from MVI-Pediatric Package Insert, Armour Pharmaceutical, 1985.

ENTERAL NUTRITION

Enteral alimentation is preferred for LBW infants, because this approach is more physiologic and associated with fewer known complications than parenteral alimentation. Initiating a tiny amount of an appropriate milk feeding is beneficial whenever possible. However, the decision to advance enteral feedings is often difficult and involves consideration of the degree of prematurity, history of perinatal insults, current medical condition, functioning of the gastrointestinal tract, respiratory status, and several other individualized concerns. Table 11–11 summarizes factors to consider before initiating or advancing enteral feedings.

Requirements

LBW infants should be fed enough to allow them to maintain homeostasis without weight loss or tissue catabolism and yet not excessively to avoid potential toxicity and superfluous fat deposition. The exact quantities of nutrients needed to reach these goals are still being defined. In general, the requirements of premature infants are higher than those of full-term babies because of shortened gestation, decreased retention

TABLE 11–11. Factors to Consider before Initiating or Advancing Enteral Feedings*

Factors to Consider	Comments
Perinatal	
Perinatal asphyxia	If severe, enteral feedings should be withheld during the first 48 hours of life and possibly longer, depending on respiratory status.
Apgar scores	Wait 24 to 48 hours before feeding if Apgar scores are less than about 3. Consider clinical condition of the infant and neurologic status in determining when to feed.
Respiratory status	
Ventilated baby with respiratory distress syndrome	May consider feedings when: Ventilatory settings are consistent and show improvement. Blood gases are adequate. Episodes of apnea and bradycardia are mild and relatively infrequent. Low risk for pneumothorax.
Medical status	
Vital signs	Note that infants with tachypnea (rapid respiratory rate) and retractions are vulnerable to aspiration of milk. Heart rate, respiratory rate, temperature, blood pressure, color, and tone should be adequate for each infant.
Acute illness (e.g., sepsis)	Acutely ill babies are medically unstable and less likely to tolerate enteral feedings. Once the acute phase has passed and the infant is responding to treatment, enteral feedings should be reconsidered.
Gastrointestinal tract	
Anomalies	Certain anomalies prohibit the use of enteral feedings (e.g., gastroschisis, omphalocele) until surgically repaired.
Patency	The inability to pass a feeding tube or the occurrence of vomiting or distention in response to enteral feedings may indicate inadequate patency of the gastrointestinal tract. Intestinal obstructions (e.g., atresia, stenosis, volvulus) may prohibit enteral feedings before surgical correction.
Functioning	Signs that indicate a functioning gastrointestinal tract should be present (e.g., normal bowel sounds, ability to pass stools).
Risk of necrotizing enterocolitis	Factors that may increase the risk for necrotizing enterocolitis include: Immaturity (<32 weeks' gestation) VLBW (<1,500 g) Episodes of hypoxia (asphyxia, respiratory disease) Inadequate perfusion of the gastrointestinal tract Patent ductus arteriosus Possibly the presence of an umbilical arterial catheter (UAC-line)
Equipment/procedures	Incubation, extubation, and so forth may be temporary barriers to enteral feedings. Any procedure that is stressful to the infant may warrant *temporary* witholding of enteral feedings.

* From O'Leary MJ: Nourishing the premature and low-birthweight infant. *In* Pipes PL: Nutrition in Infancy and Childhood, 4th ed. St Louis, CV Mosby, 1989.

and utilization of nutrients for physiologic and metabolic reasons, and increased needs associated with stress, illness, and use of certain medications. In addition, a greater portion of the total nutrient intake of preterm infants is needed for synthesis of new tissue and for more rapid growth. It is also important to keep in mind that the enteral nutrient requirements are different from parenteral requirements for most nutrients.

Energy

The energy requirement of premature babies varies with individual biologic and environmental factors. It has been estimated that 60 to 80 kcal/kg/day are required to meet maintenance energy needs, compared with 100 to 120 kcal/kg/day to provide adequate energy for growth as shown in Table 11–12. However, energy needs may be increased by stress and rapid growth or decreased in a neutral thermal environment and when absorptive loss is eliminated with parenteral nutrition. To estimate the energy needs of individual infants, it is important to consider the dynamic biologic and environmental factors that alter their needs. To evaluate the accuracy of the estimate, it is important to consider the infants' growth progress in relation to their average energy intakes. Some premature infants may need at least 130 to 150 kcal/kg/day to sustain an appropriate rate of growth. To achieve these high caloric intakes in babies with limited capacities to tolerate large fluid volumes, it may be necessary to concentrate the feedings to provide more than 20 kcal/oz.

TABLE 11–12. Energy Requirements of Low-Birthweight Infants*

	kcal/kg/day
Basal metabolic rate	50
Activity	15
Cold stress	10
Total maintenance	75 (range 60–80)
Specific dynamic action	8
Fecal loss	12
Growth	25
Total additional requirements	45
Total energy needs for growth	120 (range 100–130)

* Adapted from Sinclair J et al: Supportive management of the sick neonate: parenteral calories, water and electrolytes. Pediatr Clin N Am 17:863, 1970.

Protein

Although much attention has been directed toward determining the enteral protein requirements of LBW infants, this is still a controversial subject. At the core of the controversy are basic questions relating to optimal postnatal growth and tissue composition changes of premature babies. Answers to these questions and data from direct clinical investigations are needed to establish precise protein requirements.

AMOUNT. One approach considers the goal to be the intrauterine rate of protein accumulation. A reference fetus model is used to determine the amount of protein that would need to be ingested to match the quantity of protein that is deposited into newly formed fetal tissue (Ziegler et al, 1976). In order to achieve these fetal accretion rates, additional protein must be supplied to compensate for intestinal losses and obligatory losses in urine and skin.

Based on this method for determining protein needs, Ziegler and associates (1981) suggested an advisable intake for protein of 3.5 to 4 g/kg/day. This amount of protein is apparently well tolerated by stable infants who are growing rapidly. There is, however, concern that this amount of protein may exceed the metabolic capacity of very immature infants or may be an additional stress to sick infants who are not growing.

TYPE. Another approach to estimating the protein needs of preterm infants considers the effect that the quality or type of protein may have on the quantitative requirement. *Whey-predominant proteins* of high biologic value for the preterm infant support sustained growth in quantities less than advisable intake estimates (Gross et al, 1983). Several studies have shown that premature infants tolerate whey better than casein. Whey protein is also more soluble than casein in gastric acid secretions and may be digested more easily by premature infants. In addition, the amino acid composition of whey protein differs from that of casein and may be more appropriate for premature infants. Because of the advantages of whey protein for premature infants, mother's milk or formulas containing whey-predominant proteins (60:40 for the whey:casein ratio) should be chosen whenever possible.

Taurine is a sulfonic amino acid that may be important for preterm infants. Human milk is a rich source of taurine, and taurine is added to most infant formulas. Preterm babies develop low plasma and urine concentrations of taurine without a dietary supply, but the clinical significance of this needs further study (Gaull, 1989).

In addition to the amount and type of protein, the distribution of protein calories (relative to carbohydrate and fat) affects the protein requirement. It is desirable that protein constitutes 7 to 16% of total calories. Less than 7% may be growth-limiting; more than 16% may be toxic with consequent azotemia and acidosis.

Lipid

AMOUNT. The growing LBW infant needs an adequate intake of well-absorbed dietary fat to help meet the high energy needs of growth, to provide essential fatty acids, and to assist absorption of other important nutrients such as the fat-soluble vitamins and calcium. However, neonates in general, and premature and SGA infants in particular, are relatively inefficient in digestion and absorption of lipid.

The percentage of total calories as fat relative to carbohydrate and protein is another important consideration. Fat should constitute 30 to 55% of total calories; fat intake greater than 60% of calories may lead to ketosis. Furthermore, a diet that is high in fat and low in protein may yield more fat deposition than is desirable for the growing LBW infant. *Linoleic acid* must comprise at least 3% of the total calories to meet essential fatty acid needs (American Academy of Pediatrics, 1985).

TYPE. Immature infants have low levels of the pancreatic enzyme lipase and consequently digest fat poorly. In addition to low lipase concentrations, premature infants also have an intraluminal concentration of bile acids that is below the critical micellar concentration and is therefore insufficient to solubilize most long-chain lipids for absorption. Because *medium-chain triglycerides (MCT)* do not require pancreatic lipase and bile acids for digestion and absorption, they have been added to the fat mixture in premature infant formulas. Initial studies showed that when MCT was added to long-chain vegetable oils, there was improved fat absorption resulting in alleviation of steatorrhea, increased weight gain, enhanced calcium absorption, and improved nitrogen retention (Tantibhedhyangkul and Hashim, 1975). One study (Hamosh et al, 1989), however, has reported that growth and fat absorption were not improved when a formula containing predominantly MCT was fed to preterm infants. Further investigation is needed to clarify these conflicting reports.

Human milk and vegetable oils contain linoleic acid; MCT oil does not. Premature infant formulas must contain vegetable along with MCT oil in order to provide this essential fatty acid.

The composition of dietary fat also has a role in the digestion and absorption of lipid. Preterm infants absorb vegetable oils more efficiently than saturated animal fats. One exception is the saturated fat in human milk. Preterm infants show better digestion and absorption of human milk fat than the saturated fat in cow's milk, or even the vegetable oil in standard infant formulas. This is because human milk naturally contains two lipases that facilitate digestion and has a special fatty acid composition that aids absorption.

Carbohydrate

Carbohydrate is an important source of energy, and the enzymes for endogenous production of glucose from carbohydrate, protein, and fat are present in LBW infants.

AMOUNT. Human milk and standard infant formulas contain approximately 40% of the total calories as carbohydrate. Too little carbohydrate may lead to hypoglycemia, whereas too much carbohydrate may provoke an osmotic diuresis or loose stools. The recommended range for carbohydrate intake is 35 to 65% of total calories.

TYPE. *Lactose* is the predominant carbohydrate in almost all mammalian milks and may be important to the neonate in glucose homeostasis. There is concern that the premature infant's ability to digest lactose may be marginal, but in practice this is an infrequent problem. Although babies born before 28 to 34 weeks of gestation have low lactase activity, lactase is an inducible enzyme and increases in activity in response to feeding lactose. *Sucrose* is another disaccharide that is found commonly in commercial infant formula products. Because sucrase activity is present at 70% of newborn levels early in the third trimester, sucrose is well tolerated by most premature infants. Both sucrase and lactase are sensitive to changes in the intestinal milieu, however, and babies afflicted by diarrhea, antibiotic therapy, or undernutrition may develop a temporary intolerance to lactose and sucrose.

Glucose polymers are an increasingly common carbohydrate in the diets of LBW infants. The polymers, consisting mainly of chains of five to nine glucose units linked together, are used to achieve the isoosmolality of certain specialized formulas. Glucosidase enzymes for digestion of glucose polymers are active in small preterm infants.

Minerals and Vitamins

Premature infants require all of the vitamins and minerals essential for full-term infants; however, LBW babies have increased requirements for several of these because of poor body stores and physiologic immaturity (American Academy of Pediatrics, 1985).

CALCIUM AND PHOSPHORUS. Adequate intakes of calcium and phosphorus are required for optimal bone mineralization by growing premature infants. The recommended intakes for these nutrients have not yet been precisely defined (Greer and Tsang, 1985).

Two thirds of the calcium and phosphorus content of the body of the full-term newborn is accumulated via active transport mechanisms during the last trimester of pregnancy. The infant born prematurely is deprived of this important intrauterine mineral deposition. When dietary intake falls short of what the fetus would have received *in utero* (120 to 150 mg of calcium/kg/day and 75 mg of phosphorus/kg/day) (Ziegler et al, 1976), preterm infants can develop *osteopenia of prematurity* (Steichen et al, 1980). This disease is characterized by demineralization of growing bones and is documented by radiologic evidence of "washed-out" bones in preterm infants. Very immature babies are particularly susceptible to osteopenia and may develop bone fractures or florid rickets if dietary deficiency is prolonged. Osteopenia of prematurity is most likely to occur in preterm infants who: (1) are fed any infant formulas other than the three designed especially for feeding to LBW infants and (2) are fed human milk that is not supplemented with calcium and phosphorus.

VITAMIN D. An oral supplement of 400 IU/day of vitamin D is currently recommended for the growing preterm infant (American Academy of Pediatrics, 1985). Larger daily supplements are probably unwarranted. Large doses are unlikely to treat or prevent osteopenia of prematurity when this disease is caused primarily by a lack of calcium and phosphorus (Tsang, 1985). There is no evidence that administration of the active vitamin D metabolites (25-hydroxy and 1,25-hydroxy vitamin D) to LBW infants is either necessary or advisable (American Academy of Pediatrics, 1985).

IRON. LBW infants are at risk for developing iron deficiency anemia because of reduced iron stores associated with premature birth. At birth, most of the available iron is in the circulating hemoglobin. Thus, frequent blood sampling further depletes the amount of iron available for erythropoiesis. Transfusions of red blood cells are often needed to treat the early physiologic anemia of prematurity (American Academy of Pediatrics, 1985).

Recommendations for iron supplementation in LBW infants have been summarized by Oski (1985). Ferrous sulfate at a dose of 2 to 3 mg/kg/day should be started at 1 to 2 months of age (American Academy of Pediatrics, 1985). Infants fed human milk should be given ferrous sulfate drops. Formulas fortified with iron usually contain sufficient supplemental iron for LBW infants on a per kilogram basis.

VITAMIN E. Preterm infants require more vitamin E than full-term infants because their tissue stores are limited at birth and because their absorption of this fat-soluble vitamin is limited. Vitamin E deficiency is exacerbated by a high intake of iron or polyunsaturated fatty acids (PUFA), each of which increases the vitamin E requirement (American Academy of Pediatrics, 1985).

An important function of vitamin E is its protection of biologic membranes against oxidative breakdown of lipids. Requirements for vitamin E increase when the level of PUFA in the diet is high. The PUFA gradually produce a change in the composition of the fatty acids in cellular and intracellular membranes. The membranes then become more susceptible to oxidative damage, which increases the requirement for the antioxidant effect of vitamin E. Because iron is a biologic oxidant, a diet high in either iron or PUFA increases the risks of vitamin E deficiency. A premature infant who has vitamin E deficiency may experience *hemolytic anemia* (oxidative destruction of red blood cells).

The fat blends in human milk and the premature infant formulas contain appropriate vitamin E:PUFA ratios to prevent the development of hemolytic anemia. Supplemental iron should not be given to preterm infants less than 2 weeks of age, and dosages should not exceed 2 to 3 mg/kg/day. Since the dietary requirement for vitamin E depends on the PUFA content of the diet, the recommended intake of vitamin E is commonly expressed as a ratio of vitamin E to PUFA. The requirement for vitamin E is 0.7 IU (0.5 mg of d-alpha-tocopherol) per 100 kcal and at least 1.0 IU of vitamin E per gram of linoleic acid (or PUFA) (American Academy of Pediatrics, 1985). It is recommended that preterm infants receive an additional 5 to 25 IU/day of vitamin E. Depending on the type of feeding, oral supplements can be adjusted to give the appropriate dose.

In the past, higher doses of vitamin E were given because of suggestions that the antioxidant nature of vitamin E may impede the development of bronchopulmonary dysplasia and retrolental fibropolasia by reducing the toxic effects of oxygen. Not only is evidence of this contradictory, but also high doses of vitamin E may increase the incidence of hemorrhagic disease in preterm infants (Phelps et al, 1987).

Folic Acid. Premature infants seem to have higher folic acid needs than infants born at term. Although serum folate levels are high at birth, they decrease dramatically soon after that. This may be a reflection of the high utilization of folic acid by the premature infant for DNA and tissue synthesis. Because the premature baby grows at a more rapid rate than the term infant, he or she may have a higher intrinsic need for folic acid.

A mild form of folic acid deficiency manifested by low serum folate concentrations and hypersegmentation of neutrophils is not unusual in premature infants. Megaloblastic anemia is much less commonly observed. A daily supplement of 60 μg is effective in preventing neutrophil hypersegmentation and in maintaining normal serum folate concentrations. Liquid multivitamin preparations for infants do not contain folic acid because of this vitamin's instability in solutions (American Academy of Pediatrics, 1985).

Sodium. LBW infants, especially those who are most premature, are susceptible to hyponatremia in the neonatal period. These babies may have excessive urinary sodium losses because of renal immaturity and inability to conserve adequate sodium. Furthermore, their sodium needs are high related to their rapid rate of growth. Dietary intake may be poor, especially for infants who consume small volumes of milk.

Daily sodium intakes of 4 to 6 mEq/kg or more may be required by some infants to avoid hyponatremia and to correct associated growth failure. Infants receiving diuretic therapy may need as much as 8 to 9 mEq/kg/day. Routine sodium supplementation of mother's milk and infant formulas is not necessary. However, it is important to consider the possibility that hyponatremia may occur and to monitor infants by frequent assessment of serum or urinary sodium concentrations. Milks can be supplemented with sodium if repletion is necessary.

Methods of Feeding

Preterm infants can be fed either by gastric gavage (tube) or by bottle nipple. When mothers have chosen to breastfeed their premature infants, it is desirable to begin nursing at the breast as soon as the infants are ready to begin nippling.

Gastric Gavage. *Oral gastric gavage* feeding is often chosen for infants unable to suck because of immaturity or insults to the central nervous system. Infants of less than 32 to 34 weeks of gestational age, regardless of birthweight, may be expected to have poorly coordinated sucking and swallowing activity related to their developmental immaturity, and consequently have difficulty with nipple feeding. Using the oral gastric gavage method, a soft feeding tube is inserted through the mouth and into the baby's stomach. The major risks of this technique include aspiration and gastric distention. Because of weak or absent cough reflexes and poorly developed respiratory muscles, the tiny baby may not be able to dislodge milk from the upper airway, causing reflex bradycardia or airway obstruction. However, with electronic monitoring of vital functions and proper positioning of the infant during feeding, the danger of aspiration from regurgitation of stomach contents is minimized. Gastric distention and vagal nerve stimulation with resultant bradycardia are potential problems when oral gastric gavage feedings are delivered on an *intermittent bolus* schedule. Elimination of the distention and vagal bradycardia may occasionally require the use of an indwelling tube for *continuous gastric gavage* feedings, instead of the intermittent bolus technique. Continuous drip feedings are sometimes preferred for tiny, immature infants whose small gastric capacity and slow intestinal motility may impede the tolerance of larger volume bolus feeds. *Nasal gastric gavage* is sometimes better tolerated than oral tube feeding. But because newborns are obligatory nose breathers, this technique may compromise the nasal airway in LBW infants with associated deterioration in respiratory function.

TRANSPYLORIC GAVAGE. Transpyloric gavage feeding is rarely indicated for LBW infants. The goal of this method is to circumvent the often slow gastropyloric motility of the immature infant by passing the feeding tube through the stomach and pylorus and by locating its tip within the duodenum or jejunum. Advantages to transpyloric feeding include the elimination of the pylorus as a barrier for adequate propulsion of milk and a reduced chance of aspiration; however, several disadvantages occur as well. Transpyloric feedings have been associated with decreased fat absorption, diarrhea, dumping syndrome, alteration of the intestinal microflora, contamination of the feeding system, intestinal perforation, and bilious fluid in the stomach. Transpyloric tubes also require considerable expertise in their placement and x-rays to determine the location of the catheter tip. Because of the problems inherent in using this technique, transpyloric feeding is now rarely used to feed LBW infants.

NIPPLE-FEEDING. Nipple-feeding may be attempted in infants whose gestational age is greater than 32 weeks. The ability to nipple-feed is usually indicated by evidence of an established sucking reflex and sucking motion. Because sucking requires effort by the infant, any stress from other causes such as hypothermia or hypoxemia will diminish sucking ability. Nipple-feeding, therefore, should be offered only when the infant is under minimal stress and has sufficient maturity and strength for a sustained sucking effort.

BREAST-FEEDING. Breast-feeding, if chosen by the mother, should be initiated as soon as the infant is ready to begin nippling (Niefert, 1988). Better coordination of sucking, swallowing, and breathing and less disruption in ventilation has been seen in premature infants who were breast-fed, compared with those who were bottle-fed (Meier, 1987).

Volume of Feeding

The appropriate amount of milk to be fed to LBW infants depends on their estimated stomach capacity. The undistended stomach volume varies with the size of the infant and may be as small as 2 to 3 ml in the 800-gram newborn or about 40 ml in the 4,000-gram newborn. Although gastric capacity increases with postnatal age, individual infants vary in their ability to tolerate enteral volumes and should be monitored by regular measurement of gastric residuals.

The poor gastrointestinal motility of preterm infants is the most limiting factor in increasing the volume of enteral feeds. Although neonatal intensive care nurseries vary in their approach to initiating enteral feedings, most nurseries introduce small enteral volumes and increase volume slowly. There is no documented advantage to feeding formula that is diluted to one-quarter or one-half strength.

Tolerance of Feedings

All LBW babies receiving enteral nutrition should be monitored consistently for signs of feeding intolerance. Vomiting of feedings usually signals the inability of the infant to retain that amount of milk. When not associated with other signs of a systemic illness, vomiting may indicate a too rapid increase in feeding volumes or excessive volume for the infant's size and maturity. A reduction in volume may be all that is needed. If this does not eliminate vomiting or if signs of a systemic illness coexist, feedings may need to be interrupted until the infant's condition has stabilized.

Abdominal distention may be caused by feeding of excessive volumes, organic obstruction, excessive swallowing of air, resuscitation, or sepsis (i.e., systemic infection). Observation of the infant for abdominal distention should be a routine practice for the nurse caring for the infant. Intermittent measurement of abdominal circumference will aid in the early detection of distention. This symptom often indicates the need for interruption of feeding until the cause of the distention is determined and the abdomen is once more soft and nondistended.

Gastric residuals are measured by aspiration of the stomach contents and should be checked routinely before each bolus gavage feeding and intermittently in all continuous drip feedings. Whether or not a residual is significant depends partly on its volume in relation to the total volume of the feeding; a residual whose volume is more than 20% of the total feeding might be a sign of feeding intolerance. When interpreting the significance of a gastric residual, however, it is important to consider that residual in light of other concurrent signs of feeding intolerance and the pattern of residuals established for that infant. Gastric residuals that are bloody or bilious are more alarming than those that appear to be undigested milk.

The *frequency and consistency of bowel movements* require constant attention when feeding LBW infants. Furthermore, routine testing of stools for reducing substances is a useful procedure that promptly detects incomplete absorption of sugars by the intestine. Although the presence of gross blood can be detected by simple inspection, occult blood is not always visible and should be investigated by a specific assay to detect small amounts of blood in the stool.

No one method of feeding is without hazards for LBW infants, and unless close attention is paid to symptoms indicative of poor feeding tolerance, serious complications may ensue. Certain diseases can be recognized clinically by determination of signs of feeding intolerance. Necrotizing enterocolitis is a serious and potentially fatal disease that is associated with signs such as abdominal distention and tenderness and abnormal gastric residuals.

Composition of Feedings

HUMAN MILK. Although human milk is considered to be the ideal food for healthy full-term infants, there is controversy over what is the optimal milk for premature neonates. It is intriguing to note that the composition of milk from mothers delivering prematurely differs from that of mothers delivering at term during the first month of lactation (Lemons, 1982). When premature infants are fed their own mother's milk, they grow more rapidly than infants fed banked breast milk (mature breast milk) and are able to attain intrauterine rates of weight gain (Gross et al, 1983).

In addition to the nutrient concentration, several other factors make the preterm mother's milk the feeding of choice for her own infant. First, it contains certain *growth factors* that apparently have an important role in the proliferation and differentiation of cells in body tissues of infants. An example is epidermal growth factor that exerts a trophic effect on developing intestinal epithelium of premature infants (Gaull et al, 1985). Second, human milk *protein is whey predominant* and has an amino acid composition that favors the LBW infant. Third, the presence of *lipase* and *amylase* in human milk contributes to the premature infant's ability to digest fat and carbohydrate and to derive the maximum caloric benefit from the feeding. Fourth, the *renal solute load* of human milk is appropriately low and does not interfere with water balance in the LBW infant. Fifth, there are *anti-infective factors:* (1) maternal immune factors such as secretory IgA and (2) antibacterial factors that cause acidification of the infant's gut and promote the establishment of a vigorous lactobacillus flora. These factors may provide protection from infection for the developing gut mucosa.

There is however, one well-documented problem associated with feeding human milk to LBW infants. Whether preterm, term or mature, human milk does not meet the calcium and phosphorus needs for normal bone mineralization in infants born prematurely. Despite increased calcium absorption found in preterm infants receiving human milk, the total calcium content of the milk is deficient for the growing preterm infant. Preterm infants who receive their mother's milk can develop hypophosphatemia and hypercalciuria (although serum calcium values are usually normal), presumably as a result of low dietary phosphorus intake (Rowe et al, 1984). For these reasons, calcium and phosphorus supplements are recommended for rapidly growing LBW infants fed predominantly human milk.

Currently two *human milk fortifiers* contain calcium and phosphorus, along with protein, carbohydrate, fat, vitamins, and minerals, and are designed to be added to expressed breast milk fed to premature and LBW infants. Similac Natural Care (Ross Laboratories) is available in liquid form, whereas Enfamil Human Milk Fortifier (Mead Johnson Nutritional Division) is available in powdered form.

Providing breast milk to the premature infant can be a very positive experience for a mother and promotes maternal involvement and interaction. Because many preterm infants are neither strong enough nor mature enough to nurse at their mother's breast in the early neonatal period, mothers usually express their milk for several days and sometimes several weeks before nursing can be established. The proper technique of expression, storage, and transport of milk should be considered. Discussion of the special considerations for nursing a preterm infant is provided by Meier (Meier and Anderson, 1985; Meier and Pugh, 1987; Neifert, 1988; and O'Leary, 1989).

PREMATURE INFANT FORMULAS. Formula preparations have been developed to meet the unique nutrient and physiologic needs of growing LBW infants. The quantity and quality of nutrients contained in these products promote growth at intrauterine rates. These premature formulas differ in many aspects from standard cow's milk-based formulas (Table 11–13). For example, they contain 24 kcal/oz instead of 20 kcal/oz in the standard formula for full-term infants. The amount of protein is increased; the type of fat is different; and there are increased concentrations of calcium, phosphorus, and other minerals, vitamins, and electrolytes.

Selection of Feeding

During the initial period of feeding, premature infants are often still adjusting to enteral nutrition and may experience concurrent stress, weight loss, and diuresis. The primary goal of enteral feeding during this initial period is to facilitate tolerance to the milk provided. Aggressive nutritional support from the onset of enteral feeding often meets with failure, because babies appear to be unable to assimilate a large volume and concentration of nutrients until adjustment has been established. Supplementation of enteral feedings with

TABLE 11–13. Composition of Human Milk, Premature Formulas, and Standard Formulas

	Caloric Density	Protein *Whey/casein*	Protein % Total Calories	Carbohydrate	Carbohydrate % Total Calories	Fat	Fat % Total Calories	Ca (*mg/l*)	P (*mg/l*)	Renal (*mOsm/l*)	Gastrointestinal (*mOsm/kg H_2O*)
Human Milk											
Mature	20 kcal/oz (0.67 kcal/ml)	60:40	7	Lactose	38	Human milk fat	55	340	169	75	300
Premature	22 kcal/oz (0.73 kcal/ml)	60:40		Lactose		Human milk fat		293	134		300
Standard Formulas											
Similac	20 kcal/oz	18:82	9	Lactose	43	Corn/coconut 60:40	48	510 520	390 438	110–120	285
SMA	20 kcal/oz	60:40	9	Lactose	41–43	Coconut/oleo/safflower/soy	48–51	420	280	105	250
Enfamil	20 kcal/oz	60:40	9	Lactose	41	Coconut/soy		460	320	134	285
Good Start	20 kcal/oz	100:0	10	Lactose, corn syrup	44	Palm/safflower/coconut	46	430	240	99	265
Premature Formulas											
Similac Special Care	24 kcal/oz (0.81 kcal/ml)	60:40	11	Lactose/glucose polymers 50:50	42	MCT/corn/coconut 50:30:20	47	1440	702	208	300
Enfamil Premature	24 kcal/oz	60:40	12	40:60	42	40:40:20	44	940	470	220	300
Premie SMA	24 kcal/oz	60:40	10	50:50	42	Coconut/safflower/oleo/soy/ MCT 27:25:20:18:10	48	750	400	175	300

parenteral fluids is often required until adequate oral volume is tolerated.

After the initial period of adjustment, the goal of enteral feeding changes to provide complete nutrition to promote growth and rapid organ development. All essential nutrients should be provided in quantities that support sustained growth in all parameters. For this effect, the following feeding choices are appropriate: (1) human milk supplemented with human milk fortifier, (2) premature formula for babies who weigh less than about 2 kg, or (3) standard infant formula for infants who weigh more than about 2 kg.

Formula Manipulations

It is occasionally desirable to increase the energy content of the formulas fed to small infants. This may be appropriate when the infant is not growing at a desirable rate and is already ingesting a maximum volume of fluid.

CONCENTRATION OF FORMULAS. One approach to providing hypercaloric formulas is to subtract water, thus concentrating all nutrients, including energy. Concentrated infant formulas with energy contents of more than 24 kcal/oz or more are available to hospitals as ready-to-feed nursettes. When using these concentrated formulas, however, it is important to consider the infant's fluid intake and fluid losses in relation to the renal solute load of the concentrated feeding to ensure that positive water balance is maintained.

CALORIC SUPPLEMENTS. Another approach to increasing the energy content of formulas employs the use of caloric supplements such as MCT oil (Mead Johnson) and glucose polymers such as Polycose (Ross Laboratories). These supplements increase the caloric density without marked alterations in solute load or osmolality. However, they do alter the relative distribution of total calories from protein, carbohydrate, and fat. Because adding even small amounts of MCT oil or Polycose adversely dilutes the percentage of protein calories while altering the percentage of calories from fat and carbohydrate, adding these supplements to human milk or standard 20 kcal/oz formula is not advised.

When a high-energy formula is appropriate, MCT oil and Polycose are added to a 24 kcal/oz base (either full-strength premature formula or a concentrated standard formula), to a maximum of 60% of total calories as fat, and a minimum of 7% of total calories as protein.

For infants weighing 2 kg or more who require energy-dense formulas (e.g., those with bronchopulmonary dysplasia), instructions for using vegetable oil and sucrose are given in Table 34–3. Unless these infants have a particular problem with fat absorption or osmotic load, use of MCT oil and Polycose is not necessary.

TABLE 11–14. Advisable Intakes of Vitamins for Low-Birthweight Infants*

Vitamins	Per Day
Vitamin A (IU)	500
Vitamin D (IU)	600
Vitamin E (IU)	30
Vitamin K (μg)	15
Vitamin C (mg)	60
Thiamin (mg)	0.2
Riboflavin (mg)	0.4
Niacin (mg)	5
B_6 (mg)	0.4
B_{12} (μg)	1.5
Folic acid (μg)	60
Pantothenic acid (mg)	2
Biotin (μg)	12

* Data from Ziegler EE, Biga RL, and Fomon SJ: Nutritional requirements of the premature infant. *In* Suskind RM (ed): Textbook of Pediatric Nutrition. New York, Raven Press, 1981, p 36.

Vitamin and Mineral Supplementation

The vitamin and mineral requirements of preterm infants are not precisely known. Estimates of advisable intakes take into account intrauterine accretion rates, full-term infants' needs, and the unique physiologic demands of LBW infants. Although these advisable intakes lack precision, they serve as guidelines until more precise empirical data are available (Table 11–14). The enteral vitamin and mineral needs of preterm infants have been summarized by Tsang (1985) and by the American Academy of Pediatrics (1985).

Usually the vitamin and mineral needs of infants less than 2 kg are met by fortified human milk or premature formulas; additional supplementation is usually not required. If oral vitamin and mineral supplementation is needed, it should be delayed until the infant has tolerated full-strength formula or breast milk for at least 48 hours at a volume sufficient to provide calories for both maintenance and growth. Because most liquid vitamin preparations have very high osmolarities, these supplements may need to be administered in divided doses and mixed with the iso-osmolar milk before feeding. This minimizes the possibility of adverse effects, such as increased gastric residuals and regurgitation.

GROWTH AND NUTRITIONAL ASSESSMENT

All neonates typically lose some weight after birth. This is true particularly for LBW infants, who are born with more extracellular water than full-term infants and benefit from some degree of fluid loss. However, postnatal weight loss should not be excessive. LBW infants who lose more than about 15 to 20% of their birthweight can be expected to have dehydration as a result of inadequate fluid intake or tissue wasting from poor energy intake. Birthweight should be regained by the first or second week of life.

During the first month of life, the growth chart of Dancis shown in Figure 11–3 is commonly used to assess weight progress (Dancis et al, 1948). This chart has the advantages of depicting daily weight changes and actual growth curves; however, the chart is based on a small sample size and data that are now nearly 45 years old. The Dancis curves should not, therefore, be interpreted to represent optimal growth, particularly for VLBW infants in modern neonatal intensive care units.

A comparison between the postnatal weight curves of premature infants with the Dancis curves showed that infants weighing more than about 1,300 grams at birth lost less weight and gained weight faster than infants followed by Dancis in the mid-1940s (Jaworski, 1974). However, the study showed no difference for VLBW infants weighing less than about 1,100 grams at birth. A similar comparison in the 1980s found that the relatively healthy, enterally fed infants in the study gained weight at a rate more than twice that of the original prediction of Dancis (Brosius et al, 1984). Although these two more recent studies indicate that healthy LBW infants can gain weight faster than the rates shown in the Dancis curves, very sick or stressed infants are still probably not able to achieve these more rapid rates of growth. Pushing unstable infants to achieve faster weight gain may only increase their stress.

Intrauterine growth curves have also been developed

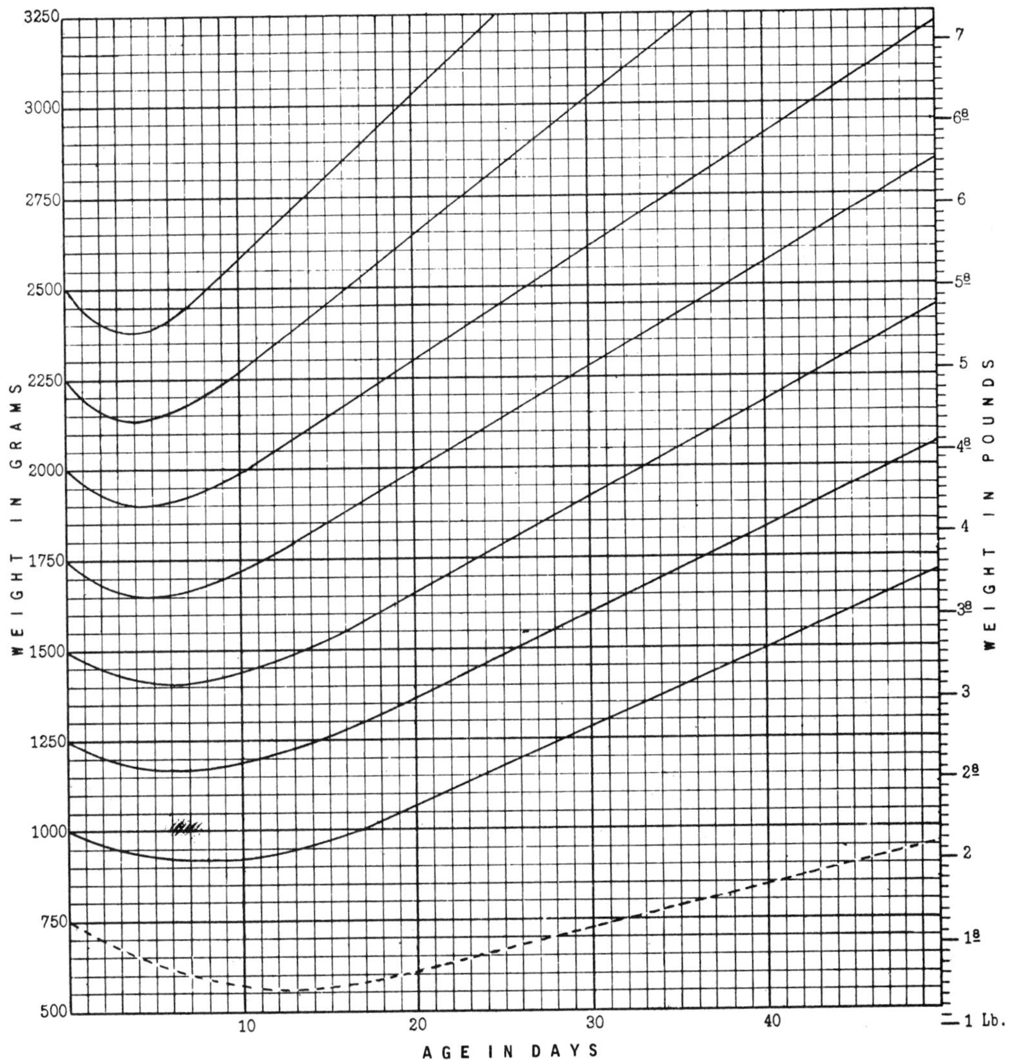

FIGURE 11–3. *Weight chart for premature infants based on actual growth data. (From Dancis J, O'Connell J, and Holt L: A grid for recording the weight of premature infants. J Pediatr 33:570, 1948.)*

using birthweight data of infants born at successive weeks of gestation. These curves do not depict the initial period of postnatal weight loss and are probably unrealistic goals for VLBW infants in the neonatal period. Once the infant's condition stabilizes and full nutrient intake is possible, the infant may be able to grow at a rate that parallels these curves (i.e., gain of 20 to 30 g/day).

Although weight is an important anthropometric parameter during the early neonatal period, weekly (or at least bimonthly) measurements of length and head circumference should be taken once the infant is stable. Growth curves, such as those shown in Figure 11–4, can be used to evaluate the adequacy of growth in all three parameters. These curves have the benefit of having a built-in correction factor for prematurity. However, they are based on data that are now about 25 years old, and the curves are drawn from a compilation of cross-sectional birthweight data (less than 40 weeks of gestation) and from data of studies on full-term infants. Reference curves for preterm infants based on a large sample of longitudinal data are not yet available.

The curves for full-term infants from birth to 3 years of age from the National Center for Health Statistics can also be used for preterm infants after 40 weeks of gestation, as long as age is corrected (or adjusted) for prematurity. For example, at 3 months' postnatal age, the growth parameters of a premature infant born at 32 weeks' gestation can be compared with those of a 1-month-old baby born at term. When using growth grids, age should be adjusted for prematurity until at least 1 to 2 years corrected age (Fig. 11–5).

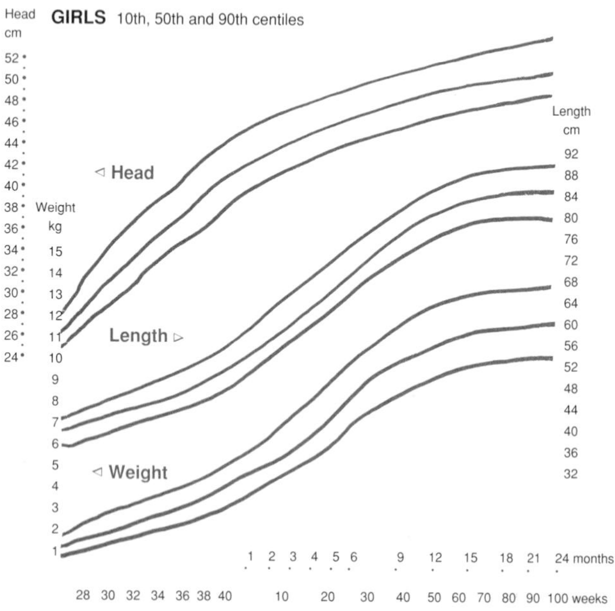

FIGURE 11–4. *An example of a chart of weight, length, and head growth of premature infants from birth to 24 months of age. This growth chart has a built-in correction factor for prematurity.*

Laboratory Indices

Several laboratory measurements have been used as indicators of nutritional status in children and adults. However, these measurements are difficult to interpret in premature infants. Reference ranges for most laboratory parameters based on data from studies in healthy, enterally fed preterm infants are not yet available. At present, laboratory indices are used primarily to evaluate the nutritional status of preterm infants who receive parenteral nutrition.

DISCHARGE CARE

Most of the criteria for discharge from the neonatal nursery involve feeding. Preterm babies must be able to (1) tolerate and in most cases nipple all of their feeds, (2) grow adequately on a modified-demand feeding schedule (usually every 3 to 4 hours during the day), and (3) maintain their body temperature outside of an incubator. In addition, it is important that any ongoing chronic illness, including nutrition problems, be able to be managed successfully at home.

Many preterm infants are discharged from the hospital weighing less than 5½ lb. Increasingly, small babies weighing only about 4 lb are sent home. Although these babies must meet discharge criteria before going home, the stress of a new environment may lead to setbacks. Small preterm infants should be followed very closely during the first month after discharge, and parents should be given as much information and support as possible.

Factors that affect the feeding skills and behavior of preterm infants are particularly important in discharge care (Blackburn and O'Leary, 1987). Physical factors such as variable heart rate, rapid respiratory rate, and tremulousness are examples of physiologic events that interfere with feeding. Infants weighing less than 5½ lb have poor muscle tone. Although this gradually improves as infants become larger and more mature, it can decline quickly in infants who are tired or weak. Feeding is often difficult for babies who have limited muscle flexion and strength and poor head and neck control to maintain good feeding posture. It helps to position these babies in a manner that supports normal body flexion and to be certain that the head and neck stay in a straight line during the course of the feeding.

Babies weighing less than 5½ lb sleep more than larger, full-term infants. It will be much easier for preterm babies to feed effectively if they are fully awake before feeding. To awaken a preterm baby, provide one type of gentle stimulation for a few minutes, then change to a different activity, and so on until the baby is fully awake. It is important to make the feeding environment as quiet as possible. Preterm babies can be

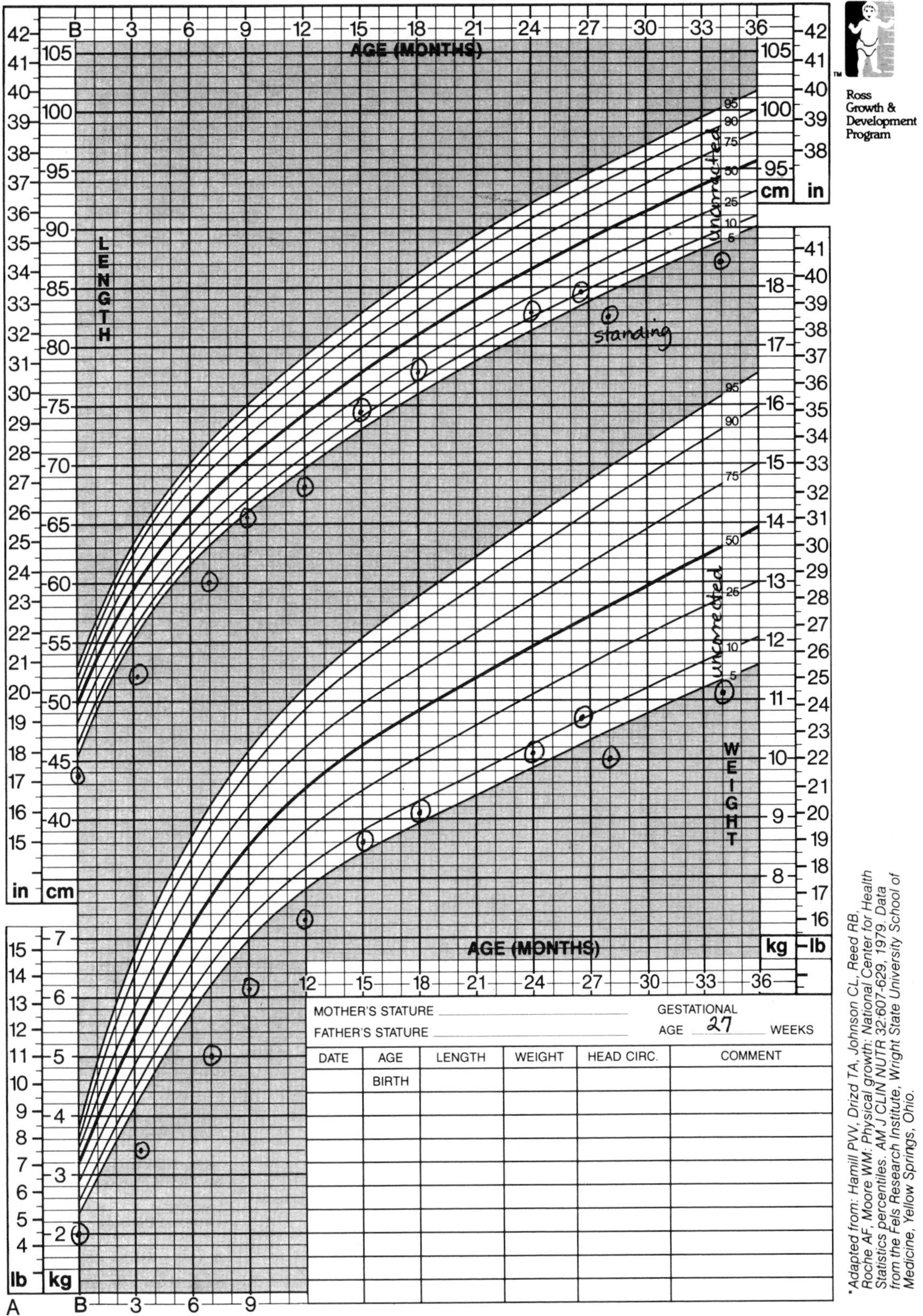

FIGURE 11–5. A, *These graphs show how A.R., a 27-week-old preemie, grew after leaving the neonatal unit 1 day before her due date and at the weight of 4½ lb. Heights and weights up to the age of 28 months were plotted on the grid at "corrected age" points and after that at "uncorrected age" points. She exhibited catch-up growth during the first 15 months.* B, *A.R.'s growth pattern is shown from the age of 2 to 6½ years. During these years she appears to be growing at the 5th percentile for weight and the 10th percentile for height. She is following channel but not exhibiting catch-up growth.*

Illustration continued on following page

GIRLS: 2 TO 18 YEARS
PHYSICAL GROWTH
NCHS PERCENTILES*

NAME A. R. RECORD #

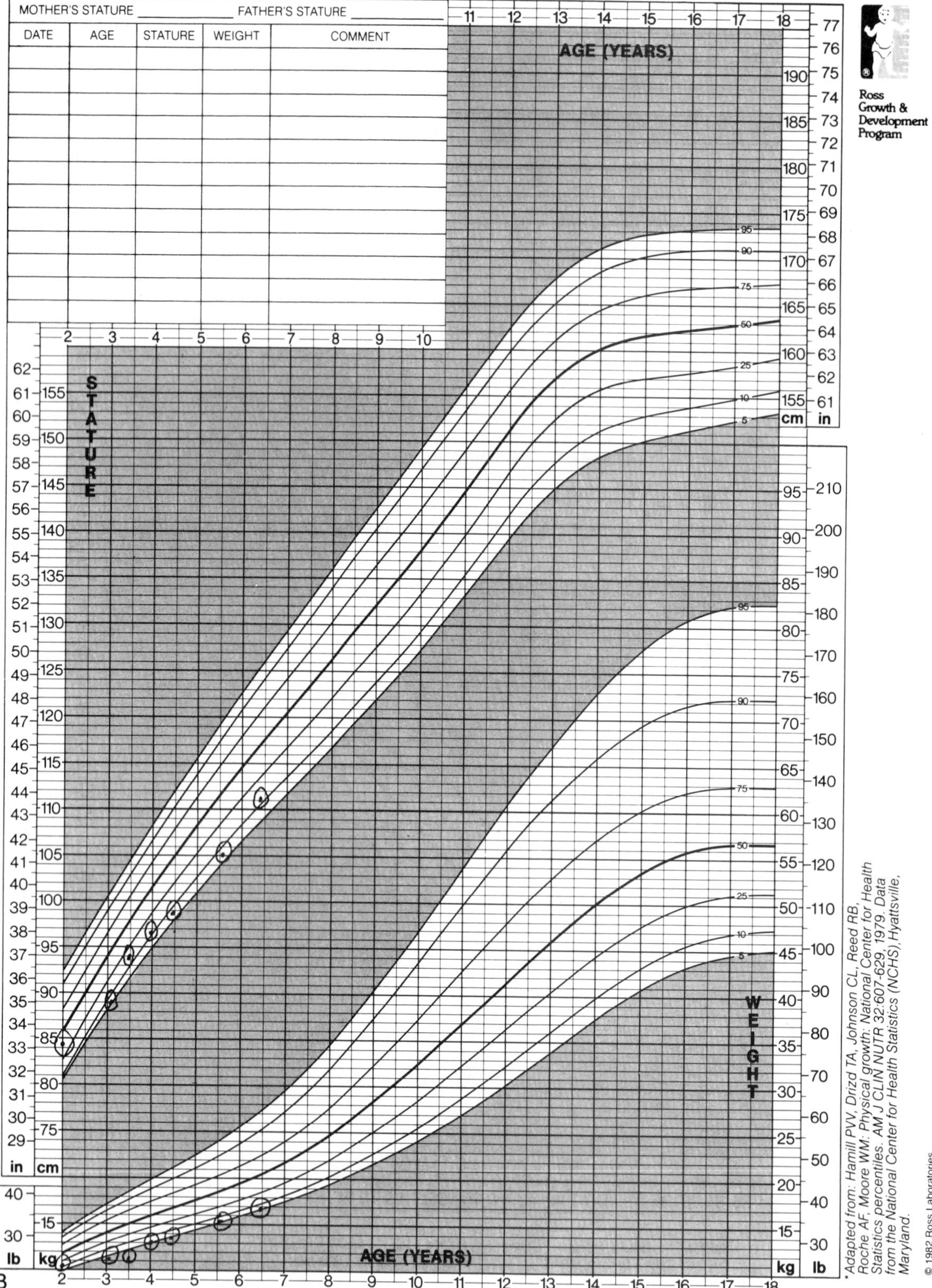

FIGURE 11–5 *Continued*

easily distracted and have difficulty with focusing on feeding when noises or movements interrupt their attention. They also tire quickly and may easily become overstimulated. When this happens, they may show only subtle signs of distress. It is important to teach parents of premature infants to recognize and understand from these subtle cues that rest or comfort is needed.

After discharge, most preterm infants need at least 165 to 180 ml/kg/day (or 2½ to 2⅔ oz/lb/day) of 20 kcal/oz breast milk or standard infant formula. This amount of milk provides 110 to 120 kcal/kg/day (or 50 to 55 kcal/lb/day). The best way to determine whether these amounts are adequate for individual infants is to compare intake with growth progress over time. In some cases, it may be necessary to concentrate feedings as described on page 582.

It is important to evaluate needs based on growth in all three parameters—weight, length, and head circumference. Patterns of growth should be assessed to determine if: (1) weight is appropriate for length, (2) growth is proportionate in all three parameters, (3) individual curves at least parallel reference curves, and (4) growth curves are not shifting inappropriately across growth percentiles.

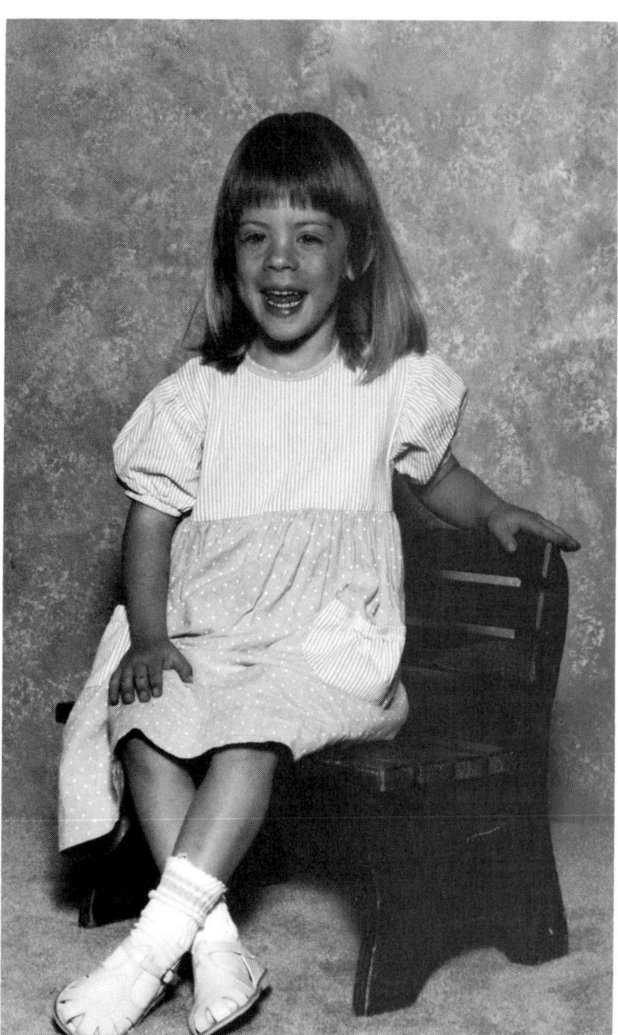

FIGURE 11–6. *This photograph shows the same A.R. as in Figure 11-2 at a healthy 3½ years of age.*

NEURODEVELOPMENTAL OUTCOME

It is apparent that it is possible to meet the metabolic and nutritional needs of premature and LBW infants in a manner sufficient to sustain life and to promote growth and development. With adequate nutritional support and recent advances in neonatal intensive care technology, more tiny, immature infants are surviving than ever before. Survival for infants of 1,001 to 1,500 grams of birthweight improved significantly during the 1970s. During this same period, survival rates nearly doubled for extremely small babies of 501 to 1,000 grams of birthweight (Horwood et al, 1982).

With increased survival of VLBW infants, there is increased concern for the short- and long-term neurodevelopmental outcome of these babies. Many questions are asked about the quality of life awaiting infants who received neonatal intensive care. Surviving LBW infants, particularly those with birthweights less than 800 grams, have an increased risk of developing central nervous system handicapping conditions of varying severity and functional impairment (Bennett, 1988). But despite this risk, many of these premature babies reach school age without evidence of any disability (Fig. 11–6).

CITED REFERENCES

American Academy of Pediatrics, Committee on Nutrition: Commentary on parenteral nutrition. Pediatrics 71:547, 1983.

American Academy of Pediatrics, Committee on Nutrition: Nutritional needs of low-birthweight infants. Pediatrics 75:976, 1985.

American Medical Association, Nutrition Advisory Group: Multivitamin preparations for parenteral use: A statement by the Nutrition Advisory Group. JPEN 3:258, 1979.

Bennett FC: Neurodevelopmental outcome of premature/low-birthweight infants: The role of developmental intervention. *In* Guthrie RD: Neonatal Intensive Care. New York, Churchill Livingstone, 1988.

Blackburn S and O'Leary MJ: Health related concerns. *In* Johnson-Crowley N and Sumner GA (eds): Nursing Systems Toward Effective Parenting—Preterm. Seattle, NCAST Publications, 1987.

Brosius KK, Ritter DA, and Kenny JD: Postnatal growth curve of the infant with extremely LBW who was fed enterally. Pediatrics 74:778, 1984.

Dancis J, O'Connell J, and Holt L: A grid for recording the weight of premature infants. J Pediatr 33:570, 1948.

Farrell PM et al: Essential fatty acid deficiency in premature infants. Am J Clin Nutr 48:220, 1988.

Gaull GE: Taurine in pediatric nutrition: Review and update. Pediatrics 83:433, 1989.

Gaull GE, Wright CE, and Isaacs CE: Significance of growth modulators in human milk. Pediatrics 75:142, 1985.

Greene HL et al: Guidelines for the use of vitamins, trace elements, calcium, magnesium, and phosphorus in infants and children receiving total parenteral nutrition: Report of the Subcommittee on Pediatric Parenteral Nutrient Requirements from the Committee on Clinical Practice Issues of The American Society for Clinical Nutrition. Am J Clin Nutr 48:1324, 1988.

Greer FR and Tsang RC: Calcium, phosphorus, magnesium and vitamin D requirements for the preterm infant. *In* Tsang RC (ed): Vitamin and Mineral Requirements in Preterm Infants. New York, Marcel Dekker, 1985.

Groh-Wargo S, Ciaccia A, and Moore J: Neonatal metabolic acidosis: Effect of chloride from normal saline flushes. JPEN 12:159, 1988.

Gross SJ et al: Growth and biochemical response of premature infants fed human milk or modified infant formula. N Engl J Med 308:237, 1983.

Hamosh M et al: Gastric lipolysis and fat absorption in preterm infants: Effect of MCT on long-chain triglyceride containing formulas. Pediatrics 83:86, 1989.

Heird WC et al: Pediatric parenteral amino acid mixture in low birthweight infants. Pediatrics 81:41, 1988.

Helms RA et al: Comparison of a pediatric versus standard amino acid formulation in preterm neonates requiring parenteral nutrition. J Pediatrics 110:466, 1987.

Helms RA et al: Enhanced lipid utilization in infants receiving oral L-carnitine during long-term parenteral nutrition. J Pediatr 109:984, 1986.

Hoehn GJ et al: Alternate day infusion of calcium and phosphate in VLBW infants: Wasting of the infused mineral. J Pediatr Gastroenterol Nutr 6:752, 1987.

Horwood SP et al: Mortality and morbidity of 500 to 1499 gram birthweight infants liveborn to residents of a defined geographic region before and after neonatal intensive care. Pediatrics 69:613, 1982.

Jaworski AA: New premature weight chart for hospital use. Clin Pediatr 13:513, 1974.

Kerner JA Jr (ed): Manual of Pediatric Parenteral Nutrition. New York, John Wiley, 1983.

Kerner JA Jr: Monitoring IV fat emulsions in neonates with fatty acid/serum albumin molar ratio. JPEN 5:517, 1981.

Kine CL et al: Rickets in premature infants receiving parenteral nutrition: a case report and review of the literature. JPEN 6:152, 1982.

Koo WK et al: Calcium, magnesium and phosphorus. *In* Tsang RC and Nichols B (eds): Nutrition in Infancy. Philadelphia, Hanley and Belfus, 1988.

Lebenthal E (ed): Total Parenteral Nutrition. New York, Raven Press, 1986.

Lemons JA et al: Differences in the composition of preterm and term human milk during early lactation. Pediatr Res 16:113, 1982.

Lima LAM: Neonatal parenteral nutrition with medium-chain triglycerides: Rationale for research. JPEN 13:312, 1989.

MacDonald MG et al: The potential toxicity to neonates of multivitamin preparations used in parenteral nutrition. JPEN 11:169, 1987.

Meier P and Anderson GC: Responses of small preterm infants to bottle-and breastfeeding. Matern Child Nurs J 12(2):97, 1987.

Meier P and Pugh EJ: Breastfeeding behavior of small preterm infants. Mat Child Nurs J 10(6):396, 1985.

Neifert M and Seacat J: Practical aspects of breastfeeding the premature infant. Perinatol-Neonatol 12(1):24, 1988.

Nutrition management of adolescent pregnancy: Technical support paper. J Am Diet Assn 89:105, 1989.

O'Leary MJ: Breastfeeding Education Materials for Preterm Infants (Pamphlets, Videotapes, and Poster), Health Sciences Center for Educational Resources, Distribution Center, SB–56, University of Washington, Seattle, Washington, 1989.

Oski FA: Iron requirements of the premature infant. *In* Tsang RC (ed): Vitamin and Mineral Requirements in Preterm Infants. New York, Marcel Dekker, 1985.

Phelps DL et al: Tocopherol efficacy and safety for preventing retinopathy or prematurity. Pediatrics 79:489, 1987.

Rowe J et al: Hypophosphatemia and hypercalciuria in small premature infants fed human milk: Evidence for inadequate dietary phosphorus. J Pediatr 104:112, 1984.

Slagle TA and Gross SJ: Effect of early low-volume enteral substrate on subsequent feeding tolerance in very low birthweight infants. J Pediatr 113:526, 1988.

Spear ML et al: Effect of heparin dose and infusion rate on lipid clearance and bilirubin binding in premature infants receiving IV fat emulsions. J Pediatr 112:94, 1988.

Steichen JJ, Gratton TL, and Tsang RC: Osteopenia of prematurity: The cause and possible treatment. J Pediatr 96:528, 1980.

Tantibhedhyangkul P and Hashim SA: Medium chain triglyceride feeding in premature infants: Effects on fat and nitrogen absorption. Pediatrics 55:359, 1975.

Tsang RC: Vitamin and Mineral Requirements in Preterm Infants. New York, Marcel Dekker, 1985.

U.S. teens have highest rate of abortions: U.N. study finds. Seattle Times Dec 14, 1988.

Ziegler EE, Biga RL, and Fomon SJ: Nutritional requirements of the premature infant. *In* Suskind RM (ed): Textbook of Pediatric Nutrition. New York, Raven Press, 1981.

Ziegler EE et al: Body composition of the reference fetus. Growth 40:329, 1976.

Zlotkin SH: Trophamine. Pediatrics 82:388, 1988.

ADDITIONAL REFERENCES

American Academy of Pediatrics, Committee on Nutrition: Use of intravenous fat emulsions in pediatric practice. Pediatrics 68:738, 1981.

Babson SG and Benda GI: Growth graphs for the clinical assessment of infants of varying gestational age. J Pediatr 89:814, 1976.

Baeckert PA et al: Vitamin concentrations in very low birthweight infants given vitamins intravenously in a lipid emulsion: Measurement of vitamins A, D, and E and riboflavin. J Pediatr 113:1057, 1988.

Berkow SE et al: TPN with Intralipid in premature infants receiving TPN with heparin. J Pediatr Gastroenterol Nutr 6:581, 1987.

Carey DE et al: Growth and phosphorus metabolism in premature infants fed human milk, fortified human milk, or special premie formula. Am J Dis Child 141:511, 1987.

Chan GM, Mileur L, and Hansen JW: Calcium and phosphorus requirements in bone mineralization of preterm infants. J Pediatr 113:225, 1988.

Chessey P et al: Calciuria in parenterally fed preterm infants: Role of phosphorus intake. J Pediatr 107:794, 1985.

Chessey P et al: Quality of growth in premature infants fed their own mother's milk. J Pediatr 102:107, 1983.

Dubowitz LMS et al: Clinical assessment of gestational age in the newborn infant. J Pediatr 77:1, 1970.

Eibl MM et al: Prevention of NEC in LBW infants by IgA–IgG feeding. N Engl J Med 319:1, 1988.

Greene HL et al: Persistently low blood retinol levels during and after parenteral feeding of very low birthweight infants: Examination of losses into intravenous administration sets and a method of prevention by addition to a lipid emulsion. Pediatrics 79:894, 1987.

Immunoglobulin feeding prevents necrotizing enterocolitis in formula-fed very-low-birthweight infants. Nutr Rev 47:186, 1989.

Jarvenpaa AL et al: Preterm infants fed human milk attain intrauterine weight gain. Acta Paediatr Scand 72:239, 1983.

Lundstrom U, Siimes MA, and Dallman PR: At what age does iron supplementation become necessary in low-birthweight infants? J Pediatr 91:878, 1977.

Mehta NR et al: Adherence of medium-chain fatty acids to feeding tubes during gavage feeding of human milk fortified with medium-chain triglycerides. J Pediatr 112:474, 1988.

Moore MC: Evaluation of a pediatric multiple vitamin preparation for TPN in infants and children. Pediatrics 77:530, 1986.

Reichman BL et al: Partition of energy metabolism and energy cost of growth in the very-low-birthweight infant. Pediatr 69:446, 1982.

Ronnholm KAR, Dostalova L, and Siimes MA: Vitamin E supplementation in very-low-birthweight infants: Long-term follow-up at two different levels of vitamin E supplementation. Am J Clin Nutr 49:121, 1989.

Schanler RJ, Abrams SA, and Garza C: Mineral balance studies in

very low-birthweight infants fed human milk. J Pediatrics 113:230, 1988.
Schanler RJ and Garza C: Improved mineral balance in very low-birthweight infants fed fortified human milk. J Pediatr 112:452, 1988.
Sturman JA: Taurine in development. J Nutr 118:1169, 1988.
Swanson JA and Berseth CL: Continuing care for the preterm infant after dismissal from the neonatal intensive care unit. Mayo Clin Proc 62:613, 1987.
Zachman RD: Retinol (vitamin A) and the neonate: Special problems of the human premature infant. Am J Clin Nutr 50:413, 1989.

CHAPTER 12

NUTRITION IN CHILDHOOD

Betty Lucas, M.P.H., R.D.

CHAPTER OUTLINE

Growth and Development
Nutrient Needs
Providing an Adequate Diet
Nutritional Concerns
Nutrition Education

KEY TERMS

ADIPOSITY REBOUND—the phenomenon of growth when the normal child increases in body fatness around 6 years of age

APPETITE—a natural desire to eat, especially when food is present

CATCH-UP GROWTH—a higher than normal growth rate to recover a previous growth curve after a period of growth suppression due to extended illness or deprivation

FOOD JAG—the refusal of previously liked foods or the requesting of a particular food at every meal; commonly seen in children who are 2 to 6 years of age

GROWTH CHANNEL—a curve of weight and height gain throughout the period of growth; stated as a percentile based on a standard growth chart

The time from 1 year of age until puberty is often referred to as the "latent" or "quiescent" period of growth, in contrast to the dramatic changes that occur in infancy and adolescence. Although physical growth may be less remarkable and more steady than during the first year, these preschool and middle school years are a time of significant growth in the social, cognitive, and emotional areas.

GROWTH AND DEVELOPMENT

Physical Growth

The rate of growth slows considerably after the first year of life. In contrast to the tripling of birthweight in the first 12 months, another year passes before birthweight is quadrupled. Likewise, birth length increases by 50% in the first year but is not doubled until approximately the age of 4. The actual increments of change are small compared with those of infancy and adolescence. Weight increases an average of 2 to 3 kg (4½ to 6½ lb) per year until the child is 9 or 10 years old, when the rate increases, an initial sign of approaching puberty. Height increments average 6 to 8 cm (2½ to 3½ in) per year from 2 years of age until the pubertal acceleration.

In general, growth is steady and slow during the preschool and school-age years, but it may be erratic in individual children. Some small children may be in an apparent "holding pattern" for several months to a year and then have a spurt in height and weight. Interestingly, these patterns usually parallel similar changes in appetite and food intake. For parents who are not knowledgeable about these trends (and even for some who are), periods of slow growth and poor appetite can cause anxiety, which may lead to mealtime struggles.

Body proportions of young children change significantly after the first year. There is little head growth; trunk growth slows substantially; and the limbs lengthen considerably to give a more mature body proportion. With increased physical activity and walking, the legs straighten while the abdominal and back muscles tighten to support the now erect child. These changes are gradual and subtle and occur over a period of years.

Body composition in preschool and school-age children remains relatively constant. Fat gradually decreases during the early childhood years and reaches a minimum at approximately 6 years of age. After that, it increases (the "adiposity rebound") in preparation for the pubertal growth spurt (Rolland-Cachera et al, 1987). Sex differences begin early, and boys have more lean body mass per centimeter of height. Girls have a higher percentage of weight as fat even in the early years, but these sex differences in lean body mass and fat do not become significant until adolescence.

Catch-Up Growth

The child recovering from an illness or undernutrition that has slowed or ceased growth will experience a greater than expected rate of recovery. This is referred to as "catch-up" growth: the body strives to catch up to the child's normal growth curve. The degree of growth suppression is influenced by the timing, severity, and duration of the insult; that is, a severe illness or deprivation for an extended time during a period of rapid growth will have the most dramatic effect.

Early studies supported the thesis that malnourished infants who did not experience immediate catch-up growth would have permanent growth retardation. However, studies in developing countries of malnourished children who were subsequently treated, as well as reports of children malnourished because of chronic diseases such as celiac disease or cystic fibrosis, have demonstrated complete catch-up growth after the first year or two of life (Barr et al, 1972; Ellis and Hill, 1975; Stoch and Smythe, 1976).

Rates of catch-up in weight gain can be 20 times faster than normal in children who are both stunted and wasted; that is, the weight deficit is greater than the length deficit. Once catch-up growth has reached an appropriate weight for length, the rate of weight gain is aproximately three times the usual rate expected for age. The catch-up in linear growth reaches its peak about 1 to 3 months after treatment starts, whereas weight gain begins immediately (Ashworth and Millward, 1986).

Nutrient requirements, especially for energy and protein, vary depending on the rate and stage of catch-up. For instance, more protein and energy will be needed during the very rapid weight gain period and in cases in which lean tissue is the major component of the weight gain. Guidelines for determining nutrient requirements are discussed in Clinical Insight, page 219.

Assessing Growth

Because children are constantly growing and changing, periodic assessment of their progress allows any problems to be detected and treated early. Many children are seen by health-care professionals only when they are ill, at which time growth and development may not be dealt with.

A complete assessment of nutritional status includes the collection of anthropometric data. This includes height and weight, weight for height (all with percentiles plotted on the National Center for Health Statistics [NCHS] growth charts as shown in Appendices 7 to 14, 23, 25, and 26), upper arm circumference, and triceps or subscapular fatfolds.

Growth measurements must be recorded at regular intervals to show growth patterns. Height and weight taken only once do not lend themselves to interpreta-

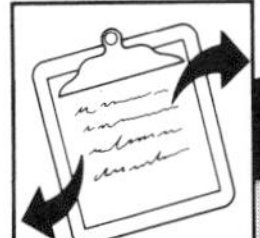

CLINICAL INSIGHT: Obtaining Optimal Catch-Up Growth

Clinical management of a child who is growth retarded owing to malnourishment, chronic disorder, or malabsorptive disease begins initially with a thorough assessment. This assessment includes determining the nature, severity, and duration of the nutritional insult, as well as the usual components of nutritional assessment—anthropometric, dietary, biochemical, clinical, and social/environmental. Growth data (height, weight, and weight/height) are important criteria to follow over time, and arm circumference and triceps fatfold can give estimates of body composition.

The nutritional goals depend on whether the child is stunted and chronically malnourished or mainly wasted (the weight deficit greater than the length deficit). The former may not be expected to gain more than 2 to 3 g/kg/day, whereas the latter may gain as much as 20 g/kg/day (Ashworth and Millward, 1986). Once a child who is wasted "catches up" in weight, dietary management changes to facilitate a slower catch up in both weight and linear growth.

The following table illustrates the varying requirements for energy and protein at different rates of weight gain. Generally, the protein need increases proportionately more than the energy need when the gain is greater.

Milk or a milk-based formula often provides the basis of the diet for young children during catch-up, along with developmentally appropriate foods. Frequent, small feedings are usually better tolerated. Because total volume and the child's stomach capacity can be limiting factors, energy and nutrients can be concentrated or adjusted by the use of commercial liquid supplements, formula concentration, increased use of fats and oils, instant breakfast products, or the addition of glucose polymers and medium-chain-triglyceride oil.

Growth and nutritional status should be monitored frequently, and dietary management can be modified as needed. In all cases, medical, social, and environmental concerns related to the growth retardation need to be resolved.

Dietary Requirements for Energy and Protein at Different Rates of Weight Gain*

Rate of Weight Gain (g/kg/day)	*Energy† (kcal/kg/day)*	*Protein‡ (g/kg/day)*	*Protein‡ (g of protein/ 100 kcal)*	Weeks Needed to Correct Wasted Child§
—	85	0.62	0.73	NA‖
1	90	0.83	0.92	50
2	94	1.04	1.11	25
5	108	1.67	1.55	10
10	130	2.72	2.09	5
20	174	4.82	2.77	2.5

* From Ashworth A and Millward DJ: Catch-up growth in children. Nutr Rev 44:157, 1986.

† Assumes intake for zero energy balance is 85.5 kcal/kg/day, and cost of weight gain is 4.4 kcal/kg, which indicates that the composition of the tissue deposited is 73.5% lean and 26.5% fat.

‡ Assumes intake for zero N balance is 100 mg N/kg/day, protein content of weight gain is 14.7%, and efficiency of dietary protein utilization for tissue deposition is 70%.

§ Assumes child has an initial weight deficit of 3 kg and an average body weight during rehabilitation of 8.5 kg.

‖ NA = not applicable.

tion of growth status. Children generally maintain their heights and weights in the same channels during the preschool and early childhood years, although the channels are not well established until after 2 years of age. Individual children sometimes grow at faster or slower rates; nonetheless, they should follow along the same channels.

The height and weight of a child should be in proportion; this can be assessed by plotting the weight for height. A gross assessment can also be made by noting the difference between the height and weight channels; a difference of more than two channels is suggestive of overweight or underweight and should be investigated further. Fat skinfold measurements yield more specific information regarding the composition of the child's weight.

Regular monitoring of growth enables trends to be identified early, and treatment is begun so that long-term growth is not compromised. Weight increasing at a rapid rate and crossing channels suggests the development of obesity. Lack of weight gain or loss of weight over a period of months may be a result of undernutrition, a severe acute illness, an undiagnosed chronic disease, or significant emotional or family problems. Figure 12-1 demonstrates these changes in growth parameters.

NUTRIENT NEEDS

Because children are growing and developing bones, teeth, muscles, and blood, they need more nutritious food in proportion to their weight than do adults. They can become at risk for malnutrition when they have a prolonged poor appetite, accept a limited number of foods, or dilute their diets significantly with nutrient-poor foods.

The Recommended Dietary Allowances (RDA) represent the current knowledge of nutrient intakes needed by children of different ages for optimal health (Food and Nutrition Board, 1989) (Table 12-1). Most of the data for children of these ages are values interpolated from data on infants and adults. Because they provide a margin of safety (except for energy) above the physiologic requirement for most children in the United States, they cannot be applied appropriately to individual children. An intake that falls below the rec-

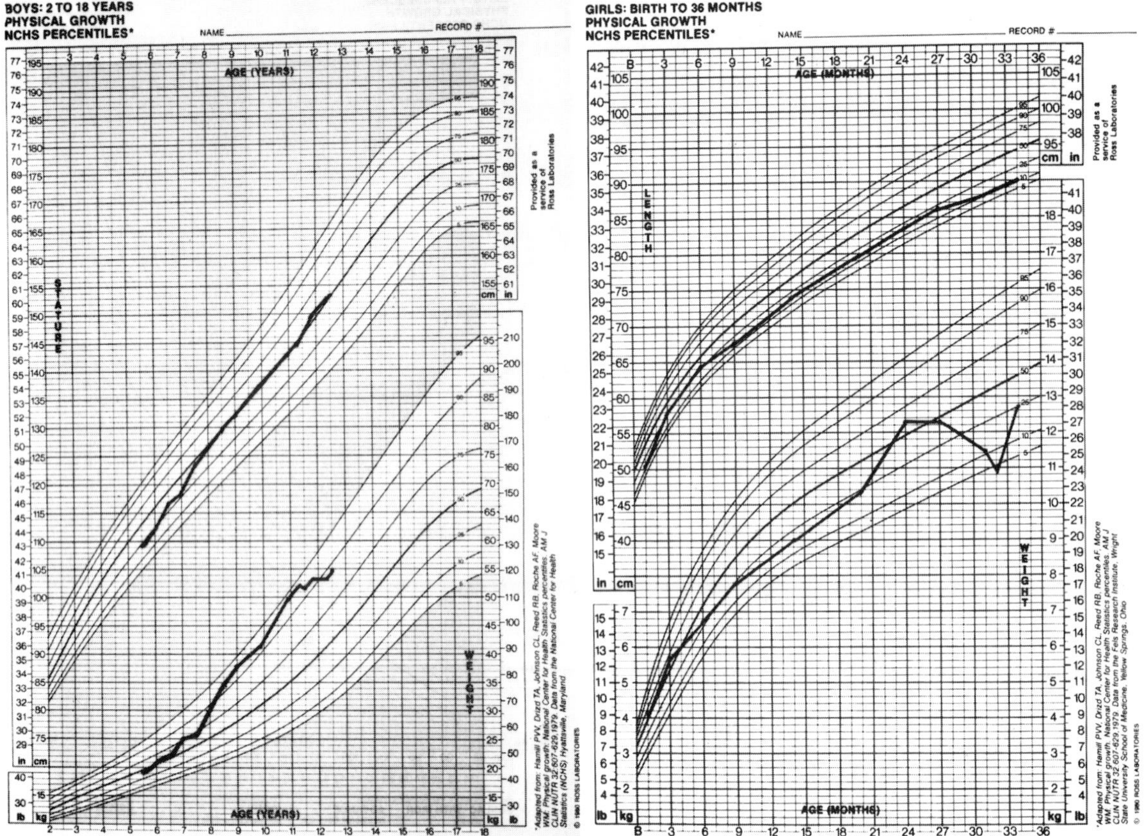

FIGURE 12–1. A, *Excessive weight gain in an 8-year-old boy after leg surgery that kept him immobilized in a body cast for 2 months. This was followed by a long period of stress due to family problems. After age 11, he became involved in a weight management clinic.* B, *Significant weight loss in a 2-year-old girl during a long period of diarrhea and feeding problems. After a diagnosis of celiac disease and the institution of a gluten-free diet, rebound weight gain was seen.*

ommended allowance does not necessarily justify the assumption that a child is inadequately nourished.

Energy

The energy needs of a child are determined by basal metabolism, rate of growth, and activity. Dietary energy must be sufficient to ensure growth and spare protein from being used for energy, without being so excessive that obesity results. A suggested proportion of energy is 50 to 60% as carbohydrate, 25 to 35% as fat, and 10 to 15% as protein.

The RDA presented in Table 12–1 should be used as a guide for determining an appropriate energy intake for a child. There are variations in energy intakes of healthy, growing children of the same age and sex depending mainly on their activity. A 7-year-old boy and a 10½-year-old girl going into puberty have significantly different factors determining their energy needs, even though they also are in the same age-and-sex category. It is useful to determine energy requirements on an individual basis using kilocalories per kilogram or per centimeter of height (Beal, 1970).

Protein

The need for protein per kilogram of body weight decreases from approximately 1.2 grams in early childhood to 1 gram in late childhood (see Table 12–1). Reported intakes from national surveys have shown that protein intakes are considerably higher, in the range of 10 to 16% of kcal (Abraham et al, 1977; Dietary Intake Source Data, 1983; Farris et al, 1986).

Protein deficiency is uncommon in American children, partly because of our cultural emphasis on pro-

TABLE 12–1. Recommended Dietary Allowances for Energy and Protein for Children*

	kcal			g of Protein	
Age	*Daily*	*Per kg*	*Per cm*	*Daily*	*Per kg*
1–3	1,300	102	14.4	16	1.2
4–6	1,800	90	16.0	24	1.1
7–10	2,000	70	15.2	28	1.0

* Reprinted with permission from *Recommended Dietary Allowances*, 10th ed., c. 1989 by the National Academy of Sciences. Published by National Academy Press, Washington, DC.

tein foods. Children most likely at risk for inadequate protein intake are those on strict vegan diets, those who have multiple food allergies, or those who have limited food selection because of fad diets, behavior problems, or limited access to food.

Minerals and Vitamins

Minerals and vitamins are necessary for normal growth and development. Insufficient intake can cause impaired growth and result in deficiency diseases, as described in Chapters 7 and 8. The RDA for different age groups are listed in Table 16–1.

The preschool child between 1 and 3 years of age is at high risk for iron deficiency anemia. The rapid growth period of infancy is marked by an increase in both hemoglobin and total iron mass. In addition, the child's diet may not be rich in iron-containing foods. Recommended intakes must take into consideration the relative absorbability as well as the quantity of iron in foods, especially those of plant origin. See Chapter 32 for further discussion.

Calcium for this age group is needed for adequate mineralization and maintenance of growing bone. Actual need depends on individual absorption rates and dietary factors, such as quantities of protein, vitamin D, and phosphorus. Because milk and other dairy products are the primary sources of calcium, children who consume none or limited amounts of these foods are at risk for calcium deficiency (Fig. 12–2).

Vitamin D is needed for calcium absorption and for deposition of calcium in the bones. Because this nutrient is also available from the action of sunlight on subcutaneous tissues, the amount required from dietary sources depends on factors such as geographical location and time spent outside. Children living in tropical areas may need no dietary vitamin D or only up to 2.5 μg (100 IU) for optimal utilization of calcium. In the temperate zones, however, some dietary source is needed, and the RDA is established at 10 μg (400 IU) daily for children. Vitamin D-fortified milk is the main source of this nutrient. Dairy products such as cheese and yogurt are not usually made from fortified milk, however.

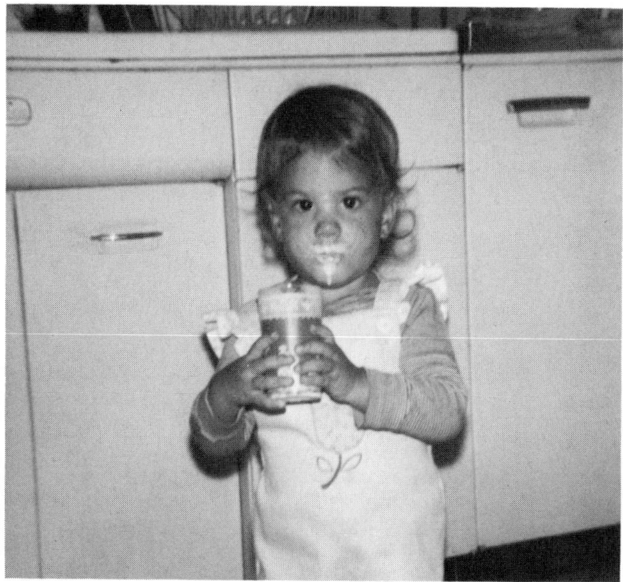

FIGURE 12–2. *Milk and other dairy products supply the preschool child with calcium needed for growing bones.*

Zinc is essential for growth; a deficiency results in growth failure, poor appetite, decreased taste acuity, and poor wound healing. An allowance of 10 mg/day of zinc is recommended, but because the best sources of available zinc are meats and seafoods, some children may regularly have a lower intake. Marginal zinc deficiency has been reported in preschool and school-aged children from both middle- and low-income families (Buzina et al, 1980; Hambidge et al, 1976). (Clinical Insight, p. 124). Diagnosis may be difficult because of variations in laboratory methods and values. A child with symptoms and dietary intake suggesting zinc depletion should undergo analysis of plasma and hair zinc content. In some cases, a careful trial of zinc supplementation may be the only conclusive way to diagnose a problem (Trace elements, 1985) (see Chapter 7).

Vitamin-Mineral Supplements

The use of supplements decreases after infancy, but approximately 37% of preschool children and 23% of school-aged children take some vitamin or mineral preparation (Bowering and Clancy, 1986). Supplements do not necessarily fulfill nutrient needs, however. For instance, calcium and iron, which are often consumed at levels below recommendations, are not commonly supplemented.

The American Academy of Pediatrics does not support routine supplementation for normal children except for fluoride in unfluoridated areas (Committee on Nutrition, 1980). Children at nutritional risk are described as those (1) from deprived families, (2) with anorexia, poor appetites, and poor eating habits, and (3) consuming vegetarian diets without adequate dairy products. The American Medical Association and the American Dietetic Association have also recommended that healthy children should receive their nutrients from food and not from supplements (American Dietetic Association, 1987; Council on Scientific Affairs, 1987).

Parents who wish to give their children a multiple vitamin or vitamin/mineral will not incur risk if the supplement contains nutrients in amounts no larger than the RDA. Megadoses should be avoided, particularly of the fat-soluble vitamins, large amounts of which can result in toxicity.

Possible Nutrient Deficiencies

Nutrients most likely to be low or deficient in children's diets are calcium, iron, zinc, ascorbic acid, and vitamin A. Clinical signs of malnutrition in American children, however, are rare. Population studies of nutritional status have reported a higher frequency of low nutrient intakes and short stature in children from low-income families (Abraham et al, 1977; Centers for Disease Control, 1972). In addition, studies of certain geographical "poverty pockets" have demonstrated a higher rate of poor dietary intake as well as biochemical and clinical signs of malnutrition (Owen and Lippman, 1977).

PROVIDING AN ADEQUATE DIET

Food and eating mean more than the provision of nutrients for body growth and maintenance. The development of feeding skills, food habits, and nutrition knowledge parallels cognitive development that takes place in a series of stages, each of which lays the groundwork for the next. Table 12–2 outlines the development of feeding skills in terms of Piaget's theory of child psychology and development.

Patterns of Intake

As physical growth is not smooth and consistent, neither is food intake. Appetite, although a subjective assessment, usually follows the rate of growth and nutrient needs. A "good" appetite in infancy often becomes a "fair to poor" appetite in the young preschool child and is a frequent cause of parental anxiety.

By the first birthday, milk consumption has declined and will continue to do so in the next year. There is a decrease in vegetable intake and an increase in desserts, starches, and sweets. Ground beef and hot dogs are preferred to meats that are harder to chew, such as roasts and steaks.

Changes in food consumption are reflected in nutrient intakes. Compared with nutrient intake in infancy, the early preschool years show a decrease in calcium, phosphorus, riboflavin, iron, and vitamin A. Most other key nutrients remain relatively stable. During the early school years, a pattern of consistent and steady increases in all nutrients is seen until adolescence.

For any age and sex group, wide variability of nutrient intake is seen in healthy children. Beal found that at any age, the maximum intake of energy, carbohydrate, fat, and protein was two to three times the minimum intake. Even wider ranges were noted in vitamin intakes; the maximum:minimum ratios in one group of well-growing children were as high as 10:1 for ascorbic acid and 20:1 for carotene (Beal, 1961).

National food consumption studies of children 1 to 5 years of age have shown changing trends in their food patterns. These include an increased use of low-fat and nonfat milk, decreased intake of whole milk, higher frequency of snacking, and more food eaten away from home (USDA, 1987).

TABLE 12–2. Piaget's Theory of Cognitive Development in Relation to Feeding and Nutrition

Developmental Period	Cognitive Characteristics	Relationships to Feeding and Nutrition
Sensorimotor (Birth–2 years)	• Progression from newborn with automatic reflexes to intentional interaction with the environment and the beginning use of symbols	• Progression is made from sucking and rooting reflexes to the acquisition of self-feeding skills • Food is used primarily to satisfy hunger, as a medium to explore the environment and to practice fine motor skills
Preoperations (2–7 years)	• Thought processes become internalized; they are unsystematic and intuitive • Use of symbols increases • Reasoning is based on appearances and happenstance • Approach to classification is functional and unsystematic • Child's world is viewed egocentrically	• Eating becomes less the center of attention than social, language, and cognitive growth • Food is described by color, shape, and quantity, but there is limited ability to classify food into "groups" • Foods tend to be classed as "like" and "don't like" • Foods can be identified as "good for you" but reasons are unknown or mistaken
Concrete operations (7–11 years)	• Child can focus on several aspects of a situation simultaneously • Cause/effect reasoning becomes more rational and systematic • Ability to classify, reclassify, and generalize emerges • Decrease in egocentricism permits child to take another's view	• Beginning realization that nutritious food has a positive effect on growth and health, but limited understanding of how or why this occurs • Mealtimes take on a social significance • The expanding environment increases the opportunities for and influences on food selection (peer influence rises)
Formal operations (11 years and beyond)	• Hypothetical and abstract thought expand • Understanding of scientific and theoretical processes deepens	• The concept of nutrients from food functioning at physiologic and biochemical levels can be understood • Conflicts in making food choices may be realized (knowledge of nutritious food vs preferences and non-nutritive influences)

Factors Influencing Food Intake

Numerous influences, some obvious and some subtle, determine the food intake and habits of children. It is well known that habits, likes, and dislikes are well grounded in the early years and carry through to adulthood, where change is often met with resistance and difficulty. The major influences on food intake in the developing years include family environment, the media, peer pressure, and illness or disease.

Family Environment

For the toddler and preschool child, the family is the primary influence in the development of food habits. Parents and older siblings are significant models for young children as they learn and imitate the individuals in their immediate environment. Food attitudes of parents have been shown to be a strong predictor of food likes and dislikes as well as diet complexity in primary school children. It is still not clear how much of the similarity between children's and their parents' food preferences is due to genetic and how much to environmental factors (Similarity . . . , 1987).

Contrary to common belief, young children do not have the innate ability to choose a balanced, nutritious diet (Further Reading, p. 191). Thus parents and other adults are responsible for offering a variety of nutritious and developmentally appropriate foods. A positive feeding relationship includes a division of responsibility between parent and children, with the parent providing safe, nutritious food as regular meals and snacks and the children deciding how much, if any, they eat (Satter, 1986).

The atmosphere around food and mealtime is also an important aspect of attitudes toward food and eating. High expectations for a child's mealtime manners, with the threat of reprimand, can make dinner a dreaded time. Arguments and other emotional stress can also have a negative effect. Meals that are rushed create a hectic atmosphere and reinforce eating too fast. A positive environment allows enough time to eat, is tolerant of occasional spills, and encourages conversation that includes all family members (see Fig. 12–3).

In recent decades, the nuclear family has changed from the traditional two-parent, one-income family. Almost half of all women are now employed outside the home. Children, therefore, eat one or more meals at

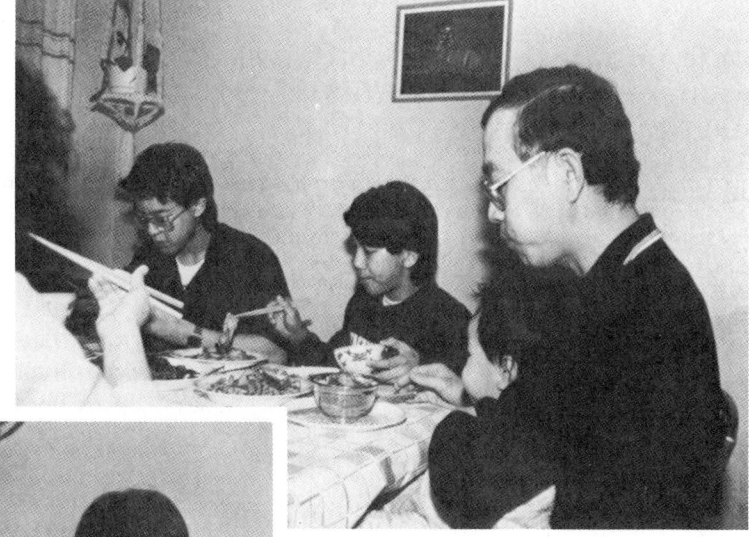

FIGURE 12–3. *The Chinese tradition of the extended family and the custom of eating a variety of authentically prepared foods gives mealtime a place of prominence in this home, not to be exchanged for "eating fast foods on the run." (From Foster RL, Hunsberger MM, and Anderson JJ: Family-Centered Nursing Care of Children. Philadelphia, WB Saunders, 1989, p G20.)*

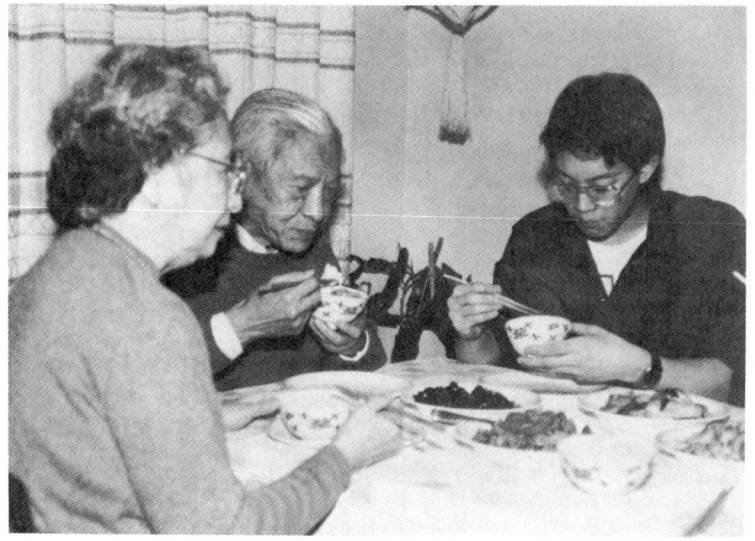

child care homes, day care centers, or schools. Because of time constraints, food purchasing and meal preparation routines are often modified to include more use of convenience or fast foods. The increasing numbers of single-parent households are mostly headed by women, which often means a lower income and less money for all expenses including food.

Media Messages

By the time the average American child has graduated from high school, he or she will have watched 15,000 hours of television and will have spent 11,000 hours in the classroom (Nielsen Company, 1985). Almost half of all commercials are for food, and the percentage is higher in children's programming (Cotugna, 1988). Most of those targeted to children are for foods high in sugar, fat, or sodium.

Preschool children are generally unable to distinguish commercial messages from the regular program, and in fact they often pay more attention to the former. As children get older, they become knowledgeable of the purpose of commercial advertising and become more critical of its validity. However, they are still susceptible to the commercial message.

Television can also be detrimental to growth and development by encouraging inactivity and passive use of leisure time. Television viewing, along with multiple media cues to eat, is documented to be a factor in excessive weight gain for children aged 6 to 17 years (Dietz and Gortmaker, 1985).

Peer Influence

As children grow, their world expands and their social contacts take on more importance. Peer influence increases with age and extends to food attitudes and choices. This may be manifested by a sudden refusal of a food or a request for a current "popular" food. Decisions on whether to participate in school lunch may be more a result of what friends do than of the menu offered. These behaviors usually represent a phase that will change. Positive aspects, such as trying new foods, can be reinforced. Parents need to set limits for undesirable influences but also to be realistic; struggles over food are self-defeating.

Illness or Disease

Children who are ill usually have a decreased appetite and limited food intake. Acute viral or bacterial illnesses are often of short duration but may require an increase in fluids, protein, or other nutrients. Chronic conditions, such as asthma, congenital heart disease, and cystic fibrosis, may make it difficult to obtain nutrients for optimal growth. Children with these types of disease are more likely to have behavior problems or family struggles around food. Children requiring special diets (e.g., those for diabetes or phenylketonuria) not only have to adjust to the limits of foods allowed but also have to deal with the issues of independence and peer acceptance as they grow older. It is not atypical to see some rebellion against the prescribed diet, especially as the child approaches puberty.

Feeding the Preschool Child

For the child from 1 to 6 years of age, this period is marked by vast development and by the acquisition of skills. The child learns to talk, run, and become a social being. The 1-year-old child primarily uses fingers to eat and may need assistance with a cup. By 2 years of age he or she can hold a cup in one hand and use a spoon well (see Fig. 10–3), but the child may still prefer to use his/her hands at times. The 6-year-old child has refined skills and is beginning to use a knife for cutting as well as for spreading.

Because growth is slower during these years, appetite also decreases, often causing parental concern. Children have less interest in food and more interest in the world around them. They develop "food jags" during this time, refusing previously accepted food or asking for one particular food at each meal. This behavior may be due to boredom with usual foods or may be a means of asserting newly discovered independence.

This is often a difficult time for parents, with their concern about the adequacy of diet and their frustration with their child's seemingly irrational food behavior. Struggles over control of the eating situation are fruitless; no child can be forced to eat. Parents need to understand that this period is developmental and temporary. They will still determine what foods are offered and set limits on inappropriate behaviors. Neither rigid control nor a laissez-faire approach is likely to succeed. The parents should continue to offer a variety of foods, including the favorite ones, and substitutions for those refused should be made within the same food group. Young children usually respond positively when offered a choice of healthy foods.

Preschool children, because of their smaller capacity and variable appetites, do best with small servings of food offered several times a day. Portion sizes are small by adult standards. A general rule of thumb is to offer one tablespoon of each food for every year of age and to serve more food according to appetite. Table 12–3 is a guide for food and portion sizes to provide an adequate diet for preschoolers. Most children eat four to six times a day, making snacks as important as meals in contributing to the total day's nutrient intake. One food consumption study indicated that approximately 76% of 1 to 5-year-old children eat more than three

TABLE 12–3. Feeding Guide for Preschool Children*†

	2- to 3-Year-Olds		4- to 6-Year-Olds		
Food	***Portion Size***	***No. of Servings***	***Portion Size***	***No. of Servings***	**Comments**
Milk and dairy products	½ cup (4 oz)	4–5	½–¾ cup (4–6 oz)	3–4	The following may be substituted for ½ cup liquid milk: ½–¾ oz cheese, ½ cup yogurt, 2½ T nonfat dry milk powder
Meat, fish, poultry, or equivalent	1–2 oz	2	1–2 oz	2	The following may be substituted for 1 oz meat, fish or poultry: 1 egg, 2 T peanut butter, 4–5 T cooked legumes
Fruits and vegetables		4–5		4–5	Include one green leafy or yellow vegetable for vitamin A, such as spinach, carrots, broccoli, winter squash
Vegetables					
Cooked	2–3 T		3–4 T		
Raw‡	Few pieces		few pieces		
Fruit					
Raw	½–1 small		½–1 small		Include one vitamin C-rich fruit, vegetable or juice, such as citrus juices, orange, grapefruit sections, strawberries, melon in season, tomato, broccoli
Canned	2–4 T		4–6 T		
Juice	3–4 oz		4 oz		
Bread and grain products		3		3	
Whole grain or enriched bread	½–1 slice		1 slice		
Cooked cereal	¼–½ cup		½ cup		The following may be substituted for 1 slice of bread: ½ cup spaghetti, macaroni, noodles, or rice; 5 saltines
Dry cereal	½–1 cup		1 cup		

* Adapted from Lowenberg M. E.: Development of food patterns in young children. *In* Pipes P: Nutrition in Infancy and Childhood, 4th ed. St Louis, CV Mosby, 1989.

† This is a guide to a basic diet. Fats, oils, sauces, desserts, and snack foods provide additional kilocalories to meet the needs of a growing child. Foods can be selected from this pattern for both meals and snacks.

‡ Do not give to children until they can chew well.

times a day (USDA, 1987). Their snacks should be chosen carefully so that they are dense in nutrients and are not limited to cookies, soda pop, and chips. Likewise, foods least likely to promote dental caries should be selected. Wholesome snacks enjoyed by many young children include fresh fruit, cheese, hard-boiled or deviled eggs, raw vegetable sticks, milk, fruit juices, whole-grain crackers, and peanut butter sandwiches.

Clinical experience suggests that fruit juices, especially apple juice, are an increasingly common beverage for young children, both at home and in group settings. These juices frequently replace water and milk in a child's diet. In addition to nutritional concerns, this practice may have other effects. One study of both healthy children and those with chronic nonspecific diarrhea found that ingestion of fruit juices often resulted in carbohydrate malabsorption (Hyams et al, 1988). Pear and apple juice were particularly implicated. This information suggests that these juices might be avoided when treating acute diarrhea with clear liquids. For children with chronic diarrhea, a trial of restricting fruit juices may be warranted before more costly diagnostic tests are done.

Other senses in addition to taste have an important part in food acceptance by young children. Extreme temperatures are generally avoided, and many children actually prefer their food lukewarm. Some foods may be rejected because of odor rather than taste. A sense of order in the food presentation is often required. Many children will not accept foods touching each other on the plate, and most casseroles and mixed dishes are not popular, except for spaghetti, macaroni and cheese, and pizza. It is not unusual for broken crackers to go uneaten or a sandwich to be refused because it is "cut the wrong way." Many young children are keenly sensitive to food palatability and can readily detect off-flavors or reject overcooked vegetables.

The physical setting of children's meals is as important as the emotional atmosphere. They should not be made to eat with feet dangling and arms reaching up to a table at chest height. Sturdy child-sized tables and chairs are ideal; if children eat at a standard table with the family, a high chair, "booster chair," or other modification should be used to make them comfortable. Bowls, plates, and cups should be nonbreakable and heavy enough to resist spilling. A shallow bowl is better than a plate for younger children to facilitate easier scooping. Thick, short-handled spoons and forks allow for an easier, less tiring grasp.

Young children usually do not eat well if they are tired, and this needs to be considered when meal and play times are scheduled. A quiet activity or rest immediately before eating is conducive to a relaxed, enjoyable meal. To stimulate a good appetite, however, children need active, large motor activity and time spent outside in the fresh air.

Group Feeding

A generation ago the food experiences of preschool children centered on home and family. Today, because of changing family lifestyles, many children spend part or most of their days in day care centers, preschools, and Head Start programs. At such places, they may consume only a snack or as much as two meals and two snacks per day, depending on the time involved. For many children, therefore, more than half of their nutrients may be provided in these settings.

Food service in group feeding settings such as day care centers and Head Start programs is regulated by federal or state guidelines, and some facilities may participate in USDA-sponsored food programs. The quality of meals and snacks can vary greatly; parents should investigate this aspect when selecting a placement for their child. In addition to providing the child with optimal nutrients, a program should offer food that is appealing and safely prepared and consider cultural and developmental patterns in planning menus.

Because of peer pressure, children usually eat well in a group setting (Fig. 12–4). These settings are also ideal environments for nutrition education programs, both at mealtimes and in various learning activities. Experiencing new foods, participating in simple food preparation, and planting a garden are all examples of activities that develop and enhance positive food habits and attitudes.

Feeding the School-Age Child

Growth during the school-age years (ages 6 to 12) is slow but steady, paralleled by a constant increase in food intake. In addition to being in school a greater part of the day, the child is also likely to begin participating in clubs and group activities, sports, and recreational programs. The influence of peers and significant adults, such as teachers, coaches, or sports idols, is greater. Friendships and other social contacts become more important. Except for severe cases, most behavioral problems connected with food have been resolved by this age, and the child enjoys eating to alleviate hunger and to obtain social satisfaction.

The school-age child may participate in the school lunch program or may carry a lunch from home. The School Lunch Program supported by the federal government provides approximately one third of the RDA for students. Children from low-income families are eligible for free or reduced-price meals. Some schools also offer a Special Milk Program or School Breakfast Program. These programs are discussed in Chapter 15.

Studies of lunches packed at home have indicated that they tend to provide fewer nutrients than the school lunch meal (Emmons et al, 1972). Favorite foods tend to be packed, and less variety is seen; limitations are set by choosing foods that travel well and do not need heating or refrigeration. Children who require diet modifications (e.g., low calorie, allergy, low sodium)

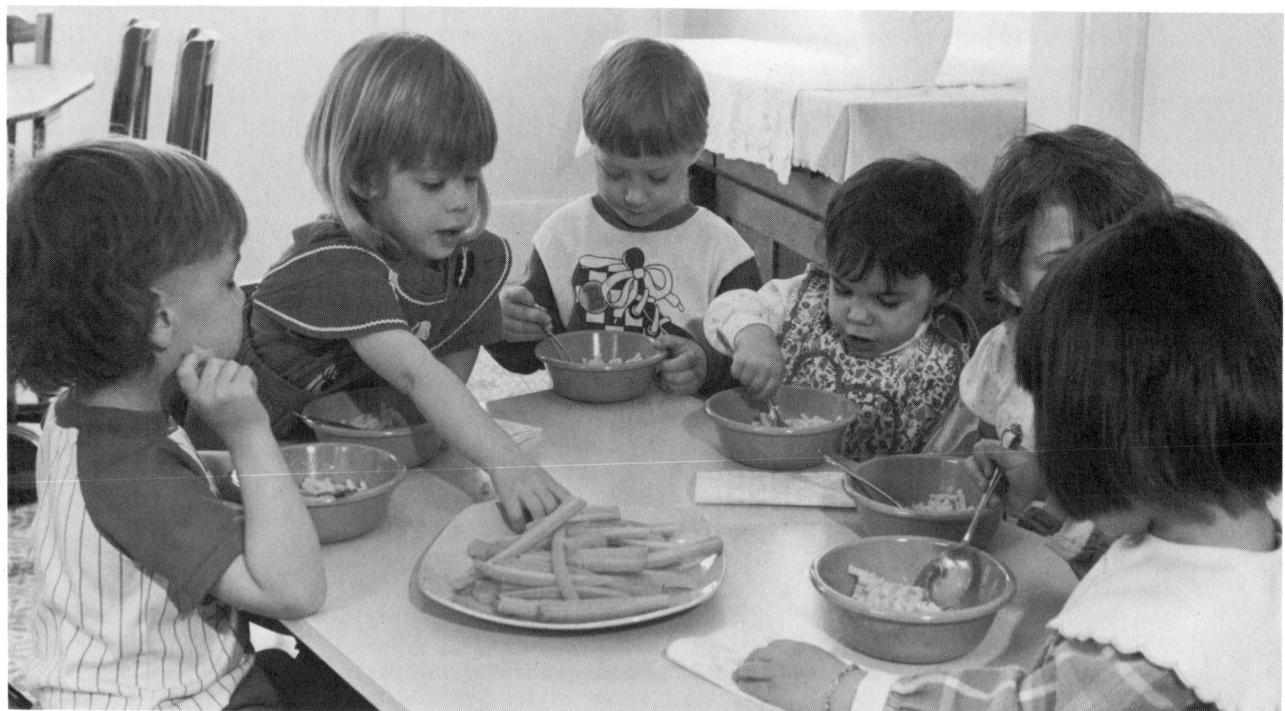

FIGURE 12–4. *Children who eat with each other in an appropriate environment often eat better than they do when alone.*

may need to bring their lunches. A typical well-balanced lunch would include a sandwich with whole-grain bread and a protein-rich filling (lean meat, egg, cheese, peanut butter), fresh fruit or vegetable, milk, and an optional cookie or other simple dessert.

Because of changes in family lifestyles, many school-age children are responsible for preparing their own breakfasts. It is not uncommon for children to skip this meal altogether, even in the primary grades. The School Breakfast Program can aid in some situations, but it is not uniformly available in all school districts. A review of nutrition and school performance suggests that children who go to school without breakfast are likely to be less attentive and more lethargic and irritable, but there is no strong documentation to support this association (Pollitt et al, 1978). A short fast may impose a greater stress on young children than on adults, because of the larger brain weight of children in proportion to glycogen storage area. The smaller musculature also limits the availability of amino acids for gluconeogenesis (Pollitt et al, 1981).

A study in a predominantly low-income school district compared academic achievement before and after introducing the School Breakfast Program. The children who received the school breakfast had significantly improved test scores and decreased tardiness compared with children who did not receive the breakfast (Meyers et al, 1989).

Snacks are commonly consumed by school-age children, primarily after school and in the evening (Fig. 12–5). Bakery products and soft drinks are the most frequently chosen snack foods (USDA, 1980). As a child grows older and has money to spend, he or she consumes more snacks from vending machines or neighborhood groceries (Fig. 12–6). Families can continue to offer wholesome snacks at home and support nutrition education efforts in the school (see Figs. 12–5 and 12–6). In most cases, good eating habits established in the first few years will carry a child through this period of decision-making and responsibility.

NUTRITIONAL CONCERNS

Obesity

The increasing prevalence of obesity in children is a significant public health problem. Comparison of skinfold data from national health surveys shows a 54% increase of obesity in 6- to 11-year-old children between the mid-1960s and the late 1970s (Gortmaker et al, 1987).

Obesity in childhood is usually not a benign condition, despite popular feelings that overweight children will "outgrow" their condition. The longer a child has been overweight, the more likely that state will continue into adolescence and adulthood; by 6 years of age and beyond the overweight status does not usually spontaneously disappear (Zack et al, 1979). Children who have their growth adiposity rebound before 5 ½ years of age are more likely to be fatter at adulthood than those who have their adiposity rebound after 7 years of age (Rolland-Cachera et al, 1987).

Determining obesity in growing children is difficult. Some excess fatness may occur at either end of this age spectrum; that is, the 1-year-old toddler and the prepubertal child may be heavier and fatter for developmental and physiologic reasons, but this is not often permanent. Height and weight alone do not allow for the highly muscled child. Triceps fatfold and body mass index (BMI) provide more valid measurements of body

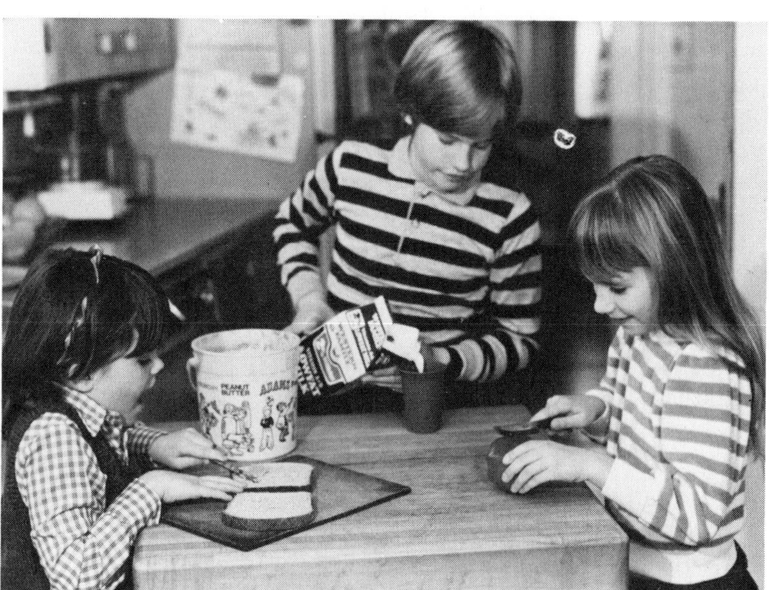

FIGURE 12–5. *These elementary school children enjoy preparing their own after-school snacks. With a selection of nutritious foods available, this independence can be encouraged.*

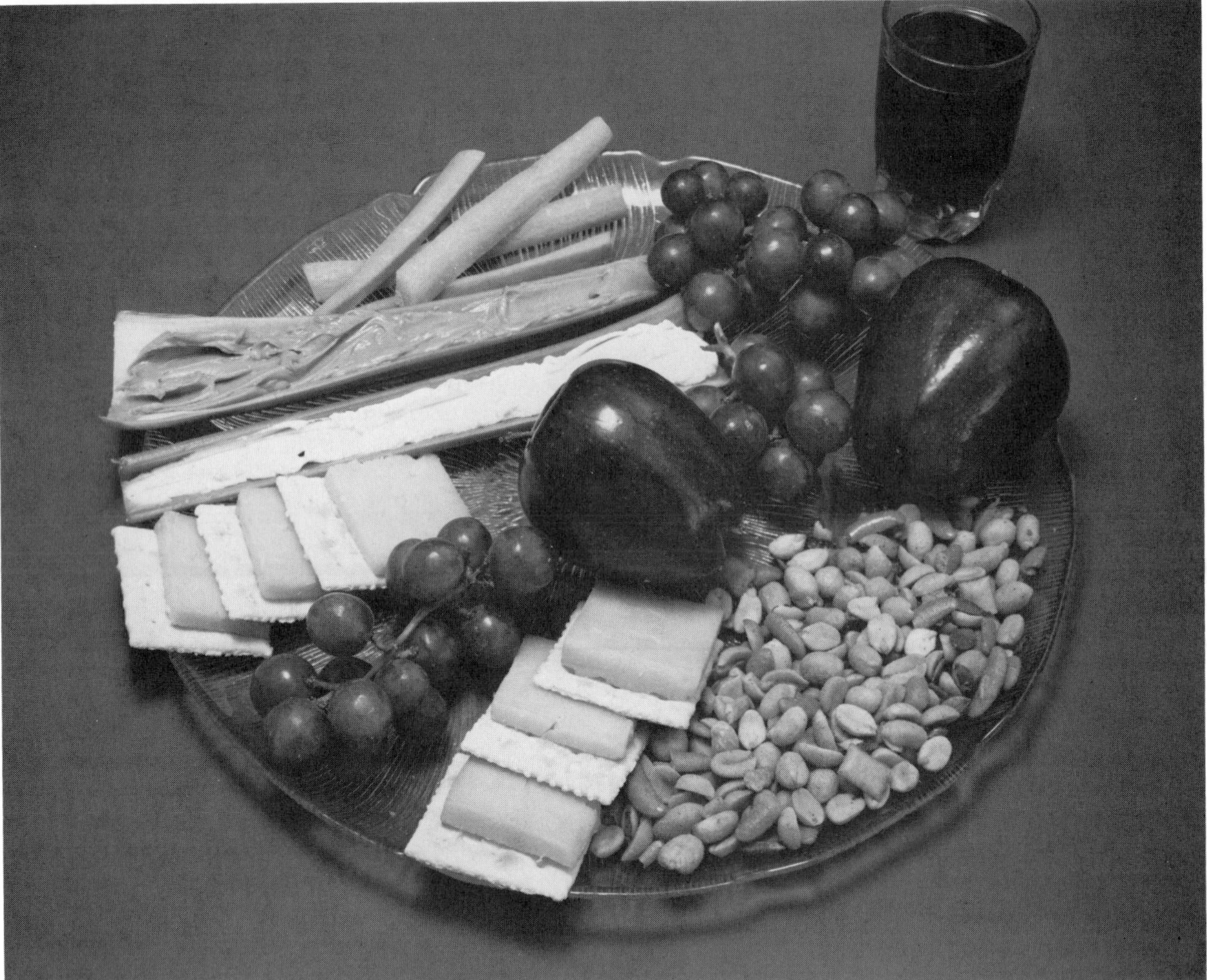

FIGURE 12–6. *A variety of nutritious snacks for school-age children.*

fat (Bandini and Dietz, 1987). Children at risk for obesity should be monitored more frequently so that early intervention can be provided. See Chapter 18 for more in-depth information about obesity.

Management of obesity in children should include nutrient needs for growth. Long-term success is most likely with a program that includes family involvement, dietary modifications, nutrition information, activity planning and behavioral components (Mahan, 1987). Depending on the child, goals for weight change may include a decrease in the rate of weight gain, a maintenance of weight, or, in severe cases, a slow weight loss (Clinical Insight, p. 333).

Underweight/Failure to Thrive

Weight loss or lack of weight gain can be caused by an acute or chronic illness, a restricted diet, a poor appetite, maternal deprivation, or a simple lack of food. Careful assessment is critical and must include the social and emotional environment as well as physical findings. If the child also has short stature, the possibility of zinc deficiency should be investigated.

Reports have documented growth failure in children as a result of contemporary lifestyle factors. Poor weight gain, short stature, and delayed puberty were seen in boys and girls 9 to 17 years of age who had deliberately restricted their energy intake in fear of becoming obese (Pugliese et al, 1983). In another report, toddlers were failing to thrive as a result of food restriction imposed by their parents' overconcern regarding obesity, atherosclerosis, or other potential health problems (Pugliese et al, 1987).

The provision of adequate energy and nutrients as well as nutrition education should be part of the management plan. Attempts should be made to increase appetite and to modify the environment to ensure an optimal intake.

Iron Deficiency

Iron deficiency is one of the most common nutrient disorders of childhood and is especially prevalent in 1- to 3-year-old children. Certain low-income populations have shown a higher incidence of iron deficiency anemia that is likely associated with factors such as parents' educational level and lack of medical care as well as dietary intake. In addition to growth and increased physiologic need for iron, dietary factors also have a role. A 1-year-old child may continue to consume a large quantity of milk to the exclusion of other foods, resulting in "milk anemia." Many young preschool children do not prefer meat, so that most of their iron is of the nonheme form that is absorbed at a lower level. Iron deficiency is less of a problem in older preschool and school-age children.

Infants with iron deficiency with and without anemia tend to score lower on standardized tests of mental development and have demonstrated a decreased attention to relevant information needed for problem-solving (Pollitt et al, 1986). However, there is not a similar association between iron deficiency and motor development. These data have clinical significance in terms of assessing the nutrient quality of individual diets, as well as policy-making in addressing the nutrition needs of low-income high-risk children.

Attention to good dietary sources of iron can help prevent iron deficiency anemia. To enhance absorbability of nonheme iron sources, education should be aimed at increasing dietary content of ascorbic acid and meat, fish, and poultry in the diet. See Chapter 32 for further discussion.

Dental Caries

Nutrition and eating habits are important factors in dental health and disease. Optimal nutrient intake is needed to produce strong teeth and healthy gums. The composition of the diet and eating habits (i.e., amount of dietary sucrose, retentiveness of foods, and frequency of eating) are significant factors in the development of dental caries. Infants and young children who drink sweetened liquids from a bottle at bedtime or frequently throughout the day are susceptible to baby bottle tooth decay, which is discussed in Chapter 23.

Because children tend to consume snacks regularly, emphasis should be placed on those that are least cariogenic. Desserts and sweet foods should be consumed less frequently and incorporated into meals to decrease cariogenicity. Parents can provide strong models for their children during this time by practicing both positive food habits and good dental hygiene. In addition, fluoride from the water or as a supplement will help to reduce the likelihood of caries.

Allergies

Food allergies usually manifest themselves in infancy and childhood and occur more frequently when there is a family history of allergies. Allergic responses most often include respiratory or gastrointestinal symptoms and skin reactions, but in some cases may be more vague, such as fatigue, lethargy, and behavior changes. Controversy exists with regard to a true definition of a food allergy, and tests for allergies to food are not specific and unequivocal. See Chapter 38 for further discussion of this topic.

Attention-Deficit Hyperactivity Disorder

Attention-deficit hyperactivity disorder (ADHD), commonly called "hyperactivity," is a clinical diagnosis based on specific criteria (i.e., excessive motor activity, impulsiveness, short attention span, low tolerance to frustration, and onset before 7 years of age). Because some dietary factors have been suggested as causes of this disorder, various dietary treatments have been promoted, such as the Feingold diet, omission of sugar, allergy elimination diets, and megavitamin therapy.

In 1973, Feingold proposed that many children were hyperactive because they were sensitive to salicylates and artificial colorings and flavorings in their food. His popular treatment was to remove those substances from the child's diet; later, the preservatives BHA and BHT were eliminated. Early reports were positive, but the studies were not controlled and the response was believed to be a placebo effect.

Studies using controlled double-blind dietary challenges and objective behavior rating scales have not supported the Feingold hypothesis (Lipton and Mayo, 1983; NIH . . . , 1982). Of the hyperactive children who seemed to respond most favorably to the diet (about 5 to 10%), most were preschoolers. One report of preschool hyperactive boys, using a total diet replacement design with crossover between experimental and control diets, suggested a more positive impact of the diet (Kaplan et al, 1989). In addition to the Feingold diet, specific foods that the family felt bothered their child were also eliminated. Almost 50% of the boys showed some improvement in behavior using accepted rating scales.

Conflicting study results could be explained in part by a placebo effect or by altered interaction between the family and the child with ADHD. For the family who wishes to try the diet, however, there is little nutritional risk. Regular nutrition counseling should be provided, and the families should be urged to consider other helpful treatments for their child's disorder, such as behavioral management, special education, and medication.

Although sugar has popularly been implicated as a cause of hyperactive behavior in children, controlled challenge studies have not demonstrated any negative behavioral effects (Ferguson et al, 1986; Wolraich et al, 1985). In one study, children were actually quieter and less active after consuming sugar than those receiving the placebo (Behar et al, 1984). Although there is little evidence to support a sugar-behavior effect, families can be reinforced for the positive benefits of decreasing sugar consumption, such as better dental health and more nutrient-dense diets.

Children who have allergies may exhibit some behaviors (irritability, poor attention) seen in children with ADHD, but it remains questionable whether elimination diets will alleviate these symptoms or alter negative behaviors. Likewise, the use of megavitamin therapy for ADHD has not been supported in controlled studies (Haslam et al, 1984).

NUTRITION EDUCATION

As children grow, they acquire knowledge and assimilate concepts by leaps and bounds. These years are ideal for providing nutrition information and promoting positive attitudes about all foods. This learning can be informal and natural, such as in the home, with parents as models and the provision of a diet from a wide variety of foods. Food can be used in daily experiences for the toddler and preschooler and can be combined with development of language, cognition, and self-help (i.e., labeling; describing size, shape, and color; sorting; assisting in preparation; and tasting).

Attempts to teach children nutrition concepts and information should take into account their developmental level. The concept of nutrients is abstract and is lost on preschoolers and on most primary school children. Some nutrition curricula are more sophisticated than children's ability to conceptualize, and modification may be necessary to make the educational experiences meaningful. Activities that concentrate on children's real-world relationship with food are more likely to yield positive results.

Because children of all ages benefit from a "hands-on" approach to learning, information about food and nutrition can be included in meals and snacks, food preparation, and activities that also focus on cognitive learning. Parental involvement in nutrition education projects can also produce more positive outcomes and carry-over into the home.

CITED REFERENCES

Abraham S et al: Dietary Intake Findings, United States, 1971–1974, DHEW Publication No. (HRA) 77-1647. Washington, DC, US Government Printing Office, 1977.

American Dietetic Association: Recommendations concerning supplement usage: ADA statement. J Am Diet Assoc 87:1342, 1987.

Ashworth A and Millward DJ: Catch-up growth in children. Nutr Rev 44:157, 1986.

Bandini LG and Dietz WH: Assessment of body fatness in childhood obesity: Evaluation of laboratory and anthropometric techniques. J Am Diet Assoc 87:1344, 1987.

Barr DGD, Shmerling DH, and Prader A: Catch-up growth in malnutrition, studied in celiac disease after institution of gluten-free diet. Pediatr Res 6:521, 1972.

Beal VA: Dietary intake of individuals followed through infancy and childhood. Am J Public Health 51:1107, 1961.

Beal VA: Nutritional intake. *In* McCammon RW (ed): Human Growth and Development. Springfield, IL, Charles C Thomas, 1970.

Behar D et al: Sugar challenge testing with children considered behaviorally "sugar reactive." Nutr Behav 1:277, 1984.

Bowering J and Clancy KL: Nutritional status of children and teenagers in relation to vitamin and mineral use. J Am Diet Assoc 86:1033, 1986.

Buzina R et al: Zinc nutrition and taste acuity in school children with impaired growth. Am J Clin Nutr 33:2262, 1980.

Centers for Disease Control: Ten-State Nutrition Survey, 1968–70, DHEW Publ. No. (HSM) 72:8130-34. Washington, DC, USHEW, HSMHA, 1972.

Committee on Nutrition, American Academy of Pediatrics: Vitamin and mineral supplementation needs in normal children in the United States. Pediatrics 66:1015, 1980.

Cotugna N: TV ads on Saturday morning children's programming—what's new? J Nutr Educ 20:125, 1988.

Council on Scientific Affairs, American Medical Association: Vitamin preparations as dietary supplements and as therapeutic agents. JAMA 257:1929, 1987.

Dietary Intake Source Data: United States, 1976–80, National Health Survey, Vital and Health Statistics Series 11, No. 231, DHHS Publ. No. (PHS) 83:1681, 1983.

Dietz WH and Gortmaker SL: Do we fatten our children at the TV set? Television viewing and obesity in children and adolescents. Pediatrics 75:807, 1985.

Ellis CE and Hill DE: Growth, intelligence and school performance in children with cystic fibrosis who have had an episode of malnutrition during infancy. J Pediatr 87:565, 1975.

Emmons L, Hayes M, and Call DL: A study of school feeding programs. II: Effects on children with different economic and nutritional needs. J Am Diet Assoc 61:268, 1972.

Farris RP et al: Macronutrient intakes of 10-year-old children. 1973–1982. J Am Diet Assoc 86:765, 1986.

Ferguson HB, Stoddart C, and Simeon JG: Double-blind challenge studies of behavioral and cognitive effects of sucrose-aspartame ingestion in normal children. Nutr Rev 44(Suppl):144, 1986.

Food and Nutrition Board, National Research Council, NAS: Recommended Dietary Allowances, 10th ed. Washington, DC, National Academy Press, 1989.

Gortmaker SL et al: Increasing pediatric obesity in the United States. Am J Dis Child 141:535, 1987.

Hambidge KM et al: Zinc nutrition of preschool children in the Denver Head Start Program. Am J Clin Nutr 29:734, 1976.

Haslam RHA, Dalby JT, and Rademaker AW: Effects of megavitamin therapy on children with attention deficit disorders. Pediatrics 74:103, 1984.

Hyams JS et al: Carbohydrate malabsorption following fruit juice ingestion in young children. Pediatrics 84:64, 1988.

Kaplan BJ et al: Dietary replacement in preschool-aged hyperactive boys. Pediatrics 83:7, 1989.

Lipton MA and Mayo JP: Diet and hyperkinesis—an update. J Am Diet Assoc 83:132, 1983.

Mahan LK: Family-focused behavioral approach to weight control in children. Pediatr Clin North Am 34:983, 1987.

Meyers AF et al: School breakfast program and school performance. Am J Dis Child 143:1234, 1989.

Nielsen Company: 1985 Nielsen Report on Television. Chicago, AC Nielsen, 1985.

NIH Consensus Development Conference: Defined diets and childhood hyperactivity, Vol 4, No 3. Washington, DC, The Institutes, 1982.

Owen G and Lippman G: Nutritional status of infants and young children: USA. Pediatr Clin North Am, 24:211, 1977.

Pollitt E et al: Iron deficiency and behavioral development in infants and preschool children. Am J Clin Nutr 43:555, 1986.

Pollitt E, Gersovitz M, and Gargiulo M: Educational benefits of the United States school feeding program: A critical review of the literature. Am J Public Health 68:477, 1978.

Pollitt E, Leibel RL, and Greenfield D: Brief fasting, stress, and cognition in children. Am J Clin Nutr 34:1526, 1981.

Pugliese MT et al: Fear of obesity: A cause of short stature and delayed puberty. N Engl J Med 309:513, 1983.

Pugliese MT et al: Parental health beliefs as a cause of non-organic failure to thrive. Pediatrics 80:175, 1987.

Rolland-Cachera M-F et al: Tracking the development of adiposity from one month of age to adulthood. Ann Hum Biol 14:219, 1987.

Satter EM: The feeding relationship. J Am Diet Assoc 86:352, 1986.

Similarity of children's and their parents' food preferences. Nutr Rev 45:134, 1987.

Stoch MB and Smythe PM: 15-year developmental study of effects of severe undernutrition on subsequent physical growth and intellectual functioning. Arch Dis Child 51:327, 1976.

Test scores improve with school breakfast. Community Nutrition Institute 18(18):2, 1988.

Trace elements. In Forbes G (ed): Pediatric Nutrition Handbook, 2nd ed. Elk Grove Village, IL, American Academy of Pediatrics, 1985.

USDA: Nationwide Food Consumption Survey, Continuing Survey of Food Intakes by Individuals: Women 19–50 years and children 1–5 years, 1 day, 1986, Report No. 86-1. Hyattsville, MD, Nutrition Monitoring Division, Human Nutrition Information Service, USDA, 1987.

USDA: Nationwide Food Consumption Survey, Spring, 1977: Food and Nutrient Intakes of Individuals in 1 day in the United States, Spring, 1977, Preliminary Report No. 2. Washington, DC, Science and Education Administration, 1980.

Wolraich M et al: Effects of sucrose ingestion on the behavior of hyperactive boys. J Pediatr 106:675, 1985.

Zack PM et al: A longitudinal study of body fatness in childhood and adolescence. J Pediatr 95:126, 1979.

ADDITIONAL REFERENCES

Birch LL et al: Mother-child interaction patterns and the degree of fatness in children. J Nutr Educ 13:17, 1981.

Committee on Nutrition, American Academy of Pediatrics: Prudent lifestyle for children: Dietary fat and cholesterol. Pediatrics 78:521, 1986.

Does zinc supplementation improve growth in children who fail to thrive? Nutr Rev 47:356, 1989.

Fomon SJ et al: Body composition of reference childen from birth to age 10 years. Am J Clin Nutr 35:1169, 1982.

Hertzler AA and Vaughan CE: The relationship of family structure and interaction to nutrition. J Am Diet Assoc 74:23, 1979.

Kneepkens CMF, Jakobs C, and Douwes AC: Apple juice, fructose, and chronic nonspecific diarrhoea. Eur J Pediatr 148:571, 1989.

Nutrition and the school-age child. Dairy Council Digest 59(2), 1988.

Rozin P and Vollmecke TA: Food likes and dislikes. Annu Rev Nutr 6:433, 1986.

Satter EM: Childhood eating disorders. J Am Diet Assoc 86:357, 1986.

Simeon DT and Grantham-McGregor S: Effects of missing breakfast on the cognitive functions of school children of differing nutritional status. Am J Clin Nutr 49:646, 1989.

Swanson-Rudd J et al: Nutrition orientations of working mothers in the North Central Region. J Nutr Educ 14:132, 1982.

CHAPTER 13

NUTRITION IN ADOLESCENCE

Jane Mitchell Rees, M.S., R.D.

CHAPTER OUTLINE

- Growth and Development
- Nutritional Requirements
- Food Habits
- Situations with Specialized Needs
- Strategies for Improving Nutritional Well-being

KEY TERMS

ADOLESCENCE—the period of life beginning with the appearance of secondary sex characteristics and ending with the cessation of somatic growth

BODY IMAGE—a mental self concept related to rate of growth and change in body proportions

EATING DISORDER—abnormal behaviors related to food and eating that may include starving, bingeing, vomiting, laxative abuse, or excessive exercise accompanied by bizarre ideas about food, unrealistic body image, and psychologic and developmental abnormalities

GROWTH SPURT—the 18- to 24-month period of adolescence when growth rate is the fastest

GYNECOLOGIC AGE—the number of years between the onset of menses and the date of conception in the pregnant adolescent

PEAK HEIGHT GAIN VELOCITY—the fastest rate of growth during the growth spurt

PUBERTY—the period during which the secondary sex characteristics begin to develop and the capability of sexual reproduction is attained

SEXUAL MATURITY RATING—a method of assessing the stage of sexual development; usually stated as Tanner's stages

TASKS OF ADOLESCENCE—the accomplishments expected in adolescence in order to achieve maturity in emotional and intellectual development

Adolescence is one of the most challenging periods in human development. Because of the extent of the physical and psychologic changes taking place, a number of important issues arise that influence the nutritional well-being of the teenager. A knowledge of the developmental process is a prerequisite to understanding the nutritional aspect of life in this period.

GROWTH AND DEVELOPMENT

Physiologic Changes

Puberty, the process of physically developing from a child to an adult, is initiated by poorly understood physiologic factors and includes maturation of the total body. Following a period of slow growth during late childhood, the change in adolescence is as rapid as that of early childhood. Figure 13–1 shows that the rate of linear growth during the teenage years compares with that for the second year of life. The child gains about 20% of adult height and 50% of weight during this period.

This growth continues throughout the approximately 5 to 7 years of pubertal development. A great percentage of this height will be gained during the 18- to 24-month period of the "growth spurt." Peak height gain velocity occurs at different ages for different individuals, as will the initiation of puberty. In general, it occurs earlier in life for girls than for boys. Factors known about the timing and milestones of pubertal development are summarized in Figure 13–2. Although growth slows following the achievement of sexual maturity, linear growth and weight acquisition continue (rarely into the late teens for females and early twenties for males). Most females gain no more than 2 to 3 inches following the onset of menses.

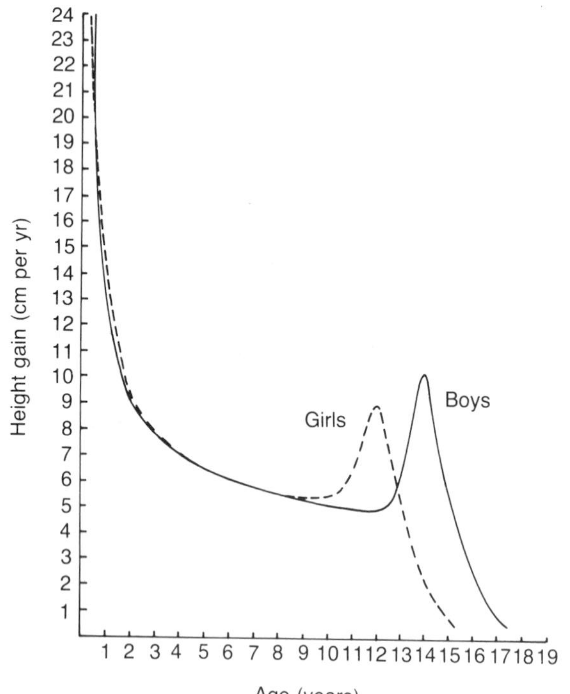

FIGURE 13–1. *Typical individual velocity curves for supine length or height in boys and girls. The curves represent the velocity of growth of the typical boy and girl at any given age. (From Tanner, JM: Foetus into Man. Cambridge, MA, Harvard University Press, 1978. Reprinted by permission.)*

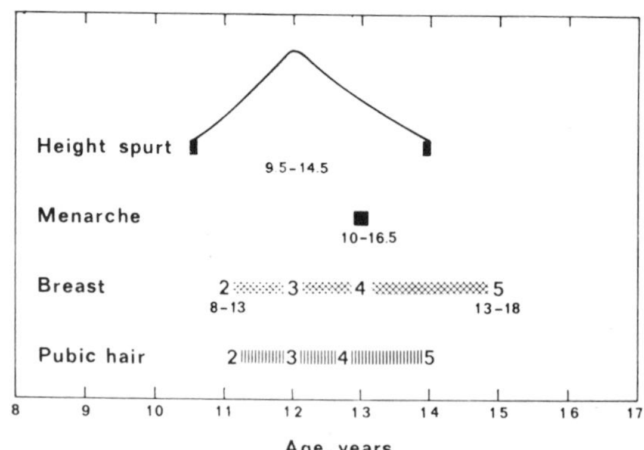

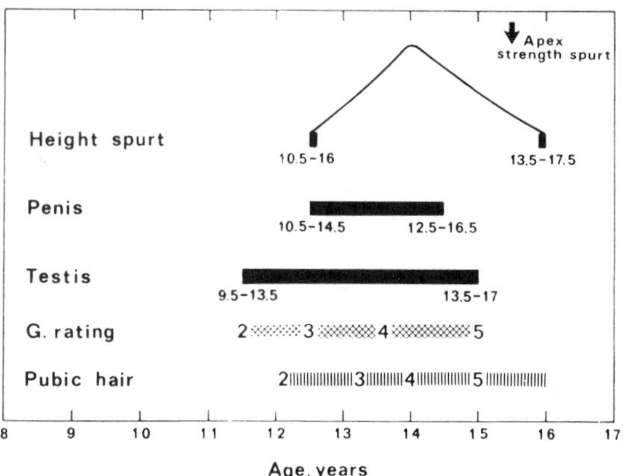

FIGURE 13–2. *Diagram of sequence of events at puberty in girls* (above) *and boys* (below). *(From Marshall WA and Tanner JM: Variations in the pattern of pubertal changes in boys. Arch Dis Child 45:13, 1970.)*

In the process of total body maturation, the composition of the body changes. In the prepubertal period the proportion of fat and muscle in males and females tends to be similar, with body fat about 15% and 19%, respectively. Females gain more fat during puberty, and in adulthood they carry about 22% of body fat compared with around 15% in males. During this time, males gain twice as much lean tissue as do females.

Assessment of Growth

Weight and height can be plotted on similar grids to determine whether an individual is keeping pace with peers or is exceeding them in total weight in a particular year. The relationship between weight and height can be evaluated by using the detailed tables of the Health and Nutrition Examination Survey (Appendix Tables 9, 10, 13, 14). For each 5-cm increment of height at a particular year of age, a range of weights is given (5th to 95th percentiles). Appropriate weights for height for

TABLE 13–1. Ratings of Sexual Maturation*

	Pubic Hair	Genitalia
Boys		
Stage 1	None present	Prepubertal
Stage 2	Small amount at outer edges of pubis, slight darkening	Beginning penile enlargement Testes enlarged to 5 ml vol Scrotum reddened and changed in texture
Stage 3	Covers pubis	Penis longer; testes to 8–10 ml Scrotum further enlarged
Stage 4	Adult type, does not extend to the thighs	Penis wider and longer Testes 12 ml; scrotal skin darker
Stage 5	Adult type, now spreads to the thighs	Adult penis, testes 15 ml
Girls		
Stage 1	None	No change from childhood
Stage 2	Small amount, downy on medial labia	Breast bud
Stage 3	Increased, darker, and curly	Larger but no separation of the nipple and the areola
Stage 4	More abundant, coarse texture	Increased size Areola and nipple form secondary mound
Stage 5	Adult, spreads to medial thighs	Adult distribution of breast tissue, continuous outline

* Adapted from Tanner JM: Growth at Adolescence, 2nd ed. Oxford, Blackwell Scientific Publications, 1962.

age and sex lie between the 25th and 75th percentiles, a range that allows for individual differences in body build (Mahan and Rosebrough, 1984). A skinfold evaluation yields a further degree of precision. For example, a low skinfold measurement in an individual above the 75th percentile weight for height indicates a state of being overweight but not overfat. An assessment of muscle and arm circumference confirms the muscular composition. However, a skinfold at the 90th percentile or greater suggests obesity. Measurement of skinfolds is further discussed in Chapter 17.

Sexual Maturity Rating

Pubertal development can be monitored by means of weight and height tables and sexual maturity ratings as described in Table 13–1. Knowledge of the relationship between these milestones and physical growth enable the clinician to assess the progress of growth in an adolescent at a particular time and give some indication of the extent of future growth.

Excessive or less-than-normal growth can be detected by plotting height changes on the grids in Appendices 9 and 13. The major cause of short stature during adolescence is genetically late initiation of puberty, although conditions such as chronic disease and skeletal and chromosomal abnormalities also account for certain children being shorter than normal. Hormonal imbalances leading to abnormal growth are rare.

Psychologic Changes

Adolescence is a period of maturation for both mind and body. Along with the physical growth of puberty, emotional and intellectual development are rapid. Gaining the ability to use abstract thinking as opposed to the concrete thought patterns of childhood enables accomplishment of the "tasks of adolescence" (Table 13–2). Many of these tasks relate to nutritional well-being.

TABLE 13–2. Developmental Tasks in Adolescence*

Developmental Task (Havighurst, Thornburg)
1. Forming more mature relationships with peers of both sexes
2. Establishing a male or female social role
3. Accepting one's physique and using one's body effectively
4. Becoming emancipated from parents and other adults
5. Preparing for marriage and family life
6. Choosing a vocation and preparing for that career
7. Developing standards and value systems as a guide to behavior
8. Developing social intelligence and a commitment to responsible citizenship
9. Developing conceptual and problem-solving, decision-making skills

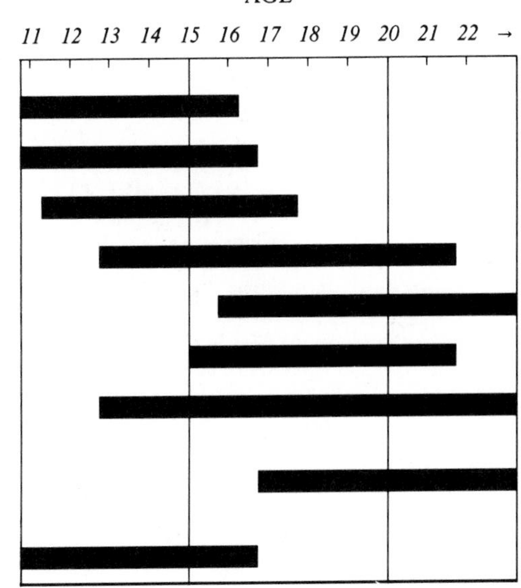

*Adapted from Mahan LK and Rees JM: Nutrition in Adolescence. St Louis, CV Mosby, 1984 and from Thornburg H: Contemporary Adolescence: Readings, 2nd ed. Monterey, CA, Brooks/Cole, 1975, p 7.

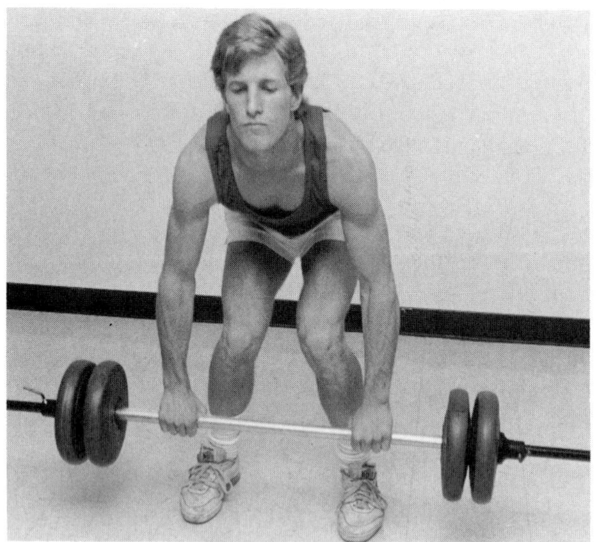

FIGURE 13–3. *Weightlifting to increase his muscular strength and endurance is a part of this older adolescent's daily routine.*

The emotional turmoil of this stage commonly affects adolescents' eating habits. For example, the drive toward independence often results in temporary rejection of the family dietary patterns.

Body Image

Developing an image of the physical self that includes an adult body is an intellectual and emotional task that is intertwined with nutritional issues. Adolescents often feel uncomfortable with their rapidly changing bodies, yet at the same time they want to be like their most perfect peers and the idols of their culture (Clinical Insight, p. 237; Fig. 13–3). Their sense of worth may be derived from feelings about their own physical attributes, a trait that causes them to be vulnerable to severe distortions if an eating disorder develops.

Desires to change rate of growth or body proportions can lead adolescents to dietary manipulations that may have negative consequences and are subject to exploitation by commercial interests. Rapid additions of weight accompanying development of secondary sexual characteristics cause many young women to unnecessarily restrict the amount of food they eat. Young men are tempted to use nutritional supplements, hoping to achieve the muscular appearance of adults.

NUTRITIONAL REQUIREMENTS

Recommendations for fulfilling the nutritional needs of adolescents arise from a small research base. Often the amounts recommended are interpolated from studies in adults or children. Part of the difficulty lies in the fact that studies of requirements must consider not only age but also stage of physical maturity. The recommended daily allowances (RDA) are therefore stated for three age groups as shown in Table 16–1. Nutrient recommendations are at levels appropriate for those growing at the most rapid rate.

Recommendations to Support Growth

Recommendations can be made more specific for individuals by dividing the recommended quantity (RDA) of a nutrient by the number of centimeters of the RDA reference individual's height. This provides an amount of nutrient per centimeter to apply to any size teenager. For example, the RDA for protein for the 11- to 14-year-old male is 45 g/day. Height of the reference adolescent is 157 cm. Thus, the recommended amount of protein would be 0.29 g/cm (Table 13–3).

Energy

The recommended range of energy intake for adolescence as shown in Table 13–3 reflects the differential needs of teenagers. Growth rate as well as level of exercise needs to be considered in determining the needs of the individual (Fig. 13–4).

TABLE 13–3. Recommended Energy and Protein Allowances*

	Height		Weight					Protein	
Age (Years)	*In.*	*Cm*	*lb*	*kg*	Kcal/day	Kcal/kg	Kcal/cm	g/day	g/cm
Females									
11–14	62	157	101	46	2,200	47	14.0	46	0.29
15–18	64	163	120	55	2,200	40	13.5	44	0.26
19–24	65	164	128	58	2,200	38	13.4	46	0.28
Males									
11–14	62	157	99	45	2,500	55	16.0	45	0.28
15–18	69	176	145	66	3,000	45	17.0	59	0.33
19–24	70	177	160	72	2,900	40	16.4	58	0.33

* Reprinted with permission from *Recommended Dietary Allowances*, 10th ed., c. 1989 by the National Academy of Sciences. Published by National Academy Press, Washington, DC.

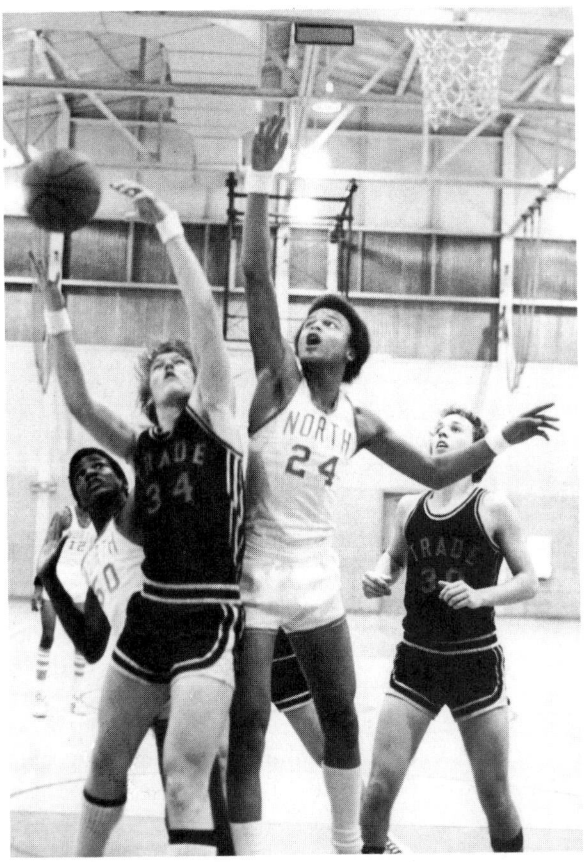

FIGURE 13–4. *Energy needs of adolescents vary according to individual growth rates. (From Marlow DR and Redding BA: Textbook of Pediatric Nursing, 6th ed, 1988.)*

Protein

Adolescent requirements for protein have been studied less than those of other age groups. Current recommendations specify that protein intake should make up to 7 to 8% of the total energy consumed. Sex, age, nutritional status, and protein quality must all be considered. The range of total protein will be from 45 to 72 grams.

Protein consumption should not be overly emphasized; sufficient protein is usually obtained in the normal diet. In situations such as chronic illness attended by nutritional depletion, protein stores should be monitored carefully and supported so that physical development will not be impaired. Assessment of protein nutriture is discussed further in Chapter 17.

Minerals

Adolescents incorporate twice the amount of calcium, iron, zinc, and magnesium into their bodies during the years of the growth spurt compared with other years.

The requirement for *calcium* in adolescence is based on needs for skeletal growth, 45% of which occurs during this period. Recommendations are therefore higher for males than for females. Both males and females have high requirements for *iron*. In males, the build-up of muscle mass is accompanied by greater blood volume, and in females iron is lost monthly with the onset of menses.

Zinc is known to be essential for growth; retention of

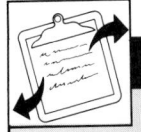

CLINICAL INSIGHT: Body Image of Adolescents

Regardless of how they look to others, adolescents are seldom satisfied with their appearance. As might be expected, girls often view their weight and body shape with disfavor, but boys also conceive enviable masculine physiques that often do not coincide with their own. This disparity between the perceived and the desired often leads to inappropriate eating behavior.

One study of approximately 1,700 adolescents and young adults aged 12 to 23 years, divided equally between the sexes, compared individual attitudes about their appearance with standards of weight appropriate for their age (Moore, 1988 and 1990). The results underscored the fairly obvious fact that many girls in this age group would like to weigh less, whereas boys are more likely to prefer weighing more. More than half of the girls who were actually of normal weight considered themselves overweight, whereas 60% of the underweight girls were satisfied with their weight. In the masculine group of normal weight, 31% were dissatisfied with their weight, of whom two thirds considered themselves to be underweight.

The attitudes of young people in each group who were actually overweight clearly reflected the disparate attitudes of society toward overweight in men and women. Although the number of overweight subjects of each sex was the same (40%), 63% of the girls who were dissatisfied with their weight thought they were overweight, whereas only 22% of the boys considered that they were overweight.

Dissatisfaction with body shape was expressed by 54% of the girls and by 33% of the boys. Girls were concerned primarily with thighs and hips, whereas boys were concerned with measurements of chest, arms, and abdomen.

Both groups reported deliberately altering eating behavior, with a higher incidence among girls than boys in such practices as attempts to lose weight (38% versus 11%), fasting for 24 hours (31% versus 12%), binge eating (30% versus 24%), and self-induced vomiting (8.5% versus 2%). Both girls (31%) and boys (11%) expressed concerns about problems with eating, usually associated with attempts at weight control.

zinc increases significantly during the growth spurt, leading to more efficient use of dietary sources (Thompson et al, 1986).

Although the role of other minerals in the nutriture of adolescents has not been studied well, the importance of *magnesium, iodine, phosphorus, copper, chromium, cobalt,* and *fluoride* is well recognized. The possibility of interactions among these nutrients cannot be overlooked. Recommendations for safe levels listed in Table 16–2 are made on the basis of the best data presently available.

Vitamins

Thiamin, riboflavin, and niacin are recommended in large amounts to meet high energy requirements. In most cases, the increased food intake demanded by higher energy needs will be accompanied by increased and adequate levels of B vitamins. Vitamin D is especially needed for rapid skeletal growth. Recommended amounts of vitamins A, E, C, folic acid, and vitamin B_6 are the same as for adults. All of these vitamins can be supplied by a well-chosen diet without the necessity of vitamin supplements.

Potential Nutritional Inadequacies

Surveys of nutrient intake have shown that adolescents are likely to obtain less vitamin A, vitamin B_6, riboflavin, iron, calcium, and zinc than recommended (Centers for Disease Control, 1973; Driskell et al, 1987; National Center for Health Statistics, 1977 and 1983). Young women are also likely to obtain less magnesium, copper, and manganese than recommended (Pennington et al, 1986).

FOOD HABITS

The growing independence, increased participation in social life, and generally busy schedules of adolescents influence their eating habits. They often eat rapidly and away from the home. They are beginning to buy and prepare more food for themselves. In fact, some advertising for prepared foods to be cooked at home is being targeted to teenagers.

Meal patterns of adolescents are often chaotic (Story, 1984). Teenagers miss more meals at home as they get older, often skipping breakfast and lunch altogether. Females tend to miss more meals than males.

Although concern has been expressed about the habit of snacking, teenagers may obtain substantial nourishment from foods eaten outside traditional meals (Fig. 13–5). Thus, the choice of foods is of more importance than the time or place of eating (Bigler-Doughten and Jenkins, 1987; McCoy et al, 1986). Emphasis should be placed on fresh vegetables and fruit and whole-grain products to complement the foods high in energy value and protein that they commonly choose.

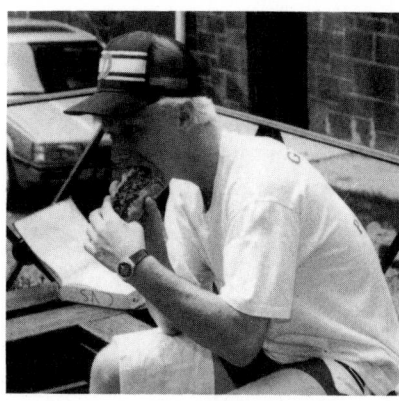

FIGURE 13–5. *The choice of foods is more important than the time or place of eating for teenagers who obtain nourishment outside traditional meals. (From Marlow DR and Redding BA: Textbook of Pediatric Nursing, 6th ed, 1988. Courtesy of F. Taylor Barnett.)*

During the time of peak growth velocity, adolescents usually need to eat often and in large amounts. They are able to use foods with a high concentration of energy; however, they need to be more careful of amounts and frequency when growth has slowed. Habits of overeating adopted during adolescence may ultimately contribute to a number of debilitating diseases.

Use of tobacco, alcohol, marijuana, and other drugs is a major public health problem. The effect of these chemicals on nutritional status depends on the amount and length of use as well as on the general state of health of the individual. Indications are that although adolescent alcohol and drug abusers are consuming adequate quantities of principal nutrients and have not developed nutrient deficiencies (Farrow et al, 1987; Story and Van Zyl York, 1987), they are obtaining nutrients from a narrower range of foods than nonabusers.

SITUATIONS WITH SPECIALIZED NEEDS

Pregnancy

Recommended weight gains during pregnancy may be slightly higher for the teenager than for the adult. One recommendation is that the adolescent should be advised to gain in the upper part of the range currently recommended for adults — 25 to 35 lb.

Pregnant adolescent women who are of young gynecologic age or are undernourished at the time of conception have the greatest nutritional needs (Rosso and Lederman, 1982). (The number of years between the onset of menses and the date of conception constitutes the gynecologic age.) A young woman who conceives soon after having her first menstrual period suffers greater risk on physiologic grounds (Zlatnick and Burmeister, 1977). Those who are more sexually mature appear to have no more physically based complications than adult women, but they are as vulnerable to psychologic stresses as adolescents of younger gynecologic age.

The assumption that pregnant adolescents need a supply of nutrients to support their own growth along with the growing fetus has been questioned. The growth that normally slows after menses may be interrupted even further by the high hormone levels that occur during pregnancy. However, preliminary studies indicate that height increases most in those of lowest gynecologic age (Scholl et al, 1988). It would appear that this group would need nutrients to support their own growth in addition to those required by pregnancy.

A clinically practical method of assuring adequacy is to encourage the pregnant adolescent to gain the recommended amount of weight by consuming nutrient-rich foods. Most important, contact with health professionals during prenatal care provides the opportunity to teach adolescents about feeding themselves and their families (Rees et al, 1989). Because of the economic instability of the pregnant adolescent, it is impossible to assume that she will have an adequate food supply, and health professionals can help with resources. Table 9–2 lists the recommended amounts of nutrients during pregnancy. Except for energy, they are the same as those for adult pregnant women.

Eating Disorders

A variety of eating disorders result in a spectrum of body shapes in the adolescent, ranging from extremely thin to extremely obese. The underlying psychologic characteristics are similar across the spectrum. This subject is discussed in more detail in Chapter 18.

Anorexia Nervosa

The adolescent with *anorexia nervosa* who has not developed a sense of self often has a distorted body image that leads to choosing lower and lower goal weights. Energy intake is reduced and output increased by excessive exercise and, at times, by self-initiated vomiting or by use of laxatives or diuretics. Eventually, the psychologic and developmental disturbances bring about a state in which the anorectic is incapable of self-care.

Bulimia Nervosa

Bulimia nervosa, a condition seen more often in older adolescents, does not usually lead to the seriously depleted nutritional state seen in anorexia nervosa. Bulimics generally maintain close to normal weight, periodically going on binges and vomiting. They tend to have unrealistic ideas about food and what is needed to sustain their bodies. However, their distortion of body size is usually less than is seen in anorexia nervosa.

Many teenagers who do not have the psychologic characteristics of the true bulimic improperly use casual vomiting as a means of weight control. It is a serious disorder when the habits become obsessional and interfere with normal education or employment.

Obesity

The obese teenager may have gained weight through a combination of psychologic, physiologic, and cultural factors as discussed in Chapter 18. It appears that the longer teenagers have been obese for any reason, the greater the chance that their bodies will be subject to processes that tend to maintain the obese state. By adolescence, they often have adopted the restricted lifestyle characteristic of the obese. Commonly they will not want to be seen in settings requiring vigorous exercise and will be subject to real or imagined social rejection.

Teenagers are vulnerable to unrealistic attitudes about the amount of time and effort necessary for effective weight management. Diet fads, drugs, and equipment appear to them to provide the quick remedy they seek. Meanwhile, realistic educational and comprehensive therapeutic programs are scarce. Thus, the obese teenager is very likely to be obese throughout life.

Education about weight control can be designed effectively for a wide range of audiences in a variety of settings, including youth programs and organizations. To be successful, therapeutic programs must include individualized dietary, fitness, and psychologically supportive components involving families as well as individuals (Mahan, 1987; Mellin et al, 1987).

Behavioral Problems and Delinquency

Nutritional status has been one of the environmental factors suspected of causing serious behavioral problems among adolescents. The popular press has given widespread attention to untested theories about the effect of nutrition on behaviors, ranging from shortened attention span to learning disorders and criminal behavior. Theories include an abundance of sugar, intoxication with heavy metals, food additives, and allergic reactions.

Knowledge that certain dietary factors will alter brain function or behavior can be therapeutically applied only in a very limited number of rare neurologic disorders. Theories that subclinical deficiencies of certain nutrients, primarily iron and the B vitamins, influence neurologic function have not led to clinically applicable intervention strategies.

There is a danger that educators and those responsible for juvenile detention facilities will expend public resources on ineffective programs based on untested theories. To demonstrate reasonable concern about nutrition, all institutions should support the teenagers they serve by making nourishing foods available. Such a policy will involve screening out less valuable foods that are tempting and commercially rewarding, such as those often sold in vending machines. Resulting improvements in nutritional health will contribute to the individual's physical well-being but at this time cannot be expected to prevent criminal behavior, attention disorders, or other behavioral problems.

Acne

Dermatologic complaints account for as many as 50% of adolescent contacts with health professionals. Acne is a normal characteristic of development that occurs in varying degrees of severity. It is initiated by the influence of testosterone on the sebaceous gland and is mediated by other factors, such as stress, stage of menstrual cycle, and make-up of the affected tissues in the individual. Dietary factors have traditionally been blamed, but carefully controlled studies have shown no correlation between the ingestion of foods and the appearance or degree of acne. Teenagers should be supported in their efforts to deal with this problem by discussion of the physiologic basis for its development and control.

Effective medications include antibiotics given orally, topical applications of benzoyl peroxide and tretinoin, and oral synthetic retinoid 13-*cis*-retinoic acid (Accutane), a vitamin A derivative. Although very effective in treating acne, 13-*cis*-retinoic acid (tretinoin) can cause an increase in serum triglycerides and total cholesterol that is reversed after medication is discontinued. Adolescents taking Accutane should have their lipid levels checked before and during treatment and appropriate diet therapy started if necessary (see Chapter 20). Women should also avoid unprotected sexual activity, because tretinoin is a teratogen and mutagen.

The role of zinc in the development and treatment of acne is confusing. If a role does exist, it may be related to the free fatty acid production of the pilosebaceous follicle (Downing et al, 1986; Rebello et al, 1986). One study found low levels of serum zinc in those suffering most from acne, suggesting that zinc deficiency exacerbates the condition (Michaelson et al, 1977).

STRATEGIES FOR IMPROVING NUTRITIONAL WELL-BEING

Assessment of Nutritional Status

Assessment of nutritional status in adolescents follows normal procedures with some exceptions. It is important to use an age-specific data base for each aspect of nutritional assessment. Standards based on stage of maturity are even more exact and should be used if available.

Nutritional assessment also includes an evaluation of the nutritional environment, including parental, peer, school, cultural, and personal lifestyle factors (Mahan and Rosebrough, 1984). The attitude of the adolescent toward food and nutrition is also a primary component of a comprehensive evaluation.

Prerequisites for Change

Especially because of their growing independence, any attempt to help adolescents improve their nutritional status will require careful planning. Before a plan can succeed, the adolescent will have to be in favor of making change. Encouraging the desire to change usually requires a great amount of attention on the part of the nutrition counselor.

Knowledge, attitude, and behavior must be addressed when guiding adolescents in the acquisition of healthful food habits. Providing knowledge or teaching can be done in a variety of settings from the classroom to a hospital bedside. A clinician needs to understand the change process and how to communicate that process in a meaningful way. Parents must be included in the process and helped to be supportive but not intrusive (Rees, 1984).

CITED REFERENCES

Bigler-Doughten S and Jenkins MR: Adolescent snacks: Nutrient density and nutritional contribution to total intake. J Am Diet Assoc 87:1678, 1987.

Centers for Disease Control: US Department of Health, Education and Welfare: Ten state nutrition survey, 1968–1970. Publ. No. (HSM) 73-8133. Atlanta, Health Services and Mental Health Administration, Centers for Disease Control, 1973.

Downing DT et al: Essential fatty acids and acne. J Am Acad Dermatol 14:221, 1986.

Driskell JA, Clark AJ, and Moak SW: Longitudinal assessment of vitamin B_6 status in Southern adolescent girls. J Am Diet Assoc 87:307, 1987.

Farrow JA, Rees JM, and Worthington-Roberts BS: Health, developmental, and nutritional status of adolescent alcohol and marijuana abusers. Pediatrics 79:218, 1987.

Mahan LK: Family-focused behavioral approach to weight control in children. Pediatr Clin North Am 34:983, 1987.

Mahan LK and Rosebrough RH: Nutritional requirements and nutritional status assessment in adolescence. *In* Mahan LK and Rees JM: Nutrition in Adolescence. St Louis, Times/Mirror Mosby, 1984.

McCoy H et al: Snacking patterns and nutrient density of snacks consumed by southern girls. J Nutr Educ 18:61, 1986.

Mellin LM, Slinkard LA, and Irwin CE: Adolescent obesity intervention: Validation of the SHAPEDOWN program. J Am Diet Assoc 87:333, 1987.

Michaelson G, Juhlin L, and Vahlquist A: Effects of oral zinc and vitamin A in acne. Arch Dermatol 113:31, 1977.

Moore DC: Body image and eating behavior in adolescent boys. Am J Dis Child 144:475, 1990.

Moore DC: Body image and eating behavior in adolescent girls. Am J Dis Child 142:144, 1988.

National Center for Health Statistics: Health and Nutrition Examination Survey, 1971–74. Vital and Health Statistics, Series 11, No. 202. Rockville, MD, Health Resources Administration, Public Health Service, 1977.

National Center for Health Statistics: Health and Nutrition Examination Survey, 1976–80. Vital and Health Statistics, Series 11, No. 231. Rockville, MD, Health Resources Administration, Public Health Service, 1983.

Pennington JAT et al: Mineral content of foods and total diets: The selected minerals in foods survey, 1982–1984. J Am Diet Assoc 86:876, 1986.

Rebello T, Atherton DJ, and Holden C: The effect of oral zinc administration on sebum free fatty acids in acne vulgaris. Acta Dermatol Venereol (Stockh) 66:305, 1986.

Rees JM: Nutritional counseling for adolescents. *In* Mahan LK and Rees JM: Nutrition in Adolescence. St Louis MO, Times/Mirror Mosby, 1984.

Rees JM, Worthington-Roberts BS, and Dixon-Doctor A: Establishing a nutritional environment supportive of reproduction: Nutrition education issues. *In* Worthington-Roberts BS, Vermeersch J, and Williams SR: Nutrition in Pregnancy and Lactation. St Louis, Times/Mirror Mosby, 1989.

Rosso P and Lederman SA: Nutrition in the pregnant adolescent. *In* Winick M (ed): Adolescent Nutrition. New York, John Wiley, 1982.

Scholl TO et al: Growth during early teenage pregnancies (Letter). Lancet 1:701, 1988.

Story M: Adolescent lifestyle and eating behavior. *In* Mahan LK and Rees JM: Adolescent Nutrition. St Louis, MO, Times/Mirror Mosby, 1984.

Story M and Van Zyl York P: Nutritional status of native American adolescent substance abusers. J Am Diet Assoc 87:1680, 1987.

Thompson P et al: Zinc status and sexual development in adolescent girls. J Am Diet Assoc 86:892, 1986.

Zlatnick FJ and Burmeister LF: Low "gynecologic age"—an obstetric risk factor. Am J Obstet Gynecol 128:183, 1977.

ADDITIONAL REFERENCES

Adams LB and Shafer M-A: Early manifestations of eating disorders in adolescents: Defining those at risk. J Nutr Educ 20:307, 1988.

Frisancho AR et al: Developmental and nutritional determinants of pregnancy outcome among teenagers. Am J Phys Anthro 66:247, 1985.

Frisch RE: Fatness of girls from menarche to age 18 years, with a nomogram. Hum Biol 48:353, 1976.

Gong E and Heald FT: Diet, nutrition and adolescence. *In* Shils ME and Young VR (eds): Modern Nutrition in Health and Disease, 7th ed. Philadelphia, Lea & Febiger, 1988.

Gong EJ and Spear BA: Adolescent growth and development: Implications for nutritional needs. J Nutr Educ 20:273, 1988.

Jacobson MF: Hey teens! This ad's for you. Nutr Action 16(7):8, 1989.

McKigney J and Munro H: Nutrient Requirements in Adolescence. Cambridge, MA, MIT Press, 1976.

Meserole LP et al: Prenatal weight gain and postpartum weight loss pattern in adolescents. J Adolesc Hlth Care 5:21, 1984.

Morgan KJ, Zabik ME, and Stampley GL: Breakfast consumption patterns of US children and adolescents. Nutr Res 6:635, 1986.

Newman B and Newman P: Adolescent Development. Columbus, OH, Merrill Press, 1986.

Position of the American Dietetic Association: Nutrition management of adolescent pregnancy. J Am Diet Assoc 89:104, 1989.

Results from the National Adolescent Student Health Survey. JAMA 261:2025, 1989.

Story M and Resnick MD: Adolescents' views on food and nutrition. J Nutr Educ 18:188, 1986.

Tanner JM: Foetus into Man: Physical Growth from Conception to Maturity. Cambridge, MA, Harvard University Press, 1978.

Thompson P et al: Zinc status and sexual development in adolescent girls. J Am Diet Assoc 86:892, 1986.

Wright LS: Physiological development in adolescence. *In* Mahan LK and Rees JM: Nutrition in Adolescence. St Louis, MO, Times/Mirror Mosby, 1984.

CHAPTER 14

NUTRITION IN AGING

Mary Podrabsky, R.D.

CHAPTER OUTLINE

KEY TERMS

ACHLORHYDRIA—absence of hydrochloric acid in gastric juice
CELLULAR THEORY—a theory that relates aging to the creation of cross-linkages between macromolecules
EDENTULOUS—without natural teeth
ERROR THEORY—a theory that relates aging to environmental damage to the DNA template, leading to errors in the genetic program
FREE-RADICAL THEORY—a theory that relates aging to cellular damage caused by free radicals
HYPOCHLORHYDRIA—deficiency of hydrochloric acid in the gastric juice
LIFE EXPECTANCY—the mean length of life projected to be remaining for a population of a given age
LIFE SPAN—the maximum potential length of life that humans may live
OLD OLD—75 years of age and older
PROGRAM THEORY—a theory of aging proposing that cells reproduce themselves for a programmed finite number of times and then die
TITLE III FUNDS—funds authorized under the 1973 Older Americans Act, providing for congregate and home-delivered nutrition programs for the elderly
YOUNG OLD—65 to 75 years of age

The past century has witnessed a challenging shift in the age makeup of the population in the United States. Primarily as a result of breakthroughs in health care, the number of persons over 65 years of age has increased from 4% of the population in 1900 to 12% in 1985 and is expected to reach 20% by the year 2030 (US Senate . . . , 1988). The most rapidly growing age bracket is the over-85 segment, which currently includes 2 million Americans (Leaf, 1988) (Fig. 14–1).

Traditionally, the age group from 65 and beyond has been said to constitute the "elderly." However, the increasing number of healthy and active people at the younger end of the aging spectrum has led to the need for more definitive age groupings. Thus the specific age groups of 65 up to 75, and 75 and over are often referred to as the "young old" and the "old old," respectively, or the "aging" and the "aged." Research continues to distinguish the sometimes wide variations between and within these two groups.

More than ever before, there is an increased interest in identifying factors that lead to healthy aging. Good nutrition throughout life is a clear factor in determining the quality of life that a person may expect to enjoy in later years.

LONGEVITY

Discussions of length of life are frequently confused because of interchanging terminology of life span and life expectancy. *Life span* defines the maximum potential length of life that humans may live. At present, the record for the longest life span belongs to a woman in Wales who died at 114 years of age; in the United States, the record is 110 years of age (Chernoff and Lipschitz, 1988).

Life expectancy, on the other hand, is the mean length of life projected to be remaining for a population of a given age. When expressed in terms of life expectancy at birth, it identifies the number of years an infant born at a particular time may expect to live, assuming that prevailing conditions remain the same.

There is no evidence that improved nutritional status contributes to an increased life potential in humans. However, by its positive effect on life expectancy, it has clearly increased the number of people who have approached the maximum life span and has moved the general population in that direction.

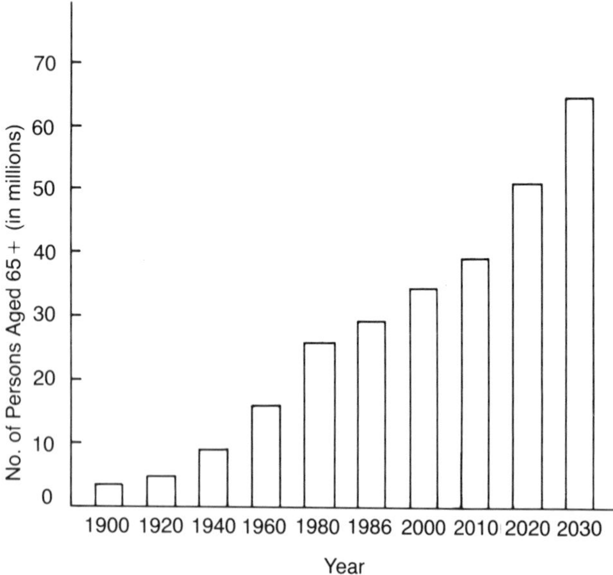

FIGURE 14–1. *Number of persons aged 65 and older from 1900 to 2030. Increments in years on horizontal scale are uneven. (Data from US Bureau of the Census.)*

Life Span (Maximum Life Span Potential)

The maximum potential life span has changed very little in recorded history (Chernoff, 1987). Environmental processes that have altered the expected length of life have failed to influence the potential, suggesting that it is determined genetically (Morrison, 1983). Ancestors of centenarians and nonagenarians have significantly longer longevity. Life spans are similar within a single species and are different among species. Some species measure life in terms of days (mayflies, 1; houseflies, 30) and some in years, from a few to many (rats, 3; dogs, 12; horses, 25; humans, 70).

Attempts are made occasionally to associate dietary practices with what appear to be extended life spans within certain population groups. These include the Hunzas of Pakistan, Vilcambabans from Ecuador, and Soviets in Georgia, Azerbaijan, and Armenia. However, repeated observations of these groups have revealed that claims for extraordinary life spans cannot be substantiated, and no data have been found that would set them apart from others of their species. Large numbers of these groups do in fact live to approximately 100 years of age. Genetic factors, continued exercise, and respected, productive roles in the community appear to be the most common factors in prolonging healthy lives in these populations. No common denominator has been identified that can associate dietary practices with extended years.

Life Expectancy

Life expectancy, or the length of life that can be expected at a particular time, is subject to environmental influences and continues to increase. Life expectancy at birth in 1985 in the United States was 74.7 years, compared with 47 years at the beginning of the century. Four of these years have been added since 1968 (Leaf, 1988; Morrison, 1983).

An increase in life expectancy can be attributed

greatly to the decrease in infant and child mortality that has occurred during the last century. Twice as many infants now survive until their first birthday. Improved living standards and progress in medical care have eliminated the threat of many childhood diseases.

More recently, the period of middle to late-middle age has been marked by increased longevity. Although those reaching 65 years of age can expect to live another 17 years (Kannel, 1988), at age 80 the odds of surviving to 81 years of age are not much greater than they were 100 years ago. With increasing age, the relative increase in life expectation decreases. The increasing number of aged over 80 years of age reflects the increase in population, not an increase in life expectancy.

Beginning in 1930 for women, but only in the last 10 years for men, an increase in life expectancy of individuals reaching middle age and beyond has been observed within technologically advanced countries (Morrison, 1983). The reduced or delayed mortality is a result of postponing development of the degenerative diseases characteristic of this age period. Factors involved in these changes include improved medical care, higher standards of living, and, to some degree, improved nutrition. Survivors of childhood are now in better health and are better able to resist disease as a result of improved nutrition, primarily reflecting the increased availability of food. The current emphasis on the relationship of diet and other lifestyle practices to the occurrence of diseases of aging may lead to further increases in life expectancy. Of the 10 leading causes of death in 1987, all except two were associated closely with diet or alcohol consumption (see Table 16-13).

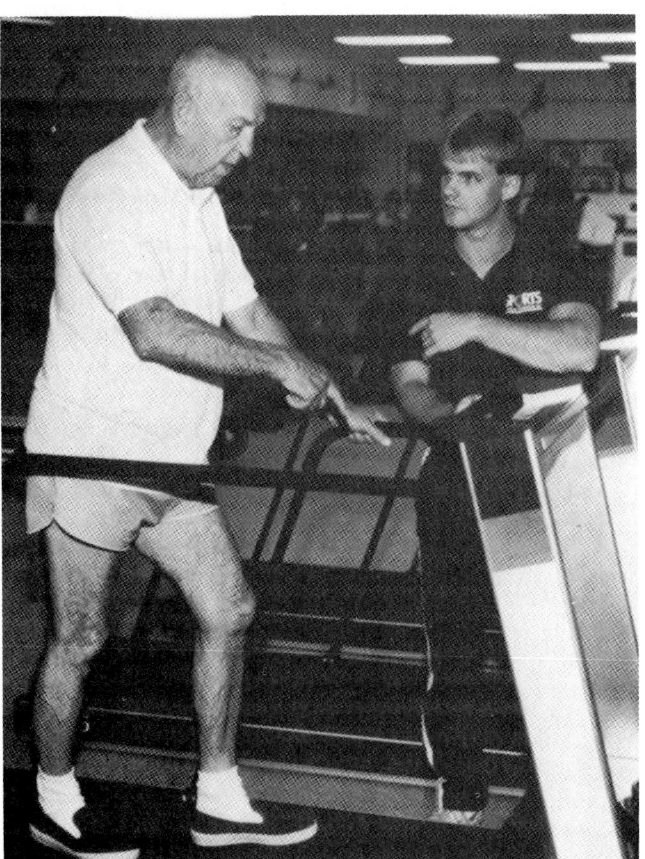

FIGURE 14-2. *Walking on a treadmill is an excellent form of moderate exercise for promoting longevity. (From Elia EA: Exercise and the elderly. Clin Sports Med 10(1): 146, 1991.)*

Since 1968 life expectancy has increased by 3 to 4 years as the result of a 30% decrease in mortality from coronary artery disease and a 50% decrease in stroke mortality (Leaf, 1988). Although this has resulted partly from improved medical treatment and care, it is attributed mainly to changes in lifestyle, including attention to nutritional factors thought to promote atherosclerosis and hypertension. Considerable epidemiologic evidence implicates nutrients as factors in certain types of cancer. The American Cancer Society estimates that as many as 35% of all cancers may be diet-related (see Chapter 36). Adequate intakes of calcium throughout life may prevent the onset of osteoporosis. National goals of reducing the incidence of obesity are also expected to reduce the occurrence of hypertension, cardiovascular disease, and non-insulin-dependent diabetes. Maintenance of normal body weight and exercise are associated with prevention of premature death (Pekkanen, 1987) (Fig. 14-2).

Theories of Aging

The degenerative changes that accompany aging are not well understood, although a number of theories have been proposed to account at least in part for the deterioration that is observed. Whether the changes are inevitably programmed into the genome or whether they occur as a result of a lifetime of exposure to environmental influences, such as stress, nutrition, or solar radiation, is not known.

Support for the *program theory* is provided by laboratory cultures of embryonic cells that reproduce themselves for a finite number of times and then die. If reproduction is halted temporarily, when resumed it continues until the established number has been reached.

Error theories suggest that environmental damage to the deoxyribonucleic acid (DNA) template results in errors in the genetic program with subsequent production of abnormal proteins that give rise to mutations and teratogens.

Cellular theories propose that environmental factors cause degenerative changes in cellular components. Cross-linkages form between macromolecules. Altering the form and function of collagen affects sensitive processes, such as passage of substances across cell membranes. Similar cross-linkages in DNA could introduce errors into the genetic program. Consonant with this "wear and tear" theory is the fact that maximum life span in different species is correlated with the metabolic level and the length of time necessary to reach reproductive maturity. Insects and shrews have extremely rapid metabolic rates and short life spans.

A challenging theory involves the continuous formation of *free radicals* as a result of exposure to oxygen, background radiation, and other environmental factors. These highly reactive substances cause damage to cellular components. A variety of antioxidants, including tocopherols, superoxide dismutase, and glutathione peroxidase, are able to repair damage caused by free radicals. It has been disappointing, however, that antioxidant therapy has failed to significantly extend the life span of mammals.

The *nutritional model,* the only model that has actually been successful in prolonging life in mammalian species, involves severe dietary restriction of energy (Masoro, 1988). The original studies in this area demonstrated that dietary restriction in rats increased longevity but with diminished sexual maturation and fertility (McCay et al, 1941). Further studies involving less severe dietary restriction (50 to 60% lower than the energy intake of animals allowed to eat ad lib) have increased longevity in rats, mice, and hamsters without the developmental abnormalities (Merry and Holehan, 1988). Susceptibility to the degenerative diseases of aging is decreased, and many age-associated physiologic changes are delayed. Although animals in these studies are leaner, the results do not support the belief that reduction of body fat is the mechanism by which food restriction extends length of life (Masoro, 1988).

The results of these experiments cannot necessarily be applied to humans. Animal studies involve change in only the single variable of energy intake, whereas human longevity is subject to a variety of interacting factors. Even if people were willing to accept the drastic restrictions in energy intake and the reduced quality of life, there is no evidence that lifelong food restriction would be safe (Masoro, 1988). Furthermore, there is nothing to suggest that such restriction would prolong life beyond the maximum life span of approximately 110 years, which is currently experienced.

THE AGING PROCESS

Aging is a normal process that begins with conception and ends at death. During periods of growth, anabolic processes exceed catabolic changes. Once the body reaches physiologic maturity, the rate of catabolic or degenerative change becomes greater than the rate of anabolic cell regeneration. The resultant loss of cells leads to varying degrees of decreased efficiency and impaired organ function.

Aging is marked by a progressive loss of lean body mass, as well as changes in most body systems. Which, if any, of these changes are the inevitable outcome of genetically programmed events, or the result of prolonged environmental influences, is a matter of debate. Although precise data on the effect of nutrition on the health of the elderly are lacking, it appears that in general the aged are subject to the same influences that govern nutritional status of the younger population.

Nutrition-Related System Changes in the Elderly

Sensory

With age, the senses of taste, smell, sight, hearing, and touch diminish at individualized rates. Atrophy of gustatory papillae beginning around 50 years of age leads to a drop in the number of taste buds per papilla from 245 in children and young adults to 88 in people 74 to 85 years old. Sensitivity to sweet and salty taste declines with age (Chauhan, 1989). Medications can change taste acuity as discussed in Chapter 25. Glossodynia (pain in the tongue) may also occur. Hearing loss, diminished olfactory sense, and impairment of short-range vision are common (Table 14–1).

Gastrointestinal

A number of changes that affect appetite and the ability to digest and absorb foods occur in the gastrointestinal system during the aging process. Loss of endogenous opioids and exaggerated effects of cholecystokinin, both involved in normal *appetite response,* may contribute to the anorexia often seen in the very old.

Although dental caries are uncommon in the elderly, *periodontal disease* or *ill-fitting dentures* frequently make eating a painful and embarrassing experience and lead to substitution of soft, low-fiber foods for whole grains, fruits, and vegetables. About 41% of per-

TABLE 14–1. Percentage of Tissue Function Remaining at Age 75 Years*

Tissue	% Remaining in a 75-year-old Man
Body water content	82
Number of glomeruli in kidney	56
Number of nerve trunk fibers	63
Brain weight	56
Number of taste buds	36

From Shock NW: The physiology of aging. Scientific American, 206:100, 1962.

sons over 65 years of age are *edentulous,* and only 60% of this group have satisfactory dentures (National Institute of Dental Research, 1987). Diminished *salivary secretion* decreases the ability to masticate and swallow food. Certain medications, such as antihypertensive drugs, cause xerostomia, or dry mouth.

The *hypochlorhydria* that frequently occurs with age, probably with loss of parietal cells, decreases absorption of calcium and nonheme iron, although it does not affect absorption of heme iron. Bacterial overgrowth of the gut may also occur as a result of the decrease in acid secretion. Some bacteria have the capacity to bind nutrients, such as vitamin B_{12}, making them biologically unavailable. Occasional lack of intrinsic factor may lead to decreased absorption of vitamin B_{12} and eventually to the development of pernicious anemia. The bacterial overgrowth can also lead to poor function of bile salts, fat malabsorption, and diarrhea (see Chapter 27).

The incidence of *gall bladder* disease increases with age. Of people over 65 years of age, 40% have some type of pancreatic insufficiency. Because of decreased motility in the large intestine and colon, *constipation* is a common problem in the elderly. Motility of the small intestine does not appear to be affected by age.

Metabolic

A decrease in glucose tolerance associated with the aging process leads to an increase in plasma glucose of 1.5 mg/dl per decade. This decrease could be the result of a diminished insulin secretion in response to a glucose challenge or a decreased tissue response to insulin action. The use of glucose tolerance curves developed for younger adults is now recognized as inappropriate for the diagnosis of diabetes in the elderly.

Basal metabolic rate decreases by 20% between the ages of 30 and 90, mainly because of the decrease in lean body mass. The tissues that remain, however, continue to produce heat at the same rate as in younger adults.

Cardiovascular

Cardiovascular disease is responsible for 70% of all deaths beyond 75 years of age, although the decline in mortality from this disease seen in the last 2 decades also includes the elderly. During the aging process blood vessels become less elastic and total peripheral resistance increases, leading to increasing prevalence of hypertension. Blood pressure continues to increase in women beyond the age of 80 but declines substantially in older men. Serum cholesterol levels in men tend to peak at 60 years of age, but total cholesterol as well as the low-density lipoprotein (LDL) fraction continue to rise in women until 70 years of age (Kannel, 1988).

Renal

Kidney function can diminish 50% between the ages of 30 and 80 years, and kidney deficiency affects 75% of the population in late adulthood. Acid-base response to metabolic challenges is slowed, and excessive amounts of protein waste products or electrolytes are handled with more difficulty. Geriatric nephropathy may be the result of chronic protein overnutrition (Rudman, 1988). The NHANES II study indicated that the average American consumption of protein is 166% of the RDA.

Musculoskeletal

Progressive replacement of lean body mass by fat and connective tissue appears to be an inevitable consequence of aging. Body protein in the healthy elderly is 30 to 40% less than that of young adults. This loss includes both muscular and visceral protein, leading to both functional and metabolic changes. Creatinine secretion rate declines, reflecting the loss of muscle protein (Welch, 1989). Fat is deposited more in the trunk and around visceral organs, and subcutaneous fat increases slightly. Bone density is diminished, and osteoporosis is a frequent complication. Shortening of the spinal column leads to a loss of stature.

Neurologic

Confusional states found in some of the elderly have numerous causes. Of great interest in this area is the experimental use of substances that serve as precursors of brain neurotransmitters involved in abnormalities such as Parkinson's disease and Alzheimer's disease—specifically, tyrosine, tryptophan, and choline. However, there is no indication that dietary inadequacies are involved in the etiology of these conditions (Hodkinson, 1988).

Immunocompetence

Immune function declines with age, and both the humoral immunity and to a great degree cell-mediated immunity are affected. These changes result in diminished ability to fight infections, leading to a prevalence of a variety of infections in the elderly. Reduced immunosurveillance may also help to explain the higher prevalence of malignancy in these people (Good and Lorenz, 1988).

Psychosocial

Some of the elderly fail to obtain an adequate diet because of social isolation (House et al, 1988). Depression often accompanies a sense of loss—loss of loved ones, productivity, a sense of worth, mobility, income, and finally, body image. If decreased sight and physical function become factors, elderly persons may be trapped by immobility. In these circumstances, shopping for food and preparing meals may become very difficult. The inability to drive safely to the local grocery store and to carry groceries often results in an inadequate food supply at home.

Elderly persons may become homebound as a result of fear of being victimized. This is a particular problem in poor, crime-ridden areas. Failing health may further increase the problem of isolation and mobility.

Retirement income is often inadequate, and elderly individuals may be forced into a lower socioeconomic status. Although an estimated two thirds of those eligible are aware of the Food Stamp program, less than 50% use it.

Nutritional Requirements of the Elderly

Energy

Although obesity in humans is associated with a shortened life expectancy, the degree involved is somewhat controversial. Some data have indicated that being underweight is associated with as high a mortality rate as moderate obesity, particularly in those over 60 years of age. Only morbid obesity, however, is a risk factor for elderly women. Moderate obesity is more of a risk factor for older men, probably because the android distribution of fat is related to the incidence of cardiovascular disease.

Energy requirements decrease with age. In addition to a normal decline in metabolism, a slackening of physical activity lowers energy needs still further. The 1989 RDA call for a reduction of average energy allowances after 51 years of age of 600 kcal/day for men and 300 kcal for women (Food and Nutrition Board, 1989). However, as demonstrated in the Baltimore Longitudinal Study on Aging (Shock et al, 1984), there is marked variability in lifestyle and health status of the elderly at all ages. Individuals over 50 years of age are more active today than in previous years.

Table 14–2 presents the recommendations of the Gerontology Research Center of the National Institute on Aging for weight ranges appropriate to increasing age. These recommendations illustrate the wide ranges of weight associated with health and longevity in the elderly and acknowledge the steady gain of weight throughout adulthood (Andres et al, 1985).

Diets that fall below 1,800 kcal/day often provide inadequate amounts of protein, calcium, iron, and vitamins and should therefore be planned to feature nutrient-dense foods.

Protein

Body protein in the healthy elderly is 60 to 70% of that of young adults, which might suggest a decreased need for dietary protein. Protein intake is related to energy intake, and although the latter tends to decrease with age, protein intake remains considerably higher than the RDA. In 1989 the Food and Nutrition Board con-

TABLE 14–2. Age-Specific Height-Weight Tables for Adults 20 to 69 Years of Age*†

		Metropolitan 1983 Weights‡ (25–59 yr)		Gerontology Research Center‡ (Age-Specific Weight Range for Men and Women)				
Height (ft and in)		*Men*	*Women*	*20–29 yr*	*30–39 yr*	*40–49 yr*	*50–59 yr*	*60–69 yr*
4	10		100–131	84–111	92–119	99–127	107–135	115–142
4	11		101–134	87–115	95–123	103–131	111–139	119–147
5	0		103–137	90–119	98–127	106–135	114–143	123–152
5	1	123–145	105–140	93–123	101–131	110–140	118–148	127–157
5	2	125–148	108–144	96–127	105–136	113–144	122–153	131–163
5	3	127–151	111–148	99–131	108–140	117–149	126–158	135–168
5	4	129–155	114–152	102–135	112–145	121–154	130–163	140–173
5	5	131–159	117–156	106–140	115–149	125–159	134–168	144–179
5	6	133–163	120–160	109–144	119–154	129–164	138–174	148–184
5	7	135–167	123–164	112–148	122–159	133–169	143–179	153–190
5	8	137–171	126–167	116–153	126–163	137–174	147–184	158–196
5	9	139–175	129–170	119–157	130–168	141–179	151–190	162–201
5	10	141–179	132–173	122–162	134–173	145–184	156–195	167–207
5	11	144–183	135–176	126–167	137–178	149–190	160–201	172–213
6	0	147–187		129–171	141–183	153–195	165–207	177–219
6	1	150–192		133–176	145–188	157–200	169–213	182–225
6	2	153–197		137–181	149–194	162–206	174–219	187–232
6	3	157–202		141–186	153–199	166–212	179–225	192–238
6	4			144–191	157–205	171–218	184–231	197–244

* From Andres R, Bierman EL, and Hazzard WR: Principles of Geriatric Medicine. New York, McGraw-Hill, 1985, p. 317. Reproduced by permission of McGraw-Hill, Inc.

† Comparison of the weight-for-height tables from actuarial data: Non–age-corrected Metropolitan Life Insurance Company and Age-Specific Gerontology Research Center recommendations.

‡ Values in this table are for height without shoes and weight without clothes.

cluded that the protein RDA of 0.75 g/kg is appropriate for adults of all ages (Food and Nutrition Board, 1989).

Protein needs increase in relation to the severity and duration of disease. Stressful physical and psychologic stimuli can induce a negative nitrogen balance. Infection, altered gastrointestinal function, and metabolic changes caused by chronic disease can reduce the efficiency of dietary nitrogen utilization.

Protein deficiency is unlikely in the American elderly population who do not have a debilitating disease (Munro et al, 1987). Protein-calorie undernutrition, however, may be a particular problem with elderly men who live alone. Such deficiencies contribute to edema, itching of the skin, chronic eczema, fatigue, muscle weakness, and tissue wastage. Wounds heal slowly, and body immune response may be impaired.

Carbohydrate

A reduced glucose tolerance renders the elderly more susceptible to temporary hypoglycemia or hyperglycemia. Insulin sensitivity may be improved by reducing the use of sugar and by increasing the amount of complex carbohydrate and soluble fiber in the diet.

Diminished lactase secretion frequently leads to a lactose intolerance.

Lipid

Coronary heart disease contributes to most deaths of older people in the United States. Serum cholesterol levels in men tend to peak during middle age and then drop slightly, whereas cholesterol levels in women continue to rise with increasing age. Reducing total dietary fat (especially the amount of saturated fat) and cholesterol in the diet can lower blood cholesterol levels and subsequent risk of heart disease (see Chapter 20). Although direct evidence that dietary changes can reduce risk of cardiovascular disease in the elderly is not available, there is no reason to believe that the same environmental factors leading to decreased risk in the younger population will not continue to be effective in later years. The recommended reduction of dietary fat to no more than 30% of total kilocalories also supports principles of weight control and cancer prevention.

Minerals

Although laboratory data or intake records frequently suggest mineral inadequacies, clinical evidence rarely supports dietary deficiencies. As lean body mass decreases with age, the requirement for trace elements needed for muscle metabolism may be reduced (Chernoff and Lipschitz, 1988). For this reason, it has been speculated that mineral requirements stated for the elderly may be too high. However, glucose intolerance may indicate increased chromium needs. Bone loss due to osteoporosis, the presence of hypochlorhydria, and the attendant failure to absorb calcium efficiently all suggest the need for increased calcium intakes. Recommendations for osteoporosis prevention specify a continued calcium intake of 800 mg/day for women 51 years of age and over. See Chapter 22 for discussion of osteoporosis and its treatment.

Nutrition-related iron deficiency anemia is not common in the elderly (Manore et al, 1989). Anemia at this age is usually related to blood loss, often from the gastrointestinal tract, and requires medical attention.

Intakes of zinc in the elderly decline in relation to the decrease in energy intake and are much lower than the recommended level of 15 mg/day for men and 12 mg/day for women. Low plasma zinc concentrations have been found in from 2 to 27% of the elderly population, depending on the study (Bogden et al, 1987; Sandstead et al, 1982). Zinc deficiency is associated with impaired immune function, anorexia, dysgeusia, delayed wound healing, and decubitus ulcers. Whether those with low plasma zinc who receive zinc supplementation will have an improvement in cellular immunity is still not confirmed (Bogden et al, 1988; Fraker et al, 1986), nor is it known whether those with low zinc intakes adapt by absorbing more efficiently.

Hypertension is common in the elderly, and recommendations for mineral intake include reducing sodium to 2 g/day and supplementing the diet with magnesium and potassium for those taking diuretics (Kannel, 1988).

Although selenium levels tend to fall with age, the RDA for selenium is the same as that for younger adults (Table 14–3).

TABLE 14–3. Recommended Dietary Allowances for Persons Aged 51 Years and Older*

	Men	Women
Energy (kcal)	2,300.0	1,900.0
Protein (g)	63.0	50.0
Vitamin A (μg RE)	1,000.0	800.0
Vitamin D (μg)	5.0	5.0
Vitamin E (mg a-TE)	10.0	8.0
Vitamin K (μg)	80.0	65.0
Thiamin (mg)	1.2	1.0
Riboflavin (mg)	1.4	1.2
Niacin (mg NE)	15.0	13.0
Vitamin B_6 (mg)	2.0	1.6
Folate (μg)	200.0	180.0
Vitamin B_{12} (μg)	2.0	2.0
Calcium (mg)	800.0	800.0
Phosphorus (mg)	800.0	800.0
Magnesium (mg)	350.0	280.0
Iron (mg)	10.0	10.0
Zinc (mg)	15.0	12.0
Iodine (μg)	150.0	150.0
Selenium (μg)	70.0	55.0

* Reprinted with permission from *Recommended Dietary Allowances*, 10th edition, c. 1989 by the National Academy of Sciences. Published by National Academy Press.

Vitamins

There is no evidence of insufficiency in the *vitamin A* nutriture of senior citizens. Adequate plasma retinol levels appear to be sustained throughout life (Garry et al, 1987). Many elderly take supplements containing vitamin A; however, the margin of safety for vitamin A intake in the elderly may not be as great as in younger individuals because liver stores are already maximal, thus reducing their ability to store excess amounts of the vitamin (Krasinski et al, 1989).

Dietary intakes of 62 to 74% of the healthy free-living elderly are below two thirds of the RDA for *vitamin D*. Whether age influences vitamin D absorption from the gastrointestinal tract is not clear. The lower levels of vitamin D in institutionalized and homebound elderly may be owing to decreased exposure to sunlight or to less efficient synthesis of vitamin D in the skin. Sunshine appears to be an important factor in maintaining appropriate vitamin D status in the elderly. Complete elimination of sunshine requires that dietary vitamin D intake be 300 IU/day (Lips et al, 1987). Some evidence suggests a decreased capacity of the aging kidney to convert vitamin D to the active $1,25(OH)_2D_3$ form. Lack of adequate vitamin D and calcium are associated with osteoporosis and osteomalacia (see Chapter 22).

Although intakes, blood levels, and tissue levels of *ascorbic acid* tend to be low in the elderly, particularly among those who are smokers or subject to stress, supplementation results in little clinical improvement. Vitamin C deficiency may present with lassitude and fatigue. Although purpura, capillary hemorrhaging, bleeding from the gums, and delayed wound healing are frequent complaints of the elderly, frank scurvy is rare, limited mainly to alcoholics and older low-income men. Encouraging the consumption of vitamin C–rich foods may be the most effective way of improving vitamin C nutriture of the elderly. Vitamin C may also have a role in cataract prevention (New Directions, see below).

Some research has indicated that intakes of vitamin B_6 and folacin are less than two thirds of the RDA; however, biochemical data supported only a deficiency of vitamin B_6 (Vaughan and Manore, 1988). Healthy elderly people appear to be able to maintain normal folate nutriture despite intakes well below the RDA. In a review of published plasma folate levels, low levels were reported in only 3 to 7% of free-living elderly (Rosenberg et al, 1982). A diet lacking unprocessed, fresh, and nutrient-dense foods is the most common cause of inadequate folate intake in the nonalcoholic elderly.

The usual cause of vitamin B_{12} deficiency is a loss of gastric intrinsic factor, although elderly people with

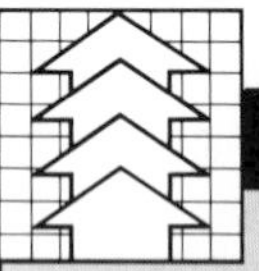

NEW DIRECTIONS: Nutrition and Senile Cataracts

Senile cataract is a major problem of the elderly around the world. In the United States it affects 18% of those aged 65 to 74 years and 46% of those aged 75 to 85 years (Taylor, 1989). Cataract repair already constitutes a significant part of health care costs and promises to increase along with the aging population. Studies suggest a possible role for nutrition in the prevention of cataracts or at least in delay of cataract occurrence.

Senile cataracts are caused primarily by oxidative stress induced by the random action of free radicals or by exposure to excessive ultraviolet light (photo-oxidation). This is in contrast to cataracts seen in diabetes and galactosemia, which are the result of osmotic stress. Senile cataracts can also form in response to the accumulation of various products of aging, which are eventually precipitated in the lens.

Lens proteins, unlike most body proteins, do not undergo rapid turnover and remain in place for decades, subject to insult from oxidation and various environmental conditions. Antioxidant enzymes are diminished in aging lenses.

Nutrients with antioxidative capabilities—primarily the carotenoids, vitamin C, and vitamin E—have been examined with respect to nutritional status of persons with cataract and the possible effectiveness of supplementation. Carotenoids, such as beta-carotene, have the capacity to perform as free-radical traps in lens tissues, and higher serum levels have been shown to correlate with a delay in cataract formation. Vitamin E, thought to be one of the best lipid-soluble antioxidants, may also have a role in maintaining the integrity of lens cell membranes.

Vitamin C, one of the most effective and least toxic of antioxidants, occurs in the lens in concentrations up to 30 times those found in plasma. However, ascorbate concentrations are lower in aged or cataractous lenses than in normal lenses, particularly in the nucleus where most senile cataracts originate. Limited studies have shown that persons with plasma ascorbate levels of 90 μmol/l have less chance of developing cataract than those with 40 μmol/l. However 500 mg/day of vitamin C are required to maintain this higher plasma level, and these excessive amounts of the vitamin are capable in themselves of increasing formation of undesirable products of aging.

Severe caloric restriction delays senile cataract in mice. Although this is an inappropriate goal for humans, understanding of the mechanisms involved may be useful in attempts to delay the onset of cataracts (Taylor, 1989).

Although specific measures to prevent or delay the onset of senile cataracts are not immediately forthcoming, the future of continued research appears promising.

hypochlorhydria or achlorhydria may also malabsorb cobalamin. Those with either of these conditions may require a higher dietary vitamin B_{12} level than is presently recommended.

Although clinical malnutrition is relatively uncommon in the healthy elderly population, a maintenance level multivitamin and mineral supplement may cure latent nutritional deficiency states that may be the basis for common complaints by some individuals. On the other hand, from recent studies it appears that 39 to 69% of elderly Americans, especially women, take vitamin or mineral supplements (Gray, 1986; Hartz et al, 1988; Stewart et al, 1985) at higher levels than the general adult population, and many are taking potentially toxic doses. Thus, they should always be asked specifically about supplement usage.

Water

Dehydration is the most common cause of fluid and electrolyte disturbances in the elderly (Phillips et al, 1984). Reduced thirst sensation and reduced fluid intake along with physiologic need and diminished water conservation by the kidneys are important contributing factors. If water intake is deficient in the presence of problems such as diarrhea or fever, it could lead to clinical dehydration requiring hospitalization in addition to aggravating other conditions, such as constipation or renal stone disease. An adequate water intake consists of 30 to 35 ml/kg ideal body weight.

Nutritional Status of the Elderly

Nutritional status of the elderly in general is satisfactory. Most maintain the eating habits established when they were younger. However, many subgroups within the aging category are at risk of malnutrition for a variety of reasons (Table 14–4). These include ignorance of appropriate nutrition, financial restrictions, physical disabilities that interfere with purchase and preparation of food, social isolation, and mental disorders. Secondary causes of malnutrition include anorexia; malabsorption arising from intestinal disease and from achlorhydria; and alcoholism, which affects the nutritional status when alcohol is substituted for nutritious foods. Alcohol may interfere with absorption of some nutrients, notably folic acid. Long-term use of certain therapeutic drugs that interfere with absorption and metabolism of nutrients may also cause malnutrition in the elderly (see Chapter 25).

TABLE 14–4. Possible Causes of Undernutrition in the Elderly

Loss of income — poverty
Social isolation
Diseases that reduce appetite, decrease absorption or utilization of nutrients, or increase requirements for nutrients
Drugs that affect food intake, or the absorption, utilization, or excretion of nutrients
Ignorance about good nutrition or food preparation
Dental problems
Depression or mental problems
Decreased physical ability to buy food or prepare a meal
Alcoholism

NUTRITIONAL CARE OF THE ELDERLY

Dietary Planning

The general principles governing the planning of a diet for the aging person are not fundamentally different from those for the mature younger adult. Modifications may be necessary because of certain characteristics inherent in the process of aging. The most important factors are that the food should be nutritious, tasty, and pleasant to eat (Fig. 14–3). Those with sensitive digestive systems should be encouraged to eat something hot at each meal. Four or five light meals are often more acceptable than three substantial ones.

Consumption of an adequate number and variety of foods from all food groups should be emphasized. When foods such as milk are voluntarily eliminated from the diet, alternatives providing the important nutrients contained in these foods should be substituted. Supplementation may be indicated if entire food groups are eliminated.

Special attention must be paid to the variety of situations that could prevent the elderly person from meeting dietary needs. If chewing is a problem, suggestions for softer, nutritious foods and for altering food textures by grinding or chopping should be explored. If shopping or meal preparation is a problem, alternatives to grocery shopping and cooking should be investigated. If arthritis prevents the elderly person from handling eating utensils comfortably, modified eating utensils can be made available.

Community Nutrition Programs

Community based programs for the elderly are administered by both public and private agencies in every section of the United States. Title III of the Older Americans Act authorizes funds for Congregate and Home-Delivered Nutrition Programs for the Elderly. Through this program, hot nutritious meals are served daily to senior citizens in group settings in more than 15,000 nutrition sites throughout the United States. A wide range of services is offered at most congregate sites, including outreach, transportation, nutrition education, recreation, and social services.

To be eligible to receive a meal at a congregate nutrition site, participants must be 60 years of age or older or

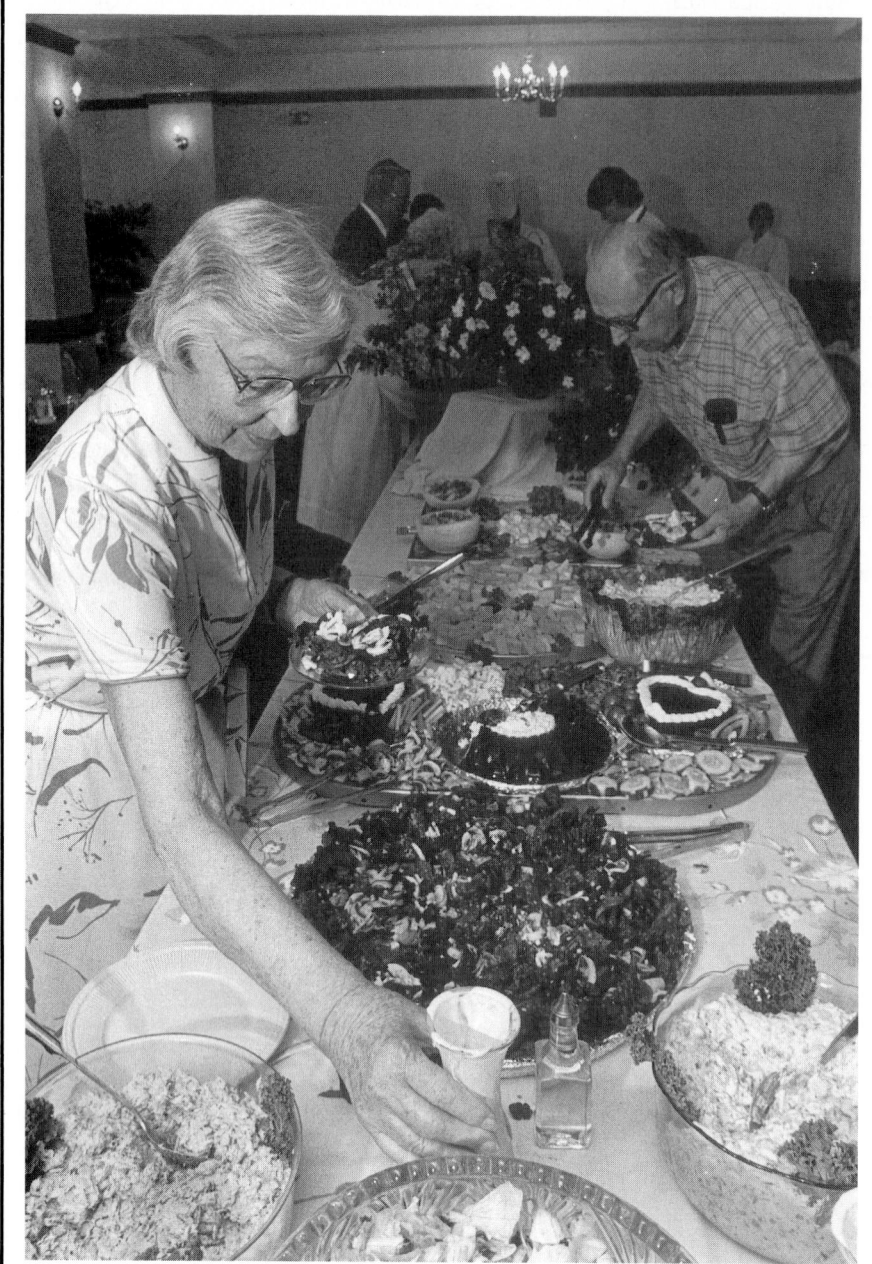

FIGURE 14–3. *A variety of nutritious foods attractively presented will tempt people of all ages. (From Matteson MA and McConnell ES: Gerontological Nursing. Philadelphia, WB Saunders, 1988, p 264.)*

the spouse or primary caretaker of an eligible participant. All meals served at the sites must meet one third of the RDA. There is often a suggested donation or opportunity to contribute for the meals, but participants decide for themselves what, if anything, they can afford to donate. Food stamps are accepted as donations for the meals.

Much of the benefits of these programs originate from the social interaction among participants. Surveys comparing food program participants with nonparticipants found that intakes of energy and protein were increased, as were intakes of vitamins and minerals, notably calcium.

The Home-Delivered Meal Program (sometimes referred to as Meals on Wheels) offers home-delivered nutritious meals to people who are 60 years of age or older and who are homebound. All home-delivered meals must meet one third of the RDA. No one is denied meals if they are unable to pay, and again food stamps are accepted as donations.

Other community resources include food banks, food co-ops, and home-delivered grocery services.

Chore services may be secured for shopping and meal preparation for senior citizens who are unable to shop or to prepare their own meals.

Nutritional Needs During Prolonged Illness

Differences in energy and nutrient requirements vary greatly with physiologic and pathologic conditions. In catabolic states associated with injury or surgery or with acute or certain chronic diseases of the elderly, such as chronic emphysema and bronchitis, cancer, organic brain syndromes, cirrhosis, and maldigestion/malabsorption syndromes, negative nitrogen balance occurs. In these conditions, negative nitrogen balance can be reduced if aggressive nutritional support is provided. Careful consideration must be given to provide for increased nutritional requirements resulting from the disease or illness process itself as well as from the compromised organ and cell functioning associated with aging. Tube feeding or parenteral nutrition may be

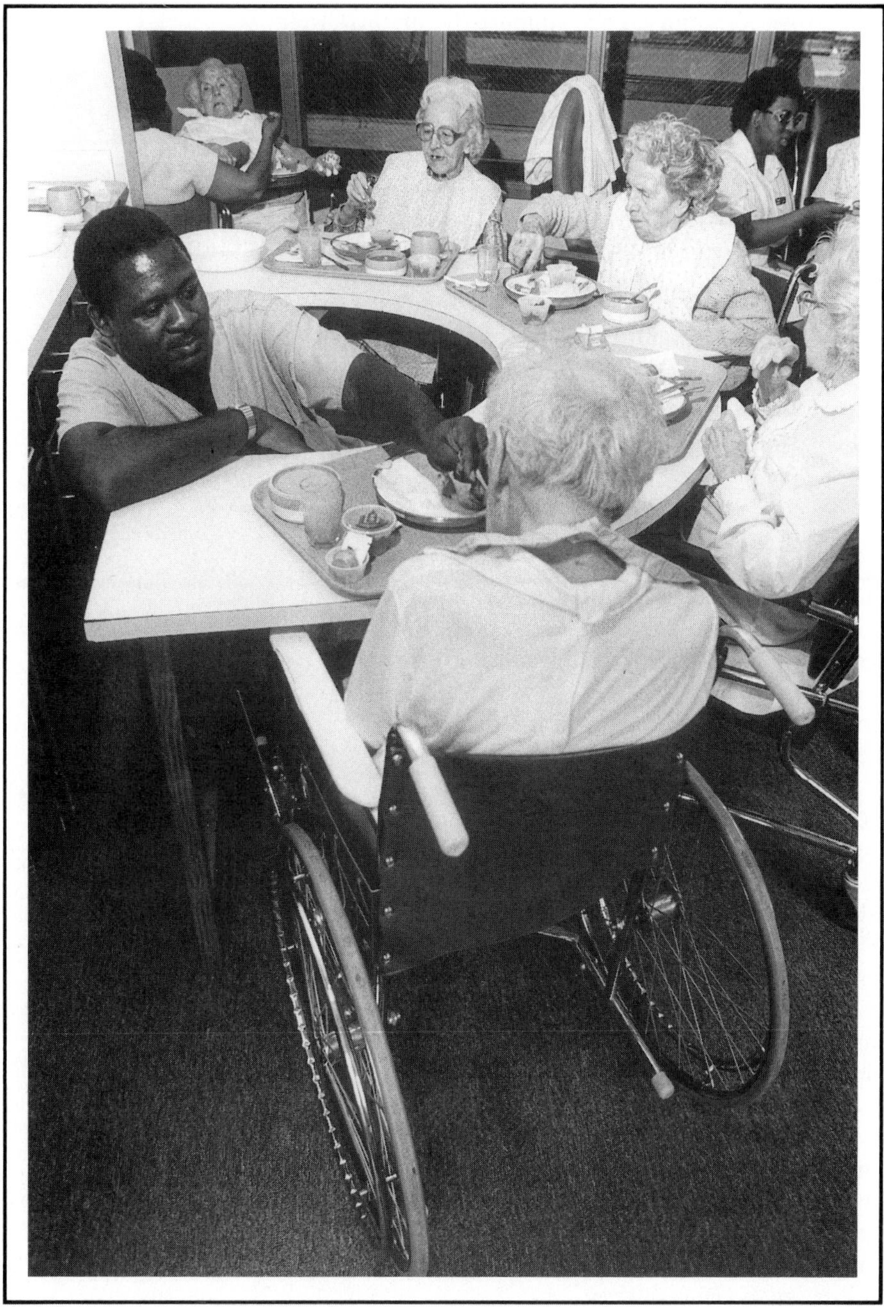

FIGURE 14–4. *The nutritional status of older persons in an institutional setting benefits greatly from special care and attention. (From Matteson MA and McConnell ES: Gerontological Nursing. Philadelphia, WB Saunders, 1988, p 621.)*

necessary because of inability to meet energy needs orally and should be given as thorough consideration as it would receive in a younger patient.

Nutritional Care in Institutionalized Settings

Approximately 5% of persons aged 65 and older are institutionalized, while the remaining 95% live independently in relatively good health (Colucci et al, 1987). Newly admitted nursing home residents are often transferred from an acute-care hospital after treatment. They are often weak, in poor health, and nutritionally depleted upon their arrival at the institution. However, data do not support the premise that institutionalization itself leads to malnutrition. In a study conducted in 15 long-term care facilities in the Boston area, subjects free from clinically apparent terminal or wasting illness were studied. Nutritional intakes were comparable with those in a simultaneously studied free-living population (Sayhoun et al, 1988). Most biochemical markers of nutritional status were equal to those of free-living populations. However, some were lower, possibly owing to a greater prevalence of chronic disease and use of medications in institutionalized groups. Another study showed an incidence of malnutrition of 52% in two urban nursing homes (Pinchcofsky-Devin and Kaminski, 1987).

Nutritional care of institutionalized elderly persons must be directed toward meeting their physiologic and psychologic needs over a long period of time. These needs change depending on the aging process, chronic and acute disease, use of medication and the emotional and mental state of the patient. Periodic reassessment of nutritional status is critical in an effort to avoid unnecessary diet restrictions or missing important unmet nutritional needs. Further discussion of nutritional assessment is found in Chapter 17.

Body weight history is an important record of nutritional status. Weights of all patients should be taken regularly and recorded. Because of gradual loss of stature (1.2 cm for each 20 years of maturity), the elderly weigh more per unit of height than younger adults. Therefore, it is important to use tables specifically developed for this age group (see Table 14–2). Observing and recording quantity and quality of fluid and food intake of residents is another important aspect of providing quality nutrition care.

Improving the dietary habits of the elderly patient requires special care and attention on the part of the nursing and dietary staff (Fig. 14–4). The service of attractive and palatable food in an environment that encourages independence in eating or provides assistance when necessary will be reflected in the nutritional well-being of the residents.

CITED REFERENCES

Andres R, Bierman EL, and Hazzard WR: Principles of Geriatric Medicine. New York, McGraw-Hill, 1985.

Bogden JD et al: Zinc and immunocompetence in the elderly: Baseline data on zinc nutriture and immunity in unsupplemented subjects. Am J Clin Nutr 46:101, 1987.

Bogden JD et al: Zinc and immunocompetence in elderly people: Effects of zinc supplementation for 3 months. Am J Clin Nutr 48:655, 1988.

Chauhan J: Pleasantness perception of salt in young vs. elderly adults. J Am Diet Assoc 89:834, 1989.

Chernoff R: Aging and nutrition. Nutr Today 22(2):4, 1987.

Chernoff R and Lipschitz DA (eds): Health Promotion and Disease Prevention in the Elderly, Vol 35 of The Aging Series. New York, The Raven Press, 1988.

Colucci R, Bell SJ, and Blackburn GL: Nutrition problems of institutionalized and free-living elderly. Comp Ther 13(1):20, 1987.

Food and Nutrition Board, National Research Council: Recommended Dietary Allowances, 10th ed. Washington, DC, National Academy of Sciences, 1989.

Fraker PJ et al: Interrelationships between zinc and immune function. Fed Proc 45:1474, 1986.

Garry PJ et al: Vitamin A intake and plasma retinol levels in healthy elderly men and women. Am J Clin Nutr 46:989, 1987.

Good RA and Lorenz E: Nutrition, immunity, aging, and cancer. Nutr Rev 46:62, 1988.

Gray GE et al: Vitamin supplement use in a Southern California retirement community. J Am Diet Assoc 86:800, 1986.

Hartz SC et al: Nutrient supplement use by healthy elderly. J Am Coll Nutr 7:119, 1988.

Hodkinson HM: Diet and maintenance of mental health in the elderly. Nutr Rev 46:79, 1988.

House JS, Landis KR, and Umberson D: Social relationships and health. Science 241:540, 1988.

Kannel WB: Nutrition and the occurrence and prevention of cardiovascular disease in the elderly. Nutr Rev 46:68, 1988.

Krasinski SD et al: Relationship of vitamin A and vitamin E intake to fasting plasma retinol, retinol-binding protein, retinyl esters, carotene, alpha-tocopherol, and cholesterol among elderly people and young adults: Increased plasma retinyl esters among vitamin A-supplement users. Am J Clin Nutr 49:112, 1989.

Leaf A: The aging process: Lessons from observations in man. Nutr Rev 46:40, 1988.

Lips P et al: Determinants of vitamin D status in patients with hip fracture and in elderly control subjects. Am J Clin Nutr 46:1005, 1987.

Manore MM, Vaughan LA, and Carroll SS: Iron status in the free-living, low income very elderly. Nutr Rep Internat 39:1, 1989.

Masoro EJ: Life span extension and food restriction. Comp Ther 14(6):9, 1988.

McCay CM et al: Nutrition requirements during the latter half of life. J Nutr 21:45, 1941.

Merry BJ and Holehan AM: Effects of diet on aging. *In* Timiras PS (ed): Physiological Basis of Geriatrics. New York, Macmillan, 1988.

Morrison SD: Nutrition and longevity. Nutr Rev 41:133, 1983.

Munro HN et al: Nutritional requirements of the elderly. Ann Rev Nutr 7:23, 1987.

National Institute of Dental Research: Oral Health of United States Adults: The National Survey of Oral Health in U.S. Employed Adults and Seniors, 1985–86, (NIH Publ. (PHS)87-2868). Bethesda, MD, USDHHS, 1987.

Pekkanen J: Reduction of premature mortality by high physical activity: A 20-year follow-up of middle-aged Finnish men. Lancet 1:1473, 1987.

Phillips MB et al: Reduced thirst after water deprivation in healthy elderly men. N Engl J Med 311:753, 1984.

Pinchcofsky-Devin GD and Kaminski MV: Incidence of protein calorie malnutrition in the nursing home population. J Am Coll Nutr 6:109, 1987.

Rosenberg IH et al: Folate nutrition in the elderly. Am J Clin Nutr 36:1060, 1982.

Rudman D: Kidney senescence: A model for aging. Nutr Rev 46:209, 1988.
Sandstead HH et al: Zinc nutriture in the elderly in relation to taste acuity, immune response, and wound healing. Am J Clin Nutr 36:1046, 1982.
Sayhoun NR et al: Dietary intakes and biochemical indicators of nutritional status in an elderly, institutionalized population. Am J Clin Nutr 47:524, 1988.
Shock NW et al: Normal Human Aging. The Baltimore Longitudinal Study of Aging, NIH Publ. No. 84-2450. Washington, DC, USDHHS, 1984.
Stewart ML et al: Vitamin/mineral supplement use: A telephone survey of adults in the United States. J Am Diet Assoc 85:1585, 1985.
Taylor A: Associations between nutrition and cataract. Nutr Rev 47:225, 1989.
US Senate Special Committee on Aging and American Association of Retired Persons: Size and growth of the older population. *In* Aging America: Trends and Projections. Washington, DC, USDHHS, 1988.
Vaughan LA and Manore MM: Dietary patterns and nutritional status of low income, free-living elderly. Food Nutr News 60(5):1, 1988.
Welch T: Nutrition-related problems in the institutionalized elderly. Dietetic Currents (Ross Laboratories) 16(1):1, 1989.

ADDITIONAL REFERENCES

Bistrian B: Nutritional support of the long-term care patient. Part II: Nutritional assessment of the elderly. Nutr Suppl Serv 8(10):17, 1988.
Bunker VW and Clayton BE: Research review: Studies in the nutrition of elderly people with particular reference to essential trace elements. Age and Ageing 18:422, 1989.
Carethers M: Diagnosing vitamin B_{12} deficiency: A common geriatric disorder. Geriatrics 43:89, 105, 111, 1988.
Chandra RK: Nutritional regulation of immunity and risk of infection in old age. Immunology 67:141, 1989.
Chauhan J et al: Age-related olfactory and taste changes and interrelationships between taste and nutrition. J Am Diet Assoc 87:1543, 1987.
Chen LH (ed): Nutritional Aspects of Aging, Vol II. Boca Raton, CRC Press, 1986.
Chernoff R: Physiologic aging and nutritional status. Nutr Clin Prac 5:8, 1990.
Chumlea WM et al: Prediction of body weight for the nonambulatory elderly from anthropometry. J Am Diet Assoc 88:564, 1988.
Daly MP: Anemia in the elderly. Am Fam Phys 39:129, 1989.
Davies L: Practical nutrition for the elderly. Nutr Rev 46:83, 1988.
Eating for your 80s. Nutr Action 14(9):4, 1987.
Fanelli MT: The ABC's of nutritional assessment in older adults. J Nutr Elderly 6:33, 1987.
Garry PJ and Chumlea WC (eds): Epidemiologic and methodologic problems in determining nutrition status of older persons. Am J Clin Nutr 50(Suppl):1121, 1989.
Garry PJ et al: Vitamin A intake and plasma retinol levels in healthy elderly men and women. Am J Clin Nutr 46:989, 1987.
Gary GE: Nutrition and dementia. J Am Diet Assoc 89:1795, 1989.
Gupta KL, Dworkin B, and Gambert SR: Common nutritional disorders in the elderly: Atypical manifestations. Geriatrics 43:87, 1988.
Halliwell B: Tell me about free radicals, Doctor: A review. J Roy Soc Med 82:747, 1989.
Harris T et al: Body mass index and mortality among nonsmoking older persons: The Framingham Heart Study. JAMA 259:1520, 1988.
Henderson CT: Approaches to nutritional care in the elderly. Comp Ther 15(6):25, 1989.
Holt V, Nordstrom J, and Kohrs MB: Changes in food preferences of the elderly over a ten year period. J Nutr Elderly 7(4):23, 1988.
Hutchinson M and Munro HN (eds): Nutrition and Aging. New York, Academic Press, 1986.
Jamison MT: Nutrition in the elderly: A descriptive study. Nutr Suppl Serv 8(5):23, 1988.
Kergoat M-J et al: Discriminant biochemical markers for evaluating the nutritional status of elderly patients in long-term care. Am J Clin Nutr 46:849, 1987.
Lehman AB: Review: Undernutrition in elderly people. Age and Ageing 18(5):339, 1989.
Masoro EJ: Food restriction research: Its significance for human aging. Am J Hum Biol 1:339, 1989.
McIntosh WA et al: The relationship between beliefs about nutrition and dietary practices of the elderly. J Am Diet Assoc 90:671, 1990.
McKay S: Who is the American food consumer? Food Nutr News 61(4):25, 1989.
Miller IJ: Human taste bud density across adult age groups. J Gerontol 43:B26, 1988.
Rammohan M, Juan D, and Jung D: Hypophagia among hospitalized elderly. J Am Diet Assoc 89:1774, 1989.
Rhodus NL: Zinc, impaired immunity and oral disease in the geriatric patient. Gerodontics 3(4):141, 1987.
Roe DA: Geriatric Nutrition, 2nd ed. Englewood Cliffs, Prentice-Hall, 1987.
Rowland M: Body mass index and mortality in the elderly. JAMA 260:183, 1988.
Russell RM: Nutritional support of the long-term care patient. Part 1: Nutritional requirements of the elderly. Nutr Supp Serv 8(10):12, 1988.
Ryan AS et al: Dietary patterns of older adults in the U.S.: NHANES II 1976–1980. Am J Hum Biol 1:321, 1989.
Ryan VC and Bower ME: Relationship of socioeconomic status and living arrangements to nutritional intake of the older person. J Am Diet Assoc 89:1805, 1989.
Senile cataract and vitamin nutrition. Nutr Rev 47:326, 1989.
Sharma R: Theories of aging. *In* Timiras PS (ed): Physiological Basis of Geriatrics. New York, Macmillan, 1988.
Soltesz KS et al: Zinc nutriture and cell mediated immunity in institutionalized elderly. J Nutr Elderly 8:3, 1988.
Swanson CA et al: Zinc status of healthy elderly adults: Response to supplementation. Am J Clin Nutr 48:343, 1988.
Taylor A: Associations between nutrition and cataract. Nutr Rev 47:225, 1989.
Tramposch TS and Blue LS: A nutrition screening and assessment system for use with the elderly in extended care. J Am Diet Assoc 87:1207, 1987.
Walford RL, Harris SB, and Weindruch R: Dietary restriction and aging: Historical phases, mechanisms and current direction. J Nutr 117:1650, 1987.
Zheng JJ and Rosenberg IW: What is the nutritional status of the elderly? Geriatrics 44(6):57, 1989.

PART 3

NUTRITION FOR HEALTH AND FITNESS

The chapters in this section reflect the evolution of nutritional science, from the identification of nutrient requirements and the practical application of this knowledge to the more recent concepts that relate nutrition to the prevention of degenerative disease.

The relation of nutrition to dental disease has long been recognized. In more recent decades, the possibility for reducing the incidence of cancer, atherosclerotic heart disease, hypertension, and osteoporosis by emphasizing appropriate nutrition has continued to accumulate supportive evidence.

Government agencies have traditionally assumed responsibility for ensuring the safety of the food supply and for making adequate nutrients available to high-risk segments of the population. The Recommended Dietary Allowances have been a part of the nutrition scene for almost 50 years. However, the setting of nutritional goals appropriate to health and fitness and specifically to prevention of degenerative diseases is a new role for government that is not universally accepted by all members of the nutrition community.

The prevention, or at least postponement, of various degenerative diseases is closely associated with physical fitness and is achieved in part through exercise and control of body weight. The opportunities for an affluent society to choose from a great variety of foods easily leads to an overabundant intake of energy, and efforts to reduce body weight, widely pursued with varying degrees of enthusiasm and diligence, are seldom successful. Although the importance of exercise is widely recognized as a major goal in a fulfilling lifestyle, current statistics do not necessarily equate agreement with actual practice of this goal. Nonetheless, the contributions of appropriate nutrition to athletic performance and general fitness will continue to achieve recognition.

CHAPTER 15

NUTRITION IN THE COMMUNITY

CHAPTER OUTLINE

KEY TERMS

ACCEPTABLE DAILY INTAKE (ADI)—the amount of chemical that, if ingested daily over a lifetime, appears to be without appreciable risk

CONTINUING SURVEY OF FOOD INTAKE OF INDIVIDUALS (CSFII)—as part of the National Nutrition Monitoring System, the first nationwide dietary intake survey designed to be conducted annually

DELANEY CLAUSE—a clause of the Food Additive Amendment that prohibits the use of any substance shown to cause cancer in animals or humans

FOOD ADDITIVE—any material natural or synthetic, other than the basic raw ingredients, used in the production of a food item to enhance the final product in some way

FOOD-BORNE DISEASE—disease, usually gastrointestinal, caused by organisms or toxins produced by them carried in ingested food; often called food poisoning

FOOD IRRADIATION—the bombardment of food with sufficient radiation to destroy insects and microorganisms; used in food preservation

FOOD STAMP PROGRAM—a federal program established in 1964 with the purpose of providing more food buying power to low-income persons or families through monthly allotments of stamps made available at a cost that translates into reduced-price groceries

GENERALLY RECOGNIZED AS SAFE (GRAS)—descriptive of 675 ingredients that were not evaluated by the prescribed testing procedure and that were already in use when the 1959 Food Additives Amendment was enacted

NATIONAL SCHOOL LUNCH PROGRAM—a program started in 1946 that makes available surplus foods and cash reimbursement so that schools can provide a lunch that meets specified nutritional requirements

NATIONAL FOOD CONSUMPTION SURVEY (NFCS)—a survey conducted approximately every 10 years with the purpose of monitoring the nutrient intake of a cross-section of the U.S. public

NATIONAL HEALTH AND NUTRITION EXAMINATION SURVEY (NHANES)—a series of surveys that include information from medical history, physical measurements, biochemical evaluation, physical examination, and dietary intake of population groups within the United States

TOTAL DIET STUDY (MARKET BASKET SAMPLE)—analysis of 234 food items representing the diets of consumers and purchased throughout the United States for comparison with acceptable daily intakes

WIC—Special Supplemental Food Program for Women, Infants, and Children with the purpose of improving the nutritional status of pregnant and lactating women and children up to 5 years of age from low-income families

The nutrition of the individual reflects to some extent the nutrition of the community. The nutrition and general health of the community are influenced by agricultural and economic systems, the safety and availability of the food supply, the accessibility of health care, the provision of education, and the monitoring and regulatory influence of governments at the local, state, and federal levels.

NATIONAL FOOD AND NUTRITION DATA SOURCES

Nutrition programs rely on data from nutrition and health surveys to identify the needs of those to be served. Although an increasing number of states have begun to conduct their own assessments on a wide variety of issues, there is still a need for national statistics. Data from national surveys are used to monitor the dietary status of the population, assess the nutritional adequacy of the food supply, measure the economics of food consumption, evaluate the effects of food assistance and regulatory programs, and provide the basis for guidance to the public about food selection. Until the late 1960s, the only information about food and nutrient consumption at a national level was provided by the surveys conducted by the United States Department of Agriculture (USDA). Since then, the proliferation of increasingly sophisticated nutrition-oriented surveys testifies to the elevated interest and concern regarding national nutritional status that has taken place in the last 20 years (Tittle-Cross, 1987).

National Health and Nutrition Examination Surveys

The first National Health and Nutrition Examination Survey (NHANES) was conducted from 1971 to 1974 by the US Department of Health, Education, and Welfare (National Center for Health Statistics, 1977) (Table 15–1). This agency, renamed in 1980 as the Department of Health and Human Services (DHHS), has continued the NHANES surveys approximately every 5 years, with NHANES II, 1976 to 1980, Hispanic HANES, 1982 to 1984, and NHANES III, 1988 to 1994 (Carroll et al, 1983; Woteki et al, 1988). The Hispanic HANES included three Hispanic subgroups—Mexican Americans, Cubans, and Puerto Ricans—living in five southwestern states, Dade County, Florida, and New York City, respectively. Except for children aged 2 to 5 years, who showed a greater prevalence of low height for age than children of the same age in the general population, the results were not appreciably different from those found for the general population (Ryan and Roche, 1990). NHANES III will study 30,000 persons with a large proportion of persons age 65 years and older. Unique to this NHANES will be the fact that there will be no upper age limit, thus making it particularly useful for the study of aging related to nutritional issues.

TABLE 15–1. Recent Food, Nutrition, and Health Surveys

Name of Survey	Timing	Agency*	Purpose/Comments
Ten State Nutrition Survey	1968–1970	DHEW	To evaluate dietary intake, nutritional, and economic status
Preschool Nutrition	1968–1970	DHEW	To evaluate dietary intake, nutritional, and economic status in children 1–6 years, in 36 states
National Health and Nutrition Examination Survey (NHANES I)	1971–1974	DHEW	First nationwide health survey to include nutrition; ages 1–74 years included
NHANES II	1976–1980	DHEW	Ages 6 months to 74 years included
Hispanic HANES (HHANES)	1982–1984	DHHS	To remedy under-reporting of Hispanics
NHANES III	1988–1994	DHHS	Ages 2 months +; to monitor health and nutrition over time, especially in the elderly
Continuing Survey of Food Intakes by Individuals (CSFII)	1985–1986	USDA/HNIS	Women 19–50 years and their children; men 19–50 years
CSFII	1989+	USDA/HNIS	US + low-income sample included
Nationwide Food Consumption Survey	1987–1988; every 10 years	USDA	US + low-income sample included
Total Diet Study	Ongoing	DHHS/FDA	Specific age-sex groups; market basket sample
Food Disappearance Data	Annual	USDA	To monitor total available food used; waste not accounted for
Cholesterol Awareness Study	1986	DHHS/NIH	To assess cholesterol knowledge of consumers
Pregnancy and Infant Feeding Survey	1988–1989	DHHS/FDA	To assess feeding practices of pregnant women and infants
Coordinated State Surveillance System	Ongoing	DHHS/CDC	Pregnant women, children included

* Agencies: CDC = Centers for Disease Control; DHEW = Department of Health, Education and Welfare until 1980, then renamed DHHS; DHHS = Department of Health and Human Services; FDA = Food and Drug Administration; HNIS = Human Nutrition Information Service; NIH = National Institutes of Health; USDA = United States Department of Agriculture.

In addition to nutrient intake data, these surveys provide information on the health status of the nation. Survey data include (1) medical history, (2) physical measurements, (3) biochemical evaluation, (4) physical signs and symptoms, and (5) diet information from food frequency questionnaires and 24-hour recalls. Reports provide a health profile of the community with respect to blood pressures and prevalence of hypertension; cholesterol levels and cardiovascular risk factors; measurements of height and weight and prevalence of overweight and obesity; levels of energy and nutrient intakes and iron status and other hematologic data.

Nationwide Food Consumption Survey

The National Food Consumption Survey (NFCS) has been conducted by the USDA approximately every 10 years since 1935. It monitors the nutrient intake of a cross-section of the American public by collecting information on food consumption of households and selected individuals. As such, it is a resource of data on national food habits and trends. The 1977 survey collected data from 15,000 households in the conterminous United States during the spring of 1977 and from 38,000 individuals during the period from April 1977 through March 1978 (Pao et al, 1982). The most recent survey was conducted in 1987 and 1988. These and similar data are the basis of programs and publications prepared by the USDA for the education of the public (Peterkin et al, 1988).

Continuing Survey of Food Intake of Individuals

In 1985 to 1986 the Continuing Survey of Food Intake of Individuals (CSFII) was added as a part of the National Nutrition Monitoring System. It is the first nationwide dietary intake survey designed to be conducted annually. These surveys have collected data on women aged 19 to 50 and their children aged 1 to 5 (1985), a similar sample of low-income women and their children aged 1 to 5 (1986), and men aged 19 to 50 years (Joint Nutrition Monitoring Evaluation Committee . . . , 1986; USDA, 1985; Nutrition Monitoring Division, 1986, 1987, and 1989). Household data are determined by calculating the nutrient content of foods reported to be used in the home during the survey week and comparing the results with the Recommended Dietary Allowances (RDA) of nutrients for persons of the same age and sex as those in the households. Data from individuals in the NFCS are obtained from 3- or 4-day records plus a 24-hour recall, and in CSFII by a single 24-hour recall, either in person or by telephone. Figure 15–1 compares the average intake of energy from protein, carbohydrate, and fat for individuals in the United States, based on 1-day and 4-day samples collected in 1977 and in 1985.

National Nutrient Data Bank

The National Nutrient Data Bank is the United States' primary resource of information on the nutrient content of foods. The data come from private industry as well as academic and government laboratories. At present more than 800,000 records are stored and 6,000 to 9,000 additions are made monthly to this data bank. The information is summarized annually to develop values for the nutritional composition of thousands of foods and is representative of food across the United States.

NATIONAL NUTRITION GUIDELINES AND GOALS

Until relatively recently, most of the nutrition education materials available to the public were produced by the USDA. The first dietary guidance pamphlet, *Food*

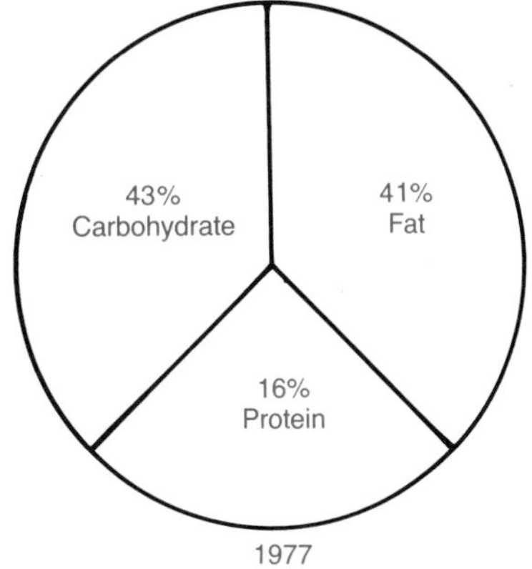

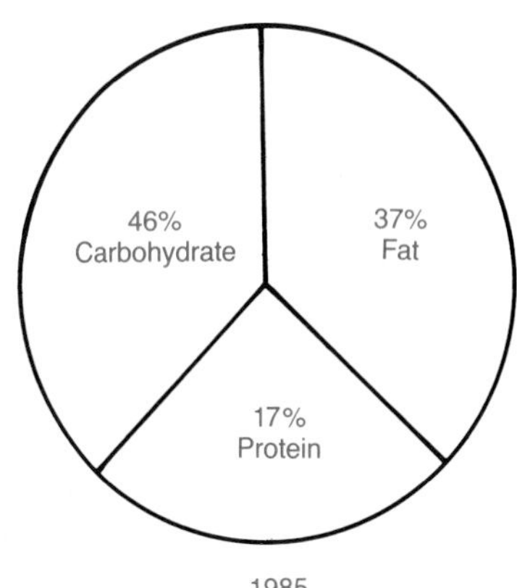

FIGURE 15–1. *A comparison of the average intake of energy from protein, carbohydrate, and fat for people in the United States in 1977 and 1985.*

For Young Children, was issued in 1916. The initial version of what eventually evolved into the Daily Food Guide based on food groups was published in 1917. It began with five food groups and evolved through seven groups to the familiar "Basic Four" groups in *Food For Fitness, A Daily Food Guide* (Haughton et al, 1987).

The Recommended Dietary Allowances were formulated in 1943 by the Food and Nutrition Board of the National Research Council, National Academy of Sciences (Food and Nutrition Board, 1989); they are discussed in detail in Chapter 16.

The first guidelines were based on achievement of optimal health through avoidance of nutrient deficiencies and on attainment of nutrient intakes as specified in the RDA; however, the distinct trend of more recent goals has been toward the prevention of nutrition-related disease (Ostenso, 1988). The Senate Select Committee on Nutrition and Human Needs presented the first *Dietary Goals for the United States* in 1977 (Senate Select Committee . . . , 1977 and 1978). In 1980 these were modified and issued jointly as *Dietary Guidelines for Americans* by the DHHS and the USDA, and revised again in 1985 and 1990 (Nutrition and Your Health, 1980 and 1990). Their emphasis on nutrient intakes and excesses reflects the increasing national concern regarding obesity, cancer, hypertension, and coronary artery disease. (The Dietary Guidelines are discussed in detail in Chapter 16.)

The first dietary guidelines based on a philosophy of preventive nutrition were formulated by the American Heart Association. Originally, these were directed toward persons at risk for hypertension and coronary artery disease; more recently, their recommendations have been extended to the general public. The National Cholesterol Education Program of the National Heart, Lung, and Blood Institute in 1987 provided specific guidelines for the identification and treatment of hypercholesterolemia (National Cholesterol Education Program, 1988). Following publication of Diet, Nutrition and Cancer (Committee on Diet, Nutrition and Cancer, 1982), the National Cancer Institute in 1988 issued the Dietary Guidelines for Cancer Prevention.

Table 15–2 lists some of the dietary reports that have influenced the development of guidelines or affected the manner in which health priorities are determined. As an example, publication of *Healthy People* (1979), the Surgeon General's first report on health promotion and disease prevention, eventually led to formulation of health objectives addressing specific issues in the priority areas identified.

Strategies for achieving the 1990 objectives were outlined in the Public Health Service publication *Promoting Health/Preventing Disease: Objectives for the Nation* (Miller and Stephenson, 1987; Promoting Health/Preventing Disease, 1980). A midcourse review of the 1990 objectives conducted in 1985 to 1986 indicated that some of the objectives were being met. These included development of a national nutrition monitor-

TABLE 15–2. History of Dietary Recommendations for the US Public

Publication	Year	Organization or Agency*	Recommendation
Food for Young Children	1916	USDA	First dietary guidance pamphlet
Food Guide	1917	USDA	5 food groups: flesh, starches, fats, watery fruits and vegetables, sweets
Food Guide	1933	USDA	12 food groups
RDA	1943	FNB/NAS	Recommended intakes for known nutrients
Food Guide	1946	USDA	"Basic 7" food groups
Food for Fitness (Daily food guide)	1958	USDA	"Basic 4" food groups based on RDA†
Dietary Goals for the US, 1st ed	1977	Senate Select Committee on Nutrition and Human Needs	First government publication to address macronutrient intake and excess
Dietary Goals for the US, 2nd ed	1978	Senate Select Committee on Nutrition and Human Needs	Refined recommendations of first edition
Nutrition and Your Health: Dietary Guidelines for Americans	1980	USDA/DHHS	Generic recommendations similar in content to the Dietary Goals without specified amounts
Toward Healthful Diets	1980	FNB/NAS	Similar to Guidelines and Goals except for fat recommendations
Various guidelines on nutrition	1980	AMA, AHA, NCI, American Society for Clinical Nutrition, NAS	Several organizations published similar recommendations
Diet, Nutrition, and Cancer	1982	Committee on Diet, Nutrition and Cancer, NRC, NAS	Dietary guidelines to reduce risk of cancer
Dietary Guidelines for Americans	1985	USDA/DHHS	2nd edition
National Cholesterol Education Program	1987	DHHS/NHLBI	Guidelines for cholesterol education
NCI Dietary Guidelines: Rationale	1988	DHHS/NCI	Recommendations to reduce risk of cancer
Nutrition and Your Health: Dietary Guidelines for Americans	1990	USDA/DHHS	3rd edition

* AHA = American Heart Association; AMA = American Medical Association; DHHS = Department of Health and Human Services; FNB = Food and Nutrition Board; NAS = National Academy of Sciences; NCI = National Cancer Institute; NHLBI = National Heart, Lung and Blood Institute; NRC = National Research Council; USDA = United States Department of Agriculture.

† RDA = Recommended Dietary Allowances; revised approximately every 5 years since 1943.

ing system, an increase in breast-feeding, and greater public knowledge of appropriate weight-loss strategies and dietary issues related to chronic disease.

The Surgeon General's Report on Nutrition and Health (The Surgeon . . . , 1988) includes comprehensive documentation of the scientific basis for the recommendations. The detailed report examines current knowledge of specific dietary practices and specific disease conditions and states the implications for the individual as well as for future public health policy decisions (Table 15–3).

FOOD ASSISTANCE AND NUTRITION PROGRAMS

The provision of guidelines and food selection information does not guarantee optimal nutrition without access to adequate food or money to buy food. An increasing variety of food and nutrition programs have become available to assist the consumer in obtaining a safe and wholesome food supply that is available continuously in adequate amounts. Over the years these programs have almost exclusively come from the USDA. Programs currently under the direction of that organization are listed in Table 15–4. A wide variety of health-related programs conducted by the DHHS also affect significantly the nutritional status of the population, from the newborn infant to the most elderly.

TABLE 15–3. Recommendations of The Surgeon General's Report on Nutrition and Health*

Issues for Most People:

- *Fats and cholesterol:* Reduce consumption of fat (especially saturated fat) and cholesterol. Choose foods relatively low in these substances, such as vegetables, fruits, whole grain foods, fish, poultry, lean meats, and low-fat dairy products. Use food preparation methods that add little or no fat.
- *Energy and weight control:* Achieve and maintain a desirable body weight. To do so, choose a dietary pattern in which energy (caloric) intake is consistent with energy expenditure. To reduce energy intake, limit consumption of foods relatively high in calories, fats, and sugars, and minimize alcohol consumption. Increase energy expenditure through regular and sustained physical activity.
- *Complex carbohydrates and fiber:* Increase consumption of whole grain foods and cereal products, vegetables (including dried beans and peas), and fruits.
- *Sodium:* Reduce intake of sodium by choosing foods relatively low in sodium and limiting the amount of salt added in food preparation and at the table.
- *Alcohol:* To reduce the risk for chronic disease, take alcohol only in moderation (no more than two drinks a day), if at all. Avoid drinking any alcohol before or while driving, operating machinery, taking medications, or engaging in any other activity requiring judgment. Avoid drinking alcohol while pregnant.

Other Issues for Some People:

- *Fluoride:* Community water systems should contain flouride at optimal levels for prevention of tooth decay. If such water is not available, use other appropriate sources of fluoride.
- *Sugars:* Those who are particularly vulnerable to dental caries (cavities), especially children, should limit their consumption and frequency of use of foods high in sugars.
- *Calcium:* Adolescent girls and adult women should increase consumption of foods high in calcium, including low-fat dairy products.
- *Iron:* Children, adolescents, and women of childbearing age should be sure to consume foods that are good sources of iron, such as lean meats, fish, certain beans, and iron-enriched cereals and whole grain products. This issue is of special concern for low-income families.

* From The Surgeon General's Report on Nutrition and Health—Summary and Recommendations. USDHHS (PHS) Publ 88-50211. Washington, DC, US Govt. Printing Office, 1988.

Among some of the landmark programs are the National School Lunch Program, the Special Supplemental Food Program for Women, Infants, and Children (WIC), and the Food Stamp Program.

National School Lunch Program

The feeding of children in the schools began to a limited degree in the early 1900s at the time when free, compulsory, and universal education was established. The first widely scattered efforts were conducted by philanthropic organizations, local school districts, and private individuals, and some of these organizations began as early as 1853. States and municipalities gradually expanded the number of feeding programs with increasing federal involvement, primarily in the form of donations from the accumulation of surplus foods. Legislation establishing the National School Lunch Program under the direction of the USDA was passed in 1946. Under the program, federal cash reimbursement and donated foods are provided to schools that serve a lunch meeting specified nutritional requirements. Modifications in 1971 specified that children from families with incomes at the poverty level must be provided a free or reduced-price lunch.

Special Supplemental Food Program for Women, Infants, and Children

The WIC program, also administered by the USDA, was established in 1974 for the purpose of improving the nutritional status of pregnant and lactating women and children up to 5 years of age from low-income families. The program involves cash grants to state health departments and comparable agencies that make available supplemental foods through participating health clinics. (See Chapter 9 for further discussion.)

Food Stamp Program

The Food Stamp Program was established in 1964 to supplement the food-buying power of needy individuals and families in a manner permitting freedom of choice. Monthly allotments of food stamps to be used for food purchase are made available at a cost that translates into reduced-price groceries. Bonus stamps are pro-

TABLE 15–4. Food Programs Administered by USDA

Program and Year Started	Eligible Individuals or Groups	Objectives of Program	Components of Program
Food Distribution Program (Donable Foods), 1930s	Supplemental food programs for mothers and infants. Elderly feeding programs. Schools and institutions.	To distribute surplus food to individuals and institutions to help agricultural support program.	Distribution of surplus food. Previously, to needy families but at present, only to eligible schools, institutions, and persons in US Trust Territories.
National School Lunch Program (NSLP), 1946	All children enrolled at participating schools, residential child care institutions, including homes for developmentally disabled up to 21 years of age, juvenile detention centers, and orphanages.	To provide a nutritious lunch (one that has as its objective to provide one third of the RDA* for a child) at a reasonable cost to school children. To provide reduced-price or free lunches to needy eligible children.	Donated food to participating schools. Federal monetary support.
Food Stamp Program, 1964	Needy families and individuals in participating counties (almost all counties).	To supplement an individual's or a family's food-buying power.	Limited monthly allotment of food stamps at a reduced price, depending upon income. Stamps are used to pay for food.
Child Care Food Program (CCFP), 1968	Preschool children in nonprofit facilities such as day care centers, Head Start centers and family day care homes.	To provide meal service for children in full-time day care centers and Head Start Programs and after-school care programs.	Federal monetary support. Cash in lieu of commodities available.
Special Milk Program†, 1968	Schools, child care centers, summer camps, and institutions.	To reduce the cost of milk to children or provide it free to children who are also eligible for free meals.	Federal reimbursement to schools or centers for all or part of the cost of the milk served.
Summer Food Service Program for Children, 1968	Public agency sponsored programs for preschool and school-age children in schools, recreation centers and summer camps, and during vacations in areas with a continuous school calendar.	To provide free lunches to children in summer programs.	Federal monetary support.
School Breakfast Program, 1973	All children enrolled in participating schools.	To provide a nutritious breakfast at a low cost to children.	Donated food to participating schools. Federal monetary support.
Supplemental Food Program for Women, Infants, and Children (WIC), 1974	Pregnant and lactating women and infants and children up to 5 years of age who are judged to be at nutritional risk because of inadequate nutrition or income.	To improve the nutritional status of pregnant and lactating women and children up to 5 years of age in low-income areas.	Cash grants to state health departments and comparable agencies who make available supplemental foods through participating health clinics. Health clinics provide specified nutritious food supplements or vouchers for these foods. Regular health examination of the mother and the children required.

* RDA = Recommended Dietary Allowances.
† If a school is on the School Lunch Program, it cannot receive the Special Milk Program and vice versa.

vided free to purchasers of food stamps under specified circumstances.

FOOD SAFETY: LAWS, REGULATIONS, AND ISSUES

Technology and Food Safety

Many changes have been made in the food supply since the days when the chores of gathering, hunting, storing, and growing food resided with those who consumed the results of their efforts. The first methods of storing foods were developed to ensure seasonal supplies as well as to protect against periods of famine. Increasingly sophisticated methods of processing have gradually made a variety of foods widely available and have not only freed large parts of the world from the threat of starvation but also removed the necessity of living close to the food supply. Release from the continuous obligation to produce food has made it possible for people to pursue other efforts that benefit themselves and society. The availability of a wide variety of processed foods has facilitated increased participation of women in the work force.

These legacies of technology have not been without a price. As human societies continued to grow in size and in areas of specialization, the consumer lost control over the direct production of foodstuffs, becoming vulnerable to the sometimes unethical provider. Guilds or fellow merchants at first regulated their own professions to ensure protection for the consumer; however, most societies soon grew too large to allow the various professions to regulate themselves. As contamination, adulteration, and false advertising of foods became increasingly common, governments were forced to regulate the producers and providers of foodstuffs. Table 15–5 summarizes the U.S. history of food regulation in this century.

Regulatory Agencies

A number of government agencies share responsibility for the safety and honest marketing of the food supply in the United States. The *Food and Drug Administration* (FDA) is authorized by the Food, Drug, and Cosmetic Act to establish standards of acceptable intake of additives and contaminants in foods and to monitor pesticide levels in commodities in intrastate shipment. The FDA also regulates labeling of packaged foods (see Chapter 16). The *Environmental Protection Agency* (EPA) establishes tolerances and approves pesticides for use. The *USDA* is responsible for the wholesomeness of meats and poultry, and the *Federal Trade Commission* (FTC) and *Federal Communications Commission* (FCC) regulate advertising and marketing.

Safety Concerns

Continuing changes in the food supply with respect to both content and manner of use introduce new safety concerns. Microwave use poses problems with migration of chemicals from packaging materials as well as inadequate pathogen destruction because of irregular

TABLE 15–5. History of Laws and Rules Regulating Food Safety and Quality in the United States

Name of Act and Date Passed	Content of Legislation
Wiley Act or "pure food and drug law." Passed 1906. The act itself was repealed 1938, but not some of amendments.	"An act for preventing the manufacture, sale or transportation of adulterated or misbranded or poisonous or deleterious foods, drugs, medicines and liquors, and for other purposes."
Meat Inspection Act, passed 1907.	Requires that "all meat and meat food products in interstate commerce be prepared under the supervision of the USDA."
Weight and Measure Amendment to Wiley Act, passed 1913.	Clarifies rules about stating the quantity of the contents of packaged foods.
Kenyon Amendment to Wiley Act, passed 1919.	Extends the weight and measure amendment to cover packaged meats.
McNary-Napes Amendment to Wiley Act, passed 1930.	Authorizes the USDA to establish minimum standards for the quality, condition, and amounts of foods in containers, to be required of all canned foods except meat and milk.
Seafood Inspection Amendment to the Wiley Act, passed 1935.	Authorizes the USDA "to provide government inspection of the packaging of any seafood which might enter into interstate commerce" for those packers desiring such inspection service.
Food, Drug and Cosmetic Act, passed 1938.	Authorizes the Food and Drug Administration (FDA) to carry out the intent of Congress to ensure that foods are safe, pure, and wholesome, are made or processed under sanitary conditions, and are honestly labeled and packaged; to carry on research and public education; to set regulations governing the definitions and standards of identity of foods, containers, and labeling; and to promote honesty and fair dealing in the interest of the consumer. Standards of identity to be obtained from the FDA free of charge. Minimum standards of quality were set for tenderness, color, and freedom from defects. Standards for enrichment were set. Products labeled "enriched" or "fortified" must contain the exact specified amount of added nutrients.
Miller Pesticide Amendment, passed 1954.	Establishes acceptable or relatively harmless levels for pesticide and chemical residues on raw agricultural commodities. The applicant must demonstrate the "usefulness" of a pesticide to the USDA's satisfaction and its "safety" to the FDA before its use.
Poultry Products Inspection Act, passed 1956.	Makes continuous inspection compulsory for fresh, frozen, ready-to-eat, and canned poultry products. Labeling regulations were established for poultry products and enforcement powers were given to the USDA.
Food Additives Amendment to the Food, Drug and Cosmetic Act, passed 1958.	Requires that the safety of chemicals used in processing be proved by industry to be safe before being sold for use in foods. Previously the government was responsible for proving a chemical unsafe *after* it was on the market, often requiring court action for removal. Chemicals in use prior to 1959 were considered Generally Recognized as Safe (GRAS) and use was allowed to continue. The Delaney Clause prohibits the use of any food additive found to produce cancer when ingested in any amount by test animals of any species.
Color Additive Amendment to the Food, Drug and Cosmetic Act, passed 1960.	Requires manufacturers to prove that their color additives are safe, and authorizes the FDA to establish and enforce tolerances for the use of color additives in foods, drugs, and cosmetics.
Fair Packaging and Labeling Act, passed 1967.	Requires prominent labels on packaged foods and the following information: (1) Statement of the food's identity must appear on the principal display panel in bold type. (2) Name and address of manufacturer, packer, and distributor must be conspicuously stated. (3) Statement of the net contents must appear in concise standard measure. No qualifying terms such as "giant quart" may appear. (4) Statement listing ingredients, when required, must appear in type of legible size on a single panel of the label. The common names of the ingredients must appear in decreasing order of predominance. These regulations include proposals for special diet foods, with particular reference to vitamin and mineral supplementation and low-calorie foods.

heating. Foods such as baked potatoes and garlic oils, not previously considered sources of food-borne illness, have led to episodes of botulism. The use of irradiation as a mode of food preservation and the areas of hormonal manipulation and bioengineering have prompted consumer concerns regarding safety. Potential problems associated with the trend toward ultrafortified foods include the possibility of toxicity and the bioavailability of the nutrients used (Greger, 1987).

Concerns about food safety are shared by both the regulatory agencies and the public, although the emphasis tends to be very different. The public worries about food additives and the residues from agricultural use of pesticides, antibiotics, and hormones (Further Reading, p. 269). However, in terms of measurable risk of illness, these actually rank low on a list that begins with microbial contamination and also includes the presence of natural toxicants in food (Table 15–6).

Microbial Contamination

Microbial contamination of food is a leading cause of illness; in addition, it can cause disability and even death. Figure 15–2 lists the most common bacterial causes of the estimated 6.4 million cases of food-borne diseases that occur annually in the United States (Archer and Young, 1988). For reasons not well understood, the incidence of enteric illness appears to be increasing. The largest salmonella outbreak in history occurred in 1985 (Ryan et al, 1987). Changing food choices that encourage consumption of more raw or partially cooked foods may be involved, as well as new methods of food preparation. For example, *Clostridium botulinum* toxin has developed in baked potatoes tightly wrapped in foil and allowed to stand for an extended period of time (Sugiyama et al, 1981).

In addition to *Salmonella, Shigella,* and *Staphylococcus,* all of which have long been recognized as major causes of food poisoning, other bacteria are now emerging as perhaps even greater threats. *Campylobacter* is considered the most frequent cause of bacterial diarrhea in the United States (Doyle, 1985). *Listeria monocytogenes* in Mexican-style soft cheese in 1985 resulted in the largest number of confirmed food-associated deaths in recent history (USDHHS, 1985).

Foods most commonly implicated in bacterial diarrhea in the United States are raw milk and undercooked poultry. Meats, dairy products, and eggs are common sources of food-borne contamination (Fig. 15–3). Transmission usually occurs through improper food handling, in which infectious organisms are introduced into foods by those responsible for preparation, either commercially or at home. Cross-contamination also occurs when pathogens from raw meat or poultry are transferred via a cutting board or utensil to other food products prepared at the same site. Although external contamination of eggs with *Salmonella* organisms has been recognized for some time, recently identified internal contamination with *S. enteritidis* suggests the route of transovarian contamination (St. Louis et al, 1988).

Symptoms of enteric disease are primarily diarrhea and vomiting; however, they may also include fever, abdominal cramps, nausea, and flatulence. Episodes of food poisoning are often misidentified as "24-hour flu" and tend to be regarded for the most part as an uncomfortable nuisance. However, these have become a matter of more concern with the knowledge that it is possible for bacteria to translocate from the gut to the blood stream, with the potential sequelae of rheumatoid conditions, especially rheumatoid arthritis, as well as renal diseases and nutritional and other malabsorptive disorders (Cohen et al, 1987).

Natural Toxicants in Food

Toxicants occurring naturally in foods are not subject to regulatory control, and many would not receive approval if they were proposed as food additives at the levels in which they occur. Some are actually carcino-

TABLE 15–6. Compounds of Toxic Capability Found in Naturally Occurring Substances*

Toxin	Food Source	Primary Toxic Effect
Hemagglutinins	Several varieties of beans	Agglutination of red blood cells
Goitrogens†	Cabbage, kale, broccoli, other brassicae	Hypothyroidism (goiter)
Hydrogen cyanide†	Kernels of stone fruits, several varieties of beans, cassava	Cyanide poisoning
Pressor amines	Bananas, pineapple, aged cheeses, wine, chocolate	Increased blood pressure
Oxalates	Spinach, rhubarb, many others	Corrosive gastroenteritis, shock, death
Myristicin	Nutmeg, parsley, carrots	Hallucinations
Falcaranol	Carrots	Neurotoxicity
Aspergillus flavus (aflatoxin)	Corn, figs, grain, sorghum, cotton seed, certain tree nuts, peanuts	Liver carcinogen
Solanine	Skin of green potatoes, sprouts on "eyes" of potatoes	Interferes with transmission of nerve impulses
Ochratoxin	Barley, corn	Nephrotoxicity

* Data from Rodricks J: Food hazards of natural origin. Fed Proc 37:2587, 1978; Larkin T: Natural poisons in food. FDA Consumer. HEW Publ. No. (FDA) 76-2009, 1975.

† Not present in plants, but formed enzymatically from nontoxic precursors during processing or ingestion.

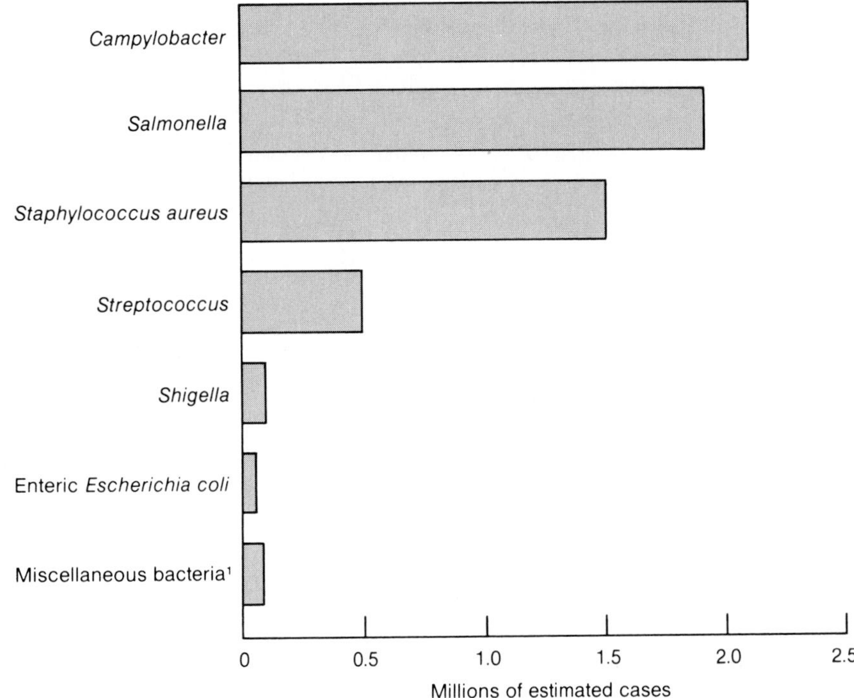

FIGURE 15–2. *Common bacterial causes of foodborne diseases. (Redrawn from Foodborne Disease. National Food Review 12[3]:52, 1989.)*

gens and would not be allowed in any amount. For example, the use of safrole, a flavoring agent from the sassafras root, is not permitted as a food additive because of its association with liver cancer; however, it is naturally present in small amounts in a number of spices normally consumed. Potatoes contain 150 chemicals, including oxalic acid (interferes with bodily absorption of calcium), solanine (an alkaloid that interferes with the transmission of nerve impulses), arsenic, and nitrates (may be converted to nitrites, which are carcinogens). Nitrates and nitrites occur naturally in green leafy vegetables and can be synthesized in the human intestine by bacteria.

Aflatoxin, a known carcinogen of high potency, is the product of a mold that occurs on peanuts and cereal grains, particularly in climates of high temperature and humidity. Herbal teas contain a number of potentially harmful substances; some of them, such as the alkaloid symphytine in comfrey tea, are carcinogens. Fortunately, none of these occur in amounts that would be harmful at normal levels of use.

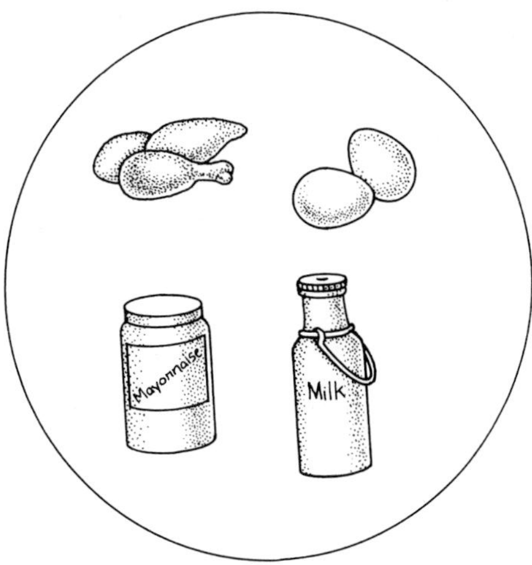

FIGURE 15–3. *Common vectors for foodborne contamination through which infectious organisms like* Salmonella, Shigella, Staphylococcus, *and* Campylobacter *are transmitted to foods.*

Intentional Additives

Food additives are widely used in food processing to improve product quality in a variety of ways (Table 15–7).

APPROVAL PROCEDURE. The 1958 Food Additives Amendment to the Food, Drug and Cosmetic Act speci-

TABLE 15–7. Functions and Uses of Common Food Additives

Functions	Additives Used	Examples of Foods in Which Additives Are Used
To improve nutritional value of certain foods	Thiamin, riboflavin, niacin, iron, vitamin A, vitamin D, ascorbic acid, potassium iodide	Wheat, flour, bread, rolls, biscuits, breakfast cereals, macaroni and noodle products, cornmeal, margarine, milk, iodized salt
To maintain appearance, palatability, and wholesomeness in certain foods (delaying undesirable changes in food caused by oxidation or microbial growth; preventing food spoilage caused by molds, bacteria, yeast)	Propionic acid, calcium and sodium salts of propionic acid, ascorbic acid, butylated hydroxyanisole (BHA), butylated hydroxytoluene (BHT), propylene glycol	Bread, pie filling, cake mixes, potato chips, crackers, cheese, syrup, fruit juices, frozen and dried fruits, margarine, shortenings, lard
To enhance flavor of certain foods	Spices (cloves, ginger, cinnamon, etc.), citrus oils, amyl acetate, carvone, benzaldehyde, monosodium glutamate, vanilla	Spice cake, gingerbread, ice cream, candy, carbonated beverages, fruit-flavored gelatins, toppings, sausage
To give characteristic color to certain foods	Annatto, carotene, cochineal, chlorophyll nitrates	Baked goods, candy, carbonated beverages, cheese, margarine, ice cream, jams, jellies, meat products
To maintain desired consistency in foods (emulsifiers and stabilizers)	Lecithin, mono- and diglycerides, gum arabic, carboxymethyl cellulose, carrageenan	Bakery products, cake mixes, salad dressings, frozen desserts, ice cream, chocolate milk, candy, beer
To control acidity or alkalinity in certain foods (leavening and neutralizing agents)	Potassium acid tartrate, tartaric acid, sodium bicarbonate, lactic acid, citric acid, adipic acid, fumaric acid	Cakes, cookies, biscuits, crackers, waffles, muffins, butter, processed cheese, cheese spreads, chocolates, carbonated beverages, confectionery
To serve as maturing and bleaching agents	Chlorine dioxide, chlorine, potassium bromate and iodate	Wheat flour (to make it white), certain cheeses
To help retain moisture (humectants), prevent caking, or act as curing agents	Glycerin, magnesium carbonate, sodium nitrate, calcium phosphate	Coconut, marshmallows, table salt, garlic and onion powder, frankfurters, sausages, dietetic foods

fied the responsibility of prior proof of safety by manufacturers seeking approval of new food additives. The required demonstrations include tests at three different levels: (1) acute toxicity tests to show the effects of a single dose given to a variety of laboratory animals; (2) short-term (90-day) toxicity studies showing the effects of feeding different concentrations to two kinds of laboratory animals; and (3) long-term toxicity studies of 2 years or more to show the effects of lifetime consumption. Approved tolerances are based on the level at which no adverse effects can be demonstrated in the test animals in long-term studies. The margin of safety is very wide—usually 1/100 to 1/1,000 of the "no effect level"—to provide for unknown differences in human and animal response and for individuals who may be more susceptible to a particular substance.

FOODS GENERALLY RECOGNIZED AS SAFE. At the time the Food Additives Amendment was enacted, some 675 ingredients not evaluated by the prescribed testing procedures were classified as generally recognized as safe (GRAS). This list includes commonly used substances, such as salt, sugar, and seasonings. Many of the items are forms of artificial flavorings. A continuing review of the entire GRAS list has resulted in the removal of some items and the specification of acceptable levels of others.

THE DELANEY CLAUSE. The Delaney Clause of the Food Additives Amendment prohibits the use in any amount of any substance shown to cause cancer in animals or humans. When the bill was introduced in 1958, substances could be detected in 100 parts per billion (ppb); anything less was considered equal to zero. Improvements in technology now permit detection of some substances in parts per trillion. Accordingly the FDA in 1986 initiated a policy based on the doctrine of *de minimis,* which holds that the law does not concern itself with trifling matters and that courts should not apply literally the terms of a statute to mandate pointless results (Curran, 1988). Under this doctrine, if a food additive or any of its metabolites or breakdown products increases the chance of developing cancer over a lifetime by less than one case per million cases of cancer, the threat is considered too small to be of concern.

Proponents of the policy hold that risks must be put into proper perspective and that the benefits of additives in improving quality, availability, and convenience of modern foods are worth what is considered to be a negligible risk. Furthermore, many toxicants and even carcinogens occur naturally in foods at levels many orders of magnitude higher than the levels approved for use by the FDA. Use of the de minimis policy has been challenged and is currently being argued in the courts.

FOOD IRRADIATION. A recent addition to the techniques available for preserving food is the process of irradiation, which for the purposes of establishing

FURTHER READING: Is It Really Organic?

The popularity of organic foods has increased in recent years, in part reflecting environmental concerns as well as response to media and other pressures that have erroneously fostered lack of trust in the safety of the food supply.

Although *organic* is a somewhat ambiguous term, in general it is understood to describe fruits and vegetables grown without the use of chemical fertilizers, herbicides, and pesticides.

It is very difficult to find produce that is absolutely free of pesticides, because traces linger in the soil and contamination from neighboring fields is common. Some states have established specific definitions governing use of the term *organic,* including in some cases the length of time that must pass since the last application of chemicals to a particular field. Most states have no laws regulating use of the term (Is organic . . . , 1989).

The absence of adequate definition and regulation leaves the consumer without any guarantee that the produce marked *organic* is truly free of chemical additives common to modern agriculture. The grocery shopper may also be at the mercy of unscrupulous dealers who can easily substitute non-organically grown produce without detection.

Although organically grown foods may provide psychological benefits to the user that justify the increased cost (from 20 to 100% above conventionally grown varieties), they fail to demonstrate advantages in taste, safety, or nutritive value. Pesticide residues exceed safe and acceptable levels in only 0.1% of conventionally grown foods, and then by very small margins. Organic fertilizers, on the other hand, may be a source of pathogenic bacteria. A legitimate concern of those who oppose the overuse of "chemical" fertilizers is contamination of ground water; however, studies have shown that this is not a significant problem to date.

safety has been classified by the FDA as a "food additive." This involves bombarding foodstuffs with ionizing radiation of sufficient energy to destroy insects and microorganisms to a degree that is related to the intensity of the radiation process. Irradiation-sterilized foods are currently in use by the United States Army as well as astronauts and some hospital patients confined to special sterilized environments, such as some transplant patients.

Lower doses of radiation that are less damaging to flavor in some foods are used to delay spoilage in highly perishable foods such as fish and shellfish, extend shelf life, delay mold growth, delay sprouting, destroy insects, reduce the number of microorganisms in spices, and destroy parasites and some types of disease-causing bacteria such as the salmonella that infest poultry. Irradiation can also replace the use of some fumigants and insecticides to destroy insects in grains and other stored foods.

Food irradiation has been approved by the World Health Organization and currently more than 30 countries have approved some form of use. Although irradiation has been in the development stage since the early 1950s, it was only recently approved for use in the United States. Because the FDA elected to classify irradiation as a food additive, individual foods subjected to this process are required to undergo the same rigorous testing procedures specified for all food additives. Final rules published in 1986 include a requirement of declaration on retail food labels of irradiated foods, with the exception of processed foods containing small quantities of irradiated ingredients (American Council on Science and Health, 1988).

Irradiation at the relatively low dosages used in food processing does not cause foods to become radioactive. Some "radiolytic" end-products are formed as a result of exposure to the ionizing radiation; however, extensive study of these products has failed to find any that differ from similar products formed in foods as the result of commonly used cooking methods employing high temperatures, such as frying, roasting, and baking (American Council on Science and Health, 1988; Hall, 1984).

PUBLIC ATTITUDES. The American public nurtures an ambivalence toward what is acceptable in terms of health risks from the food supply. In one incident in 1989, misleading information about pesticide residues prompted rejection of all apples and apple products from entire school districts. A very different response developed in 1977 when the FDA proposed a ban on saccharin, as required by the Delaney Amendment, when Canadian researchers found that this artificial sweetener caused urinary bladder cancer in animals. The public outcry was so great that Congress declared a moratorium on the ban that continues to be extended.

It is possible that many substances currently considered safe are carcinogenic when administered in massive doses to susceptible laboratory animals. The question becomes one of risks versus benefits.

Agricultural Residues

PESTICIDES

Tolerances and Risk Assessment. The EPA approves the use of and establishes tolerances for pesticides at both the commodity/field level and the processed food level. The FDA monitors and enforces the tolerances.

To obtain approval of a particular pesticide, the manufacturer must supply the EPA with data from toxicologic studies, residue data, and justification of use in terms of economics and an adequate food supply. A risk-benefit analysis leads to rejection or acceptance and establishment of a legal tolerance. Approval is granted only for the specific commodity application requested. For example, a chemical approved for use on lettuce would be considered in violation if used on cabbage or any other food. Unfortunately, tolerances are frequently sources of consumer concern when they are misinterpreted to mean the levels of residue that may be expected in the marketplace.

Surveillance Sampling. The FDA is responsible for surveillance of both imported and domestic foods (Fig. 15–4). When possible, samples are collected close to the point of production so that crops in violation of tolerances can be intercepted and destroyed. Of the more than 14,000 samples examined in 1987, more than half contained no detectable residues, and except for the less than 1% in violation of regulatory limits, the remainder contained residue at low levels. Most of these violations were in the category of use in food crops in which tolerances had not been established for a particular pesticide/ commodity combination.

Total Diet Study (Market Basket Sample). The FDA also routinely surveys table-ready foods. Four times each year, 234 food items representing the diets of American consumers are purchased in different cities around the United States. These are prepared as they would be in the home, and then analyzed for actual levels of pesticides, industrial chemicals, heavy metals, radionuclides, and essential minerals. The intakes for eight age-sex groups are compared with the acceptable daily intakes (ADI) as established by the Food and Agriculture Organization/World Health Organization of the United Nations. (The *ADI* is the *acceptable daily intake* of a chemical that, if ingested over a lifetime, appears to be without appreciable risk.) Twenty-five years of data have reported levels of pesticide residue consistently lower than the ADI. Actual pesticide intakes as determined by the Total Diet Studies are usually considerably lower than the ADI (Table 15–8).

ANTIBIOTICS. Subtherapeutic use of antibiotics to improve growth in food animals has been a matter of consumer concern because of the potential for development of resistant strains of bacteria. However, in response to a request to establish levels of risk for antibiotic use, the Institute of Medicine of the National

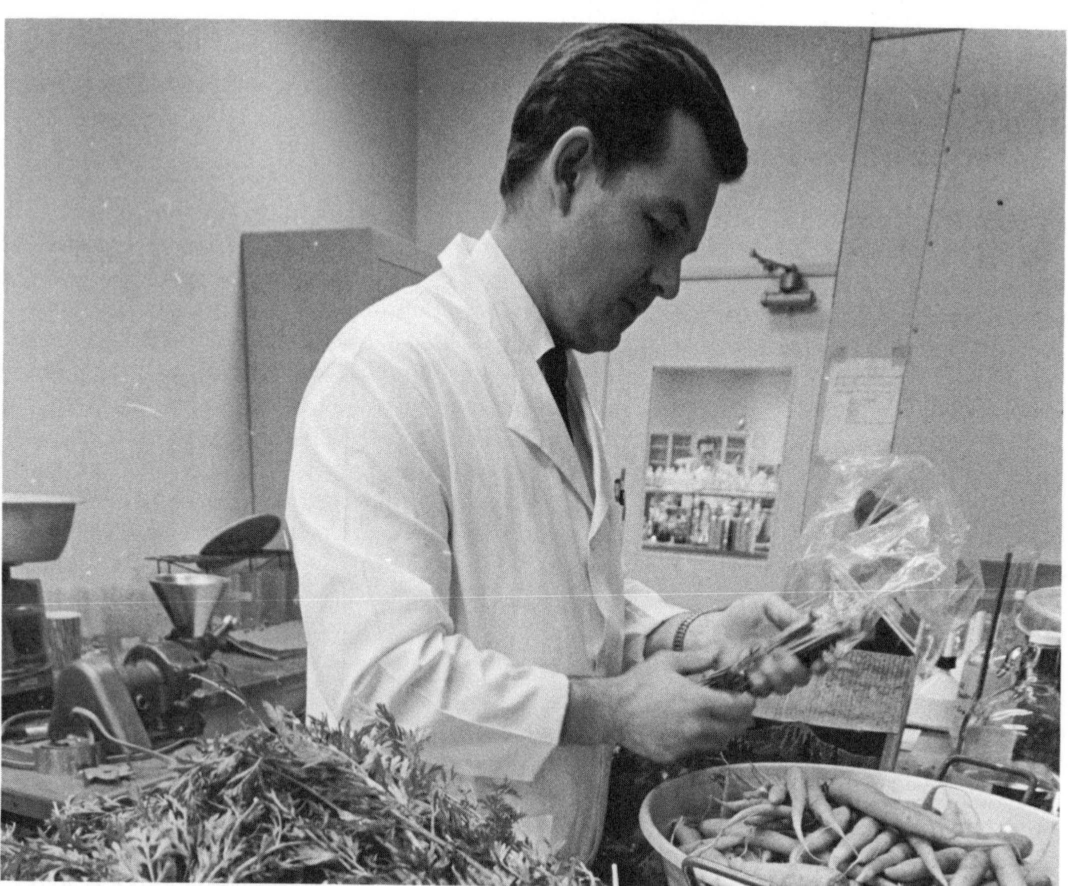

FIGURE 15–4. *The FDA monitors and enforces tolerances for residue levels of pesticides.*

TABLE 15-8. Selected Pesticide Intakes (μg/kg body weight/day) Found in Total Diet Analyses in 1987*

Pesticide	FAO/WHO ADI†	Intake		
		6-11 months	14-16 yr M‡	60-65 yr F§
Captan	100	0.0194	0.0088	0.0244
Carbaryl	10	0.1550	0.0173	0.0227
Dimethoate	10	0.0092	0.0009	0.0024
Malathion	20	0.1395	0.1193	0.0710
Methamidophos	0.6	0.0092	0.0087	0.0215
Parathion	5	0.0062	0.0007	0.0016

* From Food and Drug Administration Pesticide Program: Residues in Foods—1987. J Assn Official Analyt Chemists 71 (Nov/Dec), 1988.

† FAO/WHO = Food and Agriculture Organization/World Health Organization; ADI = Acceptable Daily Intake, usually expressed as mg/kg body weight/day but expressed here as μg/kg body weight/day for ease of comparison.

‡ M = male.

§ F = female.

Academy of Sciences reported in 1989 that it had been unable to find data implicating subtherapeutic antibiotics in human illness and was unable to formulate a numeric definition of risk. Except for penicillin and tetracycline, antibiotics presently added to animal feeds are not prescribed for human use.

HORMONES. The use of hormones in cattle feed has also been a source of concern for consumers. The use of such additives is permitted when residues do not occur in meat and milk as they arrive at the marketplace. The use of the estrogen diethylstilbestrol (DES) was discontinued when the increased precision of analytic techniques enabled the identification of extremely small amounts in some meat products. Use of bovine growth hormone (somatotropin or gonadotropin) has resulted in significant increases in milk (20 to 40%) and meat (10 to 20%) production. Growth hormones from other species are inactive in humans. In addition, because of its protein nature, this hormone is inactivated and digested by enzymes in the stomach.

CITED REFERENCES

American Council on Science and Health: Irradiated Foods. New York, American Council on Science and Health, 1988.

Archer DL and Young FE: Contemporary issues: Diseases with a food vector. Clin Microbiol Rev 1:377, 1988.

Carroll MD, Abraham S, and Diesser CM: Dietary Intake Source Data: United States, 1976-80. Vital and Health Statistics, Series 11, No. 231 (DHHS Publ No (PHS) 83-1681) Hyattsville, MD, National Center for Health Statistics, Public Health Service, USDHHS, 1983.

Cohen JI, Bartlett JA, and Corey GR: Extra-intestinal manifestations of *Salmonella* infections. Medicine (Baltimore) 66:349, 1987.

Committee on Diet, Nutrition and Cancer, National Research Council: Diet, Nutrition and Cancer. Washington, DC, National Academy Press, 1982.

Curran WJ: Cancer-causing substances in food, drugs, and cosmetics: The "de minimis" rule versus the Delaney Clause. N Engl J Med 319:1262, 1988.

Doyle MP: Food-borne pathogens of recent concern. Annu Rev Nutr 5:25, 1985.

Food and Nutrition Board, National Research Council, NAS: Recommended Dietary Allowances, 10th ed. Washington, DC, National Academy Press, 1989.

Greger JL: Food, supplements, and fortified foods: Scientific evaluations in regard to toxicology and nutrient bioavailability. J Am Diet Assoc 87:1369, 1987.

Hall RL: The ripple of the future. Nutrition Today 19(4):12, 1984.

Haughton B, Gussow JD, and Dodds JM: An historical study of the underlying assumptions for U.S. food guides from 1917 through the Basic Four Food Group Guide. J Nutr Educ 19:169, 1987.

Healthy People. The Surgeon General's Report on Health Promotion and Disease Prevention. Washington, DC, USDHHS, Public Health Service, 1979.

Is organic the way to go? Tufts Univ Diet and Nutr Letter 6(11):1, 1989.

Joint Nutrition Monitoring Evaluation Committee Report—May, 1986: Nutritional status of the U.S. population. Nutrition Today 21(3):23, 1986.

Miller SA and Stephenson MG: The 1990 National Nutrition Objectives: Lessons for the future. 87:1665, 1987.

National Center for Health Statistics: Health and Nutrition Examination Survey, 1971-74. Vital and Health Statistics, Series II, No 202 (DHEW Publ No [HRA] 77-1647). Rockville, MD, Health Resources Administration, Public Health Service, 1977.

National Cholesterol Education Program: Report of the Expert Panel on Detection, Evaluation, and Treatment of High Blood Cholesterol in Adults. NIH Publ No 88-2925, NHLBI, USDHHS, Public Health Service, Bethesda, MD, National Institutes of Health, 1988.

Nutrition and Your Health. Dietary Guidelines for Americans. Home and Garden Bulletin No 232. Washington, DC, USDA and USDHHS, 1980.

Nutrition and Your Health. Dietary Guidelines for Americans, 3rd ed. Home and Garden Bulletin No 232. Washington, DC, USDA and USDHHS, 1990.

Nutrition Monitoring Division, Human Nutrition Information Service: USDA Nationwide Food Consumption Survey: Continuing Survey of Food Intakes by Individuals—1985. Nutrition Today 21(3):18, 1986.

Nutrition Monitoring Division, Human Nutrition Information Service: USDA Nationwide Food Consumption Survey: Continuing Survey of Food Intakes by Individuals—1986, Nutrition Today 22(5):36, 1987.

Nutrition Monitoring Division, Human Nutrition Information Service: USDA Nationwide Food Consumption Survey: Continuing survey of food intakes by individuals—1986. Nutrition Today 24(5):35, 1989.

Ostenso G: Nutrition—policies and politics. J Am Diet Assoc 88:833, 1988.

Pao EM et al: Foods Commonly Eaten by Individuals: Amount Per Day and Per Eating Occasion. Home Economics Research Report No 44, Human Nutrition Information Service. Hyattsville, MD, USDA, 1982.

Peterkin BB, Rizek RL, and Tippett KS: Nationwide Food Consumption Survey, 1987. Nutrition Today 23(1):18, 1988.

Promoting Health/Preventing Disease: Objectives for the Nation. Washington, DC, USDHHS, 1980.

Ryan AS and Roche AF (eds): Growth of Mexican-American Children: Data from the Hispanic Health and Nutrition Examination Survey (1982–1984). Proceedings of a Symposium, April 7, 1989. Am J Clin Nutr (Suppl)51:897s, 1990.

Ryan CA et al: Massive outbreak of antimicrobial-resistant salmonellosis traced to pasteurized milk. JAMA 258:3269, 1987.

St Louis ME et al: The emergence of grade A eggs as a major source of *Salmonella enteritidis* infections. JAMA 259:2103, 1988.

Senate Select Committee on Nutrition and Human Needs: Dietary Goals for the United States. Publ No 052-070-03913-2. Washington, DC, US Government Printing Office, 1977.

Senate Select Committee on Nutrition and Human Needs: Dietary Goals for the United States, 2nd ed. Publ No 052-070-04376-8. Washington, DC, Government Printing Office, 1978.

Sugiyama H et al: Production of botulinum toxin in inoculated pack studies of foil-wrapped baked potatoes. J Food Protection 44:896, 1981.

The Surgeon General's Report on Nutrition and Health. Summary and Recommendations. USDHHS (PHS) Publ No 88-50211. Washington, DC, US Government Printing Office, 1988.

Tittle-Cross, A.: Politics, poverty and nutrition. J Am Diet Assoc 87:1007, 1987.

USDA: Nationwide Food Consumption Survey. Continuing Survey of Food Intakes by Individuals: Women 19–50 Years and Their Children 1–5 Years, 1 Day. Report No 85-1, USDA, NFCFS, CSFII, Nutrition Monitoring Division, Human Nutrition Information Service, Hyattsville, MD, USDA, 1985.

USDHHS: Listeriosis outbreak associated with Mexican-style cheese — California. MMWR 34:357, 1985.

Woteki CE et al: National Health and Nutrition Examination Survey — NHANES. Plans for NHANES III. Nutrition Today 23(1):25, 1988.

ADDITIONAL REFERENCES

Ames BN, Magow R, and Gold LS: Rating of possible carcinogenic hazards. Science 236:271, 1987.

Archer DL: The true impact of foodborne infections. Food Tech 42:53, 1988.

Expert Panel on Food Safety and Nutrition, Institute of Food Technologists: The risk/benefit concept as applied to food: A scientific status summary. Food Technology 42:119, 1988.

Franco DA: *Campylobacter* species: Considerations for controlling a foodborne pathogen. Journal of Food Protection 51:145, 1988.

Holmberg SD, Solomon SL, and Blake PA: Health and economic impacts of antimicrobial resistance. Rev Infect Dis 9:1065, 1987.

Kenney J and Fallert D: Livestock hormones in the United States. National Food Review 12:21, 1989.

Kuchler F, McClelland J, and Offutt SE: Regulating food safety: The case of animal growth hormones. National Food Review 12:25, 1989.

Nestle M: Promoting health and preventing disease: National Nutrition Objectives for 1990 and 2000. Food Tech 42:103, 1988.

Pennington JAT, Young BE, and Wilson DB: Nutritional elements in U.S. diets: Results from the Total Diet Study, 1982–1986. J Am Diet Assoc 89:659, 1989.

Petersen B and Chaisson C: Pesticides and residues in food. Food Tech July, 1988, p 59.

Rogan A and Glaros G: Food irradiation: The process and implications for dietitians. J Am Diet Assoc 88:833, 1988.

CHAPTER 16

GUIDELINES FOR DIETARY PLANNING

CHAPTER OUTLINE

KEY TERMS

DIETARY GUIDELINES FOR AMERICANS—dietary recommendations to promote health specifically with respect to prevention or delay of onset of chronic diseases

ESTIMATED SAFE AND ADEQUATE DAILY DIETARY INTAKES (ESADDI)—recommended ranges of appropriate intake of those nutrients for which not enough information is available to establish Recommended Dietary Allowances

NATIONAL CHOLESTEROL EDUCATION PROGRAM—a nationwide program to educate the public and health providers about the risks of an elevated serum cholesterol and to make recommendations regarding methods to lower it

RECOMMENDED DIETARY ALLOWANCES (RDA)—recommendations for the average amounts of nutrients that should be consumed daily by healthy people in the United States

RECOMMENDED NUTRIENT INTAKES (RNI)—the Canadian RDA

REFERENCE MEN AND WOMEN—men and women of designated heights and weights as determined from actual medians from NHANES II, which form the basis of the RDA for adults

US RECOMMENDED DAILY ALLOWANCE (US RDA)—used for labeling purposes only; based on the 1968 RDA for protein, five vitamins, and two minerals

An appropriate diet is one that is both adequate and balanced and recognizes individual variations, such as age and stage of development, taste preferences, and food habits. It also reflects the availability of foods, socioeconomic conditions, storage and preparation facilities, and cooking skills.

An adequate and balanced diet is one that meets all the nutritional needs of an individual for maintenance, repair, the living processes, and growth or development. It includes all nutrients in proper amounts and in proportion to each other. The presence or absence of one essential nutrient may affect the availability, absorption, metabolism, or dietary need for others. The increasing recognition of nutrient interrelationships emphasizes the principle of maintaining variety in foods in order to provide the most complete diet.

DETERMINING NUTRIENT NEEDS

A number of standards are available to serve as guides for planning and evaluating diets and food supplies for individuals and population groups. Many countries have issued guidelines appropriate to their individual circumstances. The Food and Agriculture Organization of the World Health Organization of the United Nations has established standards in many areas of food quality and safety (Joint FAO/WHO Expert Committee, 1984a, 1984b, and 1985).

Recommended Dietary Allowances

The basic American standard is the Recommended Dietary Allowances (RDA), established by the Food and Nutrition Board (FNB) of the National Research Council/National Academy of Sciences (NRC/NAS), first published in 1943 and most recently revised in 1989 (Food and Nutrition Board, 1989) (Table 16–1). Revisions approximately every 5 years incorporate the most recent research findings. The evolution of the RDA is shown in Table 16–2.

Definition

The RDA are recommendations for the average amounts of nutrients that should be consumed daily over a period of time by healthy people in the United States; they are intended to be met by a diet of a wide variety of foods.

The nutrient requirements of individuals vary greatly and are usually unknown. For this reason, the RDA for most nutrients are established at levels exceeding the requirements of most individuals, thus ensuring that the needs of almost all in the population are met. Intakes below the recommended allowance for a nutrient are not necessarily inadequate, but the *risk* of inadequacy increases whenever intakes fall below recommended levels.

Nature of Target Population

RDA are recommendations established for healthy populations. Special needs for nutrients arising from problems such as premature birth, inherited metabolic disorders, infections, chronic diseases, and the use of medications require special dietary and therapeutic measures and are not covered by the RDA.

Age-Sex Groups

Because needs for nutrients are highly individualized depending on age, sexual development, and the reproductive status of women, the RDA are listed in 15 groups based on age, and beyond 10 years of age they are divided according to sex. Recommendations for pregnancy and lactation are also included.

Reference Men and Women

Because the requirement for many nutrients is based on body weight, the RDA shown in Table 16–1 are listed in terms of *reference men* and *women* of designated height and weight. These values for age-sex groups over 19 years of age are based on actual medians obtained for the American population by the second National Health and Nutrition Examination Survey (NHANES II), 1976 to 1980. Although this does not necessarily imply that these weight-for-height values are ideal, at least they make it possible to define recommended allowances appropriate for the largest number of people. Recommended energy intakes for median heights and weights are shown in Table 16–3.

Estimated Safe and Adequate Daily Dietary Intakes

A number of nutrients are known to be essential to life and health, but available data are insufficient to establish a recommended intake. These are listed as *Estimated Safe and Adequate Daily Dietary Intakes* (ESADDI) in Table 16–4. Most intakes are shown as ranges to indicate not only that specific recommendations are not justified at this time but also that at least the upper and lower limits of safety should be observed. Safe and adequate ranges for sodium, potassium, and chloride have not been included because "they are difficult to justify" (Food and Nutrition Board, 1989). Estimated minimum requirements for these electrolytes are listed in Table 16–5.

TABLE 16–1. Recommended Dietary Allowances*†

Designed for the Maintenance of Good Nutrition of Practically All Healthy People in the United States

Category	Age (Yrs) or Condition	Weight‡ (kg)	Weight‡ (lb)	Height‡ (cm)	Height‡ (in)	Protein (g)	Fat-Soluble Vitamins: Vitamin A (μg RE)§	Vitamin D (μg)‖	Vitamin E (mg α-TE)¶	Vitamin K (μg)	Water-Soluble Vitamins: Vitamin C (mg)	Thiamin (mg)	Riboflavin (mg)	Niacin (mg NE)**	Vitamin B_6 (mg)	Folate (μg)	Vitamin B_{12} (μg)	Minerals: Calcium (mg)	Phosphorus (mg)	Magnesium (mg)	Iron (mg)	Zinc (mg)	Iodine (μg)	Selenium (μg)
Infants	0.0–0.5	6	13	60	24	13	375	7.5	3	5	30	0.3	0.4	5	0.3	25	0.3	400	300	40	6	5	40	10
	0.5–1.0	9	20	71	28	14	375	10	4	10	35	0.4	0.5	6	0.6	35	0.5	600	500	60	10	5	50	15
Children	1–3	13	29	90	35	16	400	10	6	15	40	0.7	0.8	9	1.0	50	0.7	800	800	80	10	10	70	20
	4–6	20	44	112	44	24	500	10	7	20	45	0.9	1.1	12	1.1	75	1.0	800	800	120	10	10	90	20
	7–10	28	62	132	52	28	700	10	7	30	45	1.0	1.2	13	1.4	100	1.4	800	800	170	10	10	120	30
Males	11–14	45	99	157	62	45	1,000	10	10	45	50	1.3	1.5	17	1.7	150	2.0	1,200	1,200	270	12	15	150	40
	15–18	66	145	176	69	59	1,000	10	10	65	60	1.5	1.8	20	2.0	200	2.0	1,200	1,200	400	12	15	150	50
	19–24	72	160	177	70	58	1,000	10	10	70	60	1.5	1.7	19	2.0	200	2.0	1,200	1,200	350	10	15	150	70
	25–50	79	174	176	70	63	1,000	5	10	80	60	1.5	1.7	19	2.0	200	2.0	800	800	350	10	15	150	70
	51+	77	170	173	68	63	1,000	5	10	80	60	1.2	1.4	15	2.0	200	2.0	800	800	350	10	15	150	70
Females	11–14	46	101	157	62	46	800	10	8	45	50	1.1	1.3	15	1.4	150	2.0	1,200	1,200	280	15	12	150	45
	15–18	55	120	163	64	44	800	10	8	55	60	1.1	1.3	15	1.5	150	2.0	1,200	1,200	300	15	12	150	50
	19–24	58	128	164	65	46	800	10	8	60	60	1.1	1.3	15	1.6	150	2.0	1,200	1,200	280	15	12	150	55
	25–50	63	138	163	64	50	800	5	8	65	60	1.1	1.3	15	1.6	150	2.0	800	800	280	15	12	150	55
	51+	65	143	160	63	50	800	5	8	65	60	1.0	1.2	13	1.6	150	2.0	800	800	280	10	12	150	55
Pregnant						60	800	10	10	65	70	1.5	1.6	17	2.2	400	2.2	1,200	1,200	320	30	15	175	65
Lactating	1st 6 months					65	1,300	10	12	65	95	1.6	1.8	20	2.1	250	2.6	1,200	1,200	355	15	19	200	75
	2nd 6 months					62	1,200	10	11	65	90	1.6	1.7	20	2.1	250	2.6	1,200	1,200	340	15	16	200	75

* From Food and Nutrition Board, National Research Council, National Academy of Sciences: Recommended Dietary Allowances, 10th ed. Washington, DC, National Academy Press, 1989.

† The allowances, expressed as average daily intakes over time, are intended to provide for individual variations among most normal persons as they live in the United States under usual environmental stresses. Diets should be based on a variety of common foods in order to provide other nutrients for which human requirements have been less well defined.

‡ Weights and heights of Reference Adults are actual medians for the U.S. population of the designated age, as reported by the National Health and Nutrition Examination Survey II. The median weights and heights of those under 19 years of age were taken from Hamill et al (1979). The use of these figures does not imply that the height-to-weight ratios are ideal.

§ RE = retinol equivalents; 1 retinol equivalent = 1 μg retinol or 6 μg β-carotene. See Chapter 6 for calculation of vitamin A activity of diet as retinol equivalents.

‖ As cholecalciferol; 10 μg of cholecalciferol = 400 IU of vitamin D.

¶ α-TE = α-tocopherol equivalents; 1 mg d-α-tocopherol = 1α-TE. See Chapter 6 for variation in allowances and calculation of vitamin E activity of the diet as α-tocopherol equivalents.

** NE = niacin equivalent; 1 NE = 1 mg of niacin or 60 mg of dietary tryptophan.

TABLE 16–2. Evolution of Recommended Dietary Allowances from 1943 to 1989

Nutrient	RDA Establishment*	Nutrient	RDA Establishment*
Protein	First established in 1943		
Vitamin A		Panthothenic acid	No RDA established, but ESADDI† established in 1980 and revised in 1989
Vitamin D		Biotin	
Thiamin		Copper	
Riboflavin		Fluoride	
Niacin		Chromium	
Calcium		Manganese	
Iron		Molybdenum	
Vitamin E	First established in 1968	Sodium	Estimated minimum requirements established in 1989
Folacin		Potassium	
Vitamin B_6		Chloride	
Vitamin B_{12}		Essential fatty acids	No RDA or ESADDI yet established
Phosphorus		Carbohydrate	
Magnesium		Choline	
Iodine		Other trace minerals	
Zinc	First established in 1974		
Vitamin K	First established in 1989		
Selenium			

* RDA = recommended dietary allowance.
† ESADDI = estimated safe and adequate daily dietary intake.

TABLE 16–3. Median Heights and Weights and Recommended Energy Intake*

		Weight		Height			Average Energy Allowance (kcal)‡		
Category	Age (Yrs) or Condition	*(kg)*	*(lb)*	*(cm)*	*(in)*	REE† (kcal/day)	Multiples of REE	Per kg	Per day§
Infants	0.0–0.5	6	13	60	24	320		108	650
	0.5–1.0	9	20	71	28	500		98	850
Children	1–3	13	29	90	35	740		102	1,300
	4–6	20	44	112	44	950		90	1,800
	7–10	28	62	132	52	1,130		70	2,000
Males	11–14	45	99	157	62	1,440	1.70	55	2,500
	15–18	66	145	176	69	1,760	1.67	45	3,000
	19–24	72	160	177	70	1,780	1.67	40	2,900
	25–50	79	174	176	70	1,800	1.60	37	2,900
	51+	77	170	173	68	1,530	1.50	30	2,300
Females	11–14	46	101	157	62	1,310	1.67	47	2,200
	15–18	55	120	163	64	1,370	1.60	40	2,200
	19–24	58	128	164	65	1,350	1.60	38	2,200
	25–50	63	138	163	64	1,380	1.55	36	2,200
	51+	65	143	160	63	1,280	1.50	30	1,900
Pregnant	1st trimester								+0
	2nd trimester								+300
	3rd trimester								+300
Lactating	1st 6 months								+500
	2nd 6 months								+500

* Reprinted with permission from *Recommended Dietary Allowances,* 10th ed., c. 1989 by the National Academy of Sciences. Published by National Academy Press.
† REE = resting energy expenditure; calculated using Food and Agriculture Organization equations, then rounded.
‡ In the range of light to moderate activity, the coefficient of variation is ±20%.
§ Figure is rounded.

TABLE 16–4. Estimated Safe and Adequate Daily Dietary Intakes of Selected Vitamins and Minerals*

Category	Age (Yrs)	Vitamins: Biotin (μg)	Vitamins: Pantothenic Acid (mg)
Infants	0–0.5	10	2
	0.5–1	15	3
Children and adolescents	1–3	20	3
	4–6	25	3–4
	7–10	30	4–5
	11+	30–100	4–7
Adults		30–100	4–7

Category	Age (Yrs)	Trace Elements†: Copper (mg)	Manganese (mg)	Fluoride (mg)	Chromium (μg)	Molybdenum (μg)
Infants	0–0.5	0.4–0.6	0.3–0.6	0.1–0.5	10–40	15–30
	0.5–1	0.6–0.7	0.6–1.0	0.2–1.0	20–60	20–40
Children and adolescents	1–3	0.7–1.0	1.0–1.5	0.5–1.5	20–80	25–50
	4–6	1.0–1.5	1.5–2.0	1.0–2.5	30–120	30–75
	7–10	1.0–2.0	2.0–3.0	1.5–2.5	50–200	50–150
	11+	1.5–2.5	2.0–5.0	1.5–2.5	50–200	75–250
Adults		1.5–3.0	2.0–5.0	1.5–4.0	50–200	75–250

* Reprinted with permission from *Recommended Dietary Allowances,* 10th ed., c. 1989 by the National Academy of Sciences. Published by National Academy Press.

† Since the toxic levels for many trace elements may be only several times usual intakes, the upper levels for the trace elements given in this table should not be habitually exceeded.

Appropriate Use

The RDA are intended to be applied to the needs of population groups; however, they can be appropriately used to estimate the risk of nutrient deficiency for individuals if intakes are averaged over a sufficient period of time (Food and Nutrition Board, 1989). It would be a mistake to assume that individuals whose diets do not meet the RDA are necessarily suffering from malnutrition, inasmuch as the RDA include a margin of safety to allow for individual variations. For this reason, arbitrary cutoff points (e.g., two thirds of the RDA, 70% of the RDA) are frequently used as the levels below which lack of individual nutrients is interpreted as introducing an element of risk.

It is equally invalid to assume that because the average nutrient intakes for a population group meet the standards of the RDA, there is no malnutrition among individuals within that group.

The Recommended Nutrient Intakes (RNI) for Canada (similar to the RDA in the United States) are presented in Table 16–6.

TABLE 16–5. Estimated Sodium, Chloride, and Potassium Minimum Requirements of Healthy Persons*†

Age	Weight (kg)	Sodium (mg)†‡	Chloride (mg)†‡	Potassium (mg)§
Months				
0–5	4.5	120	180	500
6–11	8.9	200	300	700
Years				
1	11.0	225	350	1,000
2–5	16.0	300	500	1,400
6–9	25.0	400	600	1,600
10–18	50.0	500	750	2,000
>18‖	70.0	500	750	2,000

* Reprinted with permission from *Recommended Dietary Allowances,* 10th ed., c. 1989 by the National Academy of Sciences. Published by National Academy Press.

† No allowance has been included for large, prolonged losses from the skin through sweat.

‡ There is no evidence that higher intakes confer any health benefit.

§ Desirable intakes of potassium may considerably exceed these values (~3,500 mg for adults).

‖ No allowance included for growth. Values for those below 18 years assume a growth rate at the 50th percentile reported by the National Center for Health Statistics and averaged for males and females.

Nutrition Labeling and the US Recommended Daily Allowances

Nutrition Labeling

To aid in the translation of nutritional requirements into foods and meals, the Food and Drug Administration (FDA) in 1973 established a system of labeling certain processed foods on the basis of their content of selected nutrients as compared with the 1968 RDA. This system is currently under extensive revision to update and expand nutrient recommendations, add data in line with current recommendations for preven-

TABLE 16–6. Recommended Nutrient Intakes (RNI), Canada, 1990, Based on Age, Energy, and Body Weight Expressed as Daily Rates*

Age	Sex	Energy (kcal)	Weight (kg)	Thiamin (mg)	Riboflavin (mg)	Niacin (NE)†	n-3 PUFA‡ (g)	n-6 PUFA (g)	Protein (g)	Vit. A (RE)§	Vit. D (μg)	Vit. E (mg)	Vit. C (mg)	Folate (μg)	Vit. B_{12} (μg)	Calcium (mg)	Phosphorus (mg)	Magnesium (mg)	Iron (mg)	Iodine (μg)	Zinc (mg)
Months																					
0–4	Both	600	6.0	0.3	0.3	4	0.5	3	12‖	400	10	3	20	50	0.3	250¶	150	20	0.3**	30	2**
5–12	Both	900	9.0	0.4	0.5	7	0.5	3	12	400	10	3	20	50	0.3	400	200	32	7	40	3
Years																					
1	Both	1,100	11	0.5	0.6	8	0.6	4	19	400	10	3	20	65	0.3	500	300	40	6	55	4
2–3	Both	1,300	14	0.6	0.7	9	0.7	4	22	400	5	4	20	80	0.4	550	350	50	6	65	4
4–6	Both	1,800	18	0.7	0.9	13	1.0	6	26	500	5	5	25	90	0.5	600	400	65	8	85	5
7–9	Male	2,200	25	0.9	1.1	16	1.2	7	30	700	2.5	7	25	125	0.8	700	500	100	8	110	7
	Female	1,900	25	0.8	1.0	14	1.0	6	30	700	2.5	6	25	125	0.8	700	500	100	8	95	7
10–12	Male	2,500	34	1.0	1.3	18	1.4	8	38	800	2.5	8	25	170	1.0	900	700	130	8	125	9
	Female	2,200	36	0.9	1.1	16	1.1	7	40	800	5	7	25	180	1.0	1,100	800	135	8	110	9
13–15	Male	2,800	50	1.1	1.4	20	1.4	9	50	900	5	9	30	150	1.5	1,100	900	185	10	160	12
	Female	2,200	48	0.9	1.1	16	1.2	7	42	800	5	7	30	145	1.5	1,000	850	180	13	160	9
16–18	Male	3,200	62	1.3	1.6	23	1.8	11	55	1,000	5	10	40††	185	1.9	900	1,000	230	10	160	12
	Female	2,100	53	0.8	1.1	15	1.2	7	43	800	2.5	7	30††	160	1.9	700	850	200	12	160	9
19–24	Male	3,000	71	1.2	1.5	22	1.6	10	58	1,000	2.5	10	40††	210	2.0	800	1,000	240	9	160	12
	Female	2,100	58	0.8	1.1	15	1.2	7	43	800	2.5	7	30††	175	2.0	700	850	200	13	160	9
25–49	Male	2,700	74	1.1	1.4	19	1.5	9	61	1,000	2.5	9	40††	220	2.0	800	1,000	250	9	160	12
	Female	2,000	59	0.8	1.0	14	1.1	7	44	800	2.5	6	30††	175	2.0	700	850	200	13	160	9
50–74	Male	2,300	73	0.9	1.3	16	1.3	8	60	1,000	5	7	40††	220	2.0	800	1,000	250	9	160	12
	Female	1,800	63	0.8‡‡	1.0‡‡	14‡‡	1.1‡‡	7‡‡	47	800	5	6	30††	190	2.0	800	850	210	8	160	9
75+	Male	2,000	69	0.8	1.0	14	1.0	7	57	1,000	5	6	40††	205	2.0	800	1,000	230	9	160	12
	Female§§	1,700	64	0.8‡‡	1.0‡‡	14‡‡	1.1‡‡	7‡‡	47	800	5	5	30††	190	2.0	800	850	210	8	160	9
Pregnancy (additional)																					
1st Trimester		100		0.1	0.1	0.1	0.05	0.3	5	100	2.5	2	0	300	1.0	500	200	15	0	25	6
2nd Trimester		300		0.1	0.3	0.2	0.16	0.9	20	100	2.5	2	10	300	1.0	500	200	45	5	25	6
3rd Trimester		300		0.1	0.3	0.2	0.16	0.9	24	100	2.5	2	10	300	1.0	500	200	45	10	25	6
Lactation (additional)		450		0.2	0.4	0.3	0.25	1.5	20	400	2.5	3	25	100	0.5	500	200	65	0	50	6

* From Recommended Nutrient Intakes for Canadians. Bureau of Nutritional Sciences, Ottawa, 1990.
† NE = Niacin Equivalents.
‡ PUFA = polyunsaturated fatty acids.
§ RE = Retinol Equivalents.
‖ Protein is assumed to be from breast milk and must be adjusted for infant formula.
¶ Infant formula with high phosphorus should contain 375 mg calcium.
** Breast milk is assumed to be the source of the mineral.
†† Smokers should increase vitamin C by 50%.
‡‡ Level below which intake should not fall.
§§ Assumes moderate physical activity.

tion of chronic disease, and make the label information easier for the public to use. In December 1990, Congress passed the Nutrition Labeling and Education Act, (NLEA) which mandated changes to take effect in May 1993. Other changes are expected to follow. (DeBruyne, 1990)

Nutrition labeling may be used by any manufacturer provided it conforms to the standards established for the US Recommended Daily Allowances. It is required when nutrients such as vitamins and minerals have been added to the food, or when a nutritional claim has been made on the label of a natural food (e.g., "high in vitamin C" on an orange juice label).

The terminology used on the label is specific as explained in Table 16–7.

The US Recommended Daily Allowances

The *US Recommended Daily Allowances* (US RDA) are for the most part based on the 1968 RDA; however, they differ from that guideline in a number of ways. Primarily because of the constraints imposed by the amount of space available on a package label, the table of US RDA is an abbreviated version of the RDA (Table 16–8).

MANDATORY LISTINGS ON FOOD LABEL. Nutrients for which the US RDA have been established and which must appear on a label include protein, five vitamins (A, C, thiamin, riboflavin, and niacin), and two minerals (calcium and iron). The nutrients contained in one "serving" of a food product are shown on the label in grams of protein, fat, and carbohydrate, and in percentage of the US RDA for protein, vitamins, and minerals. Energy value is listed in kilocalories/serving (see Fig. 16–1). In conformity with the NLEA extensive changes in label information will be specified.

SIZE OF SERVING. A "serving" of the food being described is defined on the label in terms of average serving size and number of servings per container. Serving sizes should not be taken for granted, because their determination is at the discretion of the manufacturer. Presumably they represent reasonable amounts, although at times they are misused, for example in implying that a particular food is low in kilocalories.

OPTIONAL LISTINGS ON FOOD LABEL. Information about sodium, cholesterol, and saturation of fat presently may be included at the option of the manufacturer. However in the labeling regulations to take effect in 1993, saturated fat and cholesterol will be mandatory. Sodium and cholesterol are listed in mg/serving and also mg/100 g of the product. Fat information may include the percentage of calories from fat in one serving, as well as g/serving of polyunsaturated and saturated fat.

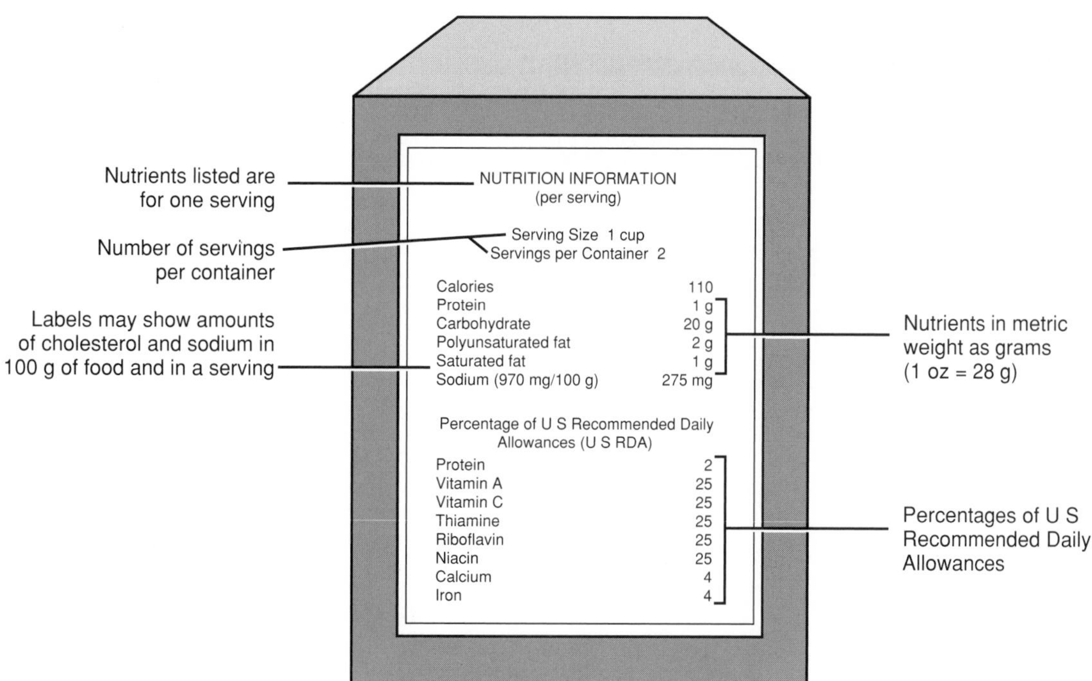

FIGURE 16–1. *Example of the present nutrition label. Mandatory changes that will appear on the label in 1993 include addition of the following per serving: grams of fat, saturated fat, cholesterol, complex carbohydrate, sugar, dietary fiber, and sodium. Grams of polyunsaturated fat will be optional. The "US RDA" will be omitted, and vitamins A and C, calcium and iron will be stated in terms of a "percentage of daily value."*

TABLE 16–7. Food Label Terminology*

Term	Nutritional Meaning	Term	Nutritional Meaning
Reduced calorie	At least one-third lower in kilocalories than regular food and not nutritionally inferior to regular food		
Lower calorie	Not more than 40 kcal/serving and not more than 0.4 kcal/g or about 11 kcal/oz; term cannot appear immediately before the product name if it is naturally low in calories		
Diet or dietetic	Can be used for both reduced-calorie and low-calorie foods, as well as foods clearly intended for other special dietary purposes, e.g., low sodium		
Lite	Not yet defined by the Food and Drug Administration and is left to the interpretation of the manufacturer		
Imitation	Resembles or substitutes for another food, but contains less than 2% of any of eight nutrients required on the label (protein, vitamin A, vitamin C, thiamin, riboflavin, niacin, calcium, iron)		
		Enriched or Fortified	Nutrients added to food to restore those lost in storage, handling and processing, to make the foods resemble traditional foods, to meet nutritional standards, or when suitable, to overcome a nutritional deficiency in a particular population group.
		Sugar-free or sugarless	Does not contain sucrose; may contain other sweeteners; implies lower or reduced kilocalories. If this is not true the label must also state, "not a reduced calorie food"
		Unsweetened	Naturally sweet with no sweeteners added

* Adapted from Hoyt JW: Selecting the right foods. *In* Powers MA: Handbook of Diabetes Nutritional Management. Rockville, MD, Aspen Publishers, 1987, p. 166, and Federal Register Vol. 43 (43259) Sept. 22, 1978 and Vol 43 (52700) Nov. 14, 1978.

Other nutrients may be listed in terms of the percentage of the US RDA if they have been added or occur naturally in significant amounts. These include vitamins B_6, B_{12}, D, and E, folic acid, biotin, and pantothenic acid, as well as phosphorus, iodine, magnesium, zinc, and copper.

AGE GROUPS. The US RDA have been established on the basis of three age groups. Most of the label information applies to adults and children over 4 years of age (see Table 16–8). The information on baby foods, formula, and vitamin-mineral supplements for infants and small children is based on the US RDA for infants and children under 4 years of age. Vitamin-mineral supplements for pregnant or lactating women conform to standards appropriate for that group.

Because the RDA for the individual categories of the adults and children groups cover a wide range, the highest value of that range is used as the single value representing the group for the US RDA. This intro-

TABLE 16–8. US Recommended Daily Allowances (US RDA)*

Vitamins and Minerals	Unit of Measurement	Adults and Children 4 or More Years of Age†	Infants and Children Under 4 Years of Age	Pregnant or Lactating Women
Protein	Grams	65‡	28	—§
Vitamin A	International Units	5,000	2,500	8,000
Vitamin D	International Units	400	400	400
Vitamin E	International Units	30	10	30
Vitamin C	Milligrams	60	40	60
Folic Acid	Milligrams	0.4	0.2	0.8
Thiamin	Milligrams	1.5	0.7	1.7
Riboflavin	Milligrams	1.7	0.8	2
Niacin	Milligrams	20	9	20
Vitamin B_6	Milligrams	2	0.7	2.5
Vitamin B_{12}	Micrograms	6	3	8
Biotin	Milligrams	0.3	0.15	0.3
Pantothenic Acid	Milligrams	10	5	10
Calcium	Grams	1	0.8	1.3
Phosphorus	Grams	1	0.8	1.3
Iodine	Micrograms	150	70	150
Iron	Milligrams	18	10	18
Magnesium	Milligrams	400	200	450
Copper	Milligrams	2	1	2
Zinc	Milligrams	15	8	15

* Based on the 1968 Recommended Dietary Allowances.

† These US RDA values appear on most nutrition labels.

‡ If protein efficiency ratio of protein is equal to or better than that of casein, US RDA is 45 g for adults and 20 g for infants.

§ Not specified because this US RDA used only in vitamin and mineral supplements for pregnant or lactating females.

TABLE 16–9. Mean Intakes of Macronutrients of Respondents-NFCS 1987–88*

Sex and Age (yr)	Calories (kcal)		Protein (g)			Fat (g)			Carbohydrate (g)			Saturated Fat (g)			Cholesterol (mg)		Fiber (g)		Sodium (mg)	
	Mean	SD	Mean	SD	% kcal	Mean	SD	% kcal	Mean	SD	% kcal	Mean	SD	% kcal	Mean	SD	Mean	SD	Mean	SD
Both sexes																				
1–2	1163	329	45.7	14.7	16	46.3	15.8	36	145	47	50	18.9	7.0	15	184	107	7.2	3.3	1866	660
3–5	1390	404	53.1	16.6	15	55.8	19.2	35	175	55	50	21.6	8.2	14	201	109	8.9	3.9	2288	746
6–11	1780	514	68.2	21.0	15	72.2	24.4	36	220	67	50	28.0	10.0	14	252	123	11.9	4.9	2956	947
Men																				
12–15	2152	716	83.2	26.3	16	87.9	32.3	37	263	103	48	33.9	12.9	14	309	147	13.8	7.1	3637	1361
16–19	2406	729	93.3	31.7	16	99.2	35.4	37	289	93	48	37.1	14.2	14	354	179	14.6	6.0	4097	1504
20–29	2228	794	89.1	33.9	16	92.8	39.9	37	252	98	46	33.6	15.6	13	358	208	14.0	6.8	3884	1531
30–39	2154	712	89.5	31.6	17	90.9	35.3	38	236	88	44	32.7	14.1	14	362	200	14.7	7.5	3764	1397
40–49	2016	673	83.6	28.2	17	85.0	32.5	38	222	92	44	29.6	12.0	13	336	180	14.3	7.0	3661	1330
50–59	1943	744	83.3	29.9	18	82.6	35.7	38	212	93	44	28.6	13.3	13	357	191	14.3	6.7	3666	1491
60–69	1890	658	81.4	27.4	18	79.1	33.3	37	210	82	45	27.0	12.7	13	333	179	15.3	7.2	3479	1262
70+	1812	545	74.0	23.9	17	72.7	26.9	36	214	74	47	25.5	10.6	12	310	164	16.0	7.5	3190	1081
Women																				
12–15	1744	532	66.1	21.5	15	71.1	24.8	36	215	70	49	27.1	10.5	14	239	120	11.1	5.1	2977	1185
16–19	1618	606	62.1	24.4	16	66.3	28.2	36	196	77	49	25.0	11.5	14	249	153	9.8	4.8	2696	1134
20–29	1524	524	62.0	23.6	16	63.2	26.2	37	177	67	47	23.0	10.3	13	248	138	9.9	4.9	2500	975
30–39	1473	512	60.7	21.6	17	61.0	24.7	37	170	68	46	22.1	9.8	13	235	130	10.4	5.1	2386	912
40–49	1419	465	58.9	20.0	17	58.6	23.5	37	164	64	46	20.5	8.7	13	232	126	10.7	5.0	2332	898
50–59	1420	459	62.3	20.4	18	58.7	23.6	37	162	59	46	20.6	9.3	13	246	124	11.7	5.7	2333	963
60–69	1410	424	61.0	18.9	18	57.0	21.8	36	166	56	47	19.6	8.2	12	236	125	12.4	5.2	2306	811
70+	1377	411	57.5	18.4	17	54.5	21.1	35	168	58	49	19.6	8.7	13	226	117	12.4	6.0	2206	817

* Adapted from Wright HS et al: The 1987–88 Nationwide Food Consumption Survey: An update on the nutrient intake of respondents. Nutr Today 26(3):21, 1991.

TABLE 16–10. Mean Intakes of Vitamins and Minerals of Respondents—NFCS 1987–88

Sex and Age (yr)	n	Vitamin A (IU)		Vitamin C (mg)		Thiamin (mg)		Riboflavin (mg)		Vitamin B_6 (mg)		Vitamin B_{12} (μg)		Folate (μg)		Vitamin E (mg-αTE)		Calcium (mg)		Iron (mg)		Zinc (mg)		Magnesium (mg)		Copper (mg)	
		Mean	SD	Mean	SD	Mean	SD	Mean	SD	Mean	SD	Mean	SD	Mean	SD	Mean	SD	Mean	SD	Mean	SD	Mean	SD	Mean	SD	Mean	SD
Both Sexes																											
1–2	285	3649	3026	72.1	51.1	1.0	0.3	1.5	0.6	1.1	0.4	3.7	2.9	154	83	4.4	3.6	953	368	9.2	4.8	6.4	2.2	161	51	0.7	0.6
3–5	415	4191	3912	77.5	52.4	1.2	0.4	1.7	0.6	1.2	0.5	4.2	3.9	185	93	5.3	4.2	781	341	10.1	4.6	7.5	2.6	183	63	0.7	0.3
6–11	818	5059	3582	88.3	52.7	1.4	0.5	2.0	0.7	1.5	0.6	4.8	3.1	229	114	6.9	4.8	936	368	12.6	5.4	9.7	3.8	226	75	0.9	0.3
Men																											
12–15	217	5705	3909	100.5	71.2	1.7	0.7	2.3	1.0	1.8	0.9	6.1	4.2	272	147	7.8	5.2	1033	460	15.4	11.6	12.2	5.1	261	102	1.1	0.4
16–19	203	6194	4612	114.4	83.4	1.9	0.8	2.4	1.1	2.0	1.0	6.7	7.8	293	174	9.6	6.7	1089	518	16.2	7.4	13.4	5.2	278	99	1.2	0.4
20–29	546	5297	5484	86.8	61.5	1.6	0.7	2.0	0.9	1.7	0.8	6.6	10.4	236	128	9.2	6.2	863	475	14.4	6.4	12.6	6.0	260	103	1.2	0.5
30–39	661	5905	5680	89.4	70.1	1.6	0.7	2.0	0.9	1.8	0.8	6.4	10.2	250	147	9.3	6.4	819	433	14.7	7.4	12.8	6.4	277	113	1.2	0.6
40–49	437	6163	5720	93.1	57.5	1.5	0.6	1.8	0.7	1.7	0.7	5.9	7.3	236	118	8.6	4.2	715	353	13.9	5.9	12.4	8.5	266	100	1.2	0.6
50–59	344	6651	5639	98.1	68.6	1.5	0.7	1.8	0.8	1.7	0.8	5.9	6.9	249	131	9.0	6.2	718	393	13.8	6.3	12.6	14.9	266	98	1.2	0.8
60–69	368	8236	7018	105.7	68.4	1.6	0.7	2.0	1.0	1.8	0.9	7.6	12.7	273	157	10.0	7.1	745	405	14.9	7.8	12.2	7.7	276	96	1.2	0.5
70+	263	7792	7587	102.7	68.4	1.5	0.6	1.9	0.8	1.7	0.8	6.2	9.9	258	133	8.9	6.6	702	321	14.2	6.8	11.4	6.4	265	90	1.3	1.0
Women																											
12–15	242	4308	3208	85.2	60.6	1.3	0.5	1.8	0.7	1.4	0.7	4.2	2.1	211	114	6.7	4.4	833	407	12.0	5.8	9.4	3.7	207	76	0.9	0.3
16–19	235	4309	4007	80.2	70.2	1.2	0.5	1.6	0.8	1.2	0.6	4.0	3.1	189	121	6.5	5.1	718	387	10.4	5.3	8.9	4.5	187	83	0.8	0.4
20–29	683	4907	5323	71.5	52.0	1.1	0.5	1.5	0.7	1.2	0.5	4.9	7.9	178	103	6.6	4.8	639	347	10.4	4.9	8.6	3.7	188	73	0.9	0.5
30–39	772	4798	4540	73.1	56.6	1.1	0.5	1.4	0.6	1.2	0.6	3.8	3.9	184	107	6.7	4.9	597	315	10.2	4.9	8.4	3.8	200	77	0.9	0.4
40–49	522	5819	7252	81.5	59.1	1.1	0.4	1.4	0.6	1.2	0.5	4.9	10.3	187	95	6.7	4.5	558	289	10.4	4.7	8.4	4.6	200	75	0.9	0.4
50–59	425	5810	5011	94.3	67.4	1.2	0.5	1.5	0.7	1.3	0.6	4.6	6.3	213	117	7.2	5.4	578	295	11.1	5.2	8.7	3.7	220	82	1.0	0.4
60–69	489	6747	5956	93.9	68.5	1.2	0.4	1.5	0.6	1.4	0.5	4.8	7.5	213	98	7.2	4.6	579	263	10.9	4.7	8.8	4.4	220	71	1.0	0.4
70+	402	6920	5775	94.0	59.7	1.2	0.5	1.5	0.6	1.4	0.7	4.3	4.4	229	124	7.5	6.4	592	284	11.7	5.8	9.1	8.7	213	75	1.0	1.0

SD = standard deviation
Adapted from: Wright, H.S. et al: The 1987–88 Nationwide Food Consumption Survey: An update on the nutrient intake of respondents, Nutr. Today, 26(3): 21, 1991.

duces a very large margin of safety, and in general, the US RDA for any individual is higher than the RDA.

Further details regarding nutrition labeling can be found in the Food and Drugs section of the Code of Federal Regulations (Code of Federal Regulations 21, 1977).

NUTRITIONAL STATUS OF AMERICANS

Food and Nutrient Intake Data

The nutritional status of Americans is determined primarily from data obtained by national surveys conducted at regular intervals as a part of the National Nutrition Monitoring System. These are the Nationwide Food Consumption Surveys (NFCS) and the NHANES. (See Chapter 15 for a discussion of these surveys.)

Status Report from Monitoring Surveys

1987–88 Nationwide Food Consumption Survey

The most recent Nationwide Food Consumption Survey (NFCS), which was conducted in 1987–88, included 8,337 respondents 1 year of age and older. Based on a 24-hour recall and a 2-day food record, the results represent the average intake for any age and sex group. These results are summarized in Table 16–9 and Table 16–10. Because of the low response rate, however, these results cannot be generalized to the United States population (Wright HS, 1991).

Notwithstanding the public awareness of the role of diet in disease that has developed over the past decade, there were few differences between the results of this survey and the 1977–78 NFCS. Protein intakes continued to exceed the RDA at 15 to 18% of total kilocalories. Dietary fats represented 35 to 37% of energy intake, of which saturated fats provided considerably more than one third. Cholesterol exceeded the standard of 300 mg for men but was within or below desirable ranges for women. Dietary fiber intakes were higher for women than men, but both were considerably lower than recommended.

In general, vitamin intakes met or exceeded the 1989 RDA, giving little reasons for concern about inadequacies. Intakes of minerals that were 75% or less of RDA in some age groups were suggestive of increased risk. These included iron and calcium in women, zinc in men, and magnesium and copper in both men and women.

Nutrition Monitoring Report

At the request of the Department of Health and Human Services (DHHS) and the US Department of Agriculture (USDA), an Expert Panel on Nutrition Monitoring was established by the Life Sciences Research Office of the Federation of American Societies for Experimental Biology (FASEB) to review the dietary and nutritional status of the American population (Expert Panel on Nutrition Monitoring, 1990). The report of the committee summarized the results of data from NHANES II, Hispanic HANES, and the NFCS and Continuing Survey of Food Intake of Individuals (CSFII) surveys described earlier. In general the committee concluded that the food supply in the United States is abundant, although some may not receive an adequate share for a variety of reasons. Nutrient intakes are most likely to be low in persons living below the poverty level. Intakes of nutrients reported to be low in the general population are even lower in the poverty group.

Among the evaluations undertaken by the committee were categorization of various food components according to the degree in which their intakes constituted public health issues (Expert Panel on Nutrition Monitoring, 1990).

FOOD COMPONENTS CONSTITUTING CURRENT PUBLIC HEALTH ISSUES

Energy. Most reported energy intakes do not exceed recommendations. In fact, intakes of 1,661 kcal by women reported in the 1985 CSFII were low enough to raise concern about adequacy of nutrient intake of the total diet. However, the reported prevalence of overweight (one quarter of all adults) indicates an energy imbalance, most probably on the side of insufficient activity. Overweight is also common in Hispanics, particularly Mexican-Americans and Puerto Ricans.

Total Fat, Saturated Fat, and Cholesterol. Intakes of fat and saturated fat are higher than recommended, and cholesterol intakes are high in adult men. Elevated levels of serum cholesterol occur in 11 to 22% of almost all adult groups aged 20 to 74. However, eating patterns suggest that people are making an effort to eat less saturated fat and cholesterol. High fat intakes in women are associated with smoking, being white, and education beyond high school.

Sodium. Sodium intakes exceed recommended levels in almost all age-sex groups.

Alcohol. Although alcohol excess does not appear to be a common problem, enough people report excessive intakes (1 oz of ethanol/day in 9% of adults) to warrant serious attention.

Iron and Calcium. Some nutrients constitute serious public health concerns in certain subgroups of the population. Lack of *iron,* primarily in young children and women of child-bearing age, remains the single most widespread nutrient deficiency in this country, although prevalence appears to be declining in children 1 to 5 years old. *Calcium* intakes of women are a concern in view of osteoporosis incidence in later life.

FOOD COMPONENTS CONSIDERED TO BE POTENTIAL PUBLIC HEALTH ISSUES. Some nutrients are considered to be po-

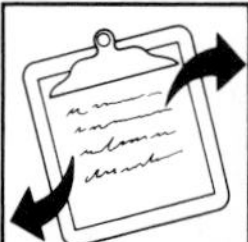

CLINICAL INSIGHT: Nutrition and Your Health: Dietary Guidelines for Americans*

Eat a variety of foods.
Maintain a healthy weight.
Choose a diet low in fat, saturated fat, and cholesterol:

- —30% or less of calories from fat
- —less than 10% of calories from saturated fat

Choose a diet with plenty of vegetables, fruits, and grain products every day:

- —3 or more servings of various vegetables
- —2 or more servings of various fruits
- —6 or more servings of grain products

Use sugars only in moderation.
Use salt and sodium only in moderation.
If you drink alcoholic beverages, do so in moderation:

- —1 drink per day for women
- —2 drinks per day for men

* From Nutrition and Your Health: Dietary Guidelines for Americans, 3rd ed. Home and Garden Bulletin No., 232. Hyattsville, MD, USDA, USDHHS, 1990.

tential problems but require further study with respect to either requirements or association with risk. These include *dietary fiber, vitamin A* in certain groups, *folacin, zinc, fluoride,* and *vitamins B_6 and C.*

NUTRIENTS NOT CONSIDERED TO BE POTENTIAL PUBLIC HEALTH ISSUES. Nutrients consumed in adequate amounts by the majority, or for which there does not appear to be risk involved in either high or low intakes, include *protein, carbohydrate, vitamins E and B_{12}, thiamin, niacin, riboflavin, phosphorus, magnesium,* and *copper.*

NATIONAL GUIDELINES FOR DIET PLANNING

Current Health Issues

Within the last 30 years, attention has been focused increasingly on the relationship of nutrition to degen-

CLINICAL INSIGHT: Nutrition Recommendations for Canadians*

The Canadian diet should provide energy consistent with the maintenance of body weight within the recommended range.

The Canadian diet should include essential nutrients in amounts specified in the Recommended Nutrient Intakes. (See Table 16–6.)

The Canadian diet should include no more than 30% of energy as fat (33 g/1,000 kcal or 39 g/5,000 kJ) and no more than 10% as saturated fat (11 g/1,000 kcal or 13 g/5,000 kJ).

The Canadian diet should provide 55% of energy as carbohydrates (138 g/1,000 kcal or 165 g/5,000 kJ) from a variety of sources.

The sodium content of the Canadian diet should be reduced.

The Canadian diet should include no more than 5% of total energy as alcohol, or two drinks daily, whichever is less.

The Canadian diet should contain no more caffeine than the equivalent of four cups of regular coffee per day.

Community water supplies containing less than 1 mg/l of fluoride should be fluoridated to that level.

* From Communications/Implementation Committee, Minister of National Health and Welfare: Action Towards Healthy Eating, Cat No H39-166/199. Ottawa, Branch Publications Unit, 1990.

erative disease. Although this interest derives to some degree from the rapid increase in size and longevity of the elderly population, it is also prompted by the desire to prevent premature deaths from causes such as cancer and cardiovascular disease.

Sixty-five per cent of deaths in the United States are caused by degenerative disease. Of the 10 leading causes of death, five are associated with diet (heart disease, stroke, diabetes, atherosclerosis, and some kinds of cancer) and three with excessive alcohol consumption (cirrhosis, accidents, and suicide) (Public Health Service, 1988) (Table 16–11). The development of current guidelines is discussed in Chapter 15.

TABLE 16–11. Ten Leading Causes of Death, United States, 1987*

Rank	Cause of Death	No.	% of Total Deaths
1†	Heart disease	759,400	35.7
2†	Cancer	476,700	22.4
3†	Stroke	148,700	7.0
4‡	Unintentional injury	92,500	4.4
5	Chronic obstructive lung disease	78,000	3.7
6	Pneumonia and influenza	68,600	3.2
7†	Diabetes mellitus	37,800	1.8
8‡	Suicide	29,600	1.4
9‡	Chronic liver disease and cirrhosis	26,000	1.2
10†	Atherosclerosis	23,100	1.1

* From Public Health Service, DHHS: The Surgeon General's Report on Nutrition and Health. DHHS (PHS) Publ No 88-50211. Washington, DC, DHHS, 1988.

† Causes of death in which diet plays a part.

‡ Causes of death in which excessive alcohol consumption plays a part.

Current Guidelines for the United States and Canada

At least 8 different organizations, mostly federal, have issued dietary guidelines within the last 10 years (Table 15–2). The specific recommendations of seven of these are compared in Table 16–12. Except for minor differences, they are all very much alike (Fig. 16–2); and when numerical goals are specified, they are surprisingly similar to those established by the Senate Select Committee in 1977 (see Table 15–2). Some, such as the Dietary Guidelines for Americans and the Nutrition Recommendations for Canadians, are deliberately general (Clinical Insight, p. 284), while others, such as the NRC/NAS Committee on Diet and Health Recommendations, are more specific (Clinical Insight, p. 287). Guidelines directed toward a particular disease state, such as the National Cancer Institute (NCI) Cancer Guidelines, contain recommendations unique to that condition (Butrum et al, 1988). Other differences reflect actual disagreement regarding amounts or even the need to include items such as cholesterol, sodium, sugar, or alcohol.

The basic universal prescription for health and fitness appears to be:

Adjust energy intake and exercise level to achieve and maintain appropriate body weight.

Eat less total fat, less saturated fat.

Increase total carbohydrate, increase complex carbohydrate.

To this can be added (from most, but not all, guidelines):

Eat less cholesterol.

Reduce intake of refined sugar.

Eat less sodium.

Eat more fiber.

Eat more fruits and vegetables.

Eat a variety of foods.

Drink alcohol in moderation or not at all.

Unique to the Cancer Guidelines:

Eat cruciferous vegetables frequently.

Eat fruits and vegetables high in vitamins A and C.

Limit the use of salt-cured, smoked, and charcoal-broiled foods.

Unique to the Canadian Guidelines:

Limit caffeine intake to the equivalent of 4 cups of coffee per day.

Included in a few recommendations:

Limit protein to twice the RDA or less.

Drink fluoridated water.

Meet the RDA for calcium, especially adolescents and women.

Meet the RDA for iron, especially children, adolescents, and women of childbearing age.

Avoid the use of dietary supplements.

IMPLEMENTING THE GUIDELINES

The task of planning nutritious meals centers on the inclusion of the essential nutrients in optimal amounts as outlined in the RDA, along with appropriate energy and limited amounts of salt, sugar, cholesterol, and fat, especially saturated fat.

Table 16–13 presents a composite of the dietary guidelines described in Table 16–12 and can be used as a basis for dietary planning. Suggestions are included to assist in meeting the specifics of the recommendations. When specific numerical recommendations differ, they are presented as ranges. For a discussion of planning a vegetarian diet, see Further Reading, page 290.

TABLE 16–12. Comparison of Recommendations of Selected Dietary Guidelines

Guideline and Date	Total Fat	Saturated Fat (% of Total Energy)	Polyunsaturated Fat	Cholesterol	Carbohydrate (% of Total Energy)	Sugar	Fiber	Sodium	Alcohol
Dietary Goals* 1977	27–33%	8–12%	8–12%	250–300 mg/day	45–51%	8–12%	Increase	Salt: 4–6 g/day Sodium: 1.6–2.4 g/day	
Dietary Guidelines for Americans† 1985	30% or less	Less than 10%		Avoid excess	Increase	Avoid excess	Increase	Avoid excess	Moderation
Cancer Guidelines‡ 1988	30% or less						20–30 g/day; 35 g max.		Moderation
Surgeon General's§ 1988 Report	30% or less	Less than 10%		Less than 300 mg/day	Increase	Limit in caries-susceptible persons	Increase	Reduce	No more than 2 drinks/day
Diet and Health‖ 1989	30% or less	Less than 10%		Less than 300 mg/day	Increase			Salt: 6 g/day	Less than 1 oz of alcohol/day
National Cholesterol Education Program¶ 1990	30%	Less than 10%	Up to 10%	Less than 300 mg/day					
Nutrition Recommendations for Canadians** 1989	No more than 30%	No more than 10%			55% of calories			Reduce	Less than 5% of total energy

* *Dietary Goals for the United States,* Senate Select Committee on Nutrition and Human Needs.
† *Dietary Guidelines for Americans,* 2nd ed, USDA/DHHS.
Eat a variety of foods.
Maintain a healthy weight.
Choose a diet with plenty of vegetables, fruits, and grain products.
‡ *Cancer Guidelines,* National Cancer Institute/DHHS.
Choose a variety of fruits and vegetables including cruciferous vegetables (broccoli, brussels sprouts, cabbage, kale, turnips, rutabagas).
Limit consumption of smoked, salt-cured, salt-pickled foods, and charcoal-broiled foods.
§ *The Surgeon General's Report on Nutrition and Health,* Public Health Service/DHHS.
Achieve and maintain desirable weight. Choose dietary pattern in which energy intake is consistent with expenditure.
Increase consumption of whole-grain foods and cereal products.
Community water systems should contain fluoride at optimal levels, or use other sources.
Adolescent girls and adult women should increase consumption of high-calcium foods.
Children, adolescents, and women of childbearing age should choose foods that are good sources of iron.
‖ *Diet and Health,* Committee on Diet and Health, FNB/NRC/NAS.
Balance food intake and physical activity to maintain appropriate weight.
Maintain protein at moderate levels.
5 or more servings of fruits and vegetables, especially green or yellow vegetables and citrus fruit.
Maintain adequate intake of calcium.
Avoid supplements in excess of RDA.
Maintain optimal intake of fluoride, particularly during years of primary and secondary tooth formation and growth.
¶ *National Cholesterol Education Program,* DHHS.
Step 1: Less than 10% of energy from saturated fat; Step 2: less than 7%. See Table 20–5 for further detail.
** *Nutrition Recommendations for Canadians.*
Caffeine: 4 cups/day.
Fluoridation: yes.

Change diet →	Reduce fats	Control calories	Increase starch and fibers	Reduce sodium	Control alcohol
Reduce risk ↓					
Heart disease	●	●		●	
Cancer	●	●	●		●
Stroke	●	●		●	●
Diabetes	●	●	●		
Gastrointestinal diseases	●	●	●		●

FIGURE 16–2. *Consistency of recommendations to reduce the risk of chronic diseases or their complications. Starch refers to complex carbohydrates provided by fruits, vegetables, and whole-grain products. Gastrointestinal diseases affected by dietary factors are primarily gallbladder disease (fat and energy), diverticular disease (fiber), and cirrhosis of the liver (alcohol). (Redrawn from McGinnis JM and Nestle M: The Surgeon General's Report on Nutrition and Health: Policy implications and implementation strategies. Am J Clin Nutr 49:23, 1989, p 26.)*

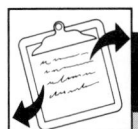

CLINICAL INSIGHT: Recommendations of the Committee on Diet and Health, National Research Council, 1989*

Reduce total fat intake to 30% or less of calories. Reduce saturated fatty acid intake to less than 10% of calories, and the intake of cholesterol to less than 300 mg/day. The intake of fat and cholesterol can be reduced by substituting fish, poultry without skin, lean meats, and low-fat or nonfat dairy products for fatty meats and whole-milk dairy products; by choosing more vegetables, fruits, cereals, and legumes; and by limiting oils, fats, egg yolks, and fried and other fatty foods.

Every day eat five servings or more of a combination of vegetables and fruits, especially green and yellow vegetables and citrus fruits. Also, increase intake of starches and other complex carbohydrates by eating six or more daily servings of a combination of breads, cereals, and legumes.

Maintain protein intake at moderate levels.

Balance food intake and physical activity to maintain appropriate body weight.

The committee does not recommend alcohol consumption. For those who drink alcoholic beverages, the committee recommends limiting consumption to the equivalent of less than 1 ounce of pure alcohol in a single day. This is the equivalent of two cans of beer, two small glasses of wine, or two average cocktails. *Pregnant women should avoid alcoholic beverages.*

Limit total daily intake of salt (sodium chloride) to 6 g or less. Limit the use of salt in cooking and avoid adding it to food at the table. Salty, highly processed salty, salt-preserved, and salt-pickled foods should be consumed sparingly.

Maintain adequate calcium intake.

Avoid taking dietary supplements in excess of the RDA in any 1 day.

Maintain an optimal intake of fluoride, particularly during the years of primary and secondary tooth formation and growth.

* From Committee on Diet and Health, Food and Nutrition Board. National Research Council: Diet and Health Implications for reducing chronic disease risk, Washington, D.C., National Academy Press, 1989.

TABLE 16–13. Composite of Selected Dietary Guidelines

General	Specific	Instruction
Reduce consumption of fat (especially saturated fat) and cholesterol.	Reduce total fat intake to 30% or less of calories. Reduce saturated fat intake to less than 10% of calories, and the intake of cholesterol to less than 300 mg/day.	Substitute extra lean ("select") beef and pork, skinless chicken and turkey, fish and shellfish (except shrimp) for high-fat meats. Eat a maximum of 7 oz animal protein daily. Use cottage, pot, ricotta, and other low-fat cheeses in place of hard chesses as much as possible. Maximal use of legumes, whole grains, vegetables and fruits. Minimal use of butter, margarine, mayonnaise, salad dressings, peanut butter, rich sauces, and gravies. Use reduced fat versions if possible. Use no more than 3 to 4 egg yolks per week.
Increase consumption of carbohydrates, especially complex carbohydrates and fiber.	Increase carbohydrate consumption to at least 55% of total calories. Limit intake of refined sugars to 10% of calories.	Every day, eat at least 5 servings of fruits and vegetables, including potatoes and those high in vitamins A (orange-yellow and dark green) and C. (See Tables 6–3 and 6–32.) Eat at least 6 servings of whole-grain breads, cereals, and/or pasta each day. Eat less of sugar-rich foods (jams, jellies, syrups, candies, rich desserts, baked goods).
Maintain protein at moderate levels.	Do not exceed two times the RDA for protein, or approximately 100 g for an adult woman and 125 g for an adult man.	Eat moderate portions of high-protein foods. Limit meat servings to 7 oz/day. (A 3-oz serving is about the size of a deck of cards and contains around 20 g of protein.) Limit dairy products to a total of 3 or 4 servings daily. One cup of milk or 1oz of hard cheese contains 8 g of protein.
Limit intake of salt (sodium chloride).	Limit daily salt intake to 6 g (1 level tsp) or less.	Do not add salt to food at the table; use only small amounts during cooking and serving. Minimal use of salty foods (chips, crackers, other salted snack foods, French fries), processed foods (canned soups, frozen entrees), salt-preserved and salt-pickled foods.
Maintain adequate calcium intake.	Meet daily RDA, particularly for adolescents and young women up to 25 years of age (1,200 mg)	Increase daily intake of nonfat or low-fat milk or dairy products to at least 2 to 3 servings (1 cup milk or equivalent). Eat tofu (calcium sulfate processed), vegetable greens, broccoli, or calcium-fortified orange juice frequently.
Emphasize dietary cancer prevention.	Reduce fat consumption to 30% of calories and use foods high in vitamins A and C (see earlier). Include cruciferous vegetables in the diet. Avoid potential dietary carcinogens.	Include broccoli, brussel sprouts, cauliflower, cabbage, kale, turnips, and rutubagas frequently. Avoid charcoal-broiled meats or eat them infrequently. Reduce fat intake as described earlier.
Children, adolescents, and women of childbearing age should consume foods that are good sources of iron.		Eat lean red meats, fish, beans, whole-grain products, and daily servings of iron-enriched cereals.
Community water systems should contain fluoride at optimal levels for prevention of tooth decay.		Drink water containing fluoride at the level of approximately 1 ppm. When fluoridated water is not available, use supplementary fluoride.
Avoid taking dietary supplements in excess of the RDA in any 1 day.		Do not take vitamins and minerals indiscriminately just because they are available.
If you do drink, do so in moderation. Pregnant women should avoid alcoholic beverages.	Limit consumption to the equivalent of less than 1 oz of pure alcohol in a single day.	Limit daily intake to two cans of beer or two small glasses of wine or two 1½ oz jiggers of distilled spirits, each of which contains 1 oz of alcohol.
Balance food intake and physical activity to achieve and maintain appropriate body weight.	Appropriate weight is 15–18% body fat for men and 20–24% body fat for women. Overweight is 120% of desirable weight or body mass index above 25.	Reduce weight slowly to appropriate level when necessary. Exercise aerobically at least three times per week.

TABLE 16–14. Food Groups and Serving Sizes

Food Group	Suggested Daily Servings	What Makes a Serving
Breads, cereals, and other grain products Whole-grain Enriched	6 to 11 servings Include several servings a day of whole-grain products.	1 slice of bread ½ hamburger bun or English muffin A small roll, biscuit, or muffin 3 to 4 small or 2 large crackers ½ cup cooked cereal, rice, or pasta 1 oz of ready-to-eat breakfast cereal
Fruits Citrus, melon, berries Other fruits	2 to 4 servings	1 piece of whole fruit such as an apple, banana, orange 1 grapefruit half 1 melon wedge ¾ cup of juice ½ cup berries ½ cup cooked or canned fruit ¼ cup dried fruit
Vegetables Dark-green leafy Deep-yellow Dry beans and peas (legumes) Starchy Other vegetables	3 to 5 servings Use all types regularly; use dark-green leafy vegetables, dry beans, and peas several times a week.	½ cup of cooked or chopped raw vegetables 1 cup of leafy raw vegetables, such as lettuce or spinach
Meat, poultry, fish, and alternates Eggs, dry beans and peas, nuts, and seeds	2 to 3 servings—total 5 to 7 oz lean	Serving sizes will vary. Amount should total 5 to 7 oz of lean meat, fish, or poultry a day. Count these alternates as 1 oz of lean meat: 1 egg ½ cup cooked dry beans 2 T of peanut butter
Milk, cheese, and yogurt	2 servings 3 servings for teenagers and women who are pregnant or breast-feeding. 4 servings for teenagers who are pregnant or breast-feeding.	1 cup of milk 8 oz of yogurt 1½ oz natural cheese 2 oz processed cheese
Fats, sweets, and alcoholic beverages	Avoid too many fats and sweets. If consumed, alcoholic beverages should be in moderation.	

- Include different foods from within the groups.
- Choose more often those foods in each group that are low in fat and sugars.
- Eat at least the minimum number of servings from each group. Those requiring more such as older children or active women, men, and teenagers should have the higher number of servings. Young children can have smaller servings except from the milk group.

FURTHER READING: What is a "Varied Diet"?

Many of the food guides and other recommendations for Americans emphasize eating "a wide variety of foods" for the purpose of achieving dietary adequacy. "Uncertainties in the knowledge base" (Food and Nutrition Board, 1989) make it impossible to establish RDA for all the known nutrients, and there is always the possibility, albeit remote, that unidentified factors may contribute to optimal nutrition. According to the Food and Nutrition Board, meeting the RDA by choosing a variety of foods will probably provide adequate amounts of those nutrients whose recommended levels have not been precisely defined.

Although it is not possible to measure the effect of a varied diet on these intangibles, it does appear that increasing the number of foods eaten over a period of time improves food choices in general. Some studies have shown that nutritional adequacy of the diet increases with a greater number of different foods. Such diets tend to include less protein, meat, and meat alternatives and more carbohydrate, fruits, and vegetables (Guthrie, 1984; Smiciklas-Wright, 1986). Diets with limited food intakes, such as weight-reduction diets, are improved in nutritional adequacy when they include a larger number of different foods.

"Variety" is obviously an arbitrary definition when applied to numbers. One Canadian study defined diets of "limited variety" as consisting of 49 or fewer different items consumed throughout 1 year (Krondl, 1982). The intake of 12.5 different food items in 1 day by Puerto Rican teenagers was described as "low" (Duyff, 1975).

The mean number of different foods consumed during a 3-day period as recorded in the 1977–78 NFCS was 26.2. Oranges, orange juice, apples, and bananas accounted for 62% of the fruit mentioned, and potatoes, tomatoes, peas, beans, corn, and lettuce accounted for 73% of the vegetables reported (Guthrie, 1984).

FURTHER READING: Vegetarian Diets

Vegetarian diets of various descriptions have enjoyed increased popularity in recent years, their use motivated by philosophical, religious, and ecologic concerns as well as what some perceive to be a more healthful lifestyle.

Considerable evidence attests to the health benefits of a vegetarian diet. Epidemiologic data, particularly from studies of Seventh Day Adventists, indicate lower rates of non–insulin-dependent diabetes mellitus, breast and colon cancer, and cardiovascular and gallbladder disease. However, data are not sufficient to prove that an omnivorous diet, planned according to recommended guidelines and combined with a healthy lifestyle, is not equally beneficial (National Institute of Nutrition, 1990).

Of the 8 to 10 million people in the United States who profess to be vegetarians, most eliminate "red" meats but include fish, poultry, and dairy products (Lessons we can learn . . . , 1988). The *lacto-vegetarian* does not eat meat, fish, poultry, or eggs, but includes milk, cheese, and other dairy products in his diet. The *lacto-ovo-vegetarian* also uses eggs. The true vegetarian, or *vegan,* shuns all foods of animal origin. The vegan program is the only one that incorporates any real risk of inadequate nutrition, and this can be avoided by careful planning.

Vegetarian diets tend to be low in iron, although the nonheme iron present in fruits, vegetables, and unrefined cereals is usually accompanied, either in the food or in the meal, by large amounts of ascorbic acid that aids in assimilation. Iron-deficiency anemia is not common among vegetarians.

Without dairy products, calcium intakes may be low, and vitamin D may be inadequate in northern latitudes. The calcium present in some vegetables is inactivated by the presence of oxalates. Phytates in unrefined cereals also can inactivate calcium; however, this is not a problem with Western vegetarians, whose diets tend to be based more on fruits and vegetables than on the unrefined cereals used in middle-Eastern cultures.

Vegans of long standing may develop megaloblastic anemia as a result of vitamin B_{12} deficiency, inasmuch as this vitamin occurs only in foods of animal origin. Curiously, this is less of a problem in areas where sanitation is poor because contaminating bacteria can serve as a source of this vitamin. The hazard of vegan diets is that the presence of high levels of folate may mask the neurologic damage of a B_{12} deficiency.

Although vegetarian diets tend to be lower in protein than those of omnivores, the levels are usually adequate and even exceed the RDA. Deficiencies of some essential amino acids in vegetable proteins require the use of careful planning to provide the complementarity necessary for adequate protein synthesis. However, it no longer appears to be necessary to provide all of the amino acids together in the same meal (American Dietetic Association, 1988) (see Chapter 5).

Because of the high bulk of a vegetarian diet, it is difficult for children and adolescents to consume enough food to provide for their energy needs. Children on such diets may grow and thrive, but they are often small for their age.

The Daily Food Guide shown in Table 16–14 offers a pattern for daily food choices based on "servings" from the six food groups. When planned to include a wide variety of foods within each food group, this pattern will result in a diet that is adequate in nutrients (Further Reading, p. 289). To achieve an eating pattern that reduces fat intake to 30% of total kilocalories, it is necessary to also incorporate the recommendations of Table 16–13 for lowering total fat and saturated fat. Tables in Chapters 6 and 7 list good food sources of individual vitamins and minerals.

A useful variation developed by the National Dairy Council provides specific guidelines for planning individualized diets that will meet the recommendation of 30% of energy from fat (see Chapter 20).

CITED REFERENCES

American Dietetic Association: Position of the American Dietetic Association: Vegetarian diets–technical support paper. J Am Diet Assoc 88:352, 1988.

Butrum RR et al: NCI dietary guidelines: Rationale. Am J Clin Nutr 48(Suppl):888, 1988.

Code of Federal Regulations 21: Food and Drugs, Parts 100 to 199. Rev April 1, 1977. Washington, DC, US Government Printing Office, 1977.

Committee on Diet and Health, Food and Nutrition Board, National Research Council: Diet and Health. Implications for Reducing Chronic Disease Risk. Washington, DC, National Academy Press, 1989.

Communications/Implementation Committee, Minister of National Health and Welfare: Action Towards Healthy Eating. Canada's Guidelines for Healthy Eating and Recommended Strategies for Implementation. Cat No H39-166/1990E. Ottawa, Minister of Supply and Services, 1990.

DeBruyne LK: The changing roles of food labels. Nutrition information and health messages, Nutr Clin 5(4):1, 1990.

Duyff R et al: Food behavior and related factors of Puerto-Rican American teenagers. J Nutr Educ 7:99, 1975.

Expert Panel on Nutrition Monitoring, Life Sciences Research Office, Federation of American Societies for Experimental Biology: Nutrition monitoring in the United States: An update report on nutrition monitoring. Nutrition Today 25(1):33, 1990.

Food and Nutrition Board, National Research Council, NAS: Recommended Dietary Allowances, 10th ed. Washington, DC, National Academy Press, 1989.

Guthrie HA: Eating trends and nutritional consequences. *In* Food and Nutrition Board, Commission on Life Sciences, National Research Council: What Is America Eating? Washington, DC, National Academy Press, 1986.

Hamill PVV et al: Physical growth: National Center for Health Statistics percentiles. Am J Clin Nutr 32:607, 1979.

Joint FAO/WHO Expert Committee on Food Additives: Evaluation of Certain Food Additives and Contaminants. Tech Report Series #710. Geneva, World Health Organization, 1984a.

Joint FAO/WHO Expert Committee on Food Safety: The Role of Food Safety in Health and Development. Tech Report Series #705. Geneva, World Health Organization, 1984b.

Joint FAO/WHO/UNU Expert Consultation: Energy and Protein Requirements. Tech Report Series #724. Geneva, World Health Organization, 1985.

Krondl M et al: Food use and perceived food meanings of the elderly. J Am Diet Assoc 80:523, 1982.

Lessons we can learn from vegetarians. Tufts Univ Nutr Letter 6(5):3, 1988.

National Institute of Nutrition (Canada): Risks and benefits of vegetarian diets. Nutrition Today 25(2):27, 1990.

Nutrition and Your Health: Dietary Guidelines for Americans, 3rd ed. Home and Garden Bulletin No 232. Hyattsville, MD, USDA, USDHHS, 1990.

Public Health Service, USDHHS: The Surgeon General's Report on Nutrition and Health. Summary and Recommendations, DHHS (PHS) Publ No 88-50211. Washington, DC, US Government Printing Office, 1988.

Smiciklas-Wright H et al: Variety in foods. *In* Food and Nutrition Board, Commission on Life Sciences, National Research Council: What Is America Eating? Washington, DC, National Academy Press, 1986.

Wright HS et al: The 1987–88 Nationwide Food Consumption Survey: An update on the nutrient intake of respondents. Nutr Today 26(3):21, 1991.

ADDITIONAL REFERENCES

American Cancer Society: Nutrition, common sense and cancer. Publ No 2096-LE. New York, American Cancer Society, 1985.

American Red Cross: Better eating for better health: Instructor's guide and participant's packet. Washington, DC, American Red Cross, 1984. Available from local Red Cross chapter.

Cronin FJ et al: Developing a food guidance system to implement the dietary guidelines. J Nutr Educ 19:281, 1987.

Cronin FJ and Shaw AM: Summary of dietary recommendations for healthy Americans. Nutrition Today 23(6):26, 1988.

Derelian D: Healthy Dividends. A Plan for Balancing Your Fat Budget, Leader's Guide and A Do-It-Yourself Approach to Lowering Fat for Life. Rosemont, IL, National Dairy Council, 1990.

Fanelli-Kuczmarski M and Wotecki CE: Monitoring the nutritional status of the Hispanic population: Selected findings for Mexican Americans, Cubans and Puerto Ricans. Nutrition Today 25(3):6, 1990.

National Center for Health Statistics, DHHS, Public Health Service: Plan and Operation of the Second National Health and Nutrition Examination Survey 1976–80. DHHS Publ No (PHS) 81–1317. Hyattsville, MD, DHHS, 1981.

Pennington JAT: Bowes and Church's Food Values of Portions Commonly Used, 16th ed. Philadelphia, JB Lippincott, 1990.

Pennington JAT, Young BE, and Wilson DB: Nutritional elements in U.S. diets: Results from the Total Diet Study, 1982–1986. J Am Diet Assoc 89:659, 1989.

Public Health Service, USDHHS, and NHLBI: National Cholesterol Education Program (NCEP), Report of the Expert Panel on Detection, Evaluation, and Treatment of High Blood Cholesterol in Adults. NIH Publ No 88-2925. NHLBI, Washington, DC, US Government Printing Office, 1988.

Public Health Service, USDHHS, and NHLBI: Report of the Expert Panel on Population-based Strategies for Blood Cholesterol Reduction. NIH Publ No 90-3046. NHLBI, Washington, DC, US Government Printing Office, 1990.

Rivers JM and Collins KK: Planning Meals That Lower Cancer Risk: A Reference Guide. Washington, DC, American Institute for Cancer Research, 1984.

Scientific Review Committee and Communications/Implementation Committee, Minister of National Health and Welfare: Nutrition Recommendations. A Call for Action. Cat No H39-162, 1990E. Ottawa, Minister of Supply and Services, 1990.

Public Health Service, USDHHS, NIH: Diet, Nutrition and Cancer Prevention: A Guide to Food Choices. Rev ed, Publ No 87-2878. Washington, DC, US Government Printing Office, 1987.

CHAPTER 17

THE ASSESSMENT OF NUTRITIONAL STATUS

Dorice M. Czajka-Narins, Ph.D.

CHAPTER OUTLINE

KEY TERMS

ANTHROPOMETRY—the science that deals with the measurement of the size, weight, and proportions of the human body

BIOELECTRICAL IMPEDANCE ANALYSIS (BIA)—a method of body composition analysis based on electrical conductance and the greater electrical conductivity of fat-free mass

BODY MASS INDEX (BMI)—weight (kg)/height (m^2); a definition of the level of adiposity

DIETARY HISTORY—a detailed dietary assessment, which may include a 24-hour recall, food frequency questionnaire, and additional information such as weight history, previous diet changes, use of supplements, and food intolerances

FOOD DIARY—a written record of amounts of all foods and liquids consumed during a time period, usually 3 to 7 days; often includes information on time, place, and situation of eating

FOOD FREQUENCY QUESTIONNAIRE—a method of dietary assessment in which the questions relate to how often foods are consumed

FUNCTIONAL TEST—a test that relates nutritional status to the performance of cells, tissues, organs, or anatomic systems

HAIR ANALYSIS—analysis of mineral content of a specific portion of the hair shaft

HYDROSTATIC WEIGHING—comparison of weight before and during submersion in water to determine body density and body fatness

NEGATIVE NITROGEN BALANCE—a catabolic state in which less nitrogen is being retained than is being excreted

NITROGEN BALANCE—the state of the body with regard to ingestion of nitrogen as protein and excretion of nitrogen in urea, feces, sweat, hair, skin, and nails in which the amount retained is equal to the amount excreted

NUTRITIONAL STATUS—a measurement of the extent to which the individual's physiologic need for nutrients is being met

POSITIVE NITROGEN BALANCE—the anabolic state in which more nitrogen is being retained than is being excreted

PROGNOSTIC NUTRITIONAL INDEX (PNI)—an equation relating several objective measures of nutritional status to the occurrence of postoperative morbidity and mortality

SENSITIVITY—the ability of a measurement to indicate an abnormality when an abnormality truly exists

SPECIFICITY—the ability of a measurement to indicate a normal state in which no abnormality exists

SUBJECTIVE GLOBAL ASSESSMENT (SGA)—a method of assessing the relationship of nutritional status to the occurrence of postoperative morbidity and mortality based on clinical judgment

24-HOUR RECALL—a method of dietary assessment in which the individual is asked to remember everything eaten during the past 24 hours

WAIST-HIP RATIO (WHR)—the ratio of the waist measurement compared with the hip measurement; a method for assessing fat distribution

WEIGHT FOR LENGTH CURVE—a standard for evaluating the growth of children that gives the percentile rankings for weight for specific heights with no attention to age

Nutritional status expresses the degree to which physiologic needs for nutrients are being met. The balance between nutrient intake and nutrient requirements is influenced by many factors, as shown in Figure 17-1.

Appropriate techniques of assessment detect nutritional deficiency in the early stages of development so that dietary intake can be improved through nutritional support and counseling before a more severe lesion appears. These techniques involve examination of physical condition, growth and development, the function of various organ systems, behavior, the urinary blood or tissue levels of nutrients, and the quality and quantity of the nutrient intake. Information on medication, stress or chronic illness, economic situation, knowledge about nutrition, cultural patterns, and living conditions is also useful because these factors influence intake and sometimes nutritional requirements.

An assessment of nutritional status should be done routinely for everyone in a health care system. However, a different type of assessment should be done on the basically healthy person than on someone who is critically ill. Persons at risk can be identified by screening tools that utilize information obtained routinely on admission to a hospital or nursing home. Information obtained in the nutritional assessment is usually used as the basis for designing the nutritional care plan, as discussed in Chapter 24. A thorough nutritional assessment makes the planning of nutritional support, nutrition education, or counseling more effective.

DEVELOPMENT OF NUTRITIONAL DEFICIENCY

Nutritional deficiency and nutritional overload are progressive phenomena. Within the safe range of intake, homeostatic mechanisms of the body appear to utilize nutrients equally effectively without a detectable advantage of a given level of intake. As nutritional deficiencies or overloads develop, adaptations are made to achieve a new steady state without any significant loss in physiologic function. As the intake departs further from the accepted range, the organism accommodates to the changing supply of nutrients by reducing functional levels or by changing the size or status of affected body compartments. By identifying the presence or absence of these adaptations, the nutritional status of an individual can be determined. For example, prior to the development of iron deficiency anemia as identified by measures of hematocrit, hemoglobin, and appropriate clinical signs, the gradually diminishing iron stores can be detected by increased iron absorption, falling serum ferritin, or evaluation of bone marrow.

Figure 17-2 illustrates the general sequence of steps leading to the development of a deficiency or overload and the points at which various components of assessment can intervene to provide for anticipating problems and preventing poor nutrition before it develops.

COMPONENTS OF NUTRITIONAL ASSESSMENT

A thorough assessment of nutritional status includes: (1) dietary history and intake data; (2) biochemical data; (3) clinical examination and health history; (4) anthropometric data; and (5) psychosocial data.

When time, money, or professional staff is limited, the assessment must be abbreviated. The minimal nutritional screening, especially for the hospitalized patient, includes measurement of height and weight, change in appetite, serum albumin, and total lymphocyte count, all of which can be measured easily in the hospital (Fig. 17-3; see also Table 24-1). As with all aspects of nutritional status assessment, findings below the standard only identify patients "at risk" of developing a clinical nutritional deficiency. Verification of a deficiency requires further evaluation.

Dietary Intake

The accurate recording and evaluation of individual dietary intakes is the most difficult and frustrating aspect of nutritional assessment. The information obtained can be very useful; however, it is important to recognize the limitations of the data. For example, the very act of recording has a tendency to influence food intake. Also, many people simply cannot remember the types or amounts of food they ate. It is particularly difficult to elicit information from children and the very elderly. Age, however, is only one of many factors; the ability to recall information also depends on intelligence, mood, attention, how important people perceive the information to be, and frequency of exposure to the process (Blake et al, 1989; Karvetti and Knuts, 1985; Lissner et al, 1989).

Converting food intake data to intake of specific nutrients is also an inexact science. This process has been made easier with the use of microcomputers and the variety of software available. However, food composition tables are neither complete nor necessarily accurate for foods that are eaten today. Many processed foods are not listed in the tables or data bases, and information must be obtained from food manufacturers, some of whom may use a different technique than the one used by the US Department of Agriculture. Analytic techniques are not all equally precise,

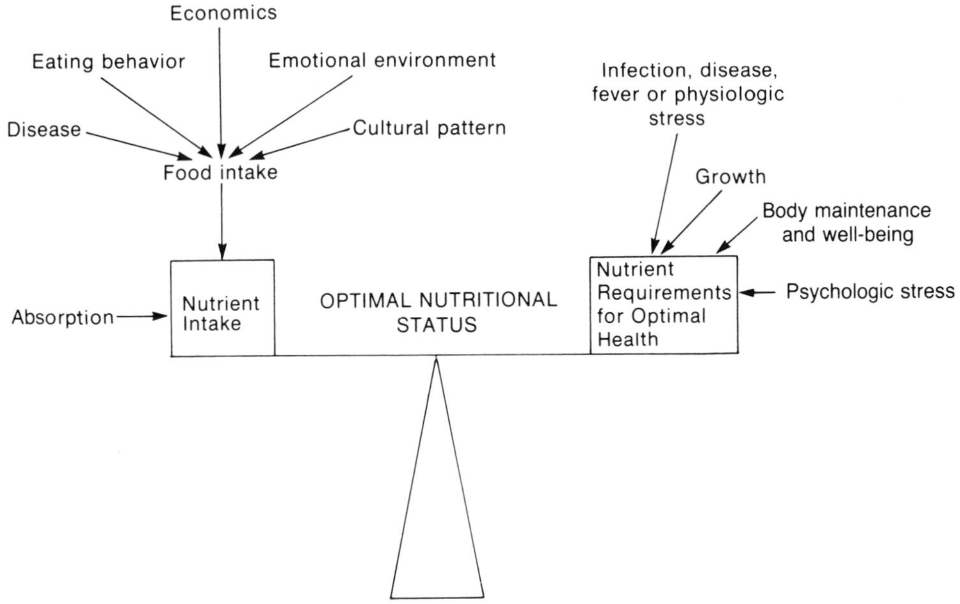

FIGURE 17–1. *Optimal nutritional status as a balance between nutrient intake and nutrient requirements.*

FIGURE 17–2. *Development of a clinical nutritional deficiency with dietary, biochemical, and clinical evaluations. (From Beaton GH and Patwardhan VN: Physiological and practical considerations of nutrient function and requirement.* In *Beaton GH and Bengoa JM [eds]: Nutrition and Preventive Medicine. Geneva, Switzerland, World Health Organization, 1973, p 445–481. [WHO Monograph Series No. 62])*

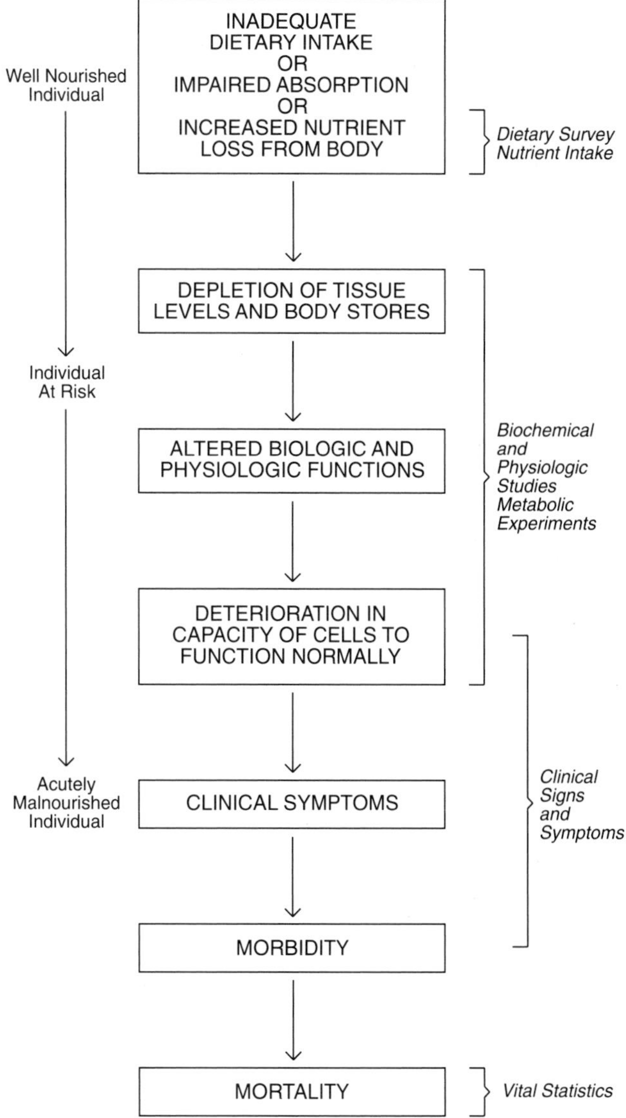

DATE ________

S	Wt. change	None	N/A	N____ V____ D____
	Appetite change	None	N/A	Special diet ________
	Dysphagia ☐ Yes ☐ No		N/A	Other ________
	Food allergies			

O	Ht____ Wt____ Usual wt____ IBW____		*Other Pertinent Information:*
	Age____ %Usual wt %IBW____		
	Serum album in____ g/dl ☐ WNL ☐ Depletion		
	Diet Order ________		
	Diagnosis ________		

A	Nutritional status:	☐ High risk	☐ Moderate risk	☐ Not compromised at this time
	Requires further R.D./D.T. intervention? ☐ Yes ☐ No			

P

☐ Provide basic nutrition care services. Re-evaluate in 3 5 7 10 days.

☐ Screening data not available. Please order:

☐ Nutritional assessment

☐ Nutrient intake analysis (NIA)

☐ Nutrition counseling / diet instruction ________

☐ Other

UH 0165 JUL 86

____

NUTRITION SCREEN

FIGURE 17–3. *University Hospital, Seattle: Reproduction of a nutritional screening form. (From DeHoog S: Nutritional screening and assessment in a university hospital. Report of the 8th Ross Roundtable on Medical Issues. Columbus, OH, Ross Laboratories, 1988.)*

TABLE 17–1. 24-Hour Recall Form and Food Group Evaluation

Food and Fluid Intake from Time of Awakening Until the Next Morning								
	Food and Drink Consumed		**Number of Servings in the Food Groups***					
Time	*Name and Type*	*Amount*	*Milk Group*	*Meat Group*	*Fruits and Vegetables*	*Breads and Cereals*	*Fats, Sweets, and Alcoholic Beverages*	
Totals								

Recommended Number of Servings Daily						
	Amount	*Milk Group*	*Meat Group*	*Fruits and Vegetables*	*Breads and Cereals*	*Fats, Sweets, and Alcoholic Beverages†*
Children aged 6 or under		2–3	2	3	4	Avoid too many
Adolescent		3–4	2–3	3–5	6–11	Avoid too many
Adult		2–3	2–3	3–5	6–11	Avoid too many
Pregnant or Lactating		3–4	2–3	3–5	6–11	Avoid too many
		Milk Group	*Meat Group*	*Fruits and Vegetables*	*Breads and Cereals*	*Fats, Sweets, and Alcoholic Beverages*
Evaluation L = low A = adequate E = excessive						

* See Table 16–14 for serving sizes for Four Food Group Plan.

† Servings of high calorie, low-nutrient items, such as sugar, candy, and soda pop. Excessive amounts in this group usually mean excessive fat, sugar, and energy intake.

and accurate and newer techniques continue to be introduced.

Biochemical variability is common among the same foods obtained from different sources or harvested at different times. For example, the amount of ascorbic acid in a potato varies substantially depending on the season. Bioavailability of nutrients may also vary in relation to the diet. In general, nutrient intake data are estimated to be accurate within 10%.

Methods for Obtaining Dietary Information

TWENTY-FOUR–HOUR RECALL. The most popular and easiest method of obtaining dietary information is the *24-hour recall,* in which the individual is asked to recall everything eaten during the last 24 hours, either by completing a questionnaire or in response to a dietitian/nutritionist or a nurse trained in dietary interviewing (Table 17–1).

Although data obtained in this manner have been shown to be statistically valid for population groups of 50 or more, in dealing with individuals this method of recall is most useful as a basis for informal communication about general eating patterns. Sources of error include: (1) inability to recall accurately the kinds and amounts of food eaten; (2) atypical intakes on the previous day; and (3) failure to obtain the truth for a variety of reasons, one of which may be embarrassment. There is a tendency to underestimate intake as portion sizes increase and to overestimate intake as portion sizes decrease. Foods are often added or omitted depending on the subject's concept of an appropriate intake. Recall can be improved by using food and portion size models and measuring cups and spoons.

FOOD FREQUENCY QUESTIONNAIRE. The food frequency questionnaire collects information on intake of particular foods or food groups on a daily, weekly, or monthly basis. This information can help to validate the accuracy of the 24-hour recall data and clarify the true food consumption pattern. The food frequency questionnaire may be either selective, with questions about foods suspected of being deficient or excessive in the diet, or general, with questions concerning all foods likely to be eaten. Examples are shown in Tables 17–2 and 17–3.

Asking for information in relation to "meals" rather than food groups may trigger responses of other foods eaten at the same time, although the fact that not everyone eats meals may be a disadvantage. Cross checking with shopping lists or weekly purchases also increases the accuracy of food frequency data.

TABLE 17–2. A General Food Frequency Questionnaire

For the frequency of food use, the following pattern of questions may be useful. However, you may have to modify questions after learning some information from the 24-hour recall. For instance, if the patient has said he or she had a glass of milk yesterday, you wouldn't ask "Do you drink milk?" but rather "How much milk do you drink?" Record answers as 1/day, 1/wk, 3/mo, for example, or as accurately as possible. It may just have to be noted as "occasionally" or "rarely."

1. Do you drink milk? If so, how much? ________ What kind? Whole ________ Skim ________ Low-fat ________
2. Do you use fat? If so, what kind? ________ How much? ________
3. How many times do you eat meat? ________ eggs ________ cheese ________ beans ________
4. Do you eat snack foods? If so, which ones? ________ How often? ________ How much? ________
5. What vegetables do you eat? (in each group) How often?
   a. Broccoli ________ green peppers ________ cooked greens ________ carrots ________ sweet potato ________
   b. Tomatoes ________ raw cabbage ________
   c. Asparagus ________ beets ________ cauliflower ________ corn ________ cooked cabbage ________ celery ________ peas ________ lettuce ________
6. What fruits and how often?
   a. Apples or applesauce ________ apricots ________ banana ________ berries ________ cherries ________ grapes or grape juice ________ peaches ________ pears ________ pineapple ________ plums ________ prunes ________ raisins ________
   b. Oranges ________ orange juice ________ grapefruit ________ grapefruit juice ________
7. Bread and cereal products
   a. How much bread do you usually eat with each meal? ________ between meals ________
   b. Do you eat cereal (daily, weekly) cooked ________ dry ________
   c. How often do you eat foods such as macaroni, spaghetti, noodles, etc. ________
   d. Do you eat whole grain breads and cereals? ________ how often? ________
8. Do you use salt? ________ Do you salt your food before tasting it? ________ Do you cook with salt? ________ Do you "crave" salt or salty foods? ________
9. How many tsp of sugar do you use/day (1 packet = 1 tsp)? ________
   (Be sure to ask patient about sugar on cereal, fruit, toast and in coffee, tea, etc.)
10. Do you eat desserts? ________ If so, how often? ________
11. Do you drink sugar-containing beverages such as soda pop? ________ How often? ________
12. How often do you eat candy or cookies? ________
13. Do you drink water? ________ How often during the day? ________ How much each time? ________ How much would you say you drink each day? ________
14. Do you use sugar substitutes in packet form or in drinks? ________ What is your use? ________ How often? ________
15. Do you drink alcohol? ________ How often? ________ How much? ________ Beer, wine, liquor? ________

TABLE 17–3. Selective Food Frequency Questionnaire

Frequency of Food Use: Record as Times/Wk or Times/Day or N = Never, R = Rare

High or Moderately High in:			*High or Moderately High in:*		
Cholesterol:	Eggs	______	**Unsaturated Fat:**	Polyunsaturated margarines	______
	Liver	______		Vegetable oils	______
	Shellfish	______	**Sodium:**	Prepared frozen foods	______
	Beef	______		Canned soups	______
	Pork	______		Sausages or franks	______
Saturated Fat:	Beef	______		Snack foods, e.g., pretzels, potato chips, crackers, salted peanuts	______
	Pork	______		Softened water	______
	Butter	______		Olives, pickles	______
	Whole milk	______		Smoked fish; canned fish	______
	Cream	______		Ham and other canned meat	______
	Pastries	______	**Iron:**	Iron supplements	______
	Gravies	______		Dark green leafy vegetables	______
	Ice cream	______		Enriched cereals	______
	Cheese	______		Dried beans	______
Sugar:	Cakes	______		Meat, fish, or poultry	______
	Pastries	______		Eggs	______
	Cookies	______		Orange juice	______
	Coke	______			
	Soda pop	______			
	Candy	______			
	Sugared cereals	______			
	Fruit candies	______			

Dietary History. The dietary history is more complete than either the 24-hour recall or food frequency questionnaire and usually includes both of these sources as well as additional information (Table 17–4). Obtaining such a history requires the talents of an experienced interviewer who recognizes the need for understanding and objectivity. Dietary habits are personal, and an individual may be unwilling to talk about them (especially if the interviewer is considered to be judgmental). Time can be saved by putting the dietary history into a questionnaire that can be filled out by the patient.

Food Diary or Record. This method requires the subject to write down everything consumed during a particular time period. The nutrient contribution for each food is calculated. The total day's intake for each nutrient is then obtained and is divided by the number of days to give an average daily intake. Three-day diaries covering 2 weekdays and 1 weekend day have been used most frequently. Because of the longer periods needed to predict usual nutrient intakes of individuals, 4-day records are now recommended (Basiotis et al, 1987; Karkeck, 1987).

Information about lifestyle, companions, and meal eating atmosphere can be obtained by asking the subject also to note the time, place, and people with whom meals are eaten. Recall can be combined with the food diary method when the nutrition counselor goes over the food record with the patient and asks for additional information regarding amounts and types of preparation of the food. A food record is usually more accurate if the food eaten is recorded throughout the day when it is consumed.

Observation of Food Intake. Although observation of food intake is the most accurate method, it is also the most time consuming, expensive, and difficult and therefore has limited use. It must be nonintrusive and is done most easily when meals are provided, such as in the case of a hospitalized patient, nursing home resident, or child at a camp or boarding school. It requires knowledge of the amount and the kind of food presented and a record of the amount actually eaten.

The ultimate in a controlled situation is available in a metabolic unit where a weighed amount of food can be presented, the amount of uneaten food reweighed, and the difference recorded as the amount eaten. In scientific studies, a duplicate meal is prepared and measured accurately, and an aliquot is taken for chemical evaluation of nutrient content.

Evaluating Dietary Information

A rapid and very general evaluation of food intake data can be made by determining the number of servings from the *four food groups* that are included in the foods consumed in 24 hours (see Table 17–1 and Chapter 16). Gross deficiencies of protein, iron, calcium, riboflavin, vitamin A, and vitamin C can be detected in this manner. It is more difficult to use this method if the diet has many food mixtures or unusual cultural foods that do not fit into one of the food groups.

Another rapid evaluation that allows the practi-

TABLE 17–4. Dietary History Information

Economics

Income—frequency and steadiness of employment
Amount of money for food each week or month and individual's perception of its adequacy for meeting food needs
Eligibility for food stamps and cost of stamps
Public aid recipient?

Physical Activity

Occupation—type, hours/week, shift, energy expenditure
Exercise—type, amount, frequency (seasonal?)
Sleep—hours/day (uninterrupted?)
Handicaps

Ethnic or Cultural Background

Influence on eating habits
Religion
Education

Home Life and Meal Patterns

Number in household (eat together?)
Person who does shopping
Person who does cooking
Food storage and cooking facilities (stove, refrigerator)
Type of housing (home, apartment, room, etc.)
Ability to shop and prepare food

Appetite

Good, poor, any changes
Factors that affect appetite
Taste and smell perception and any changes

Attitude Toward Food/Eating

Disinterest in food
Irrational ideas about food, eating, and body weight
Parental interest in child's eating

Allergies, Intolerances, or Food Avoidances

Foods avoided and reason
Length of time of avoidance
Description of problems caused by foods

Dental and Oral Health

Problems with eating
Foods that cannot be eaten
Problems with swallowing, salivation, food sticking

Gastrointestinal

Problems with heartburn, bloating, gas, diarrhea, vomiting, constipation, distention
Frequency of problems
Home remedies
Antacid, laxative, or other drug use

Chronic Disease

Treatment
Length of time of treatment
Dietary modification—physician prescription?, date of modification, education, compliance with diet

Medication

Vitamin and/or mineral supplements—frequency, type, amount
Medications—type, amount, frequency, length of time on medication

Recent Weight Change

Loss or gain
How many pounds, over what length of time
Intentional or nonvolitional

Dietary or Nutritional Problems (As Perceived by Patient)

tioner to identify dietary excesses is to compare the intake with the Dietary Guidelines discussed in Chapter 16. An assessment of kilocalories, protein, fat, and carbohydrate can also be derived by quantifying the food intake in terms of *diabetic exchanges* (see Table 31–10).

A more accurate evaluation can be obtained by *calculating the amounts* of each nutrient in the foods consumed, either by hand or with the aid of an appropriate computer program, and comparing the totals with the values in the Recommended Dietary Allowances (RDA). Nutrient values can be obtained from several publications (Adams, 1988; Gebhardt and Matthews, 1981; Pennington, 1989; USDA, 1976–1986) as well as from nutrition labels and information supplied by food manufacturers.

STANDARDS FOR EVALUATION OF NUTRIENT INTAKE. The RDA have been established with a "safety factor" for most nutrients to provide for members of the population with the greatest needs and are appropriate for assessing the nutritional adequacy of diets consumed by population groups (see Chapter 16). However, because inclusion of the safety factor may erroneously indicate that intakes of specific nutrients are insufficient, they are not accurate in assessing intakes of individuals. Some authorities use 70 or 75% of the RDA as an appropriate standard for comparison.

It is important to recognize that intake values lower than the RDA are not indicators of nutrient deficiency. At best they are suggestive of nutritional risk, the extent of which can only be evaluated by biochemical and clinical assessment. In addition, the RDA were designed to apply only to healthy individuals. Nutritional requirements have not been established for various disease states. Therefore, the RDA are the only standards available, but they must be used with discretion.

INTERPRETATION OF DIETARY INTAKE DATA. Energy and protein intake should be evaluated on the basis of body weight, or in the case of the underweight or overweight, on the basis of height or ideal weight. This increases the usefulness of the RDA in individual assessment, especially with children who at any particular age may differ greatly in size. Table 12–1 shows how the RDA are interpreted on the basis of height and how an individual intake is compared with the RDA.

Biochemical Measurements

Biochemical tests are the most objective measures of nutritional status. However, their precision and accuracy are vulnerable to the methods used. In addition, their sensitivity and specificity are reduced by the overlap in populations as described in Further Reading, p. 302. Other factors that affect the validity of these measurements are as follows:

1. No single biochemical indicator is diagnostic. The combined use of several indicators provides a much better measure of status. For example, iron status is frequently defined by three tests: serum ferritin, hematocrit, and free erythrocyte protoporphyrin.
2. Individual variability in measured response to every measured function or chemical component results in a range of values considered to be normal.
3. What is "normal" is affected by age, gender, physiologic state, and possibly race, as well as by environmental circumstances. All of these factors affect hemoglobin levels, for example.
4. Some blood concentrations reflect immediate nutrient intake while others reflect true status; therefore, all of the factors that affect concentration must be taken into account.
5. Some biochemical tests are affected by non-nutrition factors. Stress or injury can increase white blood cell counts and decrease serum protein concentration.
6. Some drugs can interfere significantly with the analysis of laboratory tests. Antibiotics, for example, interfere with the microbiologic assay for folate; fluorescent drugs such as tetracycline interfere with the determination of riboflavin by fluorescence.
7. Daily or weekly variations in the indicator may occur, so that a single measurement should not be considered definitive. Serum cholesterol is one of the measurements that exhibit unexplained fluctuations.
8. Different tests may give different information; thus a battery of tests may be preferable to delineate the changes that mark the development of a deficiency of a nutrient.
9. A biochemical value for one nutrient can be influenced by the intake or body level of another nutrient. For example, serum folate is influenced by the status of other B vitamins.

At present, biochemical measurements for evaluation of all nutrients are not available. Furthermore, there are still questions about the meaning of abnormal values for certain tests. To detect nutritional problems at all stages of development, tests that respond to changes in nutrient intake are needed. These tests should be influenced minimally by exercise, infection, physical or emotional stress, and trauma.

Tests for biochemical evaluation of various nutrients are listed in Table 17-5. Guidelines by which to evaluate biochemical measurements and nutritional status are given in Appendix Table 30.

TABLE 17-5. Biochemical Measurements of Nutritional Status

Nutrient	Test
Protein	Serum thyroxine-binding prealbumin Serum retinol-binding protein Serum transferrin
Lipids	Serum cholesterol—high-and low-density lipoprotein Serum triglycerides Serum lipoproteins
Vitamin A	Serum retinol Serum retinol-binding protein
Vitamin D	Serum 25-OH D_3 Serum 1,25 OH_2 D_3 Serum alkaline phosphatase
Vitamin E	Hydrogen peroxide erythrocyte hemolysis test Serum or plasma vitamin E
Vitamin K	Plasma vitamin K Plasma clotting factors II, VII, IX, X Prothrombin time
Thiamin	Erythrocyte transketolase activity Thiamin pyrophosphate effect
Riboflavin	Plasma riboflavin Erythrocyte glutathione reductase activity Urinary riboflavin
Nicotinic acid	Urinary N_1-methylnicotinamide Urinary 6-pyridone
Vitamin B_6	Tryptophan load test—xanthurenic acid Plasma pyridoxal phosphate Erythrocyte transaminase—serum glutamic-oxaloacetic transaminase (SGOT) and serum glutamic-pyruvic transaminase (SGPT)
Folic acid	Red blood cell folate Serum folate
Vitamin B_{12}	Serum vitamin B_{12} Schilling test
Pantothenic acid	Blood pantothenic acid Urinary pantothenic acid
Biotin	Urinary biotin
Vitamin C	Plasma ascorbic acid Buffy coat (leukocyte and platelet) ascorbic acid Urinary ascorbic acid
Iron	Iron deposits in bone marrow % transferrin saturation Total iron-binding capacity Serum ferritin Protoporphyrin heme Serum iron Hemoglobin Hematocrit Thin blood film Mean corpuscular volume (MCV)
Iodine	Serum iodide Radioiodine uptake
Calcium	Serum alkaline phosphatase
Phosphorus	Serum phosphorus Urinary phosphorus
Zinc	Serum zinc Tissue zinc Urinary zinc Hair zinc
Magnesium	Serum magnesium
Copper	Ceruloplasmin

Sources of Biochemical Data

Biochemical data relating to nutritional status can be obtained from examination of plasma, red blood cells, white blood cells, and urine, or from tissues, such as liver, bone, and hair.

FURTHER READING: Misclassification of Risk

Fixed cutoff points are commonly used to determine *normal* in the case of biochemical tests and *adequate* in the case of dietary intake. The placing of these cutoff points determines the number of people who are properly classified in terms of risk. The *sensitivity* of a measurement is its ability to indicate abnormality when abnormality truly exists. *Specificity* is a measurement's ability to indicate normal where there is no abnormality. As the number of laboratory tests increases, the probability of getting an abnormal value where there is no abnormality also increases.

Rather than use absolute cutoff points to evaluate adequacy, a probability approach has been suggested. This approach is particularly useful in evaluating dietary intake. We cannot assume that the person with the low usual intake will necessarily have the low requirement, nor on the other hand can we assume that the person with the high usual intake will have a high requirement. A probability of inadequacy can be assigned to any observed level of usual intake. A probability of risk curve is specific to a particular class of people, such as menstruating females. Applying this probability approach to the data of the 1977 to 1978 USDA Nationwide Food Consumption Survey revealed an estimated prevalence of inadequate intake of iron to be 23% as compared with more than 95% for whom intake falls below the US RDA of 18 mg/day. An important advantage of this method is that an estimate of prevalence of inadequate intake can be better compared with the prevalence of depletion or deficiency assessed by biochemical or clinical means (Subcommittee . . . , 1986).

Hair Analysis. Although hair analyses are done frequently, they are often misused. For example, hair analysis is valid only with respect to mineral status; it is useless as an indicator of vitamin status. The analytic techniques for hair analysis are sensitive and specific; however, the degree of contamination of the hair sample is frequently unknown and ignored. For example, more than a dozen elements, mostly metals, are components of shampoos and other grooming products and could interfere with analysis (Klevay et al, 1987). Age, sex, place of residence, physiologic state, and presence of disease alter status of some minerals. Inasmuch as there is little agreement on what constitutes normal concentrations of trace elements in hair, any interpretation is somewhat subjective (New Directions, p. 303).

Functional Measurements

Functional measurements of nutritional status may be more clinically relevant because the true significance of a deficiency is impairment of physiologic function. Such indicators relate nutritional status to optimal performance of cells, tissues, organs, or anatomic systems. Many functional indicators of nutritional status are still in the research phase or require unconventional laboratory equipment. These include breath pentane analysis as an index of lipid peroxidation (a functional test for vitamin E status) and measures of dark adaptation (a functional test for vitamin A status).

Hand Grip Strength. Hand grip strength using a dynamometer is a measure of skeletal muscle function that can be used to assess the effects of starvation or predict postoperative complications by measuring the extent of protein catabolism (Kalfarentzos et al, 1989; Webb et al, 1989).

Immunologic Measurements. Malnutrition is associated with depressed immune competence manifested by decreased lymphocyte count and decreased, delayed cutaneous hypersensitivity (DCH). DCH is evaluated by response to five recall antigens, usually *Candida,* streptokinase-streptodornase (SK-SD), coccidioidin, mumps, and purified protein derivative (PPD). Lack of response or redness and induration of less than 5 mm indicate that the individual lacks the ability to mount an immune response.

A wide variety of medical treatments and metabolic abnormalities, including trauma, sepsis, malignancy, and edema, can interfere with the skin reactions. For this reason responses to skin tests are usually used as one of several factors in nutritional prognostic indices rather than alone. Total lymphocyte count can be affected by an acute stress response or by the presence of a large wound.

Nitrogen Balance. A good measure of the adequacy of protein intake and maintenance of lean body mass is the determination of nitrogen balance. Problems with this technique include the 24-hour urine collection as well as the several days required for analysis before the test results are returned.

The *nitrogen balance* is a measure of the extent of protein utilization. By comparing the amount of nitrogen that enters the body in the form of food protein with the amount that is lost in the excreta, the nitrogen status of the individual can be determined.

Because most proteins contain around 16% nitrogen, the amount of nitrogen in a food can be calculated

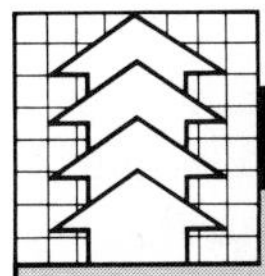

NEW DIRECTIONS: Hair Analysis

Hair analysis for the assessment of minerals such as sodium, magnesium, phosphorus, potassium, calcium, iron, and iodine is not useful inasmuch as there already are fairly good measures for evaluating body functions related to these minerals. However, hair analysis may have a place in assessing status of the trace elements zinc, copper, chromium, and manganese, for which measurements of functional status are not well developed, and for cadmium and lead, which have negative biologic effects. To be clinically useful, hair analysis procedures will need to be refined and standardized and "normal" values for hair mineral content defined and accepted. Currently hair analysis is more useful in experimental efforts than in clinical medicine. It is most useful when it is done for a single element rather than several elements at one time, where the probability of finding an abnormal result increases as the specificity of the test drops.

Even if a hair analysis value could be judged abnormal, it is still not known whether it reflects an abnormal exposure to the element and thus a cause of the disease, or whether the abnormal value is the result of the disease. Lastly, there is no evidence that nutritional therapy based on the hair analysis will have any benefit.

by dividing the chemically determined protein content by the factor of 6.25. Excreted nitrogen is primarily in the form of urea, although small amounts are also lost in feces and sweat as well as in hair, skin, and nails. These losses are usually estimated by a standard figure.

Nitrogen consumed in the form of food protein is primarily in the form of amino acids. These amino acids may be used in activities involving production of new tissue, or if their amount is in excess of body needs, they may be broken down and the nitrogen portion excreted in the form of urea. Excreted nitrogen may also be derived from processes that result in breakdown of body tissue with subsequent destruction of amino acids.

In addition, nitrogen is continuously being accumulated and lost through the ongoing homeostatic replacement of protein tissues in the body. Breakdown of the amino acids involved in this turnover releases nitrogen for excretion. An equal amount of food protein nitrogen is retained for replacement.

If the amount of nitrogen excreted is equal to the amount of nitrogen consumed, an individual is said to be in *nitrogen balance.* Replacement nitrogen is equal to the amount of nitrogen excreted in the normal turnover process of repair and maintenance of protein tissues. Nitrogen consumed in excess of body needs is excreted and does not contribute to an imbalance. A rough estimation of nitrogen balance can be made by using the following formula:

$$\text{Nitrogen intake} = \frac{\text{(protein intake in g/24 hr)}}{\text{(6.25 g protein/g of nitrogen)}}$$

$$\text{Nitrogen output} = \text{urinary urea nitrogen in g/24 hr} + 4 \text{ g of nitrogen}$$

$$\text{Nitrogen balance} = \text{nitrogen intake} - \text{nitrogen output}$$

An individual in *positive nitrogen balance* is retaining more nitrogen than is being excreted. This circumstance, prompted by the synthesis of new protein tissue, is seen in growing children, pregnancy, lactation, muscle development of athletes, and recovery from injury, surgery, or malnutrition.

Negative nitrogen balance often involves destructive catabolic processes, such as those accompanying the trauma of burns, surgery, or injury, which cause more protein to be lost than is retained. Adequate protein may be consumed, but the cells are incapable of converting it into new tissue. A diet without sufficient protein to meet the needs of normal maintenance will also result in negative nitrogen balance, as will a diet so low in calories that protein tissues must be destroyed to meet energy needs. Protein-calorie malnutrition, weight-reduction programs, emotional stress, and high fevers are marked by negative nitrogen balance. Bedridden invalids and astronauts in the weightlessness of zero gravity lose nitrogen from inactivated muscles.

Clinical Examination

The clinical examination includes a complete physical examination and a medical history. Examination of hospitalized patients should give special attention to loss of subcutaneous fat in the triceps and chest areas and loss of muscle over the quadriceps and deltoids. The presence of edema or ascites should also be noted. Special attention should be given to the areas where signs of nutritional deficiencies appear—skin, hair, teeth, gums, lips, tongue, eyes, and the genitalia in men. Hair, skin, and mouth are susceptible because of the rapid cell turnover of epithelial tissue. Mucosal changes of the gastrointestinal (GI) tract are reflected in problems such as diarrhea. The patient should be questioned regarding GI symptoms, such as diarrhea and anorexia, as well as about changes in dietary habits related to mastication and swallowing.

The clinical examination for nutritional assessment in many hospitals includes bedside assessment of energy expenditure. This procedure of indirect calorimetry is further discussed in Chapter 2.

Table 17–6 lists some physical signs of possible nutritional significance. The clinical terms in this table are further defined in Appendix Table 31. Clinical symptoms are seldom diagnostic for specific nutritional deficiencies and require confirmation by means of diet histories and biochemical tests. Clinical symptoms frequently reflect the presence of more than one nutritional deficiency.

TABLE 17–6. Physical Signs Indicative or Suggestive of Malnutrition

	Normal Appearance	Signs Associated with Malnutrition	Possible Disorder or Nutrient Deficiency	Possible Non-nutritional Problem
Hair	Shiny; firm; not easily plucked	Lack of natural shine; dull and dry Thin and sparse Dyspigmented Flag sign Easily plucked (no pain)	Kwashiorkor and, less commonly, marasmus	Excessive bleaching of hair Alopecia
Face	Skin color uniform; smooth, healthy appearance; not swollen	Nasolabial seborrhea (scaling of skin around nostrils) Swollen face (moon face) Paleness	Riboflavin Kwashiorkor	Acne vulgaris
Eyes	Bright, clear, shiny; no sores at corners of eyelids; membranes a healthy pink and moist; no prominent blood vessels or mound of tissue or sclera	Pale conjunctiva Bitot's spots Conjunctival xerosis (dryness) Corneal xerosis (dullness) Keratomalacia (softening of cornea) Redness and fissuring of eyelid corners Corneal arcus (white ring around eye) Xanthelasma (small yellowish lumps around eyes)	Anemia (e.g., iron) Vitamin A (Bitot's spots through keratomalacia) Riboflavin, pyridoxine Hyperlipidemia (corneal arcus, xanthelasma)	Bloodshot eyes from exposure to weather, lack of sleep, smoke or alcohol
Lips	Smooth, not chapped or swollen	Angular cheilosis (white or pink lesions at corners of mouth)	Riboflavin	Excessive salivation from improper fitting dentures
Tongue	Deep red in appearance; not swollen or smooth	Magenta tongue (purplish) Filiform papillae atrophy or hypertrophy—red tongue	Riboflavin Folic acid Niacin	Leucoplakia
Teeth	No cavities; no pain; bright	Mottled enamel Caries (cavities) Missing teeth	Fluorosis Excessive sugar	Malocclusion Periodontal disease Health habits
Gums	Healthy; red; do not bleed; not swollen	Spongy, bleeding Receding gums	Vitamin C	Periodontal disease
Glands	Face not swollen	Thyroid enlargement (front of neck swollen) Parotid enlargement (cheeks become swollen)	Iodine Starvation Bulimia	Allergic or inflammatory enlargement of thyroid
Nervous system	Psychological stability; normal reflexes	Psychomotor changes Mental confusion Sensory loss Motor weakness Loss of position sense Loss of vibration Loss of ankle and knee jerks Burning and tingling of hands and feet (paresthesia) Dementia	Kwashiorkor Thiamin Thiamin (sensory loss through paresthesia) Niacin, vitamin B_{12}	

Anthropometry

Assessment of growth and development is an important part of the clinical examination. The common failure to measure weight and, more often, height hampers nutritional assessment of growth and change. Anthropometric data is most valuable when accurately measured and recorded over a period of time. Measurements such as height and head circumference reflect past nutrition or chronic nutritional status. Others, such as midarm circumference, weight, and skinfold thickness, reflect present nutritional status. Ethnic, familial, birth weight, and environmental factors affect growth and should be taken into account when anthropometric measurements are being taken.

Height and Weight

Height and weight are the measurements made most frequently, but because of failure to appreciate their significance, they are frequently measured without care or omitted entirely. Height is a measure of chronic nutrition. Growth failure should arouse suspicion of malnutrition.

Techniques for measuring height and weight are shown in Clinical Insight, p. 306. When height cannot be measured directly, alternatives have been suggested. Arm span and knee height have been used for individuals with scoliosis, cerebral palsy, or muscular dystrophy, and with the elderly (Gleason, 1983; Mitchell and Lipschitz, 1982). Sitting height has also been used to measure growth of children who cannot stand.

HEIGHT. Children under 2 years of age should be measured in the recumbent position (crown-heel length) (Fig. 17–4). Recumbent length is generally greater than stature by about 2 cm or almost 1 inch. Length should then be plotted on the chart appropriate for children who are 1 to 36 months of age. If height is taken when the child can cooperate and stand appropriately (usually at 24 months), then the measurements should be plotted on the chart for 2- to 18-year-old children. Plotting standing height on the birth-to-36-months chart or recumbent length on the 2- to 18-year chart can introduce error into the evaluation (Murphy and Trahms, 1981; Trahms, 1982).

Regular tables show attained growth, which is affected by growth during all preceding periods. Incremental growth, or growth during a particular time interval (usually 6 months), is more sensitive to change because it does not depend as directly on previous attainment. Incremental growth tables have been published for weight and stature from birth to 18 years and for head circumference and recumbent length for birth to 3 years (Baumgartner et al, 1986). Further discussion of growth assessment in children can be found in Chapters 12 and 13.

Adults should be measured using the same technique that is used with children, although standing up straight may be difficult for some people. Because

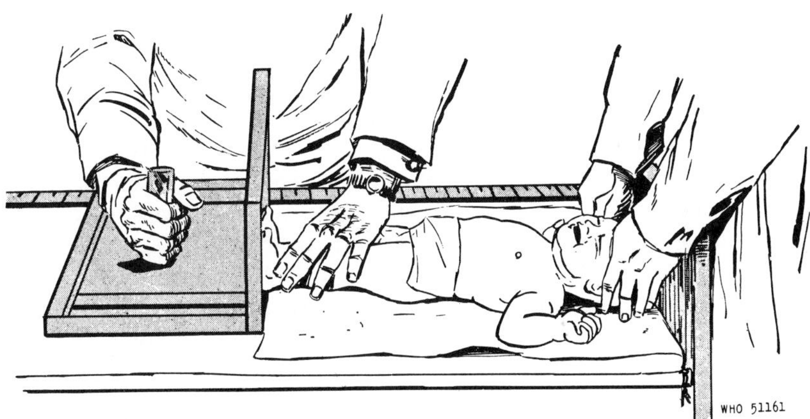

FIGURE 17–4. *Measurement of length of an infant. Crown-heel length should be measured in children 36 months and younger in the following manner: (1) The child is laid on a ruled board that has an attached piece of wood at one end and a movable piece at the other. (2) Make sure that the child is stretched out on the board to give the most accurate measurement. This usually requires two people. The top of the child's head is placed against the immovable end. (3) The movable end is placed so that it is flat against the bottom of the child's foot, and the length is read from the side of the board. (From Jelliffe DB: The Assessment of the Nutritional Status of the Community. WHO Monograph No. 53. Geneva, Switzerland, World Health Organization, 1966.)*

CLINICAL INSIGHT: Measurement of Height and Weight

HEIGHT

1. Height should be measured without shoes.
2. Feet should be together with the heels against the wall or measuring board.
3. The subject should stand erect, neither slumped nor stretching, looking straight ahead, without tipping the head up or down. The top of the ear and outer corner of the eye should be in a line parallel to the floor (the "Frankfort plane").
4. A horizontal bar, a rectangular block of wood, or the top of the statiometer should be lowered to rest flat on the top of the head.
5. Height should be read to the nearest 1/4 inch or 0.5 cm.

WEIGHT

1. Use a beam balance scale, not a spring scale, whenever possible.
2. Periodically calibrate the scale for accuracy, using known weights.
3. Weigh the subject in light clothing without shoes.
4. Record weight to the nearest 1/2 lb or 0.2 kg for adults, and 1/4 lb or 0.1 kg for infants. Measurements above the 90th or below the 10th percentiles warrant further evaluation.

adults begin losing height after the fourth decade, the measured height is usually shorter than the "known" or "remembered" height.

WEIGHT. Weight in children is a sensitive measure of growth and can be an early clue to nutritional inadequacy. It reflects more recent nutrition than does length or height. Regular weight measurements are particularly important in the presence of chronic illness.

Bedridden patients in hospitals can be weighed by using a special scale. Prediction equations for weight of the nonambulatory elderly have been developed using arm and calf circumferences, subscapular skinfold, and knee height (Chumlea et al, 1988).

INTERPRETATION OF HEIGHT AND WEIGHT. Reference standards in current use for evaluating anthropometric data are based on a statistical sample of the population of the United States. Therefore, an individual measurement shows how the subject stands relative to the total population, not to an absolute standard.

Children. Height and weight measurements are evaluated by comparing them with various norms. For children, the height and weight are recorded as a percentile, which reflects the percentage of the total population of children of the same sex at or below that height or weight at that age. This allows the child's growth at each age, or growth "curve," to be followed. This is done using Appendix Tables 7 and 11 for infants and Appendix Tables 9 and 13 for children and adolescents.

Most percentile charts or tables place the child within a broad range, for example "between the 25th and 50th percentile." A method of evaluating growth that does not relate the child's performance to "normal" children is *percentage-of-median.* This allows quantification of nutritional improvement, as for a child whose weight has improved with nutrition therapy from 30 to 45% of the median. Standard deviation units (Z-scores) can also be used but are not as easy for health professionals and parents to relate to.

Weight and height can also be evaluated with respect to each other by using the *weight-for-standard-length curve* for prepubescent children only (males less than 11.5 years of age and no more than 145 cm [57 inches] in height, and females less than 10 years of age and no more than 137 cm [54 inches] in height). For most children a weight for height between the 25th and 75th percentiles is appropriate. Children whose weight for height percentile is above or below this should be evaluated further by using skinfold measurements or other anthropometry. Use of this weight for height table allows the clinician to evaluate whether a child's weight is appropriate. It also has the advantage of not needing to know the child's exact age. When height for age is above the 10th percentile but weight for height is less than the 5th percentile, acute or chronic illness or nutritional deficiency is suggested (see Appendices 8, 10, 12, and 14).

Evaluation of weight and height measurements as well as growth in pregnancy, prematurity, infancy, childhood, and adolescence is further discussed in Chapters 9 through 13.

Adults. Height and particularly weight are also useful in determining nutritional status in adults. Both should be measured if at all possible because there is a tendency to overestimate height and underestimate weight, resulting in underestimation of relative weight. Weight loss reflects the immediate ability to meet nutritional requirements and thus may indicate nutritional risk. Determination of per cent weight loss according to the formula

$$\% \text{ weight loss} = \frac{\text{usual weight} - \text{present weight}}{\text{usual weight} \times 100}$$

is highly reflective of the extent of illness. Another useful calculation is present weight as a percentage of usual weight.

Weight loss after surgery is generally proportional to the degree of trauma and is usually less than that which occurs with total starvation. It is generally accepted that a loss of up to 10% does not jeopardize convalescence. With severe trauma and sepsis, weight loss can equal that seen in starving patients and can be fatal (see Chapter 29).

Reference Standards. To determine whether an adult's weight is appropriate for height, the weight is usually compared with a reference standard. The most common is the Metropolitan Life Insurance (MLI) table, as shown in Appendix Table 17. This table gives weight ranges for men and women at 1-inch increments of height for three body frame sizes.

Several problems are involved in the use of these tables to determine appropriate body weight: (1) The stated weight ranges merely reflect the weights of those with the lowest mortality of insured persons, which may not be representative of the American population. (2) Weight ranges for lowest mortality do not necessarily reflect optimal weight for height. (3) There is no agreement on how best to measure frame size.

Determining Frame Size. Proper use of these tables requires the assessment of frame size. However, to date, there is no accepted method for determining this measurement. Two different methods, elbow breadth and wrist circumference as related to height, are presented in Appendix Table 18. Once frame size is determined, the range of recommended weight can be more specific.

Body Mass Index (Quetelet Index). The *body mass index (BMI)* or *Quetelet Index* accounts for differences in body composition by defining the level of adiposity according to the relationship of weight to height and eliminates dependence on frame size (Stensland and Margolis, 1990).

$$\text{BMI} = \text{weight (in kilograms)} / \text{height (in meters)}^2$$

$$\text{BMI} = \text{weight (in pounds)} / \text{height (in inches)}^2 \times 705$$

This index has the least correlation with body height and the highest correlation with independent measures of body fatness for adults, including the elderly (Keys et al, 1972). A score of 20 to 25 is associated with the least risk of early death. Obesity is categorized according to three grades: Grade I (25 to 29.9), Grade II (30 to 40), and Grade III (40+). In general, a BMI of 27 or greater indicates obesity and increasing risk of developing health problems (Bray et al, 1976) (Fig. 17–5).

BMI values increase with increasing age; therefore, age-specific guidelines for BMI to be used for the elderly have been suggested (Bray, 1987) (see Chapter 14). Appendix 19 gives the BMI for most heights and weights. The appropriate BMI for age categories presented by Bray is given at the bottom of the table.

Body Composition

Differences in skeletal size and in proportion of lean body mass can contribute to variations in body weight among individuals of similar height. Athletes, for example, with extensive muscle development may be classified as overweight secondary to excess muscle mass rather than adipose mass.

Subcutaneous Fat (Skinfold Thickness). The fatfold or skinfold thickness measurement is practical for use

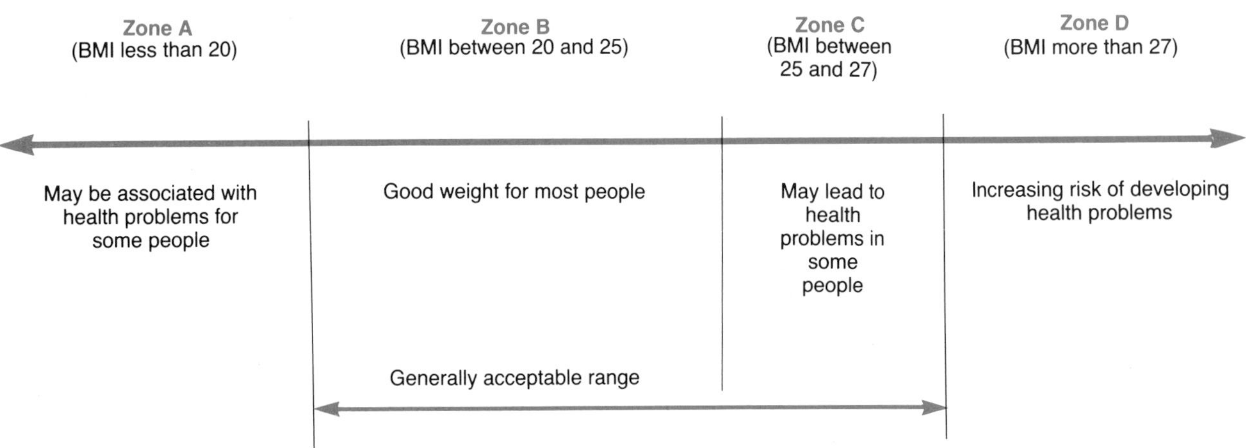

FIGURE 17–5. *Canadian guidelines for healthy weights (for adults 20 to 65 years old). (From Expert Group, Health Promotion Directorate, Health Services and Promotion Branch: Canadian Guidelines for Healthy Weights. Cat. No. H39-134/1989 E. Ottawa, Canada, Minister of National Health and Welfare, 1989.)*

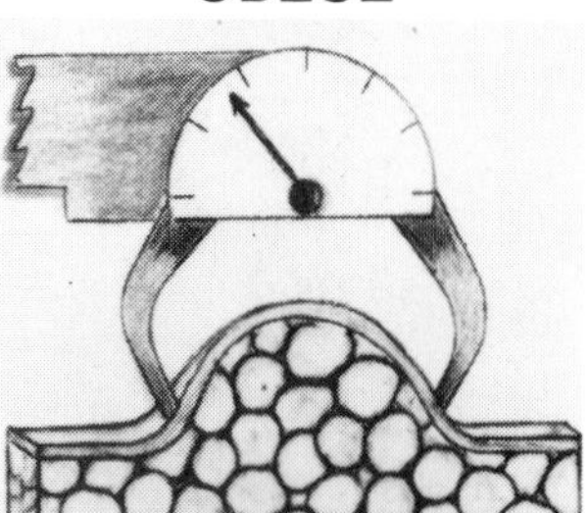

FIGURE 17–6. *Skinfold calipers measure in millimeters the thickness of the subcutaneous fat tissue. This gives a rough measurement of adiposity. (Diagram courtesy of Dorice Czajka-Narins, Ph.D.)*

in a clinical setting, although validity depends upon accuracy of the measuring technique (Fig. 17–6). Estimates of total body fat by this measurement are based on the assumption that 50% of body fat is subcutaneous. Accuracy decreases with increasing obesity. Skinfold sites identified as most reflective of body fatness are over the triceps, biceps, below the scapula, suprailiac (above the iliac crest), and upper thigh. The triceps and subscapular measurements are the most useful because the most complete standards and methods of evaluation are available for these sites. Figures 17–7 and 17–8 illustrate these measurements.

The technique outlined by Durnin and Womersley may be one of the best tools for estimation of body fat in a clinical setting, assuming accurate skinfold measurements at the correct sites (see Appendix Table 28). Appendices 23 and 24 give the percentiles for triceps skinfold thickness for youths aged 1 to 17 years and adults.

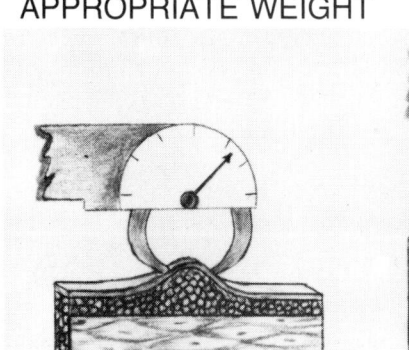

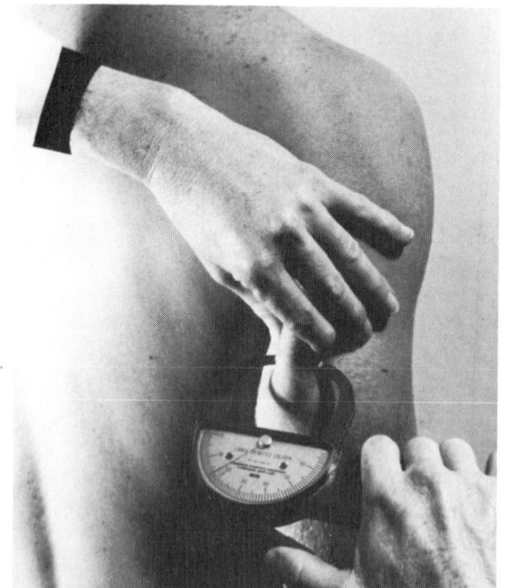

FIGURE 17–7. *The triceps skinfold measurement is made at a point over the triceps muscle midway between the acromion and olecranon processes on the posterior aspect of the arm; the arm is held vertically, with the skinfold running parallel to the length of the arm.*

Hydrostatic Weighing. Hydrostatic weighing is a measure of body density based on the principle that lean tissue is more dense than adipose tissue. Weight is recorded with the subject completely submerged and with only residual air remaining in the lungs after complete expiration. The difference between this weight and an out-of-water weight gives a measure of adipose tissue or percentage body fat.

Electrical Conductance Techniques. *Total body electrical conductivity (TOBEC)* and *bioelectrical impedance analysis (BIA)* are based on electrical conductance and on the fact that fat-free mass, with its richer electrolyte content, has a much greater conductivity than does fat, thus allowing the development of a relationship between conductance and fat-free mass. Accuracy of these methods requires adequate hydration of the patient. BIA is more widely used because it is less expensive and easy to operate, is portable, and requires only the removal of one shoe and stocking (Fig. 17–9).

Research Methods. A variety of sophisticated techniques are available to determine the percentage of body fat with a high degree of accuracy. However, because of expense or the requirement for highly skilled technicians, or both, some of these are appropriate only for use in research. These techniques include ultrasound, potassium body counter, computed tomography, magnetic resonance imaging, and neutron activation. Ultrasound is able to measure large fat layers with more accuracy than is possible with skinfold calipers.

Circumference Measurements

If more complete information on actual body composition is needed, additional anthropometric data can be obtained. These usually include additional skinfold measurements and circumference measurements.

Waist and Hip Circumference Ratio. With the recognition of fat distribution as an indicator of risk, circumferential measurements have once again become

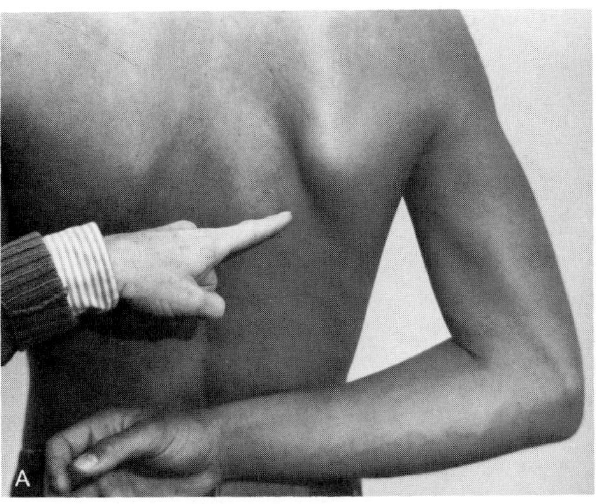
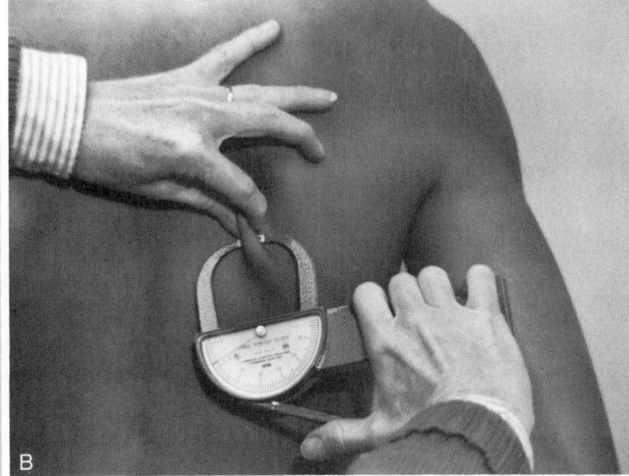

FIGURE 17–8. *Measurement of the subscapular skinfold thickness.*

important (see Chapter 18). The most frequently used measure of adiposity currently is the *waist-to-hip ratio (WHR),* also called the *abdominal/gluteal ratio,* which differentiates between android and gynoid obesity. A WHR of 1.0 or greater in men (0.8 or greater in women) is indicative of android obesity and increasing risk for obesity-related diseases. This also appears to be true in children (Freedman et al, 1989). Circumferences are easy to measure with either plastic or steel measuring tapes, which are relatively inexpensive. A spring-loaded, constant tension tape improves accuracy and reliability. Difficulty in determining where the waist is located, because it moves up and down with change in weight and muscle tone, is resolved by using the smallest circumference. The hip circumference is defined as the largest circumference between the waist and the knees. Like many other measures including weight itself, WHR denotes a combination of lean and fat tissues, especially in the mid-ranges. Appendix 20 presents a nomogram for determining the WHR.

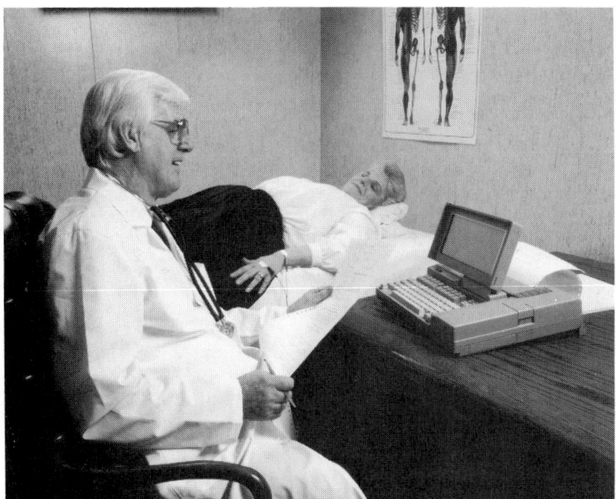

FIGURE 17–9. *Bioelectrical impedance analysis (BIA). (Courtesy of Danninger Medical Technology, Inc., Columbus, Ohio.)*

MID–UPPER ARM CIRCUMFERENCE. Mid–upper arm circumference, as shown in Figure 17–10, is measured halfway between the acromion process of the scapula and the tip of the elbow. Standards for arm circumference are given in Appendix Tables 25, 26, and 27.

Combining the mid–upper arm circumference with the triceps skinfold thickness measurement enables indirect determination of the arm muscle area and arm fat area (Fig. 17–11). Bone-free arm muscle area is calculated by using the same formulas as in Figure 17–11, except that in men the factor 10 is subtracted from the arm muscle area and in women the factor 6.5 is subtracted (Frisancho, 1984).

The arm muscle area or the bone-free arm muscle area is a good indication of the lean body mass and thus the skeletal protein reserves. This is important in growing children and is especially valuable in evaluating the person who may be protein-energy–malnourished as a result of chronic illness, stress, multiple surgeries, or inadequate diet (see Chapter 30). Nomograms for determining arm muscle and fat areas for children and adults without lengthy calculations appear in Appendices 21 and 22. Norms for arm muscle and arm fat areas are given in Appendix Table 26.

HEAD CIRCUMFERENCE. The measurement of head circumference is useful in children under the age of 3 as an indicator primarily of non-nutritional abnormalities. Undernutrition must be very severe to affect head circumference.

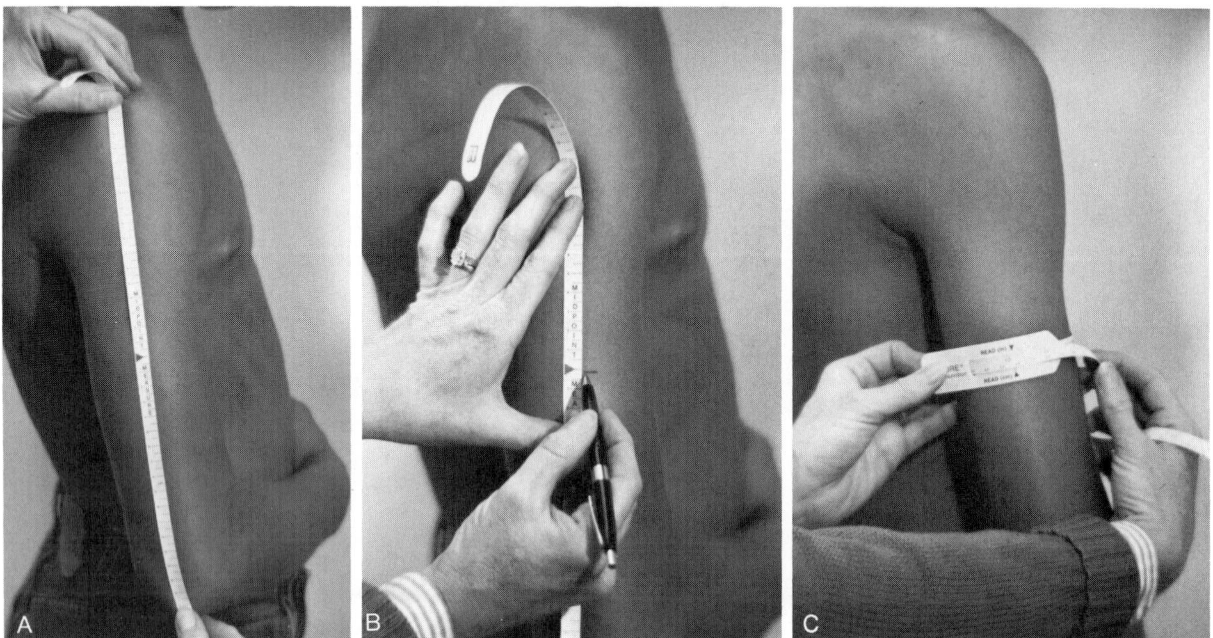

FIGURE 17–10. A, *Measurement of the midpoint between the acromion process at the shoulder and the olecranon process at the elbow.* B, *Marking of the midpoint.* C, *Measurement of the arm circumference in centimeters at the midpoint.*

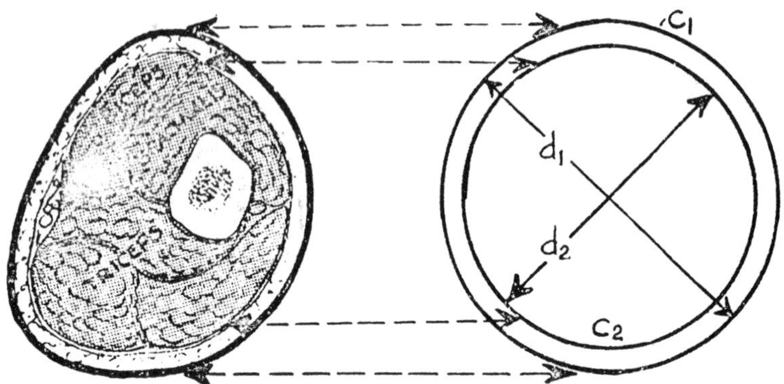

FIGURE 17–11. *Upper arm area (AA), upper arm muscle area (AMA), and upper arm fat area (AFA) are derived from measures of upper arm circumference. (C_1) and triceps skinfold (T) in millimeters.*

$$AA\ (mm^2) = \frac{\pi}{4} \times d_1^2 \text{ where } d_1 = \frac{C_1}{\pi}$$

$$AMA\ (mm^2) = \frac{(C_1 - \pi T)^2}{4\pi} = \frac{(C_1 - \pi T)^2}{12.56}$$

$$AFA\ (mm^2) = AA - AMA$$

$$\text{bone-free } AMA = AMA - 10 \text{ for males}$$
$$= AMA - 6.5 \text{ for females}$$

Arm area and muscle area can also be determined using the nomograms in Appendix Tables 21 and 22.

FURTHER READING: Malnutrition in Hospitals

In a landmark article in 1974, Butterworth showed that malnutrition could indeed be found in the United States—in hospitals, where it was frequently not recognized. Over the course of the next few years, malnutrition was found in many hospitals and there were attempts to evaluate its severity and reverse its course. Since that time there have been periods of heightened awareness and periods of minimal awareness. With only weak programs in nutrition (weak being defined as having nutrition courses either spread through the curriculum or having very few contact hours, not weak in terms of the quality of the teachers) in most medical schools, the majority of physicians graduate with very little knowledge about nutrition. Not surprisingly, this results in decreased physician awareness of malnutrition. In one acute medical service only 12.5% of the patients were correctly identified as at risk for malnutrition before an educational program in contrast to 100% after the program (Roubenoff, 1987). To maintain a high level of awareness, physician education programs in nutrition should be conducted regularly.

NUTRITIONAL ASSESSMENT FOR HOSPITALIZED AND STRESSED PATIENTS

The most likely problem of physically stressed, ill, or traumatized patients is protein-calorie malnutrition (PCM) (Further Reading, p. 311). Under all circumstances, PCM is a multinutrient problem because the foods that are good sources of protein and energy are also sources of many other nutrients. Although repletion obviously requires provision of all nutrients in the amounts needed, the major need is for energy and protein (see Chapters 29 and 30). Chapter 2 describes methods for determining energy requirements, and Chapter 5 discusses the determination of protein needs.

Indicators of protein status are especially important in stressed individuals. Serum albumin, transferrin, prealbumin and retinol-binding protein measurements have been used in this assessment. Prealbumin (transthyretin) and retinol-binding protein have very short half-lives (1 to 2 days and 10 hours respectively) and are therefore sensitive to protein status change. However, the assays are sophisticated and may be less available than those for serum albumin and transferrin. Table 17–7 lists the measures commonly used to assess the presence of PCM.

TABLE 17–7. Variables Commonly Used in Assessing Protein-Calorie Malnutrition

Anthropometry	Comments
Height	
Weight	
Usual weight	
Weight as % of usual weight	
Weight as % of ideal weight	Appendix 17
Triceps skinfold (mm)	
Triceps skinfold % of norms	Appendices 23 and 24
Arm circumference (cm)	
Arm muscle circumference (cm)	
Arm muscle circumference (% of norms)	Appendix 25
Biochemical/Immunologic	**Comments**
Serum albumin (g/dl)	3 g/dl acceptable
Serum transferrin (mg/dl)	170 mg/dl acceptable
Serum thyroxine-binding prealbumin (transthyretin) (mg/dl)	Consult laboratory
Total lymphocytes (#/mm^3)	1,200/mm^3 acceptable
Skin test results	

Prediction of Postoperative Morbidity and Mortality

In an attempt to correlate various methods of nutritional assessment with the occurrence of postoperative morbidity and mortality, several equations have been developed. The one most frequently used is the *Prognostic Nutritional Index (PNI)* (Buzby et al, 1980; Mullen et al, 1980):

$$\text{PNI} = 158 - 16.6\ (\text{Alb}) - 0.78\ (\text{TSF}) - 0.20\ (\text{TFN}) - 5.8\ (\text{DH})^*$$

The higher the PNI, the greater the risk of operative complications due to nutritional factors that could be reduced by appropriate nutritional support.

In contrast to methods of assessment that employ objective biochemical and anthropometric measurements is the *Subjective Global Assessment* (SGA) of nutritional status. Table 17–8 lists the features of SGA. This is an "eyeball" technique that requires good clinical judgment. Guidelines for health professionals are set forth by the developers of this technique (Detsky et al, 1987). The correlations to clinical outcome are similar to those obtained using more objective

* Alb = serum albumin concentration (g/dl); TSF = triceps skinfold (mm); TFN = serum transferrin concentration (mg/dl); DH = delayed hypersensitivity (graded 0 = nonreactive; 1 = <0.5 mm induration; 2 = >0.5 mm induration).

TABLE 17–8. Subjective Global Assessment of Nutritional Status*

Features of Subjective Global Assessment (SGA)

(Select appropriate category with a checkmark, or enter numerical value where indicated by "#.")

A. History
1. Weight change
   Overall loss in past 6 months: amount = # __________ kg; % loss = # __________
   Change in past 2 weeks: __________ increase
   __________ no change
   __________ decrease
2. Dietary intake change (relative to normal)
   __________ No change
   __________ Change __________ duration = # __________ weeks
   __________ type: __________ suboptimal solid diet __________ full liquid diet
   __________ hypocaloric liquids __________ starvation
3. Gastrointestinal symptoms (that persisted for >2 weeks)
   __________ none __________ nausea __________ vomiting __________ diarrhea __________ anorexia
4. Functional capacity
   __________ No dysfunction (e.g., full capacity)
   __________ Dysfunction __________ duration = # __________ weeks
   __________ type: __________ working suboptimally
   __________ ambulatory
   __________ bedridden
5. Disease and its relation to nutritional requirements
   Primary diagnosis (specify) ______________________________
   Metabolic demand (stress): __________ no stress __________ low stress
   __________ moderate stress __________ high stress

B. Physical (for each trait specify: 0 = normal, 1+ = mild, 2+ = moderate, 3+ = severe)
   # __________ loss of subcutaneous fat (triceps, chest)
   # __________ muscle wasting (quadriceps, deltoids)
   # __________ ankle edema
   # __________ sacral edema
   # __________ ascites

C. SGA rating (select one)
   __________ A = well nourished
   __________ B = moderately (or suspected of being) malnourished
   __________ C = severely malnourished

* From Detsky AS et al: What is subjective global assessment of nutritional status? J Parenter Enter Nutr 11:8, 1987.

measures. This type of evaluation has been found to be extremely useful and cost-effective (Nutritional Assessment Present and Future, 1988).

CITED REFERENCES

Adams CF: Nutritive Value of American Food. Agriculture Handbook No 456. Washington, DC, ARS, USDA, 1988.

Basiotis PP et al: Number of days of food intake records required to estimate individual and group nutrient intakes with defined confidence. J Nutr 117:1138, 1987.

Baumgartner RN, Roch AF, and Himes JH: Incremental growth tables: Supplementary to previously published charts. Am J Clin Nutr 43:711, 1986.

Blake AJ, Guthrie HA, and Smiciklas-Wright H: Accuracy of food portion estimation by overweight and normal-weight subjects. J Am Diet Assoc 89:962, 1989.

Bray GA: Overweight is risking fate: Definition, classification, prevalence and risks. Ann NY Acad Sci 249:14, 1987.

Bray GA et al: Evaluation of the obese patient. I: An algorithm. JAMA 235:1487, 1976.

Buzby GP et al: Prognostic nutritional index in gastrointestinal surgery. Am J Surg 134:160, 1980.

Chumlea WC et al: Prediction of body weight for the nonambulatory elderly from anthropometry. J Am Diet Assoc 88:564, 1988.

Detsky AS et al: What is subjective global assessment of nutritional status? J Parenter Enter Nutr 11:8, 1987.

Freedman DS et al: Relation of body fat patterning to lipid and lipoprotein concentrations in children and adolescents: The Bogalusa Heart Study. Am J Clin Nutr 50:930, 1989.

Frisancho AR: New standards of weight and body composition by frame size and height for assessment of nutritional status of adults and the elderly. Am J Clin Nutr 40:808, 1984.

Gebhardt SE and Matthews RH: Nutritive Value of Foods. Home and Garden Bulletin No 72. Washington, DC, HNIS, USDA, 1981.

Gleason C: Nutritional assessment of boys with physical deformities: Stature estimation (Abstract). Fed Proc 42:1044, 1983.

Kalfarentzos F et al: Comparison of fore arm muscle dynamometry with nutritional prognostic index, as a preoperative indicator in cancer patients. J Parenter Enter Nutr 13:34, 1989.

Karkeck JM: Improving the use of dietary survey methodology. J Am Diet Assoc 87:869, 1987.

Karvetti RL and Knuts JR: Validity of the 24-hour dietary recall. J Am Diet Assoc 85:1437, 1985.

Keys A et al: Indices of relative weight and obesity. J Chronic Dis 25:329, 1972.

Klevay LM et al: Hair analysis in clinical and experimental medicine. Am J Clin Nutr 46:233, 1987.

Lissner L et al: Body composition and energy intake: Do overweight women overeat and underreport? Am J Clin Nutr 49:320, 1989.

Mitchell CO and Lipschitz DA: Arm length measurement as an alternative to height in nutritional assessment of the elderly. J Parenter Enter Nutr 6:226, 1982.

Mullen JL et al: Reduction of operative morbidity and mortality by combined preoperative and postoperative nutritional support. Ann Surg 192:604, 1980.

Murphy S and Trahms C: Assessment of Children: A Guide for Weighing and Measuring. Seattle, Child Development and Mental Retardation Center, University of Washington, 1981.

Nutritional Assessment Present and Future. Nutr Supp Serv 8:7, 1988.

Pennington JA: Bowes and Church's Food Values of Portions Commonly Used, 15th ed. Philadelphia, JB Lippincott, 1989.

Roubenoff R et al: Malnutrition among hospitalized patients. Arch Intern Med 147:1462, 1987.

Stensland SH and Margolis S: Simplifying the calculation of body mass index for quick reference. J Am Diet Assoc 90:856, 1990.

Subcommittee on Criteria for Dietary Evaluation, National Research Council, NAS: Nutrient Adequacy. Washington, DC, National Academy Press, 1986.

Trahms C: Rate Yourself Measurement Techniques. Seattle, Child Development and Mental Retardation Center, University of Washington, 1982.

USDA: Composition of Foods—USDA Handbook No 8 Series. Washington, DC, US Government Printing Office, 1976–1986.

Webb AR et al: Hand grip dynamometry as a predictor of postoperative complications: Reappraisal using age standardized grip strengths. J Parenter Enter Nutr 13:30, 1989.

ADDITIONAL REFERENCES

Barrett S: Commercial hair analysis: Science or scam? JAMA 254:1041, 1985.

Beal VA: The nutritional history in longitudinal research. J Am Diet Assoc 51:426, 1967.

Bistrian B: Nutritional support of the long-term care patient. II: Nutritional assessment of the elderly. Nutr Supp Serv 8(10):17, 1988.

Burke BS: The dietary history as a tool in research. J Am Diet Assoc 23:1041, 1947.

Chumlea WC, Roche AF, and Steinbaugh ML: Estimating stature from knee height for persons 60 to 90 years of age. J Am Geriatr Soc 33:116, 1985.

Dwyer JT et al: The problem of memory in nutritional epidemiology research. J Am Diet Assoc 87:1059, 1987.

Falciglia G, O'Connor J, and Gedling E: Upper arm anthropometric norms in elderly white subjects. J Am Diet Assoc 88:563, 1988.

Frisancho AR: Nutritional anthropometry. J Am Diet Assoc 88:553, 1988.

Grant A and DeHoog S: Nutritional Assessment and Support, 4th ed. Seattle, Grant/DeHoog Publications, 1991.

Guthrie HA: Interpretation of data on dietary intake. Nutr Rev 47:33, 1989.

Hamill PV and Moore WM: Contemporary growth charts: Needs, construction and application. Dietetic Currents 3(5):1, 1976.

Himes JH et al: Parent-specific adjustments for assessment of recumbent length and stature, Vol 13. Monogr Paediatr, Basel, S Karger, 1981.

Jeejeebhoy KN: Bulk or bounce—the object of nutritional support. J Parenter Enter Nutr 12:539, 1988.

Katch VL and Freedson PS: Body size and shape: Derivation of the "HAT" frame size model. Am J Clin Nutr 36:669, 1982.

Kenny JJ et al: Applied kinesiology unreliable for assessing nutrient status. J Am Diet Assoc 88:698, 1988.

Kohrs MB et al: Factors affecting the nutritional status of the elderly. *In:* Munro HN and Danford DE (eds): Nutrition, Aging and the Elderly. New York, Plenum Press, 1989.

Krall EA et al: Factors influencing accuracy of dietary recall. Nutr Res 8:829, 1988.

Lohmann TG et al (eds): Anthropometric Standardization Reference Manual. Champaign, IL, Human Kinetics Publishers, 1988.

Lopes J et al: Skeletal muscle function in malnutrition. Am J Clin Nutr 36:602, 1982.

Lukaski HC: Methods for the assessment of human body composition: Traditional and new. Am J Clin Nutr 46:537, 1987.

McLaren DS: Color Atlas of Nutritional Disorders. London, Wolfe Medication Publications, 1981.

Medlin C and Skinner JD: Individual dietary intake methodology: A 50-year review of progress. J Am Diet Assoc 88:1250, 1988.

Segal KR: Lean body mass estimation by bioelectrical impedance analysis: A four-site cross-validation study. Am J Clin Nutr 47:7, 1988.

Solomons NW and Allon LH: The functional assessment of nutritional status. Principles, practice and potential. Nutr Rev 41:33, 1983.

Stewart AW: Underestimation of relative weight by use of self-reported height and weight. Am J Epidemiol 125:122, 1987.

Todd KS et al: Food intake measurement: Problems and approaches. Am J Clin Nutr 37:139, 1983.

Tramposch TS: A nutrition screening and assessment system for use with the elderly in extended care. J Am Diet Assoc 87:1207, 1987.

Weinsier RL et al: Handbook of Clinical Nutrition, 2nd ed. St Louis, CV Mosby, 1989.

Willett WC et al: The use of a self-administered questionnaire to assess diet four years in the past. Am J Epidemiol 127:188, 1988.

Young CM: Subjects' estimation of food intake and calculated nutritive value of the diet. J Am Diet Assoc 29:1216, 1953.

CHAPTER 18

WEIGHT MANAGEMENT

CHAPTER OUTLINE

KEY TERMS

ANDROID FAT DEPOSITION—deposition of fat around the waist and upper abdomen; "apple-shape" fat distribution

ANOREXIA NERVOSA—an eating disorder characterized by refusal to eat, a loss of at least 25% of body weight and body image, sense of control, and family and social relationship abnormalities

BEHAVIOR MODIFICATION—a technique that uses self-monitoring to identify unacceptable behavior, develop stimulus control, and self-reward as a consequence following more acceptable behavior

BROWN ADIPOSE TISSUE (BAT)—fat located in the scapular area that is involved in heat production for cold adaptation and possibly burning off excess energy

BULIMIA NERVOSA—an eating disorder that is characterized by periods of bingeing and purging, unrealistic ideas about food, and distortion of body image

ESSENTIAL FAT—the body fat located in specific sites that is necessary for survival; about 4 to 7% of body weight

GASTRIC BYPASS—a surgical procedure in which the size of the stomach is reduced by a stapling procedure, and the small intestine is connected to the smaller stomach pouch through a new opening

GASTROPLASTY—a surgical procedure in which the size of the stomach is reduced with a row of staples across the top half of the stomach and a small opening is left into the distal stomach

GYNOID FAT DISTRIBUTION—deposition of fat in the thighs and buttocks; "pear-shape" fat distribution

HORMONE-SENSITIVE LIPASE (HSL)—an enzyme in the adipose cell that is responsible for the hydrolysis of triglyceride into fatty acids and glycerol that then leave the adipose cell and enter the circulation

HYPERPLASIA—increase in tissue size by an increase in the number of cells

HYPERTROPHY—increase in tissue size by an increase in cell size

LEAN BODY MASS (LBM)—the total of all body components except storage lipid

LIPOPROTEIN LIPASE (LPL)—an enzyme on the luminal side of the capillary that facilitates transport of lipid from the blood and into the adipose cell

LIPOSUCTION—aspiration of fat deposits by means of a small incision through which a tube is fanned out into the adipose tissue

MORBID OBESITY—a state of adiposity in which body weight is 100% above the ideal; a body mass index of 45 or greater

OBESITY—a state of adiposity in which body fatness is above the ideal; a body mass index greater than 25

OVERWEIGHT—a state in which weight exceeds a standard based on height

STORAGE FAT—the fat that accumulates under the skin and around internal organs

UNDERWEIGHT—a body weight 15 to 20% below the accepted weight standard; a body mass index of less than 20

VERY LOW CALORIE DIET (VLCD)—a diet providing 200 to 800 kcal/day

WHITE ADIPOSE TISSUE—repository for triglyceride; a cushion to protect body organs and an insulator to preserve body heat

YO-YO EFFECT—the process of losing and gaining weight several times throughout a lifetime; characterized by a greater fatness after each cycle

Most adults maintain a constant body weight, owing to a complex system of neural, hormonal, and chemical mechanisms that keeps the balance between energy intake and energy expenditure within fairly precise limits. Abnormalities of these mechanisms, many of which are not completely understood, result in exaggerated fluctuations in weight. Of these, the most common are overweight and obesity. The inability to gain weight can be a problem, although this is usually secondary to another disease state. The eating disorders of anorexia nervosa and bulimia nervosa, which are becoming more common in both men and women, are frequently life-threatening.

Approximately 34 million American adults (24% of men and 27% of women) are overweight, and the numbers continue to increase in children as well as in adults. Prevalence of overweight was highest in the Midwest, especially in Wisconsin and Indiana, and was lowest in the West, with the lowest prevalence in New Mexico (Prevalence . . . , 1989).

Although the total energy intake in the United States has decreased by 10% since 1900, the extent of obesity has doubled since then (Pi- Sunyer, 1988). The 1971 to 1974 NHANES reported 28.8 million obese in the United States, of whom 8.4 million were classified as being severely obese. According to NHANES II, these numbers had increased between 1976 and 1980 to 34 million obese, of whom 13 million were severely obese. "Obese" was defined as being 20% above desirable weight and "severely obese" as being 40% above desirable weight (Council on Scientific Affairs, 1988).

Obesity is more common in women than in men, in black women than in white women, in middle-aged black men than in white men of the same age, in women in poverty than in well-to-do women, and in affluent men than in men in lower income brackets. The percentages of overweight for age, sex, and race categories are shown in Figure 18–1.

Obesity is associated with a large number of disease states and is related in degree to levels of mortality. Perhaps equally devastating is the negative cosmetic effect perceived in current society, which leads to the widespread attitude that obesity is a disgrace. Young children at the age of 6 to 9 have already adopted the disparaging attitudes of their parents toward the obese (Feldman et al, 1988).

Although society is gradually being exposed to the concept that fatness is a more complex issue than a matter of self-control, the obese — particularly women, adolescent girls, and the morbidly obese — continue to encounter discrimination in areas such as college placement, employment, and social opportunities. Victims typically are caught up in a vicious cycle of low self-esteem, depression, overeating for consolation, increased fatness, social rejection, and further self-defeating actions.

Among health professionals at least, the simplistic view of obesity as a reflection of controllably excessive intake or inadequate physical activity is gradually being abandoned in favor of recognizing the physiologic and metabolic factors, to some extent genetically endowed, that lead to an undesirable physical state.

COMPONENTS OF BODY WEIGHT

Body weight is the sum of bone, muscle, organs, body fluids, and adipose tissue. Some or all of these components are subject to normal change as a reflection of growth, reproductive status, variations in exercise levels, and the effects of aging. Water, which makes up 60 to 65% of body weight, is the most variable compo-

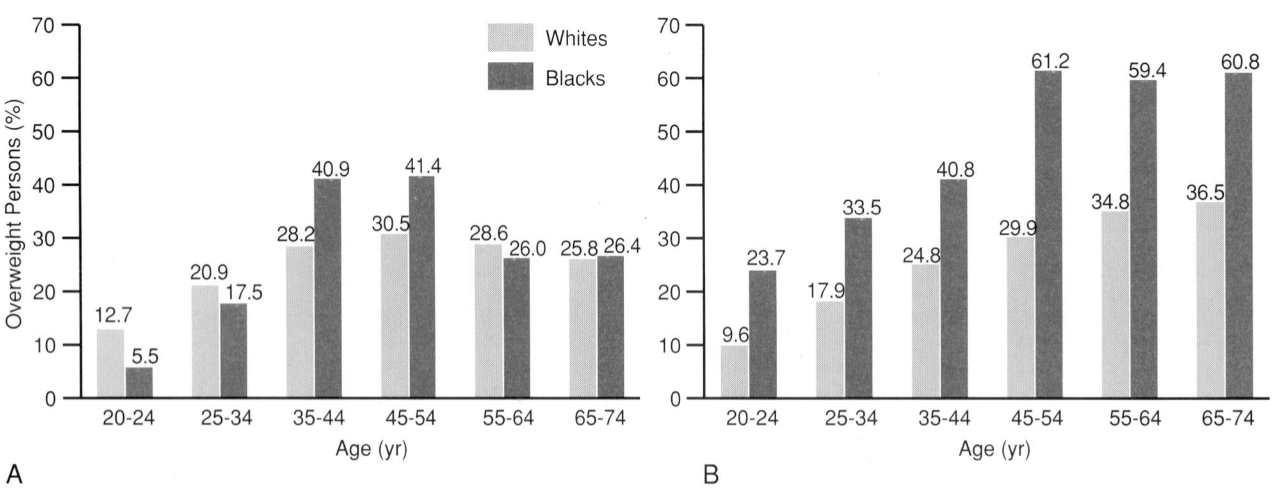

FIGURE 18–1. *Data from the National Center for Health Statistics (NHANES II) show the percentage of overweight men* (A) *and women* (B) *by age and race using the 85th percentile of weights for height of 20- to 24-year-olds as the upper limits for weight. (Redrawn from Bray EA and Gray DS: Obesity, Part I: Pathogenesis. West J Med 149:429, 1988, p 433; Van Itallie TB: Health implications of overweight and obesity in the United States. Ann Intern Med 103:983, 1985. Reproduced with permission.)*

nent, and the state of hydration can induce fluctuations of several pounds. Muscle and even skeletal mass adjust to some extent to support the changing burden of adipose tissue. However, true weight loss and excessive gain are associated primarily with a change in the size of the fat depots.

Nonadipose tissue is frequently described in terms of *lean body mass (LBM).* Measures of *fat-free mass (FFM),* or tissue devoid of all extractable fat, are available only by direct carcass analysis, whereas LBM can be determined clinically. LBM is higher in men, increases with exercise, and is lower in women and in the aging; it is the major determinant of the resting metabolic rate (see Chapter 2).

ADIPOSE TISSUE: THE FAT DEPOT

Fat, the primary energy reserve of the body, is stored as triglyceride in depots made up of adipose tissue. Appropriate body fatness for a woman is 20 to 27% of body weight, and about 12% is *essential fat* (Fig. 18–2). In women, the essential fat includes an extra 5 to 9% *sex-specific body fat* in the breasts, pelvic regions, and thighs. It is not clear whether this fat is expendable or whether it is a reserve store. In men, appropriate body fatness is 12 to 15% of body weight, and approximately 4 to 7% is essential fat. This essential fat in both sexes includes fat stored in bone marrow, heart, lung, liver, spleen, kidneys, intestines, muscles, and lipid-rich tissues in the nervous system and is necessary for normal physiologic functioning. *Storage fat* is the fat that accumulates in the adipose tissue under the skin and around internal organs to protect them from trauma. Body fatness below the level of essential fat appears to be incompatible with good health.

The totality of fat stores is capable of extensive variation, thus allowing for changing requirements of growth, reproduction, and aging, as well as fluctuations in environmental and physiologic circumstances such as the availability of food and the demands of physical

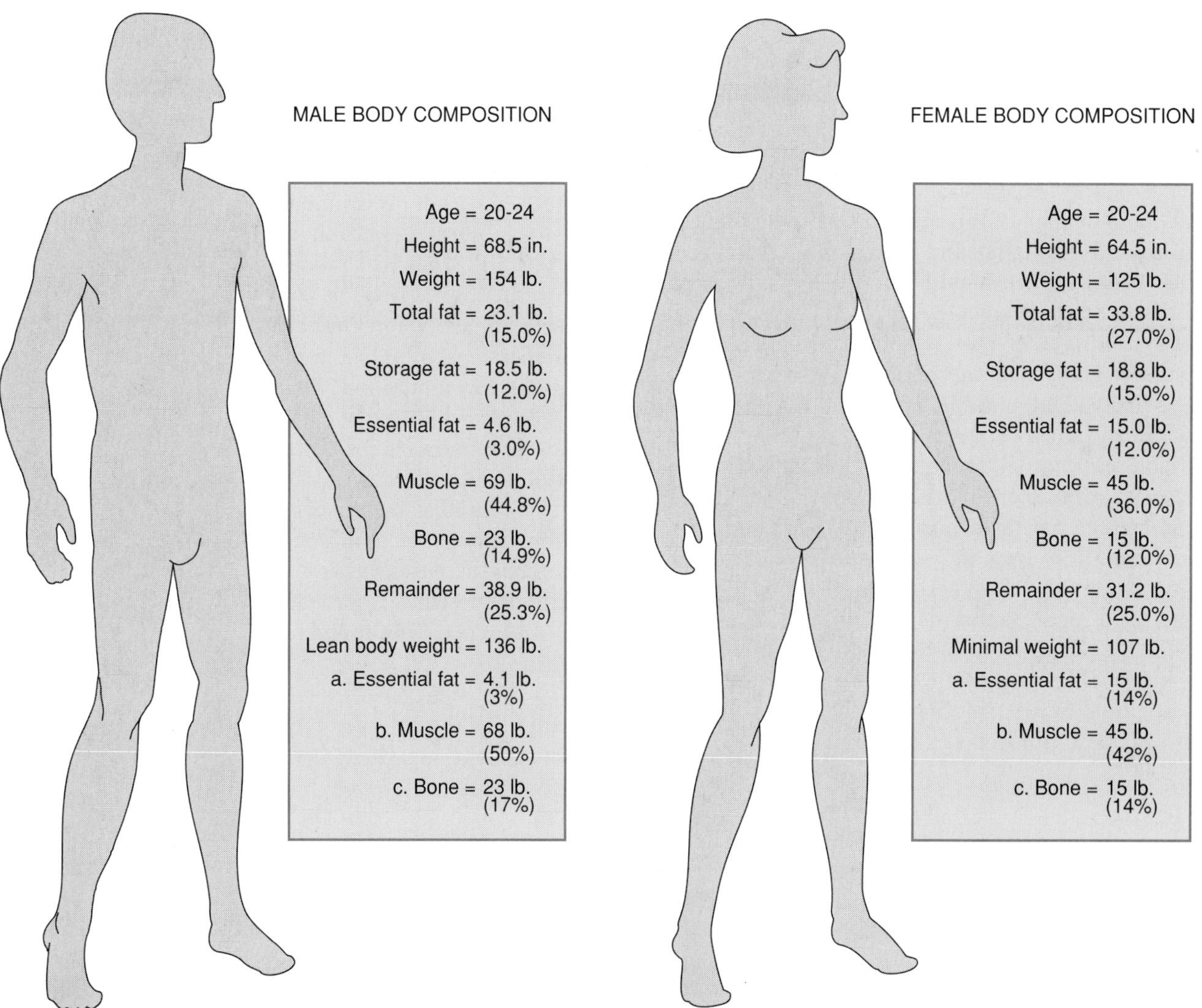

FIGURE 18–2. *Behnke's theoretical body composition model for a man and woman. (Redrawn from McArdle WD, Katch FI, and Katch VL: Exercise Physiology. Energy, Nutrition and Human Performance, 2nd ed. Philadelphia, Lea & Febiger, 1986, p 485.)*

exercise. This variability is a function of the fat cells, or *adipocytes,* which are able to increase and decrease in size as well as increase (and possibly decrease) in number.

Structure

Adipose tissue is located primarily under the skin, in the mesenteries and omentum, and behind the peritoneum. *White adipose tissue* serves as a repository for triglycerides, a cushion to protect abdominal organs, and an insulator to preserve body heat. The slightly yellow color is caused by carotene. *Brown adipose tissue (BAT),* seen in infants and in very small amounts in adults, occurs primarily in the scapular and subscapular areas. The brown color is due to extensive vascularization. It has been studied most extensively in animals, where it appears to be involved in heat production as a means of adapting to cold and possibly of dissipating excess energy.

Regional Distribution

Regional patterns of fat deposit are controlled genetically and differ between, and among, men and women. The *gynoid type* common to women is characterized by the "pear shape" that is created by heavier deposits of fat around the thighs and buttocks. Deposits of fat in these areas are presumably energy reserves to support the demands of pregnancy and lactation. Women with the gynoid type of obesity do not develop the impairments of glucose metabolism seen in obese women of the same weight who carry their fat in an android distribution (Greenwood and Pittman-Waller, 1988).

The *android* or "apple shape" typical of men features fat around the waist and upper abdomen. This type of regional fat deposit is characterized by rapid mobilization of free fatty acids and is associated with significant risk for hypertension, cardiovascular disease, and non-insulin dependent diabetes mellitus (NIDDM) (Bjorntorp, 1987). Combinations of the two types are also seen, particularly in women.

Regional fat distribution defines risk of hyperlipidemia in obese children as it does in adults (Freedman et al, 1989).

Adipocytes

The mature adipocyte consists of a large central lipid droplet surrounded by a thin rim of cytoplasm, which contains the nucleus and the mitochondria. Adipocytes store fat in quantities equal to 80 to 95% of their volume.

Hypertrophy and Hyperplasia

Adipose tissue increases either by adding lipid to increase the size of cells already present *(hypertrophy)* or by increasing the number of cells *(hyperplasia).* Weight gain may be the result of hypertrophy, hyperplasia, or a combination of the two. Obesity is always characterized by hypertrophy, but only some forms of obesity also involve hyperplasia (Bray, 1990).

The fat depots can expand as much as 1,000 times through hypertrophy alone, a process that can occur at any time as long as space is available in the adipocytes (Bjorntorp, 1987). Hyperplasia occurs primarily as a part of the growth process during infancy and adolescence, but it can also occur in adulthood when the fat content of existing cells has reached the limit of their capacity. When weight is reduced due to trauma, illness, starvation, or changes in diet and exercise, fat cell size decreases.

Weight loss is more difficult to achieve in hypercellular obesity and is regained more easily than in obesity of the hypertrophic type.

Fat Cell Development

The greatest level of fatness in normal growth (approximately 25%) occurs at the age of 6 months. In lean children, fat cell size then decreases; however, this decrease does not occur in obese children. At the age of 6 years in normal children, a gradual increase in fatness occurs ("adiposity rebound"), the increase being greater in girls than in boys (Fomon et al, 1982). An early adiposity rebound occurring before 5.5 years is predictive of a higher level of adiposity at 16 years of age and in adulthood, a relationship that appears to occur regardless of the child's adiposity at 1 year of age. A later rebound is correlated with normal adult weight (Rolland-Cachera et al, 1984 and 1990).

Cell number increases in both lean and obese children throughout childhood into adolescence, but the number increases faster in obese than in lean children. After adolescence, increases in body fat occur primarily by an increase in fat cell size.

Fat Storage

Source of Lipid in Fat Cells

Most depot fat comes directly from dietary triglycerides, as is evidenced by the fact that fatty acid composition of adipose tissue mirrors the fatty acid composition of the diet. Excess carbohydrate and protein are also converted to fatty acids in the liver, by means of a comparatively inefficient process. Almost 25% of the energy available in the glucose molecule is used in conversion of carbohydrate to triglyceride, whereas only 3% of lipid energy is used in the process of depositing triglycerides in adipose tissue (Danforth, 1985). Therefore, extra kilocalories in the diet provided by fat are eight times as "lipogenic" as excess kilocalories from carbohydrate.

Role of Lipoprotein Lipase

Dietary triglyceride is transported to the liver as a part of chylomicrons and is removed from the blood by the enzyme *lipoprotein lipase (LPL),* which sits on the luminal side of the capillary and facilitates removal of lipid from the blood and entry through the capillary wall into the adipose cell. Triglyceride synthesized in the liver from free fatty acids travels attached to *very low density lipoprotein (VLDL)* particles and is removed in the periphery by LPL. This enzyme hydrolyzes triglycerides into free fatty acids and glycerol. Glycerol proceeds to the liver; fatty acids enter the adipocyte, where they are re-esterified into triglyceride. When needed by other cells, the latter are hydrolyzed once again to fatty acids and glycerol through the action of *hormone-sensitive lipase (HSL)* and re-enter the circulation.

Hormones affect LPL activity in different adipose tissue regions. *Estrogens* appear to stimulate LPL activity in the gluteofemoral adipocytes and thus promote fat storage in this area, an effect that is seldom seen in obese men. This may be for the specific purpose of providing for childbearing and lactation. However, in the abdominal region, estrogen appears to stimulate lipolysis. The "postmenopausal stomach" may thus be explained in terms of estrogen decrease (Rebuffe-Scrive et al, 1985).

LPL increases during periods of weight gain in both the obese and nonobese. After weight is lost, LPL returns to normal levels in the nonobese; however, in the reduced-obese, the LPL does not decrease and in fact increases. This increase is obviously a major factor in the rapid weight regain that is so common (Elliot et al, 1987). LPL is also higher in smokers and does not decrease at cessation of smoking (at least not at first) and may be a factor in the weight gain that is common after "quitting." Levels of LPL are also characteristically high in genetically obese rats.

REGULATION OF BODY WEIGHT

A variety of regulatory systems exist to maintain body weight at some predetermined point. The answer to how or on what basis this point is determined, or even whether it exists, is not known. However, studies with both animals and humans have demonstrated the existence of controls.

Regulatory systems involving neurotransmitters in the brain govern feeding activities in response to signals originating in affected body tissues. The catecholamines norepinephrine and dopamine are released by the sympathetic nervous system (SNS) in response to dietary intake. These neurotransmitters mediate the activity of areas in the hypothalamus that govern feeding behavior. Fasting and semistarvation lead to a decrease in SNS activity and an increase in adrenal medullary activity with a consequent increase in epinephrine, which fosters substrate mobilization (Katzeff et al, 1986; Vasselli and Maggio, 1988).

Set-Point Theory

Fat storage in nonobese adults appears to be regulated in a manner that preserves a specific body weight. In both animals and humans, deliberate efforts to starve or overfeed are followed by a rapid return to the original weight, as though the latter constituted a set point that is amenable to physiologic influences. If this is true, then some forms of obesity could be the result of an abnormally established set point.

A classic study of volunteer prisoners in Vermont involved deliberately inducing obesity in men of normal weight by overfeeding. At the conclusion of the study, when they were allowed to eat as much as they pleased, most men returned to their normal weight without any particular effort (Sims et al, 1968).

Short- and Long-Term Regulation

Some evidence suggests that regulation takes place on both a short-term and long-term basis. Short-term regulation governs consumption of food from meal to meal; long-term regulation is regulated by the availability of adipose stores (Bray, 1987).

Short-Term Controls

Short-term controls are concerned primarily with factors governing hunger, appetite, and satiety. *Satiety* is associated with the postprandial state when excess food is being stored. *Hunger* is associated with the postabsorptive state when those stores are being mobilized. There may not be such a thing as a stimulus for hunger; rather, the presence or absence of feelings of satiety (Stricker, 1984).

THERMOGENESIS. The components of energy expenditure are the resting energy expenditure (REE) expressed as resting metabolic rate (RMR), the energy expended in voluntary activity, and the thermogenic effect of food. These concepts are discussed in detail in Chapter 2.

RESTING METABOLIC RATE (RMR). When the body is suddenly deprived of adequate energy, such as in accidental or deliberate starvation or semistarvation, the RMR adapts to conserve energy against an unpredictable future by dropping rapidly—as much as 15% in 2 weeks. When adequate food intake is restored, the RMR returns to normal levels per kilogram of body weight (Wadden, 1990).

Thermogenic Effect of Food (TEF). The TEF is made up of an obligatory component related to the energy value of food consumed and an additional adaptive component that presumably responds to overeating by eliminating the excessive energy in the form of heat (see Chapter 2). The existence of the adaptive component has been demonstrated in animals, primarily in the BAT. However, the amount of BAT in adults is not sufficient to account for adaptive thermogenesis. Whether a blunting of the adaptive component is a significant factor in the obese is controversial; nonetheless, it is an attractive theory to account for the ability of the nonobese to adjust without effort to excessive intake and for the failure of obese persons to maintain leaner weight levels.

Gut Peptides. Mechanical contact of food with the mucosa of the muscles of the stomach and small intestine stimulates secretion of *gut peptides,* which have an immediate effect on satiety. Among those that have been identified is *cholecystokinin (CCK),* which causes cessation of eating when injected into animals. Some of the gut peptides are also found in the brain, where they both stimulate and inhibit eating.

Thyroid Hormones. Thyroid hormones modulate the tissue responsiveness to the catecholamines secreted by the SNS. A decrease in T_3 lowers the response to SNS activity and consequently diminishes adaptive thermogenesis. Such a subtle defect could be one of the factors predisposing some of the obese to excessive weight gain.

Insulin. Peripheral administration of *insulin* leads to an acute increase in food intake. This response is attributed to peripheral hypoglycemia, which is a potent stimulus for eating. Impaired insulin activity may lead to reduced SNS activity and thus to impaired thermogenesis.

Fasting insulin levels increase proportionately with the degree of obesity. However, many obese individuals demonstrate insulin resistance, impaired glucose tolerance, and associated hyperlipidemia. These sequelae can usually be corrected with weight loss.

Long-Term Regulation

A feedback mechanism has been proposed involving a signal from the *adipose mass* that is released when "normal" body composition is disturbed, possibly when the lipid content of fat cells has reached a certain level. The signal has not been identified although serum insulin has been suggested, as well as blood levels of glycerol or free fatty acids released from the adipose tissue during lipolysis.

WEIGHT IMBALANCE: OBESITY

Overweight is a state in which weight exceeds a standard based on height; *obesity* is a condition of excessive fatness, either general or localized. It is possible to be obese at a weight within normal limits according to standard tables, just as it is possible to be overweight without being obese; however, in most people, overweight and obesity tend to parallel each other.

Assessment

Assessment of underweight and obesity is made in a variety of ways, depending on the necessity for accuracy. The tables of the Metropolitan Life Insurance Company (MLI) are widely used in establishing a standard of *ideal body weight (IBW).* The more preferred methods are: (1) the *body mass index (BMI),* or Quetelet Index ($BMI = W/H^2$ in which W is weight in kilograms and H is height in meters), and (2) the *waist-hip ratio,* which compares the circumference measurements of waist and hip to identify android and gynoid body types. These methods and others of assessment of body fatness are discussed in detail in Chapter 17.

Tables for determination of BMI and W/H ratios are presented in Appendix Tables 19 and 20, respectively. The MLI tables appear in Appendix Table 17. Overweight and obesity are defined in terms of IBW and BMI in Table 18–1.

Risk

Obesity is associated with a large number of disease states. A National Institutes of Health Consensus Development Panel, convened in 1985 to assess the

TABLE 18–1. Classification of Overweight and Obesity*

	Men		Women	
Classification	*% IBW*†	*BMI (kg/m²)*	*% IBW*	*BMI (kg/m²)*
Super obese	225	>50	245	>50
Morbidly obese	200	45	220	45
Medically significant obesity	160	35	170	35
Obese	135	30	145	30
Overweight	110	25	120	25
IBW	100	20–25	100	20–25

* Adapted from Forse A et al: Morbid obesity: Weighing the treatment options—surgical options. Nutr Today 24(5):10, 1989, p 11.
† IBW = ideal body weight.

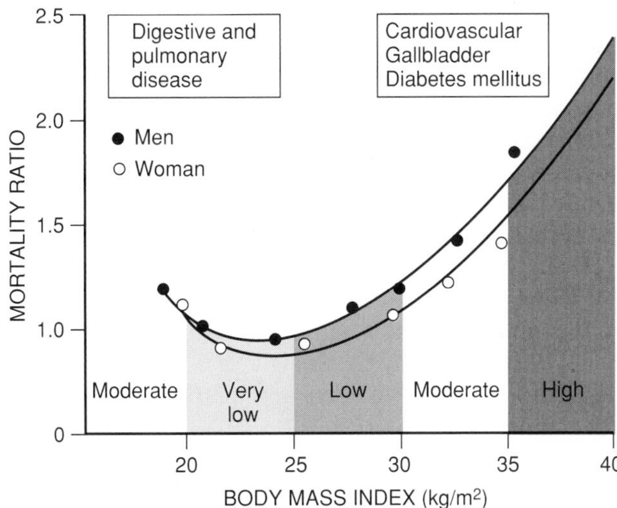

FIGURE 18–3. *Body mass index and mortality risk. Data from the American Cancer Society study have been plotted for men and women to show the relationship of body mass index to overall mortality risk. At a body mass index below 20 kg/m² and above 30 kg/m², there is an increase in relative mortality. The major causes for this increased mortality are listed, along with a division of body mass index groupings into various levels of risk. (Redrawn from Bray GA and Gray DS: Obesity. Part I: Pathogenesis. West J Med 149:429, 1988, p 436. Originally adapted from Lew EA and Garfinkle L: Variations in mortality by weight among 750,000 men and women. J Chronic Dis 32:563, 1979.)*

current status of knowledge about obesity, determined that a 20% increase in body weight substantially increases the risk for hypertension, coronary artery disease, lipid disorders, and NIDDM. Obesity is also considered a risk factor for some kinds of cancer and is associated with joint disease, gallstones, and respiratory problems.

Data from a large American Cancer Society study show that mortality risk increases with a BMI of 25 or greater and at a BMI of 20 or less (Lew and Garfinkle, 1979). Death at the lower weights is primarily from digestive and pulmonary disease (Fig. 18–3). Pooled information from insurance companies covering 750,000 men and women between 1959 and 1972 found the lowest mortality in persons who weighed 10 to 20% below average, whereas those 30 to 40% above average weight had 50% greater mortality and the mortality rate in those over 40% of average weight was 90% greater.

Etiology

The nature and causes of obesity are the subject of intensive and continuing research. Both environmental and genetic factors are involved in a complex interaction of variables, which include psychologic and cultural influences as well as physiologic regulatory mechanisms.

Over the years many hypotheses have evolved to explain why some people become fat while others remain lean, and why it is so difficult for the reduced-obese to maintain the weight loss that is achieved so painstakingly. The fact that no single theory can completely explain all manifestations of obesity, or applies consistently to all individuals, only underscores the complex nature of this condition. Few have been completely rejected, but many of those recognized as being too simplistic have evolved into more complex rationales. Theories suggesting imbalances of energy input are generally related to factors influencing hunger and appetite or satiety. Theories relating to imbalances of energy output are concerned primarily with TEF, physical activity, and the RMR. Heredity and environment influence both the input and output of energy.

Heredity

Many of the hormonal and neural factors involved in normal weight regulation are determined genetically. These include the short- and long-term signals that determine satiety and feeding activity. Small defects in their expression or interaction could contribute significantly to weight gain. Number and size of fat cells, regional distribution of body fat, and resting metabolic rate are also determined genetically.

Evidence for a *genetic component* as high as 67% in some types of obesity has been obtained with studies of twins and adoptees (Stunkard et al, 1990). Body weights and fat distribution of monozygotic twins correlate more strongly than dizygotic twins (Stunkard et al, 1986a; Bouchard et al, 1988). Weights of 540 Danish adoptees were found to correlate with their biologic parents across all weight classes, from very thin to very fat, whereas no such relationship was seen with the adoptive parents (Stunkard et al, 1986b).

Factors Affecting Weight Gain

Obesity is the consequence of an imbalance of energy intake with reference to energy output. Excessive energy intake would appear to be the result of *hyperphagia;* however, many studies indicate that the obese do not eat more than the nonobese and that they often eat less. In the process of becoming obese, however, hyperphagia is indeed a factor. Animal studies demonstrating excessive eating in response to foods high in fat or sugar or to "cafeteria diets" may have meaning when applied to human eating circumstances (Bennett, 1987).

An *externality theory* proposed that some people respond more to external rather than to internal cues and that once confronted with appetizing food they are unable to resist the opportunity to overeat (Schachter, 1968; Stunkard and Kaplan, 1977), whereas bland, tasteless foods in unstimulating surroundings can actually lead to underconsumption.

Failure to reliably demonstrate this theory in all cases has led to the *restraint theory,* which suggests that continued dieting eventually oversensitizes some individuals to the smell, taste, or sight of food. As reduced-obese, their time is mainly spent suffering through prolonged periods of restraining the impulse to eat, but occasionally unforeseen events release the restraints and lead to periods of bingeing.

Considerable evidence supports the *"pull" theory* which holds that excessive fatness comes first and leads to the hyperphagia, which causes excessive overweight. Genetically obese rats become overfat before they begin to overeat. When restricted by pair-feeding to the intake of their litter-mate controls, they become obese. When fasted to normal weight, they retain higher content of body fat than equal weight controls, and when reduced to their pre-experiment weight they continue to be overfat (Greenwood and Pittman-Waller, 1988).

A *defect in thermogenesis* has been proposed as a factor in excessive weight gain. A blunting of the thermogenic effect of food after meals has been seen in some, but not all, obese. Whether a form of adaptive thermogenesis actually exists has not been fully established, but it is still an attractive theory (see Chapter 2).

TISSUE ADAPTATION TO WEIGHT LOSS

Tissue response to starvation, or even semistarvation of the kind encountered in most weight loss programs, is one of adaptation to an anticipated period of deprivation. The classic starvation studies done by Keys (1950) found that during the first 10 days of a fast and after utilization of glycogen stores, approximately 8 to 12% of the energy expenditure is from protein with the balance from fat. As starvation progresses, up to 97% of energy expenditure is from stored triglyceride. Use of fat, with more than twice the kilocalories of protein, is not only more efficient but also spares vital protein tissues. However, even when the body has adjusted completely, 5% of weight loss is still from protein in muscle supporting adipose tissue (Bray and Gray, 1988a).

Plateau Effect

A common experience in weight-reduction programs is arrival at a weight plateau, when weight remains at the same level for a period of time. Eventually, weight loss halts completely. One theory is that interim plateaus reflect a reduction of lipid in individual adipocytes to some signal-triggering level that demands metabolic adjustment and weight maintenance.

Any weight loss, whether fast or slow, results in a loss of the extra muscle that has developed to support the excess adipose tissue. Because this extra LBM has contributed to an increased metabolic rate, the RMR decreases as the LBM is lost. The fact that the RMR decreases very rapidly at the onset of a weight-reduction diet—by as much as 15% within 2 weeks— indicates that other adaptations to the lower weight as well as to the threat of deprivation are taking place.

Other factors join the decrease in RMR to limit effectiveness of the restricted energy intake. A decrease in the total kilocalories ingested results in a decrease in TEF. Because a body that weighs less requires less expenditure of energy to move around, the cost of physical activity is also less.

A state of equilibrium is eventually reached at which the energy intake is equal to energy expenditure. Unless a change is made in either diet or physical activity, weight loss will stop at this point.

Weight Cycling

Many obese people reduce and gain weight several times throughout their lifetimes (i.e., *the yo-yo effect*). With each turn of the cycle, it takes longer to lose the same amount of fat and, conversely, less time to regain it. Typically, more weight is regained than was lost, and the regained weight is higher in fat in proportion to LBM than at prediet levels (Blackburn et al, 1989). Weight instability is positively related to higher waist-to-hip ratios with consequent risk of coronary heart disease and possibly other diseases (Rodin et al, 1990; Saris, 1989).

Maintenance after a period of significant weight reduction is said to require 25% fewer calories than at the beginning of the program. This suggests a downward revision in the RMR, caused by the reduction in LBM that accompanies the fat loss plus other metabolic adjustments in adapting to periods of semistarvation. Although it is true that RMR per kilogram of body weight drops significantly during weight loss, most studies indicate that it returns to prediet levels very rapidly.

MANAGEMENT OF OBESITY

In 1985, 44% of American women and 25% of American men were dieting (Blackburn et al, 1989). Weight-reduction programs with the most promise of success integrate diet, exercise, and behavior modification. Pharmacologic treatment and surgical intervention are appropriate in some circumstances.

Goals of Treatment

Although achieving desirable or ideal weight is usually the goal of treatment, this may not always be realistic or desirable, and under some circumstances it may not be appropriate at all (Blackburn, 1987). Depending on the type and severity of the existing obesity and on the age and lifestyle of the individual involved, successful weight reduction can vary from a relatively simple matter to virtually impossible. For those who successfully reduce weight, regardless of the method, the evidence for successful maintenance of the new weight for more than a few years, if that long, is sparse. Continued episodes of loss and gain are associated with increasing metabolic adaptation to lower and lower intakes, and each reduction becomes even more difficult.

On the other hand, the risks with respect to other diseases are considerable and are associated with relatively low levels of obesity. Some conditions, such as hypertension, respond to even a moderate degree of weight reduction. Mild and moderate obesity can be treated by integrated weight reduction programs, although to date no approach appears to guarantee success in the long term. Morbid obesity is of sufficiently life-threatening nature that more drastic measures are indicated.

Although achievement of ideal weight may be an appropriate endpoint for many of the mildly obese, a program of management that simply maintains present weight without further gain is the most that can be expected for many people and is preferable to continued weight cycling. It has been suggested that because obesity is essentially incurable, it should be treated on a continuing basis like any other chronic illness.

Rate and Extent of Weight Loss

Reduction of body weight involves loss of both protein and fat, in amounts determined to some degree by the rate of weight reduction. Steady losses over a longer period favor reduction of fat stores, limit the loss of vital protein tissues, and avoid the sharp decline in RMR that accompanies rapid weight reduction. One approach designed to minimize the decrease in RMR recommends loss of ½ to 1½ lb/week, leading to a weight reduction at the end of the first year of 10 to 15% of body weight (Blackburn, 1987). After a period of adjustment to the lower weight, the year-long program can be repeated.

Final goals should be individualized and chosen realistically. For example, neither the hyperplastic obese nor the gynoid types will be able to maintain large weight losses. Female role models of dress sizes 6 to 10 and male models with 30- to 34-inch waists "may not be appropriate to the obese population," and in fact even BMIs of 25 are unreasonable goals for many dieters (Blackburn, 1988).

Even with the same caloric intake, rates of weight reduction vary. Men reduce weight faster than women of similar size because of their higher LBM and RMR. The heavier person, who because of his or her higher weight expends more energy than one who is less obese, will reduce faster on a given intake.

Dietary Modification

Weight loss programs with any degree of success integrate diet with exercise, frequently with behavior modification, and always with nutritional education and possibly psychologic support. When these approaches fail to bring about the desired reduction in weight, medication may be added to the program and, in the case of morbid obesity, surgical intervention may be required.

Recommendations

A Consensus Panel of the International Congress on Obesity has recommended that a weight-loss program should combine a nutritionally balanced diet with exercise and behavior therapy at the least possible expense. The diet should furnish 500 kcal/day less than maintenance requirements (about 850 kcal/m^2 for women; about 900 kcal/m^2 for men). This daily deficit should provide a loss of 0.45 kg (1 lb)/wk (National Institutes of Health, 1985).

Another formula proposes using the value of 22 kcal/kg actual weight to determine energy needs and then designing a diet that will provide a deficit of 1,000 kcal/day. Such a diet would result in a loss of 1 kg (2.2 lb)/wk (Bray and Gray, 1988b).

Brownell proposes that in many cases dieters should simply follow a low-fat diet combined with a regular exercise program and "let the weight take care of itself" (Brownell, 1988) (see Chapter 20).

Restricted-Energy Diets

Moderate Energy Restriction. A balanced energy controlled diet is the most widely prescribed method of weight reduction. The diet should be nutritionally adequate except for energy, which is decreased to the point where fat stores must be mobilized to meet daily energy needs. The energy level varies with the individual's size and activities, but as a general rule it should not be less than 800 kcal. Most adults can reduce weight on an intake of 1,200 to 1,300 kcal/day.

The diet should be relatively high in carbohydrates, primarily starch (55% of kcal) with generous protein (0.8 to 1.2 g/kg ideal weight, around 12 to 15% of kcal) to allow for conversion of some dietary protein to energy. The inclusion of extra fiber is recommended to reduce caloric density, promote satiety by delaying stomach emptying time, and decrease to a small degree the efficiency of intestinal absorption.

Because fat provides more than twice as much energy per gram as either protein or carbohydrate (9 kcal vs 4 kcal), an effective diet is one that controls this nutrient to as large an extent as possible (20 to 30% of kilocalories). Fat also has a lipogenic quality apart from and in addition to its energy content.

With a restricted food intake, it becomes necessary to choose foods of high nutrient density. Alcohol and foods high in sugar should be limited as unnecessary sources of energy; however, small amounts can be included for palatability. Artificial sweeteners (discussed in Chapter 31) and fat substitutes (discussed in Chapter 4) may improve the acceptability of limited food intakes for some people.

Vitamin and mineral supplements are usually recommended with weight reduction programs that provide for less than 1,200 kcal.

Exchange System Diets. A popular and easily manipulated method for planning a diet program tailored to the individual is the Exchange System, which is discussed in detail in Chapter 31. A 1,200-kcal diet based on this system is shown in Table 18–2 and Figure 18–4. The energy content of the diet can be increased by adding midafternoon and evening snacks, or by increasing the number of servings from various groups. Non-nutritious, high-energy foods, such as sweets, desserts, or alcohol, can be added sparingly.

Formula Diets. Formula diets are supplied by pharmaceutical and food-processing companies in a variety of forms. The recommended daily quantity of the drink or powder supplies approximately 900 kcal distributed as 20% protein, 30% fat, and 50% carbohydrate. At this energy level, and with vitamins and minerals to meet the Recommended Dietary Allowances, these formulas are considered to be safe. Quantities of formula equivalent to a single meal are used successfully as substitutions for a meal at times when it is difficult to obtain

TABLE 18–2. 1,200-kcal Diet—22% of Kilocalories from Fat

Food	Food Exchanges* (No.)	Carbohydrate (g)	Protein (g)	Fat (g)
Milk, skim	2	24	16	—
Vegetables	3	15	6	
Fruits	4	60		
Bread	5	75	10	
Meat,† lean	5		35	15
Fat	3			15
	Totals	174	67	30

Sample Meal Plan

Breakfast

Fruit, 1 exchange
Bread, 2 exchanges
Milk, skim, 1 exchange

Lunch or Supper

Vegetables, 1 exchange
Bread, 2 exchanges
Meat, lean, 2 exchange
Fruit, 1 exchange
Milk, skim, 1 exchange

Dinner or Supper

Meat, lean, 3 exchanges
Vegetable, 2 exchanges
Bread, 1 exchange
Fat, 1 exchange
Fruit, 2 exchanges

Sample Menu

Breakfast	*Lunch*	*Dinner*
½ grapefruit	Sandwich:	Bouillon
1 slice of whole-wheat toast	2 slices of rye bread	1 parsley potato (2-in. diameter)
1 glass (8 oz) of skim milk	2 oz of sliced turkey	3 oz of roast veal, lean
¾ cup of dry cereal	2 stalks of celery	½ cup of peas and carrots
Coffee or tea as desired	1 carrot	1 green salad
	1 peach (medium)	2 tsp salad dressing
	1 glass (8 oz) of skim buttermilk	½ cup applesauce (unsweetened)
		1 small banana
		Tea or coffee as desired

* From exchange lists, Table 31–10.
† Lean meat with visible fat removed is used, reducing the fat content from 5 to 3 grams per Meat Exchange.

1200 kCAL DIET

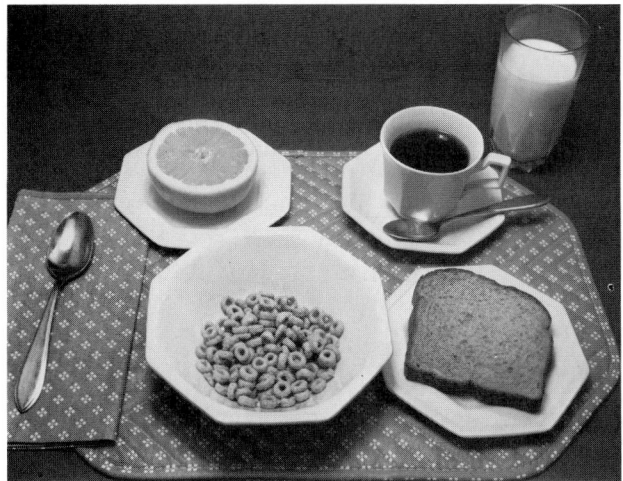

BREAKFAST

½ grapefruit (small)
1 slice whole-wheat toast
1 glass (8 oz) skim milk
¾ c dry cereal
Coffee

TYPICAL AMERICAN DIET

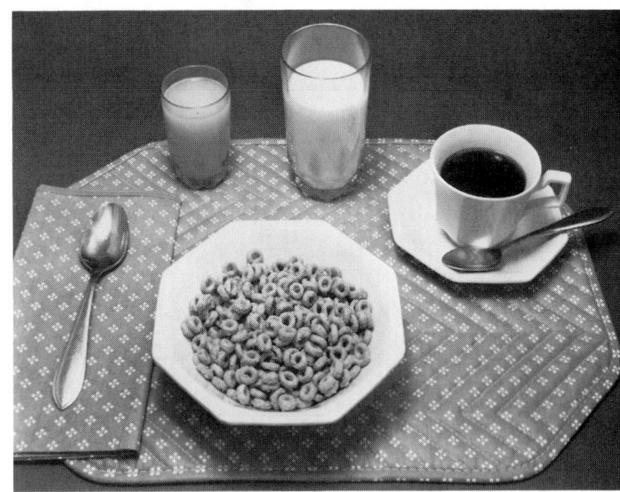

BREAKFAST

1½ c Cheerios
¾ c orange juice
1 c 2% milk
Coffee

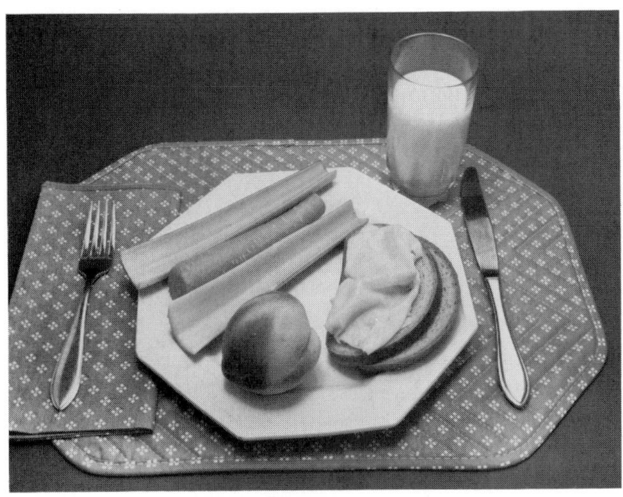

LUNCH

Sandwich:
  2 slices rye bread
  2 oz sliced turkey
2 stalks celery
1 carrot
1 medium peach
1 glass (8 oz) skim buttermilk

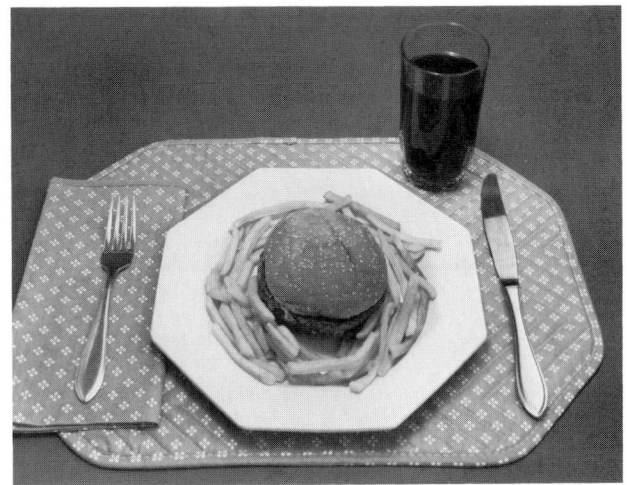

LUNCH

1 quarter-pound cheeseburger, lettuce, tomatoes
French fries
8 oz diet soda

FIGURE 18–4. *Sample daily menu for a 1,200-kcal diet—22% of kcal from fat.* Illustration continued on following page

foods appropriate to a weight-reduction program. Negative aspects of the formula diets include dependence on a particular featured product, and failure to develop new, appropriate long-term eating habits.

Commercial Programs. Millions of Americans use commercial weight loss programs to lose weight (Table 18–3). Most offer diets that are well balanced and safe, except for the problems associated with rapid weight loss. Unfortunately, there are little data to support the long-term effectiveness of these programs and the attrition rate is high. Some of these provide a low-calorie eating plan (about 500 to 800 kcal) and require daily "weigh-ins" for a cost based on the amount of weight needing to be lost. Others require the use of their prepackaged low-fat meals. Some provide classes on behavior modification and nutrition. Prepackaged diets

1200 kCAL DIET

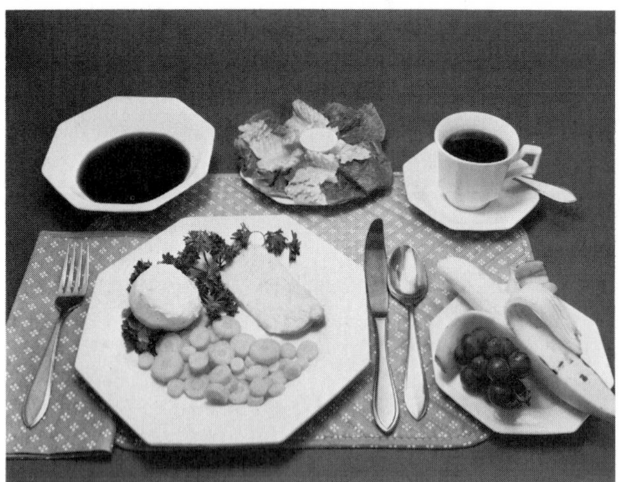

DINNER

Bouillon
1 parsley potato (2 in. diameter)
3 oz roast veal, lean
½ c carrots
1 green salad, 2 tsp salad dressing
15 grapes
1 small banana
Coffee

TYPICAL AMERICAN DIET

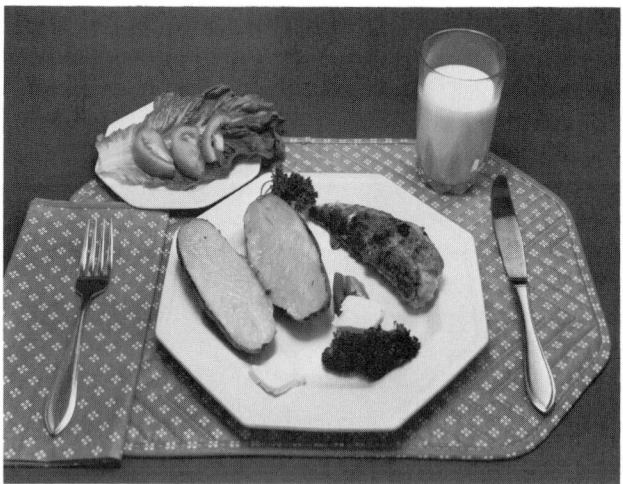

DINNER

1 baked potato with margarine
1 broiled chicken breast (4 oz after cooking)
1½ c 2% milk
½ c broccoli, margarine
2 c salad (lettuce, tomatoes, 2 T creamy dressing)

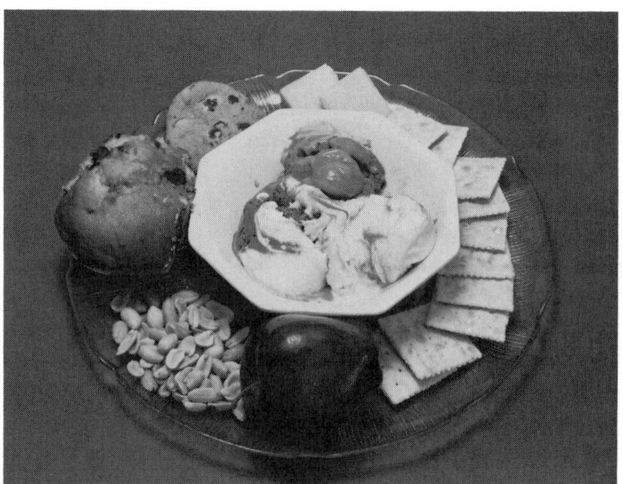

SNACKS

1 large blueberry muffin
Coffee
8 oz 2% milk
1 cookie
10 saltines
1 apple
2 oz cheese
1¼ c ice cream
¼ c peanuts

FIGURE 18–4. Continued

appeal to some people because they allow them to avoid making decisions about food choices. However, even though such programs are effective for weight reduction, they may actually limit long-term weight maintenance because there is no learning of the food choice skills needed for permanent change (Fatis et al, 1989).

Fad Diets. A continuous supply of new and often bizarre approaches to weight reduction is available to the consumer through the popular press. Although some of the programs are sensible and appropriate, most tend to emphasize fast results with a minimum of effort. Often the proposed diets would lead to nutri-

TABLE 18–3. Popular Commercial Diet Programs

Name	Foods or Products	Education	Teachers/Counselors	Maintenance
VLCD* Programs				
Medifast	Special drink; physician supervised	Weekly individual sessions Weekly group meetings	Physician or designates	Weekly meetings for 5 months
Optifast	Special drink; physician supervised	Weekly individual sessions w/MD 1½-hr weekly group meetings 1 meeting w/RD	Health professionals	7 weekly meetings; 26 biweekly meetings
HMR	Special drink; multidisciplinary team	1½-hr weekly group meetings w/RD	Health professionals	Weekly meetings for 18 months
Diet Programs				
Weight Watchers	Regular food	45 min weekly group meetings	Program graduates	Weekly meetings for 6 weeks; free meetings if maintain goal weight
Jenny Craig	Prepackaged foods	14 1-hr video group classes; weekly individual sessions	College graduates	Monthly meetings for 1 year
Nutri/System	Prepackaged foods	30 min weekly group meetings; 10 min weekly individual sessions	College graduates	1-year transition diet—program and regular foods
Diet Workshop	Regular food	1 hr weekly group meetings	Program graduates	Weekly meetings for 4 weeks
Weight Loss Clinic	Regular food	10 min daily individual sessions	RN, LPN, RD, or trained staff	Biweekly meetings for 6 weeks; 6 additional monthly meetings

* VLCD = very low calorie diet.

tional deficiencies over an extended period; however, the potential health risks are seldom realized because the diets are usually abandoned after a few weeks. On the other hand, fad diets encourage unrealistic expectations, thus setting the dieter up for failure, subsequent guilt, and feelings of helplessness at ever managing the weight problem.

Variations of a *low-carbohydrate, high-fat diet* were popular for many years. Carbohydrate was severely restricted, but protein and fat intakes were unlimited. Protein obtained from animal sources meant that fat, saturated fat, and cholesterol levels were also high. Although these diets featured production of large numbers of ketones, their only value was to suppress appetite to a minor degree. Even with total fasting, converting fats to ketones lowers the energy value of the diet by only 100 kcal/day. The initial rapid weight loss from diuresis was secondary to the carbohydrate restriction.

A *high-carbohydrate, low-fat diet,* known as the *Pritikin diet,* restricts fat to 10% of total kilocalories with the carbohydrate level at 80% of calories. The diet produces rapid weight loss and is nutritionally adequate as formulated, although highly restrictive.

EXTREME ENERGY RESTRICTION. Extreme energy restricted diets provide less than 800 kcal/day, whereas starvation or fasting diets provide less than 200 kcal/day (Bray and Gray, 1988b).

Fasting. Fasting is seldom prescribed as a treatment for obesity. However, it is frequently invoked by individuals as a part of religious or protest regimes or in a personal effort to lose weight. Under these circumstances, it is seldom continued long enough to produce the serious neurologic, hormonal, and other side effects that accompany prolonged starvation. Over 50% of the rapid weight reduction is fluid, which often leads to serious hypotension problems. Accumulation of uric acid can precipitate episodes of gout.

Very Low Calorie Diets. Diets providing 200 to 800 kcal are classified as *very low calorie diets (VLCD).* Their major advantage is the rapid weight loss, which typically amounts to 20 kg (44 lb) in 12 weeks, the recommended length of the program (Fisler and Drenick, 1987). Because of potential side effects, prescription of these diets is reserved for the moderately to morbidly obese for whom other diet programs have been unsuccessful.

The VLCD that first became popular in the early 1970s resulted in several deaths (Further Reading, p. 328). However, improved formulation, particularly with respect to protein quality, has led to wide acceptability for those whose obesity is potentially life-threatening. Currently most VLCD are in one of two forms. The *protein-sparing modified fast* contains 1.5 g of protein/kg of ideal body weight in the form of lean meat, fish and poultry, no carbohydrate, and only the fat contained in the protein sources. The second form uses *commercially formulated liquid diets* based on milk or egg protein. These typically contain 33 to 70 grams of protein, 30 to 45 grams of carbohydrate, and a small amount of fat.

FURTHER READING: History of Protein-Sparing Modified Fast Diets

The first protein-sparing modified fast (PSMF) diets were developed after observing that during total fasts, popular for weight reduction in the late 1950s and early 1960s, dieters lost large amounts of potassium and protein. The first PSMF diets were developed to add protein to the fasting regime. Protein in the early formulas was exclusively in the form of hydrolyzed collagen, which was a protein lacking tryptophan, an essential amino acid. The formulas were not supplemented with vitamins, minerals, or electrolytes and were not necessarily supported by medical supervision. The products were used by more than 100,000 people, among whom 60 diet-related deaths had been reported to the Centers for Disease Control by the end of 1977.

The diet was directly implicated as the basis for the cardiac arrhythmias causing 17 deaths (Isner et al, 1979). Of the 17 deaths, those with the highest percentage of body fat prior to beginning the diet were better able to preserve body protein, especially that in the myocardium (Van Itallie and Yang, 1984). A common feature of 9 of the 17 victims was an abnormal electrocardiogram, possibly owing to deteriorating cardiac muscle or to potassium depletion.

The hazardous products were removed from the market. PSMF formulas currently contain complete protein and some carbohydrate; are supplemented with vitamins, minerals, and electrolytes; and are usually used as part of a complete multidisciplinary program.

Proper use of VLCD requires careful instruction and follow-up. Long-term effectiveness is improved when they are combined with behavior modification, increased exercise, and particularly nutritional counseling to facilitate maintenance of weight loss. When used alone, their long-term effectiveness is no greater than that of other diet programs. One study compared three treatment programs — a VLCD, behavior therapy, and a combined approach using both treatments. The group with the combination approach achieved significantly higher weight loss, but at the end of 1 year had regained one third of the original weight loss. However, this was considerably better than the two thirds regained by the diet-only group (Wadden and Stunkard, 1986).

VLCD promote rapid weight loss, averaging 0.78 kg/day (12 lb/wk) during the first week, owing to sodium loss and diuresis, and 0.28 kg/day (4 lb/wk) by the third week of the fast (Fisler and Drenick, 1987). Risks include potassium loss as well as loss of body protein, which is proportionately greater (20 g/kg of weight lost) in the less obese compared with the more obese (Forbes, 1987). Serum electrolytes need to be monitored and supplemented when necessary. VLCD can lead to an increase of urinary ketones that interfere with the renal clearance of uric acid, resulting in increased serum uric acid levels that are often manifested in gout. Higher serum cholesterol levels resulting from mobilization of adipose stores pose a risk of gallstones. Other risks that may be nothing more than uncomfortable side effects of rapid weight loss are cold intolerance, fatigue, light-headedness, nervousness, euphoria, constipation or diarrhea, dry skin, thinning reddened hair, anemia, and menstrual irregularities. Some of these are typical of triiodothyronine (T_3) deficiency. The greatest risk, however, is the inability of most rapid dieters to maintain the reduced state.

The American Dietetic Association has outlined the criteria that should be followed in using the VLCD in weight management (American Dietetic Association, 1990) (Clinical Insight, p. 330).

Behavior Modification

Behavior modification programs focus on three components: self-monitoring, stimulus control, and techniques for self-reward. *Self-monitoring* with daily records of place and time of food intake, as well as accompanying thoughts and feelings, helps to identify the physical and emotional settings in which eating occurs. It also provides feedback on progress and places the responsibility for change and accomplishment on the patient. Self-monitoring also gives clues to the occurrence of relapses and consequent guilt and how they can be prevented. *Stimulus control* involves modification of: (1) the settings or the chain of events that precede eating, (2) the kinds of foods consumed when eating does occur, and (3) the consequences of eating. Some of these techniques are listed in Table 18–4. The last component includes *self-reward* for eating control.

Behavior modification in weight control appears to be most effective for the mildly obese (20 to 40% overweight). The low attrition rate averages 13.5% compared with 25 to 75% in most other programs (Bray and Gray, 1988b). Patients can lose 20 to 25 lb and can successfully maintain the weight loss if they continue to practice the techniques and exercise regularly. It also appears that the longer programs are the most successful (Buckmaster and Brownell, 1988). Most programs usually last for 15 weeks and result in an average weight loss of 1.2 lb/wk. Average weight reduction at the end of the program is 20 lb (Foreyt, 1989).

Evaluations of long-term effectiveness of behavior modification in achieving and maintaining weight reduction are conflicting. One study, which involved two

TABLE 18-4. Behavioral Modification Strategies*

Elimination of Eating Cues
Eat only sitting down at one designated place.
Sit in a different seat at the table.
Leave the table as soon as eating is done.
Do not combine eating with other activities, such as reading or watching television.
Do not put bowls of food on the table.
At a restaurant, pass the rolls to the other end of the table or ask the waitress to take them away or bring them later.
Do not keep inappropriate foods at home.
Keep all food in cupboards where it cannot be seen.
Shop for groceries from a list after a full meal.
Limit the amount of money taken when shopping.
Plan meals and snacks.
Plan for special events, parties, and dinners.
Discard leftovers in the garbage so that they are not eaten later.
Negotiate with the family to not eat inappropriate foods when around
Ask others to monitor eating patterns and provide positive feedback.
Substitute other activities for snacking.
Behaviors to Prolong Eating and Reduce the Amount of Food Eaten
Eat slowly and savor each mouthful.
Put down the fork between bites.
Delay eating for 2 to 3 minutes and converse with others.
Postpone a desired snack for 10 minutes.
Serve food on a smaller plate.
Leave 1 or 2 bites of food on the plate.
Divide portions in half so that another portion can be permitted.

* Adapted from Holli BB: Using behavior modification in nutrition counseling. J Am Diet Assoc 88:1530, 1988.

or more annual follow-up periods during a period of 5 years, measured weight regained at each visit and found that less than 3% of 152 subjects had maintained post-treatment weight at the end of 4 years whereas 40% had gained up to the original weight or above (Kramer et al, 1989).

On the other hand, when behavior modification techniques are used in conjunction with VLCD programs to enhance long-term weight maintenance, they appear to improve the outcome (Stunkard, 1987).

Exercise

Exercise is an important part of a weight management program. By increasing LBM in proportion to fat, exercise helps to balance the loss of LBM and reduction of RMR that inevitably accompany even a well-managed weight reduction program (Pavlou et al, 1989a). By lowering glycogen stores, aerobic exercise promotes the use of fat for fuel. Numerous positive side effects include strengthening cardiovascular integrity as well as increasing sensitivity to insulin. Possibly the most valuable contributions of exercise are the relief of boredom, increased sense of control, and improved sense of well-being (Fig. 18-5).

Increased exercise can result in an energy deficit, and even without diet, exercise alone can be expected to lower weight around 2.5 kg (Bray and Gray, 1988b; Gwinup, 1975) depending on the intensity, duration, and type of exercise. Dieters with hypertrophic obesity lose more fat during an exercise program than the very obese with hyperplastic obesity (Bjorntorp, 1983). This may account for the observation that although the moderately obese lose body fat during physical training, it is difficult to demonstrate this result in the massively obese.

Some studies of programs combining diet and exercise have shown that although there is no increase in weight loss in the exercising group over diet alone, an increased loss of body fat does occur (Hill et al, 1987; Van Dale et al, 1987). A decrease in body fat does not necessarily mean a decrease in body weight. Initially, physical exercise increases muscle mass, and because LBM is more dense than the fat it replaces, body weight may not change. With continued exercise, the limited capacity of muscle mass to increase is overcome by the decrease in fat, resulting in a net decrease in body weight. A minimum of 2 months is needed to obtain any reduction of adipose tissue with adequate training programs (Bjorntorp, 1976).

The RMR is elevated during aerobic exercise, but the effect does not appear to persist for more than 40 minutes after exercise has stopped. Energy expenditure during this period represents replacement of muscle glycogen as well as the effects of hormonal changes and the increase in metabolic processing of fuel stores. Whether exercise has an effect on TEF remains unresolved.

Contrary to popular belief, spot reduction is not possible with exercise; fat is removed from the largest concentrations of adipose tissue. Another misconception is that exercise is counterproductive because it increases the desire to eat. Although lean individuals usually

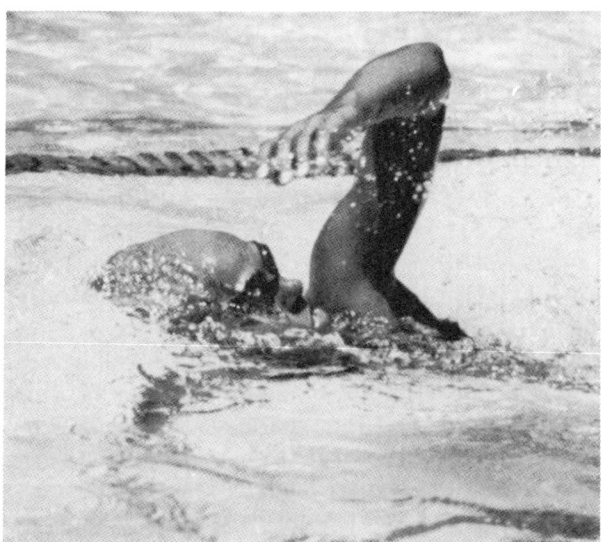

FIGURE 18-5. *Swimming is an excellent aerobic activity to include in a weight reduction program. (From Richardson AR: The biomechanics of swimming. Clin Sports Med 5:103-113, 1986.)*

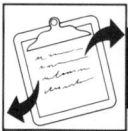

CLINICAL INSIGHT: American Dietetic Association Criteria for Use of Very Low Calorie Diets

Whereas very low calorie diets (VLCD) promote rapid weight reduction and may be beneficial for certain individuals, such diets have health risks and should be undertaken only with the supervision of a multidisciplinary health team with monitoring by a physician and nutrition counseling by a registered dietitian (American Dietetic Association, 1990).

The VLCD is only one part of a weight reduction program and in order to be most effective, should be combined with nutrition education, psychologic counseling, exercise, and behavior therapy.

The following criteria should be used in selecting candidates for a VLCD program:

1. At least 30% overweight with a minimum BMI of 32.
2. Free from contraindicated medical conditions: pregnancy or lactation, active cancer, hepatic disease, renal failure, active cardiac dysfunction, or severe psychologic disturbances.
3. Committed to establishing new eating and lifestyle behaviors that will assist the maintenance of weight loss.
4. Committed to taking the time to complete both the treatment and the maintenance components of a program.

The VLCD should be preceded by 2 to 4 weeks on a well-balanced 1,200-kcal diet that allows time for the body to adjust to the caloric deprivation and promotes a gradual diuresis.

The VLCD should be limited to 12 to 16 weeks to reduce the risk of adverse complications related to body protein losses, in particular cardiac problems. Dieters should be closely monitored.

The VLCD should be followed by a gradual refeeding period of 2 to 4 weeks during which time food, especially simple sugars, are reintroduced slowly to prevent a rapid fluid weight gain.

Dieters should continue a follow-up or maintenance program for at least 12 months, or until they can demonstrate voluntary restriction of eating particularly during times of stress, a normal eating pattern, and a sense of well-being.

Some dieters will require ongoing support even after the maintenance program has ended, and all dieters will need to continue with regular aerobic exercise for long-term weight reduction success.

compensate for energy expended in physical activity by increasing their food intake, obese persons do not, possibly because the exercise level is less strenuous (Pi-Sunyer, 1988).

Adherence to an exercise program is necessary for the benefits to be realized, but this is especially difficult for many obese individuals. Programs that involve supervision or regular participation within the structure of a social group appear to be the most successful in the long-term (Pavlou et al, 1989b). Socioeconomic circumstances can be an important factor. Many exercise programs are expensive, and it is not always possible or even safe to indulge in brisk walking, for example, in some neighborhoods. Whatever the exercise it needs to be readily available, pleasant, inexpensive, and easy to do.

Pharmaceutical Management

Appetite-suppressing drugs act on the central nervous system through catecholamine and serotonin neurotransmitters. Amphetamines and their derivatives, which have been in use for decades, are often useful during the initiation period but lose their effectiveness with time. They tend to be addictive and can cause cardiovascular side effects as well as insomnia, dysphoria, dizziness, tremor, dry mouth, and confusion. Newer drugs (e.g., fenfluramine and phenylpropanolamine) are not addictive and are equally effective. Thermogenic drugs, currently in the development stage, increase energy expenditure through excess heat production. Among these are ephedrine, beta-agonists, and thyroid hormone.

Surgical Procedures

Morbid obesity is often treated surgically. This treatment is preferably reserved for those who are at least 100% above ideal weight (BMI of 45). Various surgical procedures have been used to decrease the amount of food entering or absorbed from the gastrointestinal tract. These include esophageal banding, gastric restrictive surgery, and jejunoileal bypass. Gastric restrictive surgery is currently the surgery of choice.

Before considering any morbidly obese person for surgery, there should be demonstrated failure of a comprehensive program including calorie restriction, exercise, behavior modification, psychologic counseling, and family involvement. Failure is defined as an inability of the patient to reduce body weight by one third and body fat by one-half, and an inability to maintain any weight loss that has been achieved. Such patients have *intractable morbid obesity* and should be considered for surgery. Prior to surgery the patient should be evaluated extensively with respect to physiologic and medical complications, psychologic problems such as depression and poor self-esteem, and the extent of motivation.

Gastric Restriction (Gastric Bypass And Gastroplasty). *Gastric restriction,* which surgically reduces the reservoir capacity of the stomach by closing off a part of that organ, is successful in achieving weight reduction in people who are morbidly obese, and at present is the only well-accepted surgery for that purpose. Of the two common procedures, the gastric bypass appears to be slightly more effective in achieving weight loss. Although gastroplasty may be minimally safer in terms of operative morbidity and mortality, long-term results appear to be more consistent with the bypass (Bray and Gray, 1988b).

Gastroplasty reduces the size of the stomach by applying rows of stainless-steel staples across the top of the stomach in a manner that leaves only a small opening (0.8 to 1 cm) into the distal stomach. This opening may be banded by a piece of mesh to prevent it from enlarging during the years after surgery. The *gastric bypass* involves reducing the size of the stomach with the stapling procedure, but then connecting a small opening in the upper portion of the stomach to the small intestine by means of an intestinal loop (Fig. 18–6). Both have the effect of reducing the amount of food that can be taken at one time and produce early satiety. The new stomach capacity may be as small as 30 ml.

The most frequent complications of gastric partitioning are bloating of the pouch, nausea, and vomiting. A postsurgical food record noting the tolerance for specific foods in particular amounts will help in devising a program to avoid these episodes. There should also be a careful postoperative feeding regimen of pureed or liquid foods for 6 weeks followed by a 3-meal-a- day regimen consisting of high nutrient-density foods. Attention to protein intake and vitamin and mineral supplementation is advised (Suchow, 1988). Patients should be counseled to eat slowly, chew food well, and avoid swallowing chunks of meat or other food that

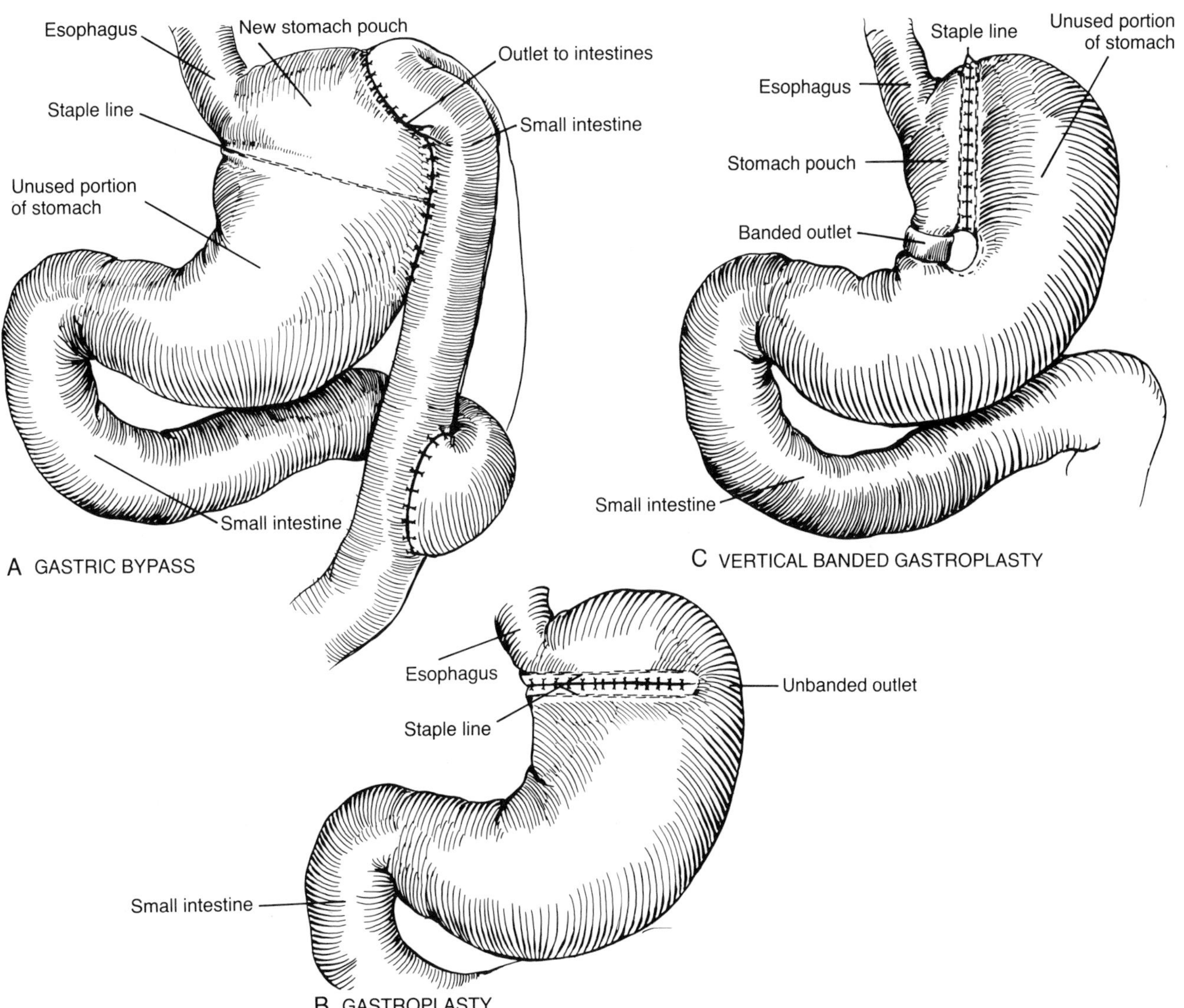

FIGURE 18–6. *Gastric surgeries for obesity.*

cannot be completely liquefied and that could block the pouch opening. Frequent small meals are important. Patients tend to choose liquids; however, weight loss can be deterred by drinking too much calorically dense liquid, such as milk shakes and soft drinks. Eventually, the pouch expands to accommodate 4 to 5 oz at a time.

Because use of the lower part of the stomach is omitted, the gastric bypass patient may also have dumping syndrome (see Chapter 27). The symptoms of tachycardia, sweating, and abdominal pain are so negative that they can further motivate the patient to make the right behavior changes and refrain from overeating.

Completion of the surgery does not end the obesity treatment; rather, it is the beginning of a 1- to 2-year period of eating and exercise behavior changes accompanied by support and by regular monitoring by an interdisciplinary team of health care professionals. Monitoring should include an assessment of body fat loss, potential anemia, and deficiencies of potassium, magnesium, folate, and vitamin B_{12}, especially in gastric bypass patients.

The results of gastric surgery are favorable and are attended by fewer complications than with the intestinal bypass surgery practiced during the 1970s. Overall the reduction of excess weight after gastric restriction surgery is about 55% (Benotti et al, 1989; Brolin, 1987; Mason et al, 1987). A realistic goal of surgery is 160% of IBW (Blackburn, 1988).

A review of more than 5,000 patients from 12 centers showed a mortality rate after gastric restriction surgery one fourth that of morbidly obese patients and equivalent to normal- weight patients of the same age (Forse, 1989). In addition, most patients report positive psychological results—improved self-esteem, and feeling more attractive and less depressed.

JAW WIRING (MAXILLOMANDIBULAR FIXATION). Wiring the jaws closed restricts eating to liquids that can be taken through a straw. Dental attention before wiring as well as oral hygiene and nutritional care while the jaws are wired are important. Counseling should include recommendations for combinations of liquids and supplements that will provide adequate nutrients. The patient should also be taught how to cut the wires if necessary and how to deal with any episode of vomiting.

This technique has been effective in producing weight reduction; however, without education and ongoing support, body weight generally returns to pretreatment levels after the wires are removed. New behaviors need to be internalized, and a sense of control must be established if weight reduction is to be maintained.

LIPOSUCTION. *Liposuction* involves aspiration of fat deposits by means of a 1- to 2-cm incision through which a tube is fanned out into the adipose tissue. The most successful operations are performed on younger persons with only small amounts of fat to be removed, where the elastic properties of the skin are able to allow tightening over the aspirated areas. It is not a weight-reduction technique but rather a cosmetic surgery, because only 5 lb of fat can be removed at a time.

Psychotherapy

Psychotherapy has been used in both individual and group situations for the treatment of obesity. The effectiveness of this therapy is not well validated, primarily because of a lack of appropriate control studies. *Cognitive restructuring*—learning how to visualize oneself at an appropriate weight and in control of eating—and increased self-esteem are goals of therapy that can lead to body weight control.

Learning techniques to change attitudes toward eating, dieting and body fat are also useful (Table 18–5). An important outcome is a change in attitude toward one's obesity and size in the event that attempts at weight reduction are unsuccessful.

Weight Management in Children

The treatment goal for the child who is overweight but has not yet reached his or her potential adult weight should be weight maintenance or a slowing of weight gain. This gives the child time to "grow into" his or her weight. If the weight appropriate for the child's anticipated adult height has already been reached, then maintenance at that weight should be the lifetime goal (Clinical Insight, p. 333). The child who already exceeds his or her optimal adult weight can safely experience a slow weight loss of 10 to 12 lb/yr until the optimal adult weight is reached.

Obviously, the child who needs to reduce weight is going to require more attention from family and health professionals, and effort on his or her part, than the child able to still gain weight, even if at a slower rate.

TABLE 18–5. Techniques for Improving Attitude in a Weight Control Program*

Weigh advantages and disadvantages of dieting	Beware of attitude traps
Realize complex causes of obesity	Stop dichotomous thinking
Distinguish hunger from cravings	Counter impossible dream thinking
Confront or ignore cravings	Focus on behavior rather than weight
Set realistic goals	Banish imperatives from vocabulary
Use the shaping concept for habit change	Be aware of high-risk situations
Counter food and weight fantasies	Distinguish lapse and relapse
Ban perfectionist attitudes	Outlast urges to eat
	Cope positively with slips and lapses

* Adapted from Brownell KD and Steen EN: Modern methods of weight control: The physiology and psychology of dieting. Phys Sports Med 15:122, 1987.

This attention should be directed to all the areas mentioned previously with strong behavior modification and exercise components. The program should be long-term over the entire growth period and perhaps longer (Mahan, 1987).

Maintenance of Reduced Weight

Prognosis for maintaining the status of the reduced-obese is very poor. Of those who do reduce weight, only 5% manage to keep from gaining weight by the end of 5 years. This population may not be representative of those who reduce weight, because the successful weight reducers do not present themselves to a medical program and are not available for follow-up and inclusion in the statistics. The typical picture, however, is one of recidivism. Continued dieting, with repeated ups and downs, leads gradually to a net increase in body fat and thus to a health risk for hyperlipidemia, hypertension, and diabetes.

Energy requirements for weight maintenance after weight reduction appear to be 25% lower than at the baseline weight. The net effect is that the reduced obese are faced with the necessity of maintaining a reduced energy intake even after the desired weight has been lost. Whether this reduced intake must be maintained for an indefinite period is not known.

It appears that *behavior modification* is a key to weight maintenance (Stunkard, 1987). This may be related to the fact that because obesity is a chronic disease, its management requires continuous treatment (modification of unacceptable behaviors) as with other chronic diseases (e.g., insulin for diabetes or medication for hypertension).

Regular planned *exercise* may be even more important in maintaining the reduced obese state over the long term (Bray and Gray, 1988b; Brownell et al, 1986; Dahlkoetter et al, 1979). In contrast to the conflicting evidence of exercise effectiveness in weight reduction, the data strongly support the addition of exercise in improved long-term maintenance of lowered body weight. A 3-year follow-up study of males who were previously 22% overweight showed that in order to be effective, exercise must be carried out at least three times per week with a 1,500-kcal/wk expenditure (Pavlou, 1989b). Maintenance of reduced body weight of those in the study who continued to exercise was almost 100%.

Support groups are invaluable for the obese who are trying to lose weight and for the reduced-obese who are maintaining a new lower weight. They help individuals facing similar problems to learn ways of staying with their programs. Two large networks of self-help support groups are Overeaters Anonymous and Take Off Pounds Sensibly (TOPS). These groups are very inexpensive, continuous, include a "buddy system," and encourage participation on a regular basis or as often as needed. The Weight Watchers program offers free lifelong maintenance classes for those who have reached and are maintaining their goal weights.

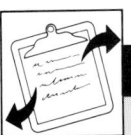

CLINICAL INSIGHT: Determining Appropriate Rate of Weight Gain in the Obese Child

From the history of family growth patterns and review of the prior growth pattern of the obese child, determine the predicted adult height of the child. He or she will probably maintain his or her present height growth channel. For example, an 8-year-old girl on the 75th percentile for height will probably maintain that growth channel and will achieve 67 in. as an adult height.

Determine a rough estimation of the appropriate weight for the anticipated adult height. Using the Hamwi equation, for women, the rule is 100 lb for the first 5 ft of height and an additional 5 lb for each inch in height over 5 ft. For men, it is 106 lb for the first 5 ft and an additional 6 lb for each inch over 5 ft. An appropriate range is ±10% on either side of this weight.

Subtract the child's present weight from the calculated appropriate adult weight. The remainder is the number of pounds that the child should gain throughout the rest of his or her growth period. This amount, divided by the number of years remaining of linear growth, is the appropriate yearly rate of weight gain for the child to achieve a normal adult weight. The number of years of growth remaining is determined based on the parental report of their own growth patterns. In the case of the 8-year-old girl, if her mother reports reaching adult height at age 15, then probably her daughter will do the same. Thus, the daughter has 7 years of growth remaining.

Example: an 8 year old who presently weighs 90 lb (over 95th percentile) and is 52 in. tall (75th to 90th percentile).
Eventual adult height = 67 in.
Appropriate weight for adult height = 100 lb + 35 lb = 135 lb (+ or − 10 lb)
Number of years of growth remaining = 15 years (age when the mother reached adult height) − 8 years (present age) = 7 years
(125 lb to 145 lb) − 90 lb (present weight) = 35 lb to 55 lb to be gained over next 7 years
Approximate rate of weight gain = 5 lb to 8 lb per year for the next 7 years

WEIGHT IMBALANCE: EXCESSIVE LEANNESS

Almost eclipsed by the attention focused on obesity is the effort of some people to gain weight. The term *underweight* is applicable to those who are 15 to 20% or more below accepted weight standards. Because underweight is often a symptom of a disease, it should be assessed medically. A BMI under 20 is associated with greater mortality risk that increases as the BMI falls (Bray and Gray, 1988b).

Undernutrition itself may lead to underfunction of the pituitary, thyroid, gonads, and adrenals. Young women with anorexia nervosa, for example, can stop menstruating when they have lost a significant amount of weight. Other risk factors include loss of energy and susceptibility to injury and infection, as well as distorted body image and other psychologic problems.

Etiology

Underweight may be caused by: (1) an intake insufficient in quantity to meet activity needs; (2) excessive activity, such as in the case of compulsive athletes in training; (3) poor absorption and utilization of the food consumed; (4) a wasting disease, such as cancer or hyperthyroidism that increases the metabolic rate and energy needs; and (5) psychologic or emotional stress.

Assessment

Assessment of the cause and extent of underweight before starting a treatment program is important. A thorough history and pertinent medical tests usually determine whether underlying disorders are a cause of the underweight. From anthropometric data such as arm muscle and fat areas, it is possible to determine whether health-endangering underweight really exists. Biochemical measurements will indicate whether malnutrition accompanies the underweight.

Assessment of body fatness is useful, especially in dealing with the patient who has an eating disorder and who needs to begin the body acceptance process (see Chapter 17).

Management

Any underlying cause of underweight must be dealt with as a first priority. A wasting disease or malabsorption requires treatment. Activity should be modified, and psychologic counseling should be started if necessary. Nutritional support and dietary change are effective along with or after treatment of the underlying disorder, or when the cause of the underweight is merely inappropriate or inadequate food intake.

HIGH-ENERGY DIETS FOR WEIGHT GAIN. A careful dietary history prior to planning a dietary program will reveal inadequacies in dietary habits and nutritional intakes. Meals at scheduled hours instead of hastily planned, bolted meals are advised. Because nervous tension often contributes to underweight in some individuals, mealtimes should be relaxed.

TABLE 18–6. Suggestions for Increasing Energy Intake

Additional Foods	kcal	Protein (g)
Plus 500 kcal (Served Between Meals)		
1. 1 cup dry cereal	110	2
1 banana	80	
1 cup whole milk	159	8
1 slice toast	60	2
1 T peanut butter	86	4
	495	16
2. 8 saltine crackers	99	3
1 oz cheese	113	7
1 cup ice cream	290	6
	502	16
3. 6 graham cracker squares	165	3
2 T peanut butter	172	8
1 cup orange juice	122	
2 T raisins	52	
	511	11
Plus 1000 kcal (Served Between Meals)		
1. 8 oz fruit flavored yogurt	240	9
1 slice bread	60	2
2 oz cheese	226	14
1 apple	87	
¼ of 14″ cheese pizza	306	16
1 small banana	81	1
	1,000	42
2. Instant Breakfast with whole milk	280	15
1 cup cottage cheese	239	31
½ cup pineapple	95	
1 cup apple juice	117	
6 graham cracker squares	165	3
1 pear	100	1
	996	50
Plus 1,500 kcal (Served Between Meals)		
1. 2 slices bread	120	4
2 T peanut butter	172	8
1 T jam	110	
4 graham cracker squares	110	2
8 oz fruit flavored yogurt	240	9
¾ cup roasted peanuts	628	28
1 cup apricot nectar	143	1
	1,523	52
2. 1 baked custard	285	13
Instant Breakfast with whole milk	280	15
1 cup dry cereal	110	2
1 banana	80	
1 cup whole milk	159	8
1 cup orange juice	122	
4 T raisins	104	
1 bagel	165	6
2 T cream cheese	99	2
2 T jam	110	
	1,514	46

In addition to the kilocalories needed to meet total energy requirements, an allowance of 500 to 1,000 additional kilocalories per day should be planned. Daily energy requirements can be calculated on the basis of the individual's present weight. If 2,400 kcal are normally needed to maintain present weight, 3,000 to 3,400 kcal would be required to achieve weight gain. The intake should be increased gradually to these levels to avoid gastric discomfort and periods of discouragement.

The energy distribution of the diet should be at least 35% of the kilocalories from fat with at least 12 to 15% of the kilocalories from protein. A vitamin and mineral supplement may be necessary depending on nutritional status revealed by the initial assessment.

The underweight person frequently must be encouraged to eat, even when not hungry. The secret is to individualize the program with readily available foods that the individual really enjoys and with a plan for regular eating times throughout the day. In addition to larger meals, snacks are usually necessary to adequately increase the energy intake. Often a liquid supplement taken with meals or between meals is effective because it is easy to prepare and consume. This is important when it is necessary to overcome a lack of interest in food and eating. A 500-kcal step-up program is outlined in Table 18–6 (Fig. 18–7).

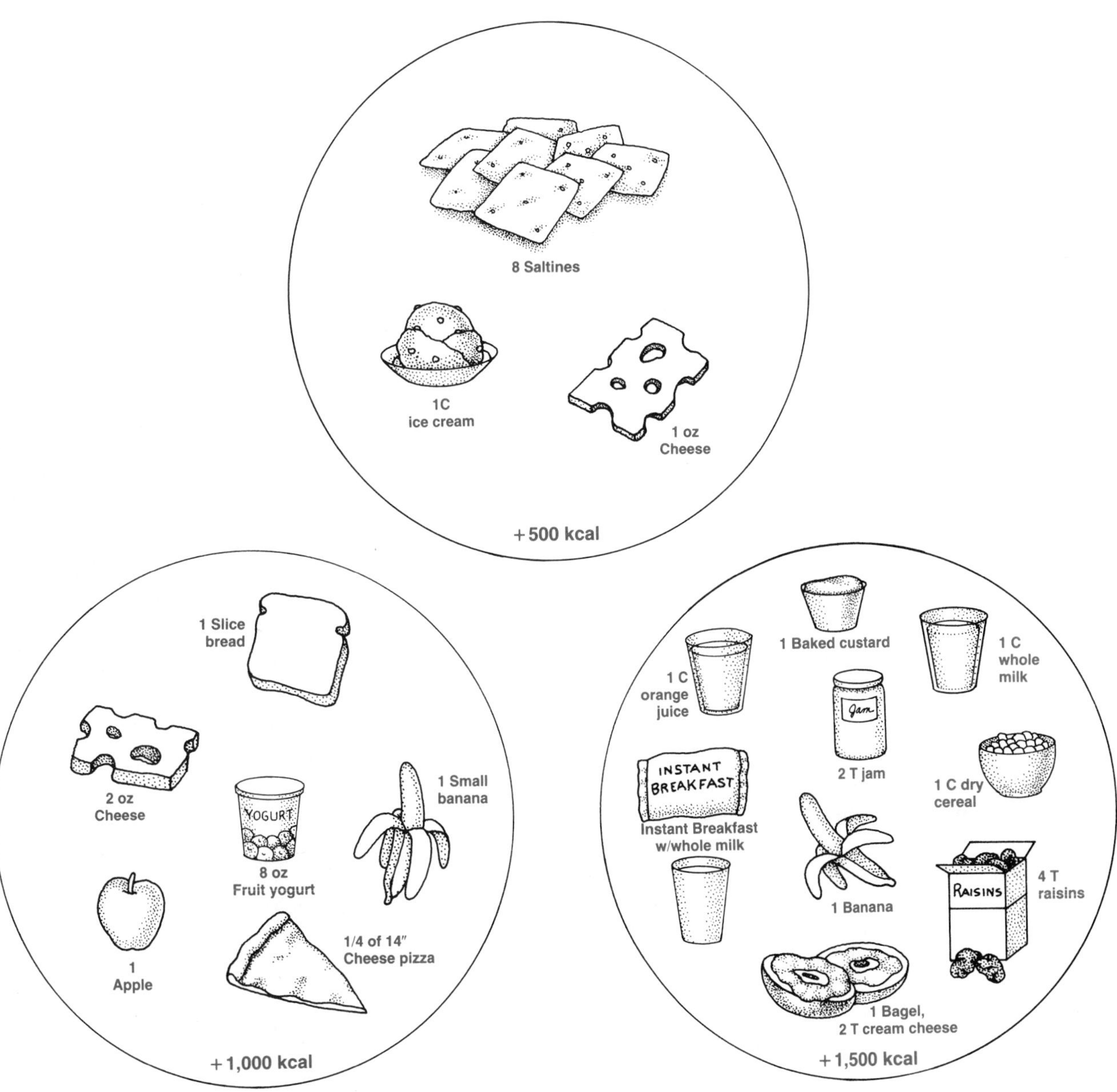

FIGURE 18–7. *Each circle illustrates the total amount of food that must be added to the diet to increase the intake by either 500 kcal, 1,000 kcal, or 1,500 kcal.*

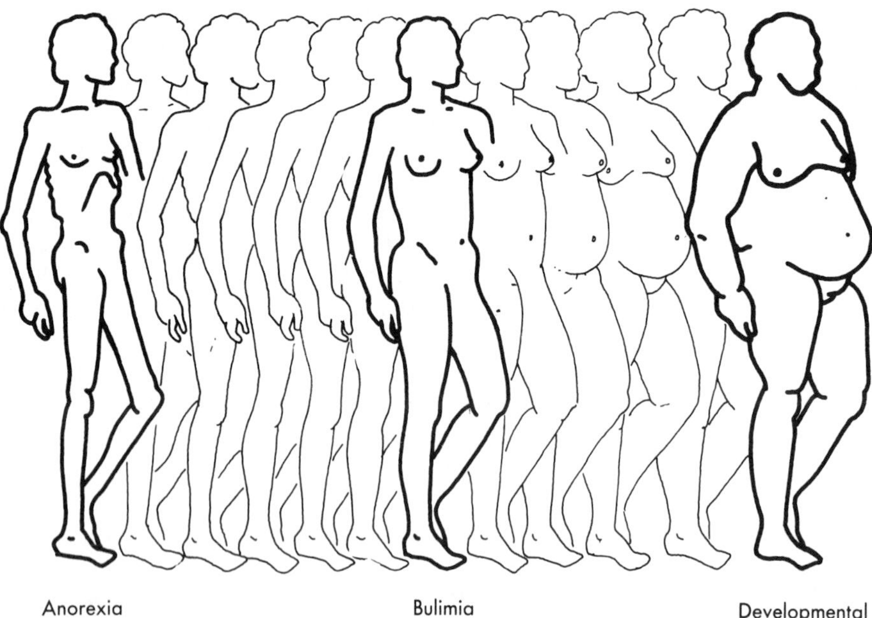

FIGURE 18–8. *Spectrum of eating disorders. Although physical conditions vary, underlying psychologic characteristics are held in common across the spectrum. (From Mahan LK and Rees JM: Nutrition in Adolescence. St. Louis, CV Mosby, 1984, p 105.)*

MANAGEMENT OF EATING DISORDERS

Jane Mitchell Rees, M.S., R.D.

Anorexia nervosa and bulimia nervosa are eating disorders whose incidence has become increasingly common in recent years. Although these abnormalities are seen chiefly in women, particularly among adolescent females, they are becoming more common in males and in females at other ages.

Occurrence

Anorexia nervosa and bulimia nervosa are seen typically in members of middle socioeconomic level families in affluent societies. Most of these families appear to be stable and happy, but a characteristic pattern of unresolved conflicts generally lies beneath the surface. The occurrence of the syndrome is reinforced in a culture in which slimness is highly valued at the same time that food is used for recreation as well as for survival and health. The developmental problems of the affected young women make them extremely vulnerable to these mixed messages.

Whereas gorging and vomiting have been seen as part of the syndrome of *anorexia nervosa,* these symptoms in combination and in the absence of starvation have recently been recognized as making up a separate syndrome known as *bulimia nervosa.* Five per cent of college women are estimated to have this disorder, while as many as 20% exhibit some bulimic symptoms. This condition seems to affect women who are slightly older and often from lower socioeconomic groups than those most often affected by anorexia nervosa (Halmi et al, 1981). About 50% of anorectic individuals develop bulimia. In fact, eating disorders seem to exist on a continuum with anorectics on one end achieving drastically low weights with energy restriction, and on the other end are obese individuals who have an eating disorder related to excessive energy intake. (Some obese do not overeat and therefore cannot be classified as having an eating disorder. They are obese for other physiologic reasons.) In the middle range are the bulimic anorectics who maintain a lower than normal body weight and the normal weight bulimics (Fig. 18–8).

Men or boys who typically develop eating disorders are those whose careers require thinness (e.g., actors, dancers, or models) or who are involved in athletic endeavors demanding continuous weight control (e.g., jockeys, runners, or wrestlers).

TABLE 18–7. Physical Signs of Anorexia Nervosa*

Physical Signs
Fat store depletion
Muscle wasting
Amenorrhea
Cheilosis
Desquamation
Dry skin
Hirsutism
Thin, dry, brittle hair
Alopecia
Degradation of fingernails
Acrocyanosis
Postural hypotension
Dehydration
Edema
Bradycardia
Bradypnea
Hypothermia
Constipation
Sleep disturbance

* From Rees JM: Eating disorders. *In* Mahan LK and Rees JM: Nutrition in Adolescence. St Louis, CV Mosby, 1984.

Characteristics

Anorectic patients initially develop bizarre food habits and refuse to eat. These people eventually lose from 25 to 35% of body weight. They usually exercise vigorously and may abuse laxatives or diuretics and voluntarily vomit (Table 18–7). Without intervention, the disorder may progress to starvation, at which time the symptoms listed in Table 18–7 will be evident (Fig. 18–9). The importance of the ability of health care professionals to recognize the symptoms of anorexia nervosa at an early stage cannot be overemphasized.

Anorectics have an abnormal fear of being fat, which is exhibited in distortions of body image and other perceptions, probably reflecting a combination of altered physical state, distorted perception, and denial of perceptions leading to self-gratification. Because they experience arrested development, they do not develop a normal sense of "self" or complex advanced patterns of thinking.

Bulimics try to restrict food intake in a way that leads to physical and psychologic urges to stuff themselves. The food is then purged by forced vomiting or laxatives. Because of their distorted concept of food, the amount of food considered a "binge" by some bulimics would be only a normal amount of food to the unrestricted eater.

Non–life-threatening physical complications include damage to the teeth, irritation of the throat, esophageal inflammation, cracked and damaged lips, broken blood vessels in the face, and calluses on the hands where they are placed on the teeth to support the

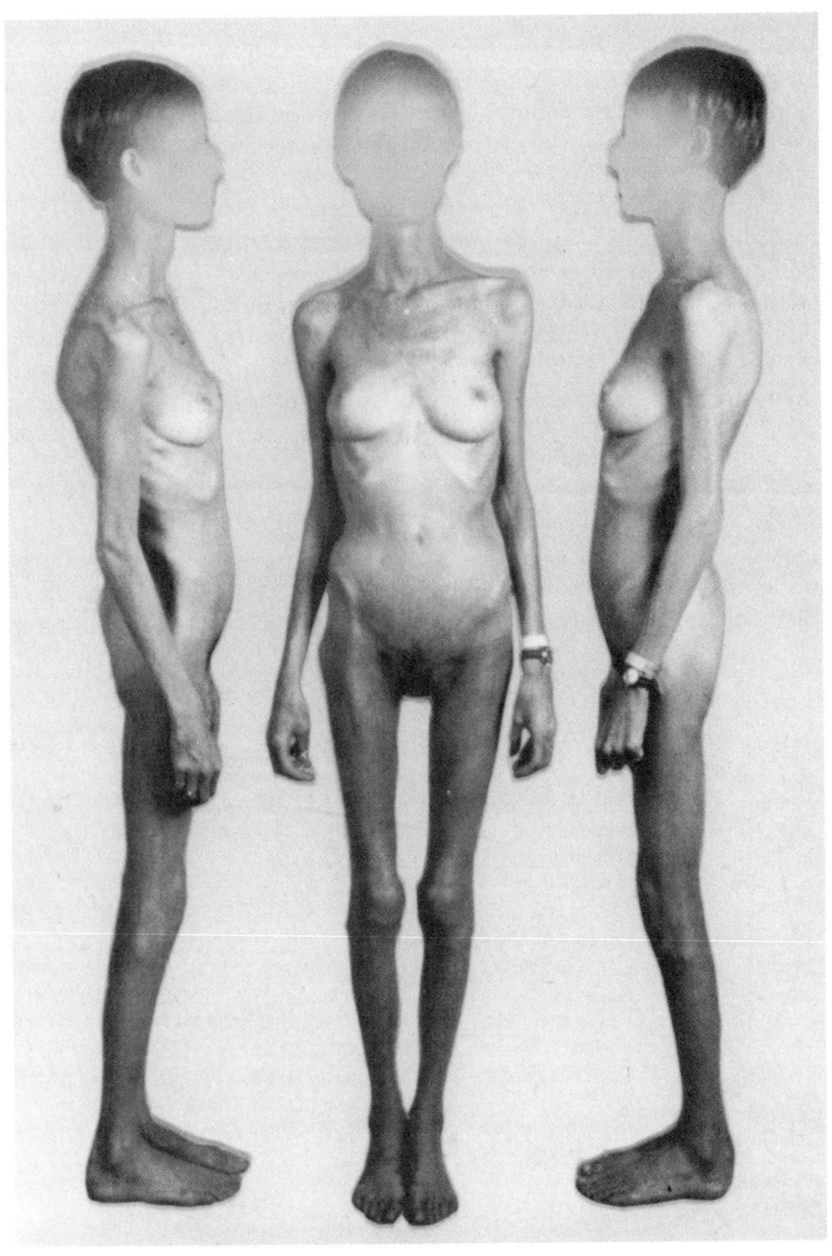

FIGURE 18–9. *Severe emaciation with characteristic findings of anorexia nervosa. (From Comerci GD: Anorexia nervosa and bulimia. Med Clin North Am 74(5):1300, 1990.)*

head while the person is vomiting. Whether the common occurrence of swollen salivary glands is the result of acidic reflux or constant stimulation is not known. Overuse of laxatives may lead to rectal bleeding. More rare and acute symptoms include dehydration and electrolyte imbalance, upper gastrointestinal fistulas, kidney damage, and reversible myopathies caused by the ingestion of emetics. Calcium deficiency as a result of long-term laxative abuse can be a specific nutritional consequence.

Although bulimics are usually close to normal weight, they are afraid of gaining weight and their feelings of self-worth are tied to feelings about their bodies. Like the anorectics, they have psychosocial problems. They are usually unable to tolerate frustration and attempt to dull various feeling states by the bingeing and purging behavior. As opposed to the anorectics, bulimics tend to have poor impulse control, misuse substances, and shoplift. One of the chief psychologic characteristics is guilt over the cycle of bingeing and vomiting that is carried out in secret, even while their lives may seem ideal to those around them. The same issues of being unable to resolve problems in their lives also exist for bulimics. Whereas the anorectic has turned away from food, the bulimic has turned to it. Some patients have been previously anorectic or obese. Bulimic individuals eat compulsively to escape painful problems and then, fearing weight gain and ashamed of their out of control behavior, they attempt to remove the food from their bodies before it can be absorbed.

Etiology

Although anorexia nervosa was first described in 1874, it is still not known if it is primarily a psychologic disorder, a physical disorder of hypothalamic or pituitary function, or a combination of both. The earliest theories proposed that disturbed sexuality was the cause. Presently, it is seen as arising from disturbed patterns of family interactions. In early life the patient has generally functioned as a cooperative participant in the "anorexigenic" family until an event or phase of life precipitated the physical manifestation of symptoms. The usual progression of this disease is shown in Figure 18–10.

Typical changes in body functions such as thermoregulation, menstruation, basal metabolic rate, and activity, have led to the speculation that the disorder may be caused by an organic cause. On the other hand, the hypothalamic dysfunction and other endocrine abnormalities may be secondary to the starvation, malnutrition, or psychiatric illness. Like anorexia nervosa, starvation is also characterized by amenorrhea, slowed heart rate, dry skin, disturbance in hair growth, and disinterest in sex (Keys, 1950). However, amenorrhea seen in these patients initially is usually a consequence of psychologic stress. There may yet be other physical factors that are not caused by malnutrition (Wakeling, 1985).

There is some suggestion that bulimics may be physiologically or genetically predisposed to this disorder because many come from families characterized by alcoholism and depression, two other psychologic conditions with physiologic components. Furthermore, some bulimics respond quickly to antidepressant medication, possibly because these drugs affect a neurotransmitter imbalance in the brain.

Lastly, the influence of the media and the image of the very thin woman as the ideal has to be considered in the etiology of eating disorders. For most women, achievement of this ideal means dieting and being hungry in order to achieve a body weight that is not compatible with their basic biology. This constant restraint can lead to bingeing and an eating disorder.

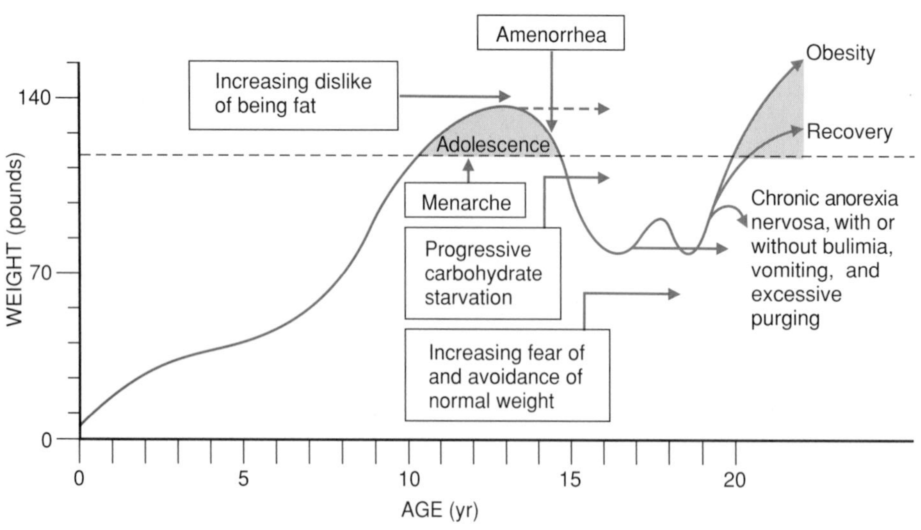

FIGURE 18–10. *Typical development of an eating disorder. (Redrawn from Crisp AH: Anorexia nervosa.* In *Silverstone T and Barraclough B [eds]: Contemporary psychiatry. Br J Psychiatry [Special Publication No. 9] 1975.)*

Management

Both anorectics and their families are very resistant to treatment, and great skill is usually needed to convince them of the need for professional help. Treatment incorporates psychotherapeutic, nutritional, and medical components.

Psychotherapy

Both family and individual psychotherapy should be initiated as soon as the disease becomes apparent. With early diagnosis, therapy can shift the focus from food to underlying interactional and developmental problems before a severe physical state develops. If the disorder has reached an advanced stage, the patient may need to be hospitalized. In the crisis of starvation, the situation will be compounded by mental dullness, apathy, and constant preoccupation with food. Although psychotherapy is not usually effective until the patient is renourished, psychologic factors are considered in the design of in-hospital treatment plans. Hospitalization may also provide needed separation of the anorectic patient and the family. Following hospitalization, long-term psychotherapy must address the developmental and psychologic problems (Bruch, 1973; Crisp, 1980; Minuchin et al, 1978).

Nutritional Care

Nutritional care consists of helping the anorectic change his or her ideas about food. This can be done only at a pace acceptable to the patient, which depends in great part on the success of psychotherapy.

If the physical state deteriorates, the need for hospitalization will be indicated by fainting spells, insufficient strength to carry out normal activities, slowed speech, and muscle wasting (see Chapter 17 for assessment of extent of muscle depletion).

The hospital atmosphere should be protective and nonpunitive. The method by which the patient is encouraged to eat varies depending on the overall protocol, but it is generally possible to succeed in oral feeding. Highly nourishing liquids may be given if the patient will not eat solid food. Parenteral, enteral, or nasogastric feeding routes are reserved for life-threatening states, and are usually unnecessary. Signs of a life-threatening state include imbalance of fluid and electrolytes, severe cardiac abnormalities in the absence of electrolyte imbalances, diarrhea, absence of ketone bodies in the urine, and concurrent infection.

The diet should be made up of foods acceptable to the patient and should be moderate in protein, carbohydrate, and fat. The goal will be to increase the dietary intake gradually while energy output is decreased, so that a positive balance is achieved. For this reason, "privileges" such as being out of bed may be combined with weight gain as contingencies in a behavior modification program. A genuine change in attitude is as important as a gain to normal weight for height as a basis for discharge from the hospital.

Following hospitalization, an anorectic will need long-term nutritional counseling regarding stabilizing weight (which tends to fluctuate widely), maintaining the menses in women, and normalizing ideas and habits related to food. The patient with bulimia nervosa may need less energy to maintain normal body weight than a person of similar size and age who was not previously bulimic (Gwirtsman, 1989).

Treatment of bulimia is similar to that for recovering anorectics, with facilitation of normal development a primary goal. Because they are often older and separated from their families, bulimics are more commonly involved in individual counseling, although the family should be included if they are living together. Bulimics are often able to make gains within group therapy.

A smaller number of bulimics than anorectics are seen in poor physical condition. Those who have cardiac or kidney irregularities, or severe fluid and electrolyte imbalances will require hospitalization.

During long-term recovery, the underlying philosophy of the bulimic about weight and food needs to be assessed and the distorted beliefs need to be replaced. Psychologic gains are accompanied by the ability to accept body configuration (including reasonable weight for height and body structure), to give up vomiting or purging, and to adopt a more physiologically normal dietary ideal (Story, 1986). An important breakthrough comes with the ability to separate the goal of ceasing to vomit from that of losing weight, a change that cannot be imposed on the patient but must come from within the patient, facilitated by skillful counseling. Disclosure appears to be an important issue for these patients, occurring when disgust with the habit and a desire to eat normally outweighs their fear of fatness.

Prognosis

Early and more knowledgeable treatment of anorexia nervosa has led to a decline in mortality from around 10 to 2% (Hsu, 1980). However, 20 to 30% will have lifelong problems with irrational dieting and food fears. Present emphasis on the broad range of treatment issues should contribute to a similar improvement in the other outcomes of the disorder. Outcome criteria encompass weight and dietary habits (including food intake, weight and shape ideation, and weight for height proportion), menstruation, and adjustment of sexual, psychologic, and social characteristics. These must be assessed for several years after a crisis in order to identify true outcome.

CITED REFERENCES

American Dietetic Association: Position of the American Dietetic Association: Very-low-calorie weight loss diets. J Am Diet Assoc 90:722, 1990.

Bennett W: Dietary treatments of obesity. Ann NY Acad Sci 499:250, 1987.

Benotti PN et al: Gastric restrictive operations for morbid obesity. Am J Surg 157:150, 1989.

Bjorntorp P: Exercise in the treatment of obesity. Clin Endocrinol Metab 5:431, 1976.

Bjorntorp P: Fat cell distribution and metabolism. *In* Wurtman RJ and Wurtman JJ (eds): Human obesity. Ann NY Acad Med 499:73, 1987.

Bjorntorp P: Physiological and clinical aspects of exercise in obese persons. Exerc Sport Sci Rev 11:159, 1983.

Blackburn GL: Guest editorial. Top Clin Nutr 2(2):viii, 1987.

Blackburn GL: Presentation. San Francisco, Am Dietetic Association Annual Meeting, 1988.

Blackburn GL et al: Weight cycling: The experience of human dieters. Am J Clin Nutr 49:1105, 1989.

Bouchard C et al: Inheritance of the amount and distribution of human body fat. Int J Obes 12(3):205, 1988.

Bray GA: Obesity. *In* Brown ML (ed): Present Knowledge in Nutrition, 6th ed. Washington, DC, International Life Sciences Institute, Nutrition Foundation, 1990.

Bray GA: Obesity: A disease of nutrient or energy balance? Nutr Rev 45:33, 1987.

Bray GA and Gray DS: Obesity. I: Pathogenesis. West J Med 149:429, 1988a.

Bray GA and Gray DS: Obesity. II: Treatment. West J Med 149:555, 1988b.

Brolin RE: Results of obesity surgery. Gastroenterol Clin North Am 16:317, 1987.

Brownell KD and Steen SN: Modern methods for weight control: The physiology and psychology of dieting. Phys Sports Med 15:122, 1987.

Brownell KD: Presentation. San Francisco, American Dietetic Association Annual Meeting, 1988.

Brownell KD et al: Understanding and preventing relapse. Am Psychol 41:765, 1986.

Bruch H: Eating Disorders. New York, Basic Books, 1973.

Buckmaster L and Brownell KD: Behavior modification: The state of the art. *In* Frankle RT and Yang M-U (eds): Obesity and Weight Control. Rockville, MD, Aspen Publishers, 1988.

Council on Scientific Affairs. American Medical Association: Treatment of obesity in adults. JAMA 260:2547, 1988.

Crisp AH: Anorexia Nervosa: Let Me Be. New York, Grune & Stratton, 1980.

Dahlkoetter JA et al: Obesity and the unbalanced energy equation: Exercise versus eating habit change. J Consult Clin Psychol 47:898, 1979.

Danforth E: Diet and obesity. Am J Clin Nutr 41:1132, 1985.

Elliot DL et al: Obesity: Pathophysiology and practical management. J Gen Intern Med 2:188, 1987.

Fatis M et al: Following up on a commercial weight loss program: Do the pounds stay off after your picture has been in the newspaper? J Am Diet Assoc 89:547, 1989.

Feldman W et al: Culture vs. biology: Children's attitudes toward thinness and fatness. Pediatrics 81:190, 1988.

Fisler JS and Drenick EJ: Starvation and semistarvation diets in the management of obesity. Annu Rev Nutr 7:465, 1987.

Foman SJ et al: Body composition of reference children from birth to age 10 years. Am J Clin Nutr 35:1169, 1982.

Forbes GB: Lean body mass-body fat interrelationships in humans. Nutr Rev 45:225, 1987.

Foreyt JP: Behavior therapy in the management of obesity. Nutr MD 15(11):1, 1989.

Forse A, Benotti PN, and Blackburn GL: Morbid obesity: Weighing the treatment options—surgical options. Nutr Today 24(5):10, 1989.

Freedman DS et al: Relation of body fat patterning to lipid and lipoprotein concentrations in children and adolescents: The Bogalusa Heart Study. Am J Clin Nutr 50:930, 1989.

Greenwood MRC and Pittman-Waller V: Weight control: A complex, various and controversial problem. *In* Frankle RT and Yang M (eds): Obesity and Weight Control. Rockville, MD, Aspen Publications, 1988.

Gwinup G: Effect of exercise alone on the weight of obese women. Arch Intern Med 135:676, 1975.

Gwirtsman H: Decreased caloric intake in normal weight patients with bulimia: Comparison with female volunteers. Am J Clin Nutr 49:86, 1989.

Halmi KA et al: Binge-eating and vomiting: A survey of a college population. Psychol Med 11:697, 1981.

Hill JO et al: Effects of exercise and food restriction on body composition and metabolic rate in obese women. Am J Clin Nutr 46:622, 1987.

Hsu LKG: Outcome of anorexia nervosa. Arch Gen Psychiatr 37:1041, 1980.

Isner JM et al: Sudden, unexpected death in avid dieters using the liquid-protein-modified-fast diet. Circulation 60:1401, 1979.

Katzeff HL et al: Metabolic studies in human obesity during overnutrition and undernutrition: Thermogenic and hormonal responses to norepinephrine. Metabolism 35:166, 1986.

Keys A: The Biology of Human Starvation. Minneapolis, University of Minnesota Press, 1950.

Kramer FM et al: Long-term followup of behavioral treatment for obesity: Patterns of weight regain among men and women. Int J Obes 13:123, 1989.

Lew EA and Garfinkle L: Variations in mortality by weight among 750,000 men and women. J Chronic Dis 32:563, 1979.

Mahan LK: Family-focused behavioral approach to weight control in children. Pediatr Clin North Am 34:983, 1987.

Mason EE et al: Super obesity and gastric reduction procedures. Gastroenterol Clin North Am 16:495, 1987.

Minuchin S et al: Psychosomatic Families: Anorexia Nervosa in Context. Cambridge, MA, Harvard University Press, 1978.

National Institutes of Health Consensus Development Panel: Health implications of obesity. Ann Intern Med 103:1073, 1985.

Pavlou KN et al: Physical activity as a supplement to a weight-loss dietary regimen. Am J Clin Nutr 49:1110, 1989a.

Pavlou KN, Krey S, and Steffee WP: Exercise as an adjunct to weight loss and maintenance in moderately obese subjects. Am J Clin Nutr 49:1115, 1989b.

Pi-Sunyer FX: Exercise in treatment of obesity. *In* Frankle RT and Yang M-U (eds): Obesity and Weight Control. Rockville, MD, Aspen Publishers, 1988.

Prevalence of overweight: Behavioral Risk Factor Surveillance System. JAMA 262:471, 1989.

Rebuffe-Scrive M et al: Fat cell metabolism in different regions in women. J Clin Invest 75:1973, 1985.

Rodin J et al: Weight cycling and fat distribution. Int J Obes 14:303, 1990.

Rolland-Cachera M-F and Bellisle F: Letter to the editor. Lancet 335:918, 1990.

Rolland-Cachera M-F et al: Adiposity rebound in children: A simple indicator for predicting obesity. Am J Clin Nutr 39:129, 1984.

Saris WHM: Physiological aspects of exercise in weight cycling. Am J Clin Nutr 49:1099, 1989.

Schachter S: Obesity and eating. Science 161:751, 1968.

Sims EAH et al: Experimental obesity in man. Trans Assoc Am Phys 81:153, 1968.

Story M: Nutrition management and dietary treatment of bulimia. J Am Diet Assoc 86:517, 1986.

Stricker EM: Biological basis of hunger and satiety: Therapeutic implications. Nutr Rev 42:333, 1984.

Stunkard AJ: Conservative treatments for obesity. Am J Clin Nutr 45:1142, 1987.

Stunkard AJ and Kaplan D: Eating in public places: A review of reports of the direct observation of eating behavior. Int J Obes 1:89, 1977.

Stunkard AJ, Foch TT, and Hrubec Z: A twin study of human obesity. JAMA 256:51, 1986a.

Stunkard AJ et al: An adoption study of human obesity. N Engl J Med 314:193, 1986b.

Stunkard AJ et al: The body-mass index of twins who have been reared apart. N Engl J Med 322:1483, 1990.

Suchow EL: Vertical banded gastroplasty as a treatment for morbid obesity: Nutritional considerations. Nutr Suppl Serv 8(6):23, 1988.

Van Dale D et al: Does exercise give an additional effect in weight reduction regimens? Int J Obesity 11:367, 1987.

Van Itallie TB and Yang M: Cardiac dysfunction in obese dieters: A potentially lethal complication of rapid, massive weight loss. Am J Clin Nutr 39:695, 1984.

Vasselli JR and Maggio CA: Mechanisms of appetite and body-weight regulation. *In* Frankle RT and Yang M (eds): Obesity and Weight Control. Rockville, MD, Aspen Publications, 1988.

Wadden TA and Stunkard AJ: Controlled trial of very low calorie diet, behavior therapy, and their combination in the treatment of obesity. J Consult Clin Psychol 54:482, 1986.

Wakeling A: Neurobiological aspects of feeding disorders. J Psychiatr Res 19:191, 1985.

ADDITIONAL REFERENCES

Andersen AE: Anorexia nervosa: Who are you? Where are you? (Editorial) Mayo Clin Proc 63:511, 1988.

Behnke AR and Wilmore JH: Evaluation and Regulation of Body Build and Composition. Englewood Cliffs, NJ, Prentice-Hall, 1974.

Bouchard C et al: The response to long-term overfeeding in identical twins. N Engl J Med 322:1477, 1990.

Bray GA: Basic considerations and clinical approaches. Dis Mon 35(7):451, 1989.

Brone RJ and Fisher CB: Determinants of adolescent obesity: A comparison with anorexia nervosa. Adolescence 23:155, 1988.

Brumberg JJ: Fasting Girls: The Emergence of Anorexia Nervosa as a Modern Disease. Cambridge, MA, Harvard University Press, 1988.

Committee on Diet and Health, National Research Council: Diet and Health: Implications for Reducing Chronic Disease Risk. Washington, DC, National Academy Press, 1989.

Connors ME and Johnson CL: Epidemiology of bulimia and bulimic behaviors. Addictive Behaviors 12:165, 1987.

Geracioti TD and Liddle RA: Impaired cholecystokinin secretion in bulimia nervosa. N Engl J Med 319:683, 1988.

Himms-Hagen J: Thermogenesis in brown adipose tissue as an energy buffer. N Engl J Med 311:1549, 1984.

Hirsch J and Knittle JL: Cellularity of obese and non-obese adipose tissue. Fed Proc 29:1516, 1970.

Kaye WH et al: Relative importance of calorie intake needed to gain weight and level of physical activity in anorexia nervosa. Am J Clin Nutr 47:989, 1988.

Kirschner MA et al: An eight-year experience with a very-low-calorie formula diet for control of major obesity. Int J Obes 12:69, 1987.

Knittle JL et al: Adipose tissue development in man. Am J Clin Nutr 30:762, 1977.

Krotkiewski ML et al: Adipose tissue cellularity in relation to prognosis for weight reduction. Int J Obes 1:395, 1977.

Leon AS et al: Effects of a vigorous walking program on body composition, and carbohydrate and lipid metabolism of obese young men. Am J Clin Nutr 33:1776, 1979.

Lissner L et al: Dietary fat and the regulation of energy intake in human subjects. Am J Clin Nutr 46:886, 1987.

Moore DC: Body image and eating behavior in adolescent girls. Am J Dis Child 142:1114, 1988.

National Center for Health Statistics: Anthropometric reference data and prevalence of overweight, U.S., 1976–1980. Pub. No. 8-1688. Hyattsville, MD, US Dept of Health and Human Services, National Center for Health Statistics, 1987.

Ravussin E et al: Reduced rate of energy expenditure as a risk factor for body weight gain. N Engl J Med 318:467, 1988.

Smoller JW et al: Popular and very-low-calorie diets in the treatment of obesity. *In* Frankle RT and Yang M (eds): Obesity and Weight Control. Rockville, MD, Aspen Publications, 1988.

Tayback M et al: Body weight as a risk factor in the elderly. Arch Intern Med 150:1065, 1990.

Turner LW: Weight maintenance and relapse prevention. Nutr Clin 5(1):1, 1990.

Wadden TA, Van Itallie TB, and Blackburn GL: Responsible and irresponsible use of very-low-calorie diets in the treatment of obesity. JAMA 263:83, 1990.

Weinsier RL: Etiology, complications and treatment of obesity. Ala J Med Sci 24:435, 1987.

CHAPTER 19

NUTRITION FOR ATHLETIC TRAINING AND PERFORMANCE

KEY TERMS

AEROBIC METABOLISM—the transfer of usable energy through oxidative phosphorylation in the respiratory chain in the presence of oxygen

ADENOSINE TRIPHOSPHATE (ATP)—a nucleotide occurring in all cells that is involved in energy transfer

ANAEROBIC METABOLISM—the transfer of usable energy without the presence of oxygen

CREATINE PHOSPHATE (CP)—an important temporary storage form of high-energy phosphate in muscle cells

ERGOGENIC AID—a substance or practice that increases energy or work output

GLYCOGEN—the form of carbohydrate storage in animals

GLYCOGEN LOADING (GLYCOGEN SUPERCOMPENSATION)— a combination of exercise and high-carbohydrate diet that enables muscles to store glycogen beyond their normal capacity

GLYCOLYSIS—the breaking down of glucose with or without the presence of oxygen into simpler compounds, chiefly pyruvate or lactate

LACTIC ACID—a product from glucose metabolism in anaerobic metabolism

METABOLIC EQUIVALENT (MET)—a multiple of the resting metabolic rate; one MET is equal to 3.6 ml of oxygen/kg of body weight per minute

MYOGLOBIN—a ferrous protoporphyrin protein that is similar to hemoglobin but with only one iron atom per molecule instead of four; it contributes to the color of muscle and acts as a store of oxygen

OXYGEN DEBT—recovery oxygen consumption; the difference between O_2 consumption during the recovery period following exercise and the O_2 consumption at rest

SPORTS ANEMIA—a transient anemia seen in heavily training athletes characterized by a decrease in the red blood cell count, hemoglobin concentration, and packed cell volume, but with normal red blood cell morphology

Vo_2MAX—a measure of maximal oxygen uptake; liters of O_2 consumed per kg of body weight per minute

Interest in physical fitness is extremely high in the United States population. Whether the individual concern is with respect to general health and the overall quality of life or with participation in athletics and possibly competition, the routes to achievement of fitness differ only in degree. Both nutrition and exercise are closely involved with the important factors of body composition, muscular competence, and respiratory and cardiovascular capabilities. Diet can influence performance, and belief in the consumption of certain foods may confer the psychologic edge that is particularly important to the athlete.

PHYSIOLOGY AND BIOCHEMISTRY OF EXERCISE

Muscle Contraction

Muscle fibers consist of collections of *fibrils,* which in turn consist of *filaments* that number many billions per fiber. The filaments consist primarily of two proteins, *myosin* and *actin,* which act together to effect contraction and relaxation. Filaments are divided into sections known as *sarcomeres,* which constitute the functional units of the muscle cell. Flexion of the muscle is stimulated by nerve impulses, which provoke complex movements of contraction and relaxation that continue until the nervous stimulus has ceased. This process is actually continuous, so that even in a state of rest the "muscle tone" is maintained at the cost of some energy expenditure.

The *sliding filament theory* proposes that muscle contraction takes place when the myosin and actin portions within the sarcomere slide across each other, with neither changing in length but in effect shortening the muscle fiber (contraction) or restoring it to its full length (relaxation). The unenergized position of the filament is in the contracted state; return of the filament to a relaxed state requires the input of energy in the form of *adenosine triphosphate (ATP).* A complex action involves attachment of the actin to cross-bridges on the myosin molecule, forming *actomyosin.* Joining ATP to actomyosin brings about its separation into actin and myosin, thus returning the two proteins to a state in which they can again respond to continuing nerve impulses. Enzymatic splitting of ATP to form *adenosine diphosphate (ADP)* and inorganic phosphorus releases the energy for this reaction. Oxygen is not required at this stage.

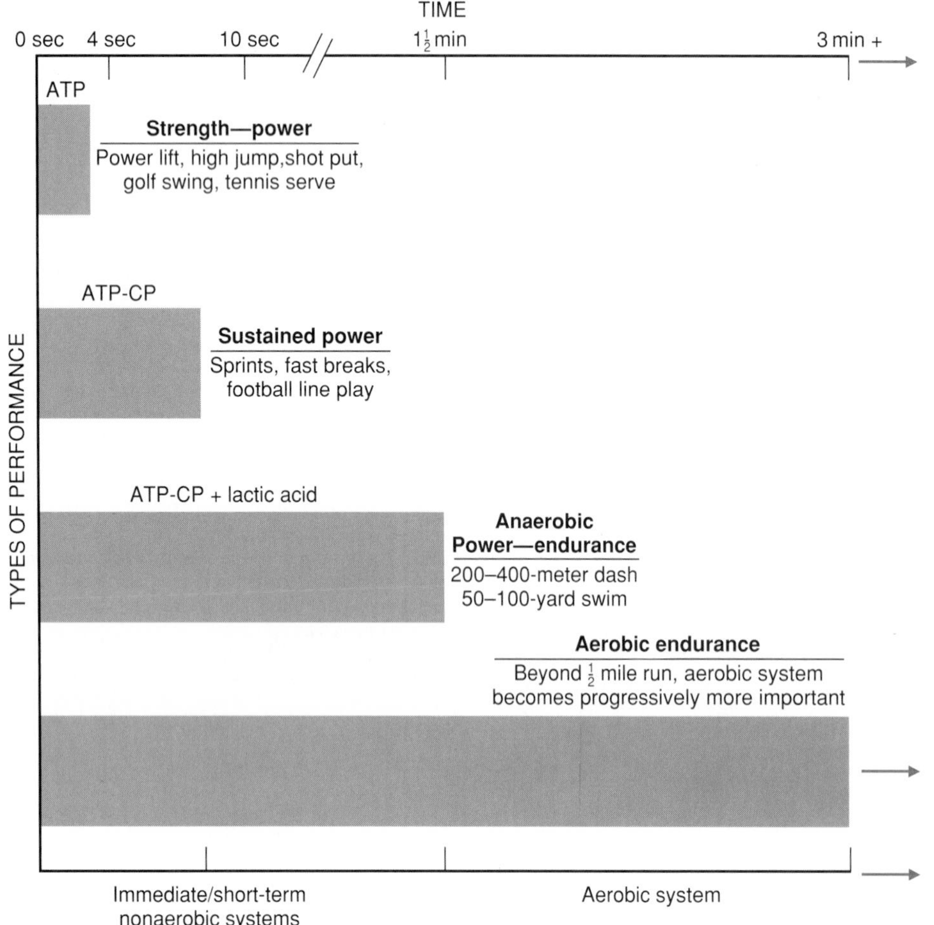

FIGURE 19–1. *Classification of activities based on duration of performance and the predominant energy pathways. (Redrawn from Katch FI and McArdle WD: Nutrition, Weight Control and Exercise, 3rd ed. Philadelphia, Lea & Febiger, 1988.)*

Phosphagen Energy Sources

The ATP present in the muscles at any one time is sufficient to power activity for several seconds, thus enabling immediate response to nervous stimuli. This response is further supported by the presence in muscle cells of *creatine phosphate (CP),* which like ATP contains a high-energy phosphate group. As ATP is split, releasing energy, the ADP thus formed is combined with enzymatically released high-energy phosphate from CP to resynthesize further ATP. There is three to five times as much CP in the cell as ATP, thus providing for a few more seconds of energy for which oxygen is not required. Further energy to sustain muscle activity must be derived from energy-containing nutrients (Fig. 19–1).

The most rapidly available mechanism for supplying ATP for more than a few seconds is the process of *glycolysis,* in which the energy in glucose is released either with or without the presence of oxygen. When the process is aerobic, *pyruvic acid* is the predominant end product; *lactic acid* is the end product of anaerobic metabolism. In either case, the amount of ATP furnished is relatively small (the process is only 30% efficient) compared with the amount yielded by mitochondrial oxidation via the Krebs cycle, which must eventually contribute energy if activity is to continue for any period of time.

Oxygen Requirements

Aerobic Metabolism

Production of ATP in amounts sufficient to support continued muscle activity requires the input of oxygen. Energy stored in nutrients is transferred to the high-energy phosphate bonds in ATP through a complex series of enzymatically guided reactions, involving separation of hydrogen atoms from the parent compounds. Vital to the continuation of these reactions is the presence of coenzymes, which act as hydrogen acceptors until the process of oxidative phosphorylation culminates with the formation of ATP. Ultimately, hydrogen is combined with oxygen to form water, and the coenzymes are thus freed to accept more hydrogen in a continuation of the process. If sufficient oxygen is not present to combine with the hydrogen, no further ATP will be forthcoming. Therefore, the oxygen furnished through the process of respiration is of vital importance (Fig. 19–2).

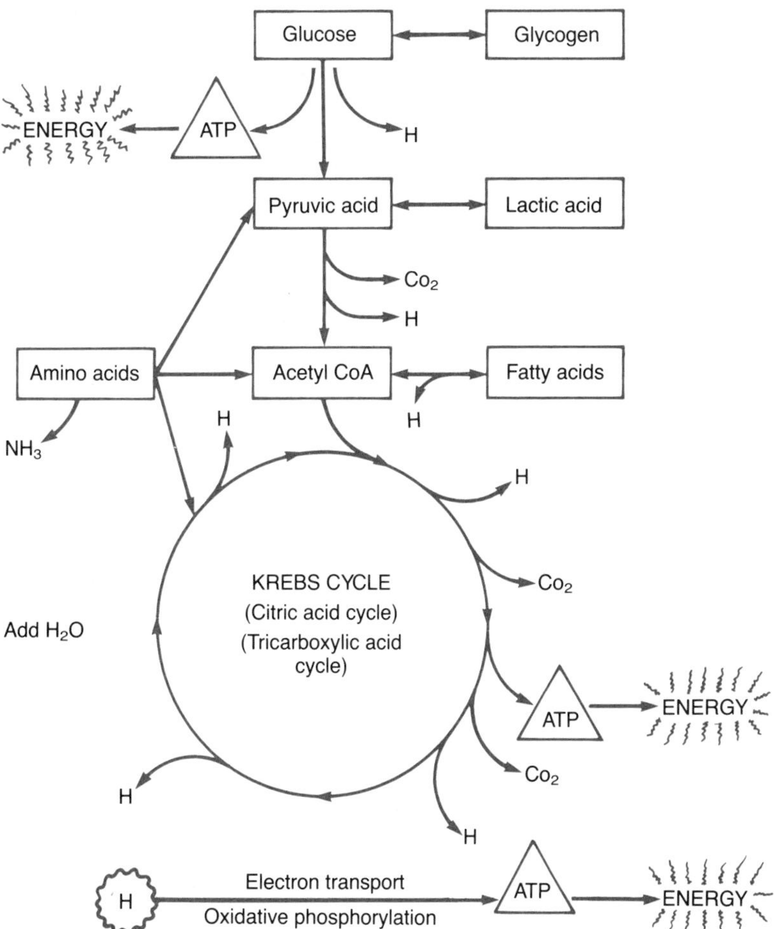

FIGURE 19–2. *Pathways of energy production (H = hydrogen atoms; ATP = adenosine triphosphate.)*

Aerobic metabolism is limited only by the availability of substrate and by a continuous and adequate supply of oxygen. At the onset of exercise and with the increase of exercise intensity, the capability of the cardiovascular system to supply adequate oxygen becomes a limiting factor.

Anaerobic Metabolism

In the absence of sufficient oxygen, such as in high-intensity, short-duration events, it is possible to temporarily obtain a supply of ATP through the eventual hydrogenation of pyruvic acid, the end product of glycolysis. With the transference of two hydrogen atoms to pyruvic acid, thus converting it to lactic acid, a vital coenzyme is freed to participate in further ATP synthesis. The lactic acid is removed rapidly from the muscle and into the blood stream. It is eventually converted to energy, either in muscle, liver, or brain, or to glycogen. This conversion to glycogen takes place in liver and to some extent in muscle, particularly among trained athletes.

Although this process provides immediate protection from the consequences of insufficient oxygen, it can only continue temporarily. As lactic acid accumulates in the blood during exercise, it eventually lowers the pH to a level that interferes with enzymatic action, leading to fatigue. Also, the amount of ATP produced through glycolysis is very small compared with that available through the Krebs cycle. Substrate for this reaction is restricted to glucose provided from blood sugar or the glycogen stores in the muscle. Liver glycogen contributes to blood sugar but is limited in amount. Muscle glycogen is not capable of transfer via the blood stream, so that the anaerobic capacity of each muscle is limited to its own glycogen content.

Beyond several minutes, aerobic metabolism predominates and oxygen consumption becomes an important factor (Fig. 19–3). The *respiratory quotient (RQ),* which compares the amount of inspired oxygen required to metabolize dietary intakes of individual nutrients with the amount of carbon dioxide expired, indicates that metabolism of carbohydrates (RQ = 1.0) is more efficient with respect to oxygen consumption than is fat (RQ = 0.70), and protein falls in between (RQ = 0.82). This is related to the fact that the number of hydrogen atoms that must eventually be combined with oxygen to form water is much greater in fats than in proteins and carbohydrates.

Oxygen Debt

During the recovery period after exercise, oxygen uptake continues at a high level for a period of time. The difference between this level and the amount that would be required for the same individual at rest is called the *oxygen debt,* or *recovery oxygen consumption.* This represents in part the oxygen required for replacement of the ATP and CP reserves used during the initial exercise phase, reoxygenation of myoglobin and hemoglobin, and conversion of lactic acid to glucose and glycogen. It also includes the oxygen participating in restoration of the physiologic changes created by the exercise in systems such as circulation, respiration, and temperature regulation. If the previous energy expenditure was primarily aerobic, the oxygen debt is repaid within several minutes after stopping exercise. How-

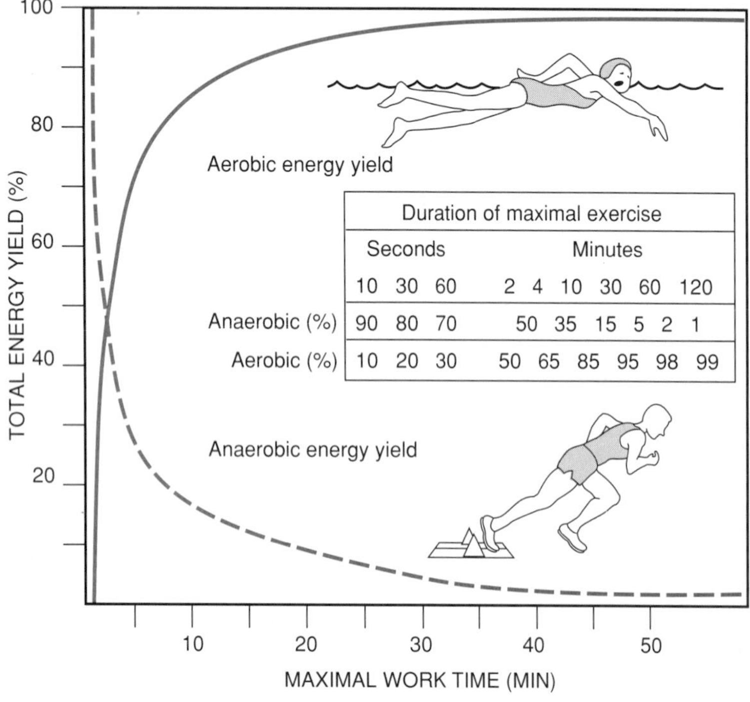

	Duration of maximal exercise									
	Seconds			Minutes						
	10	30	60	2	4	10	30	60	120	
Anaerobic (%)	90	80	70	50	35	15	5	2	1	
Aerobic (%)	10	20	30	50	65	85	95	98	99	

FIGURE 19–3. *Relative contribution of aerobic and anaerobic energy during maximal physical activity of various durations. Note that 1½ to 2 minutes of maximal effort requires 50% of the energy from each of the aerobic and anaerobic processes. (Redrawn and modified from Astrand P and Rodahl K: Textbook of Work Physiology. New York, McGraw-Hill, 1970.)*

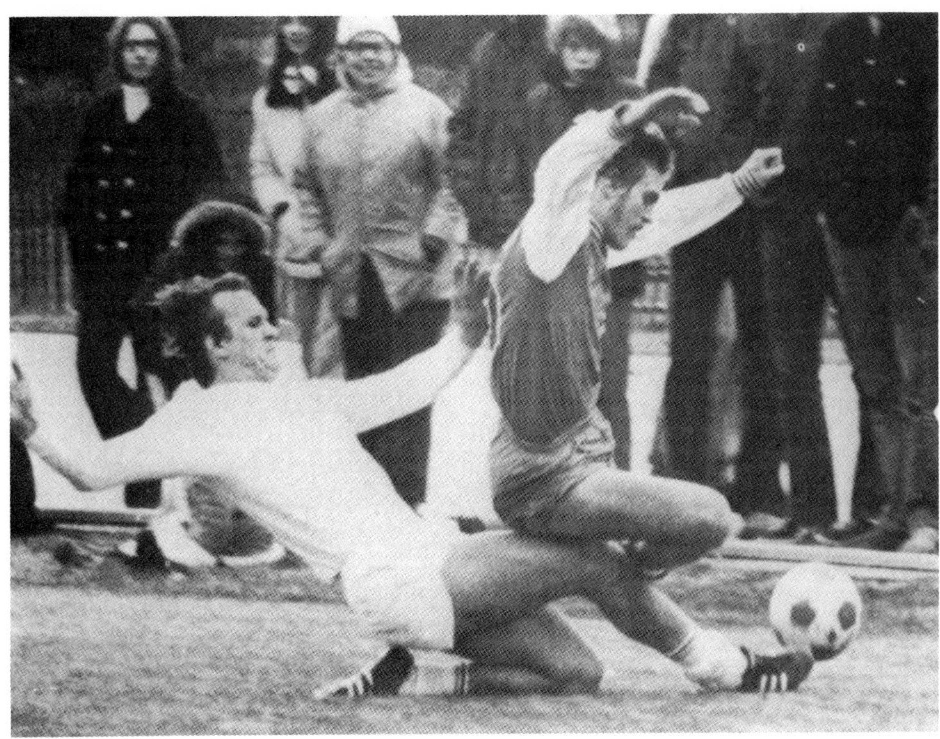

FIGURE 19–4. *In a strenuous form of exercise like soccer, players are pushed to a high level of anaerobic metabolism from which they may not fully recover in brief rest periods. After aerobic activities, however, the oxygen debt is repaid within several minutes after stopping exercise. (From Kuprian W [ed]: Physical Therapy for Sports. Philadelphia, WB Saunders, 1982, p 117.)*

ever, after high-intensity strenuous exercise with lactic acid build-up and body temperature increase, it may take several hours to 1 day to recover the oxygen debt. This can be a problem in sports such as basketball, hockey, soccer, or volleyball in which players are pushed to a high level of anaerobic metabolism and may not fully recover in the brief rest periods between points, time outs, half-time breaks, or even rest periods between games (Fig. 19–4).

Fuel of Muscle Contraction

Sources of Fuel

Proteins, fats, and carbohydrates are all possible sources of fuel for muscle contraction. The glycolytic pathway is restricted to glucose, which can originate in dietary carbohydrates or can be synthesized from the carbon skeletons of certain amino acids through the process of gluconeogenesis. The Krebs cycle is fueled by three-carbon fragments of glucose, two-carbon fragments of fatty acids, and carbon skeletons of specific amino acids, primarily alanine. Which of these nutrient substrates is used depends on the intensity and duration of the exercise.

Choice of Fuel

As already mentioned, carbohydrate is the most efficient fuel with respect to oxygen consumption. However, available carbohydrate is limited to the blood sugar and the glycogen stores in liver and muscle, which provide approximately 600 kcal. In contrast, the potential supply of fatty acids in the adipose stores is essentially unlimited.

In general, both glucose and fatty acids provide fuel for exercise, in proportions depending on the intensity and duration of the exercise and the fitness of the athlete. Exertion of very high intensity and short duration draws primarily on reserves of ATP and CP. High-intensity exercise that continues for more than a few seconds depends on anaerobic glycolysis. During exercise of low to moderate intensity ($<60\%\dot{V}o_2max$), energy is derived mainly from fatty acids. Carbohydrate becomes a larger fraction of the energy source as intensity increases until at an intensity level of 85 to 90% $\dot{V}o_2max$, carbohydrate from glycogen is the principal energy source and the duration of activity is limited.

The length of time that use of fatty acids can be sustained is related to athlete conditioning. In addition to improving cardiovascular systems involved in oxygen delivery, training increases the number of mitochondria and levels of enzymes involved in aerobic synthesis of ATP, thus increasing capacity for fatty acid metabolism.

NUTRITIONAL REQUIREMENTS OF EXERCISE

Fluid and Electrolytes

Fluid

The importance of fluid replacement during exercise is well documented. The cell conducts its activities in an aqueous medium. Water transports nutrients and waste products to and from the cells via the blood stream, and adequate blood volume is essential to the body's ability to dissipate heat through dilation of skin blood vessels and sweat during exercise.

Depletion of body water occurs through sweating and respiration. Much of the water lost through sweating comes from the blood, leading to a reduction of blood volume to a level that may threaten cardiovascular function. When fluid losses reach a significant level, sweating and blood flow to the skin are diminished and core temperatures are elevated. Even partial dehydration impairs performance; a water loss of 4 to 5% reduces work capacity by 20 to 30%, while a 10% loss threatens circulatory collapse (see Fig. 8–2).

The amount of fluid lost during exercise depends on the intensity and duration of the effort and especially on the atmospheric temperature and humidity. Without exercise, an individual produces 500 to 700 ml/day of sweat, whereas prolonged exercise in a humid environment may result in 8 to 12 l/day of sweat. Some marathon runners lose in excess of 5 liters during competition, which amounts to 6 to 10% of body weight.

The evaporation of 1 gram of sweat removes about 0.6 kcal of heat, and sweat glands can deliver 30 g/min of sweat. Thus, under ideal temperature conditions, all excess heat could be dissipated via sweat evaporation. In cool weather, much of the heat generated during exercise is liberated by radiation and by convection from the exposed skin. In warm temperatures, when the difference between air temperature and body temperature is less, not as much heat is released by convection and radiation and the evaporation of sweat is necessary for dissipation of heat. The hotter the temperature, the more important is sweating for body heat dissipation.

During long strenuous exercise, particularly in hot climates, athletes should replace water lost in amounts sufficient to maintain their pre-exercise weight. Thirst is not always a dependable indicator of fluid requirement. In some situations of strenuous exercise, such as soldiers marching in the heat or athletes running in summer marathons, drinking ad lib does not replace all fluid losses. Fluid losses should be monitored with body weight measurements and urine color. One pound loss is equal to two cups of fluid that should be replaced. Dark yellow urine can indicate dehydration. Continuous replacement is necessary both during and after exercise, and further rehydration is required afterwards.

Electrolytes

Sweat, which contains sodium, chloride, magnesium, and potassium, is hypotonic compared with body fluids. Even with prolonged sweating (as much as 9 lb of body weight loss), electrolyte losses do not jeopardize performance. Sweating always causes a loss of more water than salt. When plasma volume gets low, aldosterone acts to conserve sodium.

During heavy training in hot temperatures, a dilute salt solution of no more than ½ tsp of salt per liter of water may be used as a rehydration drink to correct excessive sweat loss (American College of Sports Medicine, 1984). Salt tablets or excessive salt intake are rarely necessary. Sodium and chloride can usually be replaced by eating salty foods and by salting foods to satisfy taste.

In the absence of vomiting or diarrhea, the daily potassium losses of an athlete are offset by a normal dietary intake of this mineral (70 to 80 mEq/day). Magnesium losses are low.

Energy

The amount of energy expended during a particular activity depends on the intensity and the duration of the activity and the individual characteristics of the

TABLE 19–1. Classification of Physical Work Based on Energy Expenditure*

Work Category	Men (kcal/min)	Women (kcal/min)	Activities
Light	2.0–4.9	1.5–3.4	Walking, reading, driving, shopping, bowling, fishing, golf, pleasure sailing
Moderate	5.0–7.4	3.5–5.4	Pleasure cycling, dancing, volleyball, badminton, calisthenics
Heavy	7.5–9.9	5.5–7.4	Ice skating, water skiing, competitive tennis, novice mountain climbing, jogging
Very heavy	10.0–12.4	7.5–9.4	Fencing, touch football, scuba diving, basketball, swimming (most strokes)
Unduly heavy	≥12.5	≥9.5	Handball, squash, cross-country skiing, paddleball, running (fast pace)

* Adapted from Katch FI and McArdle WD: Nutrition, Weight Control and Exercise, 3rd ed. Philadelphia, Lea & Febiger, 1988, p 111.

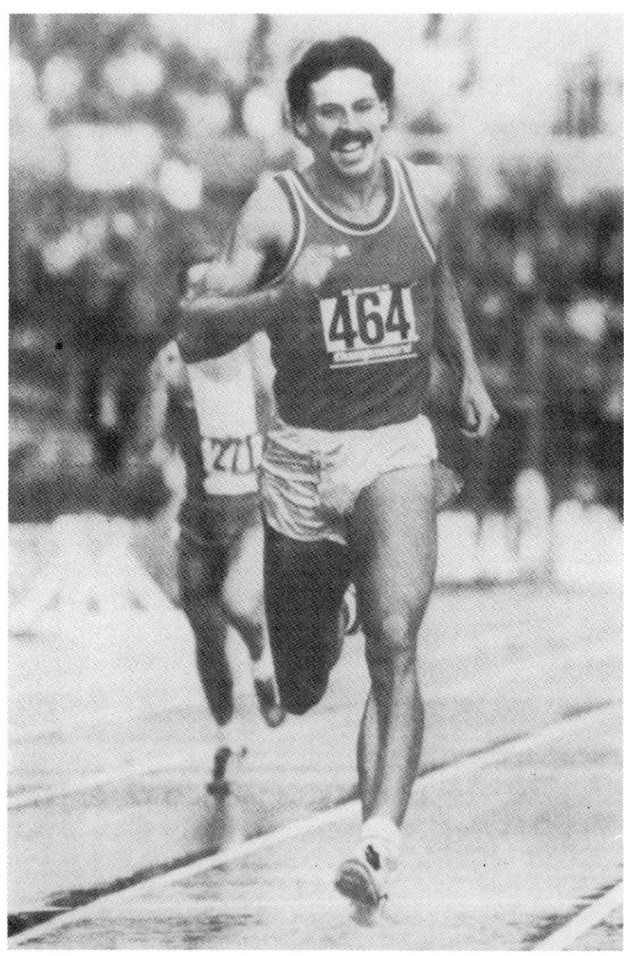

FIGURE 19–5. *Sports like running, rowing, and swimming require repetitive muscle contractions and thus use more energy than those involving more muscle contraction maintenance, such as gymnastics and golf. (From Kuprian W [ed]: Physical Therapy for Sports. Philadelphia, WB Saunders, 1982, p 114.)*

athlete, such as sex, age, size, state of maturation, and level of training. Table 19–1 categorizes the energy expenditure associated with different kinds of physical work on the basis of intensity of effort. Because more energy is needed to initiate a muscle contraction than to maintain it, sports requiring repetitive muscle contractions (such as running, rowing, and swimming (Fig. 19–5) use more energy than those involving more muscle contraction maintenance (such as gymnastics and golf; Fig. 19–6 and Appendix Table 36.) Some athletes in heavy aerobic training may require as much as 4,000 to 6,000 kcal/day or more.

Fit individuals use more energy with a lower heart rate. When the level of fitness and the pulse rate are known, the energy expenditure per minute of an individual can be determined by means of the data in Figure 19–7. Because oxygen uptake is related to the heart rate, it is also possible to determine the energy expenditure of an individual performing an activity by measuring the heart rate during that activity. Metabolic equivalents (MET) are also used to classify activity levels (Clinical Insight, p. 351).

Carbohydrate

The first source of glucose for the exercising muscle is its own glycogen store. When this is depleted, glycogenolysis and then gluconeogenesis (both in the liver) maintain the glucose supply.

Exhaustion is correlated with depletion of glycogen stores and the consequent failure to provide enough blood glucose for the exercising muscle. After 3 hours of continuous exercise at 70 to 80% of maximal oxygen uptake, athletes tire owing to hypoglycemia. At this stage, carbohydrate is still providing 50 to 60% of the energy being used, but it is coming from blood glucose because muscle glycogen stores are depleted. (This is the rationale for the sugar-containing sports drinks.) Liver glycogen is insufficient to maintain blood glucose for prolonged periods at high work intensities. Depletion can occur during a long distance event, as seen when the athlete "hits the wall." It can also develop after consecutive days of heavy training, when the time between work-outs is insufficient for complete glycogen resynthesis. This situation, known as "staleness," in which even the smallest amount of exercise can cause fatigue, can be avoided by increasing dietary carbohydrate and by timing the intake to improve its availability. To allow for maximal repletion of glycogen, most athletes should consume a diet in which 50 to 70% of the kilocalories are from carbohydrate. This amounts to about 500 to 600 g/day of carbohydrate.

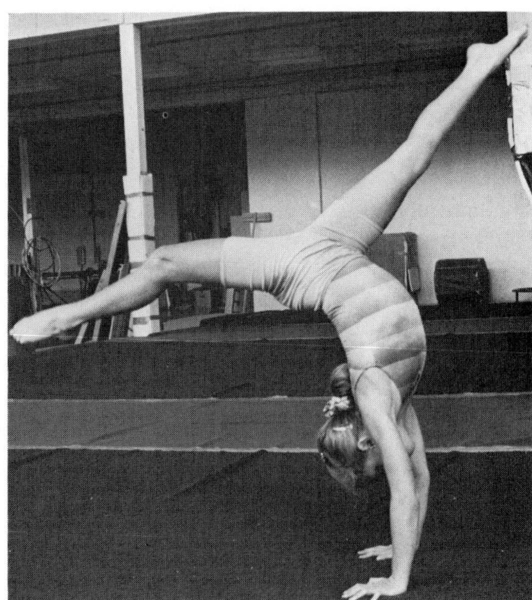

FIGURE 19–6. *Gymnastics, a moderate form of exercise, requires a moderate amount of energy.*

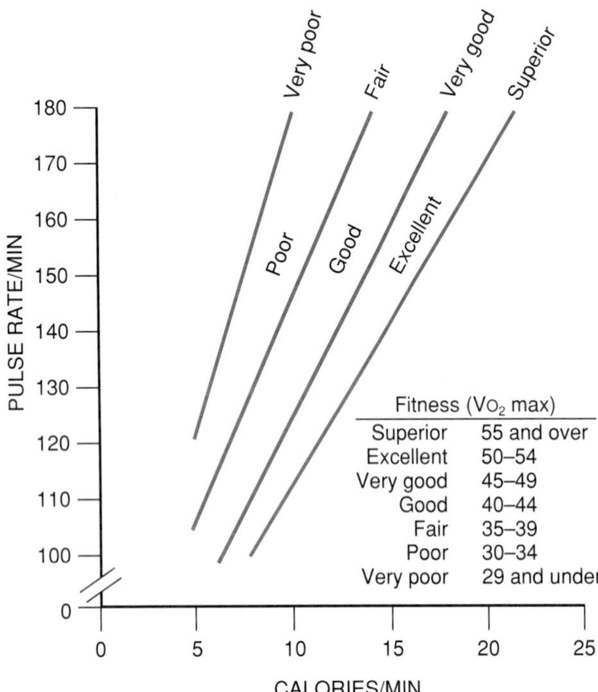

FIGURE 19–7. *Predicting calories burned during physical activity from pulse rate. (From Sharkey BJ: Physiology of Fitness, 2nd ed. Champaign, IL, Human Kinetics Publishers, 1984, p 310.)*

Glycogen Loading

In the 1960s, Swedish physiologists demonstrated by means of a muscle biopsy technique that the duration of intense, prolonged aerobic exercise is limited by the extent of muscle glycogen stores. By means of appropriate training and diet manipulation, they were able to increase muscle glycogen to at least twice the normal amount, thus doubling the capacity for aerobic activity (Bergstrom and Hultman, 1967). The program consisted of three stages: depletion of glycogen stores by a hard work-out of the affected muscles, accompanied by a diet low in carbohydrate; followed by a very high carbohydrate diet during a period of 3 days of light work-out, during which the muscles were allowed to replenish glycogen; and, finally, no exercise at all with a high-carbohydrate intake during the day before the event.

Practically, however, the phase of glycogen depletion that combines an extremely low-carbohydrate diet (maximum of 100 g/day of carbohydrate) with 3 to 4 days of heavy training results in hypoglycemic athletes. A modified "depletion taper" regimen, which appears to be almost as effective in raising muscle glycogen levels as the original program (Sherman, 1987), involves a long, hard work-out on the seventh day before the event, followed by 4 days during which the carbohydrate intake is increased gradually to a maximum of 500 to 600 g/day (50 to 70% of kcal). Training is decreased during this period, and the athlete does not exercise during the day before the event. Such a regimen increases glycogen stores 20 to 40% above normal.

After a hard work-out and glycogen depletion, it takes 12 to 24 hours to replete glycogen levels and up to 48 hours for supercompensation. Because 60% of the total glycogen storage occurs within the first 10 hours after depletion, carbohydrate intake immediately after a training session or competition is very important. Athletes should consume 100 grams of carbohydrate within 15 to 30 minutes after exercise followed by an additional 100-gram feeding every 2 to 4 hours thereafter. Glycogen resynthesis is proportional to the amount of carbohydrate consumed; however, the contribution of intakes in excess of 600 g/day appears to be negligible. The carbohydrate should be mainly in the complex form (starches).

Glycogen loading is recommended only for athletes participating in long events of 1 hour or more, but it may be useful for athletes competing in several short events in 1 day, such as during a track, swim, or gymnastics meet. There is no value in loading glycogen stores prior to athletic events involving events of short-term or of low to moderate intensity, because these events do not make heavy demands on the glycogen supply.

Storage of glycogen is accompanied by storage of 2.7 ml of water per gram of glycogen. This leads to both weight gain and muscle tightness. Although this effect may be desirable for football players who want to gain weight before a game or body builders who want to improve muscle size and definition, it can be detrimental to athletes for whom excess weight is a handicap.

Fat

Fat is the fuel best suited to low to moderate activity because of its extensive availability in adipose stores. With prolonged exercise, free fatty acids are released from adipose stores for uptake by muscle to be used as fuel. However, this does not mean that the diet should necessarily contain large amounts of this nutrient. The 30% of kilocalories from fat recommended for the average diet is also appropriate for the athlete.

Protein

Although it has long been a popular belief among athletes that additional protein increases strength and enhances performance, it is generally held by nutritionists and some exercise physiologists that data are not available to support this thesis. Noting that the small amount of protein required for muscle development during training is easily met by the average diet, the 1989 RDA for protein do not specify intakes for work or

CLINICAL INSIGHT: $\dot{V}O_2$max and Metabolic Equivalent

$\dot{V}O_2$max is a measure of maximal oxygen intake reported in terms of liters of oxygen consumed per kg body weight per min. It is synonymous with cardiorespiratory endurance and is the best single measure of aerobic fitness. It represents the capacity for aerobic resynthesis of ATP.

A **metabolic equivalent (MET)** is a multiple of the resting metabolic rate. One MET is equal to a resting oxygen consumption rate of 3.6 ml of oxygen/kg of body weight/min. It is a measure of oxygen consumed and thus energy expended. One liter of oxygen used is equal to an energy expenditure of about 5 kcal. The oxygen uptake is related to the heart rate; thus it is possible to determine the energy expenditure of an individual doing a certain activity by measuring the heart rate during that activity. Work at 2 MET requires twice the energy of resting metabolism, whereas 3 MET is three times the resting metabolism.

training that are any different from those indicated for adults.

Some studies have suggested that the current RDA for protein, even with its built-in safety factor, is insufficient for both strength and endurance athletes and that the actual requirement is higher, perhaps by 50 to 100% (Lemon, 1987). Endurance athletes may need additional protein for the repair of damaged muscle fibers and as an additional energy source. For strength athletes it may be more related to maintenance of a highly positive nitrogen balance, so that the hypertrophic stimulus of resistance exercise, known to increase the uptake of amino acids, is maximized. These athletes may need to 1.2 to 2 grams of protein per kilogram of body weight (Lemon, 1989).

Protein can be an important energy source during events of long duration in which the availability of muscle glycogen becomes a significant factor. Depending on whether glycogen stores are optimal or depleted before the beginning of the exercise, the proportion of the energy requirement supplied by protein has been estimated at 5 to 20% (Evans et al, 1983; Lemon and Mullin, 1980). Increased protein turnover during and after exercise appears to be related to the glucose-alanine cycle of gluconeogenesis and to the possible use of branched chain amino acids — leucine, isoleucine, and valine — for energy (Lemon, 1987). Since the amino acids involved are most easily recruited from liver and muscle tissue, use of protein for gluconeogenesis can compromise muscle structure.

Table 19 – 2 estimates the requirements of the athlete whose protein needs are greatest — a growing male adolescent in rigorous training in a warm climate. This very liberal allowance is for about 104 g/day of protein or 1.5 g/kg. Although greater than the RDA of 0.85 g/kg for the adolescent male, this is still easily within the range of intake of most male teenagers and athletes. Many studies of athletes' diets indicate that their protein intakes are two to three times as high as the RDA.

In meeting his energy needs, the athlete described would probably be consuming at least 3,500 kcal. Considering the usual composition of diets in the United States, this would provide 10 to 15% protein, or 87 to 131 g/day. Thus there is generally no need to recommend additional protein unless this nutrient fails to make up at least 12% of the energy intake when the energy intake is adequate for weight maintenance. Protein at levels beyond 15% of total kilocalories can lead to ketosis, dehydration, calcium loss, gout, and possible stress to the kidney.

Minerals and Vitamins

It has usually been assumed that if the athlete meets requirements for increased energy, the vitamin and mineral requirements will also be satisfied. Although this may be true in most cases, one study of triathletes indicated low levels of selenium, molybdenum, iron, copper, and biotin even though the athletes were consuming energy at levels two to three times the RDA (Green et al, 1989). The authors speculated that be-

TABLE 19 – 2. Liberal Estimate of Protein Requirement for a 70-kg Male Adolescent Athlete*

28.7 g	Replacement of obligatory nitrogen loss in urine, feces, skin, and other sites assuming largest loss
8.6 g	30% allowance for individual variation
4.8 g	Allowance for growth assuming most rapid growth
7.5 g	Replacement of nitrogen lost in sweat during 4 hours of vigorous exercise in the heat
6.3 g	Allowance for increased muscle mass, as during some kinds of training
8.6 g	Allowance for loss of efficiency of standard protein
39.5 g	Allowance for use of protein for energy during rigorous exercise†
104 g	Total estimated protein requirement = 1.5 g/kg

* Data from *Energy and Protein Requirements:* Report of Joint FAO/WHO Ad Hoc Expert Committee; WHO, Tech. Sys. Series, No. 522, WHO, Geneva, Switzerland, 1973 and Durnin JVGA: *Nutrition, Physical Fitness, and Health.* Baltimore, MD, University Press, 1978.

† Determined using an energy expenditure during activity of an average of 12 kcal/min and exercising time daily of 240 minutes, and the assumption that 5.5% of the total energy expenditure during exercise is from protein.

cause of training and work schedules, athletes seldom eat three balanced meals but rely heavily on snacking to maintain their energy levels.

Iron

Iron performs several functions vital to muscle activity. As a component of hemoglobin, it is instrumental in transporting oxygen from the lungs to the tissues. It performs a similar role in myoglobin, which acts within the muscle as an oxygen acceptor to hold a supply of oxygen readily available for use by the mitochondria. Iron is also a vital component of the cytochrome enzymes involved in the production of ATP.

It thus follows that iron-deficiency anemia limits aerobic endurance and the capacity for work. However, partial depletion of iron stores in the liver, spleen, and bone marrow as evidenced by low serum ferritin levels, can have a detrimental effect on exercise performance, even when anemia is not present. For example, depletion of iron-containing enzymes provokes an increase in anaerobic metabolism with corresponding elevations in blood lactate levels (Schoene et al, 1983).

Although iron-deficiency anemia is not frequently seen among athletes, suboptimal stores as assessed by serum ferritin levels are relatively common (Rowland et al, 1987; Wilmore and Freund, 1986). Athletes at risk for developing low iron stores are the rapidly growing male adolescent, the female with heavy menstrual losses, the athlete with an energy-restricted diet, distance runners who may have increased gastrointestinal iron loss (Stewart et al, 1984), and those training heavily in hot climates with heavy sweating (sweat contains about 0.13 mg/l) (Paulev et al, 1983).

If the athlete has true iron-deficiency anemia, then iron supplementation along with vitamin C is appropriate to enhance its absorption. Oral iron therapy has prevented diminished endurance exercise performance in runners who are deficient in iron but are not anemic (Rowland et al, 1988).

SPORTS ANEMIA. Heavy training can cause a transient "sports anemia," which is characterized by a significant decrease in red blood cell (RBC) count, hemoglobin concentration, and packed cell volume. However, the RBC morphology remains normal, and performance does not appear to deteriorate. Possible causes include a hemodilution effect of expanded blood volume and an increased rate of RBC destruction owing to intravascular hemolysis. At present the data do not support the value of iron supplementation either in treating or in preventing "sports anemia." However, testing serum ferritin may be useful to assess iron stores in athletes. If true iron depletion is present, then iron supplementation is appropriate.

Calcium

Many female athletes, especially long-distance runners, dancers, or gymnasts who must also maintain a low body weight, become amenorrheic. Amenorrhea leads to a reduction in bone mineral content, and this is discussed further in Chapter 22. These amenorrheic athletes should be encouraged to eat a diet which meets the RDA for calcium, but there is no evidence that increasing calcium intake above the RDA will offset the loss in bone mass. However, reduction of training and possibly a gain in body fat mass to promote a return of menstruation does lead to an increase in bone density (Drinkwater, 1986).

B-Vitamins

Increased energy metabolism creates a need for more of the B-vitamins that serve as the functioning part of coenzymes involved in the energy cycles. However, when dietary intakes are expanded to meet increased energy needs, the extra foods consumed usually provide enough B-vitamins to enable the release of that energy. There is no evidence that supplementing the well-nourished athlete with B-vitamins will increase performance (Belko, 1987). A short-term deficiency in B-vitamins leads to a decrement in aerobic endurance. For some athletes, such as wrestlers who are consuming low-calorie diets for long periods of time, a B-vitamin supplement to meet the RDA may be appropriate (Williams, 1989).

Vitamin C

Many athletes use large amounts of vitamin C in an attempt to prevent fatigue. However, studies of the efficacy of ascorbic acid supplementation on physical working capacity, oxygen consumption, pulmonary function, exercise, and recovery heart rates are equivocal. Adolescent male athletes with marginal vitamin C status have benefited from intakes of 80 mg/day, although no further benefit was observed with increased levels of supplementation (Buzina et al, 1984). There is no evidence to support vitamin C supplementation in the individual who is already replete with vitamin C.

Vitamin E

Vitamin E is used widely as a supplement on the theory that by preventing lipid peroxidation it reduces the amount of oxygen used during exercise. However, studies have failed to support a contribution of vitamin E to performance (Haymes, 1983). Whether this vitamin has a protective chemical effect during exercise in polluted environmental conditions is unclear (Dillard et al, 1978).

NUTRITIONAL CONSIDERATIONS FOR AN EVENT

Pre-Event Meal

The pre-event meal is an important source of energy. However, it is frequently overemphasized, because the energy demanding effort is performed not only on the morning's intake but also on the intake of the 2 or 3 days preceding the event. However, the ritualistic aspects of the pregame meal can have considerable psychologic value and should not be ignored.

The pregame meal should be eaten 1 to 4 hours before an event and should provide 100 to 200 grams of carbohydrate. By allowing time for partial digestion and absorption, this provides for a final addition to muscle glycogen, additional blood sugar, and also for relatively complete emptying of the stomach. Prior to long-term aerobic events, the meal should be extra rich in carbohydrate. In fact, additional carbohydrate feedings up to 1 hour before the event may also be useful. However, individuals who are sensitive to a lowering of blood glucose concentration may not benefit from pre-exercise carbohydrate feedings, because an insulin-mediated drop in blood glucose concentration may occur early in the exercise. Fat should be limited, because it delays stomach emptying time and takes longer to digest. A low-protein meal minimizes the load of protein-breakdown products that must be excreted by the kidney and thus leads to less water loss through urination. Fluid intake should be generous to ensure that the body is well hydrated.

Commercial liquid formulas providing an easily digested high-fluid, high-carbohydrate meal are popular with athletes. Other appropriate pregame meals might be toast with jelly, a baked potato, spaghetti with tomato sauce, cereal with skim milk, or low-fat yogurt with fruit-sugar flavorings.

Within 15 minutes prior to a long event, the athlete should drink 400 to 600 ml of water (12 to 20 oz) of fluid. This prehydration allows for maximal absorption of fluid and will not necessitate urination. After exercise begins, the kidney slows down the making of urine to compensate for water loss.

Nutrition During Performance

The requirement for fluid and nutrient supplementation during an event depends on the intensity and duration of the event and on the ambient temperature. Humans have a very poor ability to take in fluids at the same rate at which they are lost. The athlete cannot depend on thirst to dictate fluid replacement during strenuous, prolonged exercise and must be told how much to drink and when. The composition of the optimal replacement drink for an athlete depends on the duration and intensity of the event and on the temperature and humidity of the environment. It appears that sodium is necessary for the most efficient rehydration and replacement of fluid losses. Rehydration with water alone dilutes the blood rapidly, increases its volume, and stimulates urine production. Blood dilution lowers both the salt- and volume-dependent part of the thirst drive, thus removing much of the drive to drink and replace fluid losses.

Carbohydrate taken during performance of endurance exercise ensures the availability of sufficient amounts during the later stages and offers an energy and performance advantage over water alone (Owen et al, 1986). The rate of carbohydrate ingestion should be about 25 to 30 g/30 min, an amount equivalent to 1 cup of a 6% carbohydrate solution taken every 15 to 20 minutes (American College of Sports Medicine, 1984).

The carbohydrate content should be between 6 and 8%. Drinks of this concentration enter the blood stream at the same rate as plain water; however, unlike water, these drinks are associated with improved performance because of the carbohydrate available (Davis et al, 1988). It is likely that a carbohydrate concentration of less than 5% is not enough to help performance, whereas solutions with a concentration greater than 10% are often associated with abdominal cramps, nausea, and diarrhea.

The type of carbohydrate in the replacement drink does not appear to influence its effectiveness with respect to cardiovascular and thermoregulatory response or to stomach emptying time (Mitchell et al, 1988; Murray et al, 1987b; Owen et al, 1986). Fructose ingestion during an event has not been associated with performance improvement, possibly because it is absorbed and metabolized more slowly. Osmotic diarrhea is a common complaint. However, fructose in a pre-exercise drink has extended the time of exercise until exhaustion. It may be that, in this respect, fructose provides a carbohydrate source to the muscles that does not stimulate the release of insulin with subsequent hypoglycemia and depression of fat utilization. Thus, fructose may be useful in long- term events (Okano et al, 1988).

Fluid replacement should be administered in a manner that will enhance movement of the fluid into the intestines where most of it is absorbed at the most efficient rate. The presence of glucose and sodium in the fluid greatly enhances its absorption (Mitchell et al, 1988; Murray, 1987a). Cold drinks move into the intestinal tract faster and, contrary to popular belief, do not cause stomach cramps (Costill and Saltin, 1974). Fairly large volumes rather than continuous little sips also seem to move faster; however, amounts should not be so large that they are retained in the stomach, because this can be uncomfortable. Drinking 250 ml (8.5 oz) every 10 to 15 minutes is a rate at which absorption is able to keep up with intake.

It is possible to replace only 800 ml of fluid/hr, which can be insufficient to meet the needs during long-term exertion where the fluid losses can exceed 2 l/hr. Rehydration must continue for several hours after an event to fully replace these losses.

Guidelines for fluid replacement are given in Table 19–3.

Post-Event Meal

Nutritional intake following the event should be focused on rehydration, repletion of glycogen stores, and restoration of electrolyte balance. The meal should be high in carbohydrate, primarily starches. Sodium can be replaced by salting food liberally and by choosing foods high in sodium. Fruits and vegetables are good sources of potassium. Rehydration is very important, especially if sweat losses have been great and competition is anticipated again the next day.

Other Considerations

Alcohol

Alcohol consumption has a detrimental effect on athletic performance, even though by reducing feelings of insecurity, tension, and discomfort it may cause the athlete to feel that he or she is performing better (Houmard et al, 1987; Williams, 1985). Perceptual motor performance is affected; however, except for some deleterious effects on prolonged endurance performance, alcohol has no effect on the physiologic processes of maximal exercise (Williams, 1985). Light social drinking (1 or 2 drinks) during the day before a competition will probably not influence athletic performance the following day.

Caffeine

Caffeine has been shown to contribute to endurance performance, apparently because of its ability to enhance mobilization of fatty acids and thus conserve glycogen stores (Weir et al, 1987). Caffeine may also exert a direct effect on muscle contractility, possibly by facilitating calcium transport. However, some believe that the glycogen-sparing effect of caffeine has not been sufficiently demonstrated to justify its recommendation to endurance athletes (Williams, 1989). The diuretic effect of caffeine could be a negative effect for athletes with excessive water needs.

TABLE 19–3. Guidelines for Proper Hydration

Weigh in before and after exercise, especially during hot weather.
For each pound of body weight lost during exercise, drink 2 cups of fluid.
Do not restrict fluids before or during an event.
Drink 2½ cups of fluid 2 hours before practice or competition.
Drink 1½ cups of fluid 15 minutes before the event.
Drink at least 1 cup of fluid every 15 to 20 minutes during training and competition.
The replacement drink should contain ⅓ tsp of salt per liter.
The fluid should contain 6 to 10% carbohydrate either as glucose, glucose polymers, or fructose.
The drink should be cool.

Ergogenic Aids

Over the years a wide variety of foods and nostrums have enjoyed popularity as contributors to athletic prowess. Among these are honey, gelatin, lecithin, wheat germ oil, and megadoses of vitamins. For the most part their effectiveness has not been conclusively supported, and some can even be harmful. An example is bee pollen, which can lead to anaphylactic shock in the bee allergic athlete.

Another agent promoted as increasing fat utilization during exercise is *carnitine,* a compound in the body that facilitates the transfer of fatty acids into the mitochondria for oxidation. No research supports increased use of fatty acids after carnitine ingestion, and no ergogenic effect has been demonstrated after its use (Williams, 1989).

Sodium bicarbonate, an alkaline salt in the blood, buffers lactic acid produced during the anaerobic phase of high-intensity exercise. This permits the production of ATP via anaerobic glycolysis to continue for a limited period without reducing the blood pH to fatigue-producing levels. Whether or not this is an effect of alkaline salt ingestion that can improve anaerobic performance is still controversial (Williams, 1989) (Table 19–4).

WEIGHT GAIN OR LOSS

In efforts to maximize performance, many athletes alter normal energy intake to either gain or lose weight. Although such efforts are sometimes appropriate, weight reduction programs in particular may involve elements of risk. For some young athletes, achievement of unrealistic light weights may jeopardize growth and development (Pugliese et al, 1983; Strauss et al, 1985). Starvation and dehydration as practiced by boxers, wrestlers, lightweight crew members, and jockeys to "make weight" can impair performance (Houston et al, 1981). Chronic dieting of female athletes, many of whom are dancers and gymnasts, can lead to eating disorders, delayed menarche, amenorrhea, and potential osteoporosis (Brooks-Gunn et al, 1987) (see Chapters 18 and 22).

The goal weight of an athlete should be determined

TABLE 19–4. Unproven Ergogenic Aids for Athletes*

Ergogenic Aid	Description	Claim
Bee pollen	Mixture of bee saliva, plant nectar, and pollen	Increases energy levels, enhances physical fitness
Brewer's yeast	Byproduct of beer brewing	Increases energy levels
Carnitine	A compound synthesized in the body from glutamate and methionine	Improves cardiovascular function and muscle strength; delays fatigue; decreases muscle pain
Choline	Precursor of the neurotransmitter acetylcholine	Improves performance
DNA/RNA	Deoxyribonucleic acid, ribonucleic acid	Tissue regeneration
Gelatin	Obtained from collagen	Improves muscle contraction
Ginseng	Extract of ginseng root	Protects against tissue damage
Glycine	An amino acid that is a phosphocreatine precursor	Improves muscle contraction
Inosine	A purine	Enhances physical strength
Kelp	Seaweed	Vitamin/mineral source
Lecithin	Phosphatidylcholine	Prevents fat gain
Octacosanol	Alcohol isolate extracted from wheat germ oil	Supplies energy and improves performance
Pangamic acid	Also referred to as vitamin B_{15}; varied composition depending on the supplier	Increases delivery of oxygen
Royal jelly	Substance produced by worker bees and fed to the queen bee	Increases strength
Spirulina	Microscopic blue-green algae	Protein source
Superoxide dismutase	Enzyme	Protects body against oxidative cell damage incurred from aerobic metabolism
Amino acid supplements	Arginine, ornithine, glycine plus lysine, predigested amino acids, branch-chain amino acids	Promotes muscle development

* From Sports Science Exchange, Gatorade Sports Science Institute at Chicago, 1989.

on the basis of body fatness. Adequate time should be allowed for a slow steady weight loss over a period of many weeks. Appropriate programs for modifying weight of athletes and others are discussed in Chapter 18.

CITED REFERENCES

American College of Sports Medicine: Position statement on prevention of heat injuries during distance running. Med Sci Sports Exerc 16:ix, 1984.

Belko AZ: Vitamins and exercise: An update. Med Sci Sports Exerc 19(Suppl 5):191, 1987.

Bergstrom J and Hultman E: A study of glycogen metabolism during exercise in man. Scand J Clin Lab Invest 19:218, 1967.

Brooks-Gunn J et al: The relation of eating problems and amenorrhea in ballet dancers. Med Sci Sports Exerc 19:41, 1987.

Buzina K et al: Vitamin C status and physical working capacity in adolescents. Int J Vitam Nutr Res 54:55, 1984.

Costill DL and Saltin B: Factors limiting gastric emptying during rest and exercise. J Appl Physiol 37:679, 1974.

Davis JM et al: Effects of ingesting 6% and 12% glucose-electrolyte beverages during prolonged intermittent cycling exercise in the heat. Eur J Appl Physiol 57:563, 1988.

Dillard CJ et al: Effects of exercise, vitamin E, and ozone on pulmonary function and lipid peroxidation. J Appl Physiol Respirat Environ Exerc Physiol 45:927, 1978.

Drinkwater BL et al: Bone mineral density after resumption of menses in amenorrheic athletes. JAMA 256:380, 1986.

Evans WJ et al: Protein metabolism and endurance exercise. Phys Sportsmed 11:63, 1983.

Green DR et al: An evaluation of dietary intakes of triathletes: Are RDAs being met? J Am Diet Assoc 89:1653, 1989.

Haymes EM: Proteins, vitamins, and iron. *In* Williams MH (ed): Ergogenic Aids in Sport. Champaign, IL, Human Kinetics Publishers, 1983.

Houmard JA et al: Effects of the acute ingestion of small amounts of alcohol upon 5 mile run times. J Sports Med 27:253, 1987.

Houston ME et al: The effect of rapid weight loss on physiological functions in wrestlers. Phys Sportsmed 9:73, 1981.

Lemon PWR and Mullin JP: Effect of initial muscle glycogen levels on protein catabolism during exercise. J Appl Physiol 48:624, 1980.

Lemon PWR: Influence of dietary protein and total energy intake on strength improvement. Sports Science Exchange 2(14):1, 1989.

Lemon PWR: Protein and exercise: Update 1987. Med Sci Sports Exerc 19(Suppl 5):179, 1987.

Mitchell JB et al: Effects of carbohydrate ingestion on gastric emptying and exercise performance. Med Sci Sports Exerc 20:110, 1988.

Murray R: The effects of consuming carbohydrate-electrolyte beverages on gastric emptying and fluid absorption during and following exercise. Sports Med 4:322, 1987a.

Murray R et al: The effect of fluid and carbohydrate feedings during intermittent cycling exercise. Med Sci Sports Exerc 19:597, 1987b.

Okano G et al: Effect of pre-exercise fructose ingestion on endurance performance in fed men. Med Sci Sports Exerc 20:105, 1988.

Owen MD et al: Effects of carbohydrate ingestion on thermoregulation, gastric emptying, and plasma volume during exercise in the heat. Med Sci Sports Exerc 18:568, 1986.

Paulev P-E et al: Dermal excretion of iron in intensely training athletes. Clin Chim Acta 127:19, 1983.

Pugliese MT et al: Fear of obesity: A cause of short stature and delayed puberty. N Engl J Med 309:513, 1983.

Rowland TW et al: Iron deficiency in adolescent endurance athletes. J Adolesc Health Care 8:322, 1987.

Rowland TW et al: The effect of iron therapy on the exercise capacity of nonanemic iron-deficient adolescent runners. Am J Dis Child 142:165, 1988.

Schoene RB et al: Iron repletion decreases maximal exercise lactate concentrations in female athletes with minimal iron deficiency anemia. J Lab Clin Med 102:306, 1983.

Sherman WM: Carbohydrate, muscle glycogen and improved performance. Phys Sportsmed 15(2):157, 1987.

Stewart JG et al: Gastrointestinal blood loss and anemia in runners. Ann Intern Med 100:843, 1984.

Strauss RH et al: Weight loss in amateur wrestlers and its effect on serum testosterone levels. JAMA 254:3337, 1985.

Weir J et al: A high carbohydrate diet negates the metabolic effects of caffeine during exercise. Med Sci Sports Exerc 19:100, 1987.

Williams MH: The Nutrition for Fitness Answer Book. Dubuque, IA, WC Brown Publishers, 1985, p 210.

Williams MH: Nutritional ergogenic aids and athletic performance. Nutr Today 24(1):7, 1989.

Wilmore JH and Freund BJ: Current concepts in nutrition. *In* Winick M (ed): Nutrition and Exercise, Vol 15. New York, Wiley & Sons, 1986, p 67.

ADDITIONAL REFERENCES

Benson JE et al: Relationship between nutrient intake, body mass index, menstrual function and ballet injury. J Am Diet Assoc 89:58, 1989.

Benardot D, Schwarz M, and Heller DW: Nutrient intake in young, highly competitive gymnasts. J Am Diet Assoc 89:401, 1989.

Coleman E: Eating for Endurance. Palo Alto, Bull Publishing, 1988.

Davis JM et al: Fluid availability of sports drinks differing in carbohydrate type and concentration. Am J Clin Nutr 51:1054, 1990.

Hargreaves M et al: I: Effects of carbohydrate feedings on muscle glycogen utilization and exercise performance. Med Sci Sports Exerc 16:219, 1984.

Jacobson BH and Kulling FA: Health and ergogenic effects of caffeine. Br J Sports Med 23(1):34, 1989.

Manore MM et al: Nutrient intakes and iron status in female long-distance runners during training. J Am Diet Assoc 89:255, 1989.

McArdle WD, Katch FI, and Katch VL: Exercise Physiology: Energy, Nutrition and Human Performance, 2nd ed. Philadelphia, Lea & Febiger, 1986.

Murray R et al: The effects of glucose, fructose and sucrose ingestion during exercise. Med Sci Sports Exerc 21:275, 1989.

Newhouse IJ et al: The effects of prelatent/latent iron deficiency on physical work capacity. Med Sci Sports Exerc 21:263, 1989.

Nieman DC et al: Supplementation patterns in marathon runners. J Am Diet Assoc 89:1615, 1989.

Nose H et al: Role of osmolality and plasma volume during rehydration in humans. J Appl Physiol 65:325, 1988.

Rucinski A: Relationship of body image and dietary intake of competitive ice skaters. J Am Diet Assoc 89:98, 1989.

Sharkey BJ: Physiology of Fitness: Prescribing Exercise for Fitness, Weight Control and Health, 2nd ed. Champaign, IL, Human Kinetics Publishers, 1984, p 102.

Simopoulos AP (ed): 1st International Conference on Nutrition and Fitness, May 21 to 26, 1988. Am J Clin Nutr 49(Suppl 5):909, 1989.

Steen SN, Oppliger RA, and Brownell KD: Metabolic effects of repeated weight loss and regain in adolescent wrestlers. JAMA 260:47, 1988.

Taylor CB: Eating disorders in athletes and dancers. Nutr and the M.D. 14(7):1, 1988.

Tired blood can slow your workout. Nutr Today 24(2):5, 1989.

Water: Can the endurance athlete get too much of a good thing? J Am Diet Assoc 89:1629, 1989.

CHAPTER 20

NUTRITION IN CARDIOVASCULAR ATHEROSCLEROTIC DISEASE

CHAPTER OUTLINE

Incidence
Pathology
Etiology
Relation of Dietary Factors to Serum Lipids
Treatment and Prevention

KEY TERMS

ARTERIOSCLEROSIS—sclerosis and thickening of the walls of the smaller arteries

ATHEROMA—mass of plaque of degenerated, thickened arterial intima occurring in atherosclerosis

ATHEROSCLEROSIS—a thickening and narrowing of the walls of the large and medium-sized blood vessels caused by the invasion of lipids, primarily cholesterol and other materials, into the intimal or inner layer to form plaque

BILE ACID SEQUESTRANT—a medication that adsorbs cholesterol-containing bile acids and prevents their absorption back into the blood stream

CORONARY HEART DISEASE (CHD) OR CORONARY ARTERY DISEASE (CAD)—disease involving the network of blood vessels that surrounds the heart and serves the myocardium

DOCOSAHEXAENOIC ACID (DHA)—an omega-3 polyunsaturated fatty acid found in fish oil; C-22:6ω3

EICOSAPENTAENOIC ACID (EPA)—an omega-3 polyunsaturated fatty acid found in fish oil; C-20:5ω3

FAMILIAL COMBINED HYPERLIPIDEMIA—a hyperlipoproteinemia due to overproduction of lipoproteins by the liver, usually characterized by an increase in serum triglyceride, cholesterol, or both

FAMILIAL DYSBETALIPOPROTEINEMIA—a rare lipoproteinemia characterized by elevated serum total cholesterol and triglycerides, but normal low-density lipoprotein-cholesterol

FAMILIAL HYPERCHOLESTEROLEMIA—a hyperlipoproteinemia with a genetic component characterized by a serum cholesterol in the 300 to 400 mg/dl range, xanthomas and CHD occurring in the 30s and 40s in men and 50s and 60s in women

FATTY STREAK—a small, flat, yellow-gray area composed mainly of cholesterol within an artery; probably an early stage of atherosclerosis

HIGH-DENSITY LIPOPROTEIN (HDL)—a plasma protein containing relatively more protein and less cholesterol and triglyceride; appears to remove cholesterol from the intima

INFARCTION (INFARCT)—an area of coagulation necrosis in a tissue due to local ischemia resulting from obstruction of circulation to the area

ISCHEMIA—deficiency of blood in a tissue, due to functional constriction or actual obstruction of a blood vessel

LIPOPROTEIN—a combination of a lipid and protein, possessing the solubility of proteins; the form of lipid transport in the blood

LOW-DENSITY LIPOPROTEIN (LDL)—a plasma protein containing relatively more cholesterol and triglyceride and less protein

SEVERE PRIMARY HYPERCHOLESTEROLEMIA—serum cholesterol levels greater than 300 mg/dl that are usually resistant to dietary change

THROMBUS—an aggregation of blood factors, primarily platelets and fibrin, frequently causing vascular obstruction at the point of its formation

***TRANS* FATTY ACIDS**—stereo-isomers of the naturally occurring *cis* fatty acids; artifacts of the hydrogenation process

VERY LOW DENSITY LIPOPROTEIN (VLDL)—a plasma protein containing relatively more triglyceride than cholesterol; the transport form of lipid from the liver to the periphery

Coronary heart disease (CHD) is the leading cause of death in this country and accounts for 80% of all cardiac deaths. The United States ranks with other industrial nations as having the highest incidence of CHD in the world (Fig. 20–1). As countries which at one time enjoyed a very low rate of death from CHD experience the change in lifestyle that accompanies increased industrialization, their death rates from this disease increase substantially.

Although most deaths from CHD occur in people over age 65 (half of these in people over 80 years), the large number of premature deaths has led to extensive research in areas of identification and prevention. A monumental literature has accumulated from epidemiologic, laboratory, clinical, prospective, and intervention studies that have sought to learn why only certain individuals are singled out for CHD, particularly when it leads to premature death.

INCIDENCE

The incidence of CHD increased from the beginning of this century to a point around 1920 when it became a major cause of death in the United States. The increase continued until the mid-1960s when it began to drop abruptly from 328 deaths per 100,000 population to 236 per 100,000 in 1983, an age-adjusted decrease in CHD mortality of 28% (Department of Health and Human Services, 1987) (Fig. 20–2). This decrease continued at a more moderate rate until 1986, the last date for which statistics are available. Beginning first on the Pacific Coast, the decrease occurred across all age, sex, ethnic, and population groups (Committee on Diet and Health, 1989). However, CHD remains the leading cause of death in the United States.

Reasons for the decrease have not been identified, although they are probably related to improved quality and availability of medical care, as well as changes in lifestyle. In a study designed to investigate causes of the decrease, men in the Framingham study who were aged 50 to 59 years in 1950 were evaluated again in 1960 and 1970 with respect to mortality from CHD. The findings of this study suggested that the improved mortality rate was related to lower serum cholesterol, lower systolic blood pressure, better management of hypertension, and reduced cigarette smoking (Sytkowski et al, 1990).

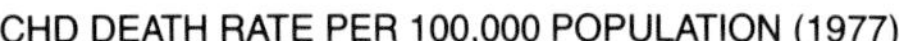

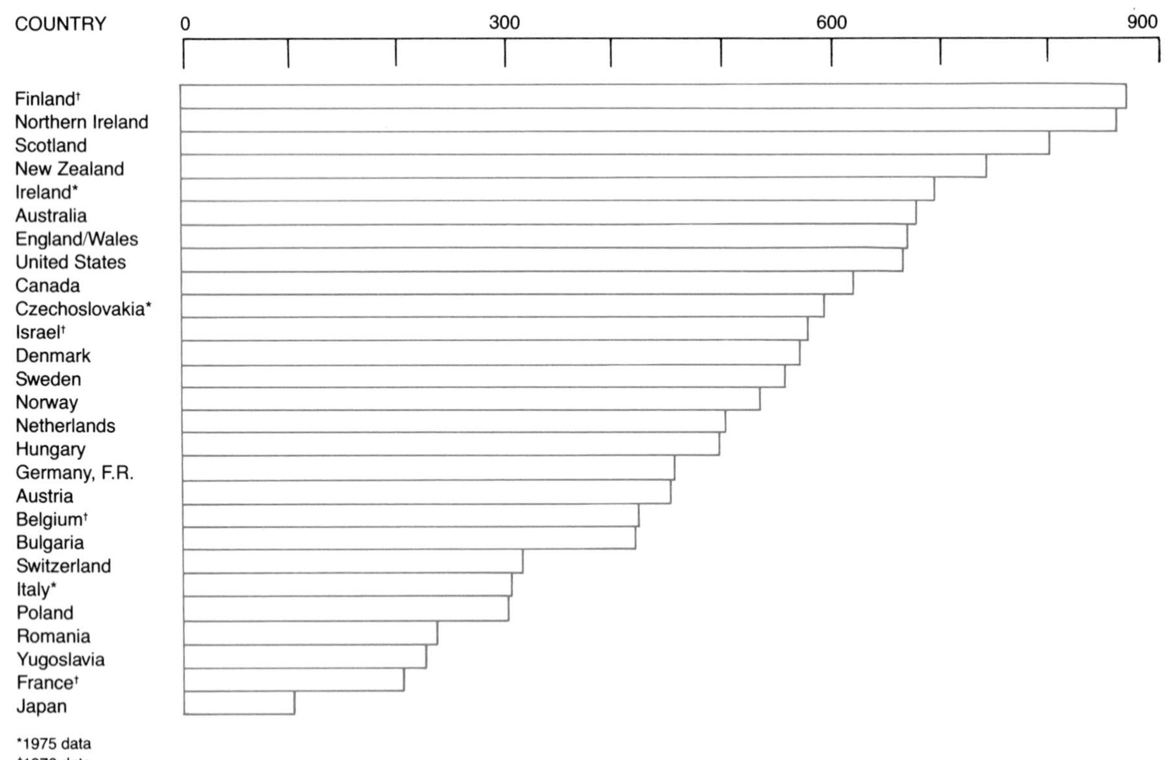

FIGURE 20–1. *Rate of deaths from CHD per 100,000 population among 35- to 74-year-old men in 1977 (except as otherwise noted) by country. (Adapted from the report of the Inter-Society Commission for Heart Disease Resources (1984). (Redrawn from Committee on Diet and Health, Food and Nutrition Board, NRC: Diet and Health. Implications for Reducing Chronic Disease Risk, Washington, DC, National Academy Press, 1989, p 100.)*

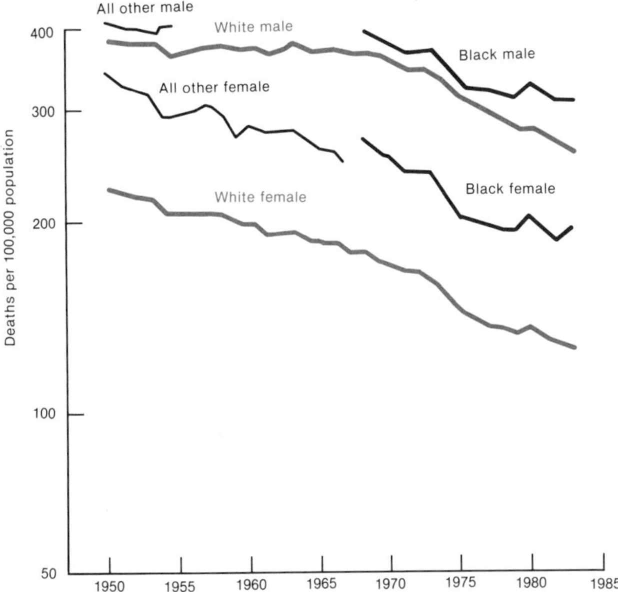

FIGURE 20–2. *Age-adjusted death rates for heart disease according to race and sex: United States 1950–83.*

PATHOLOGY

Coronary heart disease involves the network of blood vessels that surrounds the heart and serves the myocardium (Fig. 20–3). Like other arteries in the body, the coronary arteries are subject to *atherosclerosis,* a thickening and narrowing of the walls caused by the invasion of lipids, primarily cholesterol, and other materials into the intimal, or inner, layer to form *plaque.* As the plaque enlarges, the artery can become so narrowed that circulation is seriously diminished, or it can become entirely occluded by a clot *(thrombus).* The clot may be formed by hemorrhage of the plaque itself or it may travel to the spot from somewhere else in the body. The artery can also suffer a muscle spasm that interferes with circulation. The resultant ischemia causes an infarction or death of the portion of the myocardium that is deprived of oxygen and nourishment. Whether the heart is able to continue beating depends on the extent of the musculature involved, the presence of collateral circulation, and the oxygen requirement.

Autopsy data on children have demonstrated that the atherosclerotic process begins with the appearance of fatty streaks at a very early age. The development of atheroma is already established in young men; however, further proliferation into atherosclerotic plaque and subsequent occlusion of the arterial lumen does not take place in the absence of risk factors (Fig. 20–4).

ETIOLOGY

Thirty years of dedicated study have failed to establish the precise cause or causes of CHD. Certainly the designation of a "multiple etiology" is appropriate and explains part of the difficulty in designing studies to clarify the factors that contribute to 500,000 cardiovascular deaths in this country every year.

Epidemiologic data gathered from surveys around the world, many of them conducted in the 1960s and 1970s, consistently identify blood lipid levels and environmental factors, particularly dietary factors, that characterize populations with a high incidence of CHD. These findings are corroborated by clinical, laboratory, and animal studies, although studies with individuals fail to give uniform results because of the heterogeneity of risk factors and their interaction. Prospective studies have established positive relationships between serum cholesterol and CHD. More recently the serum concentrations of high-density lipoproteins (HDL) and low-density lipoproteins (LDL) have been identified as predictive of heart disease risk. Obesity and lack of exercise have also been incriminated. Although at one time coronary-prone ("type A") behavior was considered a major risk factor, lack of controls for other risk factors has clouded the results of earlier studies and subsequent work has failed to establish this relationship (Committee on Diet and Health, 1989).

Uncontrollable Risk Factors

Among the known uncontrollable risk factors for CHD are age, gender, race, and heredity. Early heart attacks occur predominantly in men; susceptibility to CHD increases linearly with age. Incidence and mortality approximately double in each 5-year period after age 24 (Committee on Diet and Health, 1989). The rates of CHD are 3 to 4 times higher in men than women during middle age, and twice as high in the elderly.

Early heart attacks occur predominantly in men. Women have relatively little cardiovascular disease, during the childbearing years, suggesting that female sex hormones are a protective factor. After menopause, however, the incidence of CHD among women prevails at a level only slightly lower than in men.

Genetic factors predisposing to CHD are probably related to genetic controls of serum cholesterol and lipoprotein concentration (Committee on Diet and Health, 1989). Members of families with a history of heart attacks are considered to be in the category of highest risk for CHD. The risk in men with a family history of CHD is 1.5 to 2 times as great as for men without such a history; the genetic factor is somewhat less of a risk in women. Blacks of both sexes are less susceptible than whites.

Nonlipid Controllable Risk Factors

Data from the original Framingham study in 1943 found the highest correlations with cigarette smoking, hypertension, and hypercholesterolemia (Further

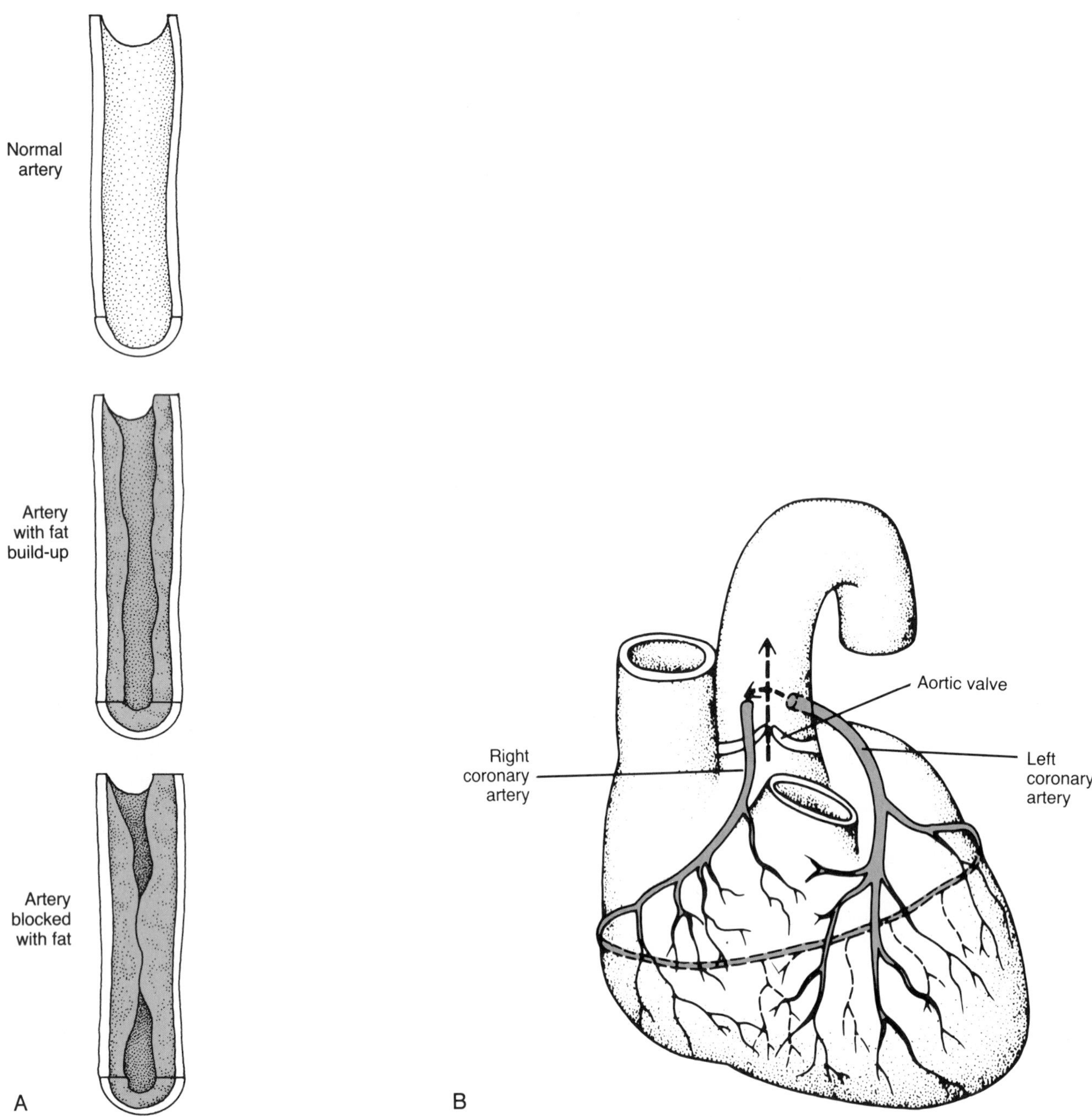

FIGURE 20–3. A, *Development of atherosclerosis.* B, *Coronary arteries.* (B, *From Guyton AC: Textbook of Medical Physiology, 8th ed. Philadelphia, WB Saunders, 1991, p. 237.)*

Reading, p. 362). Together these three factors account for 50% of CHD- related deaths (Council for Agricultural Science . . . , 1986). Glucose intolerance, obesity, and lack of physical activity have also been identified as risk factors.

Cigarette Smoking

In populations where the average diet is high in saturated fatty acids and cholesterol and where serum cholesterol levels are high, cigarette smoking is a major risk factor for CHD (Pooling Project Research Group, 1978; Stamler et al, 1986). The risk increases with the number of cigarettes smoked each day. Quitting smoking can reduce risk as much as 50% (Committee on Diet and Health, 1989).

Hypertension

Hypertension appears to aggravate the atherosclerotic process, possibly by weakening the artery walls at points of highest pressure, thus inviting invasion of

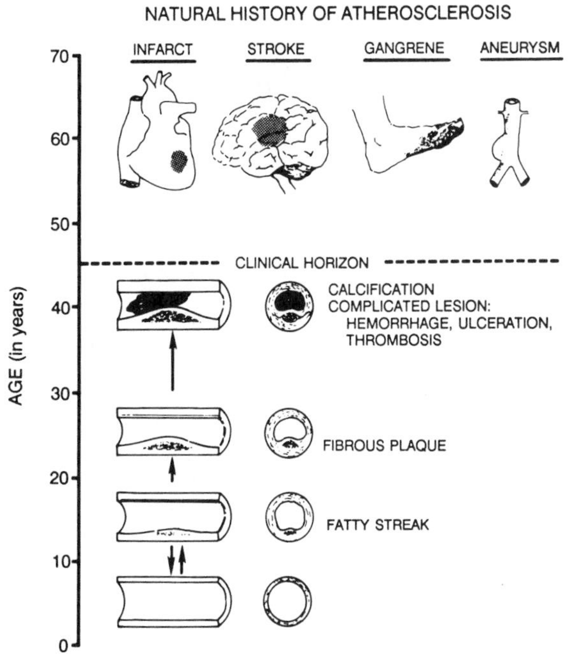

FIGURE 20–4. *Natural progression of atherosclerosis. (Redrawn from NRC, Diet and Health: Implications for Reducing Chronic Disease Risk. Report of the Committee on Diet and Health, Food and Nutrition Board, Washington, DC, National Academy Press, 1989, p 530; From McGill HC et al: Natural history of human atherosclerotic lesions.* In *Sandler M and Bourne GH [eds]: Atherosclerosis and Its Origin. New York, Academic Press, 1963.)*

cholesterol and other lipids (see Chapter 21). HDL-cholesterol levels are lower in hypertension.

Obesity

Obesity is an independent risk factor for CHD when evaluated in studies of long duration with an adequate number of subjects. The mechanism of this effect is not clear, but may be related to the fact that levels of atherogenic lipoproteins (very low density lipoproteins [VLDL] and LDL) are elevated and HDL decreased in obesity. The obese produce 20% more endogenous cholesterol per unit of body weight than the nonobese (Council for Agricultural Science . . . , 1986; Committee on Diet and Health, 1989).

Obesity is also associated with CHD morbidity and mortality as a secondary risk factor through its relationship to the development of hypertension, diabetes, and hypercholesterolemia.

It is estimated that 40% of CHD in all women and 70% in obese women is related to overweight. The risk of coronary death is markedly increased at weights 140% of ideal or body mass index of 30 and above. However, a study of 115,886 middle-aged women showed that although the incidence of CHD and fatal myocardial infarction (MI) was 3 times as high in the heaviest weight category, the risk of CHD was increased by even mild or moderate overweight (Manson et al, 1990). Some data indicate that weight distribution (upper-body or abdominal versus lower-body) is even more predictive of CHD risk (Despres et al, 1988) (see Chapter 18).

Inactivity

Data relating inactivity to CHD are conflicting. A strong relationship has not been established between exercise and the incidence of CHD even though exercise is known to elevate serum levels of HDL-cholesterol, possibly through a reduction of hepatic lipase activity that is also seen during weight reduction (Wood et al, 1988). It has also been theorized that the increased vascularity of the myocardium resulting from exercise potentiates the evolution of collateral circulation that contributes to survival following a heart attack.

One study comparing the results of dieting versus exercise as a means of reducing weight found that although the dieters lost more weight, both groups lost the same amount of fat and the effect on serum lipids was the same for both methods. The HDL were increased and the triglycerides decreased, both significantly, while total cholesterol and LDL remained the same (Wood et al, 1988). Another study has positively associated fitness, as measured by response to treadmill testing, with a lower risk of death from CHD in clinically healthy men (Ekelund et al, 1988). An extensive review by the Centers for Disease Control of data relating inactivity and CHD found a statistically significant association equal to that of the major CHD risk factors. In view of the fact that approximately 59% of Americans fail to exercise regularly (3 times or more per week for 20 minutes or more at a time), these authors believe that lack of exercise may be one of the foremost risk factors for CHD (Centers for Disease Control, 1987).

Epidemiologic data, however, fail to corroborate these findings. The Seven Countries study found no correlation between heart disease and the amount of activity involved in habitual occupations. Those with the most activity ranged from the country with the highest level of CHD (Finland) to the one with the lowest (Japan) (Keys, 1970).

Serum Lipids As Risk Factors

A considerable amount of epidemiologic data from countries around the world has emphasized the relationship between serum cholesterol levels and the incidence of CHD. Clinical and laboratory data, including studies with primates, support the relationship of serum cholesterol levels to heart disease. More re-

FURTHER READING: Framingham Heart Study

Of the many extensive studies that have endeavored to identify the risk factors leading to coronary heart disease (CHD), a unique and most productive one has been the Framingham Heart Study. This prospective and noninvasive study, which was initiated in 1949 under the direction of Dr. William Castelli, involved every other adult between the ages of 30 and 62 years living in the manufacturing town of Framingham, Massachusetts. Of the original 5,209 participants, all of whom agreed to return for check-ups and data collection at regular intervals for the rest of their lives, 2,500 were still living in 1985 (NIH, 1985).

Among the CHD risk factors positively identified by this study for the first time were high blood pressure, elevated cholesterol level, and cigarette smoking. Also associated were obesity and the protective effect of exercise. Later, the relationships of the different cholesterol fractions were clarified. The study was also the first to identify high blood pressure as the major cause of stroke.

In 1972, a companion study was initiated to measure the influence of heredity and environment on the offspring of the original participants (Wilson et al, 1989). Dietary practices, which were not followed in the initial study, were included along with more sophisticated measurements of physical status. This cohort of 5,000, which also includes spouses of the offspring, appears to date to be more health conscious than the older generation as reflected in less smoking, lower blood pressure, and lower cholesterol levels than seen in their parents at the same age. It will be interesting to see what this means in terms of CHD morbidity and mortality in this second generation.

cently, a number of large intervention studies have been conducted to corroborate these findings. Although the results have been inconclusive or contradictory to some degree, the preponderance of information associates high levels of serum lipids with the incidence of atherosclerosis and the morbidity and mortality from CHD. The National Research Council (NRC) Committee on Diet and Health defined the relationship as "strong, continuous, positive" and "established unequivocably" (Committee on Diet and Health, 1989, p 166). Although triglycerides have also been implicated, the testimony of these data has led primarily to the *lipid hypothesis,* which holds that lowering elevated levels of serum cholesterol will reduce the probability of CHD.

Hypercholesterolemia

Cholesterol has been implicated in the etiology of atherosclerosis ever since Anitschkow in 1913 induced atheromatous plaques in rabbits and identified cholesterol as their major component. Most data have been obtained in terms of total serum cholesterol. However, it is now apparent that levels of the lipoprotein transport fractions, LDL and HDL, are more significant in terms of cause, prevention, and prediction.

Cholesterol Transport. Cholesterol is absorbed from the small intestine in the company of other lipids in *chylomicrons* and transported to the liver, where triglycerides are removed through the action of *lipoprotein lipase (LPL).* The chylomicron fragments are cleared by the liver and the cholesterol is repackaged for transport in the blood in VLDL. The VLDL, which are predominantly triglyceride, circulate to the periphery where they evolve into LDL as the action of LPL removes some of the triglyceride for use by the cells (see Chapter 4). The LDL are the primary transport vehicle for lipids, including cholesterol and triglyceride (Fig. 20–5). The atherogenic effect of LDL-cholesterol (LDL-C) is readily apparent in genetic diseases characterized by high levels of this cholesterol fraction.

HDL are a separate group of lipoproteins which contain less cholesterol than LDL. Of the several classes of HDL, HDL-2 (larger, more lipid-rich) and HDL-3 (smaller, denser) predominate in human plasma.

Lipoprotein Roles in CHD. LDL appear to be involved in transport of cholesterol into the arterial wall. Some studies suggest that the uptake of LDL by macrophages into the intimal layer precedes the development of the fatty streak.

Although the relationship of LDL-C with atherosclerosis has been known for some time, an inverse relationship of HDL-cholesterol (HDL-C) to CHD has been recognized more recently. This "protective" effect has been confirmed by other studies, including the Helsinki Heart Study, in which simultaneous increases in HDL-C and decreases in LDL-C during gemfibrozil therapy were accompanied by 34% reduction in rates of MI (Frick et al, 1987; Gordon and Rifkind, 1989). The inverse relationship of HDL-C to CHD suggests that these lipoproteins remove cholesterol from the intima, or at least carry serum cholesterol away to the liver before it can be deposited in plaque. Inasmuch as a direct role for HDL-C has not been identified, it has been suggested that HDL-C *per se* may not be actively involved in preventing the accumulation of plaque cholesterol, but that higher levels only reflect a healthy transportation system that does not lead to atheroscle-

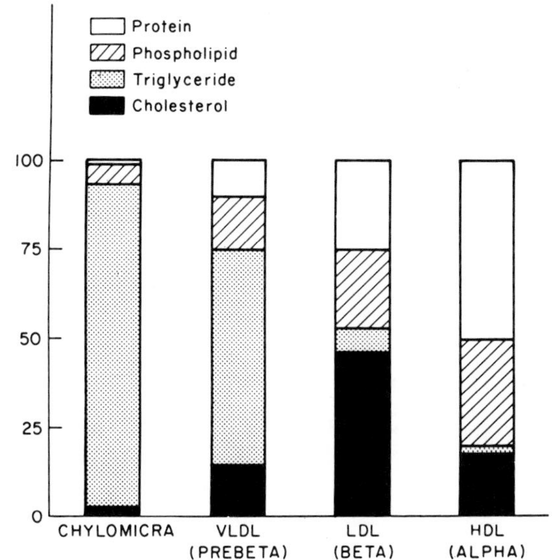

FIGURE 20–5. *Composition of the lipoproteins. (VLDL = very low density lipoproteins; LDL = low-density lipoproteins; HDL = high-density lipoproteins.)*

rosis (Eisenberg, 1984). Although the cholesterol involved in these two transport forms is popularly referred to as "good" or "bad" cholesterol, it is of course the lipoprotein form rather than the cholesterol being transported that is associated with CHD.

LEVELS OF LDL-C AND HDL-C. LDL levels are elevated by diets high in saturated fat and cholesterol. These dietary fats are thought to interfere with clearance of LDL-C from plasma by suppressing activity of LDL receptors in the liver (Blum and Levy, 1989). LDL-C levels are also high in obesity, and high levels are associated with diabetes, hypothyroidism, and familial types of hyperlipidemia. Estrogen decreases LDL-C concentration in varied degrees depending on the ratio of estrogen to progestin (National Center for Health Statistics, 1987).

Children of both sexes have similar levels of HDL-C until puberty, after which the levels of females consistently run 10 to 20 mg/dl higher than those of men throughout life (Levy, 1986). Blacks have slightly higher levels of HDL than whites, a factor that may be involved in the lesser incidence of CHD in this group. HDL-C increases with exercise (Wood et al, 1988), loss of excess weight, and moderate consumption of alcohol (Levy, 1986). It is lowered by obesity, lack of exercise, heavy cigarette smoking (20 cigarettes per day), androgenic and related steroids, beta-adrenergic blocking agents, hypertriglyceridemia, and genetic factors (Quit smoking . . . , 1978; Science News, 1979).

The fact that HDL-C is lowered somewhat by diets high in carbohydrate and low in fat has led to the suggestion that fats should not be reduced below the level that will provide 30% of total kilocalories (Levy, 1986).

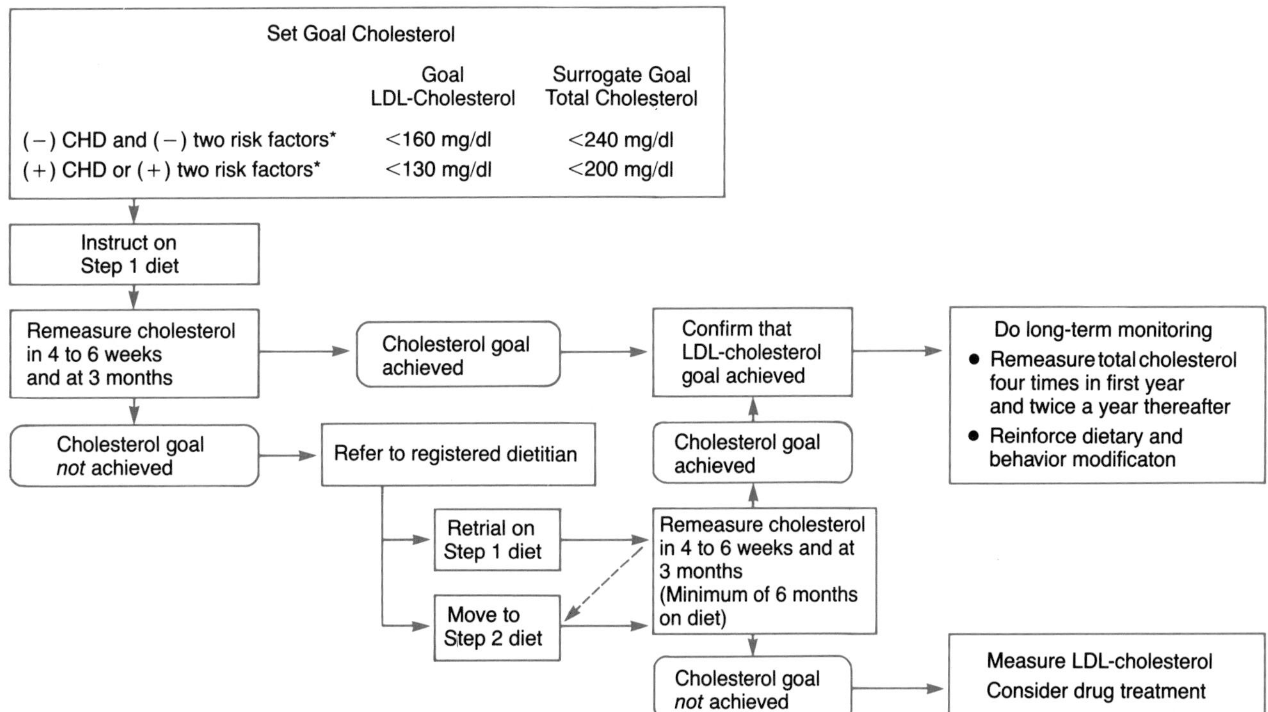

FIGURE 20–6. *Dietary treatment of hypercholesterolemia. (From Expert Panel on Detection, Evaluation and Treatment of High Blood Cholesterol in Adults: High Blood Cholesterol in Adults, National Cholesterol Education Program, NIH Publ. No. 89-2925, NIH. PHS, USDHHS, 1989, p 45.)*

Risk. Population correlations between total cholesterol (TC) and LDL-C cholesterol are strong. Lipoprotein levels considered to be at risk for CHD are (1) LDL-C above 130 mg/dl, (2) HDL-C below 35 mg/dl, and (3) TC above 200 mg/dl (Fig. 20–6). Ratios of both TC and LDL-C to HDL-C are used as points beyond which diet therapy should be instituted to reduce CHD risk (Liebman, 1990; McNamara, 1990). Ideally, TC : HDL-C should be less than 3.5; risk increases between 3.5 and 4.5. When TC is between 200 and 400 mg/dl, the TC : HDL-C ratio is a 3 to 4 times better predictor of heart disease risk than LDL-C alone and 5 to 6 times better than TC alone (Liebman, 1990).

Reduced HDL-C in the presence of elevated LDL-C favors the use of drugs for treatment (Expert Panel . . . , 1989). Patients should be advised to quit smoking, reduce body weight if obese, increase exercise if sedentary, and avoid use of anabolic steroids (e.g., athletes). Major causes of reduced HDL-C are listed in Table 20–1.

Measurement. Most studies in the past have measured TC. Even though current emphasis is on the lipoprotein forms of cholesterol transport, TC continues to be measured to a large degree because the test is simpler, less expensive, and does not require fasting before the test. Because the large part of TC is made up of LDL cholesterol, these two measurements are usually parallel. However, it has been observed that HDL-C and LDL-C are independent risk factors and that combining them into a single number conceals possibly useful information (Expert Panel . . . , 1989).

Determination of LDL-C requires measurement of TC, triglycerides (TG), and HDL-C. Although cholesterol can be determined in the nonfasting state, TG must be measured after a 12-hour fast to allow time for exogenous chylomicrons to clear. Therefore, a complete lipid profile requires that the person be fasting. The formula for calculating LDL-C is as follows:

$$\text{LDL-C} = \text{TC} - \text{HDL-C} - (\text{TG}/5)$$

where LDL-C = low-density lipoprotein cholesterol; HDL-C = high-density lipoprotein cholesterol; TC = total cholesterol; and TG = triglycerides.

Reference values for plasma lipid levels in the adult U.S. population are shown in Table 20–2, and corresponding levels of lipids in mg/dl and mmol/l are indicated in Clinical Insight, page 366. HDL-C below 35 mg/dl is considered to be an independent risk factor. Reference plasma lipid levels for children and adolescents are given in Clinical Insight, page 366.

TABLE 20–1. Causes of Low Serum HDL–Cholesterol

Cigarette smoking
Obesity
Inactivity
Androgenic and related steroids
Androgens
Progestational agents
Anabolic steroids
Beta-adrenergic blocking agents
Hypertriglyceridemia
Genetic factors

Hypertriglyceridemia

Hypertriglyceridemia is caused by an increase in VLDL resulting in a fasting plasma triglyceride level over 500 mg/dl. Higher levels of 750 to 1,000 mg/dl and over also involve accumulation of chylomicrons and a "milky" appearing plasma. At extreme levels, the condition is characterized by xanthomas and abdominal pain, with pancreatitis a risk at levels above 1,000 mg/dl. Most borderline cases are caused by exogenous or secondary factors that raise the triglyceride level, such as obesity, uncontrolled diabetes, untreated hypothyroidism, chronic renal disease, liver disease, and excessive alcohol intake. Triglyceride levels below 250 mg/dl with normal cholesterol are not associated with risk of disease (Expert Panel . . . , 1989).

Data associating high levels of plasma TG levels with CHD are conflicting. Prospective data from the Lipid Research Clinic Prevalence Study indicated that TG levels are strong predictors of death from CHD, particularly among men with lower levels of LDL-C. The Consensus Panel concluded that plasma TG levels are not an independent risk factor; however the Framingham study found them to be a risk factor in women (Expert Panel . . . , 1989).

Other Hyperlipidemias

Several relatively rare forms of hyperlipidemia have strong genetic components. (Terminology in parentheses is from an earlier classification that may still be in use to some degree.)

Familial hypercholesterolemia (Type 2a hyperlipoproteinemia) occurs in either a heterozygous form (1 in 500) or a homozygous form (extremely rare) and is diagnosed in the first or second year of life. The LDL receptors on the cells are either absent or nonfunctional. TC usually exceeds 300 mg/dl and LDL-C exceeds 200 mg/dl. Tendon xanthomas, corneal arcus, premature CHD, and a strong family history of hypercholesterolemia are common. Affected males develop CHD in their 40s, 30s or earlier; in women, CHD often occurs in the 50s and 60s. Drug treatment is combined with diet therapy at the step 2 level (see later) when diet

TABLE 20–2. Reference Values for Plasma Lipid Levels*

Total Plasma Cholesterol (mg/dl)

White Male							*White Female*						
			Percentiles							*Percentiles*			
Age (Yrs)	*Number*	*Mean*	*5*	*75*	*90*	*95*	*Age (Yrs)*	*Number*	*Mean*	*5*	*75*	*90*	*95*
0–19	5,749	155	115	170	185	200	0–19	5,470	160	120	175	190	200
20–24	882	185	125	185	205	220	20–24	1,566	170	125	190	215	230
25–29	2,042	180	135	200	225	245	25–34	4,340	175	130	195	220	235
30–34	2,444	190	140	215	240	255	35–39	2,012	185	140	205	230	245
35–39	2,320	200	145	225	250	270	40–44	2,050	195	145	215	235	255
40–44	2,428	205	150	230	250	270	45–49	2,149	205	150	225	250	270
45–69	7,710	215	160	235	260	275	50–54	1,992	220	165	240	265	285
70+	850	205	150	230	250	270	55+	4,478	230	170	250	275	295

Plasma LDL-Cholesterol (mg/dl)

White Male							*White Female*						
			Percentiles							*Percentiles*			
Age (Yrs)	*Number*	*Mean*	*5*	*75*	*90*	*95*	*Age (Yrs)*	*Number*	*Mean*	*5*	*75*	*90*	*95*
5–19	713	95	65	105	120	130	5–19	652	100	65	110	125	140
20–24	118	105	65	120	140	145	20–24	199	105	55	120	140	160
25–29	253	115	70	140	155	185	25–34	646	110	70	125	145	160
30–34	403	125	80	145	165	185	35–39	299	120	75	140	160	170
35–39	371	135	80	155	175	190	40–44	318	125	75	145	165	175
40–44	385	135	85	155	175	185	45–49	326	130	80	150	175	185
45–69	1,162	145	90	165	190	205	50–54	256	140	90	160	185	200
70+	119	145	90	165	180	185	55+	688	150	95	170	195	215

Plasma HDL-Cholesterol (mg/dl)

White Male						*White Female*					
			Percentiles						*Percentiles*		
Age (Yrs)	*Number*	*Mean*	*5*	*10*	*95*	*Age (Yrs)*	*Number*	*Mean*	*5*	*10*	*95*
5–14	438	55	35	40	75	5–19	666	55	35	40	70
15–19	299	45	30	35	65	20–24	199	55	35	35	80
20–24	118	45	30	30	65	25–34	649	55	35	40	80
25–29	253	45	30	30	65	35–39	298	55	35	40	80
30–34	403	45	30	30	65	40–44	318	60	35	40	90
35–39	371	45	30	30	60	45–49	328	60	35	40	85
40–44	383	45	25	30	65	50–54	256	60	35	40	90
45–69	1,182	50	30	30	70	55+	668	60	35	40	95
70+	119	50	30	35	75						

Plasma Triglycerides (mg/dl)

Male						*Female*					
			Percentiles						*Percentiles*		
Age (Yrs)	*Number*	*Mean*	*5*	*90*	*95*	*Age (Yrs)*	*Number*	*Mean*	*5*	*90*	*95*
0–9	1,491	55	30	85	100	0–9	1,304	60	35	95	110
10–14	2,278	65	30	100	125	10–19	4,166	75	40	115	130
15–19	1,980	80	35	120	150	20–34	5,906	90	40	145	170
20–24	882	100	45	165	200	35–39	2,012	95	40	160	195
25–29	2,042	115	45	200	250	40–44	2,050	105	45	170	210
30–34	2,444	130	50	215	265	45–49	2,149	110	45	185	230
35–39	2,320	145	55	250	320	50–54	1,992	120	55	190	240
40–54	6,862	150	55	250	320	55–64	2,768	125	55	200	250
55–64	2,526	140	60	235	290	65+	1,710	130	60	205	240
65+	1,600	135	55	210	260						

* From Rifkind BM and Segal P: Lipid Research Clinics Program: Reference values for hyperlipidemia and hypolipidemia. JAMA 250:1869–1872, 1983.

CLINICAL INSIGHT: Corresponding Levels of Lipids in mg/dl and mmol/l

Cholesterol		Triglycerides	
mg/dl	*mmol/l*	*mg/dl*	*mmol/l*
35	0.9	250	2.8
130	3.4	400	4.5
160	4.1	500	5.6
190	4.9	1000	11.3
200	5.2		
240	6.2		

therapy alone is not successful (Expert Panel . . . , 1989).

Familial combined hyperlipidemia is caused by hepatic overproduction of lipoproteins. It occurs in about 15% of CHD patients before 60 years of age. Several lipid phenotypes may occur in the same family, two thirds of which will be in one of two forms: (1) increase in VLDL only, with TG levels of 400 to 1,000 mg/dl and TC normal or elevated (Type 4 hyperlipoproteinemia, familial endogenous hypertriglyceridemia) or (2) increase in LDL only, with TG normal, TC 300 to 600 mg/dl (Type 2a hyperlipoproteinemia, familial hypercholesterolemia). The remainder occur as (1) increase in VLDL and LDL, with TG 150 to 1,000 mg/dl and TC 300 to 600 mg/dl (Type 2b hyperlipoproteinemia, familial combined hypercholesterolemia), (2) increased VLDL and chylomicrons with TG over

CLINICAL INSIGHT: NCEP Recommendations for Detection and Management of Hypercholesterolemia in Children and Adolescents

In April 1991 the NCEP made recommendations for management of hypercholesterolemia to be applied to adolescents and children over the age of about 2 years (Report, 1991). This is the first time that there has been consensus among pediatric experts, lipid researchers, and nutrition and health care communities on this subject (Timely, 1991).

For the general population of children and adolescents in the U.S., NCEP recommended that there be adoption of eating patterns to meet the following criteria:

Nutritionally adequate, varied diet

Adequate energy intake to support growth and development and maintain appropriate body weight

Saturated fat—less than 10% of total calories

Total fat—an average of no more than 30%

Dietary cholesterol—less than 300 mg/day

To implement these patterns means involvement of the entire community—parents, in selection and preparation of food; schools, in modification of school food service; health care clinics, in health education; government, in improvement of food labeling; and the food industry, in development of low-saturated-fat, low-fat foods appealing to children.

NCEP also aims to identify and treat individual children and adolescents who have hypercholesterolemia and a family history of premature cardiovascular disease, or whose parents have hypercholesterolemia. For this group the NCEP recommends:

Blood cholesterol screening of children and adolescents whose parents or grandparents, at 55 years or younger, were found to have coronary atherosclerosis; suffered myocardial infarction, peripheral vascular disease, cerebrovascular disease, or sudden death; or underwent invasive cardiac therapy (balloon angioplasty or coronary artery bypass surgery)

Blood cholesterol screening of offspring of a parent with a blood cholesterol of 240 mg/dl or greater

Appropriate levels for TC and LDL-C (see Table A)

For children with levels above these, dietary change is recommended

TABLE A. Levels of Blood Total and LDL Cholesterol in Children and Adolescents

Category	Total Cholesterol	LDL-Cholesterol
Acceptable	<170 mg/dl	<110 mg/dl
Borderline	170–199 mg/dl	110–129 mg/dl
High	≥200 mg/dl	≥130 mg/dl

The Step 1 Diet is used for 3 months and blood cholesterol is reassessed. If the desired cholesterol level is not reached, the Step 2 Diet should be implemented for at least another 6 months. If after 6 months to 1 year of dietary therapy there is insufficient blood lipid lowering, drug therapy can be considered in children over 10 years of age.

1,000 mg/dl (Type 5 hyperlipoproteinemia, mixed hyperlipemia), and (3) increased LDL-apolipoprotein-b (apo-b) with normal LDL-cholesterol (hyperapobetalipoproteinemia).

Diagnosis is through testing of first-degree relatives and by identification of multiple lipoprotein phenotypes in a single family. All of these forms involve increased risk of CHD. Diet and physical exercise resulting in the loss of even a few pounds of excess weight may lower plasma lipid levels. Therapy with nicotinic acid, which interferes with lipoprotein formation, may be required (Expert Panel . . . , 1989).

Familial dysbetalipoproteinemia (Type 3 hyperlipoproteinemia) is relatively uncommon (1 in 5,000 persons in the United States). Catabolism of VLDL remnants and chylomicrons is delayed due to a basic abnormality in the structure of apolipoprotein E. TC levels are elevated, and TG levels are even higher. LDL-C rarely is increased. There is increased risk of premature CHD and peripheral vascular disease. Treatment involves weight reduction, control of hyperglycemia and diabetes, and dietary restriction of cholesterol and saturated fat. If diet is not effective, drug therapy is recommended.

Severe primary hypercholesterolemia occurs in about 1% of the adult population. TC levels persistently over 300 mg/dl pose considerable risk for CHD. This form is often resistant to diet and must be managed with drugs (Expert Panel . . . , 1989).

Diabetic dyslipidemia and *hyperlipidemia of pregnancy and lactation* are discussed in Chapters 9 and 31, respectively.

RELATION OF DIETARY FACTORS TO SERUM LIPIDS

Dietary Fats

Data associating dietary fats with the incidence of CHD originated in epidemiologic studies showing that populations with relatively little heart disease consumed diets that were low in total fat, saturated fat, and cholesterol. On a worldwide basis, no population subsisting on a low-fat diet has been found to have high cholesterol levels or a high frequency of heart attacks (Keys, 1970). These data have been verified by clinical studies, although the results tend to be conflicting when applied to individuals.

Total fat intakes are related to obesity, which in turn is involved with major risk factors for atherosclerosis. However the primary influence of fat on CHD is associated with the effect of dietary fatty acid components and cholesterol on serum cholesterol, particularly LDL-C.

Saturation of Fatty Acids

The influence of fatty acids on development of serum cholesterol is measured in terms of their variable degrees of saturation, which influence the levels of LDL-C and HDL-C in different ways. Reaction of individuals to different saturation levels is by no means uniform, however.

SATURATED FATTY ACIDS. In general, *saturated fatty acids (SFA)* tend to elevate both LDL-C and HDL-C. However, the effect appears to be limited to fatty acids of chain length between 10 and 18 (C-10 and C-18) (Hegsted et al, 1965; Keys et al, 1965) (see Chapter 4). The most atherogenic SFA are myristic (C-14) and palmitic (C-16), and possibly lauric (C-12). Stearic acid (C-18) is an exception in that it is desaturated to oleic acid so rapidly that it does not have a cholesterol-raising effect (Grundy et al, 1988). Stearic acid is the most common saturated fatty acid in beef (20%), coconut oil, and cocoa butter. However, because these foods also contain palmitic acid (C-16), they continue to raise serum cholesterol. Some people appear to be "SFA sensitive," responding to SFA with much higher elevations of serum cholesterol than is generally seen.

POLYUNSATURATED FATTY ACIDS

Omega-6 Polyunsaturated Fatty Acids. For many years the use of the ω-6 form of *polyunsaturated fatty acids (PUFA)* has been encouraged because of their ability to lower serum cholesterol levels when substituted for SFA. Enthusiasm for PUFA diminished to some degree when they were associated with incidence of cancer, but evaluation of existing data appears to have cleared them of that stigma (Committee on Diet and Health, 1989). In recent years, however, as knowledge of the different lipoprotein cholesterol forms became more sophisticated, it was realized that when substituted for SFA, ω-6 PUFA lower both LDL- C and HDL-C. Further, eliminating SFA is twice as effective in lowering serum cholesterol levels as increasing PUFA (Grande et al, 1972; Kuske and Feldman, 1987).

Omega-6 PUFA are widespread in foods, but the major source is in vegetable oils, the consumption of which has almost doubled in the past 90 years. Table 20–3 gives the fatty acid content of major fats and oils in the American diet.

Omega-3 Polyunsaturated Fatty Acids. *Omega-3 polyunsaturated fatty acids (ω-3 PUFA)* became the focus of widespread interest when attention was drawn to Eskimo populations in Greenland, whose high intakes of fish oils were associated with low incidence of CHD. A study in the Netherlands found lowered incidence of

TABLE 20–3. Fatty Acid Composition of Fats and Oils* †

Product (1 T)	Saturated Fatty Acids (g)	Cholesterol (mg)	Polyunsaturated Fatty Acids (g)	Monounsaturated Fatty Acids (g)
Canola oil	0.9	0	4.5	7.6
Safflower oil	1.2	0	10.1	1.6
Sunflower oil	1.4	0	5.5	6.2
Peanut butter, smooth	1.5	0	2.3	3.7
Corn oil	1.7	0	8.0	3.3
Olive oil	1.8	0	1.1	9.9
Hydrogenated sunflower oil	1.8	0	4.9	6.3
Margarine, liquid, bottled	1.8	0	5.1	3.9
Margarine, soft, tub	1.8	0	3.9	4.8
Sesame oil	1.9	0	5.7	5.4
Soybean oil	2.0	0	7.9	3.2
Margarine, stick	2.1	0	3.6	5.1
Peanut oil	2.3	0	4.3	6.2
Cottonseed oil	3.5	0	7.1	2.4
Lard	5.0	12	1.4	5.8
Beef tallow	6.4	14	0.5	5.3
Palm oil	6.7	0	1.3	5.0
Butter	7.1	31	0.4	3.3
Cocoa butter	8.1	0	0.4	4.5
Palm kernel oil	11.1	0	0.2	1.5
Coconut oil	11.8	0	0.2	0.8

* From USDHHS: Eating to Lower Your High Blood Cholesterol. NIH Publ No 89-2920. Washington, DC, NCEP, NHLBI, 1989.

† Sources: Composition of Foods: Fats and Oils—Raw · Processed · Prepared, Agriculture Handbook 8-4. United States Department of Agriculture, Science and Education Administration (June 1979); Composition of Foods: Legumes and Legume Products—Raw · Processed · Prepared, Agriculture Handbook 8-16. United States Department of Agriculture, Human Nutrition Information Service (December 1986).

CHD in populations eating fish at least 3 times per week (Kromhout et al, 1985).

Omega-3 PUFA appear to reduce levels of plasma triglyceride, probably by inhibiting synthesis of VLDL. Any effect of lowering LDL-C is related to their displacement of SFA; simply adding ω-3 PUFA to a diet without simultaneously reducing SFA has no effect. These highly unsaturated fatty acids (*eicosapentaenoic* and *docosahexaenoic*) are precursors of the prostaglandins that interfere with blood clotting (see page 47). Excessive intakes result in prolonged bleeding times, a condition common to Eskimo populations with high dietary intakes.

MONOUNSATURATED FATTY ACIDS. A large body of data has accumulated over the years attesting to the neutrality of *monounsaturated fatty acids (MUFA)* in elevating serum cholesterol levels. However more recent studies have shown that when substituted for SFA, MUFA also lower serum cholesterol levels, in particular LDL-C, while HDL-C remains unchanged. Some studies have demonstrated lowering serum cholesterol by substituting MUFA for SFA at total fat levels similar to those currently consumed by the American public (Mensink et al, 1989). When compared with a diet high in SFA, a diet of 20% fat lowered TC and LDL-C but raised TG and significantly decreased HDL-C, whereas a diet containing 40% of kilocalories from fat, 43% of which was MUFA, lowered TC and LDL-C but had no effect on TG or HDL-C (Grundy, 1986). If supported by further studies, these findings provide the heartening possibility of formulating diets less restrictive in fat content and therefore more palatable.

Dietary monounsaturates occur almost exclusively in the form of oleic acid, which constitutes nearly one half (45%) of the fat in the American diet. Some vegetable oils, namely olive oil and canola (rapeseed) oil, are very high in MUFA. Dietary intakes of people on the island of Crete, where the incidence of CHD is very low and the olive oil content of the diet is very high, provide 40% of total energy from fat, only 8 per cent of which is saturated (Keys, 1970) (see Table 20–3).

Dietary Cholesterol

The intake of cholesterol has been positively related to the risk of CHD after adjusting for other risk factors such as age, blood pressure, serum cholesterol, and cigarette smoking.

Because of the endogenous feedback system that responds to dietary intakes of cholesterol by regulating liver synthesis, dietary cholesterol tends to have a minor effect on serum cholesterol compared with the intake of SFA. However, some people appear to have less sensitive feedback systems and therefore respond to higher cholesterol intakes with rapidly elevated serum levels.

To reduce TC significantly by lowering dietary cholesterol alone would require a daily intake of less than 150 mg/dl, a requirement that would essentially eliminate all animal products. The average daily intake of cholesterol is between 400 and 500 mg/dl (Council for Agricultural Science . . . , 1986).

Other Dietary Factors

Some people are sensitive to a *high carbohydrate* load and may respond with a temporary increase in serum triglycerides and lower HDL-C (Blum and Levy, 1989). This response appears to be related to obesity, diabetes mellitus, and impaired glucose tolerance (Committee on Diet and Health, 1989). Starches are less atherogenic than sugars, however, probably because of the difference in insulin response.

Although soluble dietary fiber can lower serum cholesterol in people with high serum lipid levels, evidence that fiber can lower risk of CHD is inconclusive. Evidence suggests that *soluble dietary fiber*—in particular, oat bran, pectin, psyllium, legume fiber, and guar gum—lowers serum cholesterol by binding with bile acids and preventing their reabsorption (Anderson and Gustafson, 1988). By increasing bulk in the large intestine, it also reduces exposure of bile salts to the mucosal cells where it is absorbed. One study suggests that the soluble fiber in oat bran is effective only to the extent that it replaces or diminishes intake of foods high in SFA (Swain et al, 1990). Insoluble fibers such as cellulose and lignin have no effect on serum cholesterol levels.

Alcohol in moderate amounts (50 to 100 g distributed throughout the week) is associated with lower risk of CHD, possibly through its effect of elevating HDL-C. However, it also increases endogenous production of triglycerides and VLDL.

A weak association of cholesterol levels with *coffee* consumption (5 to 6 cups/day) has been seen in some studies but the results are inconsistent (Rosemarin, 1989). Boiled coffee appears to raise cholesterol levels more than filtered coffee (Bak and Grobbee, 1989).

Animal proteins in the diet of experimental animals generally lead to higher blood cholesterol levels and more atherosclerosis than plant proteins (Council for Agricultural Science . . . , 1986). This may be important and reason to promote more consumption of plant proteins.

Trans fatty acids, stereo-isomers of the naturally occurring *cis* fatty acids, are artifacts of the hydrogenation process widely used in the food industry, particularly in the production of margarines and shortenings. Some evidence has linked these fatty acids with elevation of serum cholesterol (Vergroesen, 1972) as well as with lowering of HDL-C (Mensink and Katan, 1990). The average intake of *trans* fatty acids is estimated to be 6 to 8 g/day (Mensink and Katan, 1990).

TREATMENT AND PREVENTION

Although the relationship between serum cholesterol levels and the morbidity and mortality from CHD appears clearly established, the role of dietary factors remains more tenuous. In particular, the definitive study that establishes a positive relationship between dietary lipids and incidence of CHD has yet to be made. Intervention studies require following unpredictable human beings over unmanageable periods of time. A plan to conduct a large-scale prospective study in the United States was abandoned when it was determined that it would require from 100,000 to 300,000 subjects followed anywhere from 10 to 30 years (Levy, 1986).

Nonetheless certain factors have emerged from epidemiologic and clinical data that appear to identify those at risk of suffering a heart attack and to suggest appropriate treatment or preventive procedures. Whether such intervention is appropriate only for those identified as being "at risk" or for the entire population continues to invite controversy.

National Cholesterol Education Program

In 1987 the National Heart, Blood, and Lung Institute initiated a program designed to reduce the national incidence of CHD. The recommendations were generated by an Expert Panel on Detection, Evaluation and Treatment of High Blood Cholesterol in Adults. These recommendations, summarized in Table 20–4, are based on periodic monitoring of TC and LDL-C for all adults over 20 years of age at intervals determined by the presence of risk factors, and with treatment by diet or medication determined by risk factors and lipid levels (Expert Panel . . . , 1989).

Recommendations for children and adolescents are presented in Clinical Insight, page 366.

Rationale

The rationale for the National Cholesterol Education Program (NCEP) stems from the extensive data accumulated over a number of years that (1) identify cholesterol as the major constituent of atherosclerotic plaque and (2) show via epidemiologic, clinical, and prospective intervention studies that serum cholesterol levels are positively associated with incidence of CHD morbidity and mortality. Proof of dietary associations

TABLE 20–4. National Cholesterol Education Program, Treatment Guidelines for Adults National Institutes of Health*

Criteria	Action
If total blood cholesterol <200	Repeat total blood cholesterol in 5 years or at physical exam. Recommend general diet.
If total blood cholesterol 200–239 and	
• No CHD and <2 risk factors†	Repeat total blood cholesterol annually; Step 1 Diet.
• CHD present or ≥2 risk factors If total blood cholesterol ≥240	Determine LDL-C.
If LDL-C <130	Repeat total blood cholesterol in 5 years. Recommend general diet.
If LDL-C 130–159 and	
• No CHD and <2 risk factors	Repeat total blood cholesterol annually; Step 1 Diet
• CHD present or ≥2 risk factors If LDL-C ≥160	Clinical evaluation; Step 1 or 2 diet. Diet goals: LDL-C <160 or LDL-C <130 if CHD present or ≥2 risk factors
CONTINUE DIETARY TREATMENT FOR 6 MONTHS. IF GOALS NOT MET, CONSIDER DRUGS.	

* Summary prepared by Health Prospects, Suite 550, 1801 Rockville Pike, Rockville, MD 20852.
† Risk Factors for Coronary Heart Disease (CHD): Male sex; family history; cigarette smoking; hypertension; HDL < 35 mg/dl; diabetes mellitus; cerebrovascular disease or occlusive peripheral vascular disease; severe obesity.

with CHD is lacking; however, considerable data support the propensity of saturated fat and cholesterol to elevate serum cholesterol levels. Although most data have been accumulated in studies of middle-aged men, the Expert Panel concluded that there was no reason to believe the results could not be broadened to cover women and the elderly. Further, although no definitive studies have actually been carried out to support the recommendation of dietary modifications for individuals at risk of CHD, it was believed that such action is justified on a public health basis (Expert Panel . . . , 1989).

Recommendations for Treatment

The objective of the NCEP is to reduce CHD by identifying and reducing elevated levels of LDL-C. The goal is to reduce total serum cholesterol to less than 200 mg/dl and LDL-C to less than 130 mg/dl.

The recommended treatment program is based on monitoring serum cholesterol, instituting diets of progressively severe fat and cholesterol restriction, and prescribing medication. Levels of TC and LDL-C, as well as presence or absence of CHD risk factors, determine the appropriate combinations of measurement frequency, dietary requirements, and necessity for medication. The program is outlined in Figure 20–6.

Dietary Modifications

Diet modifications specified by the NCEP consist of recommendations for lowering total fat, saturated fat, and cholesterol and adjusting energy intake to achieve appropriate weight (Table 20–5). The *Step 1 Diet* contains less than 30% of total kilocalories from fat, less than 10% of kilocalories from saturated fatty acids, and less than 300 mg/day of cholesterol. The *Step 2 Diet* contains the same percentage of total kilocalories from fat, but SFA are reduced to less than 7% of kilocalories and cholesterol to less than 200 mg cholesterol per day.

The cholesterol lowering that can be expected to be achieved from the Step 1 Diet is an average reduction in

TABLE 20–5. Comparison of Step 1 and Step 2 Diets with Average American Diet*

Nutrient	Average American Diet		Step 1 Diet		Step 2 Diet	
Saturated fatty acids	15–20%	35–40% fat	<10%	<30% fat	<7%	<30% fat
Monounsaturated fatty acids	14–16%		10–15%		10–15%	
Polyunsaturated fatty acids	7%		up to 10%		up to 10%	
Carbohydrate	About 47%		50–60%		50–60%	
Protein	About 16%		up to 20%		Up to 20%	
Cholesterol	350–450 mg/day		<300 mg/day		<200 mg/day	
Total calories			To achieve and maintain weight			

* Adapted from Eating to Lower Your High Blood Cholesterol. National Cholesterol Education Program. NIH Publ No 89-2920. Washington, DC, NHLBI, NIH, USDHHS, 1989.

TABLE 20–6. Recommended Diet Modifications to Lower Blood Cholesterol: The Step 1 Diet*

Food Group	Choose	Decrease
Fish, chicken, turkey, and lean meats	Fish, poultry without skin, lean cuts of beef, lamb, pork or veal, shellfish	Fatty cuts of beef, lamb, or pork, spare ribs, organ meats, regular cold cuts, sausage, hot dogs, bacon, sardines, roe
Skim and low-fat milk, cheese, yogurt, and dairy substitutes	Skim or 1% fat milk (liquid, powdered, evaporated), buttermilk	Whole milk (4% fat): regular, evaporated, condensed; cream, half and half, 2% milk, imitation milk products, most nondairy creamers, whipped toppings
	Nonfat (0% fat) or low-fat yogurt	Whole-milk yogurt
	Low-fat cottage cheese (1% or 2% fat)	Whole-milk cottage cheese (4% fat)
	Low-fat cheeses, farmer or pot cheeses (all of these should be labeled no more than 2–6 g fat/oz)	All natural cheeses (e.g., blue, roquefort, camembert, cheddar, swiss)
	Low-fat or "light" cream cheese Low-fat or "light" sour cream	Cream cheeses, sour cream
	Sherbet Sorbet	Ice cream
Eggs	Egg whites (2 whites = 1 whole egg in recipes), cholesterol-free egg substitutes	Egg yolks
Fruits and vegetables	Fresh, frozen, canned, or dried fruits and vegetables	Vegetables prepared in butter, cream, cheese, or other sauces
Breads and cereals	Homemade baked goods using unsaturated oils sparingly, angel food cake, low-fat crackers, low-fat cookies	Commercial baked goods: pies, cakes, doughnuts, croissants, pastries, muffins, biscuits, high-fat crackers, high-fat cookies
	Rice, pasta	Egg noodles
	Whole-grain breads and cereals (oatmeal, whole wheat, rye, bran, multigrain, etc.)	Breads in which eggs are a major ingredient
Fats and oils	Baking cocoa	Chocolate
	Unsaturated vegetable oils: corn, olive, canola oil, safflower, sesame, soybean, sunflower	Butter, coconut oil, palm oil, palm kernel oil, lard, bacon fat, cocoa butter
	Margarine or shortening made from one of the unsaturated oils listed above	
	Diet margarine	
	Mayonnaise, salad dressings made with unsaturated oils listed above	Mayonnaise, dressings made with egg yolk
	Low-fat dressings and mayonnaise Seeds and nuts	Coconut

* Adapted from Expert Panel on Detection, Evaluation and Treatment of High Blood Cholesterol in Adults: High Blood Cholesterol in Adults. National Cholesterol Education Program, NIH Publ No 89-2925, Washington, DC, NHLBI, USDHHS, NIH, 1989.

cholesterol levels of 30 to 40 mg/ dl. The Step 2 Diet may lower these levels another 15 mg/dl. Most of the reduction is in the LDL-C fraction and response may be variable (Expert Panel . . . , 1989).

Reducing the average fat intake of the American diet to 30% (from 35 to 40%) of the total kilocalories means an approximate reduction of one fifth of the fat in the diet. Reducing the average saturated fat intake from 15 to 10% of total kilocalories means an approximate reduction of one third of the saturated fat in the diet. Reducing the cholesterol intake from 450 to 300 mg means reducing it by one third.

Following are three methods that may be used to achieve the goals of the Step 1 and Step 2 Diets.

Method I: The guidelines in Table 20–6 can be used to assist individuals in making food choices for the Step 1 Diet only. They are particularly appropriate for those who do not need to lose weight.

Method II: Table 20–7 gives the suggested number of servings of foods grouped by similar nutrient, especially fat content, for diets containing 30% of their calories from fat. Numbers of servings are presented for four energy levels—1,200, 1,600, 2,000, and 2,500 kcal. Adjustments for other levels can be made by adding or eliminating servings from food groups.

The serving sizes of foods in each of the food groups are presented in Table 20–8. The sweets/alcohol group includes only choices that are very low in fat. However,

Text continues on p. 376

TABLE 20–7. Eating Plans for Step 1 and Step 2 Diets

	Daily Portions—Step 1 Diet			
Food Group	***1,200 kcal***	***1,600 kcal***	***2,000 kcal***	***2,500 kcal***
Fats and oils	3	4	6	8
Fish, poultry, meat	6 oz	6 oz	6 oz	6 oz
Egg yolks	3/wk	3/wk	3/wk	3/wk
Dairy foods	2	3	3	4
Bread, beans, grains, and starches	3	4	7	10
Fruit	3	3	3	5
Vegetables	4	4	4	4
Sugars, sweets, alcohol	0	2	2	2
	Daily Portions—Step 2 Diet			
Food Group	***1,200 kcal***	***1,600 kcal***	***2,000 kcal***	***2,500 kcal***
Fats and oils	3	5	7	8
Fish, poultry, meat	6 oz	6 oz	6 oz	6 oz
Egg yolks	1/wk	1/wk	1/wk	1/wk
Dairy foods	2	2	2	3
Bread, beans, cereals, and starches	4	5	8	10
Fruit	3	3	4	7
Vegetables	4	4	4	5
Sugars, sweets, alcohol	0	2	2	2

TABLE 20–8. Choices and Serving Sizes for Step 1 and Step 2 Diets*

Fats and Oils

Notes: 1 serving = 5 g fat, 0 mg cholesterol, 45 calories.
Remember to count all the hidden teaspoons of fat in baked goods, in cooking, in sauces and salad dressings, as well as those added to other foods such as breads and vegetables.

Foods to Include	*Serving Size*
Oil	1 tsp
Recommended oils: safflower, sunflower, corn, soybean, sesame, olive, canola, walnut, or peanut	
Margarine	1 tsp
Margarines listing a liquid oil as the first ingredient	
Reduced-calorie margarines listing one of the aforementioned oils as the first ingredient.	2 tsp
Salad dressings and mayonnaise, prepared with a recommended oil	1 tsp
Reduced-calorie salad dressings and mayonnaise	4 tsp
Nuts and seeds	1 T, chopped
Avocado	1 T or ⅛
Olives	10 small or 5 large
Peanut butter	2 tsp
Nondairy creamer made with unsaturated oils	3 T liquid

Fats and Oils to Avoid

Fats
- Butter
- All margarines not listed above
- Lard, tallow, suet, shortening, bacon and meat drippings, gravies made from meat fat
- Coconut, coconut oil, cocoa butter, palm or palm kernel oil (usually used in commercial products such as baked goods, other nondairy creamers, whipped toppings, candy, fried foods)
- "Vegetable shortening" or "vegetable oil" when listed as the main source of fat in the list of ingredients
- "Hydrogenated fat"

Dressings
- Roquefort, blue cheese, green goddess, and others made with sour cream or cheese
- Dips made with cream cheese or sour cream

Nuts
- Macadamia

TABLE 20–8. Choices and Serving Sizes for Step 1 and Step 2 Diets *Continued*

Fish, Poultry, Meat

Notes: Weights are of cooked portions with fat trimmed.
Portions of seafood may be larger as they are low in saturated fat.
If any fats are added in preparation, be sure to count them in daily goal for fats and oils.

Choices	*Saturated Fat/oz (g)*		*Kinds of Fish, Poultry, Meat*
Best Choices: (lowest fat; lowest saturated fat)	0–0.5 g	Fish:	Cod, catfish, flounder, haddock, red snapper, halibut, perch, rock fish, sole, tuna.
		Seafood:	Crab, mussels, clams, oysters, lobster, scallops.
		Poultry:	Turkey or chicken—light meat, without skin. Turkey—dark meat, without skin. Turkey ham.
Good Choices:	0.6–1.5 g	Fish:	Albacore tuna, rainbow trout, salmon, mackerel.
		Poultry:	Chicken—dark meat, no skin; turkey bologna.
		Veal:	Loin, cutlet, or rib.
		Beef:	Lean round, loin, sirloin, chuck (well trimmed), venison, wild game.
		Pork:	Lean ham, loin, shoulder, or leg.
		Lamb:	Lean leg, loin, or rib.
Fair Choices:	1.6–2.5 g	Beef:	Flank, porterhouse, lean and extra lean ground beef (well cooked and drained).
		Lamb:	Lean leg, loin, or rib.
		Turkey:	Frankfurters.
Poor Choices: Avoid or limit to occasional use.	>2.5 g	Beef:	Brisket, highly marbled cuts.
		Pork:	Rib chops.
		Luncheon meats with more than 4 g of fat/oz.	
Choices to Avoid:		Regular ground beef, pork, lamb. Hot dogs, sausage, canned or packaged luncheon meats. Fried meats (unless with allowed oil). Poultry skin, salt pork, bacon, domestic duck or goose.	
High-cholesterol foods, low in fat		Limit to 3 servings or less per week: Egg yolk, organ meats, squid, shrimp, sardines	
Cholesterol Free!	Use as desired—Egg whites, fat-free egg substitute, tofu. —2 egg whites can be used in place of 1 egg in many foods. —¼ cup of egg substitute will replace 1 whole egg.		

Bread, Beans, Grains, and Starches

Note: 1 serving = 0–2 g fat (70–100 kcal)

Important: To help lower cholesterol, goal is to use *at least 2 servings per day* of the high-fiber foods.

High-Fiber Foods	*Serving Size*
Beans: navy, northern, lima red, pinto, black-eyed peas, garbanzo beans	½ cup, cooked
Dried peas, lentils	½ cup, cooked
Oat bran muffin	1 muffin
Oat bran	3 T, dry or ½ cup, cooked
Baked beans (no added meat or fat)	½ cup, cooked
Low-fat soups made with dried peas/beans	1 cup
Moderate-Fiber Foods	
Green peas, winter squash	½ cup
Corn	1 small ear or ⅓ cup
Sweet potatoes or yams	¼ cup
White potatoes, with skin	1 small or ½ cup
Cooked cereals such as oatmeal, Roman Meal	½ cup
Dry cereals such as Cheerios, Wheaties	¾ cup
Whole grain, rye, or pumpernickel bread	1 slice
Brown rice, cooked	½ cup
Popped corn, air popped, no oil	3 cups

Table continued on following page

TABLE 20–8. Choices and Serving Sizes for Step 1 and Step 2 Diets *Continued*

Low-Fiber Foods	*Serving Size*
White flour breads	1 slice
English muffin, bagel, pita bread, hamburger bun	½
Low-fat crackers	6 small
Pretzels	1 large or 12 small
Low-fat soups made with pasta or vegetables	1 cup
Tortilla, corn	1 small (6″)
Dry cereals such as Corn Flakes, Kix	¾ cup
Refined cooked cereals such as farina	½ cup
Pasta or white rice	½ cup
Pancakes or waffles made from fat-free ingredients	1 small

Foods to Avoid

Commercial doughnuts, sweet rolls, biscuits, pastries (unless made with appropriate fat), croissants, cheese bread.
Muffins, granola and granola bars, unless made with unsaturated oil.
Commercial crackers made with coconut, palm oil, or palm kernel oil, or if label says only "vegetable shortening" and does not specify the type.
Chow mein noodles.
"Ramen" type noodles.
Potatoes cooked in animal fat or hydrogenated oil.

Dairy Foods

Use of 2–3 servings of dairy products per day is encouraged. Nonfat milk and other low-fat dairy products are very low in cholesterol but high in protein, calcium, vitamins, and other minerals.

Notes: 1 Serving = 0–2 g fat
approximately 100 calories
0–30 mg cholesterol

When reading food labels choose low-fat dairy products, look for those with 2 g fat or less per serving.

	Good Choices	*Serving Size*
Milk:	Skim (nonfat) or 1% milk	1 cup (8 oz)
	Buttermilk made from skim or 1% milk	1 cup (8 oz)
	Nonfat or low-fat dry milk	⅓ cup powder
	Evaporated skim milk	½ cup undiluted
Yogurt:	Nonfat or low-fat	1 cup
Cheese:	Skim milk cheese	1 oz
	Dry curd or low-fat cottage cheese	½ cup
	Regular cottage cheese	¼ cup
	Ricotta cheese	1 oz
Other items:	Ice milk or soft-serve ice milk	½ cup
	Frozen low-fat yogurt	½ cup
	Sherbert	½ cup
	Puddings or cocoa made with skim milk	¾ cup
	Fudgesicle	1

Foods to Avoid

Buttermilk made from whole milk
Cheese made with whole milk/cream
Chocolate milk (whole milk)
Condensed or evaporated milk
Cream cheese and Neufchatel cheese
"Light cream cheese"
Half and half
Ice cream
Sour cream
Whole or 2% milk
Nondairy coffee creamers, sour cream, or whipped toppings (unless made with acceptable oils)
Whipping cream
"Gourmet" yogurt made from whole milk

TABLE 20–8. Choices and Serving Sizes for Step 1 and Step 2 Diets *Continued*

Fruit

Note: 1 serving = 0 g of fat, 0 mg of cholesterol, 60 calories

When cutting back on high-fat foods, increase intake of fruit—especially fresh whole fruits. Try some new varieties. Look for fruits in season. There's nothing better for dessert! Try:

—Sliced pineapple, papaya, and berries
—Blueberries with fat-free yogurt and brown sugar
—Broiled grapefruit halves with honey
—Melon with lemon wedge
—Mixed fruit with honey and lime juice dressing

One serving is 1 medium sized piece of fruit or ½ cup fruit or juice.
One serving of dried fruits is about 2–4 T.

Remember to count avocado and olives as fat. Avoid coconut.

Vegetables

Note: 1 serving = 0 g of fat, 0 mg of cholesterol, 25 calories

One serving = ½ cup cooked vegetable
1 cup lettuce or other leafy uncooked greens
½ cup vegetable juice
¼ cup condensed vegetable such as tomato sauce

Eating vegetables is essential in the new way of eating. Try new varieties. Be creative. Learn to enjoy the crunch and nutritional value provided by these naturally low calorie foods.

—Make it habit to include at least one vegetable at both lunch and dinner.
—Combine your favorite vegetables to make a luscious stir fry.
—Cook vegetables only to the "crisp-tender" stage. Soggy vegetables lack both eye and taste appeal.
—Say "no, thanks" to added fats and sauces.

Starchy vegetables such as potato, corn, peas, yams, and winter squash should be considered as servings of bread or starch.

Sugars

Note: 1 serving = 0 g of fat, 0 mg of cholesterol, 60 calories

Choice	*Serving Size*
Honey, sugar, jam, jelly, syrup	1 T
Carbonated beverages, lemonade (sweetened)	6 oz
Flavored, sugar sweetened gelatin	½ cup
Popsicle	1
Hard candies, licorice, jelly beans, gummies	1 oz
Dessert sauces: caramel, strawberry, pineapple, low-fat chocolate	2 T

Limit: Chocolate or carob candies. Carob or cocoa *powder or syrup* are acceptable.

Alcohol

Note: 1 serving = 0 g of fat, 0 mg of cholesterol, 100 calories

Choice	*Serving Size*
Beer, regular	12 oz
Red or white table wine	4 oz
Sweet dessert wine	3 oz
Whiskey, gin, rum, etc.	1.5 oz

* From Northwest Lipid Research Clinic, University of Washington, Seattle, Washington.

because this is an area where people prefer the option of occasional choices to help make lifestyle/eating changes more permanent, an additional list of the fat content of sweets, desserts and snacks is presented in Table 20–9. Tables 20–10 and 20–11 illustrate menus for Step 1 and Step 2 Diets (Fig. 20–7).

Method III: The third method is appropriate for those who take on the new eating program as a "project" and are interested in detailed information on the fat content of food. The "grams of fat" method involves determining the energy content of the diet and then calculating how many grams of fat can be included daily to provide 30% of total kilocalories, with saturated fat at levels of 10% (Step 1) or 7% (Step 2) (Table 20–12). After determining the daily fat allowance in grams, the patient chooses foods that will conform to that allowance by using Table 20–13, which lists the fat content of popular foods. Appendix Table 1 is then used to determine the saturated fat content of the foods. Table 20–14 is used to maintain the cholesterol content at 300 mg/day (Step 1) or 200 mg/ day (Step 2). The limitation of this method is that only fat and cholesterol are listed, and no guidelines for food choices are included to encourage appropriate levels of other nutrients.

With all three approaches, an increase in soluble fiber intake should be encouraged. This can be achieved by frequent use of oat bran, beans, fresh fruits, and fibrous vegetables. Appendix Table 2 gives the fiber content of various foods.

TABLE 20–9. Fat and Cholesterol Content of Sweets and Snacks* †

The following foods within each category (beverages, candy, cookies, cakes and pies, snacks, and pudding) are ranked from low to high saturated fat. To reduce the saturated fat, select the products from the upper portion of each category.

Product	Saturated Fatty Acids (g)	Cholesterol (mg)	Total Fat‡ (g)	% Calories from Fat §	Total Calories
Beverages					
Ginger ale, 12 oz	0.0	0	0.0	0	125
Cola, regular, 12 oz	0.0	0	0.0	0	160
Chocolate shake, 10 oz	6.5	37	10.5	26	360
Candy (1 oz)					
Hard candy	0.0	0	0.0	0	110
Gum drops	tr	0	tr	tr	100
Fudge	2.1	1	3.0	24	115
Milk chocolate, plain	5.4	6	9.0	56	145
Cookies					
Vanilla wafers, 5 cookies, 1¾" diameter	0.9	12	3.3	32	94
Fig bars, 4 cookies, 1⅝" × 1⅝ × ⅜"	1.0	27	4.0	17	210
Chocolate brownie with icing, 1½" by 1¾" by ⅞"	1.6	14	4.0	36	100
Oatmeal cookies, 4 cookies, 2⅝" diameter	2.5	2	10.0	37	245
Chocolate chip cookies, 4 cookies, 2¼" diameter	3.9	18	11.0	54	185
Cakes and Pies					
Angel food cake, 1/12 of 10" cake	tr	0	tr	tr	125
Gingerbread, 1/9 of 8" cake	1.1	1	4.0	21	175
White layer cake with white icing, 1/16 of 9" cake	2.1	3	9.0	32	260
Yellow layer cake with chocolate icing, 1/16 of 9" cake	3.0	36	8.0	31	235
Pound cake, 1/17 of loaf	3.0	64	5.0	41	110
Devils food cake with chocolate icing, 1/16 of 9" cake	3.5	37	8.0	31	235
Lemon meringue pie, ⅙ of 9" pie	4.3	143	14.0	36	355
Apple pie, ⅙ of 9" pie	4.6	0	18.0	40	405
Cream pie, ⅙ of 9" pie	15.0	8	23.0	46	455
Snacks					
Popcorn, air-popped, 1 cup	tr	0	tr	tr	30
Pretzels, stick, 2¼", 10 pretzels	tr	0	tr	tr	10
Popcorn with oil and salted, 1 cup	0.5	0	3.0	49	55
Corn chips, 1 oz	1.4	25	9.0	52	155
Potato chips, 1 oz	2.6	0	10.1	62	147
Pudding					
Gelatin	0.0	0	0.0	0	70
Tapioca, ½ cup	2.3	15	4.0	25	145
Chocolate pudding, ½ cup	2.4	15	4.0	24	150

* From USDHHS: Eating to Lower Your High Blood Cholesterol. NIH Publ No 89-2920. Washington, DC. NCEP, NHLBI, 1989.

† Source: Home and Garden Bulletin. Nutritive Value of Foods. No. 72. United States Department of Agriculture. Human Nutrition Information Service (1986).

‡ Total fat = saturated fatty acids plus monounsaturated fatty acids plus polyunsaturated fatty acids.

§ Percent calories from fat = (total fat calories divided by total calories) multiplied by 100; total fat calories = total fat (g) multiplied by 9; tr = trace.

TABLE 20–10. Sample Menu for Step 1 Diet*

1600 Calories	
Meal	*Food Group Portions*
Breakfast:	
Grapefruit (½)	1 Fruit
Bagel (1) with	2 Breads
Margarine (1 tsp)	1 Fat
Milk, 1% (1 cup)	1 Dairy
Lunch:	
Broiled chicken thigh (2 oz)	2 Meats
Tossed salad	
Lettuce (1 cup)	Free
Tomato wedges (1 tomato)	1 Vegetable
Mushroom slices (4 mushrooms)	Free
Oil and vinegar dressing	
Olive oil (1 tsp)	1 Fat
Vinegar (2 tsp)	Free
Saltine crackers (6)	1 Bread
Nectarine (1)	1 Fruit
Milk, 1% (1 cup)	1 Dairy
Dinner:	
Braised pot roast (4 oz) with	4 Meats
Tomatoes, canned (½ cup)	1 Vegetable
Green pepper strips (½ cup)	Free
Diced onion (2 T)	Free
Steamed broccoli spears (½ cup)	1 Vegetable
Carrot-raisin salad	
Shredded carrot (½ cup)	1 Vegetable
Raisins (2 T)	1 Fruit
Mayonnaise (1 tsp)	1 Fat
Roll (1) with	1 Bread
Margarine (1 tsp)	1 Fat
Gingersnap cookies (4)	2 Optional
Milk, 1% (1 cup)	1 Dairy

Nutrient Analysis

1615 Calories (distributed as follows)
24% Protein
46% Carbohydrate
30% Fat
9% Saturated fatty acids
207 mg Cholesterol†
1,775 mg Sodium

* From American Heart Association: Dietary Treatment of Hypercholesterolemia: A Manual for Patients, 1988, p 36.
† Cholesterol is less than 300 mg because an egg is not included.

TABLE 20–11. Sample Menu for Step 2 Diet*

1600 Calories	
Meal	*Food Group Portions*
Breakfast:	
Grapefruit juice (½ cup)	1 Fruit
Oatmeal (½ cup) with	1 Bread
Milk, skim (1 cup)	1 Dairy
Whole wheat toast (1 slice) with	1 Bread
Margarine (1 tsp)	1 Fat
Lunch:	
Tuna salad on lettuce	
Tuna, canned in water (½ cup)	2 Meats
Diced celery (¼ cup)	Free
Mayonnaise (2 tsp)	2 Fat
Lettuce (1 leaf)	Free
Relishes	
Broccoli flowerettes (1 cup)	1 Vegetable
Tomato wedges (1 tomato)	1 Vegetable
Saltines (6)	1 Bread
Apple (1)	1 Fruit
Dinner:	
Broiled sirloin steak (4 oz)	4 Meats
New potatoes (½ cup) with parsley and	1 Bread
Margarine (1 tsp)	1 Fat
Steamed green beans (½ cup)	1 Vegetable
Steamed carrot strips (½ cup)	1 Vegetable
Watermelon chunks (1¼ cups)	1 Fruit
French bread (1 slice) with	1 Bread
Margarine (1 tsp)	1 Fat
Gingersnap cookies (4)	2 Optional
Milk, skim (1 cup)	1 Dairy

Nutrient Analysis

1603 Calories (distributed as follows)
22% Protein
49% Carbohydrate
29% Fat
7% Saturated fatty acids
135 mg Cholesterol†
1,684 mg Sodium

* From American Heart Association: Dietary Treatment of Hypercholesterolemia: A Manual for Patients, 1988, p 60.
† Cholesterol is less than 200 mg because an egg is not included.

Pharmacologic Management

The combination of diet and drugs can produce a 30% reduction in serum cholesterol. The drugs of choice are cholestyramine and cholestipol, sequestrants that adsorb and combine with bile acids in the intestine to form insoluble complexes that are excreted in the feces. Adversely, sequestrants bind some drugs and may interfere with the absorption of fat-soluble vitamins. Constipation and unpalatability are common complaints.

Bile acid sequestrants tend to increase triglyceride levels; therefore when hypertriglyceridemia is also

Text continues on p. 385

TABLE 20–12. Fat Content of Step 1 and Step 2 Diets at Different Kilocalorie Levels*

Calorie Level	Total Fat (g)	Step 1 Saturated Fatty Acid (g)	Step 2 Saturated Fatty Acid (g)
1,200	40	13	9
1,500	50	17	12
1,800	60	20	14
2,000	67	22	16
2,200	73	24	17
2,500	83	28	19
3,000	100	33	23

* From American Heart Association: Dietary Treatment of Hypercholesterolemia: A Manual for Patients, 1988, p 64.

STEP TWO DIET

TYPICAL AMERICAN DIET

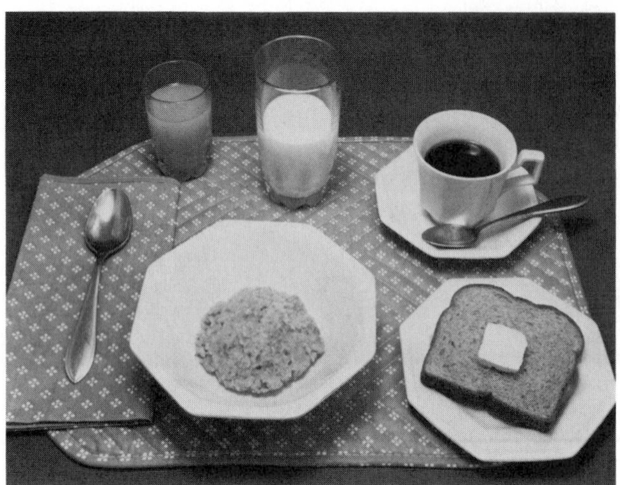

BREAKFAST

½ c grapefruit juice
½ c oatmeal
1 c skim milk
1 slice whole-wheat toast, 1 tsp margarine

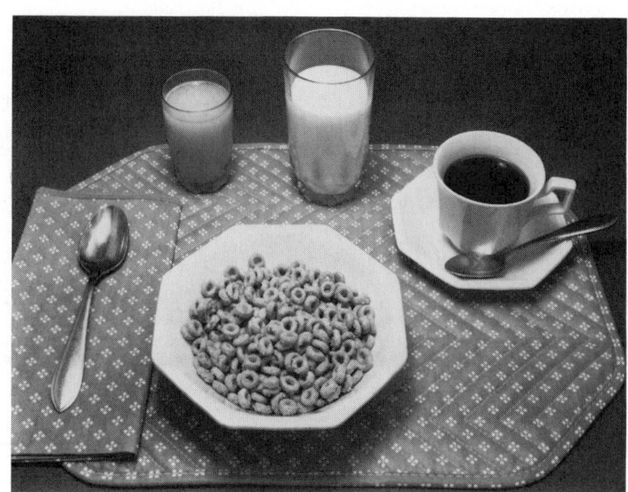

BREAKFAST

1½ c Cheerios
¾ c orange juice
1 c 2% milk
Coffee

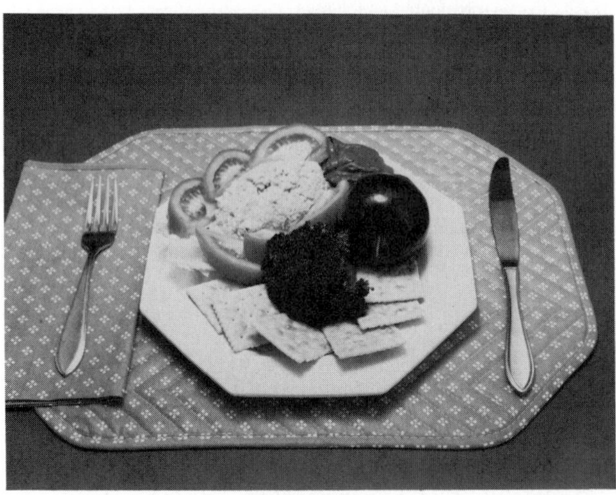

LUNCH

Tuna salad on lettuce (½ c tuna in water,
¼ c diced celery, 4 tsp mayonnaise, 1 lettuce leaf)
1 c broccoli
1 tomato (in wedges)
6 saltines
1 apple

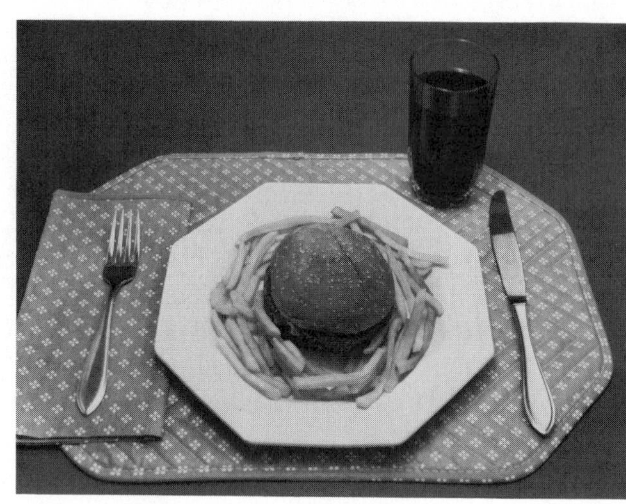

LUNCH

1 quarter-pound cheeseburger, lettuce, tomatoes
French fries
8 oz diet soda

FIGURE 20–7. *Comparison of Step 2 Diet and a typical American diet menu.*

STEP TWO DIET

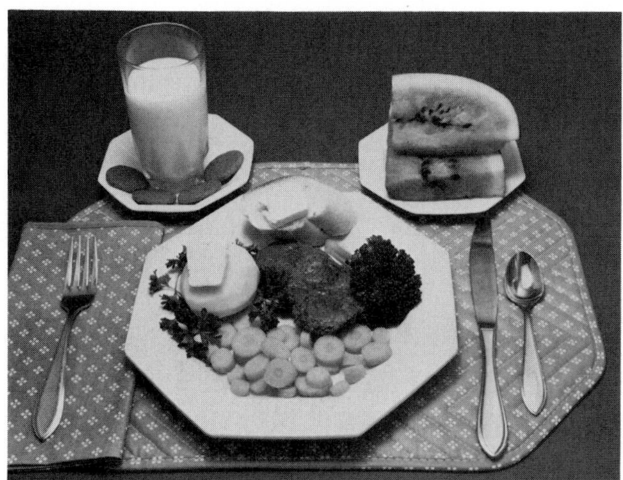

DINNER

4 oz broiled sirloin steak
1 small parsley potato, 1 tsp margarine
½ c steamed broccoli
½ c steamed carrots
1¼ c watermelon
1 slice French bread, 1 tsp margarine
2 gingersnap cookies
1 c skim milk

TYPICAL AMERICAN DIET

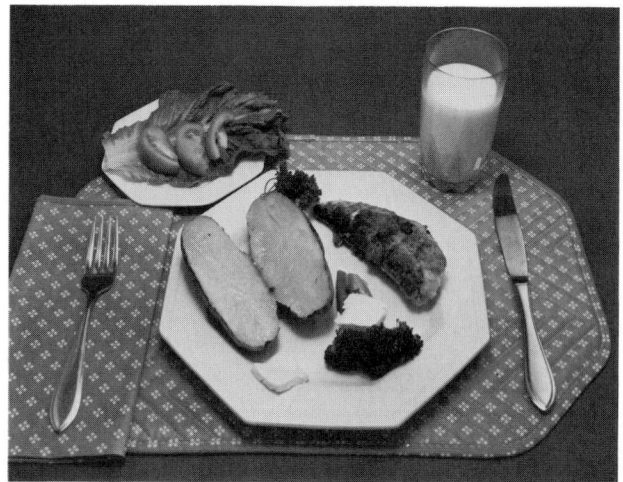

DINNER

1 baked potato, 1 tsp margarine
1 broiled chicken breast (4 oz after cooking)
1½ c 2% milk
½ c broccoli, 1 tsp margarine
2 c salad (lettuce, tomatoes, 2 T creamy dressing)

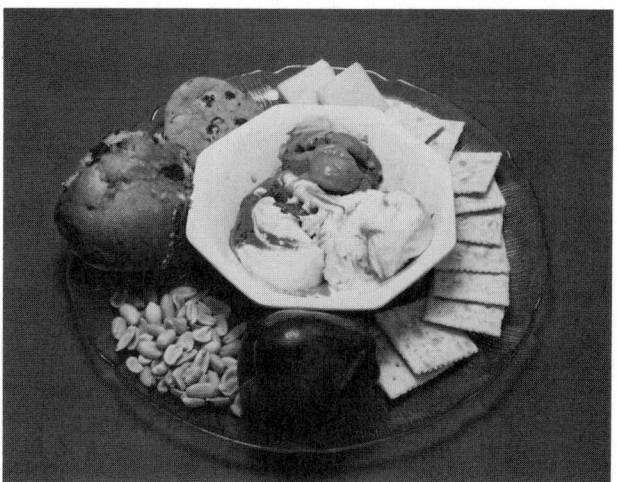

SNACKS

1 large blueberry muffin
Coffee
8 oz 2% milk
1 cookie
10 saltines
1 apple
2 oz cheese
1¼ c ice cream
¼ c peanuts

FIGURE 20–7. *Continued*

TABLE 20–13. Fat Content of Popular Foods

Food Group	0 Grams	1 Gram	3 Grams	5 Grams	10 Grams	15 Grams	20 Grams	25 Grams	30 Grams	35 Grams
Milk Group	Milk, nonfat dry (1 cup) Milk, skim (1 cup) Yogurt, plain, nonfat (1 cup)	Cheese, cottage, 1% low-fat (½ cup) Yogurt, frozen, plain (½ cup)	Buttermilk (1 cup) Cheese, cottage, 2% low-fat (½ cup) Cheese, parmesan, grated (1 T) Ice milk, hardened (½ cup) Ice milk, soft serve (½ cup) Milk, 1% low-fat (1 cup) Yogurt, fruit-flavored, low-fat (1 cup)	Cheese, cottage, creamed (½ cup) Cheese, mozzarella (1 oz) Cheese, mozzarella, part skim (1 oz) Ice cream, hardened, 10% fat (½ cup) Milk, 2% low-fat (1 cup) Milk, chocolate, 2% low-fat (1 cup) Pudding, cooked (½ cup) Pudding, instant (½ cup) Yogurt, plain, low-fat (1 cup)	Cheese, American (1 oz) Cheese, brick (1 oz) Cheese, cheddar (1 oz) Cheese, Monterey (1 oz) Cheese, Muenster (1 oz) Cheese, parmesan, grated (1 oz) Cheese, Swiss (1 oz) Ice cream, premium, hardened, 16% fat (½ cup) Ice cream, soft serve (½ cup) Milk, chocolate, whole (1 cup) Milk, whole (1 cup) Milkshake (10 fl oz)					
Meat Group	Black-eyed peas, dried, cooked†(½ cup) Egg, hard-cooked, white only (1 egg) Pinto beans, dried, cooked† (½ cup)	Black-eyed peas, canned† (½ cup) Flounder/sole, baked (3 oz) Navy beans† (½ cup) Refried beans, canned (½ cup) Shrimp, boiled (3 oz)	Chicken, roasted, without skin (3 oz) Halibut, baked (3 oz) Perch, baked (3 oz) Tuna, canned in water (3 oz)	Bologna, turkey (1 oz) Canadian bacon (2 slices) Chicken, fried flour coated (3 oz) Chicken, roasted with skin (3 oz) Egg, fried (1 egg) Egg, hard-cooked (1 egg) Egg, scrambled (1 egg) Ham, 5% fat (3 oz) Ham, turkey (3 oz) Pork roast (3 oz) Roast beef, lean only (3 oz) Salmon, canned, fish and bones (3 oz)	Bacon (3 slices) Bologna, beef (1 oz) Chicken, fried, batter dipped (3 oz) Fish sticks, oven-heated (3 oz) Ham, 11% fat (3 oz) Hot dog, chicken (2 oz) Salmon, baked (3 oz) Sausage, link (2 links) Sausage, patty (1 patty) Shrimp, breaded and fried (3 oz) Steak, rib eye, broiled (3 oz) Steak, sirloin, broiled (3 oz)	Ground sirloin/round, broiled (3 oz) Hot dog, beef (2 oz) Kentucky Fried Chicken's Original Recipe Chicken (3 oz) McDonald's Chicken McNuggets (6 pieces) Peanut butter (2 T) Pork chop, broiled (3 oz) Roast beef, lean and fat (3 oz) Sunflower seeds, dry-roasted (¼ cup)	Bratwurst (3 oz) Ground beef, broiled (3 oz) Italian sausage (3 oz) Kentucky Fried Chicken's Extra Crispy Chicken (3 oz) Peanuts, dry-roasted (¼ cup) Peanuts, oil-roasted (¼ cup) Sunflower seeds, oil-roasted (¼ cup)	Polish sausage (3 oz) Spareribs (3 oz)		

Food Group	0 Grams		1 Gram	3 Grams	5 Grams	10 Grams	15 Grams	20 Grams	25 Grams	30 Grams
				Tofu (½ cup) Tuna, canned in oil (3 oz) Turkey (3 oz)	Steak, T-bone, broiled (3 oz)					
Fruit-Vegetable Group	Apple (1 medium) Applesauce (½ cup) Broccoli (½ cup) Cabbage (½ cup) Cantaloupe (¼ melon) Carrots (1 carrot) Cauliflower (½ cup) Celery (1 stalk) Corn, frozen, cooked (½ cup) Fruit cocktail (½ cup) Grapefruit (½ medium) Grapes (½ cup) Green beans (½ cup) Green peas (½ cup) Green pepper (½ pepper) Greens (½ cup) Lettuce (½ cup) Orange (1 medium Orange juice (½ cup)	Peaches (½ cup) Pears (½ cup) Pineapple (½ cup) Potato, baked (1 large) Prunes, dried, cooked (½ cup) Prunes, dried, uncooked (½ cup) Raisins (¼ cup) Snow peas (½ cup) Spinach (½ cup) Strawberries (½ cup) Sweet potato, baked (½ medium) Tomato juice (½ cup) Tomato, fresh (1 tomato) Tossed salad, without dressing (½ cup) Watermelon (½ cup) Zucchini (½ cup)	Banana (1 medium) Corn on cob, fresh, cooked (1 ear) Corn, canned, cream style (½ cup) Pear (1 medium) Winter squash, fresh, baked (½ cup)	Coleslaw (½ cup) Sweet potato, candied (½ medium)	Potatoes, french-fried, oven-heated (10 strips) Potatoes, mashed (½ cup)	Potatoes, French-fried, (10 strips) Potatoes, hashed brown (½ cup)	Avocado, sliced (½ medium)	Avocado, puréed (½ cup)		

(Prepared without added fat)

Food Group	0 Grams	1 Gram		3 Grams	5 Grams	10 Grams	15 Grams	20 Grams	25 Grams	30 Grams
Grain Group	Corn flakes (1 oz) Cream of wheat, cooked (½ cup) Grits, cooked (½ cup) Macaroni, plain (½ cup) Macaroni, protein-fortified (½ cup) Macaroni, vegetable (½ cup) Rice, white (½ cup) Rice, wild (½ cup)	Bagel, plain (½ bagel) Bran flakes (1 oz) Bread, cracked wheat (1 slice) Bread, pita (½ pita) Bread, pumpernickel (1 slice) Bread, rye (1 slice) Bread, white (1 slice) Bread, whole wheat (1 slice)	Crackers, saltines (4 crackers) Egg noodles, cooked (½ cup) Hamburger bun (½ roll) Hard roll (½ roll) Hot dog bun (½ roll) Muffin, English, plain, toasted (½ muffin) Oatmeal, instant, cooked (½ cup) Raisin bran (1 oz)	Biscuit, from mix (1 biscuit) Biscuit, from refrigerated dough (1 biscuit) Crackers, whole wheat (2 crackers) Dinner roll (1 roll) Pancake, buckwheat (4″ pancake) Pancake, plain (4″ pancake)	Crackers, snack (4 crackers) Croissant, plain (½ roll) Granola (1 oz) Muffin, blueberry (1 small) Muffin, bran (1 small) Muffin, corn (1 small)	Waffle, homemade (7″ waffle)				

Table continued on following page

TABLE 20–13. The Content of Popular Foods *Continued*

Food Group	0 Grams	1 Gram	3 Grams	5 Grams	10 Grams	15 Grams	20 Grams	25 Grams	30 Grams	35 Grams
	Sugar frosted flakes (1 oz)	Crackers, graham (2 crackers) Crackers, rye (2 crackers)	Rice, brown (½ cup) Tortilla, corn (6″ tortilla)	Tortilla, flour (8″ tortilla) Waffle, frozen (4″ waffle)						

Food Group	0 Grams	1 Gram	3 Grams	5 Grams	10 Grams	15 Grams	20 Grams	25 Grams	30 Grams	35 Grams
Combination Foods		Baked beans (½ cup) Soup, chicken noodle, dehydrated (1 cup)	Soup, chicken noodle, canned (1 cup) Soup, clam chowder, with water (1 cup) Soup, cream of tomato, with water (1 cup)	Burrito, bean (1 burrito) Pizza, cheese (¼ of 12″) Soup, clam chowder, with whole milk (1 cup) Soup, cream of tomato, with whole milk (1 cup)	Beef and vegetable stew (1 cup) Burrito, bean and meat (1 burrito) Burrito, beef (1 burrito) Chili (1 cup) Chow mein, chicken (1 cup) Macaroni and cheese, frozen, cooked (1 cup) McDonald's Egg McMuffin (1 sandwich) Pizza, cheese and pepperoni (¼ of 12″) Pizza, cheese, meat, and vegetables (¼ of 12″) Spaghetti with meat balls, canned (1 cup) Spaghetti with meat balls, homemade (1 cup)	Arby's roast beef sandwich (1 sandwich) Chef's salad, without dressing (1½ cups) Chop suey, beef and pork (1 cup) Dairy Queen's hot dog (1 sandwich) Lasagna, without meat (2.5″ × 2.5″) Peanut butter and jelly sandwich, on white bread (1 sandwich) Roast beef sandwich, on bun (1 sandwich) Wendy's single hamburger, plain (1 sandwich)	Burger King's Croissan'wich (1 sandwich) Cheeseburger, regular (1 sandwich) Chicken stir fry, with rice (1½ cup) Dairy Queen's chili dog (1 sandwich) Enchilada, cheese (1 enchilada) Enchilada, cheese and beef (1 enchilada) Lasagna, with meat (2.5″ × 2.5″) Macaroni and cheese, homemade (1 cup) Quiche, without bacon (⅛ pie) Taco (1 small)	Burger King's Whaler (1 sandwich) Chicken pot pie, frozen, baked (1 pot pie) Chicken pot pie, homemade (¼ of 9″) Chicken salad (½ cup) Fish sandwich (1 sandwich) McDonald's Filet-O-Fish (1 sandwich) Quiche, with bacon (⅛. pie) Wendy's broccoli and cheese potato (1 potato)	Fish sandwich, with cheese (1 sandwich) McDonald's Big Mac (1 sandwich) McDonald's biscuit with sausage (1 sandwich) Pizza Hut's supreme personal pan pizza (1 pizza)	Arby's roast chicken club (1 sandwich) Burger King's Whopper (1 sandwich) Cheeseburger, large (1 sandwich) Wendy's Big Classic (1 sandwich)

					Submarine sandwich, with cold cuts and cheese (3–4″ sub) Taco Bell's bean burrito (1 burrito) Taco Bell's taco (1 taco) Tuna salad (½ cup) Turkey sandwich on whole wheat bread (1 sandwich) Wendy's chili (9 oz)			
"Others" Category	Angel food cake (1/12 cake) Barbeque sauce (1 T) Beer (12 fl oz) Catsup (1 T) Coffee (1 cup) Gelatin, flavored (½ cup) Honey (1 tsp) Ice tea (12 fl oz) Jelly (1 tsp) Maple syrup (1 T) Pickle (1 pickle) Popcorn, air popped, unbuttered (1 cup) Soft drink, cola, low calorie (12 fl oz) Soft drink, cola, regular (12 fl oz) Sugar (1 tsp) Tea (1 cup) Wine (3.5 fl oz)	French dressing, low calorie (1 T) Gravy, beef, canned (¼ cup) Mustard (1 T) Pretzels (1 oz)	Coffee whitener, nondairy, liquid (1 T) Cream, half-and-half (1 T) Popcorn, oil popped, unbuttered (1 cup) Sour cream (1 T) Sour half-and-half (1 T)	Brownie, with nuts (1 small brownie) Brownie, with nuts and frosting (1 small brownie) Butter (1 tsp) Chocolate chip cookies (2 small cookies) French dressing, regular (1 T) Granola bar, plain (1 oz) Italian dressing (1 T) Margarine (1 tsp) Neufchatel cheese (1 oz) Popcorn, oil popped, buttered (1 cup)	Chocolate cake (1/16 cake) Chocolate candy bar, plain (1 oz) Chocolate candy bar, with almonds (1 oz) Corn chips (1 oz) Cream cheese (1 oz) Doughnut, cake-type, plain (1 doughnut) Mayonnaise (1 T) Oil and vinegar dressing, homemade (1 T) Pie, chocolate cream (⅛ of 9″ pie) Potato chips (1 oz) Tortilla chips (1 oz)	Doughnut, yeast, glazed (1 doughnut) Pie, apple (⅛ of 9″ pie) Sweet roll, cinnamon (1 roll) Sweet roll, fruit (1 roll)	Cheesecake (1/12 of cake)	Pie, pecan (⅛ of 9″ pie)

* From *Healthy Dividends Consumer Booklet.* Courtesy of National Dairy Council®.
† Without fat seasoning.

TABLE 20–14. Cholesterol and Fat Content of Animal Products* †

Source	Cholesterol Content mg/3 oz	Total Fat Content g/3 oz	Source	Cholesterol Content mg/3 oz	Total Fat Content g/3 oz
Red Meats (lean)			Fish		
Beef	77	8.7	Salmon	74	9.3
Lamb	78	8.8	Tuna, light, canned in water	55	0.7
Pork	79	11.1	Shellfish		
Veal	128	4.7	Abalone	90	0.8
Organ Meats			Clams	57	1.7
Liver	270	4.0	Crab meat		
Pancreas (sweetbreads)	400	2.8	Alaskan king	45	1.3
Kidney	329	2.9	Blue crab	85	1.5
Brains	1,746	10.7	Lobster	61	0.5
Heart	164	4.8	Oysters	93	4.2
Poultry			Scallops	35	0.8
Chicken (without skin)			Shrimp	166	0.9
light	72	3.8	Dairy		
dark	79	8.2	Cheese, cheddar (1 oz)	30	9.4
Turkey (without skin)			Cheese, cottage, 2% fat (½ cup)	19	2.2
light	59	1.3	Mozzarella, part-skim (1 oz)	15	4.9
dark	72	6.1	Cream, sour, 1 T	6	2.5
Egg, 1 large	211	5.6	Milk, 2%, 1 cup	22	4.7

* Adapted from Expert Panel on Detection, Evaluation and Treatment of High Blood Cholesterol in Adults: High Blood Cholesterol in Adults, National Cholesterol Education Program, NIH, Publ No 89-2925. Washington, DC, PHS, USDHHS, 1989, p 40.

† 3 oz portions (cooked).

TABLE 20–15. Summary of the Major Lipid-Lowering Drugs*

Drugs	Reduce CHD Risk†	Long-Term Safety	Maintaining Adherence	LDL-Cholesterol Lowering	Special Precautions
Cholestyramine Colestipol	Yes	Yes	Requires considerable education	15–30%	Can alter absorption of other drugs. Can increase triglyceride levels and should not be used in patients with hypertriglyceridemia.
Nicotinic acid	Yes	Yes	Requires considerable education	15–30%	Test for hyperuricemia, hyperglycemia, and liver function abnormalities.
Lovastatin	Not proven	Not established	Relatively easy	25–45%	Monitor for liver function abnormalities and possible lens opacities.
Gemfibrozil‡	Yes	Preliminary evidence	Relatively easy	5–15%	May increase LDL-cholesterol in hypertriglyceridemic patients. Should not be used in patients with gallbladder disease.
Probucol	Not proven	Not established	Relatively easy	10–15%	Lowers HDL-cholesterol; significance of this has not been established. Prolongs QT interval.
Clofibrate	Not proven	Not established	Relatively easy	None	Lowers triglycerides to reduce risk of pancreatitis.

* Adapted from Expert Panel on Detection, Evaluation and Treatment of High Blood Cholesterol in Adults: High Blood Cholesterol in Adults. National Cholesterol Education Program, NIH Publ No 89-2925. Washington, DC, NIH, PHS, USDHHS, 1989, p 51.

† CHD = Coronary heart disease.

‡ Not FDA approved for routine use in lowering cholesterol. The results of the Helsinki Heart Study should be available soon to define the effect on CHD risk and long-term safety.

present (triglycerides equal to or over 250 mg/dl), nicotinic acid is the medication of choice. Lovostatin is another possibility although it has more problematic side effects than nicotinic acid. Gemfibrozil, probucol, and clofibrate are used primarily for lowering TG (Table 20–15).

Related Programs

Among the major risk factors for CHD are hypertension and cigarette smoking. Obesity and lack of exercise are also important contributors. Dietary modifications for prevention and control of hypertension are outlined in Chapter 21 and information on sodium restriction appears in Chapter 33. Weight-reduction programs are discussed in Chapter 18.

CITED REFERENCES

Anderson JW and Gustafson NJ: Hypocholesterolemic effects of oat and bean products. Am J Clin Nutr 48(Suppl):749, 1988.

Bak AAA and Grobbee DE: The effect on serum cholesterol levels of coffee brewed by filtering or boiling. N Engl J Med 321:1432, 1989.

Blum CB and Levy RI: Current therapy for hypercholesterolemia. JAMA 261:3582, 1989.

Centers for Disease Control: MMWR 36:426, 1987.

Committee on Diet and Health, Food and Nutrition Board. National Research Council: Diet and Health. Implications for Reducing Chronic Disease Risk. Washington, DC, National Academy Press, 1989.

Council for Agricultural Science and Technology (CAST): Diet and coronary disease. Nutrition Today 21(2):26, 1986.

Department of Health and Human Services: Monthly Vital Statistics Report, Vol 36, The Advance Report of Final Mortality Statistics, 1985. DHHS Publ No (PHS) 87-1120. Hyattsville, MD, NCHS, PHS, USDHHS, 1987.

Despres J-P et al: Abdominal adipose tissue and serum HDL-cholesterol: Association independent from obesity and serum triglyceride concentration. Int J Obes 12(1):1, 1988.

Eisenberg S: High density lipoprotein metabolism. J Lipid Res 25:1017, 1984.

Ekelund L-G et al: Physical fitness as a predictor of cardiovascular mortality in asymptomatic North American men. The Lipid Research Clinics Mortality Follow-up Study. N Engl J Med 319:1379, 1988.

Expert Panel on Detection, Evaluation, and Treatment of High Blood Cholesterol in Adults: High Blood Cholesterol in Adults. National Cholesterol Education Program, NHLBI, USDHHS, NIH Publ No 89-2925. Washington, DC, NIH, 1989.

Frick MH et al: Helsinki Heart Study: Primary-Prevention Trial with Gemfibrozil in middle-aged men with dyslipidemia. N Engl J Med 317:1237, 1987.

Gordon DJ and Rifkind BM: High-density lipoprotein—the clinical implications of recent studies. N Engl J Med 321:1311, 1989.

Grande F, Anderson JT, and Keys A: Diets of different fatty acid composition producing identical serum cholesterol levels in man. Am J Clin Nutr 25:53, 1972.

Grundy SM: Comparison of monounsaturated fatty acids and carbohydrates for lowering plasma cholesterol. N Engl J Med 314:745, 1986.

Grundy S et al: The effect of dietary stearic acid on plasma cholesterol and lipoprotein levels. N Engl J Med 318:1244, 1988.

Hegsted DM et al: Quantitative effects of dietary fat on serum cholesterol in man. Am J Clin Nutr 17:281, 1965.

Keys A (ed): Coronary heart disease in seven countries. Circulation 41(Suppl 1):1, 1970.

Keys A, Anderson JT, and Grande F: Serum cholesterol response to changes in the diet. Metabolism 14:747, 1965.

Kromhout D et al: The inverse relation between fish consumption and 20-year mortality from coronary heart disease. N Engl J Med 312:1205, 1985.

Kuske TT and Feldman EB: Hyperlipoproteinemia, atherosclerosis risk and dietary management. Arch Intern Med 147:357, 1987.

Levy RI: Changing perspectives in the prevention of CAD. Am J Cardiol 57:17G, 1986.

Liebman B: The HDL/Triglycerides trap: An interview with William Castelli, M.D., Director of the Framingham Heart Study. Nutrition Action 17(7):1, 1990.

Manson JE et al: A prospective study of obesity and risk of coronary heart disease in women. N Engl J Med 322:882, 1990.

McNamara DJ: Coronary heart disease. *In* Brown ML (ed): Present Knowledge in Nutrition, 6th ed. Washington, DC, International Life Sciences Institute—Nutrition Foundation, 1990.

Mensink RP and Katan MB: Effect of dietary trans fatty acids on high-density and low-density lipoprotein cholesterol levels in healthy subjects. N Engl J Med 323:439, 1990.

Mensink RP et al: Effect of monounsaturated fatty acid v. complex carbohydrates on serum lipoproteins and apoproteins in healthy men and women. Metabolism 38:172, 1989.

National Center for Health Statistics—National NHLBI Collaborative Lipid Group: Trends in serum cholesterol levels among U.S. adults aged 20 to 74 years. JAMA 257:937, 1987.

NIH: Prevention: Framingham's legacy. *In:* Momentum Toward Health. Washington, DC, NIH, PHS, USDHSS, 1985, p 65.

Pooling Project Research Group: Relationship of blood pressure, serum cholesterol, smoking habit, relative weight and ECG abnormalities to incidence of major coronary events: Final report of the Pooling Project. J Chron Dis 31:201, 1978.

Quit smoking—or suffer low blood HDL levels. JAMA 239:690, 1978.

Report of the Expert Panel on Blood Cholesterol in Children and Adolescents. National Cholesterol Education Program, NHLBI, USDHHS, NIH Publ. Bethesda, MD, NIH, 1991.

Rosemarin PC: Coffee and coronary heart disease: A review. Prog Cardiovasc Dis 32:239, 1989.

Science News 116:376, 1979.

Stamler J et al: Is relationship between serum cholesterol and risk of premature death from coronary heart disease continuous and graded? Findings in 356,222 primary screenees of the Multiple Risk Factor Intervention Trial (MRFIT). JAMA 256:2823, 1986.

Swain JF et al: Comparison of the effects of oat bran and low-fiber wheat on serum lipoprotein levels and blood pressure. N Engl J Med 322:147, 1990.

Sytkowski PA et al: Changes in risk factors and the decline in mortality from cardiovascular disease: The Framingham Heart Study. N Engl J Med 322:1635, 1990.

Timely statement on NCEP report on children and adolescents. J Am Diet Assoc 91:983, 1991.

Vergroesen AJ: Dietary fat and cardiovascular disease: Possible modes of action of linoleic acid. Proc Nutr Soc 31:323, 1972.

Wilson PF et al: Impact of national guidelines for cholesterol risk factor screening: The Framingham Offspring Study. JAMA 262:41, 1989.

Wood PD et al: Changes in plasma lipids and lipoproteins in overweight men during weight loss through dieting as compared with exercise. N Engl J Med 319:1173, 1988.

ADDITIONAL REFERENCES

An alternative fiber source. Psyllium for hypercholesterolemia? Nutr MD 15(1):4, 1989.

Austin MA: Plasma triglyceride as a risk factor for coronary heart disease: The epidemiologic evidence and beyond. Am J Epidemiol 129:249, 1989.

Connor SL et al: The cholesterol-saturated fat index for coronary prevention: Background, use, and a comprehensive table of foods. J Am Diet Assoc 89:807, 1989.

Dart AM et al: Effects of Maxepa on serum lipids in hypercholesterolemic subjects. Atherosclerosis 80:119, 1989.

Diehl AK et al: The relationship of high density lipoprotein subfrac-

tions to alcohol consumption, other lifestyle factors, and coronary heart disease. Atherosclerosis 69:145, 1988.
Fish oil supplements and hypertriglyceridemia. Nutr MD 15(9):3, 1989.
Gordon DJ et al: High-density lipoprotein cholesterol and cardiovascular disease: Four prospective American studies. Circulation 79:8, 1989.
Green MH: A perspective on dietary fats, plasma cholesterol and atherosclerosis. Nutrition Today 24(3):6, 1989.
Grundy SM: Trans monounsaturated fatty acids and serum cholesterol levels (Editorial). N Engl J Med 323:480, 1990.
Grundy SM et al: The place of HDL in cholesterol management: A perspective from the National Cholesterol Education Program. Arch Intern Med 149:505, 1989.
Harris WS: Fish oils and plasma lipid and lipoprotein metabolism in humans: A critical review. J Lipid Res 30:785, 1989.
Hegsted DM and Ausman LM: Diet, alcohol and coronary heart disease in men. J Nutr 118:1184, 1988.
Kendler BS: Garlic (Allium sativum) and onion (Allium cepa): A review of their relationship to cardiovascular disease. Prev Med 16:670, 1987.
Keys A: Serum cholesterol response to dietary cholesterol. Am J Clin Nutr 40:351, 1984.
Lauer RM, Lee J, and Clarke WR: Factors affecting the relationship between childhood and adult cholesterol levels: The Muscatine Study. Pediatrics 82:309, 1988.
Mattson FH: A changing role for dietary monounsaturated fatty acids. J Am Diet Assoc 89:387, 1989.
Merz B: New studies fuel controversy over universal cholesterol screening during childhood. JAMA 261:814, 1989.
Moderate alcohol consumption increases plasma HDL cholesterol. Nutr Rev 45:8, 1987.
Nash HL: Reemphasizing the role of exercise in preventing heart disease. Phys Sportsmed 17:219, 1989.
Nicklas TA et al: Dietary factors related to cardiovascular risk factors in early life. Bogalusa heart study. Arteriosclerosis 8:193, 1988.
Palm oil. Nutr MD 15(9):4, 1989.
Palumbo PJ: Cholesterol lowering for all: A closer look. JAMA 262:91, 1989.
Paul O: Background of the prevention of cardiovascular disease. II. Arteriosclerosis, hypertension, and selected risk factors. Circulation 80:206, 1989.
Shekelle RB et al: Diet, serum cholesterol, and death from coronary heart disease — The Western Electric Study. N Engl J Med 304:65, 1981.
Toward healthy blood cholesterol levels: A dietary approach. Official position of The Canadian Dietetic Association. J Can Diet Assoc 49:216, 1988.
USDHHS: Eating to Lower Your High Blood Cholesterol. NIH Publ No 89-2920. Washington, DC, NCEP, NHLBI, 1989.

CHAPTER 21

NUTRITION IN HYPERTENSION

CHAPTER OUTLINE

KEY TERMS

ESSENTIAL HYPERTENSION—hypertension of unknown etiology

HYPERTENSION—persistently high arterial blood pressure; a systolic blood pressure of 140 mm Hg or greater and a diastolic blood pressure of 90 mm Hg or greater

SALT-SENSITIVE HYPERTENSIVE—a hypertensive whose blood pressure appears to respond to salt intake

SECONDARY HYPERTENSION—hypertension secondary to some other disease state

Hypertension, or high blood pressure, contributes to the etiology of a number of degenerative diseases, many of them associated with the development of atherosclerosis. Recent programs of aggressive identification and treatment have lowered the incidence of this disease, a consequence that may or may not have contributed to the steady decrease in coronary artery disease that has marked the past decade (National Research Council, 1989). Increasing interest in nonpharmacologic therapy has suggested an expanding role for diet in the prevention and treatment of hypertension and related diseases.

DEFINITION AND CLASSIFICATION

Hypertension is identified by a systolic blood pressure (SBP) of 140 mm Hg or above and a diastolic blood pressure (DBP) of 90 mm Hg or above. "Mild" hypertension is defined by an SBP between 140 and 160 mm Hg and a DBP between 90 and 104 (Joint National Committee, 1988). (Systolic pressure is related to cardiac stroke volume; diastolic pressure measures peripheral resistance.)

Approximately 10 to 20% of Americans have hypertension—usually *essential* hypertension, so-called because the cause is unknown. In 68% of these cases, the hypertension is *mild* (Department of Health and Human Services, 1986). It is primarily the inclusion of mild hypertensives in the treatment program that has lowered the incidence of this disease in recent years (Joint National Committee, 1988).

Secondary hypertension, which affects 4 to 8% of the hypertensive population, is the outcome of other disease states, such as endocrine disease, liver disease, or, most commonly, renal disease. It is potentially reversible depending on the status of the organs involved (Einhorn and Landsberg, 1988).

PHYSIOLOGY

Blood pressure levels are determined by the push of blood into the arteries from the contractions of the heart, the volume of fluid in the vascular system (which depends on the sodium concentration of the blood), and the resistance of the muscular walls of the arterioles. A variety of mechanisms interact to maintain blood pressure at normal levels, including the kidney with its hormonal secretions and adjustment of water and sodium excretion, and the sympathetic nervous system (SNS). When these controls are not functioning or cannot compensate, hypertension develops.

Hypertension ultimately involves a rise in blood pressure in response to increased smooth muscle tone of the arterioles, which accentuates normal resistance to blood flow. Narrowing of the arterioles forces the left ventricle of the heart to increased effort in pumping blood through the system, leading eventually to *congestive heart failure* (see Chapter 33). Hypertension also encourages the development of *atherosclerosis,* possibly by weakening the arterial wall with exertion of pressure at susceptible points and opening it to invasion by lipids and other materials. Because of its association with atherosclerosis, hypertension is a high risk factor for the development of stroke, kidney disease, and coronary artery disease. Data from the Framingham study show that persons with hypertension are 3 to 4 times as likely to develop coronary heart disease and 7 times as likely to suffer a stroke as those whose blood pressure is normal or controlled (Dannenberg et al, 1988). The risk of major coronary disease increases 30% for every 10 mm Hg increase in blood pressure (National Research Council, 1989).

RISK FACTORS

A genetic predisposition to hypertension appears to interact with obesity, lifestyle, dietary components, and other factors to produce the elevated blood pressures characteristic of the condition.

Physiologic Risk Factors

Although hypertension is not confined to any particular segment of the population, it most severely affects *blacks, males,* and the *elderly.* Hypertension occurs twice as often in blacks, develops earlier, and becomes more severe in this population (Hypertension Prevalence . . . , 1984). *Heredity* is the most important risk factor and to a large degree identifies those who will suffer from essential hypertension.

Obesity is a major risk factor for hypertension, although the mechanism that brings about this relationship is not understood. A body weight 20% or more above ideal is associated with a frequency of hypertension twice that of the nonobese (Havlik et al, 1983). The waist-to-hip girth ratio appears to have a better correlation with blood pressure than other measures of adiposity inasmuch as centrally-deposited fat increases the risk for hypertension (Selby et al, 1989; Williams et al, 1987) (see Chapter 18). Weight gain during adult life, especially during the third and fourth decades, is associated with increased blood pressure (Stamler, 1975). In the Framingham study, an increase in relative weight of 10% was predictive of a 7 mm Hg rise in blood pressure, suggesting that weight gain itself rather than absolute body weight is the risk factor (Einhorn and Landsberg, 1988). The mechanism for the relationship may be the increase in SNS activity that follows excessive energy intake (Schwartz et al, 1983), inasmuch as the SNS can elevate blood pressure by direct vasoconstriction. Increased energy intake is also associated with elevated plasma insulin, a potent natriuretic factor causing increased sodium reabsorption by the kidney with consequent blood pressure elevation.

Environmental Risk Factors

Hypertension occurs most frequently among individuals with lower levels of income and education (Einhorn and Landsberg, 1988). This may be related to the acknowledged role of *stress* in the development and course of this disease. Moves of so-called primitive people to more sophisticated societies, as well as moves of individuals from rural to urban areas are accompanied by increases in blood pressure.

Dietary Risk Factors

Intakes of a number of nutrients have been associated both positively and negatively with the incidence of hypertension, although evidence supporting causative roles remains elusive. Even the role of sodium, which has been studied extensively, is not universally recognized.

Sodium

Exactly how sodium contributes to a rise in blood pressure is not clear. An inherited or acquired defect in the kidneys' ability to excrete excess sodium may lead to elevated levels of sodium, chloride, and water in the blood. Normally an increase in plasma volume prompts secretion of the *natriuretic hormone (atrial natriuretic peptide),* enabling the kidney to void some of the excess sodium in the urine. In some hypertensives, the kidneys may be unable to excrete normal amounts of sodium at normal blood pressures due to a "natriuretic handicap," one factor of which may be plasma insulin, which has been associated with increased sodium reabsorption by the kidney (Blaustein and Hamlyn, 1984).

Another hypothesis proposes that increasing intercellular sodium could inhibit sodium-calcium exchange and cause accumulation of calcium in the vascular musculature, leading to increased muscle tone and increased resistance, thus raising blood pressure (Resnick, 1987).

Much of the evidence in favor of a role for sodium in the development of hypertension comes from epidemiologic data. Primitive societies where the intake of sodium is as low as 1,600 mg/day compared with American intake of 4,000 to 5,800 mg/day experience very little hypertension, and the blood pressure increase with age, common in industrialized societies, does not occur (Fregly, 1985; Page, 1979). As members of these developing societies adopt more sophisticated living patterns or move to other countries, the incidence of hypertension increases. In countries such as Japan, where the sodium intake is extremely high (9 to 12 g/day), hypertension is prevalent and stroke is the leading cause of death among adults (New Directions, p. 390).

These data are largely supported by animal experiments, initiated primarily by Dahl (1972). Evidence from animal studies is not consistently supported by studies in people however, nor are comparisons between societies supported by studies of people within those societies. This failure may be due to the fact that the average sodium intake in the industrialized nations is so universally high that minor changes will not produce recognizable effects. It may also be that only a percentage of hypertensives who are salt sensitive will respond to alterations in dietary sodium chloride intake. Notwithstanding, it was the conclusion of the Committee on Diet and Health of the National Research Council that "Blood pressure levels are strongly and positively correlated with the habitual intake of salt" (National Research Council, 1989).

Habitual high salt intake may increase the risk of developing hypertension in certain segments of the population. However, no good method for identifying these "salt-sensitive" individuals is available. It appears that blacks and the elderly (perhaps due to diminished renal function) have enhanced susceptibility to the hypertensive effects of sodium chloride (Beretta-Piccoli et al, 1982; Einhorn and Landsberg, 1988).

Recent studies have suggested that it is not sodium per se but rather the combination of sodium with chloride that is associated with increases in blood pressure. For example, in some but not all studies, sodium citrate fails to have the same blood-pressure elevating effect as sodium chloride (Kurtz et al, 1987).

Other Minerals

CALCIUM. Data implicating inadequate dietary intakes of calcium in the development of hypertension were derived from an analysis of data from the Framingham study involving 10,000 subjects aged 18 to 74 years. In a comparison of intakes of 17 nutrients with hypertension incidence, the highest correlation was a negative one with calcium (McCarron et al, 1984). Although these results have been supported by epidemiologic and intervention studies, the relationship has not been clarified to a point justifying higher intakes of calcium for the purpose of preventing hypertension. Calcium is involved with many physiologic processes that influence blood pressure, but it has not been shown to what extent these mechanisms are affected by dietary calcium. It may be that only a minor group of "calcium-sensitive" hypertensives respond to an increased calcium intake (Kaplan, 1989).

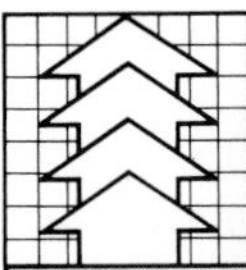

NEW DIRECTIONS: Effects of Migration on Disease

Migration of population groups to new locations where they are assimilated into new cultures and new physical environments underscores the influence of these factors on the incidence of certain types of disease.

Studies of Japanese in their native country, in Hawaii, and in the continental United States are an excellent example. Incidence of cardiovascular disease and of some types of cancer increases as emigrants move into increasingly westernized societies. Increased incidence of these diseases becomes apparent within a few years in the Issei (first generation Japanese immigrants) and is the same as that of the general American population in their children (Nisei) and grandchildren (Sansei).

Dramatic changes in lifestyle have also accompanied the industrialization and subsequent westernization of Japan, leading to a population that has been described as "migrants in time" (Lands et al, 1990). Increased consumption of dietary fats, with less of the omega-3 fatty acids present in a high fish diet, is associated with a rise in cardiovascular disease. The amount of fat in the Japanese diet at this time varies with location from 10% of kilocalories in the traditional diet to 40 to 50% of kilocalories in the Western-style diet.

With respect to hypertension, the reverse has been true. Movement of Japanese to the United States has been accompanied by a decreased level of hypertension, probably due to a lower sodium intake in the United States. In Japan, where the incidence of hypertension and stroke was at one time among one of the highest in the world, the traditional diet was extremely high in salt, derived from condiments and particularly from foods preserved with salt. In recent years, nationwide efforts in Japan to reduce salt intake have achieved dramatic results in reducing the incidence of hypertension and stroke caused by cerebral bleeding.

POTASSIUM. In several epidemiologic studies, blood pressure is inversely related to potassium intake, but controlled clinical trials have yielded conflicting findings. It may be the ratio of dietary potassium to sodium that is important in lowering or maintaining a lowered blood pressure (Khaw and Barrett-Connor, 1988; Krishna, 1989). Effects of potassium intake on blood pressure include direct arteriolar dilatation, increased loss of water and sodium from the body, suppression of renin and angiotensin secretion, decreased adrenergic tone, and stimulation of the sodium-potassium pump activity (Luft, 1989). The higher the sodium intake, the better will be the blood pressure response to increased potassium (Tobian, 1988).

In animal studies, potassium appears to protect against stroke. It has been hypothesized that a diet high in potassium protects the endothelial cells under tension from high blood pressure, thus preventing the artery wall lesions leading to cerebral hemorrhage and infarcts (Tobian, 1988).

One study of a large population-based cohort, in which 24-hour recalls of potassium intake were correlated with stroke-associated mortality during a 12-year period, found a 10 mEq/day increase in potassium intake—the equivalent of one full extra serving of fruit, citrus juice, vegetable, or potato—to be related to a 40% decrease in the incidence of stroke-related deaths. This effect appeared to be unrelated to any change in blood pressure (Khaw and Barrett-Connor, 1988). Dietary surveys consistently report American intakes of potassium to be well below dietary standards (USDA, 1986 and 1987). American blacks average a lower potassium intake than whites, which may be relevant to the higher rate of hypertension in this group (Tobian, 1988).

MAGNESIUM. An inverse relationship between serum magnesium and blood pressure has been reported (Kesteloot, 1984; Sangal and Beevers, 1982). However, there is no clear association between dietary intake of magnesium and blood pressure.

Magnesium is a potent inhibitor of vascular smooth muscle contraction and may play a role in blood pressure regulation as a vasodilator. It may also act by influencing the renin-angiotensin system, intravascular volume, or the synthesis and release of neurotransmitters (Einhorn and Landsberg, 1988).

Lipids

Polyunsaturated fatty acids (PUFA) are precursors of prostaglandins, whose actions affect renal sodium excretion and relax vascular musculature. Diets of restricted fat with PUFA: saturated fatty acid (SFA) ratios of 1.0 or more have lowered blood pressure in hypertensives; however, they have not been effective in those with either normal or only mildly elevated blood pressure, nor has their use been supported by large dietary intervention studies (Sacks, 1989).

Large doses of fish oils (50 ml daily with 15 g ω-3 fatty acids) have lowered blood pressure in mildly hypertensive men (Knapp and Fitzgerald, 1989). However, because even small doses are hazardous with respect to their effect on bleeding time and other parameters, supplementation with ω-3 fatty acids is not recommended at this time.

Vegetarians are subject to hypertension to a lesser degree than consumers of animal products, although their salt intake is not significantly different. A major distinction of their diets is the high ratio of polyunsaturated to saturated fats. The difference could also be related to a component of animal foods or to the increased potassium levels that accompany higher intakes of fruits and vegetables.

Alcohol

Five per cent of the hypertension in the population is due to alcohol consumption. Three drinks per day (a total of 3 oz of alcohol) is the most common cause of reversible hypertension (Kaplan, 1989). The condition affects from 30 to 60% of alcoholics, and women are more susceptible than men (Klatsky et al, 1986; Witteman et al, 1990).

Medications

A number of medications either raise blood pressure or interfere with the effectiveness of antihypertensive drugs. These include oral contraceptives, steroids, nonsteroidal anti-inflammatory agents, nasal decongestants and other cold remedies, appetite suppressants, cyclosporin, tricyclic antidepressants, and monoamine oxidase inhibitors (see Chapter 25).

MANAGEMENT

Pharmacologic Treatment

The standard treatment for hypertension is with diuretics and antihypertensive drugs. Various agents are employed—alone and in combination—including those that act centrally, those that produce ganglionic blockage, those that exert peripheral sympatholytic and adrenolytic effects, and those that act on the renin-angiotensin system.

The Hypertension Detection and Follow-Up Program demonstrated that aggressive treatment of hypertension, primarily pharmacologic, lowered total mortality by 17% as compared with a regular care approach. Treatment was particularly effective for those with mild hypertension, in whom a 20% reduction in mortality was achieved (Friedewald, 1982). Although drug therapy for this group protected against stroke, congestive heart failure, and progression of hypertension, the results with coronary artery disease were limited (Kaplan, 1985; Medical Research Council . . . , 1988).

Diuretics lower blood pressure in some patients by promoting volume depletion and sodium loss. However, thiazide diuretics increase urinary potassium excretion, especially in the presence of a high salt intake, thus leading to potassium loss and possibly hypokalemia. Except in the case of a potassium-sparing diuretic such as spironolactone or triamterene, additional potassium usually is required.

Nonpharmacologic Treatment

Pharmacologic treatment is not without hazard. Furthermore, medication is only palliative and usually must be continued for a lifetime. The finding that intensive treatment of mild hypertensives reduces mortality has raised the question of the advisability of putting millions of adults not previously treated on drugs that must be continued indefinitely (Stamler et al, 1989). Alternative interventions of proven value for mild hypertension are being recommended, either independently or as adjuncts to pharmacologic therapy. These interventions include weight reduction, sodium restriction, moderation of alcohol, isotonic exercise, and stress therapy.

The Joint National Committee on Detection, Evaluation, and Treatment of High Blood Pressure recommends:

1. Weight reduction to within 15% of desirable weight.
2. Alcohol restriction to no more than 1 oz/day, the amount in 2 oz of 100-proof whiskey, 8 oz of wine, or 24 oz of beer.
3. Sodium restriction to 1.5 to 2.5 g/day (4 to 6 g salt).

Weight Management

The effectiveness of weight reduction has been well documented in both mild and severe hypertensives (Hypertension Prevention . . . , 1990). Massive amounts of weight loss are not necessary, and positive results are seen with energy restriction alone. This effect may be related to metabolic adaptations to hypocaloric feeding such as reduced activity of the SNS, a system that plays a major role in blood pressure regulation (Kopopeschaar et al, 1983). The goal, particularly in individuals with a family history of hypertension, should be weight reduction to within 15% of desirable weight.

Sodium Restriction

Reducing intake of dietary sodium has some value in the regimen of hypertension management. However, except in the one fifth to one half of hypertensives who are truly salt-sensitive, the effect may be limited to enhancing the effectiveness of anti-hypertensive drugs. It is difficult to predict which hypertensives will respond positively to sodium restriction. Half of the patients with whom sodium restriction has been tried do not experience any reduction in blood pressure (Huttunen et al, 1985).

Evidence for the effectiveness of reduced sodium intakes in lowering blood pressure was obtained in the 1940s, prior to the availability of modern pharmacologic treatment. Kempner's highly restrictive "rice diet," which was low in fat and sodium and high in carbohydrate and potassium, effectively lowered blood pressure in 64% of his patients (Kempner, 1948). The diet consisted of 10 oz of dry rice (approximately 1,050 kcal), with an additional 900 to 1,000 kcal supplied by liberal quantities of sugar and fresh or preserved fruits. Fluids were limited to 700 to 1,000 ml of fruit juices. Weight reduction or the high potassium : sodium ratio may have also been factors in the dramatic blood pressure drops. In any case, the drastic nature of the diet made it realistically impossible to follow for an indefinite period.

Although evidence in support of decreasing blood pressure by lowering sodium intake is limited, most authorities agree that a moderate restriction is appropriate. Reducing intakes to 70 to 100 mEq/day (approximately 1.5 to 2.5 g of sodium or 4 to 6 g of salt) can be effective in reducing the need for medication, even in those patients who are taking only diuretics. (The typical American sodium intake is 150 to 250 mEq/day.) Anything less than 50 mEq is not only impractical but may also stimulate the renin-angiotensin system to a degree that will limit the antihypertensive and potassium-sparing effects of the sodium restriction (Kaplan, 1985) (see Chapter 33).

Other Dietary Modifications

MINERALS. Although some data strongly suggest a benefit in increased intakes of potassium, calcium, and magnesium, the information available at this time is insufficient to support a specific recommendation for increased levels of intake other than to meet the Recommended Dietary Allowances for calcium and magnesium and to increase intakes of fruits and vegetables when possible.

Potassium intakes of 120 to 175 mEq/day are somewhat effective in lowering blood pressure. However, the taste of potassium supplements is objectionable and they are expensive. Their use is contraindicated in patients with impaired renal function, as well as in those who are taking potassium-sparing diuretics or angiotensin-converting enzyme medications, all of which could contribute to hyperkalemia.

Appendix Table 1 and Table 35–7 list the potassium content of foods.

LIPIDS. Current recommendations for modifying lipid composition of the diet to increase the PUFA : SFA ratio while limiting total fat are also appropriate for treating hypertension (Kaplan, 1985). Fish oil supplementation is not recommended, although increased consumption of fish is recommended.

Exercise

The long-term effect of aerobic, endurance-type regular exercise is to lower blood pressure, even though the immediate effect during and shortly after exercise is blood pressure elevation. Exercise also has other beneficial effects with respect to coronary artery disease (Fig. 21–1; see Chapter 20).

PREVENTION

The National High Blood Pressure Education Program of the National Heart, Lung and Blood Institute of the National Institutes of Health has established a goal of identifying and treating 95% or more of all persons with high blood pressure with a goal of reducing the death rate from stroke, hypertension-associated heart disease, and renal disease.

Although the effectiveness of advising normotensives who are not apparently at risk to reduce their sodium intakes has not been documented, it is recognized that it is difficult if not impossible to identify all of those who will eventually become hypertensive. For this reason, most dietary guidelines recommend lowering sodium intakes from the present high level common to the American population to those achieved by cooking with as little salt as possible, refraining from adding salt at the table, and avoiding highly salted processed foods (see Chapter 33). The issue remains controversial.

Early identification of children as potential hypertensives has been recommended. In a major study in American children, blood pressure was found to increase gradually with age (Voors et al, 1979). However, the relationship between blood pressure in childhood and the development of hypertension is not clear. Two studies have shown a strong relationship between body size and blood pressure during growth but no clear relationships between blood pressure and intakes of sodium or any other nutrient (Berenson et al, 1980; Lauer and Clarke, 1980). The estimated safe intake of sodium is exceeded at age 6 months by 66% of infants, at age 1 to 10 years by 90 to 100% of children, and at age 13 to 17

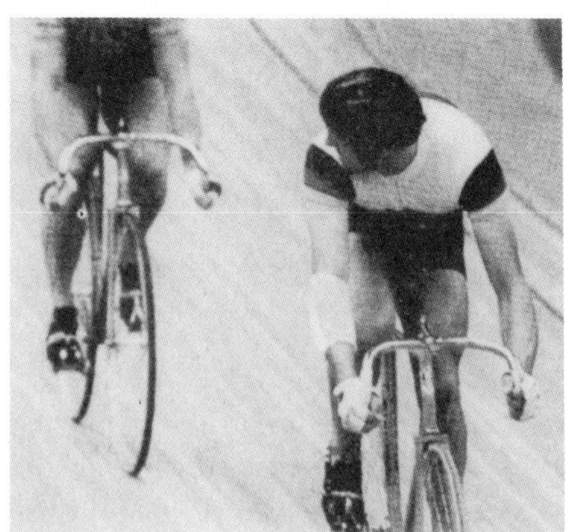

FIGURE 21–1. *Bicycling, an aerobic, endurance-type form of exercise, lowers blood pressure. (From Kuprian W [ed]: Physical Therapy for Sports. Philadelphia, WB Saunders, 1982, p 117.)*

years by 60 to 65% of teenagers. At the same time a much smaller percentage of children surpass the estimated safe intake for potassium and only 50% of children aged 7 to 10 years meet the recommended range. Intakes of calcium and magnesium tend to be low (Frank et al, 1988).

It appears that the best advice for preventing the development of hypertension is to promote normal weight gain and prevent obesity.

CITED REFERENCES

Berenson GS et al: Importance of blood pressures in children. *In* Kesteloot H and Joossens JV (eds): Epidemiology of Arterial Blood Pressure: Developments in Cardiovascular Medicine, vol I. The Hague, Martinus Nijhoff, 1980.

Beretta-Piccoli C et al: Relation of arterial pressure with body sodium, body potassium, and plasma potassium in essential hypertension. Clin Sci 63:257, 1982.

Blaustein MP and Hamlyn JM: Sodium transport inhibition, cell calcium, and hypertension: The natriuretic hormone/Na Ca exchange/hypertension hypothesis. Am J Med 77:45, 1984.

Dahl LK: Salt and hypertension. Am J Clin Nutr 25:231, 1972.

Dannenberg AL et al: Incidence of hypertension in the Framingham Study. Am J Public Health 78:676, 1988.

Department of Health and Human Services: Blood Pressure Levels in Persons 18–74 Years of Age in 1976–80, and Trends in Blood Pressure from 1960 to 1980 in the United States. Data from the National Health Survey, Ser 11, No 234, DHHS Publ No (PHS) 86-1684. Hyattsville, MD, National Center for Health Statistics, Public Health Service, USDHHS, 1986.

Einhorn D and Landsberg L: Nutrition and diet in hypertension. *In* Shils ME and Young VR (eds): Modern Nutrition in Health and Disease, 7th ed. Philadelphia, Lea & Febiger, 1988.

Frank GC et al: Sodium, potassium, calcium, magnesium, and phosphorus intakes of infants and children: Bogalusa Heart Study. J Am Diet Assoc 88:801, 1988.

Fregly MJ: Attempts to estimate sodium intake in humans. *In* Horan MJ et al (eds): NIH Workshop on Nutrition and Hypertension. Proceedings from a Symposium, March 12–14, 1984. Bethesda, Biomedical Information Corp, 1985.

Friedewald WT: Current issues in hypertension. J Am Diet Assoc 80:17, 1982.

Havlik RJ et al: Weight and hypertension. Ann Intern Med 98(Part 2):855, 1983.

Huttunen JK et al: Dietary factors and hypertension. Acta Med Scand 701(Suppl):72, 1985.

Hypertension Prevalence and the Status of Awareness, Treatment, and Control in the United States. Final Report of the Subcommittee on Definition and Prevalence of the Joint National Committee on Detection, Evaluation, and Treatment of High Blood Pressure. Bethesda, MD, National Heart, Lung, and Blood Institute, 1984.

Hypertension Prevention Trial Research Group: The Hypertension Prevention Trial: Three-year effects of dietary changes on blood pressure. Arch Intern Med 150:153, 1990.

Joint National Committee: The 1988 Report of the Joint National Committee on Detection, Evaluation, and Treatment of High Blood Pressure. NIH Publ No 88-1088. Washington, DC, Government Printing Office, 1988.

Kaplan NM: Non-drug treatment of hypertension. Ann Intern Med 102:362, 1985.

Kaplan NM: Nonpharmacological control of high blood pressure. Am J Hypertension 2(Suppl):55S, 1989.

Kempner W: Treatment of hypertensive vascular disease with rice diet. Am J Med 4:545, 1948.

Kesteloot H: Urinary cations and blood pressure—population studies. Ann Clin Res 43(Suppl 16):72, 1984.

Khaw K-T and Barrett-Connor E: The association between blood pressure, age, and dietary sodium and potassium: A population study. Circulation 77:53, 1988.

Klatsky AL, Friedman GD, and Armstrong MA: The relationships between alcoholic beverage use and other traits to blood pressure: A new Kaiser Permanente study. Circulation 73:628, 1986.

Knapp HR and Fitzgerald GA: The antihypertensive effects of fish oil. N Engl J Med 320:1037, 1989.

Kopopeschaar HP et al: The effect of modified fasting on blood pressure and sympathetic activity: A correlation? Int J Obesity 7:569, 1983.

Krishna GG et al: Increased blood pressure during potassium depletion in normotensive men. N Engl J Med 320:1177, 1989.

Kurtz TW, Al-Bander HA, and Morris C: "Salt-sensitive" essential hypertension in men: Is the sodium ion alone important? N Engl J Med 317:1043, 1987.

Lands WEM et al: Changing dietary patterns. Am J Clin Nutr 51:991, 1990.

Lauer RM and Clarke WR: Immediate and long-term prognostic significance of childhood blood pressure levels. *In* Lauer RM and Shekelle RB (eds): Childhood Prevention of Atherosclerosis and Hypertension. New York, Raven Press, 1980.

Luft FC: Dietary sodium, potassium and chloride intake and arterial hypertension. Nutrition Today 24(3):9, 1989.

McCarron DA et al: Blood pressure and nutrient intake in the United States. Science 224:1392, 1984.

Medical Research Council Working Party on Mild Hypertension: Coronary heart disease in the Medical Research Council trial of treatment of mild hypertension. Br Heart J 59:364, 1988.

National Research Council: Diet and Health. Implications for Reducing Chronic Disease Risk. Washington, DC, National Academy Press, 1989.

Page LB: Hypertension and atherosclerosis in primitive and acculturating societies. *In* Hunt JC (ed): Hypertension Update, Vol 1. Lyndhurst, NJ, Health Learning Systems, 1979.

Resnick LM: Dietary calcium and hypertension. J Nutr 117:1806, 1987.

Sacks FM: Dietary fats and blood pressure: A critical review of the evidence. Nutr Rev 47:291, 1989.

Sangal AK and Beevers DG: Serum calcium and blood pressure. Lancet 2:493, 1982.

Schwartz JH, Young JB, and Landsberg L: Effect of dietary fat on sympathetic nervous system activity in the rat. J Clin Invest 72:361, 1983.

Selby JV et al: Precursors of essential hypertension. The role of body fat distribution pattern. Am J Epidemiol 129:43, 1989.

Stamler J et al: Relationship of multiple variables to blood pressure—findings from four Chicago epidemiological studies. *In* Paul O (ed): Epidemiology and Control of Hypertension. New York, Stratton Intercontinental Medical Book Co, 1975.

Stamler R et al: Cardiac status after four years in a trial on nutritional therapy for high blood pressure. Arch Int Med 149:661, 1989.

Tobian L: Potassium and hypertension. Nutr Rev 46:273, 1988.

USDA: Nationwide Food Consumption Survey. Continuing Survey of Food Intakes by Individuals. Men 19–50 Years, 1 Day, 1985. Report No 85-3, Nutrition Monitoring Division, Human Nutrition Information Service. Hyattsville, MD, USDA, 1986.

USDA: Nationwide Food Consumption Survey. Continuing Survey of Food Intakes by Individuals. Women 19–50 Years and Their Children 1–5 Years, 4 Days, 1985. Report No 85-4, Nutrition Monitoring Division, Human Nutrition Information Service. Hyattsville, MD, USDA, 1987.

Voors AW et al: Time-course studies of blood pressure in children—The Bogalusa Heart Study. Am J Epidemiol 109:320, 1979.

Williams PT et al: Associations of dietary fat, regional adiposity, and blood pressure in men. JAMA 257:3251, 1987.

Witteman JC et al: Relation of moderate alcohol consumption and risk of systemic hypertension in women. Am J Cardiol 65:633, 1990.

ADDITIONAL REFERENCES

Beauchamp GK, Bertino M, and Engelman K: Modification of salt taste. Ann Intern Med 98(5):763, 1983.

Fortmann SP et al: Effects of weight loss on clinic and ambulatory blood pressure in normotensive men. Am J Cardiol 62:89, 1988.

Friedman GD et al: Precursors of essential hypertension: Body weight, alcohol and salt use, and parental history of hypertension. Prev Med 17:387, 1988.

Intersalt Cooperative Research Group: Intersalt: An international study of electrolyte excretion and blood pressure. Results for 24-hour urinary sodium and potassium excretion. Br Med J 297:319, 1988.

Kaare H et al: Effect of eicosapentaenoic and docosahexaenoic acids on blood pressure in hypertension. A population-based intervention trial from the Tromso study. N Engl J Med 322:795, 1990.

Kaplan NM: Dietary aspects of the treatment of hypertension. Annu Rev Public Health 7:503, 1986.

Keil U, Chambless L, and Remmers A: Alcohol and blood pressure: Results from the Luebeck Blood Pressure Study. Prev Med 18:1, 1989.

Khaw K-T and Barrett-Connor E: Dietary potassium and stroke-associated mortality. A 12 year prospective population study. N Engl J Med 316:235, 1987.

Knapp HR: Omega-3 fatty acids, endogenous prostaglandins, and blood pressure regulation in humans. Nutr Rev 47:301, 1989.

Knochel JP: Cardiovascular effects of alcohol. Ann Intern Med 98:849, 1983.

Leaf A and Weber PC: Cardiovascular effects of ω-3 fatty acids. N Engl J Med 318:549, 1988.

Liebman BF and Langford HG: Hypertension and sodium salts. Science 228:351, 1985.

Lind L et al: Blood pressure is lowered by vitamin D (alphacalcidol) during long-term treatment of patients with intermittent hypercalcemia: A double-blind, placebo-controlled study. Acta Med Scand 222:423, 1987.

Luft FC: Dietary sodium restriction in patients with hypertension. Nutr MD 15:1, 1989.

McCarron DA and Morris CD: Blood pressure response to oral calcium in persons with mild to moderate hypertension: A randomized, double-blind, placebo-controlled, crossover trial. Ann Intern Med 103:825, 1985.

Reisin E et al: Cardiovascular changes after weight reduction in obesity hypertension. Ann Intern Med 98:315, 1983.

Salonen JT et al: Blood pressure, dietary fats, and antioxidants. Am J Clin Nutr 48:1226, 1988.

Tipton CM: Exercise, training and hypertension. Exerc Sport Sci Rev 12:245, 1984.

Weinberger MH: Antihypertensive therapy and lipids: Paradoxical influences on cardiovascular disease risk. Am J Med 80(Suppl):64, 1986.

Weinberger MH et al: Dietary sodium restriction as adjunctive treatment of hypertension. JAMA 259:2561, 1988.

Weinsier R: Recent developments in the etiology and treatment of hypertension: Dietary calcium, fat and magnesium. Am J Clin Nutr 42:1331, 1985.

Wittemen JC et al: A prospective study of nutritional factors and hypertension among US women. Circulation 80:1320, 1989.

CHAPTER 22

NUTRITION AND BONE HEALTH

CHAPTER OUTLINE

Bone Physiology
Osteoporosis

KEY TERMS

AGE-ASSOCIATED OSTEOPOROSIS (TYPE II)—a loss of density in both cortical and trabecular bone that occurs in elderly of both sexes after age 70; characterized by wedge fractures of the thoracic vertebrae that lead to back pain, loss of height, and "dowager's hump"

BONE REMODELING—the process by which bone is continually dismantled and reformed in order to repair itself, grow, adapt to stresses and strains, and furnish calcium for other body needs

CORTICAL BONE—the compact bone of the shaft that surrounds the medullary cavity

ESTROGEN REPLACEMENT THERAPY (ERT)—administration of synthetic estrogen to replace the natural hormone, which declines after menopause

HYDROXYAPATITE—a crystalline structure composed of calcium phosphate and calcium carbonate in an organic collagen matrix that gives strength and rigidity to bones and teeth

OSTEOBLAST—a bone cell associated with the formation of bone

OSTEOCLAST—a bone cell associated with the resorption and removal of bone

OSTEOMALACIA—a condition of impaired mineralization caused by vitamin D and calcium deficiency

OSTEOPOROSIS—a loss of bone density to the point that the skeleton is unable to sustain ordinary stresses and fractures develop

POSTMENOPAUSAL OSTEOPOROSIS (TYPE I)—a loss of density primarily involving the trabecular bone and characterized by fractures of the distal radius and crush fractures of the lumbar vertebrae

PRIMARY IDIOPATHIC OSTEOPOROSIS—a loss of bone density that affects premenopausal women and young or middle-aged men

SECONDARY OSTEOPOROSIS—a loss of bone density secondary to another disease

TRABECULAR BONE (CANCELLOUS BONE)—the spongy bone in the knobby ends of the long bones, the iliac crest, scapula, and vertebrae

Nutrition holds promise as a preventive measure in the area of bone health. Although diseases of the bone, like many other diseases, have complex etiologies, the development of some can be minimized by provision of adequate nutrients at appropriate periods during the life cycle. Of these diseases, *osteoporosis* is the most common and the most destructive of productivity and quality of life. With the increased longevity of the American population, the tragedy of this disease becomes more significant as a contributor to morbidity and mortality in the elderly. Whether provision of bone-building nutrients is effective after onset of the disease remains questionable; however, ample evidence supports aggressive attention to adequate calcium intake during the active period of bone growth and development.

BONE PHYSIOLOGY

Composition of Bone

Bone consists of an organic matrix, primarily collagen fibers, in which are deposited salts of calcium and phosphate in combination with hydroxyl ions in crystals of hydroxyapatite. The tensile capacity of collagen and the compressional ability of calcium salts combine to give bone its great strength.

Kinds of Bone

The largest part of the skeleton (80%) is made up of compact *cortical bone.* Shafts of the large bones are primarily cortical bone. The remainder is *trabecular,* or *cancellous bone,* which occurs in the knobby ends of the long bones, the iliac crest of the pelvis, the wrists, scapulas, and vertebrae. Trabecular bone is spongy and less dense than cortical bone and is characterized in some areas by long spicules of apatite that are exposed to circulating fluids.

Calcium Homeostasis

Although 99% of the body calcium is found in the skeleton, the remaining 1% is critical to a great variety of indispensable life processes. Levels of calcium in extracellular fluids are regulated by complex mechanisms that balance calcium intake and excretion with bodily needs. When calcium intake is inadequate, homeostasis is maintained by drawing on mineral from the bone to maintain the serum calcium ion concentration at normal levels. Depending on the amount required, this can be accomplished by drawing from readily mobilizable calcium salts in the bone fluids or, through the process of remodeling, from the bone itself.

Bone Remodeling

Bone is continually undergoing the process of remodeling in order to support a growing body, adapt to changes in lifestyle that impose different stresses and strains, maintain appropriate calcium levels in extracellular fluids, and repair microscopic fractures that occur over time. Formation of new bone occurs continually in all living bone, with about 4% of surfaces involved at any given time.

Both types of bone are subject to the remodeling process, although the largest part occurs in the trabecular bone, which is located in areas subject to the greatest weight-bearing stresses. Remodeling of cortical bone is in response to the microscopic fractures that occur with the gradual deterioration of cells forming the organic matrix.

Bone remodeling is a process in which bone is continuously dismantled and reformed through the action of highly specialized cells, the *osteoclasts* and the *osteoblasts.* Osteoclasts resorb both the mineral and organic components of bone, forming small cavities on the inner and outer bone surfaces, which are then refilled with new bone by action of the osteoblasts. In normal young adults, the resorption and formation phases are tightly coupled and bone mass is maintained. Bone loss involves an uncoupling of the phases of bone remodeling with an increase in resorption over formation.

The first step of the remodeling process is hormonal *activation* of cells that line the bone surfaces. These clump together to uncover the bone surface, which is then invaded by osteoclasts. Interleukin-1, a lymphokine that activates lining cells, is involved in this phase. Acids and proteolytic enzymes released by the osteoclasts then *resorb* bone mineral and matrix, eroding a minute tunnel in cortical bone or a lacuna on the surface of trabecular bone. The *rebuilding* stage involves secretion of collagen and ground substance by the osteoblasts. Collagen polymerizes to form fibers, resulting in *osteoid tissue.* In a few days, salts of calcium and phosphorus begin to precipitate on the collagen fibers and develop into crystals of hydroxyapatite.

Resorption is accomplished in approximately 2 weeks. The osteoblasts replace resorbed bone and fill the resorption cavities over a period of 2 to 3 months (Raisz, 1988).

The action of *parathyroid hormone (PTH)* in promoting activity of the osteoclasts is countered by *estrogen,* which reduces bone tissue response to PTH stimuli. *Calcitonin* inhibits osteoclast activity.

Bone Mass

Accumulation

During the growth periods of childhood and puberty, and beyond into young adulthood, deposition outstrips the resorption of bone. Peak bone mass is reached around the age of 25 to 35 years. The long bones stop growing in length around age 20, but mass continues to accumulate for a few more years. Cortical bone continues to be formed until age 35 (NIH Consensus Conference, 1984).

Peak Bone Mass

Peak bone mass is greater in men than in women because of their larger frame size. Both bone mass and bone density are normally lower in women. One study demonstrated a 15% lower bone density and a 30% lower bone mass in women than in men after completion of skeletal growth (Mazess, 1982).

Bone density is also greater in blacks and Hispanics as compared with whites and Asians, a factor that may be related to larger muscle mass. A strong *hereditary component* is also related to the development of bone mass (Pollitzer and Anderson, 1989; Pocock et al, 1987). Premenopausal daughters of osteoporotic mothers have demonstrated reduced bone mass in the spine and femoral neck compared with daughters of normal mothers (Seeman et al, 1989).

Peak bone mass is also related to dietary calcium intakes and the extent of weight-bearing exercise during the growth and development period.

Loss of Bone Mass

Age is an important determinant of bone density. If the age of a woman is known, her vertebral bone mass often can be predicted within 10% (Clinical Insight, p. 398).

Around age 40, bone mass begins to gradually diminish in both sexes, with a continuous loss over adult life at a mean rate of 1.2%/yr. Loss of bone mass is the result of changes in the mechanisms governing osteogenesis. The processes of resorption and deposition are uncoupled to a degree that interferes with the ability of osteoblast action to keep pace with osteoclast activity.

Cortical bone and trabecular bone have different patterns of aging. Loss of cortical bone eventually plateaus and may even cease late in life (Peck et al, 1987; Riggs and Melton, 1986). Trabecular bone, however, begins to diminish in both sexes as early as 35 years. Premenopausal loss in women is much greater in trabecular bone than in cortical bone. Loss of both kinds of bone accelerates in women after the menopause, although trabecular bone is lost at a much higher rate (Fig. 22–1).

The accelerated rate of 2 to 3%/yr continues in women for around 5 to 10 years after menopause and then declines gradually to a rate leading to a postmaturity loss of 0.25 to 1%/yr. However, there is a subgroup of postmenopausal women who lose bone at an even faster rate (Christiansen, 1987). Throughout a lifetime, women lose up to 45 to 50% of bone mass (35% of cortical bone and 50% of trabecular bone) and men 20 to 30% (NIH Consensus Conference, 1984; Peck et al, 1987; Riggs and Melton, 1986).

The bone loss that occurs with aging amounts to 300 mg of calcium/day that is lost in the stool and must be replaced daily. Calcium absorption is governed to a large extent by need, so that the body can adapt to a wide range of intakes in maintaining calcium homeostasis. However, the action of hormones and other factors responsible for maintaining calcium homeostasis

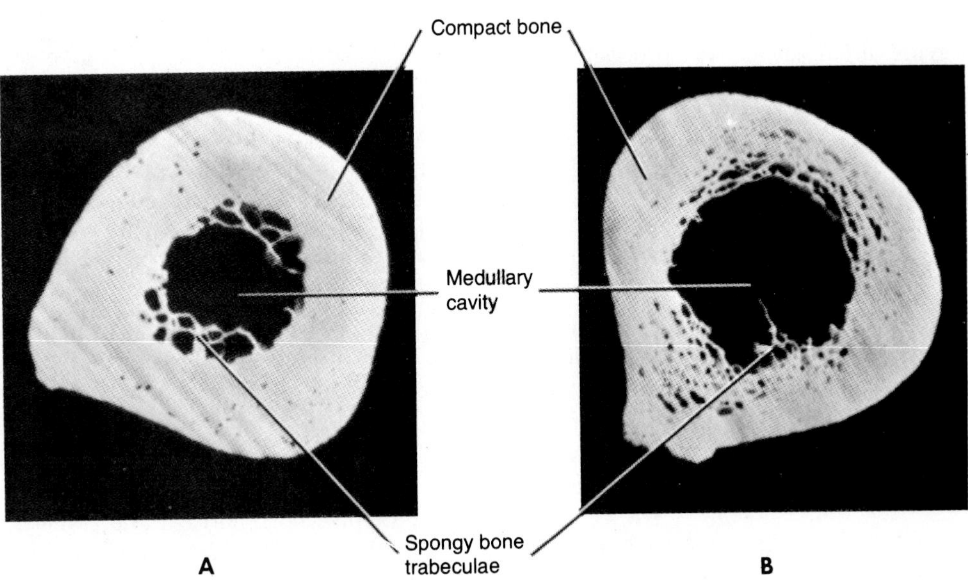

FIGURE 22–1. *Osteoporosis. Photographs of a cross section of the femur from* (A) *a normal female aged 25 and* (B) *a female with osteoporosis, aged 82. In* (B) *note the decreased thickness of the compact bone of the diaphysis, the increase in the diameter of the medullary cavity, and the thinning of the spongy bone trabeculae. (From Tortora GJ: Principles of Human Anatomy. New York, Harper & Row, 1983.)*

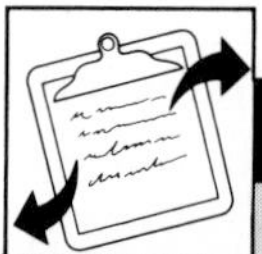

CLINICAL INSIGHT: Bone Mineral Density Measurement

Inasmuch as at present there is no safe and effective treatment to replace bone that is already lost, it seems to be important to identify the women who are at risk for developing osteoporosis as early as possible so that preventive measures can be taken to prevent further bone loss. Since low bone mass is a major risk factor for osteoporosis, its assessment appears to be clinically useful.

Assessment of bone mass based on the existence of risk factors of age, height, weight, smoking status, alcohol consumption, calcium intake, exercise, frame size, and some biochemical parameters is not clinically accurate enough. Measurement of bone mineral density (BMD), also called bone densitometry, is clinically available at a reasonable cost and is safe, precise, and accurate.

Bone densitometry measures bone mass on the basis of tissue absorption of photons produced by a radionuclide or an x-ray tube. Results are expressed as grams of mineral per cubic centimeter of bone. A committee of the National Osteoporosis Foundation has recommended several situations in which bone densitometry is appropriate, two of which are (1) estrogen deficiency and (2) long-term glucocorticoid therapy. A BMD measurement in estrogen-deficient females can identify those who also have low bone mass and help physicians and patients make decisions about ERT. In those on long-term glucocorticoid therapy a BMD measurement can indicate needed adjustments in medication.

If BMD is measured it appears that the results from any site are suitable for predicting the risk of fracture (Johnston, et al, 1991).

—as well as the absorption of calcium—becomes less efficient with age. The decreased absorption in both sexes can lead to negative calcium balance.

The normal bone loss that occurs with aging in both sexes is related to deterioration of the collagen forming the organic matrix of bone as well as to gradual uncoupling of the remodeling process. Acceleration of the process that occurs in women after menopause is directly related to the lack of estrogen (Anderson, 1990). Bone loss in men also accelerates in later years, but about 10 years later than in women, and it may be related to loss of androgen.

Age-related changes may also be associated with impaired regulation of osteoblast activity and protein anabolism, and diminished calcitonin and PTH activity. Also implicated are impaired calcitriol production and decreased levels of somatomedin C, a growth factor that stimulates osteoblast activity.

OSTEOPOROSIS

Definition and Occurrence

The bone loss that begins in adult life and continues into old age is a normal process. Bone composition is unchanged, but mass and density are decreased. *Osteoporosis* occurs when loss of bone density becomes so acute that the skeleton is unable to sustain ordinary stresses, a condition marked by the occurrence of fractures.

Osteoporosis affects from 15 to 20 million people, including 1 out of every 3 people over the age of 65. It is 8 times more prevalent in women than in men (Turner and Whitney, 1989).

The physical cost of this disease is measured in 1.3 million fractures each year. Half of these involve the vertebrae; 200,000 are fractures of the hip, which result in incapacitation, long-term nursing care, and frequently death (National Center for Health Statistics, 1988; Riggs and Melton, 1986). It is estimated that the proportion of Americans over 65 years of age will double from 12% in 1988 to 24% in 2020 (Sanborn, 1990). Because virtually all elderly are affected, the increasing longevity of this population emphasizes the need for prevention of osteoporosis early in life.

Classification

The two forms of primary, or involutional osteoporosis, are distinguished in general by sex, the age at which fractures occur, and the kinds of bone involved.

Type I, postmenopausal osteoporosis, is seen in elderly women within 15 to 20 years of menopause and it primarily involves trabecular bone. It is characterized by fractures of the distal radius (Colles' fractures) and painful and deforming "crush" fractures of the lumbar vertebrae. Bone mass in the lumbar spine of women with postmenopausal osteoporosis has been measured at levels 33% lower than in age-matched nonosteoporotic controls (Seeman et al, 1989). Other areas with a preponderance of trabecular bone such as the pelvis and the proximal end of the femur are also involved.

Type II, or *age-associated osteoporosis,* occurs around age 70 and beyond. It affects both sexes and may involve both cortical and trabecular bone. Fractures of both hip and vertebrae continue to rise with aging, with a dramatic increase in hip fractures occurring late in life. Wedge fractures of the thoracic vertebrae lead to back pain, loss of height, and spinal deformity (especially kyphosis, or "dowager's hump") (Fig.

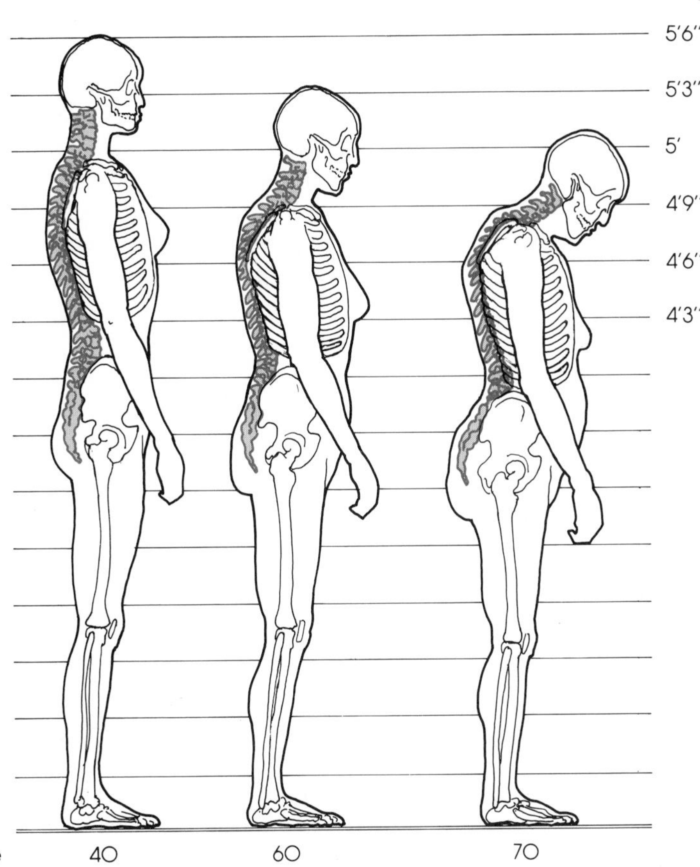

FIGURE 22-2. *Normal spine at age 40 and osteoporotic changes at ages 60 and 70. These changes can cause a loss of as much as 6 to 9 in. in height and can result in the so-called dowager's hump* (far right) *in the upper thoracic vertebrae. (From Ignatavicius D and Bayne MV: Medical-Surgical Nursing: A Nursing Process Approach. Philadelphia, WB Saunders, 1991, p 739.)*

22-2). It is not unusual for patients to lose between 4 and 8 inches in height. The most common symptom is back pain, which may be mild or severe and may last for days or weeks before receding and then recurring. Such a fracture can occur after some ordinary activity such as lifting a sack of groceries.

Although age-associated osteoporosis affects both sexes, women are the most severely affected because they suffer not only the degenerative effects of aging common to both sexes but also the skeletal deterioration that characterizes the postmenopausal period. Hip fractures affect nearly 20% of postmenopausal women up to age 80 and almost 50% of those beyond that age (Anderson, 1990).

A rare type of *primary idiopathic osteoporosis* affects premenopausal women and young or middle-aged men. *Secondary osteoporosis* results when an identifiable drug or disease process causes loss of bone tissue (Table 22-1).

Etiology

Osteoporosis is a complex heterogeneous problem of unknown etiology. Why otherwise normal processes lead in some people to bone density inadequate to support the body is not known. Although the fracture-precipitating condition of inadequate bone mass is common to all types of osteoporosis, the processes by which this end is reached probably result from etiologies distinctive to each type.

Possible Causes

Loss of bone mass to a degree that results in fractures can result from (1) an excessive acceleration of loss and (2) a peak bone mass so low that with the passage of enough time of exposure to normal attrition, the bones eventually become fragile and susceptible to fracture.

TABLE 22-1. Common Drugs That Increase Calcium Loss

Phenytoin (Dilantin)
Phenobarbital
Thyroid hormone
Corticosteroids
Methotrexate
Cyclosporin
Lithium
Tetracycline
Aluminum-containing antacids
Heparin
Phenothiazine derivatives

Risk Factors

Risk factors for osteoporosis are age, race, sex, body build, family history, premature menopause, nulliparity, limited lifelong calcium intake, limited exercise, use of cigarettes, alcohol consumption, and prolonged use of excess exogenous thyroid (Table 22–2). *Whites* and *Asians* suffer more osteoporotic fractures than blacks and Hispanics, who have a greater bone density (Cohn et al, 1977). *Petite or thin* women, particularly of Northern European extraction, are more susceptible to osteoporosis (Peck et al, 1987).

MENSTRUAL STATUS. Menstrual status is a major determinant of osteoporosis risk in women. Acceleration of bone loss coincides with the menopause, either natural or surgical, at which time the ovaries stop producing estrogen.

Any interruption of menstruation for an extended period results in bone loss. The amenorrhea that accompanies excessive weight loss as seen in anorexia nervosa or as a consequence of excessive exercise, has the same effect on bones as the menopause. Bone mass in amenorrheic athletes has been measured at levels 25 to 40% below control levels. When menses were resumed in these athletes, bone mass increased, but eventually plateaued at a level lower than that of sedentary women (Drinkwater et al, 1986).

TABLE 22–2. Risk Factors for Developing Osteoporosis

Family history of osteoporosis
Female
White or Asian
Slight body build
Estrogen depletion
- Menopause
- Early oophorectomy in women
- Hypogonadism in men
- Hypogonadism in women with excessive exercise

Age: Especially after age 60.
Lack of exercise
Prolonged use of certain medications
- Aluminum-containing antacids
- Steroids
- Tetracycline
- Anticonvulsants
- Exogenous thyroid

Diseases or conditions that result in negative calcium balance
- Hyperthyroidism
- Diabetes
- Chronic renal failure
- Chronic diarrhea or malabsorption
- Parathyroid disease
- Chronic obstructive lung disease
- Subtotal gastrectomy
- Hemiplegia

Underweight or underfat
Cigarette smoking
Excessive alcohol consumption
Excessive fiber consumption
Excessive caffeine consumption
Inadequate calcium or vitamin D intake

CALCIUM INTAKE. The density of bone mass attained at the time growth is complete determines to some degree what will be left after years of gradual loss. Although peak bone mass is determined by a number of factors, calcium intake from birth through adolescence is a major contributor. The influence of calcium intake during adulthood is not known, but available evidence indicates that those with a lifetime history of adequate calcium intake are less susceptible to osteoporosis at advanced ages (Matkovic et al, 1979).

LACK OF EXERCISE. *Immobility* in varying degrees is well recognized as a cause of bone loss (Fig. 22–3). Maintenance of healthy bone requires exposure to weight-bearing pressures. Stresses from muscle contraction and maintaining the body in an upright position against the pull of gravity stimulate osteoblast function. Bones not subjected to normal use rapidly lose mass. Invalids confined to bed or persons unable to move freely are commonly affected. Astronauts living in conditions of zero gravity for only a few days experience so much bone loss that appropriate exercise is a feature of their daily routines. To a lesser degree lack of exercise and a sedentary mode of living that continue over a lifetime, can also contribute significantly to bone loss, although their most important influence is probably with respect to the inadequate accumulation of bone mass.

MEDICATIONS. A number of *medications* contribute to osteoporosis, either by interfering with calcium absorption or by actively promoting calcium loss from bone (see Table 22–1). Steroids, for example, affect vitamin D metabolism and can lead to bone loss. Excessive amounts of exogenous thyroid hormone, even in very low amounts, can promote loss of bone mass over a period of time.

OTHER RISK FACTORS. *Cigarette smoking* and *alcohol consumption* are risk factors for developing osteoporosis, probably because of toxic effects on osteoblasts. Other dietary factors associated with bone loss include excessive *fiber intake,* which can interfere with calcium absorption. High *sodium* levels, particularly in association with a low calcium intake, can contribute to type II osteoporosis because urinary sodium excretion is accompanied by calcium excretion (Wardlaw and Barden, 1989). *Caffeine* consumption also increases urinary excretion of calcium, an effect possibly related to prostaglandin production (Dietary Caffeine . . . , 1988; Massey and Wise, 1984). A high *protein intake* without an increase in phosphorus also influences calcium balance, leading to increased urinary calcium excretion and possibly loss of skeletal calcium (Schuette and Linkswiler, 1982).

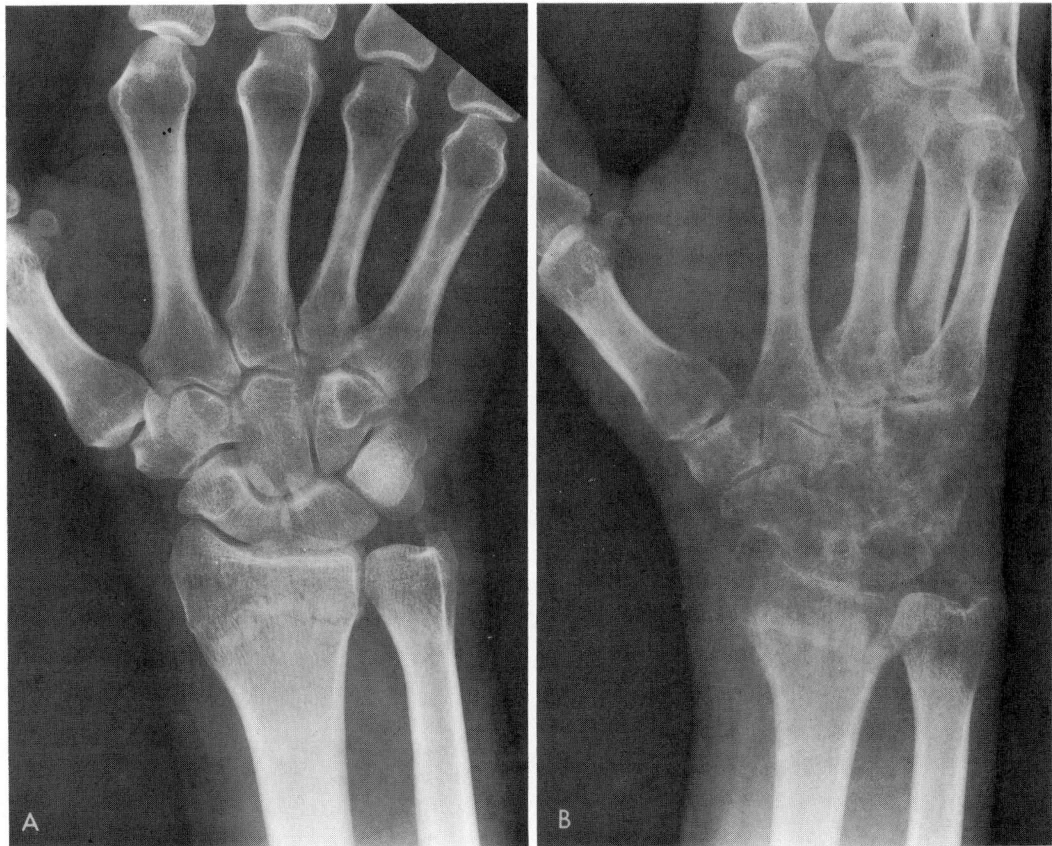

FIGURE 22–3. A, *Roentgenogram of the carpal area shortly after fracture of the distal radius. The part was immobilized by a plaster cast.* B, *Roentgenogram of the same area several weeks after immobilization. Note the disuse atrophy of the carpal bones. (From Aegerter EE and Kirkpatrick JA: Orthopedic Diseases: Physiology, Pathology, Radiology, 4th ed. Philadelphia, WB Saunders, 1975, p 32.)*

Prevention and Treatment

Estrogen Replacement Therapy

Estrogen replacement therapy (ERT) is the best-documented method for reducing bone resorption and arresting postmenopausal bone loss in women (Christiansen et al, 1980). It is most effective when used during the first 5 to 15 years after menopause (Peck et al, 1987). If estrogen is started a few years after menopause, it can even reduce the fracture rate (Jensen et al, 1982). ERT is not recommended for women who have already lost considerable bone because there is no evidence that it rebuilds or replenishes bone.

Hazards of ERT include the possible risk of endometrial cancer; however, adding progestin lowers the risk. Return of the menses discourages its use with some women. Some concerns about association with breast cancer remain to be answered. A smaller dose of estrogen may be effective in women who are also taking in 1,500 mg of calcium daily (Ettinger et al, 1987). However, a high calcium intake will not substitute for ERT in blunting postmenopausal bone loss.

Exercise

Weight-bearing exercise that involves the pull of muscle against bone and both against gravity protects against loss of bone mass by stimulating osteoblast activity. Such exercise includes walking, skiing, jogging, hiking, dancing, cycling, and weightlifting. Although one study of male swimmers showed increased bone density over nonexercising counterparts, the difference was modest compared with the effects of weight-bearing exercise (Orwoll et al, 1987).

Strenuous forms of exercise are inappropriate for the elderly, particularly those already suffering from osteoporosis. However, moderate walking is beneficial, and swimming is a nontraumatic form of exercise that can aid bone density to some degree. Patients in wheelchairs show improvement from simple exercises such as raising their arms above their heads.

In addition to arresting the loss of bone mass, exercise leads to increased fitness, with an improvement in muscle control that can prevent falls or at least make falls less traumatic.

Calcium

Recommended Intakes. Calcium therapy in the treatment of osteoporosis has received much attention, particularly since the recommendation of the 1984 NIH Consensus Conference on Osteoporosis that premenopausal women consume 1,000 mg/day of calcium and postmenopausal women 1,500 mg (NIH Consensus Conference, 1984). Other recommendations have been even higher: 1,500 mg/day for adolescents aged 12 to 18 years, 1,000 to 1,200 mg/day for those aged 18 to 40 years, 800 to 1,000 mg/day for women aged 40 through menopause, increasing 5 years after menopause to 1,500 mg/day (Heany, 1989).

Another view is reflected in the recommendations of the National Research Council, which in 1989 failed to increase the Recommended Dietary Allowances (RDA) for adults from the previous level of 800 mg/day. In reflection of their concern with maximizing bone mass during the growth period, the Council did however, increase the RDA for adolescents and young adults up to the age of 25 from 800 to 1,200 mg/day (Food and Nutrition Board, 1989).

Very few studies have evaluated the effect of increasing the calcium intake beyond the period when peak bone mass is attained. A retrospective study in Yugoslavia that compared two populations on the basis of dairy product consumption demonstrated the value of lifelong calcium intake in preservation of bone mass (Matkovic et al, 1979). Two other studies of the effect of postmenopausal supplementation with calcium in amounts of from 1,000 to 2,000 mg/day showed decreased loss of bone, primarily of cortical bone (Riis et al, 1987; Smith et al, 1989). Others feel that the value of calcium supplements in preventing loss of bone mass during the postmenopausal years has not been demonstrated (Riggs et al, 1987).

Even though the effectiveness of increasing calcium intakes at or beyond the menopause in reducing the incidence of osteoporotic fractures remains a matter of considerable controversy, it does seem reasonable to encourage all elderly persons to maintain as positive a calcium balance as possible by at least meeting the RDA.

Part of the conflict regarding the value of supplements may depend on whether bone mass or calcium balance is being measured. The daily intakes recommended by the NIH Consensus Conference of 1,000 and 1,500 mg for premenopausal and postmenopausal women, respectively, appear to be based on calcium balance data.

Calcium from Supplements. In 1985 the average daily calcium intake from food was around 650 mg for American women (USDA, 1985). Although this was an improvement from 570 mg/day in 1970, meeting the recommendation of 800 mg/day still requires extensive changes in dietary habits, mostly involving increased consumption of low-fat dairy products.

Although all recommendations specify that calcium is best utilized if obtained from food, many women who are making an effort to increase their intakes are turning to the use of calcium supplements — in the 1980s, a $318 million industry (Not all . . . , 1988).

Calcium carbonate, which is 40% elemental calcium, yields the highest amount of calcium per tablet at the least expense. In persons with low acid secretion, it is better absorbed if taken with meals than in the fasting state. Forty per cent of the elderly have no acid present in an empty stomach, and 10% suffer from achlorhydria. Calcium citrate and calcium citrate malate may be absorbed more effectively in this group (Recker, 1985). Calcium carbonate can have a constipating effect that may be minimized by dividing the dose or changing the preparation. There is some evidence that calcium supplements can reduce the absorption of nonheme iron by 40 to 45%, but the clinical significance of this is not known (Peck et al, 1987). Table 22-3 lists other potential risks of calcium supplementation.

Some calcium preparations are ineffective because they are poorly dissolved in the stomach. The method of preparation or compression is important. Comparisons of generic versus proprietary forms have found that the former were less likely to pass the test of dissolving within 30 minutes when placed in vinegar.

In view of the importance to adolescents of an adequate calcium intake, some authorities have advocated the addition of calcium to carbonated beverages and other fruit juices. Calcium is currently being added to orange juice — about 160 mg per ¾ cup of juice.

Other Treatment Modalities

Calcitonin is a hormone that inhibits bone resorption by blocking the stimulatory effects of PTH. Impaired production of this hormone in the elderly may contribute to age-related bone loss. Calcitonin therapy decreases the rate of bone loss in osteoporotic women; however it is most effective if given early. It must be given by subcutaneous injection, which limits its clinical usefulness, although other forms are being developed. There is no evidence that calcitonin reduces the

TABLE 22-3. Risks Associated with Excessive Calcium Supplementation

Contamination of bone meal or dolomite supplements with cadmium, mercury, arsenic, or lead
Urinary tract stones in susceptible individuals
Hypercalcemia from extremely high intakes (4,000 mg/day or more)
Milk alkali syndrome from extremely high intakes (4,000 mg/day or more)
Iron deficiency resulting from decreased iron absorption
Exacerbation of constipation

recurrence of fractures in patients with osteoporosis (Lindsay, 1990).

Dramatic increases in bone mass, especially in trabecular bone, follow treatment with *sodium fluoride.* However, incorporating fluoride into hydroxyapatite alters the size and structure of the crystals and may decrease the mechanical competence of the bone. Although bone mass is increased, fracture rates are not reduced. Side effects include irritation of the gastric mucosa and lower extremity pain. Fluoride therapy has so far not been approved by the Food and Drug Administration, and fluoride must still be regarded as experimental (Riggs et al, 1990).

Studies of *calcitriol* have so far failed to support administration of this hormone in the treatment of osteoporosis (Ott and Chestnut, 1989; Wardlaw, 1989). However, maintenance of an adequate dietary intake of vitamin D (100 IU or 5 μg of *cholecalciferol*) is important for the many housebound elderly who fail to get adequate exposure to sunlight.

Fractures of the hip or wrist, the most common fractures in osteoporotic elderly persons, almost always result from trauma, usually a fall. *Preventing falls* through education and attention to the environment of the very old is an important measure.

CITED REFERENCES

Anderson JJB: Dietary calcium and bone mass through the lifecycle. Nutrition Today 25(2):9, 1990.

Christiansen C, Riis BJ, and Rødbro P: Prediction of rapid bone loss in postmenopausal women. Lancet 1:1105, 1987.

Christiansen C et al: Prevention of early postmenopausal bone loss: Controlled 2-year study in 315 normal females. Eur J Clin Invest 10:273, 1980.

Cohn SH et al: Comparative skeletal mass and radial bone mineral content in black and white women. Metabolism 26:171, 1977.

Dietary caffeine and calcium excretion. Nutr Rev 46:232, 1988.

Drinkwater BL et al: Bone mineral density after resumption of menses in amenorrheic athletes. JAMA 256:380, 1986.

Ettinger B et al: Postmenopausal bone loss is prevented by treatment with low-dosage estrogen with calcium. Ann Intern Med 106:40, 1987.

Food and Nutrition Board, National Research Council: Recommended Dietary Allowances, 10th ed. Washington, DC, National Academy Press, 1989.

Heany RP: Nutritional factors in bone health in elderly subjects: Methodological and contextual problems. Am J Clin Nutr 50(Suppl):1182, 1989.

Jensen GF et al: Fracture frequency and bone preservation in postmenopausal women treated with estrogen. Obstet Gynecol 60:493, 1982.

Johnston CC, Slemenda CW, and Melton LJ: Clinical use of bone densitometry. N Engl J Med 324:1105, 1991.

Lindsay R: Fluoride and bone—quantity versus quality (Editorial). N Engl J Med 322:845, 1990.

Massey LK and Wise KL: The effect of dietary caffeine on urinary excretion of calcium, magnesium, sodium, and potassium in healthy young females. Nutr Res 4:43, 1984.

Matkovic V et al: Bone status and fracture rate in two regions of Yugoslavia. Am J Clin Nutr 32:540, 1979.

Mazess RB: On aging bone loss. Clin Orthop 165:239, 1982.

National Center for Health Statistics. 1987 Summary: National Hospital Discharge Survey. Advance Data from Vital and Health Statistics, No 159. DHHS Publ No (PHS)88-1250. Hyattsville, MD, National Center for Health Statistics, 1988.

NIH Consensus Conference: Osteoporosis. JAMA 252:799, 1984.

Not all calcium pills provide calcium. Tufts Univ Diet Nutr Letter 6:1, 1988.

Orwoll ES et al: The effect of swimming exercise on bone mineral content (Abstract). Clin Res 35:194A, 1987.

Ott SM and Chestnut CH III: Calcitriol treatment is not effective in postmenopausal osteoporosis. Ann Intern Med 110:267, 1989.

Peck WA, Riggs BL, and Bell NH: Physician's Resource Manual on Osteoporosis. Washington, DC, National Osteoporosis Foundation, 1987.

Pocock NA et al: Genetic determinants of bone mass in adults: A twin study. J Clin Invest 80:706, 1987.

Pollitzer WS and Anderson JJB: Ethnic and genetic differences in bone mass: A review with an hereditary vs. environmental perspective. Am J Clin Nutr 50:1244, 1989.

Raisz LG: Local and systematic factors in the pathogenesis of osteoporosis. N Engl J Med 318:818, 1988.

Recker RR: Calcium absorption and achlorhydria. N Engl J Med 313:70, 1985.

Riggs BL and Melton LJ III: Involutional osteoporosis. N Engl J Med 314:1676, 1986.

Riggs BL et al: Dietary calcium intake and rates of bone loss in women. J Clin Invest 80:979, 1987.

Riggs BL et al: Effect of fluoride treatment on the fracture rate in postmenopausal women with osteoporosis. N Engl J Med 322:802, 1990.

Riis B, Thomsen K, and Christiansen C: Does calcium supplementation prevent postmenopausal bone loss? N Engl J Med 316:173, 1987.

Sanborn CF: Exercise, calcium and bone density. Sports Sci Exch (Gatorade Sports Science Institute, Chicago, IL) 2:1, March 1990.

Schuette SA and Linkswiler HM: Effects on Ca and P metabolism in humans by adding meat, meat plus milk, or purified proteins plus Ca and P to a low protein diet. J Nutr 112:338, 1982.

Seeman E et al: Reduced bone mass in daughters of women with osteoporosis. N Engl J Med 320:554, 1989.

Smith EL et al: Calcium supplementation and bone loss in middle-aged women. Am J Clin Nutr 50:833, 1989.

Turner LW and Whitney EN: Nature vs. nurture: The calcium controversy. Nutr Clin 4:1, 1989.

USDA: Nationwide Food Consumption Survey: Continuing Survey of Food Intakes by Individuals, Women 19 to 50 years and Their Children, 1 to 5 years, 1 day, 1985. NFCS, CSFII, Report No 85-1. Human Nutrition Information Service, Nutrition Monitoring Division, November 1985.

Wardlaw GM and Barden HS: Osteoporosis—Summary of the 19th Steenbock Symposium. Nutrition Today 24(5):30, 1989.

ADDITIONAL REFERENCES

Behlen PM: Calcium in women's diets. National Food Rev. Washington, DC, USDA, Summer 1986, p 16.

Consensus development conference: Prophylaxis and treatment of osteoporosis. Br Med J 295:914, 1987.

Deehr MS et al: Effects of different calcium sources on iron absorption in postmenopausal women. Am J Clin Nutr 51:95, 1990.

Eriksen EF et al: Trabecular bone resorption depth decreases with age: Differences between normal males and females. Bone 6:141, 1985.

Estrogen receptors in bone. Nutr Rev 47:15, 1989.

Hall FM, Davis MA, and Baran DT: Bone mineral screening for osteoporosis. N Engl J Med 316:212, 1987.

Howat PM et al: The influence of diet, body fat, menstrual cycling and activity upon the bone density of females. J Am Diet Assoc 89:1305, 1989.

LaCroix AZ et al: Thiazide diuretic agents and the incidence of hip fracture. N Engl J Med 322:286, 1990.

Mickelsen O and Marsh AG: Calcium requirement and diet. Nutrition Today 24:28, 1989.

Nordin BEC and Morris HA: The calcium deficiency model for osteoporosis. Nutr Rev 47:65, 1989.

Resnick NM and Greenspan SL: "Senile" osteoporosis reconsidered. JAMA 261:1025, 1989.

Rodysill KJ: Postmenopausal osteoporosis—Intervention and prophylaxis: A review. J Chron Dis 40:743, 1987.

CHAPTER 23

DENTAL HEALTH

CHAPTER OUTLINE

KEY TERMS

DENTAL CARIES—a disease in which acid produced by bacterial metabolism of carbohydrate leads to demineralization of enamel and destruction of the tooth structure

DENTIN—chief tissue of the tooth that surrounds the pulp and is covered by enamel on the crown and by cementum on the roots

ENAMEL—the white, compact, and very hard substance that covers and protects the dentin of the tooth

FLUORAPATITE—the form in which fluoride is incorporated into dentin and enamel along with calcium and phosphorus

FLUOROSIS—a condition caused by exposure to excessive amounts of fluoride, which is characterized by dentin and enamel changes that in the extreme are manifested as mottling

GINGIVAE—the part of the oral mucosa overlying the crowns of unerupted teeth and encircling the necks of those that have erupted; the gums

GINGIVAL SULCUS—a shallow V-shaped space around the tooth that is bounded by the tooth surface on one side and by the epithelium lining the gingiva on the other

MOTTLED ENAMEL—a chronic form of hypoplasia of the enamel of permanent teeth resulting from ingestion of excessive amounts of fluoride during the period of enamel calcification; characterized by dull chalky white marks in the enamel

PLAQUE—a sticky, colorless film of microorganisms, salivary proteins, inorganic components, and polysaccharides that adheres to teeth and gums

STREPTOCOCCUS MUTANS—an oral bacteria implicated in the formation of dental caries

TARTAR (CALCULUS)—a hard stone-like concretion that forms on the teeth through calcification of dental plaque

Tooth decay and periodontal disease are widespread among populations throughout the world. Although dental caries is the most prevalent chronic disease in the United States and is the leading cause of tooth loss before 35 years of age, incidence in the United States and other westernized nations has declined by 50% in the last 15 to 20 years (Jenkins, 1984). This is not true of periodontal disease, however, which affects 80% of the adult population and is the leading cause of tooth loss in people over 35 years of age.

NUTRITIONAL FACTORS IN TOOTH DEVELOPMENT

Primary tooth development begins at 2 to 3 months of gestation, and permanent teeth are beginning to form several months before birth. Maternal nutrients must therefore supply the pre-eruptive teeth with the appropriate building materials. Animal studies have shown that severe nutrient deficiencies during pregnancy can result in the development of mouth malformations and teeth that are more susceptible to caries. However, the level of malnutrition required to produce such deficiencies is not usually seen in the United States or other developed countries (Shaw, 1987).

Teeth are formed by mineralization of a protein matrix. In the case of dentin, the protein is collagen, which is dependent on vitamin C for normal synthesis. Only 0.05% of enamel consists of protein, which is in a form similar to keratin and thus requires vitamin A for its formation. Vitamin D is essential to the process by which calcium and phosphorus are deposited in crystals of hydroxyapatite. Fluoride confers unique caries-resistant properties in both prenatal and postnatal developmental periods. Once teeth are formed, there is little change in their composition throughout life.

DENTAL CARIES

Dental caries is a disease of teeth in which the acid produced by the metabolism of microorganisms leads to gradual demineralization of enamel followed by rapid proteolytic destruction of the tooth structure.

Etiology

If dental caries is to develop, three factors must be present simultaneously: (1) bacteria in the dental plaque or the oral environment; (2) an appropriate substrate for bacterial metabolism; and (3) a susceptible tooth.

Microorganisms

Bacteria are an essential part of the decay process. Animals raised in a germ-free environment do not develop caries. A number of microorganisms are capable of fermenting dietary carbohydrates; environmental factors determine those that will predominate in the oral cavity. The type of carbohydrate in the diet encourages proliferation of specific bacteria. *Streptococcus mutans* is the most prevalent type because it prefers sucrose as a substrate, and this is the most common sugar consumed. Other bacteria in the oral flora are also able to metabolize carbohydrates and produce acid at levels sufficient to erode enamel.

The oral cavities of infants are germ-free at birth but are rapidly infected with the microorganisms prevailing in the local environment. The mother is a major source of oral infection for her infant, and children of mothers with heavy infections of *S. mutans* also have heavy infections of the same microorganism.

Substrate

The carious process depends on a substrate that is appropriate for bacterial metabolism. This substrate consists primarily of fermentable carbohydrate. Primitive populations have remained essentially caries-free until sugars or processed cereal grains have been introduced into their diet, after which they often have explosive tooth decay.

Sucrose appears to be slightly more cariogenic than other sugars, but glucose, fructose, maltose, and lactose also encourage bacterial activity. Of these, lactose is the least cariogenic. All dietary forms of sugar including honey, molasses, brown sugar, and corn syrup solids have strong cariogenic potential. The sugar alcohols xylitol and sorbitol have low cariogenic potential, and noncarbohydrate sweeteners such as saccharin, cyclamate, and aspartame are noncariogenic. Saccharin, like xylitol, may even have an anticariogenic effect (Tanzer and Slee, 1983).

Starch cannot initiate the caries process without a prolonged opportunity for bacteria to adapt to starch metabolism (Shaw, 1987). Given sufficient time, as with food particles lodged between the teeth, salivary amylase makes more substrate available as it hydrolyzes starch to maltose. Modern processing techniques make some starches rapidly fermentable, either by partial hydrolysis or by reducing particle size, thus increasing availability to amylase action. Prolonged depression of pH in plaque and saliva accompanies the addition of small amounts of sugar to flour products, such as in baked foods like cookies, cakes, and doughnuts, which are popularly used as snack foods (Bibby et al, 1986).

Susceptible Tooth

In addition to bacteria and appropriate substrate, development of dental caries requires the presence of a tooth that is vulnerable to attack. Composition of enamel and dentin, location of teeth in the jaw and with respect to each other, and the presence and extent of pits and fissures in the crown are some of the factors that govern susceptibility. Composition of the saliva is also important. Although abnormalities in teeth and saliva may be the result of environmental factors during development, they may also be the products of genetic determinants. However, it is difficult to separate the effects of shared host and family factors of food selection, eating patterns, and oral hygiene from possible inherited characteristics.

Decay Process

The carious process begins with the production of acids as a by-product of bacterial metabolism taking place in the dental plaque. Decalcification of the surface enamel continues until the buffering action of the saliva is able to raise the pH above the critical level (Fig. 23–1).

Plaque Formation

Plaque is a sticky, colorless mass of microorganisms, salivary proteins, and polysaccharides that adheres to teeth and gums. It harbors the acid-forming bacteria and keeps the organic products of their metabolism in close contact with the enamel surface. As a cavity develops, the plaque shields it to some extent from the buffering and remineralization action of the saliva. In time, the plaque combines with calcium and hardens to form tartar or calculus. In this state it becomes a local irritant to the gingiva and is a significant factor in the development of periodontal disease.

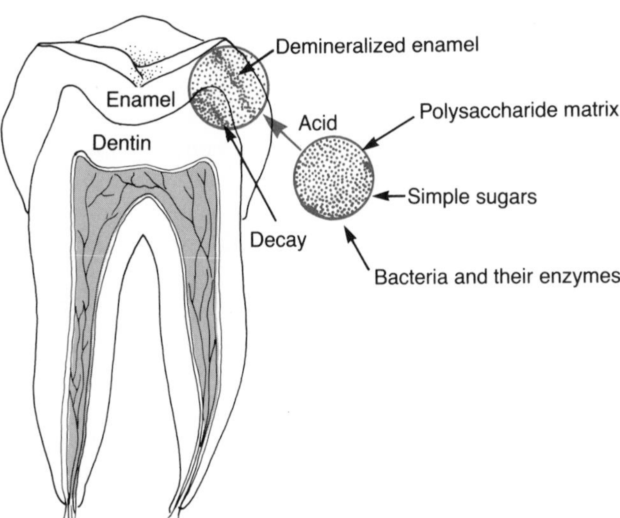

FIGURE 23–1. *Formation of dental caries.*

Acid Production

In the absence of food, the pH of plaque stays relatively constant. When food or drink containing fermentable carbohydrate is ingested, the pH of the plaque drops, although probably not until the meal is finished and saliva is no longer being produced. At a pH below 5.5 (the critical pH), the acid begins to dissolve tooth enamel. This process continues for 20 or 30 minutes until the buffering effect of saliva neutralizes plaque acidity. In "sheltered" plaques between the teeth or in the fissures on occlusal surfaces, the pH may drop to as low as 4.0 and acid production may continue for 1 hour or more (Jenkins, 1984).

Saliva Function

Salivary flow clears food debris from the oral cavity and provides the buffering action that neutralizes the action of plaque acids. Mastication promotes saliva production and probably accounts for the reduced cariogenicity of fermentable carbohydrates when consumed with a meal. In addition, saliva has antibacterial activity (Shaw, 1987).

Saliva is supersaturated with calcium and phosphorus, and at the point when buffering action has restored plaque pH above the critical point, remineralization takes place in the eroded area. If fluoride is present in the saliva, the minerals are deposited in the form of fluorapatite, which is more resistant to erosion. However, if the acid challenge is too frequent or continues for too long, the enamel is completely decalcified, and demineralization and proteolytic degradation of the dentin quickly follow.

Decreased salivary production occurs during sleep, as a symptom of disease, or as a side effect of fasting or medication (Handelman et al, 1986). Rampant caries frequently follows damage of salivary function and is seen in radiotherapy for oral cancer.

Factors Affecting Cariogenicity of Food

Although foods containing fermentable carbohydrate are the basis for bacterial action, their individual cariogenicity varies widely depending on the form in which they occur, the time at which they are eaten with respect to meals, and the presence of anticariogenic factors in either the food or the accompanying meal.

Physical Characteristics

A variety of studies have demonstrated that the total amount of sugar contained in a food is not as important as the opportunities that it provides for bacterial activity to take place.

The *frequency* with which a cariogenic food is consumed determines the number of opportunities for acid production. If pH depression lasts for 20 to 30 minutes regardless of how much sugar is present, then a single exposure to a large amount of sugary food is less cariogenic than multiple exposures of small amounts of sugar spread throughout the day. Several cookies eaten at once, preferably followed by brushing or rinsing the mouth with water, are less damaging than one cookie eaten several times throughout an afternoon.

Adherence to the surface of the tooth also determines the length of time available for cariogenic activity. Sticky candies, dried fruits, and particularly sweetened flour products adhere to the surfaces and crevices of the teeth.

The *retention time* of carbohydrate is determined by the rate at which carbohydrate and other bacterial substrate are cleared from the mouth and tooth surfaces. In this respect liquids are preferable to solids, and coarse particles are preferable to finely divided particles that more easily penetrate surface fissures and crevices between teeth. Carbonated beverages are rapidly cleared from the mouth, although their high acid content can contribute to enamel erosion when consumed in large quantities. Stimulators of salivary secretion, such as cheese, salt, and raw fruits and vegetables help to limit oral retention of cariogenic foods.

An extreme example of abnormal retention time is *baby bottle tooth decay.* This syndrome is found commonly in children who are given a bottle of milk or sugared liquid to nurse during the day or when they go to bed. The position of the tongue against the nipple causes liquid to be continually in contact with the maxillary incisors, and as the child falls asleep, unswallowed liquid spreads over the upper and lower back teeth, providing a medium that encourages the growth of bacteria. Rampant decay involving the upper front teeth begins as the teeth erupt and, if uncontrolled, will spread throughout the upper jaw. The lower front teeth are usually spared by the protective position of the lip and tongue (Fig. 23–2). The syndrome has also been reported in breast-fed infants who nurse for extended periods (Rolfes and Whitney, 1987) (Further Reading, p. 409).

Cariogenicity of Individual Foods

Sophisticated testing methods have enabled an evaluation of the cariogenicity of specific foods, primarily those commonly consumed between meals as snacks. Acid produced within dental plaque is measured endogenously by electrodes mounted in special appliances that remain in the mouth for several days until plaque is formed. Exogenous studies measure the extent of acid production and enamel erosion when pulverized bovine enamel is mixed with human saliva containing a dried and powdered sample of a particular food and a bacterial culture, and then incubated at oral temperature.

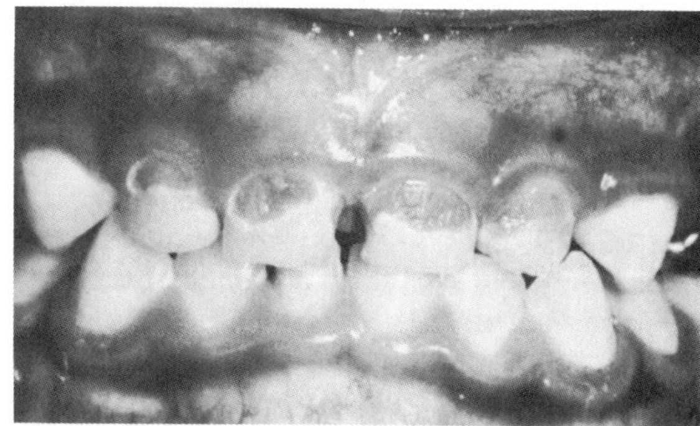

FIGURE 23–2. *Baby bottle tooth decay. (From Levine N [ed]: Current Treatment in Dental Practice. Philadelphia, WB Saunders, 1986, p 447.)*

Results of such studies have demonstrated that the amount of acid formed from a food on fermentation by salivary bacteria is not proportionate to its sugar content, nor does the amount of demineralization necessarily parallel the amount of acid produced from the food. This observation may reflect the formation of different types of fermentation products or the presence in the food of substances that retard or accentuate the caries-producing action of the sugar content.

Anticariogenic Factors

Fats decrease the cariogenic potential of carbohydrates by forming a protective film over the surface of the tooth. Cheeses, especially aged cheddar, are powerful stimulants of saliva flow. When taken immediately after eating sugar, they can almost completely prevent drop of the pH to the critical level (Rugg-Gunn et al, 1975). Thus, a piece of cheese at the end of a meal may reduce the cariogenicity of the meal. Chewing gum sweetened with xylitol or sorbitol has also been shown to arrest the drop in pH and return it to resting levels (Jensen, 1986).

Caries in laboratory animals has been reduced successfully by the addition of phosphates to their diet; however, efforts to repeat this effect in humans have been disappointing.

In summary, a food with low cariogenic potential has a relatively high-protein content, a moderate fat content to facilitate oral clearance, a minimal concentration of fermentable carbohydrate, a strong buffering capacity, a high content of calcium and phosphorus, and a pH greater than 6 (Table 23–1). In addition, it

FURTHER READING: Cultural Aspects of Baby Bottle Tooth Decay

Baby bottle tooth decay (BBTD) is the term adopted in 1986 by the *Healthy Mothers Healthy Babies Oral Health Coalition* to describe the decay of primary maxillary incisors that accompanies prolonged bottle feeding in young children. The national incidence of BBTD has been reported from 4 to 20%. However, few surveys have been done, no standard index is available to define this condition, and therefore any incidence data are only broad approximations.

BBTD occurs extensively in the American Indian and Alaska Native communities. A 1985 survey found that incidence of BBTD among Head Start children in Alaska and Oklahoma ranged from 17 to 85%. Seventy per cent of the Cherokee and Navajo Head Start students were affected (Kelly and Bruerd, 1987).

A 1989 survey of five Alaskan regions included 708 Head Start children aged from 3 to 5 years, of whom 70% were Native Alaskans and 51% lived in urban areas. BBDT was found in 40% of the Native Alaskans and 8% of the non-Native Alaskan children. Incidence was higher in the rural villages and varied significantly on a statewide basis. Overall, oral health was related to race, community, employment, and education of the mother. Although all water supplies were fluoridated, drinking water was commonly obtained from wells, springs, lakes, rain, and melted ice, while tap water was used for washing and household chores (Jones, in press).

The high incidence of BBTD among Alaskan Native children is associated closely with cultural factors. Allowing continued use of a bottle, usually containing water sweetened with something like Tang or Kool Aid, is a form of indulgence that characterizes the highly permissive attitude of parents toward young children in this society. Children are highly cherished and, at least until they go to school, are allowed to do very much as they please. (Conventional routines of daily living do not always apply in an environment that features near or total darkness for part of the year and continuous daylight for the rest of the year.) Mothers are reluctant to take away the favorite bottle that accompanies the child to nap and bedtime and is usually available throughout the day. Breast-fed babies are often weaned to a bottle.

BBTD is so common among Native Americans that decayed front teeth are not considered harmful to health and may not prompt community response. When questioned about prolonged bottle-feeding, mothers often recognize the potential harm involved. Although it is difficult to reverse the practice, a community educational project in 12 Native American communities has demonstrated encouraging success (Bruerd et al, 1989).

should stimulate saliva flow. Certain cheeses, meats, and nuts have many of these characteristics.

Fluoride

Fluoride contributes to decay-resistant teeth in a variety of ways. When incorporated into enamel and dentin along with calcium and phosphorus, it forms *fluoroapatite,* a compound less vulnerable to acid challenge than hydroxyapatite. Fluoride in the saliva promotes remineralization following erosion by plaque acids. It also exerts a small bactericidal action (Jenkins, 1984; Shaw, 1987).

TABLE 23–1. Characteristics of a Low Cariogenic Food

Characteristics
Relatively high protein content
Moderate fat content
Minimal concentration of fermentable carbohydrate
Strong buffering capacity
High concentration of calcium and phosphorus
pH greater than 6
Strong saliva stimulating capacity
Some Examples
Cheese
Potato chips
Peanuts
Meat
Eggs

Fluoride consumed in food and drink enters the systemic circulation and influences the formation of teeth prior to eruption. Fluoride in the oral cavity exerts an exogenous effect by combining with hydroxyapatite in the surface layer of enamel to form fluoroapatite. Occlusal surfaces formed in this manner are flatter and contain fewer of the pits and fissures that are highly susceptible to decay.

For some time it has been a matter of controversy whether fluoride supplementation is appropriate during pregnancy. The Food and Drug Administration does not currently permit manufacturers to claim that supplements taken during pregnancy will prevent caries. One series of studies has shown that children of mothers drinking fluoridated water and who were supplemented with 1 mg/day of fluoride during pregnancy had caries-free teeth at ages 5 and 6 (Glenn et al, 1984). However, further study is indicated, including the issue of whether the higher fluoride levels reached by supplementation plus fluoridated water place the fetus at risk in any manner.

Extensive epidemiologic studies have demonstrated that fluoride at the level of 1 part per million (1 mg/l) taken during the first 12 years of life will reduce the incidence of dental caries by as much as 50 to 70%. Drinking water containing fluoride at this level was available either naturally or by means of fluoridation to approximately 123 million people in 1983, approximately half the population of the United States. In places where fluoridated water is not available, fluoride drops can be added to drinking water and topical applications of fluoride preparations can be administered in a dentist's office. A significant source is the dentifrices used for brushing teeth, 85 to 90% of which contain fluoride.

Except for tea, which contains 0.1 mg/cup, most foods are poor sources of fluoride. However, fluoride is appearing in the food chain in increasing amounts, leading to some concern that levels in some areas may be sufficient to produce mild fluorosis (Kumar et al, 1989). The content of the diet in communities with fluoridated water has been shown to be three times that found in communities without (Leverett, 1982). Fluoride is unintentionally added to the diet in a number of ways, including the use of fluoridated water in the processing of foods and beverages. Because bones are repositories of fluoride, bone meal, fish meal, and gelatin made from bones are potent sources of the mineral. Mechanically deboned meat, which may contain minute chips of bone, adds fluoride to foods such as frankfurters and strained chicken.

Dental Status and Nutritional Intake

Dental status is sometimes reflected in general health. Poorly formed, missing, or painful teeth or improperly fitted dentures may result in the consumption of a soft, possibly nutritionally inadequate diet, because meat and fresh fruits and vegetables are often avoided. Food may be swallowed unmasticated and lead to choking and possibly impaired digestion. However, many people adapt very well to the lack of teeth, and there are no good data that support the belief that edentulousness leads to major changes in food intake.

Prophylactic Care

Although current knowledge of the cariogenicity of foods is far from complete, it suggests that attention to between-meal eating practices is potentially worthwhile. If sugary foods are consumed between meals, then they should be eaten in one small meal, preferably followed by brushing or at least by rinsing the mouth with water. Practices to avoid are sipping carbonated beverages, nibbling sugary foods throughout the day, or holding pieces of candy or sugared mouth fresheners in the mouth for extended periods. Ideally, between-meal eating should be restricted to raw fruits and vegetables.

If sugary foods and mixtures of flour and sugar are to be eaten, they should be taken with meals. A piece of cheese at the end of a meal or after eating sugared foods should be considered. Acid foods, such as apples, should not be eaten immediately before going to bed when salivary flow is insufficient.

Sticky sweets that adhere to teeth and gums, such as chewy candies, dried fruits, and sweetened baked goods, should be avoided as much as possible. Although coarse foods such as raw carrots, celery, and apples do not actually cleanse tooth surfaces, they require vigorous chewing and provoke saliva flow.

Infants and young children should not be given a bottle with milk or sweetened liquid to nurse in bed or to use as a pacifier during the day.

Fluoridated water and fluoridated dentifrices should be used, and a regular program of brushing, flossing, and dental care should be a routine.

PERIODONTAL DISEASE

Over half of the adults over age 45 are affected by gum disease. Unlike dental caries, which is closely associated with Western civilization and consumption of refined carbohydrates, periodontal disease is seen frequently in malnourished, underprivileged populations (Allukian, 1982).

Etiology

The primary etiologic factor in the development of periodontal disease is plaque. When it progresses to dental calculus, it acts as a local irritant to the periodontium, which becomes inflamed. Plaque in the gingival sulcus produces toxins that destroy tissue and permit loosening of the teeth. Several host factors, such as age, faulty tooth restorations, poor tooth alignment, and traumatic occlusion of the teeth, are also important. It is essential that immunologic, nutritional, and endocrinologic status remain optimal in order to maintain resistance of the periodontium.

The defense mechanisms of the gingival tissue, epithelial barrier, and saliva can be affected by nutritional intake and status. Healthy epithelial tissue prevents the penetration of bacterial endotoxins into subgingival tissue. Deficiencies of vitamin C, folate, and zinc in animals increase the permeability of the gingival barrier at the gingival sulcus, making the animals more susceptible to periodontal disease. Morbid deterioration of the gingiva is typical of scurvy; however, the results of treating gingivitis with vitamin C have been disappointing.

When periodontal disease results in gingival recession, carious lesions may appear on newly exposed root surfaces. The prevalence of root caries may increase as people live longer with retention of teeth until later in life (Shaw, 1987).

Nutritional Care

Each patient should be evaluated individually, and evaluation of host factors should include assessment of nutritional status as described in Chapter 17. The oral cavity should be assessed carefully because many nutritional states are reflected in tongue and gum changes.

Nutritional care is particularly important in preparation for and after periodontal surgery, when adequate nutrients are needed to regenerate tissue and to maintain an immune response to prevent infection. The adequacy of vitamin C, vitamin A, zinc, and protein should be ensured. If the procedure or the wound prevents normal dietary intake for an extended period, a complete, nutritional liquid diet should be designed and recommended for the patient (see Appendix 33).

CITED REFERENCES

Allukian M: Dentistry at the crossroads: The future is uncertain, the challenges are many. Am J Public Health 72:653, 1982.

Bibby BG et al: Oral food clearance and the pH of plaque and saliva. J Am Dent Assoc 112:333, 1986.

Bruerd B, Kinney MB, and Bothwell E: Preventing baby bottle tooth decay in American Indian and Alaska Native communities: A model for planning. Public Health Rep 104:631, 1989.

Glenn FB, Glenn WD, and Duncan RC: Fluorides: Prenatal fluoride tablet supplementation and the fluoride content of teeth: Part VII. J Dent Child 51:344, 1984.

Handelman SL et al: Prevalence of drugs causing hyposalivation in an institutionalized geriatric population. Oral Surg Oral Med Oral Pathol 62:26, 1986.

Jenkins N: Diet and dental caries. Food Nutr News 56(5):1, 1984.

Jensen ME: Effects of chewing sorbitol gum and paraffin on human interproximal plaque pH. Caries Res 20:503, 1986.

Jones DB, Schlife C, and Phipps K: An oral health survey of Head Start children in Alaska. J Publ Health Dent (in press).

Kelly M and Bruerd B: The prevalence of baby bottle tooth decay among two Native American populations. J Public Health Dent 47:94, 1987.

Kumar JV et al: Trends in dental fluorosis and dental caries prevalences in Newburgh and Kingston, N.Y.. Am J Public Health 79:565, 1989.

Leverett DH: Fluorides and the changing prevalence of dental caries. Science 217:26, 1982.

Rolfes SR and Whitney EN: The nutrition and oral health picture. Nutr Clin 2(5):1, 1987.

Rugg-Gunn AJ et al: The effect of different meal patterns upon plaque pH in human subjects. Br Dent J 139:351, 1975.

Shaw JH: Causes and control of dental caries. N Engl J Med 317:996, 1987.

Tanzer JM and Slee AM: Saccharin inhibits tooth decay in laboratory models. J Am Dent Assoc 106:331, 1983.

ADDITIONAL REFERENCES

Alvarez JO and Navia JM: Nutritional status, tooth eruption, and dental caries: A review. Am J Clin Nutr 49:417, 1989.

American Dietetic Association: Position of the American Dietetic Association: The impact of fluoride on dental health. J Am Diet Assoc 89:971, 1989.

Broderick E: Baby bottle tooth decay in Native American children in Head Start centers. Public Health Rep 104:50, 1989.

Grenby TH et al: Laboratory studies of the dental properties of soft drinks. Br J Nutr 62:451, 1989.

Grobler SR and Blignaut JB: The effect of a high consumption of apples or grapes on dental caries and periodontal disease in humans. Clin Prev Dent 11:8, 1989.

Grobler SR, Senekal PJC, and Kotze TJ: The degree of enamel erosion by five different kinds of fruit. Clin Prev Dent 11:23, 1989.

Gustafsson BE et al: The Vipeholm dental caries study: The effect of different levels of carbohydrate intake on caries activity in 436 individuals observed for five years. Acta Odontol Scand 11:232, 1954.

Johnsen D and Nowjack-Raymer R: Baby bottle tooth decay (BBTD): Issues, assessment, and an opportunity for the nutritionist. J Am Diet Assoc 89:1112, 1989.

Trautner K and Einwag J: Influence of milk and food on fluoride bioavailability from NaF and Na_2FPO_3 in man. J Dent Res 68:72, 1989.

PART 4

NUTRITIONAL CARE IN DISEASE

Nutrition plays a primary role in growth, development, health, and fitness. As we have seen, the maintenance of appropriate nutrition throughout life can also prevent, or at least delay, the onset of some nutrition-related diseases. The importance of nutritional care in the treatment of established disease is recognized in this section.

As the knowledge base expands, the list of diseases amenable to nutrition intervention increases. Availability of sophisticated feeding and nourishment procedures places increased responsibility on those who provide nutritional care. Much of the material in this section has been provided by nutrition professionals who are experts in their specific fields.

Most of the nutrition-related diseases included here are not preventable by changes in dietary practices, at least on the basis of current knowledge. Exceptions, such as some forms of neoplastic disease, are discussed both in terms of the evidence for prevention as well as the appropriate nutritional care in established disease.

CHAPTER 24

NUTRITIONAL CARE PROCESS

CHAPTER OUTLINE

- Nutritional Care Process
- Nutritional Intervention: Diet Modification
- Nutritional Care for the Hospitalized Patient

KEY TERMS

CLEAR LIQUID DIET—a diet consisting of clear liquids that is nutritionally inadequate and should be used only for a short time

DIET PRESCRIPTION—part of the implementation of nutritional care; designates the type, amount, frequency of feeding, and the amounts and forms of protein, carbohydrate, fat, fluid, vitamins, and minerals

FULL LIQUID DIET—diet composed of foods that are liquid at room or body temperature; can be nutritionally adequate

NUTRITIONAL ASSESSMENT—the process by which the nutritional status of the individual is determined; usually includes dietary history and intake data, biochemical data, clinical examination and health history, anthropometric data, and psychosocial data

NUTRITIONAL CARE PROCESS—the process of meeting nutritional needs of the individual

NUTRITIONAL CARE RECORD—written documentation of the nutritional care process, including the interventions and educational activities to meet the nutritional objectives

NUTRITIONAL INDEX (NI)—an objective evaluation of the extent to which the patient's nutritional needs are being met; actual intake of nutrient—desirable intake × 100/desirable intake of nutrient

NUTRITIONAL SCREENING—a standard, easy, efficient procedure to identify those at nutritional risk who would require a nutritional assessment

PATIENT-CENTERED OBJECTIVE—a goal that is stated in terms of what the patient will achieve or be able to do when the objective is met

QUALITATIVE DIET—an eating plan based on the type of food allowed (e.g., soft, high-fiber, tube feeding)

QUANTITATIVE DIET—an eating plan based on the amount of the food constituents (i.e., 1,800-kcal diet or 400-mg calcium diet)

SOFT DIET—an adequate diet that is moderately low in cellulose, connective tissue, and residue and is planned for conditions in which mechanical ease in eating or digestion is desired

NUTRITIONAL CARE PROCESS

Nutritional care is the process of meeting changing nutritional needs. The type of care depends on the presence of disease or potential disease, the environment, and the state of growth and development of the individual. The *nutritional care process* is made up of (1) assessment of nutritional status, (2) identification of nutritional needs or problems, (3) planning and prioritizing of objectives of nutritional care to meet these needs, (4) implementation of nutritional activities necessary to meet the objectives, and (5) evaluation of the nutritional care.

Nutritional care for a healthy person may mean only an assessment of nutritional status, identification of adequate nutritional health, and possibly education regarding eating habits that will help to prevent the development of disease.

Nutritional care for the ill or hospitalized patient is more complex and means more than simply providing a tray of food three times each day. It should include an assessment of the adequacy of nutritional intake, manipulation of the diet when necessary, provision of enteral or parenteral support when appropriate, and intervention in the form of counseling or education.

Thorough nutritional care involves many disciplines, and thus many hospitals have developed nutritional support teams (NST) that consist of physicians, dietitians, nurses, and pharmacists who can benefit from each others' expertise and who can be responsible for appropriate action. Coordinating the activities of these health care professionals requires written documentation of the process and regular discussions of patients to allow for proper communication and the interaction necessary for complete nutritional care.

Identification of Nutritional Risk

Because of the need to control hospital costs, many hospitals have adopted *nutritional screening* procedures to distinguish patients who are not at nutritional risk from those who require more thorough *nutritional assessment.* These are usually related to diagnosis-related group (DRG) requirements. Nutritional screening should be done on every patient within 3 days of the patient's entering the hospital, nursing home, or clinic; nutritional assessments are reserved for those identified from the screening to be at risk. Nutritional screening should be repeated every 7 to 14 days, because nutritional risk increases in patients hospitalized for 2 weeks or longer (Pichcofsky-Devon and Kaminski, 1985). Without such evaluation, as many as 50% of the malnourished patients could be missed in a typical hospital (Christensen and Gstundtner, 1985).

Nutritional screening should be quick (5 to 10 minutes), simple, and capable of being administered by dietetic technicians, assistants, or even personnel in other departments. Table 24–1 gives the information to be included in a nutritional screen. The most important determination is the percentage of change from usual weight, because this provides a good estimate of the impact of the disease process on dietary intake and nutritional status over the previous weeks or months. A weight loss of 10% of usual body weight usually indicates the need for further assessment.

TABLE 24–1. Nutritional Screening Information

Age
Height
Usual weight
Ideal weight
Present weight
Percentage weight change from the ideal or usual weight
Change in appetite
Dysphagia or difficulty with chewing
Presence of nausea, vomiting, or diarrhea
Serum albumin
Hemoglobin and hematocrit
Total lymphocyte count

Nutritional Care Plan

The nutritional care plan consists of a nutritional assessment, the identification of nutritional problems, the setting of objectives, education and other intervention activities, and the means for evaluation of the results.

Assessment

The identification of nutritional problems (present and potential) evolves naturally from a thorough nutritional assessment. This includes pertinent anthropometric, biochemical, clinical, dietary, and psychosocial information as summarized in Table 24–2. A complete discussion of nutrition assessment appears in Chapter 17.

An assessment of nutritional status is made from these data, and any problems or needs are identified, prioritized, and entered into the medical record. Each problem is then numbered, and future notes are identified by the same number. This procedure facilitates record keeping and allows a quick review of the patient care being provided. Additional notes regarding details of nutritional management can be kept by the dietitian.

The following is an example of a nutritional assessment and identification of nutritional problems:

PATIENT

DA is a 20-year-old white woman. From the health record, laboratory data, anthropometric data, and nutritional history, the following information serves as the database:

TABLE 24–2. Nutritional Assessment*—The Data Base in the Nutritional Care Process

Anthropometric

Weight, height, and weight changes. Growth parameters in infants, children, and adolescents, including head circumference
Skinfold thicknesses: triceps, subscapular, abdominal, etc.
Arm circumference and arm muscle circumference
Skeletal radiographic information

Biochemical

Blood, serum, plasma measurements
Urine measurements
Tissue assays or biopsies

Clinical Examination

Findings indicative of nutritional status
Findings indicative of disease that may affect nutritional status
Pertinent medical history—effect of disease, medications, recent surgery, radiation, chemotherapy, or other treatments on nutritional intake, requirements, and losses

Nutritional History

Dietary intake
- 24-hour recall
- Food frequency questionnaire

Nutrition-related information
- Use of vitamin and mineral supplementation
- Allergies, food intolerances
- Nutrition knowledge
- Physical activity

Psychosocial Information

Cooking and eating atmosphere
Attitudes toward food and eating
Economic factors
Pertinent social history
Ethnic background

* See Chapter 17 for a complete discussion of nutritional assessment.

Laboratory Data

Elevated fasting blood sugar—193 mg/dl
Glycosylated hemoglobin—9.6%
Ketosis
Daily episodes of hypoglycemia—50–60 mg/dl

Anthropometric Data

108 lb—down 10% from usual weight of 118 lb
Below-standard triceps skinfold thickness—12 mm
Height = 65″

Dietary Data

Caloric intake below energy needs—1,400 kcal/day
Irregular meals throughout the day, coffee frequently

Medical History

Diagnosed 1 year ago as having insulin-dependent diabetes mellitus; was given little instruction about diet and has hypoglycemia
Taking two injections of insulin daily—28 units NPH and 4 units regularly in the morning and 6 units NPH and 4 units regularly in the evening

Psychosocial Data

DA lives at home, attends college, and has a part-time job; rarely eats a "meal"

NUTRITIONAL ASSESSMENT

DA, although diagnosed 1 year ago as having diabetes, is not in good control of her condition, does not completely understand her diet, and does not take much interest in it because of her numerous other activities. She has been consuming fewer calories than she requires and does not follow a regular dietary pattern. Her medical problem can be described as insulin-dependent diabetes mellitus in poor control. More specifically, her nutritional problems consist of (1) hypoglycemic episodes related to poor control of diabetes mellitus, (2) weight loss, and (3) inadequate knowledge or understanding of proper dietary management.

Objectives for Nutritional Care

Identification of nutritional problems leads to formulation of a plan for dealing with each one individually, with the greatest attention being paid to the problems of highest priority. If the nutrition information is not complete, the first objective would be to collect the necessary data. For example, one objective might be to find out when DA's hypoglycemic attacks occur.

The objectives should be in behavioral form, stated in terms showing what the patient will achieve if the objectives are met. For example, a *patient-centered* objective would be: "DA will be able to select a 2,000- kcal diet from the hospital menu after 3 days of instruction," rather than "I will teach DA how to select a 2,000-kcal diet from the hospital menu." Stated in the latter way, the objective identifies what needs to be done but does not make the clinical dietitian, nurse, or even DA responsible for learning.

Objectives should be realistic and should be appropriate to the educational level as well as the economic and social resources of the patient and her family. They should also be in quantifiable terms to facilitate an evaluation of her achievement. Notations in the medical record should have the same number for each objective as the problem that is being addressed.

The objectives for the three nutritional problems identified for DA might be as follows:

PROBLEM 1. Hypoglycemic episodes.
Objectives: (1) The timing and cause of hypoglycemic attacks will be identified by DA and by the nutrition counselor. (2) DA will demonstrate an understanding of hypoglycemia through a verbal explanation of why it happens, what her body needs when it does happen, and how it can be prevented. (3) DA will modify her diet in such a manner that hypoglycemia will be avoided.

PROBLEM 2. Weight loss.
Objective: (1) DA will stop losing weight, begin to slowly gain weight up to 118 lb, and will demonstrate this by check-ups at 1, 2, and 3 months, 6 months, 9 months, and 1 year.

PROBLEM 3. Lack of knowledge about proper diet for diabetic control.

Objective: (1) DA will demonstrate understanding of the principles of her eating plan by selecting the proper foods from the hospital menu to meet her dietary requirements and by describing how she will select foods when she is back at home.

Implementation of Nutritional Care

This part of the nutritional care process includes all of those activities or interventions that will enable the patient to meet the defined objectives. Appropriate activities include the diet prescription, nutritional counseling and education, provision of food and necessary nutritional supplements, and advice on financial or food resources.

Interventions or activities are numbered to correspond with the objective that they are designed to meet. They should be complete and should include the specifics of "what, where, when, and how" so that the entire health team (including the patient) will know what is being done, especially at times when the primary care providers are not available. Information about the treatment and progress of a patient should be accessible to the health team from a central record.

Referring again to DA, the nutritional interventions for each objective might be stated as follows:

FOR OBJECTIVE 1 OF PROBLEM 1: The timing and cause of hypoglycemic attacks will be identified by DA and by the nutrition counselor.

Intervention 1–1: DA will learn self-blood glucose monitoring (SBGM), will perform it at least 4 times per day especially when she feels "shaky," and she will be able to interpret the results.

FOR OBJECTIVE 1 OF PROBLEM 2: DA will maintain her weight and begin to slowly gain to her usual weight of 118 lb.

Intervention 2–1: Energy intake will be increased to 2,000 kcal/day, and DA will maintain a 3-day food record for analysis of adequacy.

FOR OBJECTIVE 1 OF PROBLEM 3: DA will demonstrate understanding of the principles of her eating plan by selecting the proper foods from the hospital menu to meet her dietary requirements and by describing how she will select foods when she is at home.

Intervention 3–1: DA will be taught how to select a 2,000-kcal diet from the hospital menu by giving her the opportunity on February 7, 8, and 9 at 10:30 A.M. to select (with supervision and discussion) a 2,000-kcal diet from the hospital menu. On February 9, DA will demonstrate that the improvements in diet can be maintained outside of the hospital by giving examples of what she would eat on a typical week or weekend day and how she will fit this into her schedule.

This process of defining interventions would be continued for every objective for each problem.

Evaluation of Nutritional Care

The last step is an evaluation of the nutritional care provided. If the objectives have been written in measurable behavioral terms, the evaluation becomes easy, because new behavior is being measured against a behavior that has already been defined. For example, "DA was not able to select a 2,000-kcal diet after 3 days of instruction because she does not understand the food exchange system." A revision in the care plan at this point might include the following: "DA will attend classes in diabetic management during the week of February 14 to 18 in order to learn the concept of a food exchange." This new intervention would be performed and again evaluated to determine whether the objective was met.

An evaluation of the extent to which the patient's nutritional requirements are being met can be done by means of the *nutritional index (NI)* (Ghadimi, 1975). This index quantifies the extent to which actual intake of a specific nutrient meets the recommended or desirable intake as defined for a particular patient. To calculate the nutritional index:

$$\text{NI} = \frac{\text{actual intake of nutrient} - \text{desirable intake} \times 100}{\text{desirable intake}}$$

If the actual daily intake exceeds the desirable intake, the nutritional index is stated as a positive percentage. If actual intake equals desirable intake, the index is stated as +1% to avoid an index of zero. If the actual intake is less than the desirable intake, then the nutritional index is stated as a negative percentage. Obviously, the goal of nutritional care is to meet the nutritional requirements or desirable intake of the patient and thus to have as many days as possible with a positive NI. Several negative NI days indicate that the objectives are not being met and that the care should be evaluated and changed.

EXAMPLE: RM, who was badly burned, requires 50 kcal/kg/day of body weight. His daily intake per kilogram for 1 week was: Monday, 30 kcal; Tuesday, 20 kcal; Wednesday, 30 kcal; Thursday, 36 kcal; Friday, 40 kcal; Saturday, 45 kcal; and Sunday, 50 kcal. The NI for Monday would be calculated as follows:

$$\text{NI} = \frac{30\text{ kcal/kg} - 50\text{ kcal/kg}}{50\text{ kcal/kg}} \times 100$$

$$\text{NI} = \frac{-20\text{ kcal/kg}}{50\text{ kcal/kg}} \times 100$$

$$\text{NI} = -0.4 \times 100 = -40\%$$

Nutritional indexes for the entire week are: Monday, −40%; Tuesday, −60%; Wednesday, −40%; Thursday, −28%; Friday, −20%; Saturday, −10%; and Sunday, +1%. The average NI for the week is −28.4%.

On the seventh day, RM finally achieved a positive NI. During the week, his average was about 28% below his desirable intake. The goal now would be to achieve equally high positive nutritional scores to offset the negative days. At the least, the indexes should remain positive. If they do not remain positive, nutritional care should be modified, and enteral or parenteral nutrition support may be necessary (see Chapter 30). The same kind of evaluation can be made for the intake of any other nutrient. The NI for each nutrient can be plotted on a graph to provide a visual evaluation as well as a percentage evaluation of the adequacy of nutritional support.

As the evaluation reveals that objectives are not being met or that new needs have arisen, the process begins again with reassessment, identification of new needs, and formulation of a new nutritional care plan. Table 24–3 summarizes the nutritional care process, including the criteria necessary for each step.

Nutritional Care Record

The nutritional care process, as applied to an individual in either a hospital or an outpatient setting, must be documented in the health record. Documentation has the following advantages:

1. It helps the patient to understand the nutritional care and to know that success will require active participation.
2. It helps to ensure that nutritional care will be relevant, complete, and effective by providing a record that identifies the problems and sets criteria for evaluating the care.
3. It allows the entire health team to understand the

TABLE 24–3. Nutritional Care Process

Steps	Components	Factors to Consider
1. Assessment of Nutritional Status Collect information (data base). Identify problems.	Dietary history Biochemical data Clinical examination findings Medical history Anthropometric data Psychosocial data	The information should be accurate, pertinent to the patient, and appropriately interpreted. The problems should be numbered the same as those in the medical record, given priority ratings in the order of their importance, related to assessment data, and should include present and potential problems.
2. Planning for Nutritional Care Set objectives.	Collection of additional necessary information Available resources Assessment of educational level of patient and family Modification of dietary intake Supplementation of nutrient intake Measures to enable patient to meet nutritional requirements Treatment of medical problems affecting nutritional status	Objectives should be patient-centered, stated in behavioral terms, realistic, measurable, designated as short- or long-term, and numbered according to the problem that they are designed to deal with.
3. Implementation of Nutritional Care Determine nutritional interventions.	Modification of intake as required to make it acceptable to the patient Teaching patient and family about the nutritional care plan Provision of necessary nutritional supplements and alternate forms of nutritional support Resolution of health problems Enrollment of the patient in food assistance programs if necessary	Interventions should be numbered according to the problem and objective, individualized for each patient, and specific in describing what, how, why, when, and where.
4. Evaluation of Nutritional Care Determine effectiveness of nutritional care and change if necessary.	Monitoring of food and fluid intake; evaluation of intake for adequacy in meeting patient's nutritional needs Assessment of nutritional knowledge as reflected in behavioral (food choice) change Monitoring of biochemical data related to nutritional status Monitoring of anthropometric data Monitoring of clinical condition	Evaluation should include a comparison between observed behavior and expected behavior, a determination of the effectiveness of intervention in meeting objectives, an explanation of the effectiveness or ineffectiveness of intervention, and suggestions for revision of the care plan based on evaluation.

rationale for nutritional care and the means by which it will be provided.
4. It allows the health team to participate in the nutritional care and to reinforce the patient's education whenever there is an opportunity.

Much of the information needed to develop a nutritional care plan is collected routinely by various health professionals: dietitians, physicians, nurses, and social workers. For example, a physician will ask about gastrointestinal disturbances and a nurse usually will weigh and measure the patient and ask about any food allergies. Social workers frequently ask about the amount of money available for food and about the patient's living conditions. The nutritional care record ensures that all aspects of nutritional care are noted in one place as part of the total health record. Parts of this information may be incorporated into the nursing care plan, which is a detailed record kept by the nurse and is summarized periodically for inclusion in the medical record.

A detailed care record may be kept by the clinical dietitian, but if this is the case, the information it contains should be summarized periodically in the permanent health record as shown in Figure 24–1. The detailed information may be important for hospital care audits, professional standards reviews, patient education, and other efforts to maintain quality health care. Figure 24–2 is an example of a nutritional care record.

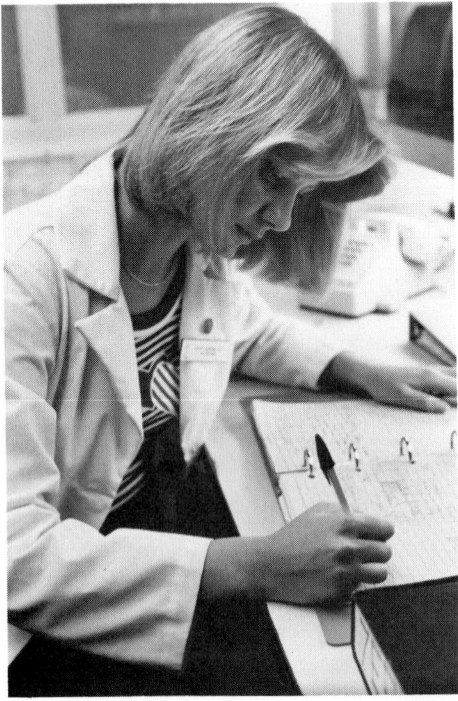

FIGURE 24–1. *Dietitian documenting nutritional care.*

NUTRITIONAL INTERVENTION: DIET MODIFICATION

Therapeutic diets are based on a normal, adequate diet that is modified as necessary to provide for individual requirements, including amount of nutrients, form of intake, digestive and absorptive capacity, alleviation of disease process, and psychosocial factors. In general, the therapeutic diet should vary from the individual's normal diet as little as possible, unless inadequacies must be remedied. Requirements for essential nutrients should be met as generously as the disease condition permits. Personal eating patterns and food preferences should be recognized, along with economic status, religious practices, and any environmental factors that influence food intake, such as where the meals are eaten and who prepares them (Clinical Insight, p. 424). In a hospital setting, attention should be paid to the individual mealtime environment.

A nutritious and adequate diet can be planned in many ways. One foundation of such a diet is the Daily Food Guide (see Table 16–8), which provides approximately 63 grams of protein and 1,200 kcal. This is a basic diet, and other foods or more of the foods listed are added to provide additional energy and increase the intake of required nutrients. Although the Recommended Dietary Allowances (RDA) are formulated for healthy persons, they are often used as a basis for evaluating the adequacy of therapeutic diets. Nutrient requirements specific to a particular disease state must always be kept in mind.

The Diet Prescription

The diet prescription in nutrition serves the same descriptive purpose as the drug prescription in the pharmacy. It designates the type, amount, and frequency of feeding based on the individual's disease process and disease management goals. It specifies an energy level based on present body weight and normal activity plus the amounts and forms of needed protein, fat, carbohydrate, minerals, vitamins, and other substances such as fluid and fiber.

Energy Allowance

The appetite regulates the weight in most normally active people with surprising accuracy. However, it cannot be depended on in disease, especially in hypermetabolic states or critical care, and thus it is frequently necessary to calculate energy needs. When possible, actual measurement of the basal or resting metabolic rate using a metabolic cart and indirect calorimetry can be very useful (see Chapter 2).

The energy requirement of an individual can also be calculated either by (1) calculating the required num-

NUTRITIONAL CARE RECORD

Rm. No.__________
Name __________
Address
and
Phone No. __________

Age __________ Sex __________

Problem List

Nutritional Care Flow Sheet: Weights, Lab Values, I&O& Dates

	Date									
Serum transferrin or serum pre-albumin or serum retinol-binding protein										
Wgt.										
Cal:N ratio										
Intake–tray pro./kcal.										
Intake–Supps. pro./kcal.										
Intake–P. Vein pro./kcal.										
Intake–C. Vein pro./kcal.										
Urine cc./24 hr.										
Stools Avg./24 hr.										

NUTRITIONAL CARE PLAN

Basal Energy Expenditure: __________ kcal.
Anabolic Req.: __________ kcal. __________ gm. pro. __________ gm. N
Maintenance Req.: __________ kcal. __________ gm. pro. __________ gm. N

Diet Calculation __________ kcal.
CHO = Pro = Fat = Na^+ =

Time					
Milk					
Meat					
Bread					
Fruit					
Fat					
Veg.					
Misc. CHO					
Total P F C	P F C	PFC	PFC	PFC	PFC

EVALUATION OF NUTRITIONAL CARE—PROGRESS NOTES

Date

RECOMMENDATIONS FOR FOLLOW-UP

FIGURE 24–2. *Nutritional care record shows assessment data, the nutritional care plan, intervention strategies, and monitoring and evaluation data.* (Figure continued)

NUTRITIONAL CARE RECORD (*Continued*)

ASSESSMENT—Data Base

Diet HX ______ Date 24 Hr. Recall	Medications/Vits. & Mins./Supplements Date / Date
	Medical HX and Clinical Findings
Allergies: Use of sugar: ______ salt: ______ Use of alcohol: ______ none ______ occas. ______ oz. ______ often Fluid intake ______	Biochemical findings Social HX
Feeding and G.I. Habits Consistency of food: Appetite: Bowel habits: Recent chngs. in eating habits: Recent wgt. chngs.: Dental condition:	Activities Occup.: ______ hr./wk. Exercise ______ Anthropometry Triceps skinfold thickness Arm circumf.: % Body fat: Arm muscle circumf.: Frame type: S M L IBW: Surface area:
Evaluation of Intake P ______ Cal. ______ ______ ______ F ______ ______ ______ ______ C ______ ______ ______ ______	Hgt: Wgt: Patient's Wgt. goal: Usual wgt: % Usual wgt.:

FIGURE 24–2. *Continued.*

ber of kcal/kg/day or (2) by calculating the percentage increase over basal metabolic demands. To make the determinations, the desirable weight based on sex, age, height, and body build (frame) is used (Appendix Table 17). Desirable current weight rather than actual current weight is used, because the latter may be abnormal as a result of undernutrition or obesity.

The basal energy expenditure (BEE) is calculated by using one of the methods described in Chapter 2. An additional factor is added depending on the activity level of the patient. Another factor is added if the patient is under physiologic stress (see Chapter 29 and Table 29–2).

Patients with mild stress, such as those with uncomplicated surgery, require additional energy up to 20% over their BEE. Those with multiple fractures or trauma are in moderate stress and may need up to 50% over BEE. Acute major infections or burns may increase the need up to 100% over basal requirements. Even the most hypermetabolic patients usually do not require more than 50 kcal/kg ideal body weight for anabolism. Table 24–4 presents the RDA for energy for unstressed patients, but the actual energy requirement should be determined from an assessment of the individual, with inquiry about usual weight and amount of weight loss or gain as a percentage of usual weight.

Determination of the energy requirement is illustrated in the following:

EXAMPLE: Suppose that DA (the patient referred to earlier in this chapter) is a 20-year-old student who has a height of 165 cm (5 ft 5 in) and a medium body build. Her weight is appropriate at 53.6 kg (118 lb). Her activity level is light. According to Table 24–4, she requires 38 kcal/ kg/day. Thus, her average calorie allowance would be 38 × 53.6, or about 2,036 kcal/day.

Protein Allowance

After the daily energy requirement is calculated, the protein fraction of the diet is determined. The RDA for protein is 0.75 g/kg of body weight for adults (see Chapter 5). The RDA is usually considered adequate for previously well-nourished individuals who are ambulatory or who require only brief periods of hospitalization.

TABLE 24–4. Recommended Energy Intakes for Children and Adults*

Category	Age (Years) or Condition	Weight (kg)	Weight (lb)	Height (cm)	Height (in)	REE (kcal/day)	Average Energy Allowance (kcal)† Multiples of REE	Per kg	Per day‡
Infants	0–0.5	6	13	60	24	320		108	650
	0.5–1.0	9	20	71	28	500		98	850
Children	1–3	13	29	90	35	740		102	1,300
	4–6	20	44	112	44	950		90	1,800
	7–10	28	62	132	52	1,130		70	2,000
Males	11–14	45	99	157	62	1,440	1.70	55	2,500
	15–18	66	145	176	69	1,760	1.67	45	3,000
	19–24	72	160	177	70	1,780	1.67	40	2,900
	25–50	79	174	176	70	1,800	1.60	37	2,900
	51+	77	170	173	68	1,530	1.50	30	2,300
Females	11–14	46	101	157	62	1,310	1.67	47	2,200
	15–18	55	120	163	64	1,370	1.60	40	2,200
	19–24	58	128	164	65	1,350	1.60	38	2,200
	25–50	63	138	163	64	1,380	1.55	36	2,200
	51+	65	143	160	63	1,280	1.50	30	1,900
Pregnant	1st trimester								+0
	2nd trimester								+300
	3rd trimester								+300
Lactating	1st 6 months								+500
	2nd 6 months								+500

*Reprinted with permission from *Recommended Dietary Allowances,* 10th ed., c. 1989 by the National Academy of Sciences. Published by National Academy Press.

†In the range of light to moderate activity, the coefficient of variation is ±20%.

‡Figure is rounded.

In the presence of malabsorption or protein loss from burns, exudates, ascites, or renal disease, an increase in protein allowance is required. For these patients in hypermetabolic states, the protein allowance is often determined on the basis of the energy:nitrogen ratio (kcal : N). Ratios of 100 to 200 kcal/g of nitrogen intake are recommended. The lower the kcal : N ratio, the greater is the protein requirement (see Chapter 29). Determination of the protein allowance is illustrated in the following:

Example: For the same 20-year-old female student previously mentioned, the protein allowance would be:

$$53.6 \times 0.75 = 40 \text{ g/day of protein}$$

Because her energy requirement is 2,036 kcal/day, the kcal : N ratio is determined by dividing these numbers by the grams of nitrogen in the diet.

40 g of protein/6.25 g of protein/g of nitrogen
= 6.4 g of nitrogen

2,036 kcal/6.4 g of nitrogen = 318 kcal/g of nitrogen

If DA was stressed or hypermetabolic, the ratio would be closer to 100 to 200 kcal/g of nitrogen because of her higher protein requirement.

Fat and Carbohydrate Allowances

Following calculation of the protein fraction, the remainder of the calories in the diet are determined and are assigned to fat and carbohydrate. The correct or optimum proportion of fat to carbohydrate varies and is discussed in each chapter dealing with a specific disease state. Current recommendations designed to decrease the risk of heart disease and cancer in Americans specify 50 to 60% of kilocalories from carbohydrate and 25 to 30% of kilocalories from fat, with no more than 10% of kilocalories from saturated fat.

A rapid and adequate method for calculating the constituents of a diet prescription consists of dividing the total energy allowance into approximately 8 to 15% protein, 25 to 35% fat, and 50 to 65% carbohydrate.

Example: Continuing with the same 20-year-old female student used in previous examples, the fat and carbohydrate needs are calculated.

Protein intake already determined: 40 g

4 kcal/g × 40 g of protein
= 160 kcal or 8% of kcal from protein

Fats make up 25 to 35% of kcal—in this case 30%.

CLINICAL INSIGHT: Cultural Factors and Nutritional Care*

When assessing the nutritional status of people, the following factors should be considered: the cultural definition of "food"; the frequency and number of meals eaten away from home; the cultural patterns; and the regularity of food consumption. The 24-hour dietary recall or 3-day food record traditionally used for assessment may be inadequate for nutrition implementation and education, because it does not include culture-specific diet information. For example, there may be vast differences in what is meant by the word "food." Certain Latin American groups do not consider greens (an important source of vitamins) to be food and thus do not list intake of these vegetables on daily food records. Dietary intake of calcium among Vietnamese refugees, although appearing low because of the low consumption of dairy products, may be adequate because the Vietnamese commonly consume pork bones and shells that are high in calcium.

An excellent way to learn about the cultural eating patterns of a people is to question them about their dietary customs. Cultural food preferences are often interrelated with religious dietary beliefs and practices, the knowledge of which permits the suggestion of improvements or modifications that will not conflict with dietary laws. A sample of some prohibited foods and beverages of selected religious groups is listed below. A more complete discussion is included in Appendix 39.

HINDUISM

- All meats

ISLAM

- Pork
- Intoxicating beverages

JUDAISM

- Pork
- Predatory fowl
- Shellfish and other water creatures (fish with scales are permissible)
- Mixing milk and meat dishes at same meal
- Blood by ingestion (e.g., blood sausage, raw meat); blood by transfusion is acceptable

Additional Notes:

Foods should be kosher (meaning "properly preserved")

All animals must be ritually slaughtered by a sochet (quickly, with the least pain possible) to be kosher

MORMONISM (CHURCH OF JESUS CHRIST OF LATTER-DAY SAINTS)

- Alcohol
- Tobacco
- Beverages containing caffeine (coffee, tea, colas, and selected carbonated soft drinks)

SEVENTH DAY ADVENTIST

- Pork
- Certain seafood including shellfish
- Fermented beverages

Additional Note:

A vegetarian diet is encouraged

* Adapted from Andrews M. *In* Jarvis C: Physical Examination and Health Assessment. Philadelphia, WB Saunders (in press).

The total kilocalorie requirement (2,036) × 0.30 = 610 kcal from fat.

$$610 \text{ kcal}/9 \text{ kcal/g fat} = 68 \text{ g of fat} = 1.3 \text{ g of fat/kg}$$

Carbohydrates make up the remainder of kcal: 62% in this case. The total kilocalorie requirement (2,036) × 0.62 = 1,262 kcal from carbohydrate (CHO).

$$1{,}262 \text{ kcal}/4 \text{ kcal/g CHO} = 315 \text{ g CHO} = 5.4 \text{ g CHO/kg}$$

The average daily food intake of a healthy or mildly stressed individual without dietary restrictions is approximately 40 to 90 grams of protein, 60 to 120 grams of fat, and 150 to 300 grams of carbohydrate.

Minerals and Vitamins

Determination of levels of minerals and vitamins for stressed individuals is difficult to make on a general basis. In times of stress, inadequacies of these nutrients may be countered with mobilization of body stores, decrease of body losses, increase in absorption, or improvement of utilization. Individual responses vary, and true deficiencies with clinical signs and symptoms usually take weeks, months, or even years to develop. Biochemical measurements capable of identifying inadequacies at early stages are still in the developmental stage.

In arriving at the appropriate vitamin and mineral intake, the following should be considered: (1) requirements for healthy individuals, (2) nature of the disease or injury, (3) body stores of specific nutrients, (4) normal and abnormal losses through the skin, urine, or intestinal tract, and (5) interactions with drugs. These are discussed further in chapters on nutritional care for various disease states. In critical care the goal is to provide at least the RDA; little is known beyond increased needs for vitamins A and C and zinc, all of which are involved in wound healing. In critical care involving tube feeding, it is important to remember that meeting the RDA for vitamins and minerals depends on the volume taken (see Chapter 30).

Fluids

Optimal convalescence demands adequate tissue hydration. A normal healthy adult at rest and not perspiring needs 1,800 to 2,500 ml/day of water to provide for urinary excretion and to replace losses from insensible perspiration. Additional fluids must be added to replace water lost by excessive sweating, vomiting, diarrhea, tube drainage, or other conditions marked by increased water loss. If sufficient water is not obtained through fluid intake and food, it must be supplied parenterally, usually along with electrolytes.

Modifications of the Normal Diet

Therapeutic diets may be defined as quantitative and qualitative modifications of the normal diet. The qualitative diet is an adequate diet adjusted according to the type of food allowed. The quantitative diet is calculated with an increase or a decrease in the amount of the food constituents. Diets for management of gastrointestinal diseases are usually qualitative, whereas diets used in managing diabetes or renal disease are usually quantitative. Some of the modifications may overlap. For example, because of acute indigestion or poor teeth a patient on a diabetic diet may also require a soft diet.

The adjustment in diet may take any of the following forms:

1. Change in consistency of foods (liquid diet, soft diet, low-fiber diet, high-fiber diet)
2. Increase or decrease in energy value of diet (weight-reduction diet, high-calorie diet during recovery from trauma)
3. Increase or decrease in type of foods (sodium-restricted diet, lactose-restricted diet)
4. Omission of specific foods (allergy diet, gluten-free diet)
5. Adjustment in the ratio and balance of proteins, fats, and carbohydrates (diabetic diet, ketogenic diet, renal diet, cholesterol-lowering diet)
6. Rearrangement of the number and frequency of meals (diabetic diet)
7. Change in delivery of nutrients such that a tube is used, either enterally or parenterally

Foods as Nutrient Sources

Correct evaluation of therapeutic diets requires a knowledge of the nutrients contained in different foods. In particular, it is helpful to be aware of the nutrient-dense foods that contribute in a major way to dietary adequacy. Table 16–16 provides some of this information. Chapters 6 and 7 give more detailed information on minerals and vitamins.

NUTRITIONAL CARE FOR THE HOSPITALIZED PATIENT

Institutional food service is important in nutritional support. Imagination and ingenuity are required in planning for a variety of foods acceptable to patients. The color, texture, composition, and temperature of food are very important, and making food taste good is an important part of nutritional care.

Standard Hospital Diets

All hospitals and institutions have some specific, basic, routine diets designed for uniformity and convenience of service. These standard diets are based on the foundation of an adequate diet pattern that is discussed in Chapter 16 and which is derived from the RDA. These diets should be as flexible as possible in order to meet the often increased nutritional needs of hospitalized individuals.

The types of standard diets are usually referred to as *general, light, soft,* and *liquid.* These diets are used routinely for patients with certain physical conditions and serve as a foundation for the diversified therapeutic diets.

General or Adequate Normal Diet

In some hospitals the general diet is also known as the "regular," "full," or "house" diet. The general diet is a basic adequate normal diet of approximately 1,600 to 2,200 kcal and usually contains 60 to 80 grams of protein, 80 to 100 grams of fat, and 180 to 300 grams of carbohydrate. All the protective foods outlined in the foundation of an adequate diet pattern are included (see Table 16–8). Larger servings or additional foods, such as margarine, desserts, salad dressing, crackers, and sugar, are added to increase energy intake and to make the diet more palatable. There are no particular food restrictions. Some hospitals have instituted general diets low in fat, saturated fat, cholesterol, sugar, and salt to be in concert with the dietary recommendations for the general population (see Chapter 16). Most hospitals have a selective menu that allows the patient a certain freedom of choice, yet controls the adequacy of the diet to some extent.

Soft or Light Diet

The soft or light diet as illustrated in Table 24–5 is used as a transition diet. It is an adequate diet that is moderately low in cellulose and connective tissue. It is

TABLE 24–5. Soft or Light Diet

Meal Plan	Sample Menu	Serving Size
	Breakfast	
Fruit	Orange juice	½ glass
Cereal	Cooked farina (cooked weight)	½ cup
Egg	Poached egg on toast	1
Bread	Toast	1 slice
Butter	Butter or margarine	1 pat
Milk	Milk	1 cup
Sugar	Sugar	3 tsp
Coffee	Coffee	2 coffee cups
	Lunch	
Soup	Tomato consommé	½ cup
Entrée	Baked macaroni and cheese	½ cup
Vegetables	Cooked asparagus tips or purée	6 spears
Bread	Light rye bread	1 slice
Butter	Butter or margarine	1 pat
Fruit	Applesauce	½ cup
Milk	Milk	1 cup
	Dinner	
Meat	Sliced chicken	3 oz
Potato	Mashed potato	½ cup
Vegetable	Buttered spinach purée	½ cup
Bread	Light rye bread	1 slice
Butter	Butter or margarine	1 pat
Dessert	Chocolate ice cream, ice milk, or frozen yogurt	1 average scoop (3½ oz or ½ cup)
Milk	Milk	1 cup

also low in residue. The soft diet is planned for conditions in which mechanical ease in eating or digestion is desired. It is appropriate for patients who have few or no teeth or ill-fitting dentures. The trend in diet planning fosters liberal interpretation of the soft diet, particularly with regard to vegetables and whole-grain breads and cereals. It is most useful when the selection of foods is guided by the patient's tolerance.

The average composition of the soft diet is 1,800 to 2,000 kcal. However, energy as well as protein, fat, and carbohydrate allowances are adjustable according to individual needs, based on activity, height, weight, sex, age, and any specific demands caused by disease.

Liquid Diets

Liquid diets are commonly ordered for patients with conditions requiring nourishment that is easily digested and consumed or that has minimal residue. They are often ordered for a brief period for patients undergoing diagnostic tests. Chewing or swallowing difficulties or dental wiring may also necessitate a liquid diet.

The two varieties of oral liquid diets are the full liquid diet and the clear or restricted liquid diet.

FULL LIQUID DIET. The full liquid diet, such as that shown in Table 24–6, is made up of foods that are liquid at room or body temperature. For example, ice cream and gelatin are both considered to be liquids. If properly designed and consumed, the diet is considered adequate for maintenance requirements except for fiber. The average composition of the diet is approximately 1,300 to 1,500 kcal with 45 grams of protein, 65 grams of fat and 150 grams of carbohydrate. By careful planning, the diet can be increased in protein and caloric value to approach the normal diet or even a high-calorie diet. This is necessary when it must be continued for an indefinite period. Protein and vitamin supplements as listed in Appendix 33 can be added to the liquids to increase the nutrient intake. However, because this diet is inadequate in fiber, constipation may result from its prolonged use. A canned fiber-containing formula (e.g., Enrich) may be useful.

Full liquid diets can be planned to meet the needs of a patient with diabetes, renal disease, or any other disorder. One of the lactose-free products should be used in place of milk as the protein source when planning a lactose-free liquid diet. A fluid restriction might neces-

TABLE 24–6. Full Liquid Diet—Sample Menu*†

A.M.

½ cup orange juice
1 cup farina with 2 tsp margarine, 1 tsp sugar, and milk
Coffee or tea with sugar
1 cup pasteurized eggnog‡

Between Meals

1 cup pasteurized eggnog‡

Noon

½ cup apricot nectar
1 cup cream of potato soup with margarine or butter
1 cup milk
½ cup Bavarian cream
Coffee or tea with sugar

Between Meals

Blenderized milkshake with 4 oz milk, 2 tsp chocolate syrup, 2 oz ice cream (plain), and 2 tsp sugar

P.M.

½ cup pineapple juice
1 cup strained cream of vegetable soup with 1 tsp margarine or butter
1 cup milk or pasteurized eggnog‡
½ cup caramel custard
Coffee or tea with sugar

Bedtime

½ cup lemon gelatin
1 cup pasteurized eggnog

*From American Dietetic Association: Handbook of Clinical Dietetics. New Haven, Yale University Press, 1981.
†To increase the calories, sugar, cream, butter, margarine or high-calorie supplements should be added whenever possible.
‡Eggnog that is prepared in powdered form and mixed with milk. This avoids the use of raw eggs, which is not recommended owing to possible *Salmonella* poisoning and avidin binding of biotin.

sitate the use of an energy-dense product that supplies 2 kcal/ml instead of the usual 1 kcal/ml.

CLEAR OR RESTRICTED LIQUID DIET. The clear or restricted liquid diet, such as that listed in Table 24–7, is frequently ordered for postoperative patients to furnish fluids, some electrolytes, and small amounts of energy prior to the return of gastrointestinal function. It is an inadequate diet composed chiefly of water and carbohydrates; therefore, it should be used for a very short time. The average clear or restricted liquid diet contains 400 to 500 kcal, 5 to 10 grams of protein, no fat, and 100 to 120 grams of carbohydrate.

The clear liquid diet composed of gelatin and sweetened beverages cannot replace the electrolytes lost in vomitus and diarrheal fluid. Electrolytes may need to be added, or they are supplied in the parenteral fluids that these patients are often also receiving at the same time.

The clear liquid diet is served at frequent intervals to supply the tissues with fluid and relieve thirst. As the name indicates, the diet consists of clear liquids, such as tea, broth, carbonated beverages, strained fruit juices, and gelatin. Milk and liquids prepared with milk are omitted as are fruit juices that do not agree with the patient. Carbonated beverages, especially ginger ale, are usually well tolerated.

When a nutritious clear liquid is needed, an appropriate liquid elemental or defined formula diet can be selected from Appendix Table 33.

Table 24–8 provides a summary of the basic hospital diets.

TABLE 24–7. Clear or Restricted Liquid Diet

Meal Plan	Sample Menu	Serving Size
	Breakfast	
Fruit juice	Orange juice (strained)	½ cup
Beverage	Coffee (decaffeinated)	2 coffee cups
Sugar	Sugar	2 tsp
	10:00 A.M.	
Fruitade	Lemonade	1 cup
	Lunch	
Soup	Consommé	½ cup
Fruit juice	Grapefruit juice (strained)	½ cup
Tea	Tea	2 teacups
Sugar	Sugar	2 tsp
	3:00 P.M.	
Carbonated beverage	Ginger ale	1 cup
	Dinner	
Soup	Chicken broth	½ cup
Gelatin	Raspberry gelatin	¼ cup
Tea	Tea	2 teacups
Sugar	Sugar	2 tsp
	8:00 P.M.	
Fruit juice	Orange juice (strained)	1 cup

Food Intake

Food served does not necessarily represent the food intake of the patient. Prevention of iatrogenic malnutrition requires frequent observation and accurate recording of patient intake. Regardless of the type of diet prescribed, it is important to check both the food served and the food left on the tray in order to obtain an accurate indication of the patient's energy and nutrient intake. Nutrient content can be determined quickly by using one of the many sophisticated computer software programs or even a programmable calculator. An approximate indication of nutrient intake can be determined manually by evaluating the intake with the use of an exchange system such as the one described in Chapter 31.

Psychologic Factors

Meals and between-meal nourishments are often highlights of the day and are anticipated with pleasure by the patient. The nurse and dietitian should therefore make mealtime as favorable an experience as possible. Food intake is encouraged in a draft-free room at a comfortable temperature, with the patient in a comfortable eating position in bed or sitting in a chair located away from unpleasant sights or unpleasant odors. Many patients prefer to wash before eating and to eat from a table that is free of other objects.

The arrangement of the tray should reflect thoughtfulness and consideration of the patient's needs and wishes. Dishes and utensils should be in a convenient location. Independence should be encouraged in those who require assistance in eating. The caregiver can accomplish this by asking patients to specify the sequence of foods to be eaten and by having them participate in eating, if only by acts such as holding their bread. Even visually impaired persons can eat unassisted if they are told where to find foods on the tray. Patients who require feeding should be fed when the foods served are still at an optimal temperature.

Rejection of meals or the prescribed diet frequently reflects a negative attitude of the patient toward the illness and hospitalization. Other reasons for poor acceptance may be unfamiliar foods and eating schedule and improper food temperatures. By giving patients an opportunity to express themselves and by accepting their attitudes, the nurse and dietitian can help patients to overcome their negative feelings and to improve their acceptance of the hospital food. Food acceptance is also improved when personal selection of menus is encouraged.

In encouraging acceptance of a therapeutic program, the attitude of the caregiver is important. The nurse who understands that the diet contributes to the restoration of the patient's health will communicate this

TABLE 24–8. Summary of Basic Hospital Diets

Food	General, Adequate, or Normal Diet	Soft or Light Diet	Full Liquid Diet	Clear Liquid Diet
Milk, cream, buttermilk	Included	Included	Included	Not included
Eggs	Raw and cooked	Included	In beverages	Not included
Cheese	All varieties	Cottage, pot, cream, mild American, Cheddar	Not allowed	Not included
Fats	All kinds	Butter, margarine, oil, mayonnaise, and French dressing	Butter, margarine, oil	Not included
Meat, fish, poultry	All included	Ground and tender beef, lamb, veal; liver, bacon, fish, poultry	Not allowed	Not included
Vegetables	All included	Cooked vegetables of low fiber; lettuce and tomato salad; potatoes boiled, mashed, baked, creamed, or scalloped; vegetable juices	Vegetable juices, vegetable purée used in soups	Vegetable water
Fruits	All included	Fruit juices, ripe bananas, cooked fruit without skin or seeds	Fruit juices, fruitades	Strained fruit juices, fruitades
Breads	All varieties	Fine whole grain, rye without seeds, enriched white, refined crackers	Not allowed	Not included
Cereals	All varieties	Refined; finely ground	Cooked gruel	Not included
Cereal products	All varieties	Cooked macaroni, spaghetti, noodles, rice	Not allowed	Not included
Soups	All varieties	Clear broth, consommé, strained cream, and vegetable soups	Clear broth, consommé; strained vegetable and cream soups	Clear broth and consommé
Beverages	All kinds	All kinds	Tea, decaffeinated coffee; carbonated beverages; eggnog	Tea, decaffeinated coffee; carbonated beverages
Desserts	All kinds	Plain puddings, yogurt, simple cakes and cookies; frozen desserts without nuts; custard, gelatin	Plain gelatin dessert, ice cream or yogurt without nuts and seeds; ices, sherbets, soft custard	Plain gelatin desserts and ices
Other			Liquid supplements listed in Appendix 33	Elemental liquids such as shown in Appendix 33

conviction by actions, facial expressions, and conversation. Patients who understand that the diet is important to the success of their medical or surgical therapy will usually accept it more willingly.

When the patient must adhere to a therapeutic dietary program indefinitely, the nurse may need to confer with the dietitian, the social worker, or the community health nurse and possibly bring the other members of the health team together to help the patient to resolve the nutritional problems. The nurse is a coordinator in this role.

During the course of patient care, the nurse comes into contact with many individuals who do not require a therapeutic dietary program. Informal opportunities for discussing nutrition principles are often available, especially with patients receiving regular diets. Nurses can also combine their skills with those of dietitians in teaching classes in normal nutrition or relating to special dietary modifications for conditions such as diabetes, hypertension, or coronary artery disease. Support groups coordinated by the nursing and dietetic staffs for patients with cancer, renal disease, ileostomies, and other debilitating conditions contribute significantly to the acceptability and success of their total care, including nutritional care.

Discharge Planning and Home Care

Nutritional care continues as a part of discharge planning when the patient returns home or goes to a long-term care facility or nursing home. Education, counseling, and mobilization of resources to provide home care and provide for nutritional support are all a part of discharge procedures. Home health care agencies are available with the expertise to provide for enteral or parenteral nutrition at home.

Care of the Terminally Ill or Hospice Patient

Comfort and the quality of life are the goals when providing nutritional care for the terminally ill patient. Dietary restrictions are rarely appropriate. Nutritional care should include techniques that may help in symptom and pain control. Recognition of the various phases of dying—denial, anger, bargaining, or acceptance—will help the dietitian or nurse to understand the patient's response to food and nutritional support. Constant communication and explanation to the family are important.

The decision with regard to when life support should

be terminated can include the issue of enteral or parenteral nutrition (Capron, 1991). Nutritional support should be continued as long as the patient is competent to make this choice and as long as it is adding to the possibility of meaningful remaining days of life. See Cited References for further discussion of ethical issues (American Dietetic Association, 1987; Gallagher-Allred, 1989; Gallagher-Allred, 1991).

CITED REFERENCES

American Dietetic Association: Position of The American Dietetic Association: Issues in feeding the terminally ill adult. J Am Diet Assoc 87:78, 1987.

Capron AM: Implications of the *Cruzan* decision for clinical nutrition teams. Nutr Clin Prac 6:89, 1991.

Christensen KS and Gstundtner KM: Hospital-wide screening improves basis for nutrition intervention. J Am Diet Assoc 85:704, 1985.

Gallagher-Allred CR: Managing ethical issues in nutrition support of terminally ill patients. Nutr Clin Prac 6:113, 1991.

Gallagher-Allred CR: Nutrition care for the terminally ill: Assessment, implementation, and evaluation. Top Clin Nutr 4:65, 1989.

Ghadimi H (ed): Total Parenteral Nutrition: Premises and Promises. New York, John Wiley, 1975, p 190.

Pichcofsky-Devon GD and Kaminski MV: Increasing malnutrition during hospitalization: Documentation by a nutrition screening program. J Am Coll Nutr 4:471, 1985.

ADDITIONAL REFERENCES

American Dietetic Association: Manual of Clinical Dietetics. Chicago, American Dietetic Association, 1988.

Bistrian BR et al: Prevalence of malnutrition in general medical patients. JAMA 235:1567, 1976.

Cooper LF: Florence Nightingale's contribution to dietetics. J Am Diet Assoc 30:121, 1954.

Cousins N: Anatomy of an illness (as perceived by the patient). N Engl J Med 295:1458, 1976.

Disbrow DD: The costs and benefits of nutrition services: A literature review. J Am Diet Assoc 89(Suppl 4):s1, 1989.

Hospital malnutrition still abounds. Nutr Rev 46:315, 1988.

How to cut hospital costs? Better nutritional care. Nutrition 4:430, 1988.

Krey SH and Murray RL (eds): Dynamics of Nutrition Support: Assessment, Implementation, Evaluation. Norwalk, CT, Appleton-Century-Crofts, 1986.

Mandel ED and Worthley JA: Skeletons in the hospital closet revisited: The management of enteral nutrition. Nutr Support Serv 6(2A):44, 1986.

Pemberton CM et al: Mayo Clinic Diet Manual, 6th ed. Philadelphia, BC Decker, 1988.

Selye H: On just being sick. Nutr Today 5:2, 1970.

CHAPTER 25

INTERACTIONS BETWEEN DRUGS AND NUTRIENTS

CHAPTER OUTLINE

KEY TERMS

ANTIVITAMIN—a substance that inactivates a vitamin or inhibits its synthesis

BIOAVAILABILITY—the degree to which a drug or other substance becomes available to the target tissue

DRUG-NUTRIENT INTERACTION—the result of the action between a drug and a nutrient that would not happen with the nutrient or the drug alone

LUMINAL EFFECTS—actions of drugs that take place in the lumen of the intestine

MIXED-FUNCTION OXIDASE SYSTEM (MFOS)—a multienzyme system in the liver responsible for the metabolism of a variety of foreign compounds and drugs

TRANSIT TIME—the interval between the time when food is ingested and when the residue of that digested food is evacuated from the rectum

TYRAMINE— a vasoactive amine found in decayed animal tissue, ripe cheese, and other foods

VASOACTIVE (PRESSOR) AMINES—organic compounds containing nitrogen that cause vasodilation and an increase in small vessel permeability

The management of many diseases requires long-term care and drug therapy, frequently involving the use of multiple drugs. Therapeutic effects or side effects of the medications may ultimately diminish nutritional status, or, conversely, the nutritional status of the patient may decrease efficacy or increase toxicity of the drug.

Drug-nutrient interactions represent a problem of potentially serious proportions. Of the top 25 prescription drugs, 19 have the potential for diet interactions of clinical significance. Drug regimens that typically lead to serious drug-nutrition interactions include (Roe, 1988):

1. Drugs taken with food
2. Drugs taken with nutrient supplements
3. Drugs taken with alcohol
4. Drugs used purposefully in order to achieve a specific drug-nutrient interaction
5. Drugs taken in multiple drug regimens in which more than one drug produces an adverse effect because of drug and diet interactions
6. Drugs that cause nutrient depletion and that are taken for long periods

The Joint Commission on Accreditation of Healthcare Organizations has placed responsibility for monitoring and preventing potential drug-nutrient interactions with pharmacists and dietitians. Standards of responsibility for dietitians, limited to date to acute care hospitals, are defined in the 1984 and 1985 Accreditation Manual for Hospitals. It is important for dietitians and pharmacists to assess the drug regimen in light of the nutritional status and intake of the patient and to recommend appropriate diet changes or nutritional supplements.

BASIC PHARMACOLOGY: NUTRITIONAL ASPECTS

A drug is a chemical that interacts with a living organism to produce a physiologic response. It modifies existing processes through interaction with functionally important molecules.

Drug action takes place in three stages: (1) the *pharmaceutical stage* (dissolution or disintegration of the drug), (2) the *pharmacokinetic stage* (absorption, transport, and elimination of the drug), and (3) the *pharmacodynamic stage* (action of the drug at its target site).

The *bioavailability* of a drug indicates the proportion passing into the systemic circulation after oral administration and reflects both absorption and metabolic degradation. The *absorption rate* can be affected by gastrointestinal motility, splanchnic blood flow, particle size and formulation, and various chemical factors relating to the nature of the drug itself. About 75% of an oral drug will generally be absorbed in 1 to 3 hours.

Drugs are *transported* either free or bound; only in the free form is a drug available for distribution to target sites, biotransformation, or excretion. The extent of binding varies widely, for example, from 40% for phenobarbital to 90% for dicumarol.

Drugs and other foreign compounds can be *metabolized* in the lungs, kidneys, intestine, skin, plasma, and to a limited extent, in the brain and adrenal cortex, but the most important organ of metabolism is the liver. Drug effects are regulated substantially by the rate of metabolism, and the activities of drug-metabolizing enzymes are dependent on the presence of nutrients and other factors.

The *mixed-function oxidase system (MFOS)* is responsible for the metabolism of many drugs and a wide variety of other foreign compounds. The components of this multienzyme system—cytochrome P-450, NADPH-cytochrome P-450 reductase, and phosphatidylcholine—use NADPH and molecular oxygen to catalyze the oxidation of a variety of substances. Nutritional components of the MFO system include protein, lipids, nicotinic acid, riboflavin, pantothenic acid, ascorbic acid, vitamins A and E, iron, copper, calcium, zinc, and magnesium.

RISK FACTORS FOR INTERACTIONS

The development of drug-induced malnutrition occurs most commonly during long-term treatment for chronic disease. Nutritional deficiency is not usually the result of a single factor. It is more likely to occur if the patient has a recent history of marginal energy or specific nutrient intake and is taking several medications. It may be precipitated by a sudden increase in nutrient requirements related to infection, surgery, or the development of disease, resulting in a rate of metabolism or excretion more likely to produce a drug-nutrient interaction. Individual differences in drug response and occurrence of adverse reactions arise in part as a result of genetic variation in activities of several drug-metabolizing enzymes.

Body composition is an important consideration in determining drug response. Distribution of fat-soluble drugs is increased in the obese and in the elderly, in whom the proportion of adipose tissue to lean body mass is greater than in younger individuals. Excessive accumulation of a drug and its metabolites in adipose tissue may result in prolonged clearance and increased toxicity. Conversely, drugs that distribute in the nonlipid water space reach higher concentrations in the elderly.

The probability of drug-drug or drug-nutrient interactions also increases in proportion to the number of drugs ingested. Both prescription drugs and over-the-counter (OTC) medications can be involved.

High-Risk Populations

The developing fetus, infants (particularly premature infants), pregnant women, the elderly, and the chronically ill are at high risk for drug-nutrient interactions. Drug reactions that lead to decreased absorption or to increased excretion of a given nutrient are more likely to affect infants and children adversely, because their higher requirements for nutrients per kilogram of body weight make them more susceptible to fluctuations of nutrient intake.

Some of the elderly metabolize drugs at the same rate as younger individuals; others do not. The elderly are very heterogeneous in their ability (as they are with many other physiologic functions) to metabolize drugs. They are also more likely to take many drugs. Approximately 70% of the elderly use medications compared with 10% of a younger population. These older Americans take a daily average of 4.5 medications at home and 5.2 medications when they are institutionalized (Beers and Ouslander, 1989).

Higher plasma concentrations of drugs may occur for different reasons. In the elderly, higher plasma concentrations of penicillin are associated with decreased kidney function, whereas excessive plasma concentrations of phenylbutazone are the result of decreased metabolism. Increased concentration of fetomaternal plasma albumin (the transport protein for most drugs) late in pregnancy leads to increased drug concentration in the fetus (Enig, 1987).

EFFECTS OF DRUGS ON NUTRITIONAL STATUS AND REQUIREMENTS

The status of almost every nutrient is potentially affected by drugs. Calcium, folate, pyridoxine, and vitamin A are particularly important because, in addition to being affected by drugs in common use, intake of these nutrients is often marginal.

Drugs That Affect Dietary Intake

Decreased nutrient intake as a result of drug use can be desirable or undesirable, either as a primary or secondary effect of drug intake. For example, weight gain as the result of increased appetite can be an undesirable side effect (Table 25–1).

Anorectic agents that diminish appetite and food consumption are sometimes used in weight reduction programs. The ideal anorectic agent should be safe, effective, and nonaddictive—characteristics that are not yet available simultaneously. Agents with low abuse potential, such as fenfluramine, mazindol, and phenylpropanolamine, have not been shown to be effective over a long period. Phenylpropanolamine is the active ingredient in many OTC weight reduction products and a component of cough medicines and nasal decongestants. Naltrexone, an opioid-blocking drug, produces an inconsistent reduction of food intake and at higher concentrations produces significant alteration of hepatic function. Because there is some evidence for a role of opioid peptides in psychiatric disorders in children, naltrexone has been tested as a treatment for autism and self-injurious behavior. The anorectic effect appears to be less in children than in adults (Herman et al, 1989).

TABLE 25–1. Some Commonly Used Drugs That Increase Appetite

Antihistamines
Cycloheptadine hydrochloride (Periactin)
Psychotropic Drugs
Chlordiazepoxide hydrochloride (Librium)
Diazepam (Valium)
Chlorpromazine hydrochloride (Thorazine)
Meprobamate (Equanil)
Amitriptyline hydrochloride (Elavil)

Numerous other drugs decrease appetite as a side effect of their action, and this factor should be appreciated when they are administered. Dextroamphetamine and the structurally related methylphenidate (Ritalin) act on the central nervous system (CNS) to depress the appetite, but hyperactivity is a side effect. Paradoxically, these compounds have a calming effect in hyperactive children. Long-term use can result in growth retardation, which is followed by "catch-up growth" when the medication is discontinued (Klein and Mannuzza, 1988). Growth retardation is even more marked with dextroamphetamine (Dexedrine). The growth effects are presumably caused by reduced food intake associated with the anorexic effect of the drugs; however, this finding has not been demonstrated conclusively. Children who are taking these medications should have frequent anthropometric measurements, including at least height and weight plotted against standard height-weight growth charts, to ensure that there are no long-term effects on growth.

Some tranquilizers, such as chlorpromazine and lithium carbonate, induce weight gain. These agents are thought to cause an increase in appetite secondary to alteration of mental status or a CNS effect. Weight gain in hospitalized patients may also be related in part to reduced activity and to the easy availability of food; therefore, patients who do gain weight should be evaluated to determine which factors are responsible.

Drugs can cause an alteration in taste sensation (dysgeusia), reduce acuity of taste sensation (hypogeusia), or leave an unpleasant aftertaste (Table 25–2). In

TABLE 25–2. Examples of Medications That Alter or Diminish Taste Perception

Acetyl sulfasalicylic acid
Amphetamines
Amylocaine
Benzocaine
Clofibrate
Dinitrophenol
5-Fluorouracil
Griseofulvin
Lidocaine
Lithium carbonate
Meprobamate
Methicillin sodium
Methylthiouracil
D-Penicillamine
Phenindione
Phenytoin
Probucol

addition to causing anorexia, penicillamine, a metal-chelating agent, reduces levels of zinc and copper, deficiencies of which can cause hypogeusia and dysgeusia. Patients who are deficient or potentially deficient in these minerals should be given supplements. Drugs used for cancer chemotherapy frequently alter taste, cause dry mouth, or provoke nausea and vomiting. Patients should be encouraged to eat well during periods when they are not receiving drugs (see Chapter 36).

Some drugs may precipitate cravings for certain foods. For example, patients taking diuretics may crave salty foods because of the increased excretion of sodium and will increase sodium intake unless counseled about avoiding it.

Drugs That Affect Nutrient Absorption

Because most drugs and nutrients are absorbed in the small intestine, drug-nutrient interactions are common in this area. The specific effects reflect complicated interrelationships that depend on the drug dosage, type and amount of food, timing, and the presence of disease or malnutrition.

In general, drugs can cause malabsorption either by exerting an effect in the intestinal lumen or by impairing the absorptive ability of the gastrointestinal mucosa. Many drugs cause malabsorption by more than one mechanism.

Luminal Effects

Drugs can reduce nutrient absorption by *influencing the transit time* of food and nutrients in the gut. Cathartic agents reduce transit time and may cause steatorrhea, both of which have been reported to cause losses of calcium and potassium.

A number of drugs *affect bile acid activity* and thus the absorption of fat, fat-soluble vitamins, carotene, and other micellar components such as cholesterol. Bile acids are sequestered by cholestyramine, clofibrate, and colestipol, which are given for the purpose of reducing cholesterol absorption, and by neomycin, which is an antibiotic used to reduce gut flora. By inhibiting the intraluminal phase of fat digestion and absorption, these drugs induce steatorrhea and interfere with absorption of fat, fat-soluble vitamins, and other micellar components. Neomycin also *inhibits the action of pancreatic lipase.*

Chronic use of mineral oil as a laxative does not appear to interfere with absorption of the fat-soluble vitamins A and E but does decrease levels of serum beta-carotene (Ballantine et al, 1986; Clark et al, 1987).

A drug may also prevent nutrient absorption by *changing the gastrointestinal environment.* Cimitidine inhibits gastric acid secretion and impairs absorption of vitamin B_{12} by reducing cleavage from its dietary binding.

Mucosal Effects

The drugs with the greatest effect on nutrient absorption are those that damage the intestinal mucosa. Damage to the structure of the villi and microvilli inhibits the brush border enzymes and intestinal transport systems involved in nutrient absorption. The result is general or specific malabsorption of various degrees. Chronic laxative abuse often has this effect, causing a mild steatorrhea. Within 6 hours of administration, neomycin causes histologic changes in the gut mucosa that lead to reversible malabsorption of fat, protein, sodium, potassium, and calcium.

Drugs that affect intestinal transport mechanisms include (1) colchicine, an anti-inflammatory agent used to treat gout; (2) para-aminosalicylic acid (PASA), an antituberculosis drug; (3) sulfasalazine, used for ulcerative colitis; and (4) trimethoprim and pyrimethamine, antibacterial and antiprotozoal agents. The first two impair absorption of vitamin B_{12}; the others are competitive inhibitors of folate transport mechanisms.

Drugs That Affect Nutrient Metabolism and Excretion

Antivitamins

Some drugs inhibit synthesis of specific enzymes by competing for the vitamins or vitamin metabolites necessary to their structure. Cancer chemotherapeutic agents operate on this principle. Two common antivitamins are the folate antagonists methotrexate (MTX), used in the treatment of leukemia and rheumatoid arthritis, and pyrimethamine, used in the treatment of malaria and ocular toxoplasmosis. Folic acid is displaced from the enzyme dihydrofolate reductase by the drugs, and the unbound folic acid is then excreted. Without folic acid, deoxyribonucleic acid (DNA) synthesis is inhibited, cell replication stops, and the cell dies.

A drug may also form a complex with a nutrient, thus making it unavailable for use by the body. Isoniazid (isonicotinic acid hydrazide, INH) functions in this manner. This drug, used in the long-term treatment of tuberculosis, forms a complex with pyridoxine and by interfering with its metabolism at several points leads to a vitamin B_6 deficiency in some patients. Some other drugs that function as vitamin B_6 antagonists are hydralazine, penicillamine, L-dopa, and cycloserine.

Other drugs that function as antivitamins are the coumarin anticoagulants that are intentional vitamin K antagonists.

Monoamine Oxidase Inhibitors

A well-known example of drug-food interaction involves monoamine oxidase inhibitors (MAOI) and the pressor amines in foods. The two classes of biologically active amines are (1) the psychoactive amines (neurotransmitters), including norepinephrine and dopamine, and (2) the vasoactive amines (pressor amines), which include tyramine, serotonin, and histamine. Biologically active amines are normally present in many foods and rarely constitute a hazard because they are deaminated very rapidly by monoamine and diamine oxidases. However, action of these oxidases is inhibited by antidepressant, antimicrobial, antihypertensive, and antineoplastic drugs (Table 25–3). Thus the tolerance for vasoactive amines (principally tyramine) in food is lowered (Clinical Insight, p. 436). Presence of the unoxidized pressor amines causes constriction of blood vessels and elevation of blood pressure. Symptoms include tachycardia, chest pains, and severe occipital headache. In severe cases, the crisis can result in intracranial hemorrhage, cardiac arrhythmias, and cardiac failure.

TABLE 25–3. Drugs That Inhibit the Action of the Oxidases

Antidepressants
Phenelzine sulfate (Nardil)
Tranylcypromine sulfate (Parnate)
Isocarboxazid (Marplan)
Antimicrobial
Furazolidone (Furoxone)
Antineoplastics
Procarbazine (Matulane)
Isoniazid (INH)

Excretion of Nutrients

Drugs act to increase the excretion of a nutrient by displacing the vitamin from its binding site on a plasma protein. An unbound vitamin will be filtered through the kidneys and excreted. For example, aspirin can alter the transport of folate in this fashion, leading to a decrease in serum folate (Lawrence et al, 1984).

D-Penicillamine is used to treat heavy metal poisoning, Wilson's disease, cystinuria, or rheumatoid arthritis by chelating with the intended metal. At the same time, it may also chelate with other metals (e.g., zinc) and increase their excretion in the urine. Ethylenediaminotetraacetate (EDTA) administered intravenously to treat lead poisoning may also lead to excessive urinary excretion of zinc.

In laboratory animals, chlorpromazine blocks the utilization of riboflavin to form the coenzyme FAD, presumably returning the vitamin to the circulation and making it available for excretion (Pinto and Riulin, 1987). Imipramine and amitriptyline also inhibit riboflavin metabolism.

Drugs can also increase the excretion of a nutrient by interfering with its reabsorption by the kidneys. Oral diuretics, such as furosemide, ethacrynic acid, and triamterene, can produce hypercalciuria by reducing calcium reabsorption to such an extent that furosemide has actually been utilized as a temporary measure to control symptoms of hypercalcemia. Because diuretics increase renal excretion of potassium, magnesium, and zinc, chronic use may result in depletion. Appendix Table 32 lists the effects of selected drugs on nutritional status. Additional readings are listed at the end of this chapter.

Summary of Nutrition-Related Action of Some Common Drugs

Anticonvulsants

Anticonvulsant drugs (ACD) such as phenytoin, phenobarbital, and primidone have been shown to induce biochemical or clinical deficiencies of folate, biotin, or vitamin D. In the latter case, the mechanism is thought to be interference with the hepatic conversion of cholecalciferol to 25-OHD_3. Clinical rickets and osteomalacia are uncommon complications of ACD, however, and usually result from factors present prior to the ACD treatment, such as highly pigmented skin and inadequate exposure to sunlight.

Megaloblastic anemia has been seen in a small percentage of patients who take ACD. Less severe folate deficiency manifested by low serum and red blood cell folate has also been seen. Even with normal serum concentrations and excretion tests, there is some evidence of cellular deficiency, suggesting a block in cellular utilization. Gingival hyperplasia and altered bone marrow function can be caused by phenytoin. The latter is par-

CLINICAL INSIGHT: Tyramine in the Diet

Tyramine, which is formed by the decarboxylation of tyrosine, occurs in variable amounts in foods, depending on differences in processing, fermentation, ripening, and location of the sample (e.g., from the middle or the edge of the cheese). Large quantities have been reported only in aged, fermented, or spoiled products. The tyramine content of foods is listed below.

Rational guidelines for dietary counseling include keeping the tyramine intake below 5 mg by preparing and consuming only fresh foods. Counseling should begin before the patient starts taking the drug, usually an MAOI. Compliance should be monitored, and the diet should be continued for 4 weeks after the cessation of drug therapy (McCabe, 1986).

The Tyramine-Restricted Diet* †

Foods That Must Be Avoided	Foods That May Be Used with Caution‡
Cheese	Avocado
Smoked or pickled fish	Raspberries
Nonfresh meat, livers	Soy sauce
Chianti and vermouth wines	Chocolate
Broad beans	Red and white wines, port wines
Banana peel	Distilled spirits
Meat extracts	Peanuts
Yeast extracts/brewer's yeast	Yogurt and cream from unpasteurized milk
Dry sausage	
Sauerkraut	
Beer and ale	
Foods with Insufficient Evidence for Restriction	
Fresh fish	Raisins
Canned figs	Tomato juice
Mushrooms	Curry powder
Cucumber	Beetroot
Sweet corn	Junket
Fresh pineapple	Boiled egg
Worcestershire sauce	Coca Cola
Salad dressings	Cookies (English biscuits)
Yeast bread	Cottage cheese
	Cream cheese

*From McCabe BJ: Dietary tyramine and other pressor amines in MAOI regimens: A review. J Am Diet Assoc 86:1059, 1986.

†Any food, especially a high-protein food, should not be used unless freshly prepared with brief shelf storage.

‡"Used with caution" means small servings (½ c/4 oz/120 ml or less).

ticularly important because it may lead to impaired immunity and resistance to disease. The mechanism of action is not known, but supplementation of patients on chronic ACD with folate suggests that phenytoin and phenobarbital may alter the uptake of folate by erythroid precursors (Collins et al, 1988).

Dermatitis and ataxia, clinical manifestations of biotin deficiency, are also side effects of therapy with ACD. An in vitro study of the effects of carbamazepine and primidone in the human intestine revealed that they are competitive inhibitors of biotin transport (Said et al, 1989). These data suggest that biotin status should be monitored in patients on ACD.

Circulating concentrations of vitamin A, retinol-binding protein, copper, and ceruloplasmin are higher than average in patients taking ACD. The clinical significance of these changes is not known.

Oral Contraceptives

Low estrogen oral contraceptives (OC) now in general use do not alter nutritional status as did the high estrogen forms used in the past. A review of the evidence (Leklem, 1986) does not support a significantly higher requirement for vitamin B_6 as had been suggested earlier. Plasma concentrations of pyridoxal phosphate in women taking OC are not indicative of deficiency. Borderline or marginal vitamin B_6 deficiency found in women from a low socioeconomic status background who had been taking OC for 1 year has been corrected by supplementation with 10 mg of vitamin B_6, which is much less than had been recommended in the past (Amatayakul et al, 1989).

Some women who take OC display lowered serum and red blood cell folate with increased excretion of formiminoglutamic acid (FIGLU), a urinary metabolite of folic acid. Whether folate deficiency develops depends mainly on the intake of folate and on the use of folate supplements. Folate replacement therapy should probably be used as a precaution before a pregnancy begins. Folate deficiency is teratogenic to laboratory animals, although there is no direct evidence of this effect in humans.

Women who take estrogen-containing OC have elevated blood concentrations of vitamin A. In laboratory animals, estrogen-containing OC stimulate hepatic synthesis of several nutrient-specific transport proteins, resulting in high circulating concentrations. These higher concentrations of circulating vitamin A could lead potentially to depletion of vitamin A stores, particularly in women who are chronically malnourished. However, in one population, use of OC for more than 1 year did not result in a significant deterioration of vitamin A status (Amatayakul et al, 1989).

Changes in plasma concentrations of minerals are thought to reflect redistribution rather than excessive excretion.

Anti-Inflammatory Drugs

Glucocorticoid drugs are widely prescribed for the treatment of chronic conditions such as asthma, rheumatoid arthritis, and systemic lupus erythematosus. Calcium absorption is reduced, and calcium excretion is increased within 8 to 10 days of starting drug therapy. Long-term administration leads to reduced bone mass in adults and to growth retardation in children. The problem is compounded by the low calcium intake typical of many women beginning at age 10 to 11 years. Calcium supplementation suppresses bone resorption without detectable suppression of bone formation and therefore is likely to result in increased bone mass. Safe and low-cost calcium is a suitable prophylactic agent for patients taking glucocorticoids (Reid and Ibbertson, 1986) (see Clinical Insight, p. 398).

Nonsteroidal anti-inflammatory agents can also cause nutritional problems. They cause irritation of the gastrointestinal tract and bleeding, fluid retention, and hyperkalemia. The bleeding can result in chronic iron deficiency anemia and some protein loss (Bjarnason et al, 1987). Although the protein loss does not appear to be clinically significant, it should be kept in mind particularly when monitoring patients whose intake has been limited for a long time. Long-term use has been linked to decreased renal function in some patients. Chloroquine, an antimalarial now also used for rheumatoid arthritis, can alter taste perception and can result in reduced appetite.

Antihypertensives

Patients with hypertension frequently take diuretics that can adversely affect mineral metabolism. Potassium deficiency is a risk in these patients, who also have low intakes of potassium and are regular users of laxatives. Calcium, magnesium, and zinc depletion may also be seen in patients on long-term diuretic therapy.

Fifty per cent of patients taking glucothiazide diuretics experience hypokalemia, and all patients should be monitored. However, half of all those with hypokalemia are also hypomagnesemic. Because magnesium is important for keeping potassium in the cell, it is impossible to replenish potassium in the presence of magnesium deficiency. Therefore, these patients should be treated with magnesium as well as with potassium.

Prolonged use of sodium-free tube feeding formulas by elderly patients on diuretics can cause sodium depletion. Hyponatremia may be overlooked in the elderly, because the mental confusion symptomatic of sodium depletion may be thought to be caused by organic brain syndrome.

Beta-adrenergic blocking drugs (beta blockers) used to lower blood pressure may cause increased serum triglycerides and decrease concentrations of HDL. Beta blockers may also impair glucose tolerance and reduce the response of diabetic patients to oral hypoglycemic agents.

EFFECT OF NUTRIENTS AND NUTRITIONAL STATUS ON THE ABSORPTION AND METABOLISM OF DRUGS

Incompatibilities with Enteral Feedings

Continuous enteral feeding is an effective method of providing nutrients to patients who are unable to eat adequately. However, the use of the feeding tube to also administer medication can cause problems such as diarrhea, binding of the drug, or blockage of the tube. The diarrhea can result from increased osmolality of the formula. Drugs that are incompatible with formulas include Dimetapp Elixir, oral Mellaril, Robitussin expectorant, pseudoephedrine (Sudafed Cough Syrup), and Thorazine concentrate. These drugs should not be given through the tube unless the formula is stopped and the tube is irrigated with water. Care should be taken when adding any drug to an enteral formula as there is not a great deal of information in this area. Some evidence suggests that the calcium caseinate used as a protein source in many formulas may bind some drugs.

Medications should not be crushed and mixed with water and forced through the feeding tube with a syringe if this can be avoided, because particles can block the tip of the tube and necessitate its removal. Sustained-release or enteric-coated medications should never be crushed. If a drug must be given through a feeding tube, the feeding should be discontinued 1 hour before and for 2 hours after the medication is given. The medication should be provided in a liquid form when possible, and the feeding tube should be flushed with 30 ml of water before and after drug administration.

Effect on Drug Absorption

The presence of food and nutrients in the lumen may reduce the therapeutic dosage of a drug by slowing and thus reducing absorption. As a result, the drug may never reach effective levels in the blood, or effects may be prolonged as the slow absorption acts as a sustained release.

The rate of gastric emptying, influenced by the presence and type of meal or food ingested, can also influence the absorption of a drug. Basic drugs that are dissolved in an acidic environment are better dissolved and absorbed when gastric emptying is delayed, because they are exposed longer to the acidic contents of the stomach. Nitrofurantoin and hydralazine are examples. On the other hand, acid-labile drugs with extended time in the stomach experience degradation and inactivation before reaching absorption sites in the small intestine. Drugs such as L-dopa and penicillin G are examples of drugs whose effectiveness is reduced by delayed gastric emptying.

Absorption can also be affected by the amount of fluid present. More dilute drug solutions are better absorbed because the large fluid volume can stimulate gastric tension receptors that stimulate gastric motility and thus movement of the drug into the small intestine where absorption takes place.

Certain nutrients can affect the absorption of drugs. Because calcium chelates tetracycline, thus preventing its absorption, tetracycline derivatives should be taken without milk or milk products. Phenytoin has a high affinity for protein, and its absorption is decreased in the presence of food proteins. In contrast, a high-fat intake increases absorption of griseofulvin, which is highly lipid-soluble, possibly by stimulating the secretion of bile.

Suspensions and solutions are much less affected by food and nutrients because they do not depend on the

TABLE 25–4. Effects of Various Foods and Beverages on Drug Action*

Food or Beverage	Drug	Effect
Beverages		
Coffee, tea, and other caffeine-containing beverages	Theophylline	Increased intake may enhance drug side effects (nervousness, insomnia)
	Neuroleptic agents (fluphenazine, haloperidol)	Increased intake may result in a large variation in plasma concentration of drug and may reduce its clinical effectiveness
Citrus juices	Quinidine	Excessive intake may increase blood levels of drug (alkalinization of urine)
Fiber		
Bran	Digoxin	May reduce drug absorption
Pectin (?) or high-carbohydrate meal	Acetaminophen	May depress rate of drug absorption
Food (in general)	Chlorothiazide	May increase drug absorption
	Propranolol	May increase drug absorption
	Nitrofurantoin	Increases bioavailability of the drug
	Cimetidine	Delayed absorption may benefit patient by maintaining blood concentration of drug between meals
	Aspirin	May decrease drug absorption and absorptive rate
	Antimicrobial agents (celphalexin, penicillin G, erythromycin stearate, penicillin V, tetracycline)	May reduce drug absorption
High-fat meal	Griseofulvin	Increases drug absorption
High-protein diets	Levodopa, methyldopa	Amino acids from dietary protein inhibit absorption of drugs
Licorice	Antihypertensive agents, diuretics	Glycyrrhizic acid in natural licorice tends to induce hypokalemia and sodium retention; ingestion in large amounts may complicate antihypertensive drug therapy
	Digoxin	Licorice-induced hypokalemia may enhance the action of digitalis and result in drug toxicity
Milk and milk products	Tetracycline	Calcium inhibits drug absorption
Protein or charcoal-broiled meats	Theophylline	High-protein or low-carbohydrate diet or ingestion of charcoal broiled meats may decrease plasma half- life of drug
Salty foods, sodium (salt)	Lithium	Increased intake of sodium may reduce therapeutic response to drug. Low-salt diets may enhance drug activity
Vegetables		
Boiled or fried onions	Warfarin	May increase fibrinolytic activity of drug
Broccoli, turnip greens, lettuce, cabbage	Warfarin	Vegetables rich in vitamin K may inhibit hypoprothrombinemic response to oral anticoagulants

*Adapted from Pemberton CM et al: Mayo Clinic Diet Manual, 6th ed. Philadelphia, BC Decker, 1988, pp 534–535.

rate of dissolution and can move from the stomach to the small intestine more easily.

Table 25–4 lists the effects of food on the absorption and serum levels of some drugs.

Effect on Drug Metabolism

Drug metabolism may be altered in states of nutritional deficiency or nutritional manipulation, because the activity of the hepatic MFOS is influenced by the intake of protein, carbohydrate, and lipid. Research results suggest that manipulation of major dietary components could be of particular clinical significance in situations such as protein increase in some weight-reduction programs or postoperative therapy using only intravenous glucose. Wheezing episodes in asthmatic children treated with the bronchodilator theophylline were less frequent with a low-protein diet because theophylline remained in the blood longer. Liver metabolism of theophylline and antipyrine was more rapid in subjects ingesting a high-protein diet (Feldman et al, 1980).

Albumin is the primary protein to which drugs are bound; however, it is the unbound form of the drug that can diffuse through the capillary wall and exert the pharmacologic action. Conditions such as malnutrition or liver disease in which serum albumin is decreased will lead to increased serum levels of the drug and heightened pharmacologic effect. Highly protein-bound drugs such as phenytoin and warfarin are most affected. Other situations that can affect the binding of a drug to serum albumin are high-fat meals and fasting, both of which lead to high serum levels of free fatty acids that compete with the drug for albumin-binding sites. The net effect is more free drug, greater pharmacologic effect, and potential toxicity.

There are other examples of drug absorption and metabolism being affected by the composition of a meal. Bioavailability of propanolol is enhanced when it is taken with a high-protein meal. A low-protein diet has been suggested as improving the response of patients with Parkinson's disease who did not respond well to standard levodopa therapy (Pincus, 1987a and b). Unfortunately, the studies were not double-blind, and the patients represented only a small subset of patients because most patients with Parkinson's disease respond well to therapy.

A number of compounds increase the activity of the MFOS, resulting in amplified metabolism of drugs. Polycyclic aromatic hydrocarbons in the environment and in charcoal-broiled foods, and compounds in vegetables such as Brussels sprouts and cabbage induce MFOS activity in the liver and intestine.

Other factors that influence the metabolism of drugs are the rate of intestinal absorption and delivery of the drug to the liver; the presence of other disease, including malnutrition; liver function; and the concomitant administration of other drugs that can either increase or decrease the metabolism of the first drug.

TABLE 25–5. Effects of Selected Drugs on Appetite*

Amphetamines	Decreased appetite, delayed onset of hunger, but tolerance develops; effect caused by blocking the uptake of catecholamines
Cocaine	Loss of appetite
Codeine	Loss of appetite with chronic use
Marijuana	Reported to enhance appetite, but not all studies agree; users appear to be more likely to lose appetite and weight
Methadone	Loss of appetite with chronic use

*Adapted from Enig MG: Pharmacologic basis of drug-nutrient interaction related to drug abuse during pregnancy. Clin Nutr 6:235, 1987.

Effect on Drug Excretion

Food and nutrient intake can affect drug excretion by changing the urinary pH. Drugs that require an acid medium are excreted more rapidly in an alkaline urine (see Chapter 35 for foods that acidify urine). Mineral drugs such as lithium carbonate are affected by body levels of other minerals. Sodium depletion provokes increased reabsorption of both sodium and lithium carbonate and increased potential for lithium toxicity. With sodium supplementation or increased fluid intake, lithium excretion is increased. Nutritional effects on renal excretion of drugs are most prominent in drugs with a narrow therapeutic range.

DRUGS OF ABUSE

Drugs of abuse is a general term that includes any compound taken legally, such as coffee, tobacco, and alcohol, or illegally, such as marijuana, cocaine, or crack. It also includes substances with recognized medical uses that are used in a nonmedical manner (e.g., barbiturates or amphetamines used for mind-altering effects or for pleasurable purposes). Although the major effects of street drugs are not nutritional, their use can induce nutritional problems, either directly by reduction of food intake during periods of altered state or indirectly by depleting all the money needed for food (Table 25–5).

CITED REFERENCES

Amatayakul K et al: Oral contraceptives: Effect of long term use on liver vitamin A storage assessed by the relative dose response test. Am J Clin Nutr 49:845, 1989.

Ballantine TVN et al: The effect of mineral oil (MO) on fat-soluble vitamin levels. JPEN 10:18S, 1986.

Beers MH and Ouslander JG: Risk factors in geriatric drug prescribing: A practical guide to avoiding problems. Drugs 37:105, 1989.

Bjarnason I et al: Blood and protein loss via small-intestinal inflammation induced by non-steroidal anti-inflammatory drugs. Lancet 2:711, 1987.

Clark JH et al: Serum beta-carotene, retinol, and alpha-tocopherol levels during mineral oil therapy for constipation. Am J Dis Child 141:1210, 1987.

Collins CS et al: Red blood cell uptake of supplemental folate in patients on anticonvulsant drug therapy. Am J Clin Nutr 48:1445, 1988.

Enig MG: Pharmacologic basis of drug-nutrient interaction related to drug abuse during pregnancy. Clin Nutr 6:235, 1987.

Feldman CH et al: Effect of dietary protein and carbohydrate on theophylline metabolism in children. Pediatrics 66:956, 1980.

Herman BH et al: Effects of acute administration of naltrexone on cardiovascular function, body temperature, body weight and serum concentrations of liver enzymes in autistic children. Dev Pharmacol Ther 12:118, 1989.

Klein RG and Mannuzza S: Hyperactive boys almost grown up. III: Methylphenidate effects on ultimate height. Arch Genet Psychiatr 45:1131, 1988.

Lawrence VA, Loewenstein JE, and Eichner ER: Aspirin and folate binding: In vivo and in vitro studies of serum binding and urinary excretion of endogenous folate. J Lab Clin Med 103:944, 1984.

Leklem JE: Vitamin B_6 requirement and oral contraceptive use: A concern? J Nutr 116:475, 1986.

McCabe BJ: Dietary tyramine and other pressor amines in MAOI regimens: A review. J Am Diet Assoc 86:1059, 1986.

Pincus JH and Barry K: Dietary methods for reducing fluctuations in Parkinson's disease. Yale J Biol Med 60:133, 1987a.

Pincus JH and Barry K: Influence of dietary protein on motor fluctuations in Parkinson's disease. Arch Neurol 44:270, 1987b.

Pinto JT and Rivlin RS: Drugs that promote renal excretion of riboflavin. Drug Nutr Interact 5:143, 1987.

Reid IR and Ibbertson HK: Calcium supplements in the prevention of steroid-induced osteoporosis. Am J Clin Nutr 44:287, 1986.

Roe DA: Diet and Drug Interactions. New York, Van Nostrand Reinhold, 1988, pp 5–6.

Said HM, Redha R, and Nylander W: Biotin transport in the human intestine: Inhibition by anticonvulsant drugs. Am J Clin Nutr 49:127, 1989.

ADDITIONAL REFERENCES

Basu TK: Drug-Nutrient Interactions. New York, Croom Helm/ Methuen, 1988.

Diuretics and hypomagnesemia. Nutr MD 14(11):4, 1988.

Folate status of patients on low-dose methotrexate therapy. Nutr Rev 47:43, 1989.

Garabedian-Ruffalo SM et al: Monitoring of drug-drug and drug-food interactions. Am J Hosp Pharm 45:1530, 1988.

Gora ML, Tschampel MM, and Visconti JA: Considerations of drug therapy in patients receiving enteral nutrition. Nutr Clin Pract 4:105, 1989.

LaFrance RJ, Miyagawa CI, and Youngs CHF: Pharmacotherapeutic considerations in enteral and parenteral therapy. *In* Lang CE: Nutritional Support in Critical Care. Rockville, MD, Aspen Publishers, 1987.

Magnesium depletion and diuretics. Nutr MD 15(12):4, 1989.

Mineral oil and absorption of fat-soluble vitamins. Nutr MD 15(3):2, 1988.

Niemec PW et al: Gastrointestinal disorders caused by medication and electrolyte solution osmolality during enteral nutrition. JPEN 7:387, 1983.

Powers DE and Moore AO: Food-Medications Interactions, 6th ed. Phoenix, AZ, Food-Medications Interactions, 1988.

Roe DA: Drug and nutrient interactions in the elderly diabetic. Drug Nutr Interact 5:205, 1988.

Roe DA: Drug-Induced Nutritional Deficiencies, 2nd ed. Westport, CT, Avi Publishing, 1986.

Roe DA: Process guides on drug-nutrient interactions for health care providers and patients. I: Overview. Drug Nutr Interact 5:131, 1987.

Roe DA: Process guides on drug and nutrient interactions in arthritics. Drug Nutr Interact 5:135, 1987.

Sulfasalazine inhibits folate absorption. Nutr Rev 46:320, 1988.

CHAPTER 26

DISEASES OF THE ORAL CAVITY, THE ESOPHAGUS, AND THE STOMACH

CHAPTER OUTLINE

KEY TERMS

ACHLORHYDRIA—absence of hydrochloric acid from maximally stimulated gastric secretions
ACHYLIA GASTRICA—absence of hydrochloric acid and pepsin in the gastric juice
ALIMENTARY HYPOGLYCEMIA—low blood glucose manifesting as weakness, perspiration, hunger, nausea, anxiety, and tremors occurring from 1 to 2 hours after a meal in people who have had gastrectomies or vagotomies
ATROPHIC GASTRITIS—chronic gastritis with atrophy of the mucous membrane and glands resulting in achlorhydria and loss of intrinsic factor
DUMPING SYNDROME—a complex physiologic response to the rapid emptying of the gastric contents into the jejunum
DUODENAL ULCER—a peptic ulcer situated in the duodenum
DYSPEPSIA (INDIGESTION)—impairment of the power or function of digestion; usually applied to epigastric discomfort following meals
EPIGASTRIC—referring to the upper middle region of the abdomen
FUNDOPLICATION—mobilization of the lower end of the esophagus and attachment of the stomach around it for the treatment of reflux esophagitis
GASTRIC ULCER—an ulcer of the gastric mucosa that is not associated with excessive gastric acid secretion but rather with disruption of the gastric mucosal barrier
GASTRITIS—inflammation of the stomach
HEARTBURN (PYROSIS)—an esophageal symptom consisting of a retrosternal sensation of warmth or burning that may be accompanied by reflux of fluid into the mouth
HIATAL HERNIA—an outpouching of a portion of the stomach into the chest through the esophageal hiatus of the diaphragm
LOWER ESOPHAGEAL SPHINCTER (LES)—the terminal few centimeters of the esophagus that prevents reflux of gastric contents into the esophagus
PARIETAL CELL VAGOTOMY—resection or removal of the portion of the vagus nerve ennervating the parietal cells such that gastric acid secretion is diminished
PEPTIC ULCER—an eroded lesion in either the esophageal, gastric, or duodenal mucosa resulting from the action of acid in gastric juice
REFLUX ESOPHAGITIS—a chronic, pathologic, potentially life-threatening disease manifested by the various sequelae associated with reflux of the stomach and duodenal contents into the esophagus
TRUNCAL VAGOTOMY—resection or removal of portions of the vagus nerve, thus decreasing the cholinergic stimulation of parietal cells and reducing the cellular response to stimulants such as gastrin
VAGUS NERVE—the tenth cranial nerve with many branches that supplies sensory fibers to the ear; tongue; pharynx; and larynx; motor fibers to the pharynx, larynx, and esophagus; and parasympathetic and visceral afferent fibers to the thoracic and abdominal viscera

DISEASES OF THE ESOPHAGUS

Physiology

The entire esophagus functions as one tissue during swallowing. As the bolus of food is moved voluntarily from the mouth to the pharynx, the upper sphincter relaxes, the food moves into the esophagus, and the lower esophageal sphincter (LES) relaxes to receive the food bolus. Peristaltic waves move the bolus down the esophagus and into the stomach.

Disorders of the esophagus are caused by obstruction, inflammation, or derangement of the swallowing mechanism. Because difficulty in swallowing *(dysphagia)* is often the result of a neurologic problem, the required nutritional care is discussed in Chapter 39. Table 26-1 gives clues in the dietary history indicative of gastrointestinal disease.

Esophagitis

Esophagitis usually occurs in the lower esophagus as a result of the irritating effect of acidic gastric reflux on the esophageal mucosa. The common symptom is *heartburn,* which is a burning epigastric substernal pain. Other symptoms are regurgitation and dysphagia.

Acute esophagitis is caused by ingestion of an irritating agent, viral inflammation, or intubation. *Chronic* or *reflux esophagitis* is a result of recurrent gastroesophageal reflux owing to a hiatal hernia, reduced LES pressure, increased abdominal pressure (as in obstructive lung disease), recurrent vomiting, or other factors. When lower esophagitis is chronic, an inflammatory stricture and eventually dysphagia can develop.

The severity of the esophagitis resulting from gastroesophageal reflux is influenced by the content of the gastric reflux, mucosal resistance, and clearing rate of the esophagus, as well as the rate of gastric emptying.

Competency of the LES is also important. The pressure of this sphincter is controlled by many factors, one of which is hormonal. LES pressures decrease during pregnancy, in women taking progesterone-containing oral contraceptives, and even in the late stage of a normal menstrual cycle. Transient reflux episodes occur for almost everyone, but prolonged reflux is a problem. Gastroesophageal reflux may be a problem in patients with chronic lung disease who aspirate during sleep.

Nutritional Care

The objectives of nutritional care are to (1) prevent irritation of the inflamed esophageal mucosa in the acute phase, (2) prevent esophageal reflux, and (3) decrease the irritating capacity or acidity of the gastric juice.

In the acute phase, the patient may prefer a liquid diet that is less abrasive to the esophagus. Orange juice and other citrus and tomato products can be irritating because of their acidity. Certain foods and factors decrease LES pressure and should be restricted or omitted. The diet should therefore be low in fat and should exclude alcohol, carminatives (peppermint and spearmint), chocolate, and caffeine-containing beverages, all of which lower LES pressure.

Obesity is a contributing factor because it increases intragastric pressure. Weight loss is an effective treatment, particularly in the presence of hiatal hernia. Table 26-2 summarizes the nutritional care for esophagitis.

Drugs and Other Treatments

Esophagitis is sometimes treated with bethanechol, a cholinergic drug that increases LES pressure; metoclopramide, a dopamine antagonist that increases LES pressure and promotes gastric emptying; and cimetidine, a histamine H_2 receptor blocking agent that decreases gastric acid production. Antacids lower gastric acidity and also raise LES pressure. Alginates (e.g., Gaviscon) provide a viscous barrier because they lie on the surface of the gastric acid pool.

Because nicotine decreases LES pressure, cigarette smoking is contraindicated (New Directions, p. 443). Medications (e.g., theophylline) that decrease LES pressure should be avoided if possible. To discourage the occurrence of nocturnal reflux, it is often helpful for the patient to sleep on a bed that has its upper portion raised 4 to 8 inches.

TABLE 26-1. Dietary History—Clues to Gastrointestinal Disease

Symptom	Possible Disorder
Ingestion of solid food causes distress but liquids do not	Esophageal stricture or tumor
Difficulty in swallowing; food sticks in the throat	Esophageal spasm; achalasia
Epigastric pain when eating	Gastric ulcer
Pain 2-5 hours after a meal, relieved after eating	Duodenal ulcer
Abdominal pain several hours after a fatty meal	Pancreatic or biliary tract disease
Cramps, distention, and flatulence 18 to 24 hours after drinking milk	Lactose intolerance probably owing to lactase deficiency
Heartburn after eating a large or fatty meal	Hiatal hernia; achalasia; esophageal motility problem

TABLE 26–2. Nutritional Care for Esophagitis

The patient with esophagitis should:

1. Avoid foods that are known to cause heartburn.
2. Eat small, frequent meals to prevent stomach distention and resultant gastric acid secretion.
3. Avoid high-fat meals and decrease fat in the diet.
4. Avoid chocolate, alcohol, and caffeine-containing beverages, such as coffee, tea, and cola drinks.
5. Avoid peppermint and spearmint oils.
6. Avoid lying down, bending over, or straining immediately after eating.
7. Avoid eating within 2 to 3 hours of going to bed.
8. Avoid tight-fitting clothing, especially after a meal.
9. Reduce weight if overweight.
10. Avoid or quit cigarette smoking.

The 5 to 10% of patients with gastroesophageal reflux who do not respond after 3 to 6 months of medical therapy should be treated surgically *(fundoplication).*

Hiatal Hernia

A common cause of gastroesophageal reflux and esophagitis is the occurrence of hiatal hernia, which is an outpouching of a portion of the stomach into the chest through the esophageal hiatus of the diaphragm. A major type of hiatal hernia, the paraesophageal hernia, is illustrated in Figure 26–1. Pressures generated by the diaphragm are sufficient to force acidic stomach contents upward into the esophagus. Patients experience most discomfort after heavy meals and when they are lying down or bending over.

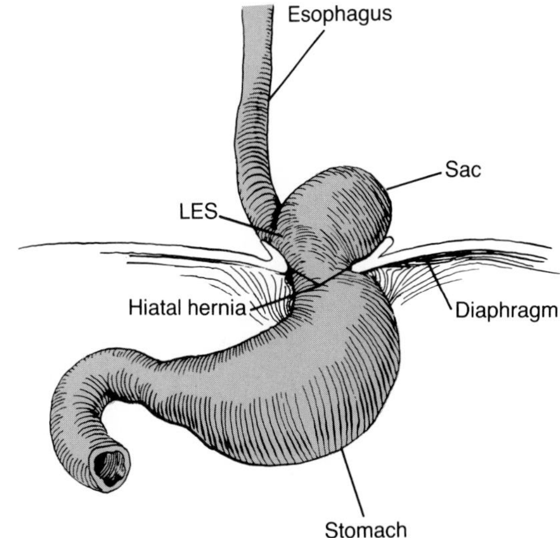

FIGURE 26–1. *Sketch of paraesophageal hiatal hernia. (Adapted from Hagarty G: A classification of esophageal hiatus hernia with special reference to sliding hernia. Am J Roentgenol 84:1056, 1960.) (LES = lower esophageal sphincter.)*

Surgery of the Mouth or Esophagus

After extensive surgery of the mouth or esophagus, it may be necessary to provide oral nutrition support in liquid form. Many nutritionally complete formulas are available (Appendix Table 33). To add variety to the diet, ordinary foods such as fruits can be puréed and mixed with water until liquefied. With more extensive oral involvement, it may be necessary to use a nasogastric tube or a gastrostomy or jejunostomy tube to provide the liquid enterally (Appendix Table 33). Enteral tube feedings can provide these formulas, or they can be made from blenderized table foods and baby foods (Table 30–2). In rare situations it may be necessary to provide nutritional support parenterally.

Tonsillectomy

Because the convalescent period following a tonsillectomy is short, the nutritional adequacy of the diet is not critical. Very cold, mild-flavored, and "non- scratchy" foods bring the most comfort to the patient and offer the most protection against bleeding of the surgical area. During the first 24 hours, foods best accepted include cold milk; milk beverages such as malted milk and eggnogs; chocolate and vanilla ice cream; fruit ice; and pear, peach, or prune juice. By the second day, warm fluids and soft foods may be started and cautiously replaced by hot foods as healing progresses and as these foods can be tolerated. A normal diet can be instituted within the next few days.

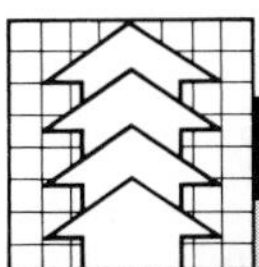

NEW DIRECTIONS: Smoking and Gastrointestinal Function

The gastrointestinal effects of smoking include the reduction of LES and pyloric sphincter pressure, increased reflux and alteration of the nature of the gastric contents, inhibition of pancreatic bicarbonate secretion, accelerated gastric emptying of liquids and lower duodenal pH (Sontag et al, 1984). The acid secretory response to gastrin or acetylcholine is considerably increased. Smoking also impairs the ability of cimetidine and other drugs to lower the overnight acid secretion that is thought to have a key role in ulcerogenesis. Lastly, smoking impairs spontaneous healing and increases the risk and rapidity of ulcer recurrence as well as the likelihood that the ulcer will perforate and require surgery.

Cancer of the Oral Cavity, Pharynx, and Esophagus

The patient with cancer of the oral cavity, pharynx, or esophagus may present with existing nutritional problems at the time of diagnosis, owing to eating problems caused by the tumor mass, obstruction, oral infection and ulceration, or coexisting alcoholism frequently associated with these tumors (see Chapter 36). This is compounded by the treatment, which commonly involves surgical resection and regional irradiation and may even include chemotherapy. Chewing, swallowing, salivation, and taste acuity are affected. Extensive dental decay, oseteoradionecrosis, and infections may occur. Chemotherapy, if given, can be expected to produce nausea, vomiting, and anorexia. Resection of the esophagus can result in fat malabsorption with varying degrees of steatorrhea (Lawrence, 1979).

Initially, nutritional support is provided via a tube feeding if the remainder of the gastrointestinal tract is functional. The extent of the resection may require long-term feeding by tube if the ability to eat cannot be regained. If oral feeding is possible after surgery, general dietary recommendations would include liquid or soft-textured moist foods for easy mastication and swallowing, and small, frequent meals of relatively high-caloric density. If steatorrhea exists, use of medium-chain triglycerides in the formula may be necessary. The use of complex carbohydrates is preferred rather than more cariogenic sugars. Periodic use of an artificial saliva solution is also helpful, as is the frequent consumption of fluids to aid the dry mouth (see Table 36–3). Normal saline rinses can help the mucositis, and application of topical anesthetics can relieve the pain. Necessary dental restorations and aggressive oral hygiene including daily use of fluoride are recommended. Oral infections at this time are usually fungal. Unfortunately, the medications used in treatment leave a metallic taste in the mouth that further compromises the patient's desire to eat.

DISEASES OF THE STOMACH

Indigestion

Indigestion, or dyspepsia, is an indefinite term used frequently to describe any discomfort occurring in the digestive tract. When possible, it is important to determine the cause, because symptoms may warn of a more serious illness.

Indigestion may originate in the stomach, or it may reflect gallbladder disease, chronic appendicitis, ulcer disease, or the derangement of some other organ such as the colon. Gastrointestinal disturbances are associated with emotions, and indigestion as a manifestation of psychoneurosis is frequently encountered. Other causes of indigestion are rapid eating, poor mastication, and overindulgence.

Nutritional Care

A therapeutic diet for simple indigestion is seldom necessary because a well-balanced diet and avoidance of rapid eating, poor mastication, and overindulgence is usually sufficient. Treating the cause, whether mental or physical, is the important factor.

Acute Gastritis

Acute gastritis, an inflammation of the gastric mucosa, is sudden and sometimes violent in onset. True gastritis is usually manifested by nausea and vomiting, hemorrhage, pain, malaise, anorexia, or headache. Attacks very often follow the eating of specific foods to which the individual is sensitive, eating too fast, or eating when overtired or emotionally upset. Acute gastritis can also result from the use of too much alcohol, tobacco (see New Directions, p. 443), and highly seasoned foods; ingestion of an infectious agent, such as *Helicobacter pylori* or a corrosive substance; or the use of aspirin or other nonsteroidal anti-inflammatory drugs (NSAID) (Fig. 26–2) (Drumm et al, 1987). Occasionally, acute gastritis follows radiation therapy, trauma, burns, surgery, hypoxia, shock, fever, jaundice, or renal failure.

The initial treatment is to remove the cause or to get rid of the offending substance as soon as possible. It may be necessary to empty the stomach by inducing vomiting, lavage, or both. Irrigation of the colon and administration of a laxative may also be valuable in hastening the cleansing process.

Nutritional Care

To allow the stomach to rest and heal, food is usually withheld for 24 to 48 hours or longer, depending on whether there is bleeding or pain. If bleeding occurs, nasogastric lavage with iced water brings homeostasis in most patients. Fluids are given intravenously.

Following the fasting period, liquids are added as tolerated. The amount of food and the number of feedings are increased according to the patient's tolerance until a full regular diet is achieved. Highly seasoned foods as well as foods shown in Table 26–3 that increase gastric acidity may need to be avoided temporarily.

Chronic Gastritis

The cause of chronic gastritis is not known. It often precedes the development of organic gastric lesions such as cancer or ulcer. It may be caused by an antral

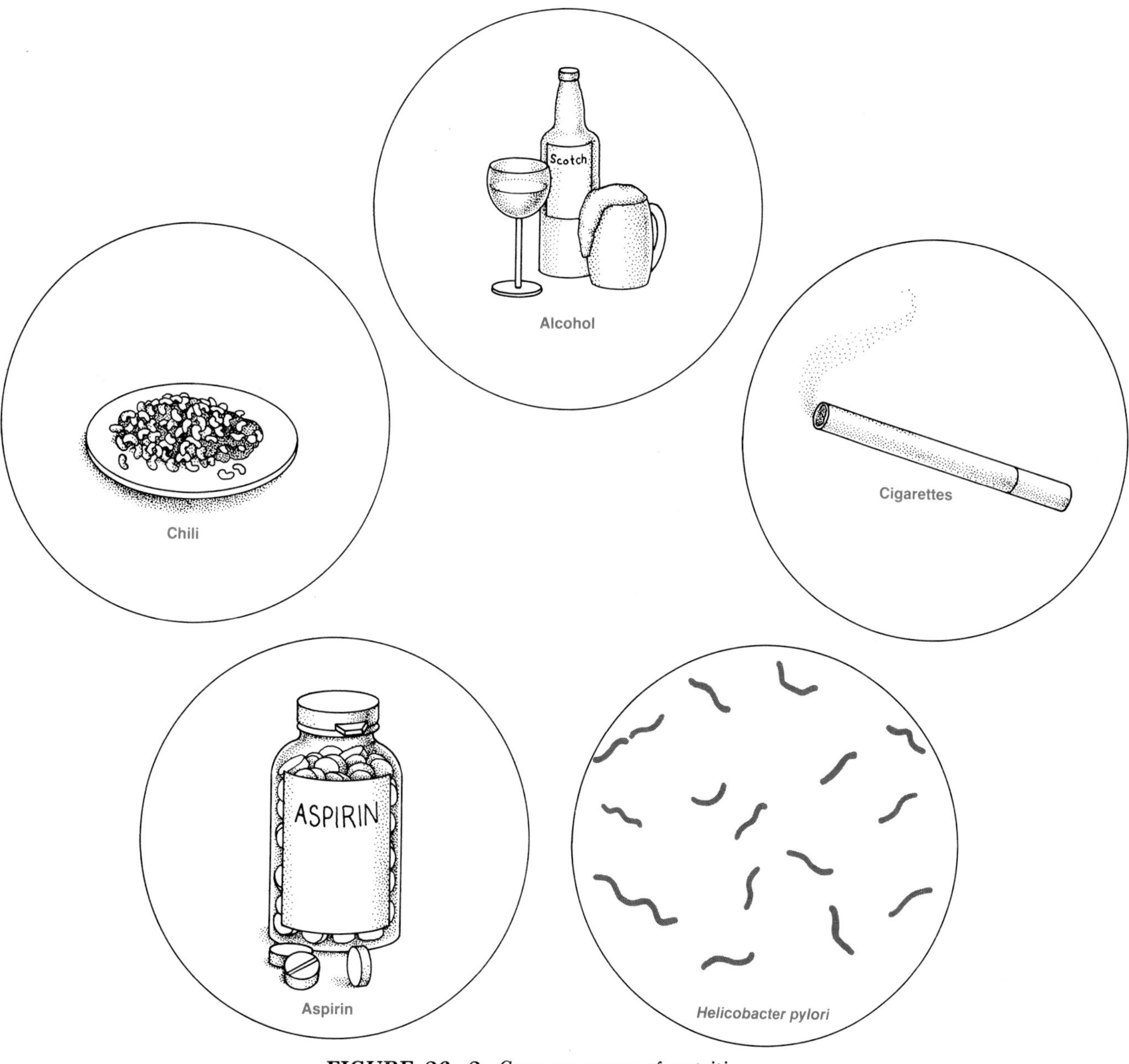

FIGURE 26–2. *Common causes of gastritis.*

infection with *H. pylori,* which leads to the inflammatory response and impaired mucosal defense (Soll, 1990). It may also be related indirectly to diseases such as tuberculosis, myocardial failure, and nephritis. Endoscopy is often used to characterize the lesion if there is one (Further Reading, p. 446). The same dietary indiscretions listed for acute gastritis are frequently associated with the chronic form. Although symptoms may be vague or absent, the most usual ones are similar to those of indigestion—loss of appetite, a feeling of fullness, belching, vague epigastric pain, and nausea and vomiting.

Nutritional Care

Because the symptoms of chronic gastritis are vague, the nutritional care must follow general principles. The prescription of individualized treatment based on foods and situations determined to cause discomfort is most important. The diet should be adequate in calories and nutrients and soft in consistency. The patient should eat at regular intervals, chew food thoroughly, and avoid foods known to cause discomfort. Highly seasoned foods are not usually tolerated well. Excess amounts of liquids with meals tend to cause discomfort

TABLE 26-3. Factors That Affect Gastric Acidity

Increase Gastric Acidity	
Cephalic Phase of Digestion	
Thought, taste, smell of food, and chewing and swallowing initiate vagal stimulation of the parietal cells in the fundic mucosa to secrete gastric acid.	
Gastric Phase of Digestion	
Effect of food in the stomach:	Distention of the fundus stimulates the parietal cells to produce acid.
	Increased alkalinity of antrum causes the release of gastrin which stimulates gastric acid secretion.
	Distention of antrum causes release of gastrin.
	Substances in food and digestive products increase acidity: i.e., coffee both with and without caffeine, alcohol, polypeptides and amino acids (products of protein digestion)
Decrease Gastric Acidity	
Gastric Phase of Digestion	
Acidification of antrum reduces gastrin release and thus gastric acid secretion.	
Food, especially protein, has an initial buffering effect.	
Intestinal Phase of Digestion	
Fat, acid, and hyperosmolarity in the small intestine stimulate release of one or more gastrointestinal hormones that inhibit gastric acid secretion.	

because of stomach distention. The principles followed in the care of ulcers are also followed in the treatment of gastritis.

Atrophic gastritis, which results in atrophy and loss of stomach parietal cells, is characterized by a loss of secretion of HCl (achlorhydria) and intrinsic factor. Vitamin B_{12} status should always be assessed in these patients, because a lack of intrinsic factor results in malabsorption of this vitamin.

Gastric Surgery

After gastric surgery, some varieties of which are shown in Figure 26-3, all fluids and foods by mouth are withheld for 3 to 5 days, and the patient is fed with a nasogastric tube. The use of total parenteral nutrition (TPN) is usually reserved for patients with poor preoperative nutritional status or postoperative complications that delay enteral feeding for an extended period.

The first type of fluids allowed by mouth are ice, which is held in the mouth, or infrequent sips of water. Some patients tolerate warm water better than iced or cold water. When vomiting ceases, larger amounts of fluids may be served. Bland foods can be started, but a more important priority is offering the patient foods that are liked and well tolerated. By the fifth to seventh postoperative day, most patients can tolerate solid foods.

Nutritional impairment frequently occurs after gastrectomy, and many patients have difficulty in regaining normal preoperative weight owing to one or both of the following: (1) inadequate food intake related in most cases to the dumping syndrome, and (2) malabsorption of ingested food, specifically fat and protein. Patients who have had a total or almost total gastrectomy often have difficulty in taking large amounts of food and may need to make a permanent habit of eating several small meals each day.

Dumping Syndrome

The dumping syndrome is a complex physiologic response to the presence of undigested food in the jejunum. Following gastric surgery, some patients who have had two thirds or more of the stomach removed (or some patients whose procedure has included a vagotomy) may experience the dumping syndrome when offered a full-diet regimen. After food is swallowed, it is "dumped" into the jejunum about 10 to 15 minutes after ingestion instead of being gradually released in small amounts. Most patients who undergo this type of surgery develop a new pouch through stretching of the remaining stomach tissue. However, many patients may continue to have chronic symptoms of the dumping syndrome.

SYMPTOMS. Some individuals complain of abdominal fullness, nausea, and, at times, crampy abdominal pain followed by diarrhea within 15 minutes after eating. Others feel warm, dizzy, weak, and faint; their pulse races, and they break into a cold sweat. Lying down

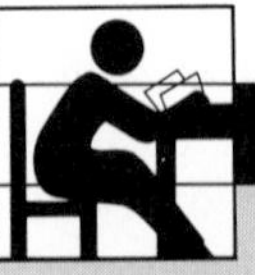

FURTHER READING: Endoscopy

The appearance of the stomach mucosa can be viewed, studied, and even photographed by means of an endoscope, a flexible tube with a light and an eye-piece that can be passed down the esophagus into the stomach. Erosions, ulcerations, changes in the blood vessels, and destruction of surface cells can be seen. These changes can then be correlated with chemical, histologic, and clinical findings when formulating a diagnosis. This kind of study is important in long-term monitoring of the patient with chronic gastritis because of the possibility that the patient will develop gastric carcinoma.

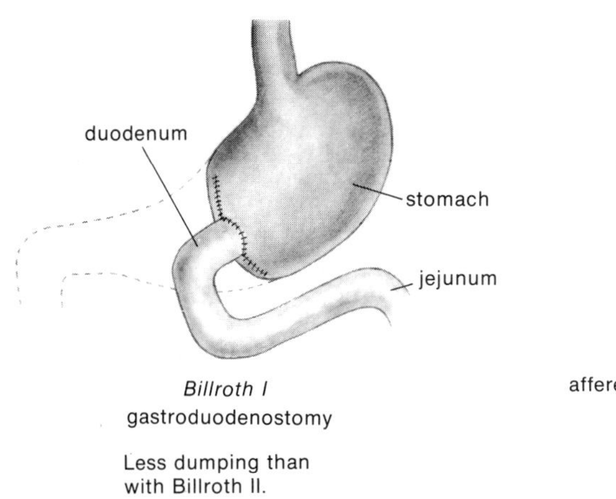

Billroth I
gastroduodenostomy

Less dumping than with Billroth II.

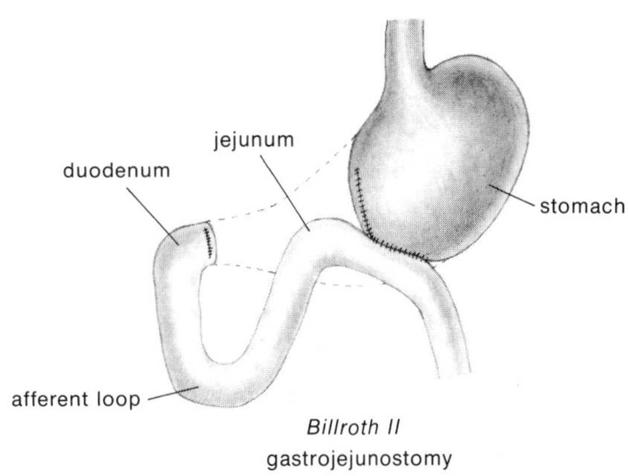

Billroth II
gastrojejunostomy

Sequelae such as steatorrhea, weight loss, dumping, vomiting and bacterial overgrowth occur more often with the Billroth II procedure.

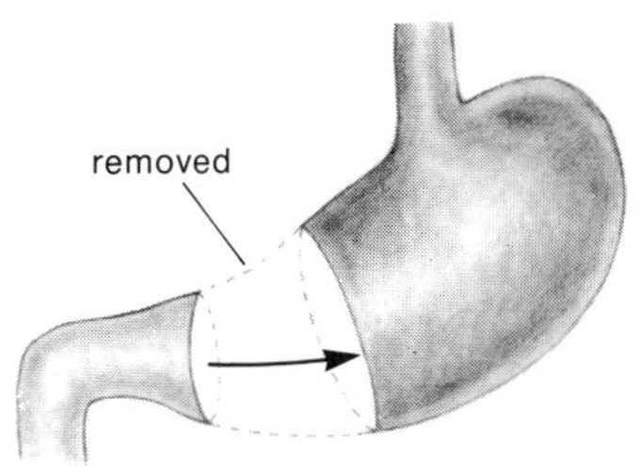

Partial Gastric Resection

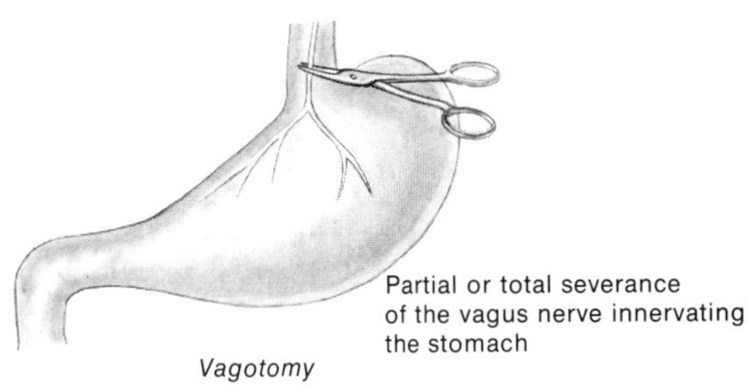

Partial or total severance
of the vagus nerve innervating
the stomach

Vagotomy

Depending on the extent of the vagotomy, HCl secretion is reduced and gastric emptying is slowed. Dumping syndrome often follows this surgery.

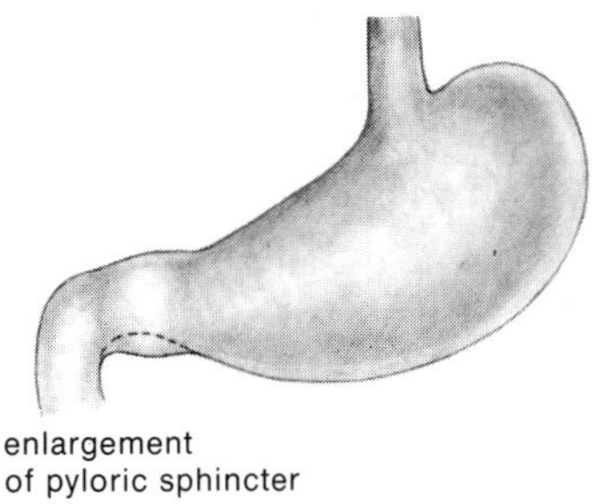

Pyloroplasty

Duodenal reflux frequently follows this surgery.

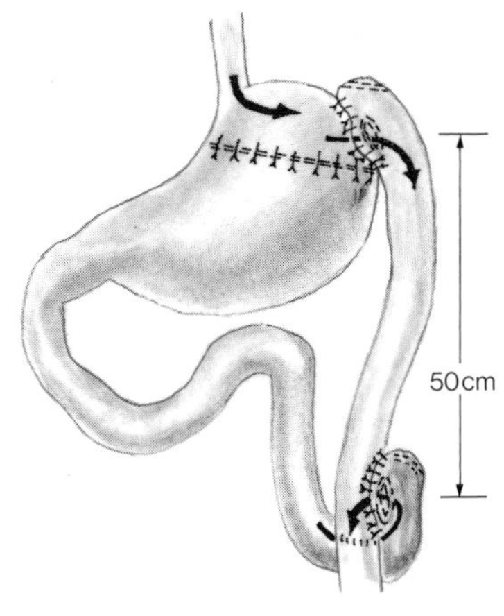

Roux-en-Y procedure

FIGURE 26–3. *Gastric surgical procedures.*

immediately after eating reduces these symptoms because food remains longer in the stomach pouch.

Rapid entry of ingested nutrients into the jejunum and their subsequent hydrolysis lead to hypertonic intestinal contents. This hypertonic material is diluted rapidly by fluid drawn from the plasma and extracellular fluid and leads to a sharp drop in circulating blood volume. A drop in blood volume, a decrease in cardiac output, and perhaps dilation of the jejunum lead to a sympathetic vasomotor response producing sweating, tachycardia, electrocardiographic changes, and weakness. Serotonin, a vasoconstrictor, and vasoactive kinins, histamine, and prostaglandins are thought to be released because of the hyperosmolarity of the jejunal chyme. These substances may be the cause of the cramping, hypermotility, and diarrhea of the dumping syndrome.

Alimentary Hypoglycemia

Symptoms of hypoglycemia, such as weakness, perspiration, hunger, nausea, anxiety, and tremors, can occur from 1 to 2 hours after a meal in patients who have had gastrectomies or vagotomies. Hypoglycemia is caused by the rapid digestion and absorption of food (especially of sugars) that has been dumped into the duodenum. The glucose rapidly enters the blood stream and causes a postprandial elevation in blood glucose and an overproduction of insulin, which results later in hypoglycemia.

Malabsorption

Following some gastric surgery, the Billroth II procedure (gastrojejunostomy) in particular, there may be steatorrhea in addition to dumping and hypoglycemia. About 10% of these patients have clinically significant steatorrhea. This is due to pancreatic insufficiency and defective digestion. Because food bypasses the duodenum, the secretion of secretin and pancreozymin by the duodenal mucosa is reduced. These two hormones stimulate the pancreas to secrete its enzymes and bicarbonate; there is little pancreatic exocrine secretion when they are not present. Furthermore, pancreatic atrophy and some fibrosis occur.

Because of the complications with the Billroth II procedure, many other procedures — including truncal, selective or parietal cell vagotomy, pyloroplasty, antrectomy, Roux-en-Y esophagojejunostomy, and loop esophagojejunostomy — have been developed as alternatives. The perfect gastric surgical treatment without complications has yet to be developed.

Anemia

Anemia may develop after gastric surgery, possibly owing to iron deficiency caused by bleeding from recurrent ulcers or by impaired iron absorption. Because of rapid stomach emptying, which prevents thorough mixing of food with gastric HCl, iron is not changed to the absorbable ferrous form. Also, because of the surgery, the iron may bypass the duodenum where 50% of iron absorption takes place. For some patients, poor iron absorption may be severe enough to require use of parenteral iron.

Vitamin B_{12} deficiency may cause the anemia. If there is a reduced amount of gastric mucosa, intrinsic factor may not be produced in quantities adequate to allow for complete vitamin B_{12} absorption, and pernicious anemia develops. Bacterial overgrowth in the proximal small bowel or in the afferent loop binds vitamin B_{12} and competes with the body for absorption. The result is a macrocytic anemia that should be treated with vitamin B_{12} injections.

Anemia can also result from folate deficiency as part of the general malabsorption syndrome (see Chapter 32).

Nutritional Care

Because of the problems that accompany eating, postgastrectomy and postvagotomy patients frequently do not eat enough; they have diarrhea from the increased intestinal activity; and they become underweight, malnourished, and frustrated. The prime objective of nutritional care is to restore nutritional status and pleasant living.

Proteins and fats are better tolerated than carbohydrates because they are hydrolyzed more slowly into osmotically active substances. Simple carbohydrates — lactose, sucrose, and dextrose — are hydrolyzed rapidly and should be limited, but complex carbohydrates (starches) can be included. Liquids enter the jejunum rapidly, and thus some patients may have problems tolerating liquids with meals. Patients who have severe problems with dumping may do better by limiting the amount of liquids taken with meals or by taking liquids only between meals, without solid food.

Pectin, the dietary fiber contained in fruits and vegetables, may be useful in treating dumping syndrome. It seems to slow down carbohydrate absorption and reduce the glycemic response and thus insulin response. An alpha-glucoside hydrolase inhibitor (acarbose), which reduces the digestion and absorption of starch, sucrose, and maltose, may also reduce the blood glucose response and subsequent hypoglycemia.

Basically, the diet is moderate in fat (30 to 40% of calories), low in simple carbohydrates, and high in protein (20% of calories), with the purpose of achieving and maintaining the optimal weight and nutritional status of the patient. The diabetic exchange lists given in Table 31 – 10 can be used to calculate the carbohydrate intake and to teach the patient about carbohydrate control.

Milk in small amounts is likely to be tolerated better than in large amounts, although some patients may not tolerate it at all. Dried skim milk or various casein hydrolysates can be used and may be well tolerated. Persons with minimal or no intake of milk or dairy products may need vitamin D and calcium supplementation.

If milk intolerance is caused by lactose intolerance, various lactose-free commercial formulas with high caloric and protein densities and low osmolalities are available. When steatorrhea is a problem, those formulas with more of the fat in the form of medium-chain triglycerides might be better tolerated. Supplemental formulas are described in Appendix Table 33. Table 26–4 gives the general nutritional care required for patients who have dumping syndrome after gastric surgery. However, each diet must be adjusted to suit the patient, based on a careful dietary and social history.

Carcinoma of the Stomach

Malignant neoplasms of the stomach can lead to malnutrition as a result of excessive blood and protein losses, or, more commonly, obstruction and mechanical interference with food intake. Most cancers of the stomach are treated by surgical resection; thus, the nutritional considerations are similar to those encountered in partial or total gastrectomy.

The etiology of carcinoma of the stomach is unknown (see Chapter 36). Symptoms are slow to manifest themselves, and the growth of the tumor is rapid so that frequently carcinoma of the stomach is overlooked until it is too late for an effective cure. Loss of appetite, loss of strength, and loss of weight frequently precede other symptoms. *Achylia gastrica* (absence of hydrochloric acid and pepsinogen) or *achlorhydria* has been shown to exist for years preceding the onset of gastric carcinoma.

Nutritional Care

The dietary regimen for carcinoma of the stomach is determined by the location of the cancer, the nature of the functional disturbance, and the stage of the disease. The patient with advanced, nonoperable cancer should receive a diet adjusted to provide comfort. Anorexia is almost always present from the early stages. Any food preferences, unless definitely harmful, are granted, and living should be made as comfortable as possible. In the later stages of the disease the patient may tolerate only a liquid diet, and it may be necessary to resort to parenteral nutrition. As long as other therapeutic procedures such as surgery, radiation therapy, or chemotherapy are being performed, the nutritional support for the patient should be equally aggressive. See Chapter 36 for a discussion of nutritional care during cancer treatment.

TABLE 26–4. Nutritional Care for Dumping Syndrome and Alimentary Hypoglycemia

Dumping Syndrome

High-protein, moderate-fat, high-calorie diet adequate for weight maintenance near IBW.* About 1.5–2 g protein per kg of IBW and 35–45 kcal/kg of IBW
Use medium-chain triglycerides if steatorrhea is present
Lie down for about an hour after eating
Avoid taking liquids with meals
Avoid those foods known to cause individual problems
Eat small meals

Alimentary Hypoglycemia

Avoid concentrated sweets such as candy, sugar, cola drinks, cookies, cakes, and ice cream unless made with sugar substitutes
Have concentrated forms of sugar available only for treatment of hypoglycemia if it occurs
Eat small meals six times each day

* IBW = ideal body weight.

GASTRIC AND DUODENAL ULCERS

A peptic ulcer is an eroded lesion in either the gastric or duodenal mucosa resulting from a variety of causes, many of which are still undefined (Fig. 26–4). Gastric ulcers occur with less frequency and are more likely to be associated with malignancy and mortality. Although duodenal ulcers are significantly more common, their incidence has decreased dramatically during the last 30 years. The same is not true for gastric ulcer disease, however, reflecting the difference in their pathogenesis. Although duodenal ulcers have in the past been primarily a disease that occurs in men, they now occur with equal prevalence in both men and women (Mulholland and Debas, 1987).

Pathogenesis of Ulcer Disease

The mucosa of the stomach and duodenum is normally protected from proteolytic action of gastric juice by the *mucosal barrier,* a coating of mucus secreted by glands located in the walls of the epithelium from the lower esophagus to the upper duodenum. The mucus contains acid-neutralizing bicarbonates, and additional bicarbonates are provided by the pancreatic juice secreted into the intestinal lumen.

Mucus production is stimulated by the action of prostaglandins. Hydrochloric acid is secreted by the chief cells in response to stimuli by acetylcholine, gastrin, and histamine.

The process of gastric digestion exposes ingested foods to pepsin and hydrochloric acid and delivers them in the form of a highly acidic liquid chyme via the pylorus into the proximal duodenum. Arrival of the acid prompts rapid secretion of pancreatic juice that contains a high level of bicarbonate and also inhibits gastric secretion and peristalsis to afford the pancreatic secretion time to reach the duodenum and act on the chyme.

Peptic ulcer results when neural and hormonal abnormalities disrupt the factors that normally maintain mucosal integrity and permit proteolytic and acidic erosion of the mucosal tissue. Most gastric ulcers occur in the lesser curve of the antrum of the stomach. Duo-

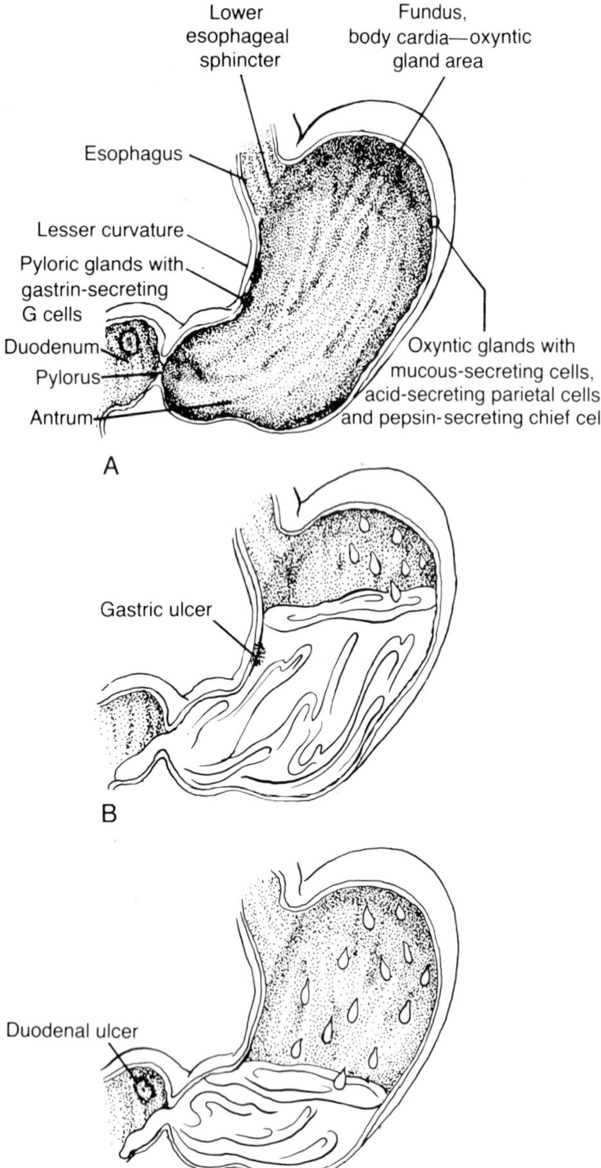

FIGURE 26–4. *Diagram showing* A, *the stomach and duodenum with eroded lesions;* B, *gastric ulcer; and* C, *duodenal ulcer.*

denal ulcers occur in a 3-cm space within the duodenal bulb in an area immediately below the pylorus where the gastric juices are not yet fully neutralized (see Fig. 26–4).

Although a chronic ulcer usually follows a typical course and produces characteristic symptoms, hemorrhage or perforation may occasionally be the first sign of the illness. Ulcers can perforate into the peritoneal cavity or penetrate into an adjacent organ (usually the pancreas), or they may erode an artery and cause a massive hemorrhage.

Etiology

A peptic ulcer is associated with a variety of genetically mediated factors such as hyperpepsinemia and increased parietal cell mass. From 20 to 50% of patients with duodenal ulcers have a family history of the disease. However, the tendency to develop either duodenal or gastric ulcers is unrelated; those with a family history of one type rarely develop the other.

Gastric Ulcer

A gastric ulcer appears to be caused by factors that disrupt the mucosal barrier, permitting hydrogen ions to diffuse into the mucosal tissue where they cause damage that leads eventually to cell destruction and subsequent ulceration. A major cause of this disruption is thought to be a defect in the pyloric sphincter that permits reflux of the duodenal contents into the antrum of the stomach, where the detergent effect of bile salts reduces mucosal resistance.

NSAID dramatically increase the risk of ulcers in those taking them. It appears that this is related to the systemic inhibition of prostaglandin production by NSAID and the resulting impaired defense against acidity by the gastric mucosa. (Soll, 1990) (Fig. 26–5).

Another major pathogenetic factor appears to be antral gastritis from *H. pylori* infection and the resulting impaired mucosal defense, leaving it vulnerable to ulceration (Soll, 1990) (see Fig. 26–5).

Gastric ulcers are not associated with excessive acid; in fact, the rate of acid secretion is normal or even low.

Duodenal Ulcer

Among the causes of duodenal ulcer are factors that either (1) increase acid secretion, (2) increase gastric emptying rates, or (3) reduce the ability of the duodenum to handle an acid load. However, these circumstances are seen in only one third of patients with duodenal ulcers, indicating that other abnormalities are involved (Isenberg et al, 1987).

Patients with duodenal ulcers frequently secrete more total acid, secrete more acid in the basal or resting state, and exhibit a more prolonged acid response to a meal (Mulholland and Debas, 1987). However, two thirds of patients with duodenal ulcers have normal acid levels. Some show less production of bicarbonate in the basal state (Isenberg et al, 1987).

The number of parietal cells in patients with duodenal ulcers is twice that seen in normal people (Mulholland and Debas, 1987). Increased secretory stimuli to the parietal cells by the secretogogues gastrin, histamine, and acetylcholine and increased sensitivity to these stimuli can further increase acid secretion. Acetylcholine is released in response to stimulation of the

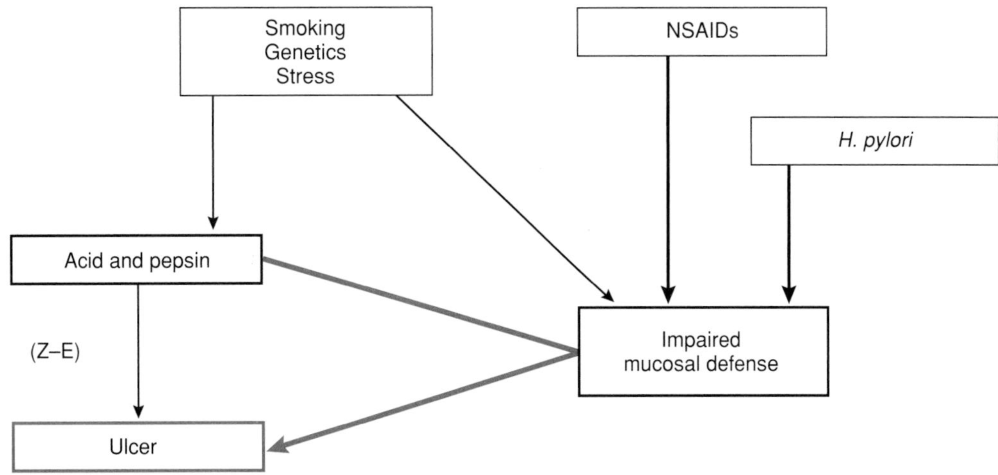

FIGURE 26–5. *A model of the pathogenesis of peptic ulcer. Acid and peptic activity overpower mucosal defense to produce ulcers most commonly when mucosal defense is impaired by exogenous factors. Two factors, nonsteroidal anti-inflammatory drugs (NSAID) and* H. pylori *infection, appear to be linked to the impairment of mucosal defense. The hypersecretion of gastric acid in the Zollinger-Ellison syndrome (Z-E) is one exception in which ulcers occur in the absence of* H. pylori *infection. In ordinary peptic ulcer disease, other risk factors are also important (smoking, genetic factors, and psychologic stress), but the evidence is conflicting about whether these factors impair mucosal defense, modulate the secretion of acid, or both. (From Soll AH: Pathogenesis of peptic ulcer and implications for therapy. N Engl J Med 322:909, 1990.)*

vagus nerve. Thus, emotional stress, particularly prolonged anxiety, is capable of initiating or aggravating ulcer disease by stimulating the vagus nerve to release increased amounts of acetylcholine (Peters and Richardson, 1983).

Failure to neutralize acid chyme in the duodenum can result from excessively rapid delivery of acid chyme without allowing the duodenum time to produce adequate buffer or from abnormalities in bicarbonate synthesis and delivery. Pancreatic output of bicarbonate is inhibited by smoking (nicotine) and by defective synthesis of prostaglandins that mediate bicarbonate secretion.

Excesses of NSAID and corticosteroids are also associated with increased risk of ulcer development (Katz et al, 1987). The pathogenetic factors in peptic ulcer disease are summarized in Table 26–5.

Management

The objectives of treatment are relief of pain, healing of the ulcer, and prevention of recurrence. Although different in etiology, gastric and duodenal ulcers are very similar in their response to therapy.

Medical Therapy

Medical treatment of peptic ulcer is directed toward (1) neutralization of acids, (2) reduction of acid secretion by the stomach, and (3) preservation of epithelial resistance to the destructive action of gastric juice. Therapy thus consists of antacids, antisecretory drugs and cytoprotective agents, limited dietary modifications, and avoidance of stressful situations. Diet therapy will probably always be secondary to drug therapy.

ANTACIDS. Antacids have long been clinically effective in reducing the pain and in encouraging the healing of peptic ulcer. It is unknown how much of the effectiveness of antacids is due to a well-recognized placebo effect and how much is due to acid neutralization or other mechanisms. Studies have shown that aluminum antacids exert a cytoprotective effect by stimulating

TABLE 26–5. Pathogenetic Factors in the Development of Peptic Ulcer Disease*

Gastric Ulcer	Duodenal Ulcer
Abnormal pyloric function	Increased acid secretory capacity
Duodenogastric reflux	Increased basal acid secretion
Defective gastric mucosal defenses	Increased parietal cell mass and sensitivity
Decreased mucosal blood flow	Prolonged meal secretory response
Decreased mucosal prostaglandin production, resulting in decreased mucosal bicarbonate production	Abnormal gastric emptying
	Abnormal duodenal mucosal defenses
	Decreased bicarbonate secretion
Decreased mucous gel layer	
Helicobacter pylori infection	

* Adapted from Mulholland MW and Debas HT: Chronic duodenal and gastric ulcer. Surg Clin North Am 67:489, 1987.

the release of mucosal prostaglandins (Holt and Hollander, 1986).

The acid-neutralizing capability of antacids varies widely. The preferred medications contain aluminum hydroxide, which has good acid-neutralizing ability and is not absorbed from the gut. However, aluminum hydroxide also binds phosphorus and prevents its absorption, which could result in a lowered serum phosphate level and phosphate-depletion syndrome that is accompanied by an extensive loss of calcium. Calcium carbonate preparations are better, despite the propensity of calcium to stimulate gastrin secretion. Magnesium is frequently added to antacid mixtures to prevent constipation. To extend their buffering effect, antacids should be taken 1 and 3 hours after meals.

OTHER DRUGS. Cimetidine (Tagamet) is an H_2 blocker that blocks acid secretion by preventing the binding of histamine to the H_2 receptors on the parietal cell surface. This drug is highly effective and is used widely in treatment of peptic ulcer disease. Many patients continue on maintenance cimetidine therapy for years to prevent the recurrence of an ulcer. The drug should not be taken simultaneously with antacids containing aluminum hydroxide, which binds with the drug and inhibits absorption. Because it may decrease B_{12} absorption, the status of this vitamin should be monitored.

Ranitidine, another H_2 blocker, also reduces gastric acid secretion. Because it does not have as many side effects as cimetidine, it is often used in patients with hepatic or renal insufficiency.

Colloidal bismuth, which has been used for decades to treat peptic ulcers, in fact also helps to eradicate *H. pylori.* However, in conjunction with an antibiotic such as tinidazole, the effect on *H. pylori* eradication is even better.

Cytoprotective agents protect the gastroduodenal mucosa from injury and promote healing without decreasing acid secretion. These medications include synthetic prostaglandins, sucralfate, arachidonic and linoleic acids (precursors of prostaglandins), gastrointestinal peptides, carbenoxolone, and sulfhydryl drugs (Holt and Hollander, 1986) (Table 26–6). Sucralsulfate protects the mucosa by forming a viscous coating over the ulcer crater. Of interest in this respect is milk, traditionally a treatment for peptic ulcer disease that more recently has fallen out of favor, which has been found to contain the prostaglandin PGE_2, a protective agent against stress-induced ulcers in rats (Materia et al, 1984).

Nutritional Care

Nutritional care aims at reduction and neutralization of stomach acid secretion, maintenance of acid resistance of gastrointestinal epithelial tissue, limitation of patient discomfort, and restoration of good nutritional status.

TABLE 26–6. Some Drugs Used in the Treatment of Peptic Ulcer Disease

Antacids	Neutralize gastric activity
Cimetidine and ranitidine	Histamine H_2 receptor antagonists; inhibit gastric acid secretion
Prostaglandins	Methyl derivatives of PGE_2; have "cytoprotective" properties
Sucralfate	Sulfated disaccharide; coats and protects ulcer base; may increase mucosal resistance
Colloidal bismuth	Coats and protects ulcer base, may increase mucosal resistance
Carbenoxolone	Licorice extract; strengthens mucosal barrier to H^+ back diffusion; may cause hypertension
Tinidazole	Antibiotic to eradicate *H. pylori*

REDUCTION AND NEUTRALIZATION OF STOMACH ACID SECRETION. Sight, smell and taste, water, and practically anything that is taken into the stomach will stimulate gastric secretions to some degree. Foods and antacids act as buffers, and the immediate effect is to lower gastric acidity. When acidity gets too low, however, a feedback mechanism in the stomach stimulates further secretion.

Beer, milk, and coffee (either regular or decaffeinated) are stimulants of gastric acid secretion. Caffeine does not appear to stimulate gastric acid secretion (McArthur et al, 1982). Factors that increase or decrease gastric acidity are listed in Table 26–3.

Protein foods buffer gastric secretions, but their buffering action is only temporary. As the products of protein digestion (amino acids and polypeptides) reach the antrum, they stimulate the secretion of gastrin and thus the secretion of gastric acid.

Fat also inhibits gastric secretion. However, the dairy fats traditionally recommended to the patient with an ulcer do not appear to be any more effective than other animal fats, vegetable oils, or foods fried in vegetable oil.

The pH of a food prior to ingestion has little therapeutic importance except for patients with lesions of the mouth or the esophagus. Most foods are considerably less acidic than the normal gastric pH of 1.6. The pH of both orange juice and grapefruit is 3.2 to 3.6. Thus on the basis of their immediate acidity, acid fruit juices should be acceptable components of the diet for patients with ulcers. However, if they are not well tolerated, they should be avoided.

FOODS THAT DAMAGE GASTROINTESTINAL MUCOSA. The knowledge of dietary factors that cause epithelial irritation and injury is limited. Neither foods that are chemically, mechanically, or thermally irritating to the mucosa nor those that are soothing have been determined with any degree of accuracy. Alcohol is known to damage the gastric mucosa independent of the acidity of the stomach contents (Tarnawski et al, 1985). Thus it is reasonable to recommend that it be avoided by patients with peptic ulcer disease, especially in concentrated amounts (40% or 80-proof).

Administration of red or black pepper directly into an empty stomach can cause superficial damage to the gastrointestinal mucosa and increased gastric acid secretion (Meyers et al, 1987). Many individuals who are not accustomed to eating spicy foods routinely report increased peptic discomfort after eating them. However, there is also evidence that even condiments such as chilies and chili powder, when taken with food, do not influence the symptoms and healing of duodenal ulcer as much as was previously thought (Kumar et al, 1984).

Patients with ulcers frequently have gas after eating particular foods. The numerous factors that influence flatulence are discussed in Chapter 27.

Diet and Eating Pattern Recommendations. Peptic ulcer disease has a long history of management by diet therapy. However, a variety of studies have failed to demonstrate that modifications of the diet either increase the healing rate or prevent a recurrence (Hollander, 1988; Lennard-Jones and Barbouris, 1965). Avoidance of certain foods sometimes diminishes discomfort, but this is a highly individual matter. Most patients prefer a little discomfort to the alternative of a very rigid diet without freedom of choice. However, there are always a few anxious patients who need a strict diet plan for emotional and psychologic reasons.

Modern dietary management of the patient who has an ulcer focuses on the individual rather than on the diet and concentrates on normal nutritional needs rather than on a special regimen (Fig. 26–6). Whether or not a food will be tolerated is best determined by trial. Patients usually avoid any food that they know from experience causes indigestion, pain, or other digestive symptoms. Regular meals with appropriate timing of antacid intake (1 and 3 hours after meals) are important. Foods should be divided into at least three meals a day; the once popular six small feedings are no longer required, because studies have found little difference in gastric acid secretion between a three- or six-meal pattern (Table 26–7).

Traditional diet therapy for peptic ulcer featured the *Sippy Diet,* which is now seldom followed. It consisted of hourly feedings of milk and cream, followed by a gradual progression to a "bland diet" that was followed for a considerable period. This diet featured six small feedings, elimination of fresh fruits and vegetables, whole-grain cereals and breads and spicy foods, and frequent ingestion of milk. Studies demonstrating that such a regimen does not hasten ulcer healing have made it possible to abandon the recommendation of this dietary program that is inadequate in fiber and many nutrients, and disturbingly high in saturated fat and cholesterol.

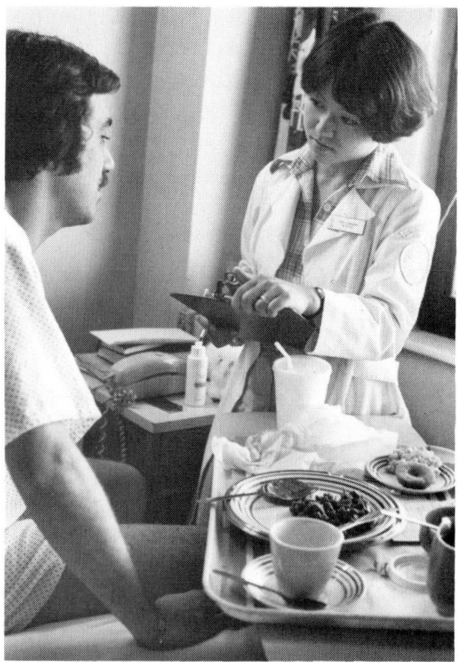

FIGURE 26–6. *Clinical dietitian and peptic ulcer patient discussing problem foods and individualizing a diet plan. (Courtesy of the nutrition staff of Lutheran General Hospital, Park Ridge, IL.)*

Surgery

Peptic ulcer is primarily a medical disease, but surgery is advised when the ulcer is complicated by hemorrhage, perforation, obstruction, or intractability or when the patient is unable to follow the medical regimen. Recurrences of ulcers are common after both medical and surgical treatment.

Vagal denervation decreases cholinergic stimulation of parietal cells and reduces cellular response to stimulants such as gastrin. A parietal cell vagotomy affects only the area of gastric acid secretion. As the antrum

TABLE 26–7. Principles of Nutritional Care for Peptic Ulcer Disease

The patient with peptic ulcer disease should:

1. Eat three regular meals daily.
2. Eat small meals to avoid stomach distention.
3. Avoid drinking coffee (decaffeinated and regular) and alcohol.
4. Cut down on or quit smoking cigarettes.
5. Avoid using large amounts of aspirin, other NSAID, or other drugs known to damage the stomach lining.
6. Avoid foods or drinks that cause discomfort.
7. Eat meals in as relaxed an atmosphere as possible.
8. Take antacids 1 and 3 hours after meals and before bedtime.

and pylorus remain innervated, gastric emptying can proceed normally. However, because the surgery is difficult and time-consuming, patients at high risk for operative morbidity and mortality would not be candidates for this procedure. A truncal vagotomy with pyloroplasty would probably be used in these circumstances. The truncal vagotomy not only interrupts innervation of the gastric parietal cells but also results in antral and pyloric dysfunction and poor peristalsis. Incorporating pyloroplasty or gastrojejunostomy permits adequate gastric emptying; however, the postoperative side effects of dumping, diarrhea, and weight loss still occur at a rate of approximately 6%. Surgery for gastric ulcer consists of removing the ulcerated area, usually by a partial gastric resection. Postoperative nutritional care is the same as that following gastric surgery.

CITED REFERENCES

Drumm B et al: Association of *Campylobacter pylori* on the gastric mucosa with antral gastritis in children. N Engl J Med 316:1557, 1987.

Hollander D: Diet therapy of peptic ulcer disease. Nutr MD 14(2):1, 1988.

Holt KM and Hollander D: Acute gastric mucosal injury: Pathogenesis and therapy. Annu Rev Med 37:107, 1986.

Isenberg JI et al: Impaired proximal duodenal mucosal bicarbonate secretion in patients with duodenal ulcer. N Engl J Med 316:374, 1987.

Katz LA, Maher E, and Horvath PJ: Primary prevention of gastrointestinal diseases. J Clin Gastroenterol 9:12, 1987.

Kumar N et al: Do chillies influence healing of duodenal ulcer? Br Med J 288:1803, 1984.

Lawrence W: Effects of cancer on nutrition: Impaired organ system effects. Cancer 43:2020, 1979.

Lennard-Jones JE and Barbouris N: Effect of different foods on the acidity of the gastric contents in patients with duodenal ulcer. Gut 6:113, 1965.

Materia A et al: Prostaglandin in commercial milk preparations. Arch Surg 119:290, 1984.

McArthur K, Hogan D, and Isenberg JI: Relative stimulatory effects of commonly ingested beverages on gastric acid secretion in humans. Gastroenterology 83:199, 1982.

Meyers BM et al: Effect of red pepper and black pepper on the stomach. Am J Gastroenterol 82:211, 1987.

Mulholland MW and Debas HT: Chronic duodenal and gastric ulcer. Surg Clin North Am 67:489, 1987.

Peters M and Richardson C: Stressful life events, acid hypersecretion and ulcer disease. Gastroenterology 84:114, 1983.

Sontag S et al: Cimetidine, cigarette smoking and recurrence of duodenal ulcer. N Engl J Med 311:689, 1984.

Tarnawski A et al: Prostaglandin protection of the gastric mucosa against alcohol injury—a dynamic time-related process. Gastroenterology 88:334, 1985.

ADDITIONAL REFERENCES

Arora A and Sharma MP: Use of banana in non-ulcer dyspepsia (Letter). Lancet 335:612, 1990.

Clark CS et al: Gastroesophageal reflux induced by exercise in healthy volunteers. JAMA 261:3599, 1989.

Dial EJ and Lichtenberger LM: A role for milk phospholipid in protection against gastric acid. Gastroenterology 87:379, 1984.

Graham DY, Smith JL, and Opekun AR: Spicy food and the stomach: Evaluation by videoendoscopy. JAMA 260:3473, 1988.

Orlando RC: Peptic ulcer: Factors influencing recurrence. J Clin Gastroenterol 9 (Suppl):2, 1987.

Schirmer BD and Jones RS: Peptic ulcer disease. Invest Radiol 22:437, 1987.

Soll AH: Pathogenesis of peptic ulcer and implications for therapy. N Engl J Med 322:909, 1990.

Tolstoi LG and Fosmire G: Milk-alkali syndrome revisited: A review of 63 years. Nutr Today 22(2):22, 1987.

CHAPTER 27

NUTRITIONAL CARE IN INTESTINAL DISEASE

CHAPTER OUTLINE

KEY TERMS

BLIND LOOP SYNDROME—a disorder of bacterial overgrowth with resultant malabsorption resulting from alterations in the anatomy of the small intestine in which a loop is disconnected from the main stream

COLOSTOMY—surgical creation of an opening into the colon to permit defecation

CONSTIPATION—a condition in which the frequency or quantity of defecation is reduced

CROHN'S DISEASE (REGIONAL ENTERITIS)—a chronic granulomatous inflammatory disease of unknown etiology involving the small or large intestine with scarring and thickening of the bowel wall

DIARRHEA—abnormal frequency and liquidity of stools

DIVERTICULITIS—inflammation of diverticulas

DIVERTICULOSIS—presence of diverticulas that are herniations of the mucous membrane through the muscular layers of the colonic wall

FISTULA—an abnormal passage between two internal organs or from an internal organ to the surface of the body

FLATULENCE—the presence of excessive amounts of gas in the gastrointestinal tract

FLATUS—gas in the gastrointestinal tract expelled through the anus

GLUTEN-SENSITIVE ENTEROPATHY (CELIAC DISEASE)—a malabsorption syndrome precipitated by the ingestion of gliadin-containing foods and characterized by a flattening of the villi of the small intestine

HIGH-FIBER DIET—a diet that contributes 25 to 50 g/day of dietary fiber

ILEOSTOMY—surgical creation of an opening into the ileum through a stoma in the abdominal wall

INFLAMMATORY BOWEL DISEASE—a general term for inflammatory diseases of the bowel of unknown etiology, including Crohn's disease and ulcerative colitis

IRRITABLE BOWEL SYNDROME (IBS)—an abnormal stooling pattern associated with symptoms of intestinal dysfunction that persists for longer than 3 months

LACTOSE INTOLERANCE—an inability to digest lactose to galactose and glucose because of a deficiency of the enzyme lactase

MEDIUM-CHAIN TRIGLYCERIDES—triacylglycerols with fatty acids of 8 to 12 carbons in length that are short enough to be absorbed directly into the portal blood

MINIMAL-RESIDUE DIET—a diet that excludes not only as much dietary fiber as possible but also foods such as milk, milk products, and connective tissue of meat that contribute to fecal residue

RESIDUE—the undigested portion of the diet that contributes to the content of the feces; includes undigested dietary fiber as well as other unabsorbed dietary constituents

SHORT-BOWEL SYNDROME—any of the malabsorption conditions resulting from massive resection of the small bowel; characterized by diarrhea, steatorrhea, and malnutrition

STEATORRHEA—excessive amounts of fat in the feces, as seen in malabsorption syndromes

ULCERATIVE COLITIS—chronic, recurrent ulceration of the mucosa and submucosa in the colon

The small and large intestines serve as organs of digestion, absorption, and excretion. Digestion is initiated in the mouth and stomach and continues in the duodenum and jejunum with the aid of secretions from the liver, pancreas, and small intestine. Absorption occurs primarily in the jejunum; the only substances absorbed in the terminal ileum are fats, bile salts, and vitamin B_{12}. The large intestine, or colon, exists for the purpose of absorbing water and excreting the fecal mass. (Digestion and absorption are discussed in detail in Chapter 1.)

PRINCIPLES OF NUTRITIONAL CARE

Many intestinal disorders involve problems of motility, absorption, and secretion and occur in the absence of recognizable pathologic conditions. Although exacerbation and remission of these disorders might be expected to reflect changes in the diet, actually it is only rarely that specific foods can be incriminated.

Dietary modifications in disorders of the intestinal tract are designed to alleviate symptoms, correct nutritional deficiencies, and, when possible, address the primary cause of difficulty. In diseased states, treatment involves attention to the primary injury of the intestinal mucosa and the secondary conditions arising as a consequence. Increased intakes of energy, protein, vitamins, minerals, and electrolytes are frequently required to replace nutrients lost as a result of impaired digestive and absorptive capacity. Consistency of the diet may also be an important factor.

Nutritional care for all patients with diseases of the intestines must be *individualized;* the principles presented here are only guidelines.

Fiber, Roughage, and Residue

Dietary fiber is defined as the portion of food that is not capable of being digested by enzymes in the human digestive tract. Although the terms "fiber" and "roughage" are sometimes used synonymously, fiber is the preferred term and includes both water-soluble and water-insoluble fractions. (See Chapter 3 for further discussion of fiber.)

Dietary fiber originates in fruits, vegetables, or cereal grains. Bran, primarily from wheat, is the most effective of the insoluble fibers in absorbing water to form soft bulky stools. Soluble fiber in fruits, vegetables, legumes, and oats forms a soft gel that slows passage of food through the intestinal tract and delays or inhibits absorption of dietary factors such as glucose and cholesterol.

Residue is the portion of the diet that contributes to the content of the feces. It includes undigested dietary fiber as well as other unabsorbed dietary constituents. Minerals such as iron and calcium, undigested starches and sugars (especially lactose), and tough meat with gristle contribute to the bulk of stools (American Dietetic Association, 1988). Sloughed gastrointestinal cells and intestinal bacteria make up a large part of the residue. Up to one half of the fecal solids accompanying typical Western diets consists of bacteria (Cummings, 1984).

Modified Fiber Diets

Restricted Fiber Diet

The restricted fiber diet outlined in Table 27–1 is used when a reduction in fecal output is necessary or when the gastrointestinal tract is blocked, as occurs after acute episodes of inflammatory bowel disease (IBD). It is often used during transition from a minimal-residue diet to a general diet. The diet contains a minimum of indigestible carbohydrates or about 10 to 15 g/day of fiber. This is achieved by avoidance of whole-grain products, cereals, nuts, seeds, and legumes and limitation of fruits and vegetables to those without skins, hulls, or seeds.

High-Fiber Diet

The high-fiber diet presented in Table 27–2 provides 30 to 60 grams of dietary fiber (see also Table 3–5). Depending on food selections, the high-fiber diet can be nutritionally adequate.

The goal of the high-fiber diet is to achieve a daily intake of at least 25 to 50 g of dietary fiber. Because most Americans consume 10 to 30 g/day of fiber, a doubling of the current intake is a reasonable goal. More than 50 g/day does not appear to improve bowel function further (Pemberton et al, 1988).

The addition of wheat or cereal bran is essential in reaching a high-fiber intake. Fiber is not destroyed by cooking, although the structure may be changed. Consumption of eight 8-oz glasses (2 quarts) of water daily is recommended to facilitate effectiveness of the high-fiber levels. Fecal impaction has been known to occur when high intakes of bran are not accompanied by sufficient fluid to soften the stool.

TABLE 27–1. Restricted Fiber Diet* †

1. Avoid all whole-grain breads, cereals, bran, and products made with these foods.
2. Avoid seeds, peanuts, other nuts, popcorn, legumes, and coconut.
3. Use only fruits and vegetables without skins, hulls, seeds, or fibrous portion.

See Appendix Table 2 and Table 3–5 for the fiber content of foods.

* Adapted from Pemberton CM et al: Mayo Clinic Diet Manual: A Handbook of Dietary Practices, 6th ed. Philadelphia, BC Decker, 1988, p 146.

† Provides less than 25 g/day of dietary fiber (usually approximately 10 to 15 g/day).

TABLE 27–2. High-Fiber Diet*

1. Include ¼ to ½ cup of wheat bran daily.
2. Increase consumption of whole-grain breads, cereals, flours, and other whole-grain products.
3. Increase consumption of vegetables and fruits, especially those with edible skins, seeds, and hulls.
4. Choose enough servings from the food groups described in Table 3–5 to provide at least 25 grams of dietary fiber.
5. Increase consumption of water to 2 quarts (64 oz) daily.

* Provides 25 to 50 g/day of dietary fiber.

At the initiation of a high-fiber diet there may be unpleasant side effects, such as flatulence and borborygmus (intestinal rumbling), cramps, or diarrhea. Gradual increase of fiber intake helps to alleviate these symptoms. Fluid intake should also be increased at the same time. Gastrointestinal disturbances associated with initial fiber ingestion usually subside within 24 to 48 hours. The high-fiber diet is most effective after several months of compliance.

Very large fiber intakes may lead to colon obstruction, but this is unusual and is most likely to occur with fiber supplements rather than with whole foods. The effect on mineral balance of a high-fiber diet does not appear to be a problem unless cereal intakes are high and mineral intakes are low (Kelsay, 1987).

Minimal-Residue Diet

The minimal-residue diet furnishes only about 8 g/day of dietary fiber and excludes not only foods of moderate- to high-fiber content but also the nonfiber foods—milk, milk products, and connective tissue of meat—that are believed to contribute to fecal residue (Joint Committee on Dieting, 1961; Watts et al, 1963) (Table 27–3). The diet is nutritionally inadequate and is intended for short-term use only. If used on a long-term basis, it should be supplemented with a low-residue formula, parenteral nutrition, or a multiple vitamin/mineral supplement. The diet is usually implemented during acute exacerbations of IBD, diverticulitis, periods of partial bowel obstruction, or before or after bowel surgery. Reducing fecal volume allows the bowel to rest, yet it is still exposed to food and the patient is able to eat.

The lowest-residue diet is a liquid low-residue formula that can be nutritionally complete if taken in large enough volume (see Table 30–2).

TABLE 27–3. Minimal Residue Diet*†

1. Avoid all whole-grain breads, cereals, bran, and products made with these foods.
2. Avoid seeds, peanuts, other nuts, popcorn, legumes, potatoes, and coconut.
3. Avoid whole fruits and vegetables, and use only vegetable and fruit juices. Do not use prune juice.
4. Avoid meat and shellfish with tough connective tissue.
5. Limit the use of milk, milk products, and foods that contain milk to 2 cups or less each day.

* Adapted from Pemberton CM et al: Mayo Clinic Diet Manual: A Handbook of Dietary Practices, 6th ed. Philadelphia, BC Decker, 1988, p 147.
† Provides less than 8 g/day of dietary fiber.

COMMON SYMPTOMS OF INTESTINAL DYSFUNCTION

Flatulence

Intestinal flatus consists primarily of N_2, O_2, CO_2, H_2, and CH_4 (methane). The normal intestine processes 7 to 10 liters of gas each day, most of which is reabsorbed into the blood. Only around 600 ml of gas are expelled, much of it insensibly, at a rate of less than 100 ml/hr. When this amount is exceeded, people frequently complain of "excessive gas." Generally, more gas is not being formed, but increased intestinal motility is causing it to be passed through the colon too rapidly to allow for normal absorption through the mucosal wall.

Excessive gas may also be the result of *aerophagia,* which is the swallowing of air while eating or drinking. However, most of this gas is *eructed* (belched) from the stomach, and only small amounts make their way as far as the colon. High N_2 and O_2 concentrations in rectal gas, both substances present in the atmosphere in large quantities, result from aerophagia. Aerophagia can be avoided by eating slowly, chewing with the mouth closed, and refraining from drinking through straws.

Although production of gas by bacterial fermentation in the colon is a normal occurrence, excessive gas may sometimes be produced from indigestible dietary residues. High amounts of H_2 and O_2 in rectal gas indicate excessive bacterial fermentation and suggest malabsorption of a fermentable substrate such as lactose. If an enzyme deficiency is the problem, the offending carbohydrates should be decreased or omitted from the diet.

The widely recognized propensity of dried beans to produce flatus has been traced to the presence of specific indigestible carbohydrates, namely stachyose and raffinose. Little research data are available regarding other so-called gas-forming foods. Possible offenders are listed in Table 27–4. Response to these foods varies widely, and trial periods of omitting individual items should be evaluated before any foods are eliminated from the diet.

Constipation

Definitions of constipation, such as "the infrequent and difficult passage of stool," tend to be highly subjective. One objective assessment defines constipation as a condition in which: (1) fewer than three stools per

TABLE 27–4. Possible Gas-Forming Foods

Vegetables	
Beans, kidney	Onions
Beans, lima	Peas, split or black-eyed
Beans, navy	Peppers, green
Broccoli	Pimentos
Brussels sprouts	Radishes
Cabbage	Rutabagas
Cauliflower	Sauerkraut
Corn	Scallions
Cucumbers	Shallots
Kohlrabi	Soybeans
Leeks	Turnips
Lentils	
Fruit	
Apples (raw)	Cantaloupe
Apple juice	Honeydew melon
Avocados	Watermelon

week are passed while a person is eating a high-residue diet, (2) more than 3 days go by without the passage of a stool, or (3) stools passed in 1 day total less than 35 grams (Devroede, 1989).

Defecation normally occurs 25 to 72 hours or more after the intake of food. Under normal conditions, the residue of food eaten one morning reaches the large bowel (but not the rectum) during the following morning. Many people who believe that it is necessary to have a daily bowel movement become disturbed when this does not occur, and may try to compensate by purging with cathartics. Evacuations every second or third day, or three evacuations in 1 day, are all within the range of normal.

Etiology

The most common causes of constipation are poor elimination habits, such as repeated lack of response to the urge for defecation and failure to establish a regular time for defecation, a lack of fiber in the diet, insufficient fluid intake, and loss of tone in the intestinal musculature. Chronic overuse of laxatives, nervous strain, and worry are common causes. Personality and behavior factors may also be involved (Tucker et al, 1981). Chronic constipation may also result from a variety of organic disorders as outlined in Table 27–5.

Treatment

Constipation is treated by developing regularity of habit through a bowel-training program and by establishing good health habits: regular meals, adequate diet providing ample fiber, regular time for elimination, rest, relaxation, adequate intake of fluids, and exercise. Patients with a laxative habit should substitute progressively milder products with an eventual goal of complete withdrawal.

Nutritional Care

An essential part of treatment for patients with constipation is the provision of a normal diet that is high in both soluble and insoluble fiber. Diets that are low in fiber result in prolonged transit time through the gut, permitting excessive water absorption and the formation of hardened stools.

The primary effect of dietary fiber on bowel function has been attributed to its water-holding capacity, which presumably led to an increase in stool bulk and caused a stretching effect on the colon, stimulating the urge to defecate. However, it now appears that the stimulatory effect is derived from the volatile short-chain fatty acids produced from fiber by the action of colonic bacteria.

The daily diet should contain at least 25 grams of dietary fiber, which can be supplied by including ample amounts of fruits, vegetables, and whole grains. Table 27–2 describes a high-fiber diet, and Appendix Table 2 lists the dietary fiber content of foods.

Wheat bran is particularly effective for promoting bulk formation and for relieving constipation. However, it should be used in moderation and should be increased gradually from 1 teaspoon/day to 4 to 6 tablespoons/day, accompanying this amount with extra intakes of water (64 oz/day).

High-fiber diets should not be used indiscriminately. When obstructive constipation continues, even with increased or large-fiber intakes, other factors such as a motility disorder or a tumor should be suspected.

TABLE 27–5. Causes of Constipation

Systemic
- Side effect of medication
- Metabolic and endocrine abnormalities, such as hypothyroidism, uremia, and hypercalcemia
- Lack of exercise
- Ignoring the urge to defecate
- Vascular disease of the large bowel
- Systemic neuromuscular disease leading to deficiency of voluntary muscles
- Poor diet low in fiber
- Pregnancy

Gastrointestinal
- Diseases of upper gastrointestinal tract
  - Celiac sprue
  - Duodenal ulcer
  - Gastric cancer
  - Cystic fibrosis
- Diseases of the large bowel that result in:
  - Failure of propulsion along the colon (colonic inertia)
  - Failure of passage through anorectal structures (outlet obstruction)
- Irritable bowel syndrome
- Anal fissures or hemorrhoids
- Laxative abuse

Laxatives

It is sometimes necessary to treat resistant constipation, as well as hemorrhoids, with substances that promote regular evacuation of soft stools. Bulking agents such as cellulose, hemicellulose derivatives, and psyllium seed are the most acceptable for this purpose. Stool softeners such as Colace are also used. Prunes and prune juice contain *dihydroxyphenyl isatin,* a chemical that stimulates intestinal motility by pharmacologic means.

Mineral oil, particularly when taken after meals, has been thought to interfere with the absorption of carotene and the fat-soluble vitamins A, D, and K. This belief is not supported by more recent evidence (Ballantine et al, 1986), although there may be some reduction in serum carotene (Clark et al, 1987).

Diarrhea

Diarrhea is characterized by the frequent evacuation of liquid stools, accompanied by the excessive loss of fluid and electrolytes — especially sodium and potassium. It occurs when excessively rapid transit of intestinal contents through the small intestine interferes with enzymatic digestion and deprives fluids and nutrients of the opportunity for complete absorption. Diarrhea also results from changes in the lumen or mucosa of the small and large intestines.

Classification and Etiology

Osmotic diarrheas are caused by the presence in the intestinal tract of osmotically active solutes that are poorly absorbed. Examples include the diarrheas accompanying the dumping syndrome and following lactose ingestion in the presence of a lactase deficiency.

Secretory diarrheas are the result of active secretion of electrolytes and water by the intestinal epithelium. Acute secretory diarrheas are caused by bacterial exotoxins, viruses, and increased intestinal hormone secretion. Unlike osmotic diarrheas, secretory diarrheas are not relieved by fasting.

Exudative diarrheas are always associated with mucosal damage, which leads to an outpouring of mucus, blood, and plasma proteins with a net accumulation of electrolytes and water in the gut. Prostaglandin release may be involved. The diarrheas of chronic ulcerative colitis and radiation enteritis are exudative.

Limited mucosal contact diarrheas result from situations of inadequate mixing of chyme and inadequate exposure of chyme to intestinal epithelium. These include the diarrhea of Crohn's disease and that following extensive bowel resection. This type of diarrhea is usually complicated by steatorrhea resulting from bacterial overgrowth and by reduced luminal concentrations of conjugated bile acids.

Nutritional Care

Because diarrhea is a symptom of a disease state, the aim of medical treatment is to remove the cause. The next priority is management of fluid and electrolyte replacement, and finally attention to nutrition concerns.

Losses of electrolytes, especially of potassium and sodium, should be corrected early by using oral glucose electrolyte solutions with added potassium. With intractable diarrhea, especially in an infant or young child, parenteral feeding is usually required. Parenteral nutrition may even be necessary if exploratory surgery is anticipated or if the patient is not expected to resume full oral intake in 5 to 7 days (see Chapter 30).

ADULTS. Besides bowel rest, the nutritional care for adults includes the replacement of lost fluids and electrolytes by increasing the oral intake of fluids, particularly those high in sodium and potassium, such as bouillon and fruit juices. Pectin is valuable in controlling diarrhea, and scraped raw apple or liberal amounts of applesauce may be given every 2 to 4 hours as tolerated.

When the diarrhea stops and the patient begins to tolerate food, the amounts given should be increased gradually as accepted, beginning with low-fiber foods (e.g., refined starches) and following with protein foods. Fat should be encouraged and should not be limited. Because the activity of the enzyme lactase may be decreased during gastroenteritis, it is wise to avoid lactose at first.

If the diarrhea becomes chronic, it may be accompanied by a number of nutritional deficiencies. Besides possible impaired absorption, heavy losses of electrolytes, vitamins, minerals, and protein occur and should be replaced. The loss of potassium alters bowel motility, encourages anorexia, and can introduce a cycle of bowel distress. Loss of iron from gastrointestinal bleeding may be severe enough to cause anemia. The nutritional deficiencies themselves cause mucosal changes, such as decreased villi height and reduced enzyme secretion, further leading to the malabsorption.

After the diarrhea begins to lessen, the addition of more fiber to the diet may be effective, because a larger stool bulk helps to restore normal bowel motility.

INFANTS AND CHILDREN. Acute diarrhea is most dangerous in infants and small children who can easily become dehydrated by the large fluid losses. In these cases, replacement of fluid and electrolytes must be aggressive and immediate. A solution of glucose and electrolytes in water has been the most effective, but sucrose can be used in place of glucose if necessary. An oral rehydration solution recommended by the World Health Organization is given in Table 27-6. Solutions containing sodium at levels between 50 and 90 mEq/l

TABLE 27–6. Oral Rehydration Solution—Composition and Recipe

Composition	
Glucose (g/100 ml)	2
Sodium (mEq/l)	90
Potassium (mEq/l)	20
Chloride (mEq/l)	80
Bicarbonate (mEq/l)	30
Osmolarity (mOsm/l)	330
Recipe	
To 1 liter of water add:	
3.5 g sodium chloride	
2.5 g sodium bicarbonate	
1.5 g potassium chloride	
20.0 g glucose	
The solution should be made up fresh every 24 hours	

From: The rehydration treatment of acute diarrhea with inexpensive oral fluids. Clin Pediatr 15:1095, 1976.

can also be effective and safe (Santosham et al, 1982). Even during acute diarrhea, the intestine can absorb up to 60% of the food eaten, and because fasting has been shown to further reduce the ability of the small intestine to absorb nutrients, the bowel should not be "rested" by omitting oral intake (Behrman et al, 1987). Folate supplementation may be useful for acute diarrhea, possibly because of its acceleration of the normal regeneration of damaged mucosal epithelial cells (Haffejee, 1988).

Steatorrhea

Steatorrhea is a consequence of malabsorption in which unabsorbed fat remains in the stool. In contrast to the 2 to 5 grams of ingested fat that normally is excreted each day, as much as 60 grams may be lost with this condition. With the exception of specific carbohydrate intolerances, almost all diseases causing malabsorption cause steatorrhea. Diagnosis is usually based on a ratio of fecal fat to ingested fat or a coefficient of absorption. A 72-hour stool is collected and analyzed for fat at the same time that a record of food intake is kept and analyzed for fat content. A diet containing 100 grams of fat is usually suggested.

Excessive fat excretion may result from (1) failure of proper digestion, such as in pancreatitis or as a consequence of gastric resection; (2) bile salt deficiency, such as in diseases of the liver and biliary tract system, blind loop syndrome, or ileal resection; (3) failure of normal absorption due to mucosal damage, such as in sprue and regional enteritis and after gastrointestinal radiation therapy; and (4) decreased fat re-esterification and decreased formation and transport of chylomicrons, which are seen in abetalipoproteinemia and intestinal lymphangiectasia. Table 27–7 lists diseases associated with malabsorption.

Nutritional Care

Because steatorrhea is a symptom and not a disease, the underlying cause of malabsorption must be determined and treated. The presence of weight loss requires an increased energy intake. Dietary protein and carbohydrate should be high, and carbohydrates and fats should be added as tolerated to meet individual needs. Multiple vitamin and mineral deficiencies necessitate supplemental therapy, with special emphasis on fat-soluble vitamins, calcium, zinc, magnesium, and iron.

MEDIUM-CHAIN TRIGLYCERIDES. Inadequate energy intake resulting from faulty digestion and absorption of fat may be alleviated by the use of *medium-chain triglycerides (MCT).* These synthetic fats are made up of fatty acids with lengths of 8 and 10 carbon atoms, compared with the 16 and 18 carbons common to most of the fatty acids that constitute dietary triglycerides. For this reason, MCT are hydrolyzed more rapidly and can rely on the small amount of intestinal lipase rather than on pancreatic lipase for digestion. The products of hydrolysis are easily dispersed and absorbed in the absence of bile acids, often the cause of fat malabsorption. Short-chain fatty acids and medium-chain fatty acids

TABLE 27–7. Diseases and Conditions Associated With Malabsorption

- Inadequate digestion
  - Pancreatic insufficiency
  - Gastric acid hypersecretion
  - Gastric resection
- Altered bile salt metabolism with impaired micelle formation
  - Hepatobiliary disease
  - Interrupted enterohepatic circulation of bile salts
  - Bacterial overgrowth
  - Drugs that precipitate bile salts
- Abnormalities of mucosal cell transport
  - Biochemical or genetic abnormalities
    - Disaccharidase deficiency
    - Monosaccharide malabsorption
    - Specific disorders of amino acid malabsorption
    - Abetalipoproteinemia
    - Vitamin B_{12} malabsorption
    - Celiac sprue
  - Inflammatory or infiltrative disorders
    - Regional enteritis
    - Ulcerative colitis
    - Amyloidosis
    - Scleroderma
    - Tropical sprue
    - Gastrointestinal allergy
    - Infectious enteritis
    - Whipple's disease
    - Intestinal lymphoma
    - Radiation enteritis
    - Drug-induced enteritis
  - Endocrine and metabolic disorders
  - Short bowel syndrome
- Abnormalities of intestinal lymphatics and vascular system
  - Intestinal lymphangiectasia
  - Mesenteric vascular insufficiency
  - Chronic congestive heart failure

are able to enter the portal venous blood for direct transport to the liver without being resynthesized into triglycerides.

MCT are available in some enteral formulas and also as MCT oil (8.3 kcal/g; 1 T = 116 kcal). Because MCT are not very palatable, most patients cannot tolerate more than 50 ml/day (equivalent to 418 kcal). MCT oil can be used as a substitute for fat in some recipes.

DISEASES OF THE SMALL INTESTINE

Celiac Sprue (Gluten-Sensitive Enteropathy)

Celiac sprue, often called *gluten-sensitive enteropathy, celiac disease, nontropical sprue,* or *adult celiac disease,* is a disease caused by a reaction to *gliadin,* the alcohol-soluble component of *gluten.* The resulting damage to the villi of the intestinal mucosa results in potential or actual malabsorption of virtually all nutrients.

The mechanism by which gliadin damages the small bowel is unknown, but it appears that both genetic and immune components are involved (Cole and Kagnoff, 1985; Ferguson et al, 1984). It is suggested that a receptor on the surface of the intestinal cell allows gliadin, or a specific amino acid sequence of gliadin, to bind to the enterocyte. This gliadin/receptor complex then becomes an immunogen capable of sensitizing T lymphocytes, which then release lymphokines that directly damage the cell (McClave, 1988).

The disease primarily affects the mucosa of the small intestine. Atrophy and flattening of the villi severely limit the area available for nutrient absorption (Fig. 27–1). The amount of small intestine compromised varies, but the proximal bowel is usually the most severely involved. Cells of the villi become deficient in disaccharidases and peptidases needed for digestion and also in the carriers needed for the transport of nutrients into the blood stream. Decreased cholecystokinin release diminishes gallbladder and pancreatic secretions, further contributing to maldigestion. Extraintestinal manifestations are listed in Table 27–8.

The diagnostic procedure consists of mucosal biopsy followed by a gluten-free diet, rebiopsy to note intestinal villi improvement, and finally a gluten challenge followed by another biopsy 6 weeks later. One-hour blood xylose or 5-hour urinary xylose tests are not as accurate in diagnosing the disease and should not be used. Determination of serum levels of IgG antigliadin and IgA antigliadin antibodies is becoming more useful along with serum folate and carotene in assessment of gastrointestinal absorption (Shanahan and Weinstein, 1988).

Institution of a gliadin-free diet reverses the process, and the intestinal mucosa reverts toward normal; however, some patients may require months or even years for maximal recovery. Gliadin must be avoided for life.

A form of celiac sprue called *refractory sprue* does not respond to the removal of gliadin or responds only temporarily. Many of these patients respond to prednisone.

The skin disorder *dermatitis herpetiformis* is associated with a mild mucosal lesion like that of celiac sprue. Evidence suggests that this disorder is also gluten-dependent and improves with gliadin withdrawal (Leonard et al, 1983). However, it takes several months to 2 years of a gluten-free diet to produce a normal-appearing skin. The diet must be followed for life.

Symptoms

Depending on the extent of small-intestine involvement, symptoms can range from devastating and life-threatening malabsorption to refractory iron deficiency anemia or evidence of osteomalacia due to malabsorption. The disease may first become apparent when an infant begins eating gliadin-containing cereals, or it may not appear until middle age when it is unmasked by gastrointestinal surgery, stress, pregnancy, or viral infection.

The most common symptoms in children 6 months to 3 years of age are diarrhea, growth failure, projectile vomiting, a bloated abdomen, and stools that are abnormal in appearance, odor, and quantity. Stool frequencies vary but can be in excess of 10 stools/day. Adults may have increased appetite, weight loss, weakness, and fatigue, or they may present with hematologic abnormalities. Diarrhea may or may not be present. Bowel movements usually are large, putty colored, and foul-smelling, with stools that tend to float because of steatorrhea (Pare et al, 1988).

Nutritional Care

Complete withdrawal of gliadin from the diet results in prompt clinical improvement. During the first few weeks of gliadin omission, the diet should be supplemented with vitamins, minerals, and extra protein to remedy deficiencies and replenish nutrient stores.

A *gliadin-free diet* omits the glutamine-bound fraction (glutenin and gliadin) of protein (Table 27–9). In this diet, wheat, rye, barley, and oats are excluded. Buckwheat, millet, amaranth, and quinoa are also excluded because of a lack of reliable information about their glutamine content. Products that can be used as substitutes are those made from corn, potato, rice, soybean, tapioca, and arrowroot. Table 27–10 provides suggestions for incorporating these substitutions into recipes.

A guarantee of a gliadin-free diet requires careful scrutiny of the labels of all bakery products and pack-

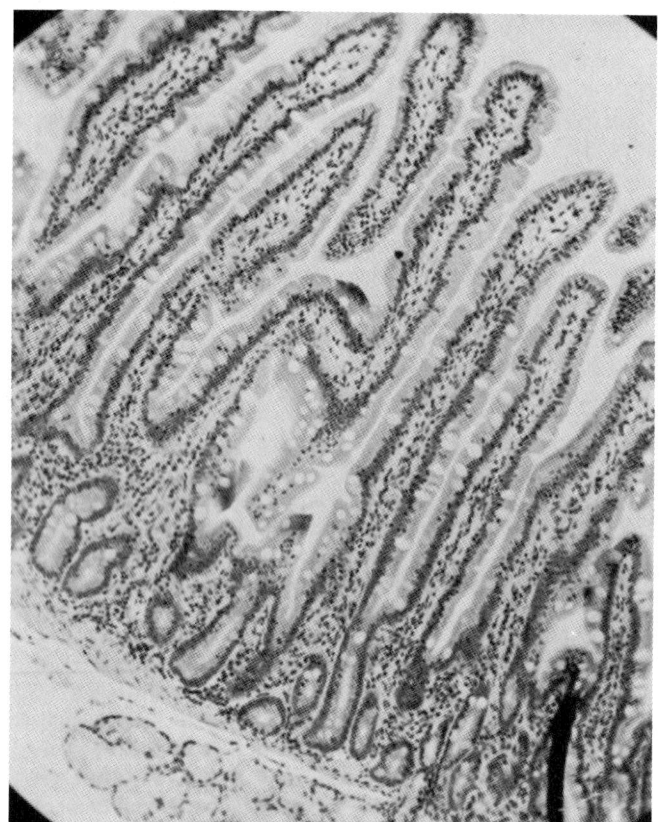

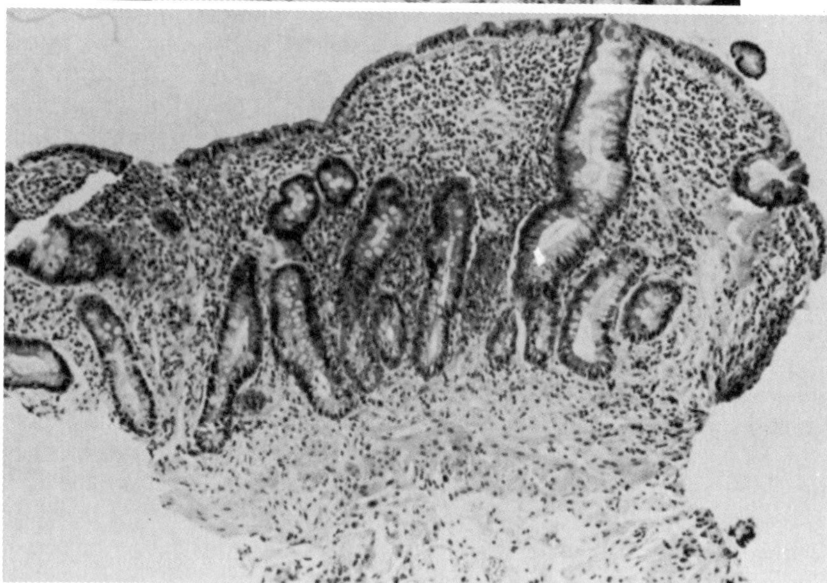

FIGURE 27-1. A, *Low-power photomicrograph (× 100) of a normal human duodenal mucosa. Note the long, thin villi.* B, *Low-power photomicrograph (× 100) of a peroral small-bowel biopsy specimen from a patient with gluten enteropathy. Note the complete loss of villi and the heavy infiltrate of white blood cells in the lamina propria. (From Floch MH: Nutrition and Diet Therapy in Gastrointestinal Disease. New York, Plenum Medical Book Co, 1981.)*

aged foods. Gliadin-containing grains may be not only a basic ingredient but may also be added during processing or preparation. Hydrolyzed vegetable protein, for example, may be made from wheat, soy, corn, or mixtures of these grains (Table 27-11).

Freedom from symptoms after eating gliadin does not necessarily mean that the villi are undamaged. The precipitating condition usually continues to exist, and gliadin causes mucosal changes within hours. However, symptoms may take 8 weeks or more to reappear. It has been observed that adults who go on and off a gliadin-free diet a number of times may eventually reach a state at which they do not respond to the diet. Complications of chronic ulcerative jejunoileitis or malignancy may develop. It is not known whether lifelong adherence to a gluten-free diet reduces the risk of developing malignancy, but it appears that it does (Holmes et al, 1989).

A lactose intolerance sometimes appears secondary

TABLE 27–8. Extraintestinal Manifestations of Celiac Sprue

Organ System	Manifestation	Probable Cause
Hematopoietic	Anemia	Iron, folate, vitamin B_{12} or B_6 deficiency
	Hemorrhage Purpura	Hypoprothrombinemia usually due to impaired intestinal absorption of vitamin K
Skeletal	Osteomalacia	Impaired absorption of vitamin D
	Osteoporosis Bone pain	Formation of insoluble calcium soaps by fatty acids in the intestinal lumen and thus defective calcium transport and absorption
Muscular	Paresthesias Muscle cramps Tetany	Calcium depletion or magnesium depletion due to poor absorption
	Weakness	Hypokalemia due to potassium loss
Neurological	Peripheral neuropathy	Deficiencies of vitamins such as thiamin and vitamin B_{12}
Endocrine	Secondary hyperparathyroidism	Calcium and vitamin D malabsorption causing hypocalcemia
	Secondary hypopituitarism	Malnutrition due to malabsorption
	Adrenocortical insufficiency	Hypopituitarism
Integumentary	Follicular hyperkeratosis	Vitamin A deficiency
	Petechiae and ecchymoses	Hypoprothrombinemia

TABLE 27–9. Gluten-Restricted Gliadin-Free Diet*

(Wheat, Rye, Oat, and Barley Free)

This diet is designed to provide adequate nutrition while eliminating wheat, rye, oats, and barley from the diet.

Gluten may be present in foods either as a basic ingredient (that is, listed as wheat, rye, oats, or barley) or added as a derivative when a food is processed or prepared. Thus, *reading labels carefully is very important.*

Since flour and cereal products are quite often used in the preparation of foods, it is important to be aware of the methods of preparation used as well as the foods themselves. This is especially true when dining out.

Food Group With Recommended Daily Intake	Foods Allowed	Foods to Avoid
Milk: 2 or more cups	Fresh, dry, evaporated or condensed milk; cream; sour cream,† whipping cream; yogurt†	Malted milk; some commercial chocolate drinks; some non-dairy creamers‡
Meat, fish, poultry: 2 or more servings	All kinds of fresh meats, fish, other seafood, poultry; fish canned in oil or brine; some prepared meat products, such as hot dogs‡ and lunch meats‡	Prepared meats that contain wheat, rye, oats or barley, such as some sausages,‡ hot dogs,‡ bologna,‡ luncheon meats,‡ chili con carne,‡ sandwich spreads‡; bread-containing products, such as: Swiss steak, croquettes; meat loaf; tuna canned in vegetable broth,‡ and turkey with hydrolyzed vegetable protein injected as part of the basting solution
Cheeses (can be used for meat and milk groups)	All aged cheeses, such as cheddar, swiss, edam, parmesan; cottage cheese,† cream cheese,† pasteurized processed cheese† ‡	Any cheese product containing oat gum as an ingredient
Eggs	Plain or in cooking	Eggs in sauce made from gluten-containing ingredients (e.g., a regular, wheat-based white sauce)
Potato or other starch: 1 or more servings Aproten, Aglutella, Ener-G	White and sweet potatoes, yams; hominy; rice; wild rice; special gluten-free noodles[a,b]; some oriental rice and bean noodles	Regular noodles; spaghetti; macaroni; most packaged rice mixes‡
Vegetables: 2 or more servings	Use all plain, fresh, frozen or canned vegetables; dried peas and beans; lentils; some commercially prepared vegetables‡	Creamed vegetables‡; vegetables canned in sauce‡; some canned baked beans‡; commercially prepared vegetables and salads‡
Fruits: 2 or more servings	All fresh, frozen, canned or dried fruits; all fruit juices; some canned pie fillings	Thickened or prepared fruits; some pie fillings‡
Breads: 3 or more servings	Specially prepared breads using only allowed flours; commercially available brands[a,b]	All others containing wheat, rye, oat, or barley flour

Table continued on the following page

TABLE 27–9. **Gluten-Restricted Gliadin-Free Diet** *Continued*

Food Group With Recommended Daily Intake	Foods Allowed	Foods to Avoid
Cereals: 1 or more servings of enriched cereal	Hot cereals made from cornmeal, cream of rice, hominy, rice; cold cereals as follows: Puffed Rice, Kellogg's Sugar Pops; Post's Fruity and Chocolate Pebbles, special cereals[a,b]	All others containing wheat, rye, oats or barley; bran, graham; wheat germ; malt; kaska; bulgar; buckwheat§; millet§, amaranth Q
Flours and thickening agents		Wheat starch (manufacturer states it contains gluten); all flours containing wheat, rye, oats, or barley
Good thickening agents	Arrowroot starch, cornstarch, tapioca starch	
Good when combined with other flours	Corn flour, cornmeal, potato flour, potato starch flour, rice bran, rice flours (plain, brown, sweet), rice polish, soy flour	
Best combined with milk and eggs in baked product	Corn flour, cornmeal, potato flour, potato starch flour, rice flours (plain, brown, sweet), rice polish, soy flour	
Grainy textured products	Corn flour, cornmeal, sweet rice flour	
Drier product than with other flours	Potato flour, potato starch flour, plain and brown rice flours	
Moister product than with other flours	Sweet rice flour	
Adds distinct flavor to product: use with moderation	Rice polish, soy flour	
Crackers and snack foods Special commercial manufacturers[a,b]	Rice wafers‡; pure cornmeal tortillas; popcorn, some crackers‡ and chips‡	All others containing wheat, rye, oats, or barley
Fats	Butter; margarine; vegetable oil; nuts; peanut butters; hydrogenated vegetable oils; some salad dressings‡; mayonnaise‡	Some commercial salad dressings‡
Soups	Homemade broth and soups made with allowed ingredients; some commercially canned soups‡	Most canned soups‡ and soup mixes‡; bouillon
Desserts	Cakes, quick breads, pastries, puddings prepared with allowed ingredients; cornstarch, tapioca, and rice puddings; gelatin desserts; custard; vanilla and coffee-flavored ice cream from: Arden, Carnation, Darigold, Foremost, Lucerne‡; some pudding mixes§; special commercial products[a,b,c]	Commercial cakes, cookies, pies, etc, made with wheat, rye, oats, or barley; prepared mixes‡; ice cream cones; pudding‡
Beverages	Instant and ground coffee; instant tea; tea; carbonated beverages‡; pure cocoa powder; wines; rums; some root beers‡; vodka distilled from grapes or potatoes	Ovaltine; malted milk; ale; beer; gin; whiskies‖; vodka distilled from grain; herbal teas containing malted barley or other gliadin-containing grains.
Sweets	Jelly; jam; honey; brown and white sugar; molasses; most syrups‡; some candy‡; chocolate; pure cocoa; coconut	Some commercial candies‡
Miscellaneous	Salt; pepper; herbs; extracts; food coloring; cloves; ginger; nutmeg; cinnamon; chili powder; tomato purée and paste; olives; pickles; rice, cider and wine vinegar; yeast; bicarbonate of soda; baking powder; cream of tartar; dry mustard; some other condiments‡; monosodium glutamate (MSG) derived from nongliadin sources.	Some curry powder‡; some dry seasoning mixes‡; some gravy extracts‡; some meat sauces‡; some catsup‡; some mustard‡; horseradish‡; some soy sauce‡; chip dips‡; some chewing gum‡; distilled white vinegar‖

* Diet developed by Elaine I. Hartsook, Ph.D., R.D. Director, Gluten Intolerance Group of N. America, former member, National Digestive Disease Advisory Board, Advisor, National Digestive Diseases Information Clearinghouse National Institutes of Health, Public Health Service, US Department of Health and Human Services.

† Check vegetable gum used.

‡ Product ingredients should be investigated.

§ Although botanically different from other gluten-containing grains, additional information is needed before this can be cleared.

‖ Distilled white vinegar uses grain as a starting material. Whiskies, including "corn whisky," use wheat, rye, oats, or barley in their mash. Gliadin-intolerant persons are advised to use rice, cider or wine vinegar in food preparations, such as making salad dressings, pickles, and in cooking. Avoid all whiskies.

[a] Dietary Specialties, Inc., P.O. Box 227, Rochester, NY 14601.

[b] Ener-G Foods, Inc., P.O. Box 84487, Seattle, WA 98124-5787.

[c] Red Mill Farms, Inc., 290 So. 5th St., Brooklyn, NY 11211.

Commercially prepared pickles, ketchup, mustard, mayonnaise, steak sauce, and other condiments are usually made with distilled grain vinegar. The maximum amount of gliadin that would be present in such products via the vinegar is probably insignificant.

TABLE 27–10. Suggestions for Substitutions for Wheat Flour in Recipes*

The following may be substituted for wheat flour in recipes:
1 cup corn flour
¾ cup coarse cornmeal
1 scant cup fine cornmeal
⅝ cup potato flour
⅞ cup rice flour
Suggestions to improve the eating quality of the final product:

1. Rice flour and cornmeal tend to have a grainy texture. A smoother texture may be obtained by mixing the rice flour or cornmeal with the liquid called for in the recipe, bringing this mixture to a boil and then cooling before adding to the other ingredients.
2. Soy flour must always be used in combination with another flour, not as the only flour in a recipe.
3. When using other than wheat flour in baking, longer and slower baking is required. This is particularly necessary when the product is made without milk and eggs.
4. When using coarse meals and flours in place of wheat flour, the amount of leavening must be increased. For each cup of coarse flour, use 2½ tsp of baking powder.
5. Muffins or biscuits, when made with other than wheat flour, are of better texture if baked in small sizes.
6. Dryness is a common characteristic of cakes made with flours other than wheat. Moisture may be preserved by (a) frosting or (b) storing in closed containers.

* From Ohlson MA: Experimental and Therapeutic Dietetics, 2nd ed. Minneapolis, Burgess Publishing Co, 1972, pp 142–143.

to the celiac sprue. A lactose-free diet in conjunction with a gliadin-free diet is useful in controlling symptoms. Once the gastrointestinal mucosa begins to heal after the omission of gliadin, the lactase usually returns and the lactose intolerance disappears. See Table 27–12 for a lactose-free diet.

If the disease has been severe, supplementation may be required. Anemia should be treated with iron, folate, or vitamin B_{12}, depending on the type. Vitamin K should be given in the presence of purpura, bleeding, or prolonged prothrombin time. Electrolyte and fluid replacement is essential in those with dehydration from severe diarrhea. Calcium and vitamin D administration may be necessary to correct osteomalacia. Vitamins A and E may be necessary to replenish stores depleted by steatorrhea. A multiple vitamin-mineral supplement should be taken regularly by those who continue to have malabsorption.

Tropical Sprue

Tropical sprue is a syndrome of unknown etiology that occurs in most tropical areas, with the exception of Africa south of the Sahara. It may be the sequela of an acute infectious diarrhea with subsequent contamination of the bowel by specific coliform bacteria. Nutritional deficiency may increase susceptibility to an infectious agent. As in celiac sprue, the intestinal villi are shortened, but the surface cell alterations are much less severe. The gastric mucosa may be atrophied and inflamed, with diminished secretion of hydrochloric acid and intrinsic factor.

Symptoms include diarrhea, anorexia, and abdominal distention as well as symptoms of nutritional deficiency, such as night blindness, glossitis, stomatitis, cheilosis, pallor, and edema. Anemia may result from iron, folic acid, and vitamin B_{12} deficiencies.

Nutritional Care

Tropical sprue responds dramatically to tetracycline and folate therapy. Folate is given as 5 mg/day orally along with intramuscular vitamin B_{12} (1,000 μg/month) and tetracycline.

TABLE 27–11. Gliadin-Containing Derivatives*

Always check the source of the following nebulous ingredients before eating any product containing them.

Ingredient (as appears on label)	Include	Avoid
"Hydrolyzed vegetable protein" (HVP)	Soy, corn	Mixtures of wheat, corn, and soya (soy)
"Flour" or "cereal products"	Rice flour, corn flour, cornmeal, potato flour, soy flour	Wheat, rye, oats, or barley
"Vegetable protein"	Soy, corn	Wheat, rye, oats, or barley
"Malt" or "malt flavoring"	Those derived from corn	Those derived from barley or barley malt syrup
"Starch"	When listed as such on an American manufacturer's ingredient list, it is *cornstarch*	
"Modified starch" or "modified food starch"	Arrowroot, corn, potato, tapioca, waxy maize, maize	Wheat starch
"Vegetable gum"	Carob bean, locust bean, cellulose gum, guar gum, gum arabic, gum acacia, gum tragacanth, xanthan gum	Oat gum
"Soy sauce" or "soy sauce solids"	Those that *do not* contain wheat, such as Chun King	Those that *contain* wheat
"Monoglycerides and diglycerides"	Those using a gliadin-free carrier.	Those that use a wheat starch carrier.

* Developed by Elaine I. Hartsook, Ph.D., R.D., Director, Gluten Intolerance Group of N. America, Seattle, Advisor, National Digestive Disease Information Clearinghouse, National Institutes of Health, Public Health Service, US Department of Health and Human Services.

These questionable ingredients must be cleared with the manufacturer before they are eaten. When writing the manufacturer, request information on the specific starting material(s) used in their nebulous ingredient. For example, when "modified food starch" appears as a labeling ingredient, ask for the specific type of starch used (i.e., potato starch, tapioca starch, etc.).

A combination of wheat, corn, and soya is primarily used as starting material for hydrolyzed vegetable protein, and thus is not allowed on a gluten-free diet. When wheat protein is "hydrolyzed," its large amino acid chains are broken down into smaller chains. Some protein researchers believe the sequence of amino acids found in these smaller chains is as toxic as the intact gliadin subfraction of the gluten protein. Thus, HVP made from wheat is not recommended for use on a gluten-free diet.

TABLE 27–12. Lactose-Free Diet*

Foods Allowed	Foods Excluded
Beverages	***Beverages***
Isomil,[a] Prosobee,[b] Pregestimil,[b] Mocha Mix,[c] meat base formulas used as milk substitutes, carbonated drinks, coffee, freeze dried coffee, fruit drinks, some instant coffees (check labels), Lidalac[d] and other lactose free milks or those treated with lactase enzymes; lactose free products such as Ensure,[a] Ensure Plus[a] Citrotrein, Nutramigen,[b] Nutri 1000 LF.[e] See Appendix Table 33. Dry or reconstituted Lacto-Free	All untreated milk of any species and all products containing milk (except lactose free milk), such as skim, dried, evaporated, or condensed milk; yogurt; cheese; ice cream; sherbet; malted milk; Ovaltine[f]; hot chocolate; some cocoas and instant coffees (read labels); powdered soft drinks with lactose curds; whey and casein milk that has been treated with lactobacilus/acidophilus culture rather than lactase, such as Nu-trish[g]
Breads and Cereals	***Breads and Cereals***
Breads and rolls made without milk, Italian bread, some cooked cereals and prepared cereals (read labels), macaroni, spaghetti, soda crackers	Prepared mixes, such as muffins, biscuits, waffles, pancakes; some dry cereals such as Total,[h] Special K,[i] and Cocoa Krispies[i] (read labels carefully); Instant Cream of Wheat[j]; commercial breads and rolls to which milk solids have been added; zwieback; French toast made with milk
Desserts	***Desserts***
Water and fruit ices; gelatin; angel food cake; homemade cakes, pies, cookies made from allowed ingredients; puddings made with water. Baked products from specialty food manufacturers[o,p,q]	Commercial cakes and cookies and mixes, custard, puddings, sherbets, ice cream made with milk; any containing chocolate, pie crust made with butter or margarine, gelatin made with carrageenan
Eggs	***Eggs***
All	Omelets and soufflés containing milk
Fats	***Fats***
Margarines and dressings that do not contain milk or milk products, oils, shortening, bacon, Rich's Whip Topping,[k] some nondairy creamers (read labels), nut butters, nuts	Margarines and dressings containing milk or milk products, butter, cream, cream cheese, peanut butter with milk solids fillers, salad dressings containing lactose
Fruits	***Fruits***
All fresh, canned, or frozen that are not processed with lactose	Any canned or frozen processed with lactose
Meat, Fish, Poultry, Etc.	***Meat, Fish, Poultry, Etc.***
Plain beef, chicken, fish, turkey, lamb, veal, pork, and ham; strained or junior meats and vegetables and meat combinations that do not contain milk or milk products; kosher frankfurters	Creamed or breaded meat, fish, or fowl; sausage products, such as wieners, liver sausage, cold cuts containing nonfat milk solids; cheese
Soups	***Soups***
Clear soups, vegetable soups, consommés, cream soups made with Mocha Mix[c] or nondairy creamers or Lact-Free[o]	Cream soups unless made with allowed ingredients, chowders, commercially prepared soups containing lactose
Vegetables	***Vegetables***
Fresh, canned, or frozen: artichokes, asparagus, broccoli, cabbage, carrots, cauliflower, celery, chard, corn, cucumber, eggplant, green beans, kale, lettuce, mustard, okra, onions, parsley, parsnips, pumpkin, rutabagas, spinach, squash, tomatoes, white and sweet potatoes, yams, lima beans, beets	Any to which lactose is added during processing; peas; creamed, breaded, or buttered vegetables; instant potatoes, corn curls, and frozen French fries if processed with lactose
Miscellaneous	***Miscellaneous***
Soy sauce, carob powder, popcorn, olives, pure sugar candy, jelly or marmalade, sugar, corn syrup, carbonated beverages, gravy made with water, baker's cocoa, pickles, pure seasonings and spices, wine, molasses, pure monosodium glutamate, instant coffees that do not contain lactose	Chewing gum; chocolate; some cocoas; toffee; peppermint; butterscotch; caramels; some instant coffees, dietetic preparations (read labels); certain antibiotics and vitamin and mineral preparations; spice blends if they contain milk products; monosodium glutamate extender; artificial sweeteners containing lactose, such as Equal,[l] Sweet n' Low,[m] Wee Cal[n]; some nondairy creamers (read labels)

* From The American Dietetic Association: Handbook of Clinical Dietetics. New Haven, Yale University Press, 1981, pp D-15–16.

[a] Ross Laboratories, Columbus, OH 43216.
[b] Mead Johnson and Co., Evansville, IN 47721.
[c] Presto Food Products, Los Angeles, CA 90021.
[d] Lidano Co., Kalunborg, Denmark.
[e] Cutter Laboratories, Berkeley, CA 94710.
[f] Ovaltine Products, Villa Park, IL 60181.
[g] Knudsen Bros., North Haven, CT 06473.
[h] General Mills, Minneapolis, MN 55435.
[i] Kellogg Co., Battle Creek, MI 49016.
[j] Nabisco, Inc., East Hanover, NJ 07936.
[k] Rich Products Corp., Buffalo, NY 14212.
[l] G.D. Searle and Co., Skokie, IL 60076.
[m] NIFDA (National Institutional Food Distributor Associates, Inc.), Atlanta, GA 30325.
[n] Domino Amstar Corporation, New York, NY 10020.
[o] Ener-G Foods, Inc., Seattle, WA 98124-5787.
[p] Red Mill Farms, Brooklyn, NY 11211.
[q] Dietary Specialties, Inc., Rochester, NY 14601.

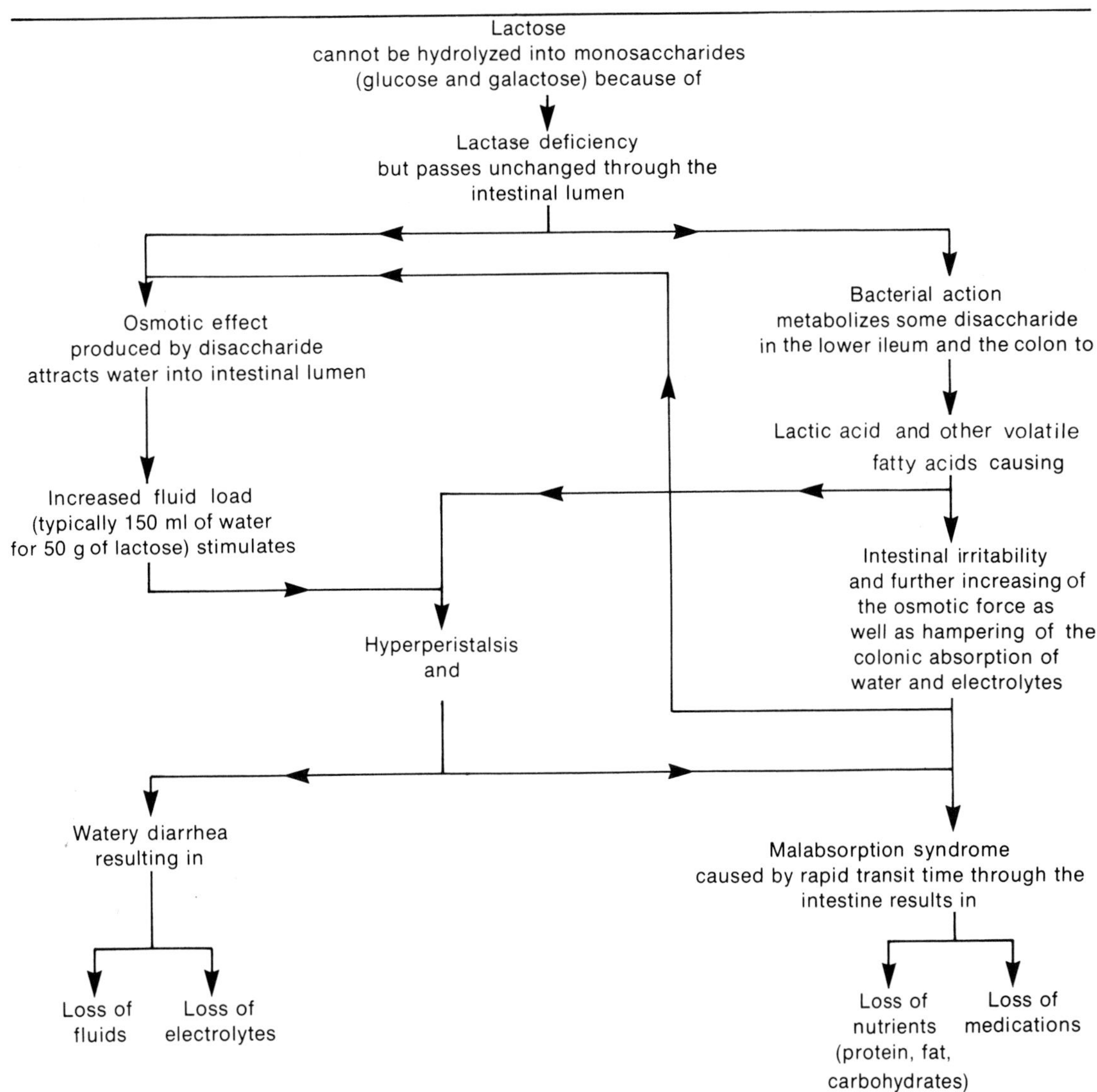

FIGURE 27–2. *Pathogenesis and clinical implications of lactose intolerance. (From Ensure Plus. Columbus, OH, Ross Laboratories, 1977, p 11.)*

Intestinal Brush Border Enzyme Deficiencies

Intestinal enzyme deficiency states involve deficiencies of the brush border disaccharidases that hydrolyze disaccharides at the mucosal cell membrane. Disaccharidase deficiencies may occur as (1) rare congenital defects, such as sucrase, isomaltase, or lactase deficiencies seen in the newborn; (2) generalized forms secondary to diseases that damage the intestinal epithelium (e.g., Crohn's disease or celiac sprue); or, most commonly, (3) a genetically acquired form (e.g., lactase deficiency) that usually appears after childhood but can appear as early as 2 years of age.

Lactase Deficiency

Intolerance to lactose is caused by a deficiency of lactase, the enzyme that digests the sugar in milk. Lactose that is not hydrolyzed into galactose and glucose remains in the gut and acts osmotically to draw water into the intestines. Bacteria ferment the undigested lactose, generating lactic acid and other organic acids, carbon dioxide, and hydrogen gas. The result is bloating, flatulence, cramps, and diarrhea (Fig. 27–2).

The condition is very prevalent in the world population, especially among blacks, Asians, and South Americans. The fact that 70% of the world's adults are unable to digest lactose has led to the proposal that lactose intolerance is the normal state, whereas lactose tolerance is the abnormal condition (Kretchmer, 1981). Although it has been suggested that the persistence of lactase is induced by the continuation of milk in the diet after weaning, there is no evidence to support this theory. More probably, the maintenance of lactase through adulthood that is common in descendants of Northern and Central European populations reflects the continuation of an ancient genetic mutation (Scrimshaw and Murray, 1988) (Further Reading, p. 468). Lactose intolerance can also develop secondary to an infection of the small intestine. Lactase activity may not return after small bowel surgery or prolonged disuse of the gastrointestinal tract, such as during total parenteral nutrition (TPN); it usually does, however, although slowly (Erickson, 1988).

Lactose deficiency is diagnosed from (1) a history of gastrointestinal symptoms that occur after milk ingestion, (2) a test for abnormal hydrogen levels in the breath, (3) an abnormal lactose tolerance test, or (4) a biopsy of the intestinal mucosa.

LACTOSE TOLERANCE TEST. The *lactose tolerance test* is based on an oral dose of lactose equivalent to the amount in 1 quart of milk (50 grams). In the presence of lactose intolerance, blood glucose increases less than 25 mg/100 ml of serum above the fasting level, and gastrointestinal symptoms may appear. In addition, there will be increased intestinal production of hydrogen, which is measured with the *breath hydrogen test.* Many patients who appear abnormal when tested have no history of intolerance to milk. These individuals appear able to tolerate smaller portions of milk in their diets but cannot accommodate the large test load of 50 grams when it is given undiluted and on an empty stomach.

NUTRITIONAL CARE. With the reduction or omission of milk and lactose-containing foods, the symptoms of lactose intolerance are alleviated. A lactose-restricted diet is described in Table 27–12. Most lactose-intolerant adults can consume some lactose without symptoms. It is presumed that in the absence of lactase, the protein, fat, vitamins, and minerals in milk are still utilized effectively. Lactose is better tolerated as part of a meal than when taken separately.

Some milk products such as aged cheese are usually well tolerated because the lactose content is low. Tolerance of yogurt may be the result of a microbial beta-galactosidase in the bacterial culture that facilitates lactose digestion in the intestine (Kolars et al, 1984; Martini et al, 1987b). This depends on the brand and processing method. Because this microbial enzyme is sensitive to freezing, frozen yogurt may not be as well tolerated (Martini et al, 1987a; Onwulata et al, 1989).

Milk and milk products treated with lactase enzyme (Lactaid) are available, as is the enzyme itself, which can be added to milk or taken orally in anticipation of a milk-containing meal. This is effective for most people (Efficacy . . . , 1988). However, *Lactobacillus acidophilus* milk is not lower in lactose and is not better

FURTHER READING: Lactose Tolerance — An Uncommon Anomaly

When lactose intolerance was first described in 1963, it appeared to be an infrequent occurrence, arising only occasionally in the Caucasian population. However, as the capacity to digest lactose was measured in people from a wide variety of ethnic and racial backgrounds, it soon became apparent that disappearance of the lactase enzyme shortly after weaning or at least during early childhood is actually the normal condition in most of the world's population. With a few exceptions, the intestinal tracts of adult mammals produce little if any lactase after weaning. (The milk of pinnipeds — seal, walrus, and sea lions — does not contain lactose.)

The exception of lactose tolerance has attracted the interest of geographers and others concerned with the evolution of the world's population. A genetic mutation favoring lactose tolerance appears to have arisen around 10,000 years ago when dairying was first introduced. It would have occurred presumably in places where milk consumption was encouraged because of some degree of dietary deprivation and in groups in which milk was not fermented prior to consumption. (Fermentation breaks down much of the lactose into monosaccharides.) The mutation would have selectively endured, because it would promote greater health, survival, and reproduction of those who carried the gene.

It is proposed that the mutation occurred in more than one location and then accompanied migrations of populations throughout the world. It continues primarily among Caucasians from northern Europe and in ethnic groups in India, Africa, and Mongolia. The highest frequency (97%) of lactose-tolerance occurs in Sweden and Denmark, suggesting an increased selective advantage in those able to tolerate lactose related to the limited exposure to ultraviolet light typical of northern latitudes. (Lactose favors calcium absorption, which is limited in the absence of vitamin D produced on skin exposure to sunlight.)

Dairying was unknown in North America until the arrival of Europeans. Thus, Native Americans and all of the non-European immigrants are among the 90% of the world's population who tolerate milk poorly, if at all. This has practical implications with respect to public feeding programs, such as school breakfasts and lunches. Fortunately, most lactose-intolerant people are able to digest milk in small to moderate amounts.

tolerated than regular milk (Newcomer et al, 1983; Savaiano et al, 1984).

The diet should be assessed for calcium, vitamin D, and riboflavin depending on the extent to which milk and milk products must be avoided, especially in children and women.

Sucrase or Alpha-Dextrinase Deficiency

Sucrose intolerance exists in the much less common circumstance of a *sucrase (alpha-dextrinase) deficiency.* Symptoms are the same as those of lactose intolerance and result from bacterial fermentation of the undigested sugar.

NUTRITIONAL CARE. A sucrose-free diet is used. This diet eliminates all table sugar and foods containing it, as well as fruits and some vegetables.

Inflammatory Bowel Disease

Etiology and Pathogenesis

Crohn's disease (regional enteritis) and ulcerative colitis are distinct forms of idiopathic inflammatory bowel disease (IBD). When an inflammatory process involves one or more lengthy segments of the small or large intestine with inflammation from the mucosa to the serosa, the disease is called *Crohn's disease.* When the inflammation is in the rectum with extension into the colon without affecting the right colon or small intestine, the disease is clearly *ulcerative colitis.* In 10 to 15% of all patients with IBD, the distinction is blurred and correct clinical diagnosis is difficult (Table 27–13). The causes of the diseases are unknown, but current theories include genetic, infectious, and immunologic factors.

IBD occurs most often in patients between the ages of 15 and 25 years, and both sexes are equally affected (Bayless, 1988; Calkins and Mendeloff, 1986). The incidence of Crohn's disease has been increasing for the past 30 years, whereas the incidence of ulcerative colitis has remained steady (Bayless, 1988). Psychologic factors are probably not primary but may be involved in flare-ups of the disease. Hepatic dysfunction associated with IBD is common.

One of the first symptoms in children may be a decrease in growth. (Children under 6 years of age appear to be resistant to Crohn's disease.) The possible causes of such failure are inadequate food intake, loss of protein into the gut lumen, fever, low-grade but chronic intestinal obstruction, malabsorption of fat and protein, and possibly secondary zinc deficiency.

TABLE 27–13. Comparison of Two Common Inflammatory Bowel Diseases*

Crohn's Disease	Ulcerative Colitis
Symptomatically similar	Symptomatically similar
Gradual insidious development of episodic diarrhea, abdominal pain, weight loss, blood, pus, or mucus in the stool	Gradual insidious development of episodic diarrhea, abdominal pain, weight loss, blood, pus, or mucus in the stool
Focal, often granulomatous inflammation in mucosal and submucosal layers in any area of the digestive tract	
Generally affects the terminal ileum and right colon, sometimes the entire bowel, rarely the entire digestive tract	Always affects the rectum, often the sigmoid and descending colon in continuity and sometimes the entire colon
Diarrhea is less common.	Diarrhea is common.
Segmental involvement is common.	Segmental involvement is rare.
Stricture formation is more common and is often a palpable mass in the lower right quadrant– thickened mucosal wall.	
Patients tend to be smokers.	Patients tend to be nonsmokers.

* From Calkins BM and Mendeloff AI: Epidemiology of inflammatory bowel disease. Epidemiol Rev 8:60, 1986.
Misclassification between the two is about 20%.

CROHN'S DISEASE. Crohn's disease is a chronic, progressive disorder. It may take a benign course and may disappear eventually, or it can become severe, with complications such as intestinal obstruction or fistula formation. When found in the small intestine, the disease is diffuse and continues to spread and damage the intestine, even after surgical resection.

Patients typically have fatigue, anorexia, variable weight loss, right lower quadrant pain or cramping, diarrhea, and fever.

ULCERATIVE COLITIS. Ulcerative colitis is a chronic inflammation and ulceration of the mucosa of the large intestine that always begins in the rectum. The intestinal musculature may also be damaged, leading to colonic dilatation *(megacolon).* It is commonly observed that individuals who develop the disease are frequently depressed, irritable, and emotionally unstable. Genetic factors may also be involved.

The disease occurs most commonly in young people aged 20 to 40 years, with a secondary peak at 50 to 60 years of age, although no age is exempt. The general characteristics are rectal bleeding, diarrhea accompanied by pain and spasm, fever, ulcerative lesions in the mucosa of the large intestine, dehydration, electrolyte imbalance, anorexia, and malnutrition. Anemia may be present as a result of blood loss. Uveitis, a feature of this disease, may bring the patient to the ophthalmologist. The inflammation can usually be suppressed by medical therapy, but in 20% of patients the colon must be removed and a colostomy, Koch or ileal pouch, and ileoanal anastomosis must be created (Bayless, 1988).

Treatment

Most important during acute periods are maintenance of fluid and electrolyte balance and the administration of an antidiarrheal agent such as salicylazosulfapyridine (sulfasalazine). Corticosteroids are given in severe cases that do not respond to other measures. Immunosuppressive agents (e.g., 6-mercaptopurine) may also be used.

Surgical removal of the diseased portion of the ileum or colon is indicated in cases of recurrent complicated IBD. The result of surgery may be an ileostomy. Emotional support is especially important, because the disease is chronic with unknown etiology and variable prognosis. Attention to cheerful surroundings and the attractive service of food, as well as efforts to inspire confidence and encouragement to eat the diet prescribed, is of primary importance to effective total therapy.

Nutritional Care

Inflammatory bowel disease easily leads to malnutrition, because of the patient's fear of eating and consequent pain and diarrhea, intolerance of certain foods, altered taste sensation, malabsorption, steatorrhea, loss of protein and blood into the gut, and use of medications that inhibit folate absorption and promote negative nitrogen balance (see Chapter 25). Therefore, restoration of good nutritional status is very important, and in some cases this alone may bring about improvement (Imes et al, 1987). Nutritional assessment is mandatory in order to determine the effectiveness of nutritional support.

During acute flare-ups of Crohn's disease, bowel rest and parenteral nutrition, along with medical treatment, can be useful, although these procedures have not been effective in ulcerative colitis (Bayless, 1988). Oral or enteral tube feeding of an elemental diet may be useful in patients who are unable to tolerate whole foods. However, the patient with IBD is usually managed on an outpatient basis, and several dietary manipulations are useful in managing symptoms and improving nutritional status.

The energy and protein content of the diet should be high (40 to 50 kcal and 1 to 1.5 grams of protein per kilogram of ideal body weight). Because the energy content is so high, frequent feedings are usually more acceptable and effective. The presence of steatorrhea necessitates a fat reduction to 25% of total kilocalories, but this also means reducing the energy content. In this situation, MCT that do not require bile for digestion are useful (see Chapter 4).

Steatorrhea promotes the loss of calcium, magnesium, and zinc from the gut so that the status of these minerals should be assessed or supplemented. Steatorrhea can also promote excessive oxalate absorption, resulting in hyperoxaluria and potential kidney stones and joint pain, thus avoidance of high oxalate foods should be recommended (see Table 35–4).

Lactase activity is usually reduced in patients with IBD, leading to lactose intolerance. It is usually not complete, thus permitting the use of some lactose daily. However, patients often improve dramatically when lactose is used in limited amounts and avoided during flare-ups.

Patients with IBD often avoid high-fiber foods because of misconceptions. Epidemiologic evidence suggests that a lack of dietary fiber may be a factor in the etiology of Crohn's disease (O'Morain, 1987). A minimal-residue diet may be helpful in acute flare-ups or when the intestinal lumen is narrowed, but long-term adherence to a low-fiber diet is probably not useful. Dietary fiber intake should be individualized, and increases should be made gradually.

Because of sulfasalazine use, loss of blood, and malabsorption, supplementation with folic acid, iron, and vitamin B_{12} may be necessary to correct anemia (Sulfasalazine . . . , 1988). Calcium and vitamin D supplements may be necessary if steatorrhea exists.

Some evidence suggests that providing a high-energy, moderate-residue diet both orally and via nasogastric tube can cause remission of the disease for as much as 9 months (Afdhal et al, 1989). With this aggressive enteral nutrition, the liver disease associated with TPN is not seen (Dolz et al, 1989).

DISEASES OF THE LARGE INTESTINE

Irritable Bowel Syndrome

Irritable bowel syndrome (IBS) is defined as an abnormal stooling pattern associated with symptoms of intestinal dysfunction that persists for longer than 3 months. It is characterized by the presence of painless diarrhea, diarrhea alternating with constipation, chronic constipation, perception of excessive flatulence, sensation of incomplete evacuation, rectal pain, and mucus in the stool (Van Ness, 1988) (Fig. 27–3). Patients usually first present in their 20s and 30s. There is no underlying pathology.

The cause of IBS is unknown, but possible mechanisms are: (1) exaggerated gastrocolic reflex, (2) abnormal colonic sensitivity to stretching, (3) psychoneurotic disorders, (4) learned illness behavior or preoccupation with bowel symptoms, and (5) dietary intolerances. Attacks are frequently associated with emotional upsets or a prolonged period of stress (Ford, 1986). Contributing causes may include excessive use of laxatives or caffeine, previous gastrointestinal illness, antibiotic therapy, and lack of regularity in sleep, rest, fluid intake, and bowel movements.

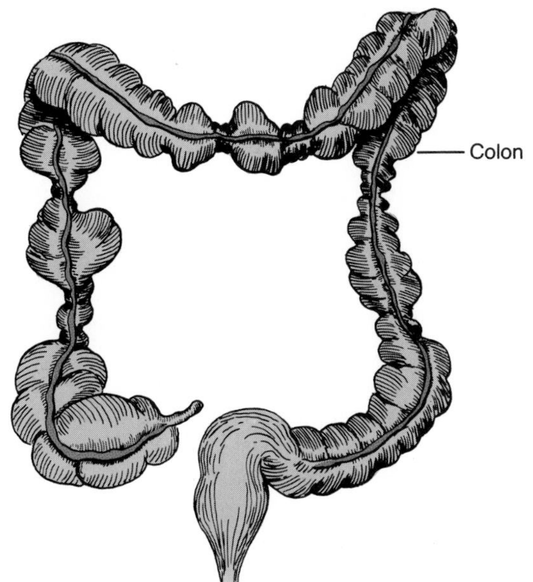

FIGURE 27–3. *Irritable bowel syndrome.*

It is important that IBS is properly diagnosed and that serious life-threatening diseases of the gastrointestinal tract (e.g., colonic carcinoma) or functional diseases are ruled out.

Nutritional Care

Persons who have IBS are frequently underweight, tense, and upset. They may be afraid to eat and are fearful of additional pain. The aim of nutritional care is to relieve the condition, nourish the patient, and bring weight back to normal. A therapeutic regimen also includes helping the patient to cope with stressful situations and to establish a healthy lifestyle.

The normal diet is recommended, with emphasis on high-fiber foods that will add bulk to the stool, thus relieving the constricting pressure and promoting normal bowel motility. When patients experience increased flatus, the amount of bran should be reduced and then slowly increased again. Twenty to 30 grams of dietary fiber is recommended (see Table 27–2). Additional fiber in the form of bulk laxatives (e.g., Metamucil or Fiberall) may also be necessary.

In patients with a strong family history of atopy, hypersensitivity to certain foods may be the cause of IBS. A trial of food elimination and challenge is probably justified under these circumstances (Zwetchkenbaum and Burakoff, 1988) (see Chapter 38).

If these measures fail to control diarrhea, then the use of anticholinergic or antidiarrheal agents may be necessary. When appropriate, psychiatric help is recommended. Biofeedback and learning techniques of relaxation and stress reduction may also be useful.

Diverticular Disease

Diverticulosis is a collection of herniations of the colonic wall. It is thought that the outpouchings result from segmentation of the colon and the resultant high intracolonic pressures as shown in Figure 27–4. These may result from a diet low in fiber. In addition, there is probably decreased strength of the colon musculature. The incidence of diverticulosis increases with aging, probably related to the gradual decrease in tensile strength of the intestinal mucosa.

Diverticulitis develops when the accumulation of fecal matter in the diverticular pockets results in infection and inflammation, sometimes causing ulceration or even perforation. Approximately 10 to 15% of patients with diverticulosis develop diverticulitis.

Nutritional Care

At one time it was thought that roughage aggravated the condition, and the classic diet therapy for diverticulosis prescribed low-roughage diets. It is now recognized that a high-fiber diet promotes soft, bulky stools that pass more swiftly, are defecated more easily, and encourage lower intracolonic pressures. Two teaspoons of bran three times daily have been found to relieve symptoms for most patients.

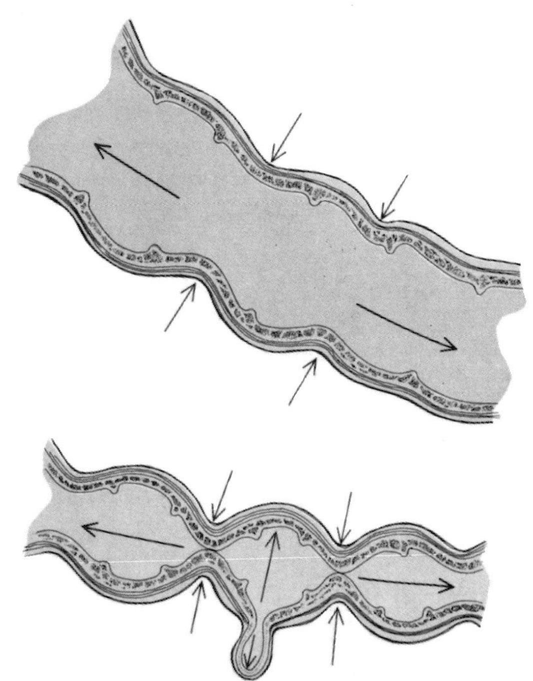

FIGURE 27–4. *Mechanism by which low-fiber, low-bulk diets might generate diverticula is shown schematically. Where colon contents are bulky* (top), *muscular contractions exert pressure longitudinally. If lumen is smaller* (bottom), *contractions can produce occlusion and exert pressure against colon wall, which may produce a diverticular "blowout."*

Patients who have followed a low-fiber diet for years may require extensive encouragement to adopt the high-fiber approach. Initially, they may have bloating or gas, but these side effects usually disappear shortly. In cases in which they cannot consume the necessary amount of bran, the bulking agents methylcellulose and psyllium have been used with good results.

For patients with an acute flare-up of diverticulitis, a low-residue or elemental diet is appropriate, followed by gradual return to a high-fiber diet.

INTESTINAL SURGERY

Small Bowel Resection — Short Bowel Syndrome

Resection of the small or large bowel is undertaken for treatment of cancer, diverticulitis, fistula, local abscess, Crohn's disease, perforation, sclerodoma, radiation enteritis, mesenteric vascular accidents, or obstruction. Removal of more than two thirds of the small bowel leads to severe metabolic problems and malnutrition. Weight loss, muscle wasting, diarrhea, rapid gastrointestinal transit time and malabsorption, diarrhea, dehydration and loss of electrolytes, and hypokalemia are common. The syndrome is commonly referred to as *short bowel syndrome.* The severity of the syndrome depends on the amount and sections of bowel remaining after surgery (Fig. 27–5). For example, a patient with an intact ileocecal valve that slows intestinal transit time can survive with less remaining bowel than if the valve has been removed. Several surgical alternatives to ensure longer transit time are being tried (Thompson and Rikkers, 1987).

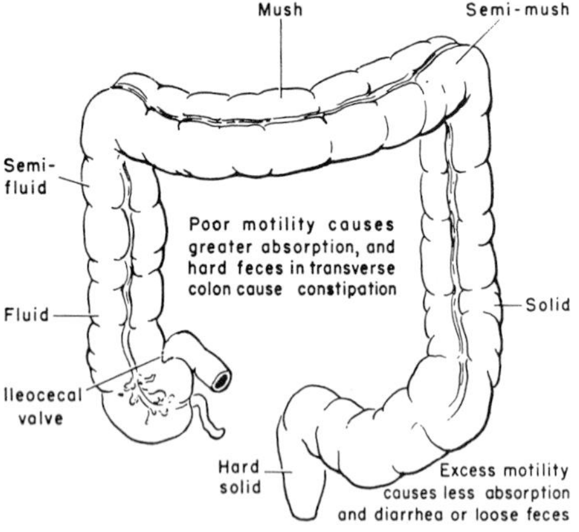

FIGURE 27–5. *As the feces move from the ileocecal valve to the anus, water is absorbed and the feces become more solid. The characteristics of the output from a colostomy depend on its location in the colon. (From Guyton AC: Textbook of Medical Physiology, 8th ed. Philadelphia, WB Saunders, 1991.)*

Effects of Decreased Intestinal Length

Absorption is decreased but gradually improves with time. Glucose and other carbohydrates are easily absorbed if adequate amounts of intestinal enzymes are present. However, carbohydrate malabsorption, particularly of lactose, is often present.

Protein nutrition is usually not a problem because protein absorption is efficient even in short lengths of otherwise normal intestine.

Fats, on the contrary, are poorly absorbed, and malabsorption may exist for some time. Besides causing steatorrhea, the unabsorbed fatty acids may saponify calcium, zinc, and magnesium in the intestine to form unabsorbable "soaps." Fat-soluble vitamins are also thought to be poorly absorbed.

The loss of ileum is more problematic than a loss of jejunum because of unique ileal functions involving vitamin B_{12} and bile salt absorption. In this case, vitamin B_{12} may have to be given as an injection or in parenteral feeding.

Other Effects

Five conditions secondary to small bowel resection also contribute to malabsorption and should be considered in planning nutritional care. (1) Hypersecretion of gastric acid occurs because the normally inhibitory small intestinal secretions are no longer present. The excessive acid injures the remaining proximal mucosa, thus reducing absorption. It also inactivates pancreatic lipase and trypsin, and the consequent maldigestion and malabsorption result in an acidic diarrheal stool. (2) Gastrointestinal motility and peristalsis are increased due to the loss of jejunal hormones cholecystokinin and secretin, which regulate bowel function. (3) Bacterial overgrowth of unknown etiology occurs in some patients. (4) Oxalate urinary stones can develop due to excessive oxalate absorption and hyperoxaluria. (5) Cholesterol gallstones can develop secondary to decreased bile salts within the enterohepatic circulation.

Adaptation of the Remaining Small Bowel

Provided that adequate nutrition is maintained both parenterally and enterally for a period of several months, the remaining small bowel increases its absorptive surface area through hyperplasia and the formation of higher villi and deeper crypts of Lieberkuhn. Nutritional support is possible with oral intake alone if at least 23 to 39 in. (60 to 100 cm) of the small bowel remains. With less than this amount, permanent parenteral nutrition will probably be required to supplement oral intake. Chapter 30 discusses permanent parenteral nutrition for patients who live at home.

Nutritional Care

In the *first stage* after surgery, nutritional support is totally by parenteral means and may be the patient's only nutritional intake for several weeks.

The *second stage* is the gradual change from parenteral to enteral nutrition. If only a small amount of intestine is available, a defined-formula liquid diet may have to be used. (See the discussion on "transitional feeding" in Chapter 30.) Lactose and sucrose may need to be avoided at first. Dilute liquid formulas are taken first and then, as the bowel adapts, the patient begins the slow return to a normal diet. Temporary setbacks will occur and will require simplification of the diet. A food not tolerated at one time should be tried again several weeks later. As the oral intake increases, parenteral nutritional support is decreased, but only to the level at which weight can be maintained. Supplements of calcium, magnesium, zinc, and iron will probably be necessary as well as supplements of the fat-soluble vitamins A, D, E, and K. Vitamin B_{12} status should also be assessed. Diarrhea and intestinal transit time are controlled with the use of antidiarrheal agents, cimetidine and sometimes cholestyramine.

Stage three defines the period within 5 months after the bowel resection, when the intestine has adapted and it is usually possible to provide the entire intake by mouth. At this point more foods are introduced into the diet. A food diary kept by the patient helps the nurse and dietitian to correlate the patient's digestive problems with possible dietary causes. Because they stimulate gastrointestinal activity, it is advisable to avoid alcohol and caffeine for at least 1 year following surgery. Six to eight small meals daily are usually better tolerated than three larger meals. Patients who do not have enough bowel adaptation to survive on enteral intake alone must resort to long-term home parenteral nutrition (see Chapter 30).

Many of these patients receive narcotics for several months postoperatively to decrease gastrointestinal motility. Requirements should decrease progressively after surgery. Excessive use manifests itself in abdominal distention, cramping, vomiting, poor dietary intake, and progressive weight loss. The situation must be differentiated from dietary intolerance and must be treated accordingly.

Blind Loop Syndrome (Bacterial Overgrowth)

Blind loop syndrome is a disorder characterized by bacterial overgrowth that results from stasis of the intestinal tract as an outcome of obstructive disease, radiation enteritis, fistula formation, or surgical repair of the intestine. Bacteria deconjugate bile salts, which besides being cytotoxic in this form are also less effective as micelle formers. Poor fat absorption and steatorrhea result. Carbohydrate malabsorption occurs because of injury to the brush border by the toxic effects of the products of bacterial catabolism and consequent enzyme loss. The expanding numbers of bacteria use available vitamin B_{12} for their own growth. Treatment is directed toward the removal of the blind loop or control of the bacterial growth with antibiotics. Use of a lactose-free diet along with MCT and parenteral vitamin B_{12} may also be useful.

Fistula Repair

A fistula is an abnormal passage between two internal organs or from an internal organ to the surface of the body. Fistulas occur as a result of prenatal developmental error or are caused by trauma or inflammatory or malignant disease processes. Fistulas of the intestinal tract can be serious threats to nutritional status, because large amounts of fluid and electrolytes are lost, and malabsorption and infection can occur. Fluid and electrolyte balance must be restored; infection must be brought under control; and aggressive nutritional support is mandatory to permit spontaneous surgical closure of the fistula and wound.

TPN or defined liquid formula diets have been used successfully (see Chapter 30). The success rate of either method depends on the location and the cause of the fistula and the overall condition of the patient.

Ileostomy or Colostomy

Patients with severe ulcerative colitis, Crohn's disease, colon cancer, or intestinal trauma frequently require the surgical creation of an opening from the body surface to the intestinal tract to permit defecation from the intact portion of the intestine. When the entire colon, rectum, and anus must be removed, an *ileostomy,* or opening into the ileum, is performed. If only the rectum and anus are removed, a *colostomy* can provide entrance to the colon. In some cases a temporary opening may be made to allow surgery and healing of more distal parts of the intestinal tract.

The opening, or stoma, eventually becomes about the size of a nickel. The output from the stoma depends on its location, as explained in Figure 27–5. The consistency of the stool from an ilestomy will be liquid, whereas that from a colostomy can range from mushy to fairly well formed. Stool from a colostomy on the left side of the colon will be firmer than that from a colostomy on the right side. Odor is a major concern of the patient with an ileostomy or colostomy; however, an ileostomy stool usually has a weakly acidic odor that is not unpleasant. A malodorous stool is usually caused by steatorrhea or by bacteria acting on particular foodstuffs to produce odorous gas. Patients learn to observe their stools to determine which foods to eliminate, and this differs with individuals. Foods tending to cause odor are corn, dried beans, onions, cabbage, highly spiced foods, fish, antibiotics, and some vitamin-mineral supplements. Persistent odor may be due to poor stoma hygiene or to an ileostomy complication that allows bacterial overgrowth in the ileum. Deodorants are available, and modern pouch appliances are odorproof. Gas production may cause the pouch to become tense and distended, and accidental dislodgment is likely. The nutritional recommendations at the beginning of this chapter for reducing flatulence may be helpful.

Ileostomy adaptation does occur, and fecal losses will lessen and stools will become firmer. This usually happens in 7 to 10 days. It does not happen to the same extent in patients who had have an ileal resection in addition to the ileostomy. Their ileal output will be about two to five times greater than that of the patient who has only an ileostomy. Patients with ileostomies need above-average intakes of salt and water to make up for excessive losses in stool. Inadequate water intake can result in small urine volumes and a proneness to renal calculi.

The patient with a normal, well-functioning ileostomy will not usually become nutritionally depleted. Those who also have an ileal resection need vitamin B_{12} supplementation. An imbalance in small bowel flora with consequent vitamin B_{12} depletion may also occur. Patients with an ileostomy often have low vitamin C intakes because of their low vegetable and fruit intakes. Ileostomates should be guided by their individual tolerance of foods, not by anecdotal reports, because many foods are probably forbidden unnecessarily (Kramer, 1987).

Because it is possible for a food bolus to get caught at the point where the ileum narrows as it enters the abdominal wall, it is important to warn the patient to avoid very fibrous vegetables and to chew all food well. Other than this, ileostomy and colostomy patients should be encouraged to follow their normal diet, omitting only particular foods known to cause them problems.

Patients with a permanent colostomy or ileostomy require considerable sympathetic understanding from the entire health team. Acceptance of the condition and the problems involved in maintaining bowel regularity is usually difficult. Plans to have these patients meet other people who have undergone similar surgery will help in making a difficult adjustment. Eventually, they are aided by the realization that in the future they will not have the multiple hospitalizations or chronic disabilities that accompanied their intestinal disease.

Rectal Surgery

Nutritional care after rectal surgery such as hemorrhoidectomy should be directed toward maintaining an intake that will allow wound repair and prevent infection of the wound by feces. The frequency of stools is minimized by the use of constipating drugs and a minimal-residue diet (see Table 27–3). Chemically defined diets are low in residue, and their use can reduce stool volume and frequency to as little as 50 grams every 6 days, making the surgical construction of a temporary colostomy unnecessary. The minimal-residue diet in Table 27–3 can be started by about the fifth day postoperatively, depending on the severity of the surgery. A normal diet is resumed after complete healing, and the patient is instructed about eating a high-fiber diet in order to avoid constipation in the future. (Table 27–2 describes a high-fiber diet.)

CITED REFERENCES

Afdhal NH et al: Remission induction in refractory Crohn's disease using a high calorie whole diet. JPEN 13:362, 1989.

American Dietetic Association: Manual of Clinical Dietetics. Chicago, The American Dietetic Association, 1988, pp 343–344.

Ballantine TVN et al: The effect of mineral oil on fat soluble vitamins. JPEN 10:18S, 1986.

Bayless TM: Ulcerative colitis. *In* Gitnick G (ed): Principles and Practice of Gastroenterology and Hepatology. New York, Elsevier, 1988.

Behrman RE, Vaughan VC, and Nelson WE (eds): Nelson Textbook of Pediatrics, 13th ed. Philadelphia, WB Saunders, 1987, p 201.

Calkins BM and Mendeloff AI: Epidemiology of inflammatory bowel disease. Epidemiol Rev 8:60, 1986.

Clark JH et al: Serum beta-carotene, retinol and alpha-tocopherol levels during mineral oil therapy for constipation. Am J Dis Child 141:1210, 1987.

Cole SG and Kagnoff MF: Celiac disease. Annu Rev Nutr 5:241, 1985.

Cummings JH: Constipation, dietary fibre and the control of large bowel function. Postgrad Med J 60:811, 1984.

Devroede G: Constipation: mechanisms and management. *In* Sleisenger MH and Fordtran JS (eds): Gastrointestinal Disease: Pathophysiology, Diagnosis, Management, 4th ed. Philadelphia, WB Saunders, 1989.

Dolz C et al: Changes in liver function tests in patients with inflammatory bowel disease on enteral nutrition. JPEN 13:401, 1989.

Efficacy of exogenous lactase for lactose intolerance. Nutr Rev 46:150, 1988.

Erickson RA: Disaccharidase insufficiency and other disorders of carbohydrate digestion. *In* Gitnick G (ed): Principles and Practice of Gastroenterology and Hepatology. New York, Elsevier, 1988.

Ferguson A, Ziegler K, and Strobel S: Gluten intolerance (celiac disease). Ann Allergy 53:637, 1984.

Ford MJ: The irritable bowel syndrome. J Psychosom Res 30:399, 1986.

Haffejee IE: Effect of oral folate on duration of acute infantile diarrhea. Lancet 2:334, 1988.

Holmes GKT et al: Malignancy in coeliac disease—effect of a gluten-free diet. Gut 30:333, 1989.

Imes S, Pinchbeck BR, and Thomson ABR: Diet counseling modifies nutrient intake of patients with Crohn's disease. J Am Diet Assoc 87:457, 1987.

Johnson JD: The regional and ethnic distribution of lactose malabsorption. *In* Paige DM and Bayless TM (eds): Lactose Digestion. Baltimore, Johns Hopkins University Press, 1981.

Joint Committee on Diet as Related to Gastrointestinal Function of

The American Dietetic Association and the American Medical Association: Diet as related to gastrointestinal function. J Am Diet Assoc 38:425, 1961.

Kelsay JL: Effects of fiber, phytic acid, and oxalic acid in the diet on mineral bioavailability. Am J Gastroenterol 82:983, 1987.

Kolars JC et al: Yogurt: An autodigesting source of lactose. N Engl J Med 310:1, 1984.

Kramer P: Effect of specific foods, beverages, and spices on amount of ileostomy output in human subjects. Am J Gastroenterol 82:327, 1987.

Kretchmer N: The significance of lactose intolerance. *In* Paige DM and Bayless TM (eds): Lactose Digestion: Clinical and Nutritional Implications. Baltimore, The Johns Hopkins University Press, 1981.

Leonard J et al: Gluten challenge in dermatitis herpetiformis. N Engl J Med 308:816, 1983.

Martini MC, Smith DE, and Savaiano DA: Lactose digestion from flavored and frozen yogurts, ice milk and ice cream by lactase-deficient persons. Am J Clin Nutr 46:636, 1987a.

Martini MC et al: Lactose digestion by yogurt beta-galactosidase: influence of pH and microbial cell integrity. Am J Clin Nutr 45:432, 1987b.

McClave SA: Celiac and tropical sprue. *In* Chobanian SJ and Van Ness MM (eds): Manual of Clinical Problems in Gastroenterology. Boston, Little, Brown, 1988.

Newcomer AD et al: Response of patients with irritable bowel syndrome and lactase deficiency using unfermented acidophilus milk. Am J Clin Nutr 38:257, 1983.

O'Morain C: Diet and Crohn's disease. Molec Aspects Med 9:113, 1987.

Onwulata CI, Rao DR, and Vankineni P: Relative efficiency of yogurt, sweet acidophilus milk, hydrolyzed-lactose milk, and a commercial lactase tablet in alleviating lactose maldigestion. Am J Clin Nutr 49:1233, 1989.

Pare P et al: Adult celiac sprue: Changes in the pattern of clinical recognition. J Clin Gastroenterol 10:395, 1988.

Pemberton CM et al: Mayo Clinic Diet Manual: A Handbook of Dietary Practices, 6th ed. Philadelphia, BC Decker, 1988, p 142.

Santosham M et al: Oral rehydration therapy of infantile diarrhea: A controlled study of well-nourished children hospitalized in the United States and Panana. N Engl J Med 306:1070, 1982.

Savaiano DA et al: Lactose malabsorption from yogurt, sweet acidophilus milk, and cultured milk in lactase-deficient individuals. Am J Clin Nutr 40:1219, 1984.

Scrimshaw NS and Murray EB: The acceptability of milk and milk products in populations with a high prevalence of lactose intolerance. Am J Clin Nutr 48(Suppl 4):1083, 1988.

Shanahan F and Weinstein WM: Extending the scope of celiac disease. N Engl J Med 319:782, 1988.

Sulfasalazine inhibits folate absorption. Nutr Rev 46:320, 1988.

Thompson JS and Rikkers LF: Surgical alternatives for the short bowel syndrome. Am J Gastroenterol 82:97, 1987.

Tucker DM et al: Dietary fiber and personality factors as determinants of stool output. Gastroenterology 81:879, 1981.

Van Ness MM: Gas, painless diarrhea, alternating diarrhea and constipation and chronic abdominal pain. *In* Chobanian SJ and Van Ness MM (eds): Manual of Clinical Problems in Gastroenterology. Boston, Little, Brown, 1988.

Watts JH et al: Fecal solids excreted by young men following the ingestion of dairy foods. Am J Dig Dis 4:364, 1963.

Zwetchkenbaum JF and Burakoff R: Food allergy and the irritable bowel syndrome. Am J Gastroenterol 83:901, 1988.

ADDITIONAL REFERENCES

Agarwal VP and Schimmel EM: Diversion colitis: A nutritional deficiency syndrome? Nutr Rev 47:257, 1989.

Bayless TM: Current Management of Inflammatory Bowel Disease. St. Louis, Mosby Times/Mirror, 1989.

Boyko EJ et al: Coffee and alcohol use and the risk of ulcerative colitis. Am J Gastroenterol 84:530, 1989.

Cook IJ et al: Effect of dietary fiber on symptoms and rectosigmoid motility in patients with irritable bowel syndrome: A controlled, crossover study. Gastroenterology 98:66, 1990.

Diet for inflammatory bowel disease. Nutr MD 14(5):7, 1988.

Food choices for ileostomy patients. Nutr MD 14(5):4, 1988.

Grimble G: Fibre, fermentation, flora and flatus. Gut 30:6, 1989.

Heaton KW, Thornton JR, and Emmett PM: Treatment of Crohn's disease with an unrefined-carbohydrate, fibre-rich diet. Br Med J 2:764, 1979.

Intestinal adaptation to massive small-bowel resection follows total parenteral nutrition supplemented with short-chain fatty acids. Nutr Rev 47:267, 1989.

Jones VA et al: Crohn's disease: Maintenance of remission by diet. Lancet 2:177, 1985.

Lee CM and Hardy CM: Cocoa feeding and human lactose intolerance. Am J Clin Nutr 49:840, 1989.

Lloyd-Still JD, Listernick R, and Buentello G: Complex carbohydrate intolerance: Diagnostic pitfalls and approach to management. J Pediatr 112:709, 1988.

Magnesium deficiency in IBD patients. Magnesium 7:78, 1988.

Marsh MN and Loft DE: Coeliac sprue: A centennial overview 1888–1988. Dig Dis 6:216, 1988.

Meshkinpour H and Glick ME: Motor function and disorders of the large bowel. *In* Gitnick G (ed): Principles and Practice of Gastroenterology and Hepatology. New York, Elsevier, 1988.

Muller-Lissner SA: Effect of wheat bran on weight of stool and gastrointestinal transit time: A meta analysis. Br Med J 296:615, 1988.

Pectin delays gastric emptying. Nutr Rev 47:268, 1989.

Roesser WW: The irritable colon: The family physician's most common gastroenterological dilemma. Can Fam Phys 34:633, 1988.

Ryan JA and Beshlian K: Nutritional significance of the small intestine. *In* Lang CE (ed): Nutritional Support in Critical Care. Rockville, MD, Aspen Publishers, 1987.

Westergaard H: The sprue syndromes. Am J Med Sci 290(6):249, 1985.

CHAPTER 28

NUTRITIONAL CARE IN DISEASES OF THE LIVER, BILIARY SYSTEM, AND EXOCRINE PANCREAS

CHAPTER OUTLINE

KEY TERMS

ALCOHOLIC LIVER DISEASE—disease resulting from excessive alcohol ingestion characterized by hepatic steatosis, hepatitis, or cirrhosis

ASCITES—accumulation of fluid, serum protein, and electrolytes within the peritoneal cavity

BILIARY DYSKINESIA—derangement of the filling and emptying mechanism of the gallbladder

BRANCHED-CHAIN AMINO ACIDS—the amino acids valine, isoleucine and leucine

CHOLECYSTECTOMY—surgical removal of the gallbladder

CHOLECYSTITIS—inflammation of the gallbladder

CHOLEDOCHOLITHIASIS—the presence of gallstones in the common bile duct

CHOLELITHIASIS—the presence or formation of gallstones

ESOPHAGASTRIC VARICES—enlarged, thin-walled veins that anastomose with tributaries of the portal vein in the lower esophagus and that occur in patients with portal hypertension

HEPATIC ENCEPHALOPATHY—a condition developing secondary to advanced liver disease; symptoms reflect abnormal exposure of the brain to nitrogenous toxins

HEPATIC FAILURE—situation when liver function is diminished to 30% or less

HEPATIC STEATOSIS—fatty liver

HEPATITIS—inflammation of the liver

HEPATITIS A—liver disease caused by the hepatitis A virus that is transmitted by the fecal-oral route

HEPATITIS B—liver disease caused by the hepatitis B virus that is transmitted primarily by the parenteral route

HEPATORENAL SYNDROME—functional renal failure without pathologic renal changes, associated with cirrhosis and ascites or with obstructive jaundice

JAUNDICE (ICTERUS)—a syndrome characterized by hyperbilirubinemia and deposition of bile pigment, resulting in yellowing of the skin, mucous membranes, and sclera

NON-A, NON-B HEPATITIS—a clinical syndrome of acute viral hepatitis occurring without the serologic markers of hepatitis A or B; commonly occurs following intravenous drug use

PANCREATITIS—inflammation of the pancreas caused by autodigestion of pancreatic tissue by its own enzymes

PANCREATODUODENECTOMY (WHIPPLE PROCEDURE)—excision of the head of the pancreas along with the encircling loop of the duodenum

PORTAL HYPERTENSION—abnormally increased blood pressure in the portal venous system, a frequent complication of cirrhosis of the liver

LIVER DISEASE

Functions of the Liver

The liver has the most varied and extensive function of any organ and is one of the most important organs involved in the metabolism of food. Most of the end products of digestion are transported directly to the liver where they are stored or resynthesized into other forms or they are transported to other parts of the body when necessary.

Hepatic cells store energy in the form of glycogen, which is made available as glucose when needed. When blood glucose concentration cannot be maintained by glycogenolysis, liver cells convert protein to glucose by means of gluconeogenesis. Triglycerides and phospholipids are synthesized in the liver and are incorporated into lipoproteins for transport to peripheral tissues for use or storage. The liver also synthesizes cholesterol and converts about 80% of it into bile salts; the remainder is transported in the form of lipoproteins. Fatty acids are oxidized to acetyl-CoA, which in turn is oxidized via the Krebs cycle to liberate energy. Before their use in protein synthesis, for energy, or conversion to carbohydrates and fats, amino acids are deaminated in the liver and the resultant ammonia is detoxified by conversion to urea. Transamination of amino acids to maintain normal blood levels of nonessential amino acids takes place in the liver, which is also the site of most plasma protein synthesis. A reserve of these proteins is maintained in the liver to replenish serum proteins when needed.

Iron and copper, both essential to hemoglobin formation, are stored in the liver, which also recovers iron from discarded red blood cells. These and several minerals and vitamins are bound within the liver to their respective carrier proteins for transport throughout the body. All the fat-soluble vitamins are stored in the liver, as well as appreciable amounts of ascorbic acid and the B-complex vitamins. Carotene is converted to vitamin A; vitamin K is converted to prothrombin; and vitamin D is converted to an active form (25-OHD_3) by the liver.

The consequences of alcohol metabolism are described in Further Reading, page 481. Drugs are metabolized and hormones are deactivated in the liver, which also detoxifies chemicals or poisons entering through food or produced in other parts of the body.

Diseases of the Liver

Acute Hepatitis

Hepatitis is an inflammation of the liver caused by a virus, toxin, obstruction, parasite, or drug. Acute viral hepatitis is caused by a known virus, of which the most common are hepatitis A (HAV) and hepatitis B (HBV), or by unidentified viruses that result in the form known as non-A, non-B (NANB) hepatitis (Fig. 28–1).

Hepatitis A, common among children and young adults, is transmitted by the fecal-oral route and is contracted through contaminated drinking water, food, or sewage. Presenting symptoms include nausea, anorexia, and right upper quadrant pain followed by dark urine and jaundice. Although most attacks are not serious, they may be severe in older people.

Hepatitis B may cause a wide variety of acute or chronic hepatic and extrahepatic diseases, including arthritis, rash, and glomerulonephritis. Acute, fulminant hepatic failure can even result. The clinical course is more variable and is usually more prolonged than that of HAV. The virus can be transmitted by transfusions from a carrier or through improperly sterilized medical instruments, dental drills, tattooing needles, or other skin-puncturing instruments that have come in contact with contaminated blood. In 3 to 10% of

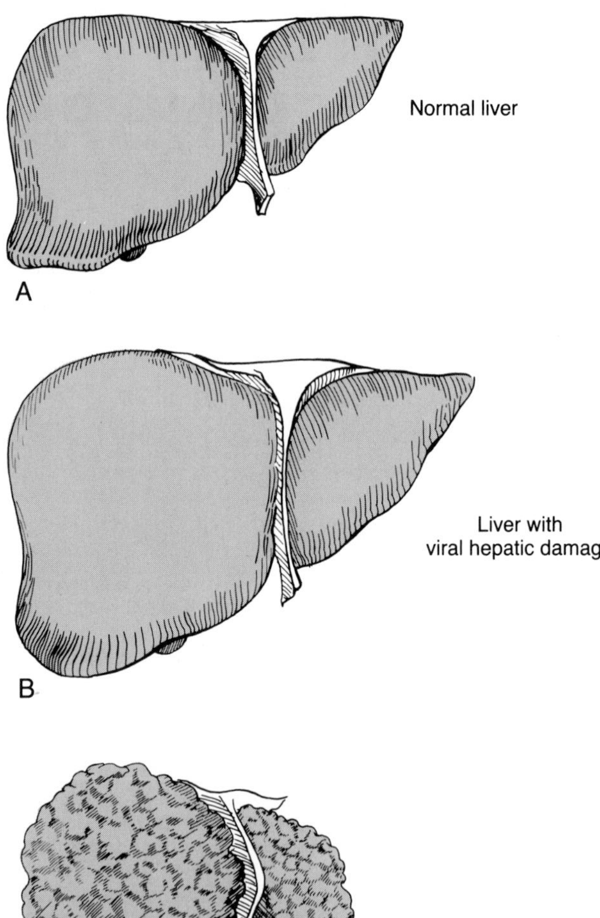

FIGURE 28–1. *Normal liver* (A); *liver with viral hepatic damage* (B); *and cirrhotic liver* (C).

cases, patients with HBV develop chronic hepatitis. Some become asymptomatic carriers of the hepatitis B antigen (HBsAg), which can transmit the disease to others through blood.

Alcoholic Liver Disease

Alcoholic liver disease (ALD) is the fourth leading cause of death among those aged 25 to 64 years in the United States (Diehl, 1988). Patients with ALD may be asymptomatic or they may be gravely ill, and there is poor correlation between liver histology and the clinical presentation of the patient.

The pathogenesis of ALD is complex and is not completely understood. It involves metabolic derangements caused by the toxic effects on mitochondrial function produced by acetaldehyde and hydrogen, the conversion products of alcohol (Fig. 28–2 and Further Reading, p. 481). Whether the alcoholic develops fatty liver (Fig. 28–3), hepatic steatosis, alcoholic hepatitis,

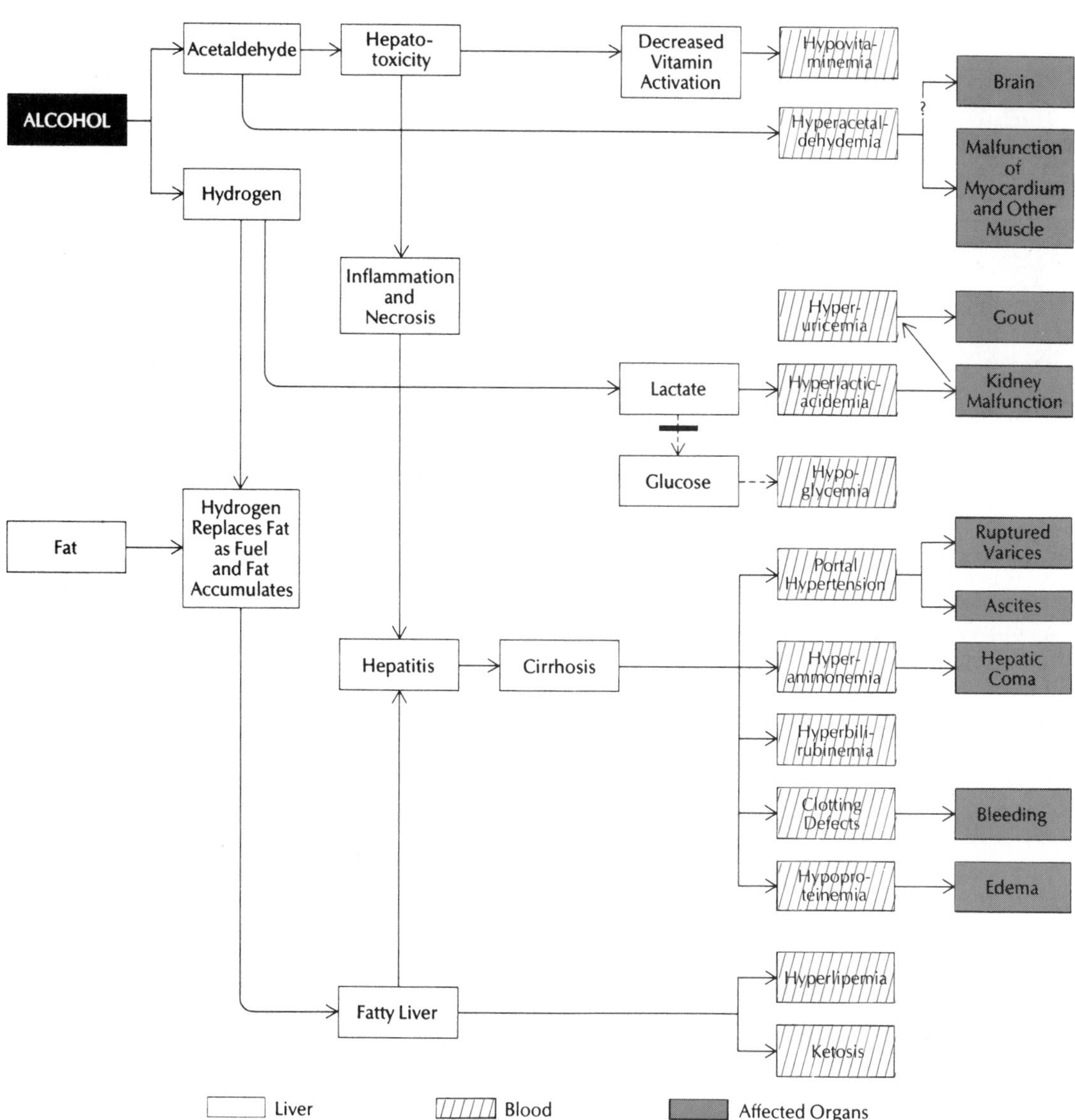

FIGURE 28–2. *Complications of excessive alcohol consumption stem largely from excess hydrogen and from acetaldehyde. Hydrogen produces fatty liver and hyperlipemia, high blood lactic acid, and low blood sugar. The accumulation of fat, the effect of acetaldehyde on liver cells, and other factors as yet unknown lead to alcoholic hepatitis. The next step is cirrhosis. The consequent impairment of liver function disturbs blood chemistry, notably causing a high ammonia level that can lead to coma and death. Cirrhosis also distorts liver structure, inhibiting blood flow. High pressure in vessels supplying the liver may cause ruptured varices and accumulation of fluid in the abdominal cavity. There are individual differences in response to alcohol; in particular, not all heavy drinkers develop hepatitis and cirrhosis. (From Lieber CS: The metabolism of alcohol. Sci Am 234:33, 1976. Copyright © 1976 by Scientific American, Inc. All rights reserved.)*

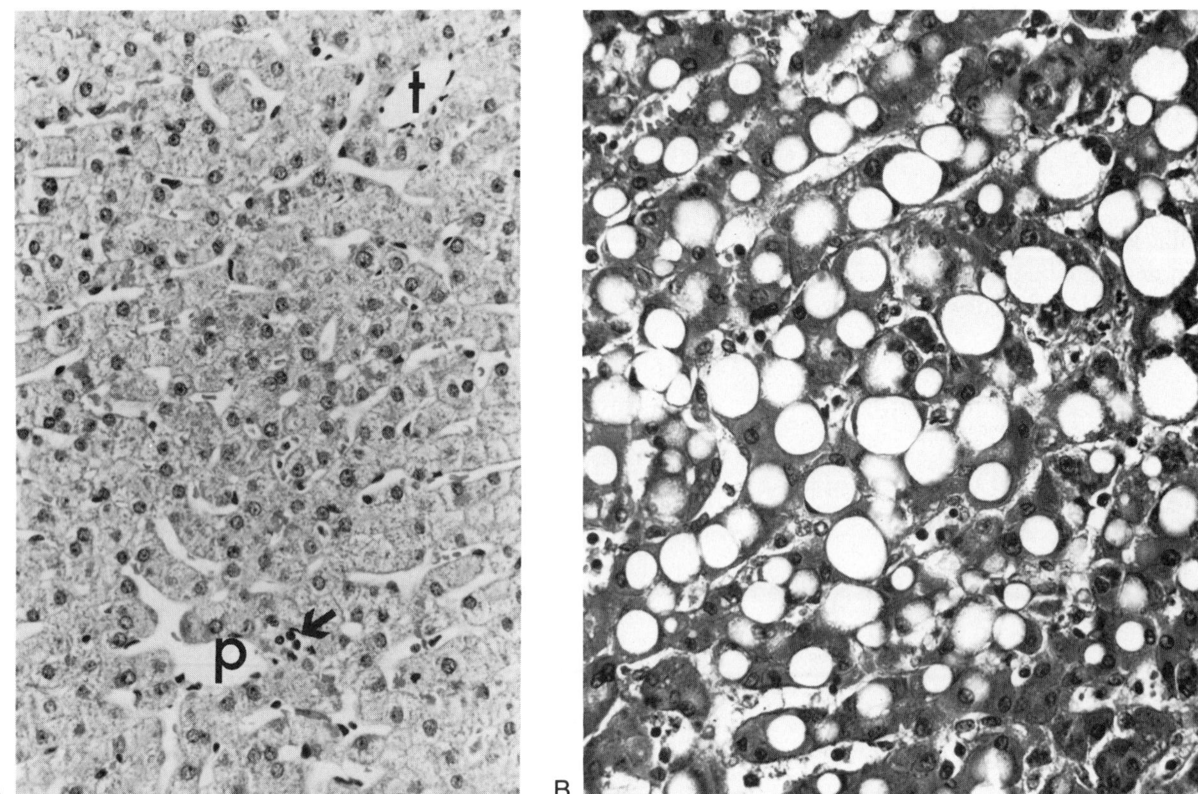

FIGURE 28–3. *Microscopic appearance of* (A) *a normal liver. (p = portal tract; t = terminal hepatic venule.)* B, *a fatty liver. (*A, *From Berk JE [ed]: Bockus Gastroenterology, 4th ed, 1985, p 2627.* B, *From Cotran et al: Robbins Pathologic Basis of Disease, 4th ed, 1989.)*

or cirrhosis depends on the duration and extent of the alcohol intake and on undefined genetic, immunologic, and possibly nutritional factors. The reason why only 17 to 30% of heavy drinkers develop alcoholic liver injury is not understood (Lieber, 1988a). Although nutritional factors may influence the hepatotoxic effect of alcohol (Diehl et al, 1985), an adequate diet does not protect against liver degeneration in the alcoholic (Lieber, 1988b).

Cirrhosis

Cirrhosis is the final stage of liver injury and degeneration and occurs in 15% of heavy drinkers (Diehl, 1988). Other causes include drug or chemical poisoning, HBV, various metabolic disorders as discussed in Chapter 41, cystic fibrosis, or biliary obstruction. Any chronic active hepatitis can lead to cirrhosis.

In this condition, normal liver tissue is gradually destroyed and replaced by inactive fibrous connective tissue (scar tissue). Regrowth of new tissue leads to the development of abnormal nodules that limit liver function by interfering with the flow of blood. In contrast to the enlarged fatty liver, the cirrhotic liver is contracted and has lost most of its function. Once the dense vascular and fibrous bands have formed, the condition is irreversible. This chronic hepatic insufficiency can be overlaid with acute episodes of exacerbation and encephalopathy.

Obstruction of the portal vein leads to high portal pressure with subsequent congestion of abdominal blood vessels and development of a collateral circulation that detours around the liver to the systemic venous circulation via the esophagus and upper stomach. A complication of these circumstances is *ascites,* which is accumulation of fluid, serum protein, and electrolytes within the peritoneal cavity. A further complication is the enlargement of the veins providing collateral circulation. Because these *esophagogastric varices* are thin-walled and subject to high pressure, they are at risk of rupture, and mortality from hemorrhage is high.

Hepatic Failure

Hepatic failure occurs when liver function is diminished to 30% or less. Among accompanying abnormalities is *hepatic encephalopathy (HE),* in which nitrogenous toxins are shunted into the circulatory system and cross an abnormally porous blood-brain barrier. The ensuing psychomotor abnormalities eventually develop into coma and finally death. Signs of severe en-

FURTHER READING: Metabolic Consequences of Alcohol Consumption

Ethanol is metabolized in the liver to form acetaldehyde, which in turn is oxidized to acetate. Acetate is converted to acetyl-CoA. Acetaldehyde inflicts liver damage by decreasing mitochondrial functions.

$$\underset{\text{ethanol}}{C_2H_2OH} + NAD \xrightarrow[\text{dehydrogenase}]{\text{alcohol}} NADH + H^+ + \underset{\text{acetaldehyde}}{CH_3{-}CHO}$$

$$\underset{\text{acetaldehyde}}{CH_3{-}CHO} + NADH + H_2O \xrightarrow[\text{dehydrogenase}]{\text{aldehyde}} NADH + H^+ + \underset{\text{acetate}}{CH_3COOH}$$

When acetyl-CoA derived from ethanol is used in energy production via the Krebs cycle, the role of oxidation of fatty acids is decreased and the synthesis of triglyceride is favored, with subsequent development of a fatty liver. Fatty acids that would normally have been used for oxidation accumulate in the liver, and excess hydrogen from the ethanol oxidation contributes to fatty acid and triglyceride synthesis. Fatty liver due to alcohol is reversible and disappears when alcohol ingestion stops.

Pyruvate metabolism is disordered because of the substitution of ethanol in energy production, and lactic acid accumulates to excessive levels. These levels can interfere with uric acid excretion and precipitate an attack of gout in susceptible individuals. In the absence of new glycogen formation, depleted reserves can lead to hypoglycemia in the malnourished alcoholic.

cephalopathy and impending hepatic coma include confusion, apathy, personality changes, asterixis ("flapping" or tremor of the hands when extended in front of the chest), and spasticity.

The primary toxin involved in HE appears to be ammonia, which is produced by action of intestinal bacteria on protein derived from dietary intake, gastrointestinal bleeding, or as a by-product of normal amino acid metabolism. The diseased liver is unable to convert ammonia into urea, and this ammonia accumulates in the blood. However, other factors are probably involved in the etiology of HE, because the correlation between blood ammonia concentration and the depth of coma or extent of neurologic changes is poor. Metabolites of methionine, mercaptans, or methanethiol (produced by bacterial metabolism of methionine) that interact with fatty acids and ammonia are probably involved (Zieve et al, 1974).

High levels of the aromatic amino acids (phenylalanine, tyrosine, and free tryptophan), normally metabolized by the liver in the presence of low levels of branched-chain amino acids (BCAA) —leucine, valine, and isoleucine—may result in production of false neurotransmitters and the precipitation of encephalopathy (Fischer and Baldessarini, 1971; Fischer and Bower, 1981; Freund et al, 1979). Increased levels of gamma-aminobutyric acid, an inhibitory neurotransmitter, have also been implicated (Schafer and Jones, 1982).

Nutritional Care in Liver Disease

The objectives of nutritional care are (1) to maintain or improve the patient's nutritional status through the provision of adequate energy and nutrients; (2) to prevent or ameliorate hepatic encephalopathy; and (3) to prevent further degeneration of the liver and enable regeneration of as much new tissue as possible.

Liver Function Tests

During the course of liver disease, liver function can change drastically, and the nutritional care must be adjusted according to the status of liver function. For example, a decrease in the serum albumin level reflects failure of protein synthesis. An elevated serum ammonia indicates that the liver is unable to synthesize urea. Table 28-1 lists common liver function tests.

Dietary Modifications in Liver Disease

MALNUTRITION IN THE ALCOHOLIC. Several factors contribute to the malnutrition that is common in chronic alcoholics with liver disease.

1. Alcohol can replace food in the diet of moderate and heavy drinkers. In light drinkers, it is usually an additional energy source (Lieber, 1988b). Although 20 oz of 86-proof liquor provides 1,500 kcal, or about 50 to 75% of the daily energy requirement, it contains no protein, vitamins, or minerals. Furthermore, although alcohol provides 7 kcal/g, its energy efficiency is not comparable with that of other nutrients.
2. By causing inflammation of the stomach, pancreas, and intestine, alcohol consumption leads to malabsorption of nutrients, particularly thiamin, vitamin B_{12}, folic acid, and ascorbic acid. Wernicke-Korsakoff syndrome from thiamin deficiency is common.
3. Alcohol and its conversion product acetaldehyde

TABLE 28–1. Common Liver Function Tests*

Diagnostic Test	Function Evaluated
Van den Bergh Icterus index Urine bilirubin Urobilinogen Fecal urobilinogen Serum bilirubin	Formation and excretion of bile
Total protein Albumin Globulin Fibrinogen	Protein metabolism and formation of albumin, globulin, fibrinogen; protein synthetic capacity
Prothrombin time	Production of prothrombin; synthetic capacity of clotting factors
Urea Uric acid Ammonia	Formation of urea and uric acids and removal of ammonia; metabolic capacity
Glucose tolerance Galactose tolerance	Carbohydrate metabolism: gluconeogenesis, glycogenesis, glycogenolysis
Serum phospholipids, triglycerides	Lipid metabolism
Cholesterol	Synthesis of cholesterol
Ketones	Formation of ketone bodies
Indocyanine green (ICG)	Detoxification; excretion of substances withdrawn from blood
Hippuric acid	Conjugation, oxidation, or reduction
Serum glutamic-oxaloacetic transaminase (SGOT) Serum glutamic-pyruvic transaminase (SGPT) Lactic dehydrogenase (LDH) Alkaline phosphatase, released with biliary obstruction Leucine aminopeptidase (LAP) 5′-Nucleotidase Cholinesterase	Enzyme production; enzymes released in liver cell damage
HAA (HB Ag) Alpha fetoprotein	Immunologic production Hepatitis Hepatocellular carcinoma Hepatic necrosis Acute hepatitis

* From Given BA and Simmons SJ: Gastroenterology in Clinical Nursing, 4th ed. St Louis, CV Mosby, 1984.

have a direct hepatotoxic effect that interferes with the metabolism and activation of vitamins A, D, B_6, and folate by liver cells.

4. The metabolism of alcohol increases the need for certain nutrients, particularly the B-vitamins and magnesium (Flink, 1986). The malnutrition-alcoholism relationship is a vicious cycle, with malnutrition initially provoked by the alcohol potentiating the hepatotoxic effects of alcohol.

ENERGY. Because there is often extreme weight loss, a high-energy diet with 35 to 45 kcal/kg of ideal body weight per day is indicated. This is approximately 150 to 175% of resting energy expenditure (Shronts, 1988). With alcohol omitted, this means much more food than the alcoholic has been accustomed to eating.

CARBOHYDRATE. Carbohydrate metabolism is deranged in hepatitis. Patients may experience fasting hypoglycemia due to decreased glycogen stores and serum insulin elevations. Glucose intolerance may also be present due to insulin resistance. Elevations of glucagon and growth hormone lead to mobilization and utilization of endogenous protein for energy. Both fasting and postprandial hyperglycemia may occur. The diet should therefore be as high as possible in complex carbohydrate; 300 to 400 g/day is recommended to spare available protein. (See Chapter 31 for exchange lists to determine carbohydrate content of diet.)

PROTEIN. Profound changes occur in the distribution and metabolism of amino acids in liver disease, and the ratio of aromatic to BCAA in the blood is abnormally high (Table 28–2). At the same time, there is an increased need for protein to provide for liver repair and to replenish protein stores if the patient is malnourished.

TABLE 28–2. Amino Acids of Importance in Liver Disease

Aromatic amino acids (AAA)
- Tyrosine
- Phenylalanine*
- Free tryptophan*

Branched-chain amino acids (BCAA)
- Valine*
- Leucine*
- Isoleucine*

Ammoniogenic amino acids
- Glycine
- Serine
- Threonine*
- Glutamine
- Histidine*
- Lysine*
- Asparagine

* Denotes indispensable amino acids.

Hepatic Encephalopathy or Hepatic Failure

At the appearance of signs and symptoms of encephalopathy or hepatic failure, the dietary intake of protein should be reduced to around 0.5 g/kg/day. However, positive nitrogen balance must be maintained because a negative balance can aggravate encephalopathy. It is difficult to maintain a positive nitrogen balance and yet prevent hepatic encephalopathy, because the protein requirement for hepatic tissue regeneration may be more than 1 g/kg/day.

Blood ammonia is frequently reduced by the oral administration of neomycin to destroy gut flora and the use of lactulose, a nondigestible carbohydrate that removes the intestinal contents by inducing diarrhea. Lactulose may also reduce colonic absorption of ammonia by lowering the luminal pH.

When encephalopathy fails to improve with protein restriction and a course of neomycin and lactulose, supplementing the protein intake with BCAA has been reported to be effective (Cerra et al, 1985; Fiaccadori et al, 1984; Hiyama and Fischer, 1988), although this is controversial (Egberts et al, 1985; Wahren et al, 1983). Defined formula diets high in BCAA are commercially available (see Appendix Table 33). More economically, BCAA powder can be added to foods, but the taste is poor (Shronts et al, 1987).

Vegetable proteins appear to be tolerated better than meat proteins, perhaps because of their lower content of methionine and aromatic amino acids and higher content of BCAA (Blendis and Jenkins, 1988). When compliance with vegetarian diets is a problem because of increased flatulence, anorexia, and early satiety, dairy protein should be used as tolerated (Fenton et al, 1966; Pemberton et al, 1988).

If the patient remains neurologically clear after about 1 week on the low-protein diet, with or without BCAA supplementation, protein intake should be increased in 10- to 15-gram increments each week until a level of 1 g/kg/day or higher is reached. If encephalopathy develops, the dietary protein must again be reduced, or BCAA or further ammonia-reducing treatments must be given.

LIPID. Cirrhosis is marked by impaired fat metabolism and malabsorption. Accumulation of fat in the liver has been reduced by lowering dietary fat to 25% of total kilocalories and also by substitution of medium-chain triglycerides (MCT) for normal longer-chain dietary fats.

Steatorrhea is found in about 50% of cirrhotic patients, whether they are alcoholics or not. Possible causes include cirrhosis-related pancreatic insufficiency, decreased amounts of bile salts, administration of neomycin or cholestyramine, and lymphatic or portal congestion. Replacement of some long-chain triglycerides with MCT oil may be useful. If MCT is used to the exclusion of other dietary fat, 4 to 7 grams of linoleic acid supplementation will eventually be required to avoid essential fatty acid deficiency (Mezitis, 1988).

When MCT use is ineffective, it may be necessary to reduce the total fat in the diet. However, food is more palatable and easier to prepare when moderate amounts of fat are allowed, especially because of the high-protein requirements. In addition, the inclusion of fats increases the energy content of the diet. Thus 40 to 70 grams of fat, or about 25 to 30% of total kilocalories, is recommended (Table 28–3). Better tolerance can occasionally be obtained with dairy fats.

VITAMINS AND MINERALS. Many vitamins need to be supplemented to repair damage and fortify the liver against stress. The most common deficiencies are of folate, thiamin, and vitamin B_{12}; however, a good source of all the B-vitamins should be prescribed.

In the presence of steatorrhea, water-soluble forms of vitamins A, D, and E may be necessary. In severe cirrhosis with problems of vitamin storage, metabolism and transport, intramuscular injections of A, D, and K may be necessary. Vitamin K should be prescribed if evidence of hypoprothrombinemia exists.

Cirrhosis is accompanied by deficient 25-hydroxylation of vitamin D in the liver. Osteopenia and osteomalacia are common. However, the value of supplemental vitamin D in preventing osteopenia has not been proved (Blendis and Jenkins, 1988). When hypocalcemia exists in the presence of steatorrhea, calcium supplementation is justified.

Primary biliary cirrhosis is accompanied by copper excess that often requires chelation with D-penicillamine. A low-copper diet can be used as adjunct therapy (Table 28–4).

Supplementation with zinc will be necessary with evidence of abnormalities of dark adaptation or taste acuity. Common vitamin and mineral deficiencies are

TABLE 28–3. Fat-Restricted Diet*

Foods Allowed	Foods Excluded
Beverages	***Beverages***
Skim milk or buttermilk made with skim milk; coffee, tea, Postum, fruit juice, soft drinks, cocoa made with cocoa powder and skim milk	Whole milk, buttermilk made with whole milk, chocolate milk, cream in excess of amounts allowed under fats
Bread and Cereal Products	***Bread and Cereal Products***
Plain, nonfat cereals, spaghetti, noodles, rice, macaroni; plain whole-grain or enriched bread	Biscuits, breads, egg or cheese bread, sweet rolls made with fat, pancakes, doughnuts, waffles, fritters, popcorn prepared with fat, muffins, natural cereals and breads to which extra fat is added
Cheese	***Cheese***
Cottage, ¼ cup to be used as substitute for 1 oz of cheese, or specially processed low-fat cheeses containing less than 5% butterfat	Whole milk cheeses
Desserts	***Desserts***
Sherbet made with skim milk; non-fat frozen yogurt; non-fat frozen non-dairy desserts; fruit ice; sorbet; gelatin; rice, bread, cornstarch, tapioca, or pudding made with skim milk; fruit whips with gelatin, sugar, and egg white; fruit; angel food cake; graham crackers; vanilla wafers; meringues	Cake, pie, pastry, ice cream, or any dessert containing shortening, chocolate, or fats of any kind, unless especially prepared using part of fat allowance
Eggs	***Eggs***
3 per week prepared only with fat from fat allowance; egg whites as desired; low-fat egg substitutes	More than 1/day unless substituted for part of the meat allowed
Fats	***Fats***
Choose up to the limit allowed among the following (1 serving in the amount listed equals 1 fat choice): 1 tsp. butter or margarine 1 T reduced-fat margarine 1 tsp. shortening or oil 1 tsp. mayonnaise 2 tsp. Italian or French dressing 1 T reduced-fat salad dressing 1 strip crisp bacon ⅛ avocado (4″ diameter) 2 T light cream 1 T heavy cream 6 small nuts 5 small olives	Any in excess of amount prescribed on diet; all others
Fruits	***Fruits***
As desired	Avocado in excess of amount allowed on fat list
Lean Meat, Fish, Poultry, and Meat Substitutes	***Meat, Fish, Poultry, and Meat Substitutes***
Choose up to the limit allowed among the following: poultry without skin, fish, veal (all cuts), liver, lean beef, pork, and lamb, all with visible fat removed—1 oz cooked weight equals 1 equivalent; ¼ cup water packed tuna or salmon equals 1 equivalent; tofu or tempeh — 3 oz equals 1 equivalent	Fried or fatty meats, sausage, scrapple, frankfurters, poultry skins, stewing hens, spareribs, salt pork, beef unless lean, duck, goose, ham hocks, pig's feet, luncheon meats, gravies unless fat-free, tuna and salmon packed in oil, peanut butter
Milk	***Milk***
Skim, buttermilk, or yogurt made from skim milk	Whole, 2%, 1%, chocolate, buttermilk made with whole milk
Seasonings	***Seasonings***
As desired	None
Soups	***Soups***
Bouillon, clear broth, fat free vegetable soup, cream soup made with skimmed milk, packaged dehydrated soups	All others
Sweets	***Sweets***
Jelly, jam, marmalade, honey, syrup, molasses, sugar, hard sugar candies, fondant, gumdrops, jelly beans, marshmallows, cocoa powder, fat-free chocolate sauce, red and black licorice	Any candy made with chocolate, nuts, butter, cream, or fat of any kind
Vegetables	***Vegetables***
All plainly prepared vegetables	Potato chips; buttered, au gratin, creamed, or fried potatoes and other vegetables unless made with allowed fat; casseroles, or frozen vegetables in butter sauce

TABLE 28–3. Fat-Restricted Diet *Continued*

Daily Food Allowances for 50-Gram Fat Diet

Food	*Amount*	*Approximate Fat Content (g)*
Skim milk	2 cups or more	0
Lean meat, fish, poultry	6 oz or 6 equivalents	18
Whole egg or egg yolks	3 per week	3
Vegetables	3 servings or more, at least 1 or more dark green or deep yellow	0
Fruits	3 or more servings, at least 1 citrus	0
Breads, cereals	As desired	0
Fat exchanges*	5–6 exchanges daily	25–30
Desserts and sweets	As desired from permitted list	0
	Total fat	46–51

* Additional fat servings are listed in Table 31–10. Fat content can be reduced further by reducing the fat exchanges. 1 fat exchange = 5 grams of fat.

TABLE 28–4. Copper Content of Foods*†

Food Groups	High 0.2 mg/portion commonly used‡	Moderate 0.1 to 0.2 mg/portion commonly used‡	Low 0.1 mg/portion commonly used‡
Meat and meat substitutes	Lamb; pork; pheasant; quail; duck; goose; salmon; all organ meats including liver, heart, kidney, brain; all shellfish, including oysters, scallops, shrimp, lobster, clams, and crab; meat gelatin; soy protein meat substitutes; tofu; all nuts and seeds	All other fish; turkey; peanut butter; chicken	Beef; cheese; cottage cheese; eggs; cold cuts and frankfurters that do not contain pork, turkey, or organ meats
Fats and oils	Avocado	Olives	All others
Milk	Chocolate; cocoa		All other dairy products; milk flavored with carob
Starch	Dried beans including soybeans, lima beans, baked beans, garbanzo beans, pinto beans; dried peas; lentils; millet; barley; wheat germ; bran breads and cereals; granola; soy flour; soy grits; fresh sweet potatoes	Whole-wheat bread; potatoes in any form; pumpkin; melba toast; whole-wheat crackers; parsnips; winter squash; green peas; instant oatmeal; instant ralston; some ready-to-eat dry cereals (check labels); dehydrated and canned soups	All others
Vegetables	Mushrooms; broccoli	Bean sprouts; beets; spinach; summer and winter squash; tomato juice and other tomato products	All others, including fresh tomatoes
Fruits	Nectarines; dried fruits including raisins, dates, and prunes (Dried fruits are permitted if dried at home)	Mango; pears; pineapple; papaya; orange juice; cranberry juice cocktail; grape juice	All others
Desserts	Desserts that contain significant amounts of any foods high in copper		All others
Sugar and sweets	Chocolate; cocoa	Licorice; carbonated beverages; syrups	All others including jams, jellies, and candies made with allowed fruits; carob; flavoring extracts
Miscellaneous	Brewers' yeast	Ketchup	
Beverages§	Instant breakfast beverages; mineral water‡; alcohol‖	Postum and other cereal beverages	All others including fruit-flavored beverages; lemonade

* From Pemberton CM et al: Mayo Clinic Diet Manual, 6th ed. Philadelphia, BC Decker, 1988.

† Data that are available on the average copper content of foods vary greatly. Estimates of the copper content of the usual American diet range from 1 mg/day to 2 to 5 mg/day. The concentration of copper in foods is affected by many factors, including soil conditions, geographic location, species, diet, processing method, and contamination in processing. The exact copper content of foods is difficult to verify. It is estimated that avoidance of high copper foods results in an intake of approximately 2 mg/day; avoidance of both high and moderate copper foods results in an intake of approximately 1 mg/day. For practical purposes, diets are designed to limit foods with a higher copper content and not to achieve a specific level of copper in the diet.

‡ Portions commonly used are those that are generally accepted as typical portion sizes in various nutrient data source manuals.

§ A water sample from the patient's home water supply should be analyzed for copper content. Demineralized water should be used if the water contains more than 100 μg/liter.

‖ Although not necessarily high in copper, alcoholic beverages are discouraged because of their action as a hepatotoxin.

listed in Table 28–5. Patients with hepatic failure are also subject to nutrient toxicities so that nutrient supplementation must be closely monitored.

FLUIDS AND SODIUM. The accumulation of fluid in ascites is reduced by restricting sodium to between 500 and 2,000 mg/day (22 to 87 mEq), depending on the rate of diuresis and on the tolerance of the patient. (See Chapter 33 for low-sodium diets.) Sodium levels should be kept as high as possible to maintain palatability because of the poor appetite characteristic of the patient with liver disease. Diuretics are also given—usually spironolactone, which inhibits the synthesis and thus renal effects of aldosterone. The goal is a gradual diuresis of 100 to 400 mg/day. When spironolactone is not effective, a loop diuretic such as furosemide can be added. Fluid intake is adjusted based on output and serum electrolytes.

Patients should be weighed and their abdomens palpated daily to check for fluid retention. Measurements of abdominal girth are also useful. Patients should also be watched for signs of hypokalemia, hyperkalemia, azotemia, hyponatremia, encephalopathy, and precipitation of *hepatorenal syndrome.* As diuresis progresses, there will be weight loss until the patient is "dry," followed by a steady, slow gain to normal levels as the nutritional status improves.

PROBLEMS IN FEEDING. Great care should be taken to serve food that is attractive and appetizing. Because the appetite is almost always poor, nutritional intake is frequently maintained with difficulty. Six to eight small feedings per day are usually more acceptable than three large meals. Because patients tend to experience nausea at the end of the day, the major part of the intake should be given in the morning.

When serving the patient with hepatitis, standard hospital procedures to avoid contamination should be followed.

Dietary Modifications in Liver Resection

Liver resection is fairly frequent now that the problem area can be located preoperatively by means of tomography and arteriography. Many patients with primary or secondary liver involvement are undernourished and if possible should be nutritionally repleted before surgery. After major hepatic resection, it is necessary to manage metabolic changes in a manner that will permit recovery and rapid regeneration of liver tissue.

Resections of 70% or more have been accompanied by severe hypoglycemia; thus, blood glucose must be monitored carefully. Hypoalbuminemia will also occur because the liver is the site of albumin synthesis. Parenteral albumin supplementation is required for 1 to 3 weeks postoperatively to prevent a progressive fall of osmotic pressure in the vascular compartment and subsequent accumulation of interstitial fluid, increased vascular load, and the danger of pulmonary edema.

Vitamin K should be administered preoperatively and postoperatively. Coagulation factors synthesized by the liver fall in the postoperative phase but will return to normal with liver regeneration.

Dietary Modifications in Liver Transplantation

Liver transplantation has become an established treatment for hepatic failure. If malnutrition is present, nutritional support is required prior to transplant (Shronts et al, 1987). A low-bacteria diet may also be used preoperatively and postoperatively. In conjunction with antibiotics, this reduces the risk of bacterial or fungal infection in the immunosuppressed patient after transplant (see Chapter 36). This diet is maintained postoperatively as long as bowel decontamination procedures are in effect (Pemberton et al, 1988). The low-bacteria diet excludes all cheese products, raw vegetables, and raw unpeeled fruits and requires the use of low-bacteria food preparation and handling practices.

TABLE 28–5. Vitamin/Mineral Deficits in Severe Hepatic Failure*

Vitamin/Mineral	Predisposing Factors	Signs of Deficiency
Vitamin A	Steatorrhea, neomycin, cholestyramine, alcoholism	Dermatitis, night-blindness
Vitamin D	Steatorrhea, glucocorticoids, cholestyramine	Osteomalacia
Vitamin E	Steatorrhea, cholestyramine	Edema, peripheral neuropathy
Vitamin K	Steatorrhea, antibiotics, cholestyramine	Bleeding
Vitamin B_6	Alcoholism	Mucous membrane lesions, dermatitis
Vitamin B_{12}	Alcoholism, cholestyramine	Megaloblastic anemia, glossitis, CNS dysfunction
Folate	Alcoholism	Megaloblastic anemia, glossitis, irritability
Niacin	Alcoholism	Dermatitis, dementia, diarrhea, inflammation of mucous membranes
Thiamin	Alcoholism, high CHO diet	Neuropathy, ascites, edema, CNS dysfunction
Zinc	Diarrhea, diuretics, alcoholism	Immunodeficiency, impaired taste acuity, wound healing, protein synthesis
Magnesium	Alcoholism, diuretics	Neuromuscular irritability, hypokalemia, hypocalcemia
Iron	Chronic bleeding	Stomatitis, microcytic anemia, malaise

* Adapted from Shronts EP: Nutritional assessment of adults with end-stage hepatic failure. Nutr Clin Prac 3:113, 1988.

Post-transplantation nutritional care appropriate to the use of cyclosporine and steroids to prevent rejection is described in Chapter 36.

GALLBLADDER DISEASE

Physiology and Function of the Gallbladder

The gallbladder is attached to the right side of the undersurface of the liver as shown in Figure 28–4. Diseases of the biliary tract and gallbladder are closely associated with liver disorders.

The main function of the gallbladder is concentration and storage of the bile, which is secreted by the liver. During the concentration process, water, and electrolytes are reabsorbed by the gallbladder mucosa. Constituents that are not reabsorbed, particularly the bile salts and lipid substances such as cholesterol, become highly concentrated in the bile. Bile assists in the digestion and absorption of fats and in the absorption of fat-soluble vitamins A, D, E, and K and the minerals iron and calcium. (See Chapter 1 for further discussion of the digestive process.)

The gallbladder is normally full and relaxed between meals, and the sphincter of Oddi is closed. During the course of digestion, food fats reaching the duodenum stimulate the production of cholecystokinin in the intestinal mucosa. This hormone causes the gallbladder to contract and the sphincter of Oddi to relax, thus releasing concentrated bile into the duodenum via the common duct located at the ampulla of Vater. This common duct also carries the digestive enzymes from the pancreas. Because of this joining of hepatic, biliary, and pancreatic ducts, diseases of these organs are often interrelated.

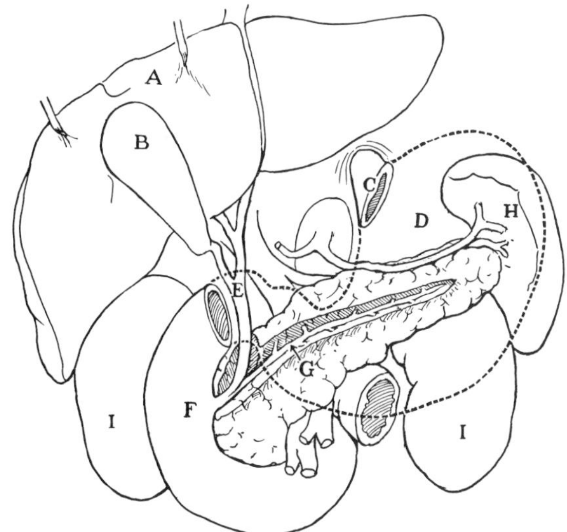

FIGURE 28–4. *Schematic drawing showing relationship of organs of the upper abdomen.* A, *liver (retracted upward);* B, *gallbladder;* C, *esophageal opening of stomach;* D, *stomach (shown in* dotted outline*);* E, *common bile duct;* F, *duodenum;* G, *pancreas and pancreatic duct;* H, *spleen;* I, *kidneys.*

Diseases of the Gallbladder

Gallbladder disease occurs in women more frequently than in men and occurs most often in obese women over 40 years of age. The common diseases of the biliary tract are biliary dyskinesia, cholelithiasis (gallstones), and cholecystitis.

Biliary Dyskinesia

Biliary dyskinesia results when the sphincter of Oddi goes into spasm and fails to open properly. The ensuing accumulation of bile increases pressure in the gallbladder, which is heralded by vague abdominal complaints.

Cholelithiasis

The formation of gallstones in the absence of infection of the gallbladder is called *cholelithiasis.* The existence of stones may cause no symptoms, and the patient may be unaware of their presence.

Choledocholithiasis develops when stones slip into the common bile duct, producing obstruction and cramps. The patient usually has severe right upper quadrant pain. Passage of bile into the duodenum is interrupted, and cholecystitis can develop. In the absence of bile in the intestine, lipid absorption is impaired and, without bile pigments, stools become light in color. If uncorrected, back-up of bile can cause liver damage, primary biliary cirrhosis, or pancreatitis. In most cases, however, the stones remain stationary and the symptoms are similar to chronic inflammation. If the gallbladder and stones are removed by surgery (cholecystectomy), most patients are cured completely. There is no evidence to suggest that a diet that is low in cholesterol will lower biliary cholesterol.

Most gallstones in the American population are unpigmented *cholesterol stones,* composed primarily of cholesterol, bile acids, and bilirubin. This type of stone can be treated by chemical dissolution, by using oral administration of bile acids (litholytic therapy), or by direct administration of methyl-tert-butyl ether (MTBE) into the gallbladder by percutaneous catheter. Risk factors for cholesterol stone formation include female sex, weight gain, overweight, high energy intake, ethnic factors (Pima Indian and Scandinavian), drugs (clofibrate, estrogens, and cholesterol sequestrants), and gastrointestinal disease (Kern, 1983; Maclure et al, 1989). Gallstones sometimes develop during dieting for weight reduction (Liddle et al, 1989).

Pigment stones typically consist predominantly of bilirubin polymers or calcium salts. In contrast to cholesterol lithiasis, risk factors associated with these stones are low body weight, a diet deficient in fat and protein, Far Eastern ancestry, bile stasis or infection, cirrhosis, sickle cell anemia, and thalassemia. Treatment involves the surgical removal of the stones or of the gallbladder. Extracorporeal shock-wave biliary lithotripsy (ESBT) can be used on these stones as well as on cholesterol stones and to fragment large stones into smaller pieces. ESBT in conjunction with chemical dissolution may prove most successful.

Cholecystitis

Inflammation of the gallbladder is known as *cholecystitis.* The primary cause is usually gallstones, which upon constriction of the gallbladder can obstruct the duct opening. Inflammation occurs as a result of the back-up of bile. The walls of the gallbladder become red and swollen, and sometimes pus collects and causes distention. During such episodes, the patient has right upper quadrant pain accompanied by nausea, vomiting, and flatulence.

Jaundice may also occur. Much of the pigment that gives the bile its greenish color is derived from the breakdown of red corpuscles. When biliary tract obstruction prevents bile from reaching the intestine, the coloring matter undergoes changes and returns to the circulation as bilirubin. The overflow of bilirubin into the general circulation causes the yellow skin pigmentation and the eye discoloration that are typical of jaundice.

Nutritional Care in Gallbladder Disease

The preferred treatment for both acute and chronic cholecystitis is surgery. However, until surgery can be performed, a low-fat diet should be recommended.

Acute Attack

An acute attack of cholecystitis occurs almost always in connection with an obstruction. When it does occur, the gallbladder should be kept as inactive as possible. Oral feedings are sometimes discontinued. However, when the patient does eat, all visible fat should be omitted, because dietary fats cause pain by stimulating the sphincter of Oddi. A formula diet low in fat can be given (see Appendix 33). Adherence to a low-fat diet (20 to 30% of kilocalories or about 50 grams of fat) is recommended until it is known whether surgical removal of the gallbladder is indicated. A combination of foods to provide this amount of fat is shown in Table 28–3.

Chronic Condition

Patients with chronic cholecystitis also require a diet that is low in fat (about 25% of total kilocalories). More strict limitation is undesirable, because fat in the intestines is important for some gallbladder stimulation and drainage of the biliary tract. The protein allowance is kept at the normal requirement, and the carbohydrate allowance is adjusted to achieve or maintain desirable weight.

The degree of food intolerance varies widely among individuals with gallbladder disease, but many commonly complain of foods they believe to be "gas-forming" or that cause them discomfort. It is best to determine from the patient any foods that should be eliminated for this reason. See Chapter 27 for a list of potentially gas-forming foods.

Because fat, and therefore the fat-soluble vitamins, is poorly absorbed, administration of water-soluble forms of vitamins A, D, E, and K may be necessary. Vitamin K has an important role in controlling bleeding in individuals afflicted with certain types of jaundice.

Although surgery is the treatment of choice for gallstones, conservative management is sometimes indicated. Chenodeoxycholic acid or ursodeoxycholic acid, normal constituents of human bile, will dissolve gallstones in most patients when given daily; however, this therapy may be necessary for 6 to 30 months. Lecithin, another component of bile, is also used to dissolve gallstones.

Gallbladder Surgery

Following gallbladder surgery, oral feedings are usually resumed with the return of bowel sounds or sometimes earlier, and the patient gradually progresses to a regular diet as tolerated. Enteral feeding by tube can begin as early as day 1 postoperatively. If enteral tube or oral feeding is not tolerated by days 5 to 7, some form of intravenous nutritional support should be started. Depending on individual tolerance, a low-fat diet is recommended for the first few weeks after surgery. Most patients tolerate a normal diet when all inflammation has disappeared. In the absence of the gallbladder, bile is stored in the large common duct connecting the liver and the small intestine. The tube stretches to perform its new function.

PANCREATIC DISEASE

Physiology and Function of the Pancreas

The pancreas is located deep in the upper abdomen, behind the stomach. Some of its cells manufacture insulin (endocrine function), and others secrete enzymes that participate in the digestion of protein, fats, and carbohydrates in the intestine (exocrine function). The duct leading from the pancreas joins a common tube through which both bile and pancreatic juices drain into the duodenum.

Pancreatitis

Pancreatitis is an inflammation of the pancreas characterized by edema, cellular exudate, and fat necrosis. It can be mild and self-limiting or severe with necrosis of pancreatic tissue. It can be acute or chronic, with pancreatic destruction so extensive that exocrine or endocrine pancreatic function is lost and steatorrhea or diabetes results.

The symptoms of pancreatitis can range from those of a mild stomach upset to severe upper abdominal pain, nausea and vomiting, distention, steatorrhea, edema, and shock, and death may result. The pain may radiate into the back and is increased by the ingestion of food.

The precise etiology of acute and chronic pancreatitis and pancreatic destruction is unknown. Possible causes include chronic alcoholism, biliary tract disease, ingestion of certain drugs, trauma, hypertriglyceridemia, and hypercalcemia. Alcohol is the leading cause of chronic pancreatitis (Hacker, 1988).

Pancreatic destruction may be caused by an obstruction to the flow of pancreatic juice. In the case of alcoholism, it is presumed that alcohol causes duodenitis and edema of the papilla of Vater. This causes the digestive juices to back up into the pancreas and to digest the organ itself. In severe cases, the enzymes move out of the pancreas and begin to digest surrounding fat tissue. When this happens, serum calcium falls to a dangerously low level, possibly as a result of "soap" formation by the calcium and the fatty acids created by fat necrosis. Movement of pancreatic amylase and lipase from the inflamed pancreas into the lymphatic system and the blood stream leads to the elevated serum levels of these enzymes, which are characteristic of pancreatic disease. The best laboratory test for confirming pancreatitis is a twofold or more elevation of total serum amylase (Steinberg, 1988). Other tests are given in Table 28-6.

TABLE 28-6. Some Tests of Pancreatic Function

Test	Significance
Secretin stimulation test	Measures pancreatic secretion, particularly bicarbonate, in response to secretin stimulation
Glucose tolerance test	Assesses endocrine function of the pancreas by measuring insulin response to a glucose load
72-hour stool fat test	Assesses exocrine function of the pancreas by measuring fat absorption that reflects pancreatic lipase secretion

Nutritional Care in Pancreatic Disease

Pancreatitis

The pain of pancreatitis is activated by the secretory activities of pancreatic enzymes and bile. The nutritional care is therefore adjusted to provide foods that will not stimulate these systems into action. During severe, acute attacks, all oral feeding is withheld and hydration is maintained intravenously.

It is a mistake to initiate feedings too soon. After 24 to 48 hours, a clear liquid diet may be given if tolerated. A defined formula diet consisting of amino acids, glucose, and a small amount of fat will not stimulate pancreatic secretions. In prolonged severe pancreatitis, total parenteral nutrition may be necessary. Fat emulsions can be used as long as the acute pancreatitis is not the basis for a hypertriglyceridemia.

In less severe attacks, easily digested, nonstimulating foods very low in fat should be given. Foods are better tolerated if divided into six small meals. The low-fat diet described in Table 28-3 can be used. However, there is also the problem of maintaining positive nitrogen balance in the presence of increased energy expenditure. Energy requirements may be as much as 150% of resting energy expenditure (Bouffard et al, 1989).

Chronic pancreatitis ensues when inflammation fails to subside or recurs at intervals. Persistent or recurrent pain is usually precipitated by meals. Large meals, fatty foods, and alcohol should all be avoided. Pancreatic enzyme replacement affords marked pain relief by decreasing exocrine secretions. Surgery is reserved for the most severe cases. Because of the nausea and vomiting provoked by pain, good nutritional status is difficult to maintain. Weight loss is common.

In long-standing pancreatitis of 5 to 6 years' duration, the pancreas has deteriorated to a point where it can no longer secrete a sufficient quantity of enzymes, resulting in maldigestion and malabsorption of protein and fat. Pancreatic enzyme replacement is mandatory.

Steatorrhea is a common occurrence, and because of malabsorption of the fat-soluble vitamins, water-soluble forms of the vitamins will be necessary. Pancrease, a pancreatic enzyme replacement administered orally after each meal, is the primary treatment for steatorrhea, but lowering the dietary fat intake to 40 to 60 g/day may bring additional benefit. In order to promote weight gain, the level of fat in the diet should be the maximum that the patient can tolerate without an increase in steatorrhea or pain. Substitution of MCT oil for dietary fat may bring further improvement in fat absorption and weight gain. Because pancreatic bicarbonate secretion will frequently be defective, bicarbonate and antacids should also be given to maintain the optimum pH level for enzyme activity. H_2 receptor antagonists that reduce gastric acid secretion may also help.

Effort should be made to cater to the patient's tolerances and preferences insofar as the diet prescription permits. However, alcohol is prohibited because it acts as an intestinal irritant and encourages recurrences.

In chronic cases with extensive pancreatic destruction, the insulin-secreting capacity of the pancreas decreases and glucose intolerance develops. Treatment with insulin and nutritional care similar to that used for a patient with diabetes mellitus is then required (see Chapter 31). These patients may also develop refractory hypoglycemia due to glucagon deficiency. Management is delicate and should have control of symptoms rather than normoglycemia as the goal.

Deficiency of pancreatic protease, necessary to cleave vitamin B_{12} from its carrier protein, frequently leads to vitamin B_{12} deficiency (Hacker, 1988). The vitamin should be given parenterally if needed. Vitamin B_{12} absorption should also improve with the administration of pancreatic enzymes.

Pancreatic Surgery

A common pancreatic surgical procedure is a *pancreatoduodenectomy* (Whipple procedure). A cholecystectomy and a vagotomy are often done at the same time. Partial or complete pancreatic insufficiency can result, depending on the surgical repair of the pancreatic stump. Even when the pancreatic duct is reanastomosed to the jejunum, there can still be pancreatic insufficiency. Nutritional care is similar to that for chronic pancreatitis.

CITED REFERENCES

Blendis LM and Jenkins DJA: Nutritional support in liver disease. *In* Shils ME and Young VR: Modern Nutrition in Health and Disease, 7th ed. Philadelphia, Lea & Febiger, 1988.

Bouffard YH et al: Energy expenditure during severe acute pancreatitis. J Parenter Enteral Nutr 13:26, 1989.

Cerra FB et al: Disease-specific amino acid infusion (FO8O) in hepatic encephalopathy: A prospective, randomized, double-blind, controlled trial. J Parenter Enteral Nutr 9:288, 1985.

Diehl AM: Alcoholic liver disease. *In* Chobanian SJ and Van Ness MM (eds): Manual of Clinical Problems in Gastroenterology. Boston, Little, Brown, 1988.

Diehl AM et al: Effect of parenteral amino acid supplementation in alcohol hepatitis. Hepatology 5:57, 1985.

Egberts EH et al: Branched chain amino acids in treatment of latent portosystemic encephalopathy. Gastroenterology 88:887, 1985.

Fenton JCB, Knight EJ, and Humpherson PL: Milk and cheese diet in portal-systemic encephalopathy. Lancet 1:164, 1966.

Fiaccadori F et al: Branched chain amino acid enriched solution in the treatment of hepatic encephalopathy: A controlled trial. *In* Capocaccia L, Fischer JE, and Rossi-Fanelli F (eds): Hepatic Encephalopathy in Chronic Liver Failure. New York, Plenum, 1984.

Fischer JE and Baldessarini RJ: False neurotransmitters and hepatic failure. Lancet 2:75, 1971.

Fischer JE and Bower RH: Nutritional support in liver disease. Surg Clin North Am 61:653, 1981.

Flink EB: Magnesium deficiency in alcoholism. Alcohol Clin Exp Res 10:590, 1986.

Freund H, Yoshimura N, and Fischer JE: Chronic hepatic encephalopathy: Long-term therapy with a branched-chain amino-acid–enriched elemental diet. JAMA 242:347, 1979.

Hacker JF: Chronic pancreatitis. *In* Chobanian SJ and Van Ness MM (eds): Manual of Clinical Problems in Gastroenterology. Boston, Little, Brown, 1988.

Hiyama DT and Fischer JE: Nutritional support in hepatic failure: Current thought in practice. Nutr Clin Prac 3:96, 1988.

Kern F Jr: Epidemiology and natural history of gallstones. Semin Liver Dis 3:87, 1983.

Liddle RA, Goldstein RB, and Saxton J: Gallstone formation during weight reduction dieting. Arch Intern Med 149:1750, 1989.

Lieber CS: Biochemical and molecular basis of alcohol-induced injury to liver and other tissues. N Engl J Med 319:1639, 1988a.

Lieber CS: The influence of alcohol on nutritional status. Nutr Rev 46:241, 1988b.

Lieber CS and Rubin E: Alcoholic fatty liver in man on a high protein low fat diet. Am J Med 44:200, 1968.

Maclure KM et al: Weight, diet, and the risk of symptomatic gallstones in middle-aged women. N Engl J Med 321:563, 1989.

Mezitis NHE: Nutritional management in liver disease. Nutr Clin Prac 3:108, 1988.

Pemberton CM et al: Mayo Clinic Diet Manual: A Handbook of Dietary Practices, 6th ed. Toronto, BC Decker, 1988, pp 174–177.

Schafer DF and Jones EA: Hepatic encephalopathy and the gamma-aminobutyric acid neurotransmitter system. Lancet 1:18, 1982.

Shronts EP: Nutritional assessment of adults with end-stage hepatic failure. Nutr Clin Prac 3:113, 1988.

Shronts EP et al: Nutrition support of the adult liver transplant candidate. J Am Diet Assoc 87:441, 1987.

Steinberg WM: Acute pancreatitis: Diagnosis and management. *In* Chobanian SJ and Van Ness MM (eds): Manual of Clinical Problems in Gastroenterology. Boston, Little, Brown, 1988.

Wahren J et al: Is intravenous administration of branched chain amino acids effective in the treatment of hepatic encephalopathy? A multicenter study. Hepatology 3:475, 1983.

Zieve L, Doizaki WM, and Zieve FJ: Synergism between mercaptans and ammonia or fatty acids in the production of coma: A possible role for mercaptans in the pathogenesis of hepatic coma. J Lab Clin Med 83:16, 1974.

ADDITIONAL REFERENCES

Achord JL: Nutrition, alcohol and the liver. Am J Gastroenterol 83:244, 1987.

Apparent per capita ethanol consumption—United States, 1977–86. MMWR 1989; 38:800; JAMA 263:354, 1990.

Bank S: Chronic pancreatitis: Clinical features and medical management. Am J Gastroenterol 81:153, 1986.

Barch DH: Vitamin deficiencies in the alcoholic patient. Nutr MD 13(10):1, 1987.

Carnitine and alcoholism. Br J Addict 84:689, 1989.

Cossack ZT, Scheinberg IH, and Sternlieb I: The efficacy of oral zinc therapy as an alternative to penicillamine for Wilson's disease. N Engl J Med 318:630, 1988.

Dietary beans: A risk factor for cholesterol gallstones? Nutr Rev 47:369, 1989.

Fraser CL and Arieff AI: Hepatic encephalopathy. N Engl J Med 313:865, 1986.

James SP: Primary biliary cirrhosis (Editorial). N Engl J Med 312:1055, 1985.

Lindeman RD: Mineral deficiencies in the alcoholic patient. Nutr MD 13(11):1, 1987.

Reuler JB, Girard DE, and Cooney TG: Wernicke's encephalopathy. N Engl J Med 312:1035, 1985.

Smithgall JM: The copper-controlled diet: Current aspects of dietary copper restriction in management of copper metabolism disorders. J Am Diet Assoc 85:609, 1985.

Taylor KB: Diet and gallstone formation. Nutr MD 12(6):1, 1986.

Uribe M et al: Treatment of chronic portal-systemic encephalopathy with vegetable and animal protein diets: A controlled crossover study. Dig Dis Sci 27:1109, 1982.

Welch CE and Malt RA: Surgery of the stomach, duodenum, gallbladder and bile ducts. N Engl J Med 316:999, 1987.

Wolfe MM and Jensen RT: Zollinger-Ellison syndrome. N Engl J Med 317:1200, 1987.

CHAPTER 29

PHYSIOLOGIC STRESS: TRAUMA, SEPSIS, BURNS, AND SURGERY

Jayne Williamson, R.D.

CHAPTER OUTLINE

Metabolic Response to Stress
Nutritional Assessment
Nutritional Care
Sepsis
Trauma of Accidental Injury
Head Injury
Extensive Burns
Surgery

KEY TERMS

ACUTE-PHASE PROTEINS—proteins needed during stress; immunoglobulins, leukocytes, lymphocytes, hemoglobin, albumin, and enzymes necessary for protein synthesis

ADRENOCORTICOTROPHIC HORMONE (ACTH) OR CORTICOTROPIN—a hormone secreted by the anterior pituitary gland that acts primarily on the adrenal cortex, stimulating its growth and secretion of corticosteroids

CYTOKINE—a nonantibody protein that is released by cells and that acts as an intercellular mediator

EBB PHASE—initial response to bodily insult characterized by lower blood pressure, cardiac output, body temperature, and oxygen consumption that results in hypovolemia, hypoperfusion, and lactic acidosis

FLOW OR ADAPTIVE PHASE—a neuroendocrine response to physiologic stress that follows the ebb phase and is characterized by hypermetabolism and hypercatabolism for the purpose of wound healing and preserving nervous system integrity

HIGH-FLOW SEPSIS—a neuroendocrine response to sepsis similar to the flow or adaptive phase response to physiologic stress; characterized by hypermetabolism, hepatic gluconeogenesis, and peripheral lipolysis and proteolysis

INTERLEUKIN-1—a protein factor produced by macrophages in response to antigenic or mitogenic stimulation that promotes fibroblast proliferation and release of proteolytic enzymes and prostaglandins in inflammatory processes; the main mediator of fever

LOW-FLOW SEPSIS—a neuroendocrine response to sepsis characterized by cardiac decompensation, inadequate tissue perfusion, and severe acidosis

LYMPHOKINE—a nonantibody protein that is released by sensitized lymphocytes on contact with antigen and which acts as a mediator of the immune response

MONOKINE—a nonantibody protein that is released by monocytes or macrophages and acts as a mediator of the immune response

SEPTIC ENCEPHALOPATHY—a clouding of consciousness similar to hepatic encephalopathy that reflects a hepatic decompensation common in sepsis

TUMOR NECROSIS FACTOR (CACHECTIN)—a hormone-like protein produced by macrophages that releases fat by reducing the concentration of enzymes required for the production and storage of fat, induces a state of anorexia, and can also produce shock

Severe physiologic stress of the kind that accompanies traumatic injury, sepsis, extensive burns, or major surgery provokes a *stress response* that is both protective and destructive. Nutrition therapy is crucial in preventing further tissue degeneration, promoting healing, and providing for anabolic recovery.

METABOLIC RESPONSE TO STRESS

Extreme physiologic stress is countered by a unique neuroendocrine response that affects a wide variety of metabolic parameters. The body does not respond to all physiologic stress situations in the same manner or with the same intensity; nonetheless, the responses are similar in many respects.

The initial reaction to severe bodily insult, sometimes referred to as the *"ebb"* phase, is primarily a reaction to shock. It is characterized by lower blood pressure, cardiac output, body temperature, and oxygen consumption and results in hypovolemia, hypoperfusion, and lactic acidosis.

The *"flow,"* or adaptive phase, represents mobilization of body resources to counteract these effects. It is a positive response but nonetheless produces a negative nitrogen balance as a necessary side effect. In contrast to the "ebb" phase, which is of brief duration, the "flow" phase lasts for several weeks or even longer. In this stage, a neuroendocrine response stimulates a state of hypermetabolism and hypercatabolism for the purpose of wound healing and preserving nervous system integrity. This is accomplished at the cost of endogenous energy stores, in particular protein tissue from skeletal muscle.

Neuroendocrine Response

Afferent nervous signals from the wound reach the hypothalamus, which in turn stimulates the anterior pituitary to release adrenocorticotropic hormone (ACTH). This hormone acts on the adrenal cortex, causing it to release cortisol, whose primary role is mobilization of amino acids from skeletal muscle. It also increases the protein and glycogen content of the liver and enhances its capacity for gluconeogenesis.

The sympathetic nervous system is sensitive to the stimuli of excitement, pain, fear, and hypovolemia, and the adrenal medulla responds by releasing epinephrine and norepinephrine. These hormones stimulate hepatic glycogenolysis, fat mobilization, and gluconeogenesis. A rise in glucagon may also be related to increased sympathetic activity.

Stress initiates the release of aldosterone, a corticosteroid that causes renal sodium retention, and antidiuretic hormone (ADH), which stimulates renal tubular water resorption. The resultant conservation of salt and water supports the circulating blood volume (Fig. 29–1).

The altered endocrine state is also mediated by secretions of mononuclear phagocytes (cytokines), of which *interleukin-1 (IL-1)* is currently the best understood. IL-1 is released by macrophages as a response to infection or inflammation from trauma. Among its effects are production of fever, hypozincemia, hypoferre-

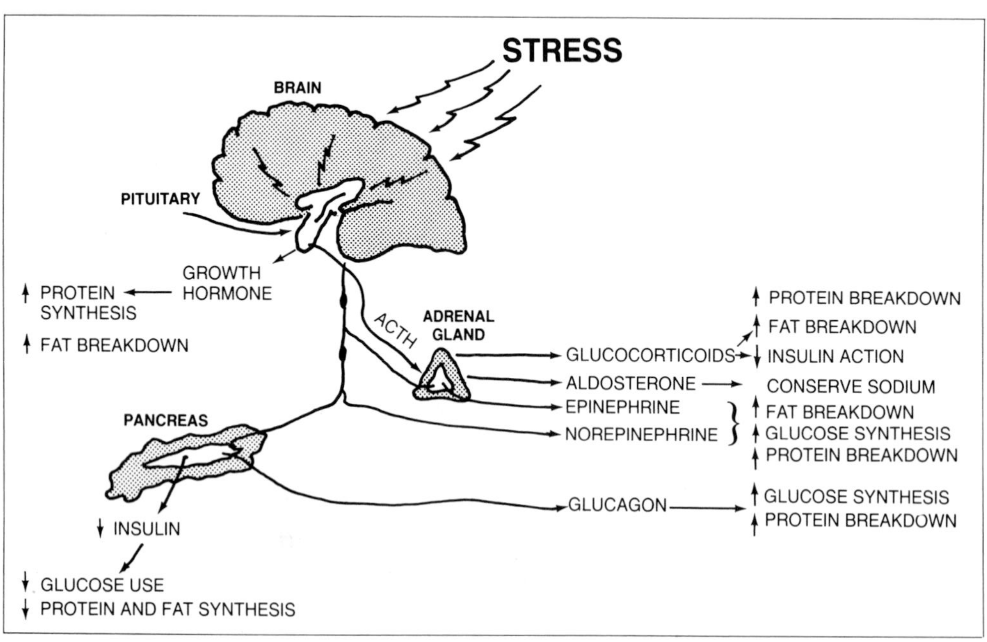

FIGURE 29–1. *Effect of stress on metabolism. (Redrawn from Berdanier CD: The many faces of stress. Nutr Today 22(2):12, 1987, p 13.)*

mia, and synthesis of acute-phase proteins (Bynoe et al, 1988; Ott et al, 1987). Another monokine, *tumor necrosis factor (TNF),* also called *cachectin,* stimulates production of the catabolic hormones (Spitzer et al, 1988). With the availability of recombinant mediators, the participation of each one can be more clearly defined. It may be possible to use them therapeutically to modify the injury response to enhance the effect of nutritional support (Pomposelli et al, 1988).

Hypermetabolic State

Energy Expenditure

Severe forms of physiologic stress are characterized by increases in basal energy expenditure (BEE) that are sometimes dramatic. Increases in BEE may range from 15 to 25% in fractures of the long bone to 100% in severe burns and injuries of the brain (Table 29–1). In this respect, stress differs considerably from a state of starvation in which the BEE actually decreases to conserve endogenous fuel supplies.

The hypermetabolic state is marked by increased blood flow and oxygen consumption in the wound area. Up to 80% of glucose consumed is used in anaerobic metabolism and production of lactate by the fibroblasts, macrophages, and leukocytes involved in wound healing.

Energy Sources

The energy requirements of heightened metabolism require rapid mobilization of endogenous fuel supplies. Glycogen stores are quickly exhausted, and lipolysis of triglyceride stores proceeds at a rapid rate. Body proteins are broken down to release amino acids that provide substrate for hepatic gluconeogenesis.

Although fatty acids are the major fuel source, the brain, nervous system, and red blood cells all require glucose for metabolism. In addition, the wound uses glucose extensively as an energy source. These primary glucose needs are met through gluconeogenesis, which takes place mostly in the liver and to some extent in the kidney. Because muscle tissue lacks a necessary enzyme, glucose-6-phosphatase, it cannot carry out gluconeogenesis; however, it does supply most of the amino acids required for this purpose. Glucose is formed from glycerol, alpha-keto acids derived from glucogenic amino acids, lactate, and pyruvate.

Protein Metabolism

Skeletal amino acids mobilized primarily through the action of cortisol are available to the liver for synthesis of new glucose, substrates for wound healing, and the "acute-phase" proteins needed during stress. The latter include immunoglobulins, leukocytes and lymphocytes to fight infection, hemoglobin and albumin to replace blood loss, and the enzymes necessary for protein synthesis.

Oxidation of branched-chain amino acids (BCAA) (leucine, isoleucine, and valine) from the skeletal muscle is increased during injury. These are deaminated, and the keto acids are converted to tricarboxylic intermediates for local metabolism. The amine groups thus released are attached to pyruvate and glutamic acid to form alanine and glutamine, which serve as a mechanism for transporting amine groups to the liver for urea synthesis and provide alpha-keto skeletons for glucose synthesis. In lactic acidosis, glutamine contributes to acid-base homeostasis by providing amine groups for combination with hydrogen ion to form ammonium ions, which are then excreted in the urine. It also serves as an oxidative fuel for the gastrointestinal tract; glu-

TABLE 29–1. Classification of Catabolism*†

Clinical Situation	Degree of Catabolism	Urea Nitrogen (g/day)	Increase of Resting Metabolic Rate Over Basic Metabolic Rate (%)	Total Energy Requirement‡ (kcal)
Person in bed	1° (Normal)	<5	None	1,800
Uncomplicated surgery	2° (Mild)	5–10	0–20	1,800–2,200
Multiple fractures or trauma	3° (Moderate)	10–15	20–50	2,200–2,700
Acute major infections or major burns	4° (Severe)	>15	50–125	2,700–4,000 or more

* Adapted from Rutten P et al: Determination of optimal hyperalimentation infusion rate. J Surg Res 18:477, 1975.

† Classification of patients according to the following: (1) obligate nitrogen loss (N obg.) expressed in grams of urea N per 24 hr; (2) energy expenditure expressed as percentage increase of the resting metabolic expenditure over calculated basal energy expenditure.

‡ This total resting metabolic requirement includes the amount needed for activity (about 20%) since these patients usually are not active, and 10% for specific dynamic action (SDA). This is a rough estimate for a 70-kg man and depends on the patient's size.

tamine consumption by the bowel and kidney is accelerated following injury.

Mobilization of amino acids results in a rapid loss of lean body mass and an increased negative nitrogen balance that continues until the cause of the stress is relieved. Breakdown of protein tissue also releases phosphorus, potassium, magnesium, and creatinine, all of which are lost in the urine. (Nitrogen balance is discussed in Chapter 17.)

Carbohydrate Metabolism

During stress response, insulin release is blocked by epinephrine at the same time that glucagon secretion is increased. The result is a rapid increase in hepatic glucose production. This, combined with a marked insulin insensitivity, results in hyperglycemia and a pseudodiabetic state called *"stress diabetes."* Insulin action is also blocked by epinephrine. A side effect of the high blood glucose level is anorexia, which is heightened by decreased peristalsis that results from the action of sympathetic nerve activity on the intestinal tract.

Lipid Metabolism

Lipolysis is accelerated following injury or stress. Fatty acids are mobilized and oxidized at an accelerated rate; however, ketosis does not develop, probably because of the continued stimulation of the sympathetic nervous system. In this manner, adaptation to the starvation of physiologic stress differs from that seen in uncomplicated starvation of voluntary fasting or food deprivation. After 1 week of such fasting, a state of ketosis develops in which ketones constitute an effective substitute for glucose, thus reducing the need for gluconeogenesis and conserving body protein to the greatest possible extent. This does not happen in the flow phase of physiologic stress.

Fluid and Electrolyte Balance

Retention of fluid and sodium as the result of aldosterone and antidiuretic hormone (ADH) action can lead to a weight gain of as much as 10 to 20% of usual weight during fluid resuscitation. This effect is much greater in the injured patient than in the postsurgical patient.

Fever

Fever accelerates cell proliferation and wound healing. The common post-trauma fever of 1 to 2° C elevation in temperature is caused by action of IL-1. About two thirds of this increase in heat production appears to be visceral, and the remainder occurs in the extremities. Alterations in superficial blood flow move heat from the visceral tissues to the wound. When the fever is not excessive and the patient is asymptomatic, the fever is usually not treated.

Acute Renal Failure

As a consequence of trauma, acute renal failure may accompany a ruptured abdomen, sepsis, multiple organ failure, or hepatorenal syndrome. It is associated with higher rates of catabolism and other metabolic imbalances. Further discussion of the particular nutritional care indicated appears in Chapter 35.

Anabolic Recovery Phase

The turning point from catabolism to anabolism does not usually occur until all wounds or burns are closed or the infection is resolved. During this "corticoid withdrawal phase," a drop in the levels of corticoids is followed by spontaneous sodium and water diuresis, a positive potassium balance, and a reduction in nitrogen excretion. The transition may last 1 or 2 days and is followed by a period of anabolism. Lean body mass and muscular strength increase, with a daily gain of 60 to 120 grams of lean tissue and about 250 grams of body weight. The total amount of nitrogen that was lost is ultimately regained; however, this process occurs at a much slower rate than that at which it was lost (Souba and Wilmore, 1988). This transition to anabolism can take place only in the presence of nutritional support.

NUTRITIONAL ASSESSMENT

At present, it is difficult to monitor the contribution of nutritional support in the progress of the traumatized patient. The traditional markers of nutritional status that are discussed in Chapter 17 are not always useful. Retention of large volumes of fluid given during resuscitative efforts may expand the volume of body water and distort anthropometric measurements. Body weight may increase as much as 10 to 20% and then fall alarmingly low when these fluids are lost during the recovery and healing phase (Souba and Wilmore, 1988). Expanded vascular volume and altered capillary permeability cause plasma markers such as serum albumin and transferrin to appear low. Skin tests measuring delayed cutaneous hypersensitivity as a means of assessing immune status (and thus protein nutriture) usually remain unresponsive for at least 10 days (Bynoe et al, 1988).

NUTRITIONAL CARE

Timing

The first emphasis of care is removal of the stress through procedures such as repairing the wound, draining the abscess, covering the burns, or treating the infection. Nutritional support should begin as soon as vital functions are stable, fluid and electrolyte and acid-base balances are achieved, and tissue perfusion is adequate to allow transport of oxygen and fuel. Nutritional support during the catabolic phase will probably not result in positive nitrogen balance, but it may slow the loss of body protein. Every day that a moderately stressed patient does not receive adequate support may require 3 to 5 days of such support for "catch up" (ASPEN Board of Directors, 1986).

Unless exogenous protein is supplied within 5 to 7 days, protein synthesis declines, and weakness, loss of immunocompetence, hypoalbuminemia, failure of wound healing, further infection, decubitus ulcers from skin breakdown, respiratory insufficiency from respiratory muscle weakness, and eventually multiple organ failure and death may result.

Route

Evidence now supports the value of early enteral feeding in maintaining gastrointestinal integrity, absorptive capacity, and immune function. Enterally fed patients develop fewer infections, probably because translocation of gut bacteria is minimized (Moore and Jones, 1986). Initially, those with pelvic fractures or multiple gastrointestinal injuries may require total parenteral nutrition (TPN); however, as long as gut continuity remains, even these patients can be fed with gastrostomies or needle catheter or standard jejunostomies. The transition from these procedures to oral feeding should be supported with enteral tube feeding to maintain optimal energy and protein intake. Complete oral feeding may be delayed by impairment of chewing, swallowing, or anorexia induced by pain-relieving medications, or post-traumatic shock and depression.

Monitoring

Monitoring of the enteral or parenteral feeding is very important to determine the effectiveness of therapy. Indirect calorimetry provides information on energy requirements, and daily weighings monitor intake and output. Serum electrolytes, blood urea nitrogen, blood glucose evaluations, and periodic nitrogen balance assessments show how well the requirements are being met (see Chapter 30).

Energy

Determination of Energy Requirements

Energy requirements may be determined either by indirect calorimetry using a bedside metabolic cart or by calculation as BEE with an added factor for activity and degree of trauma. As a rule, energy and protein needs are proportional to the degree of trauma.

A method for determining energy requirements using the Harris-Benedict formula and the activity and injury factors developed by Long (Long et al, 1979) is given in Table 29–2.

Recent data accumulated by the use of metabolic carts to measure O_2 and CO_2 have demonstrated that patients do not need two to three times their BEE as has been advocated in the past (Bynoe et al, 1988). For most patients requiring critical care, provision of 40 to 45 kcal/kg ideal body weight (IBW) is sufficient to achieve anabolism and rehabilitation. For most other patients, 30 to 35 kcal/kg IBW is adequate for maintenance and preservation of nitrogen balance (Bynoe et al, 1988). The rule of thumb is 35 to 40 kcal/kg.

Source of Energy: Glucose Versus Fat

Large quantities of glucose, once thought to avert gluconeogenesis during the hypermetabolic phase, have the following disadvantages: potential for thrombophlebitis (if given parenterally), hyperglycemia with osmotic diuresis, hyperinsulinemia with impaired mobilization of lipid from fat stores, and increased CO_2 production due to the carbohydrate metabolism. Insulin is shunted into peripheral tissues at the expense of visceral organs. A more appropriate energy source is a mixture of lipid and glucose in which 30 to 40% of the energy is provided by lipid. Because the maximal rate of glucose utilization is 4 to 5 mg/kg/min (400 to 500 g/day in a 70-kg adult) and 2 mg/kg/min at rest, dextrose concentration is usually a 15 to 20% solution.

TABLE 29–2. Determination of Energy and Protein Requirements in Stress

Total energy requirement = basal energy expenditure (BEE) × activity factor × injury factor

BEE (male) = 66.47 + 13.75W + 5.0H − 6.76A

BEE (female) = 655.1 + 9.56W + 1.85H − 4.68A

W = weight in kg; H = height in cm; A = age in years.

BEE is calculated using the Harris-Benedict formula explained in Chapter 2.

*Activity Factors**	*Injury Factors**
1.2 Confined to bed	1.2 Minor operation
1.3 Out of bed	1.35 Skeletal trauma
	1.6 Major sepsis
	2.1 Severe burn

Protein requirement

Method 1:

16% of total energy requirement = kilocalories from protein

Kilocalories from protein/4 kcal/g of protein = grams of protein

Method 2:

Cal : N ratio of 150 : 1

Total energy requirement/150 = grams of nitrogen

Grams of nitrogen × 6.25 = grams of protein

* Activity and injury factors are from Long CL et al: Metabolic response to injury and illness: Estimation of energy and protein needs from indirect calorimetry and nitrogen balance. J Parenter Enteral Nutr 3:452, 1979.

Protein is added to stimulate tissue synthesis. Glucose is usually well tolerated at a rate of 2 to 3 mg/kg/min (Bynoe et al, 1988) (see Chapter 30).

Protein

Determination of Protein Requirements

The goal of nutritional support is to supply enough protein to promote anabolism, along with sufficient calories to ensure that protein will not be used as a source of energy. The rate of nitrogen excretion varies for different trauma states, thus nitrogen balance should be monitored to assess the adequacy of protein and the energy intake.

Protein needs may be determined by calculation using standard values or by means of a nitrogen balance study. Although the latter method is more precise, it requires more laboratory support than is usually available. Nitrogen output is commonly estimated by measuring the urea in a 24-hour urine sample and by adding a factor of 4 grams to account for nonurea nitrogen as well as fecal and integumental losses (see Chapter 17).

Calorie-to-nitrogen ratios of 100 to 200 kcal/g of nitrogen or a nonprotein calorie-to-nitrogen ratio of 75 to 175 kcal/g of nitrogen are appropriate. In most cases, the moderately stressed patient requires 1 to 1.5 grams of protein per kilogram of body weight per day, and the severely stressed patient requires 1.5 to 2 g/kg (see Table 29–2).

The optimal protein intake for depleted, stressed adults is 14 to 20% of total energy. This level, in the presence of 40 to 45 kcal/kg, promotes positive nitrogen balance and the restoration of lean body mass and protein reserves. At this protein intake, the kilocalorie to nitrogen ratio is 100 to 150 : 1. It is therefore possible to approximate the nitrogen requirement in grams by dividing the total energy requirement in kilocalories by 100 or 150. The protein requirement (in grams) can then be determined by multiplying the grams of nitrogen by 6.25. Dividing the kilocalories by 16 for a 100 : 1 kcal to nitrogen ratio and by 24 for a 150 : 1 kcal to nitrogen ratio gives the same results. See Clinical Insight, below.

Initial weight gain with the achievement of positive nitrogen balance is really a reflection of body water retention, because water is incorporated into new muscle tissue and glycogen is restored. After the initial weight gain, further gain is minimal despite the continued positive nitrogen balance, because spontaneous diuresis keeps body water level down. Restoration of lean tissue and fat usually occurs at the rate of 250 grams or ½ lb/day with optimal nutritional support. Rates greater than this reflect undesirable water retention.

Vitamins

Vitamin requirements are probably increased during stress, but it is not known to what extent. In most cases the patient is receiving increased amounts of energy, and this is usually accompanied by increased amounts of vitamins.

Because ascorbic acid is required for the formation of collagen, a deficiency is associated with the delay or prevention of wound healing and with chronic, nonhealing cutaneous ulcers. The amount of this vitamin to supplement remains controversial. Megadoses of vitamin C have been associated with diarrhea, renal calculi, and lowered serum B_{12} levels. It is suggested that levels of 100 to 300 mg/day will maintain adequate plasma levels postoperatively.

Vitamin A deficiency may also interfere with wound healing, because this vitamin is necessary for normal epithelialization. It may also help to prevent gastric stress ulceration.

Vitamin K is of particular interest in surgery, be-

CLINICAL INSIGHT: Determining Energy and Protein Requirements

Example: Ms L has had a long bout with ulcerative colitis, followed by surgery with a resulting ileostomy.

Basal energy expenditure (BEE):

1,400 kcal (determined from Harris-Benedict formula)

Total energy expenditure (EE):

BEE + (BEE × 1.3 [activity factor]) + (BEE × 1.3 [injury factor])

1400 + 420 + 420 = 2240 kcal

Protein requirement:

16% of EE: 2,240 × 0.16 = 358.4 kcal

358 kcal/4 kcal/g protein = 89.5 g protein

OR

kcal : N ratio of 150 : 1

2,240 kcal/150 = 14.9 g nitrogen

14.9 × 6.25 = 93.3 g protein

cause a deficiency is characterized by a decrease in prothrombin content of the blood with a resultant defect in clotting. An increased prothrombin time may be an indicator for vitamin K supplementation.

Three B vitamins (thiamin, riboflavin, and niacin) provide essential coenzyme factors to metabolize carbohydrate and protein and can be rapidly depleted after major trauma. It is believed that their requirements are increased in hypermetabolic states, but the extent of the increase is uncertain. It appears that thiamin deficiency during wound healing impairs collagen synthesis and decreases the breaking strength of the wound (Alvarez and Gilbreath, 1982; Thiamin . . . , 1982). However, the exact mechanism is not known.

SEPSIS

Two physiologic patterns evolve in response to sepsis: (1) a hyperdynamic high-flow response characterized by increased cardiac output and hyperperfusion of tissues, and (2) a low-flow response with cardiac decompensation, inadequate tissue perfusion, and severe acidosis. The latter is difficult to reverse and usually results in death.

The catabolic response of high-flow sepsis is characterized by fever, hypermetabolism, and alterations in glucose, protein, and fat metabolism similar to those seen in other forms of physiologic stress. Hepatic gluconeogenesis as well as peripheral lipolysis and proteolysis are increased (Fig. 29–2). Hypermetabolism may increase the total BEE by 20 to 60%. Return to normal metabolism and a positive nitrogen balance depends on the elimination of sepsis.

The nutritional status of the host influences the function of its immune system; thus, the susceptibility, severity, and outcome of infection are all worsened by malnutrition. Infections in malnourished children are more frequent and develop rapidly and with morbid intensity; for example, measles in children with protein-energy malnutrition can be fatal.

Fever

Part of the hypermetabolism experienced in sepsis is the result of fever, which is usually present with infection. For each degree Celsius of elevation, the metabolic rate increases from 10 to 13% (7.2% per degree Fahrenheit). Such an increase can be as high as 40% in a patient with a temperature of 104° F (40° C). If the patient is restless, delirious, or coughing, the total energy need is increased further.

IL-1 is the main polypeptide mediator of fever. This monokine fills a number of roles in the stress response to infection, some of which can be considered beneficial. Conversely, the enormous energy demand that fever inflicts on the host may adversely affect the outcome. The function of IL-1 appears to be decreased in the malnourished host, possibly by a mechanism for reducing the energy demands of fever (Chandra, 1988; Keenan et al, 1982).

Septic Encephalopathy

Septic encephalopathy is a clouding of consciousness similar to hepatic encephalopathy and reflects a hepatic decompensation common in sepsis. The plasma amino acid pattern is similar to that described in liver disease and, because BCAA appear to be effective in managing hepatic encephalopathy, it is suggested that

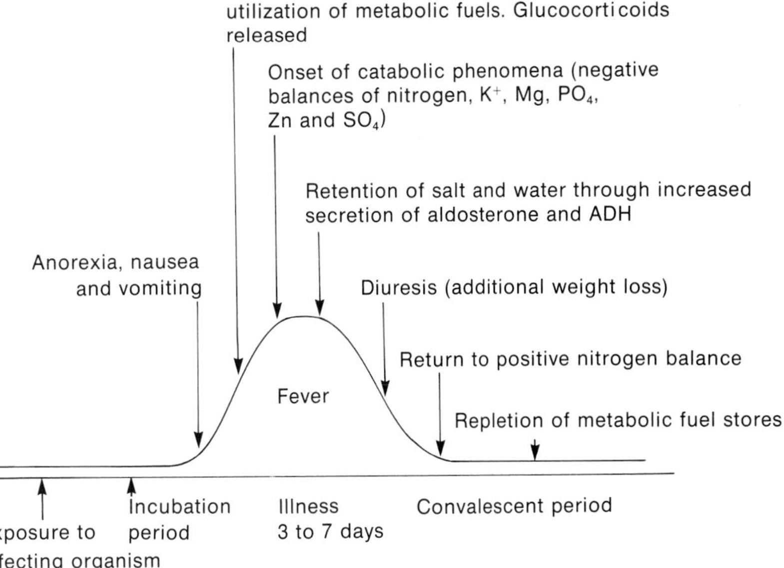

FIGURE 29–2. *Timing of catabolic response to infection. (Adapted from Beisel WR: The influence of infection or injury on nutritional requirements during adolescence. In McKigney JI and Munro HN [eds]: Nutrient Requirements in Adolescence. Cambridge, MA, MIT Press, 1976, p 259.)*

they may also be effective in managing or preventing septic encephalopathy. However, reports are not conclusive (Bower et al, 1986).

Nutritional Care

The goal of nutritional care in sepsis should be support of the beneficial aspects of changed protein metabolism (increased hepatic protein synthesis and enhanced activity of the host defense mechanisms) rather than prevention of the negative aspects of increased muscle proteolysis and negative nitrogen balance.

Fluids

Fluids are of major importance in the treatment of infections. Often 3 to 4 liters of liquid are required daily to achieve optimal hydration. Very sweet liquids tend to be unappealing and frequently cause gastric disturbance as well as abdominal distention. Less-sweet lemonade and carbonated beverages such as ginger ale are better tolerated. Protein-containing fluids such as some supplements are preferable because they help to spare body protein. If the patient is nauseated and vomiting and is too ill to take fluids by mouth, fluid may be given parenterally.

Energy and Protein

During the acute phase of infection, it is almost impossible to achieve positive nitrogen balance because of the catabolic stress response and the anorexia that typically accompanies infection. However, nutritional support can reduce the protein loss. Positive nitrogen balance can usually be achieved during the anabolic phase with protein levels of 1.2 to 2 g/kg, about 20% of the kilocalories (Blackburn, 1989). Energy levels of 35–45 kcal/kg and nitrogen to kilocalorie ratios of 100:1 are usually appropriate. BCAA may be beneficial in promoting hepatic protein synthesis and reducing insulin resistance (Bower, 1986; Blackburn, 1989). Hepatic usage of protein in sepsis is optimal when 20–30% of the calories are administered as fat. However, intravenous fat emulsions should not exceed 30 g/day (Blackburn, 1989). During the acute phase, provision of more than 1.2 grams of protein/kg does not result in improved nitrogen balance but only increases resting energy expenditure (REE), O_2 consumption, and CO_2 production as it is oxidized (Grieg et al, 1987).

Fifty to 55% of the energy is provided as glucose (Blackburn, 1989) and the remainder as lipid.

Vitamins

Vitamin supplements are usually advised. Requirements for thiamin, riboflavin, and niacin parallel increased energy needs. Antibiotics and other drugs may interfere with intestinal synthesis of the B-complex vitamins (see Chapter 25).

Minerals

Loss of potassium, phosphate, and magnesium accompany the proteolysis and negative nitrogen balance during the acute phase of illness. At the same time, there is a retention of sodium and water. The serum levels of these electrolytes should be monitored. Spontaneous diuresis occurs as the infection abates.

The anemia sometimes seen in infection is not caused by deficient intake of iron but rather by increased hepatic uptake. The removal of iron as well as zinc from the blood deprives bacteria of nutrients necessary for their proliferation and is a host defense mechanism. Supplemental iron is contraindicated because increased serum levels might worsen the infection (Loggie and Hinchey, 1984).

Zinc may be required during a prolonged infective illness, because it is not sequestered as well as iron and is lost in the urine in increasing amounts. However, serum levels do not reflect a zinc deficiency.

Serum copper levels rise during the course of an infection, sometimes as much as threefold, owing to the increased hepatic outpouring of ceruloplasmin. This acute-phase protein is thought to serve a specific protective function during infection (see Chapter 7).

Meal Plan

Frequent small liquid feedings are usually best tolerated in the acute stage. When the intake is expanded, it is important that special attention be given to the selection of food, because most patients with fevers have poor appetites. An attempt should be made to make foods appealing through the careful choice of color, temperature, and texture.

Table 30–1 illustrates incorporation of increased protein and energy into the daily meal plan in 500-kcal steps. The choice of food for the addition of energy is governed by the preference and tolerance of the patient.

When the appetite is very poor, small meals and a concentrated supplement are tolerated best, because patients are often overwhelmed by the quantity of food served on the high-calorie, high-nutrient diets. When the patient cannot consume enough food to meet the increased energy and protein requirements, supplemental or complete enteral or parenteral tube feeding should be used.

TRAUMA OF ACCIDENTAL INJURY

Trauma from motor vehicle accidents, gunshot, or stab wounds or other severe injury is the major cause of death in individuals between the ages of 5 and 35 years

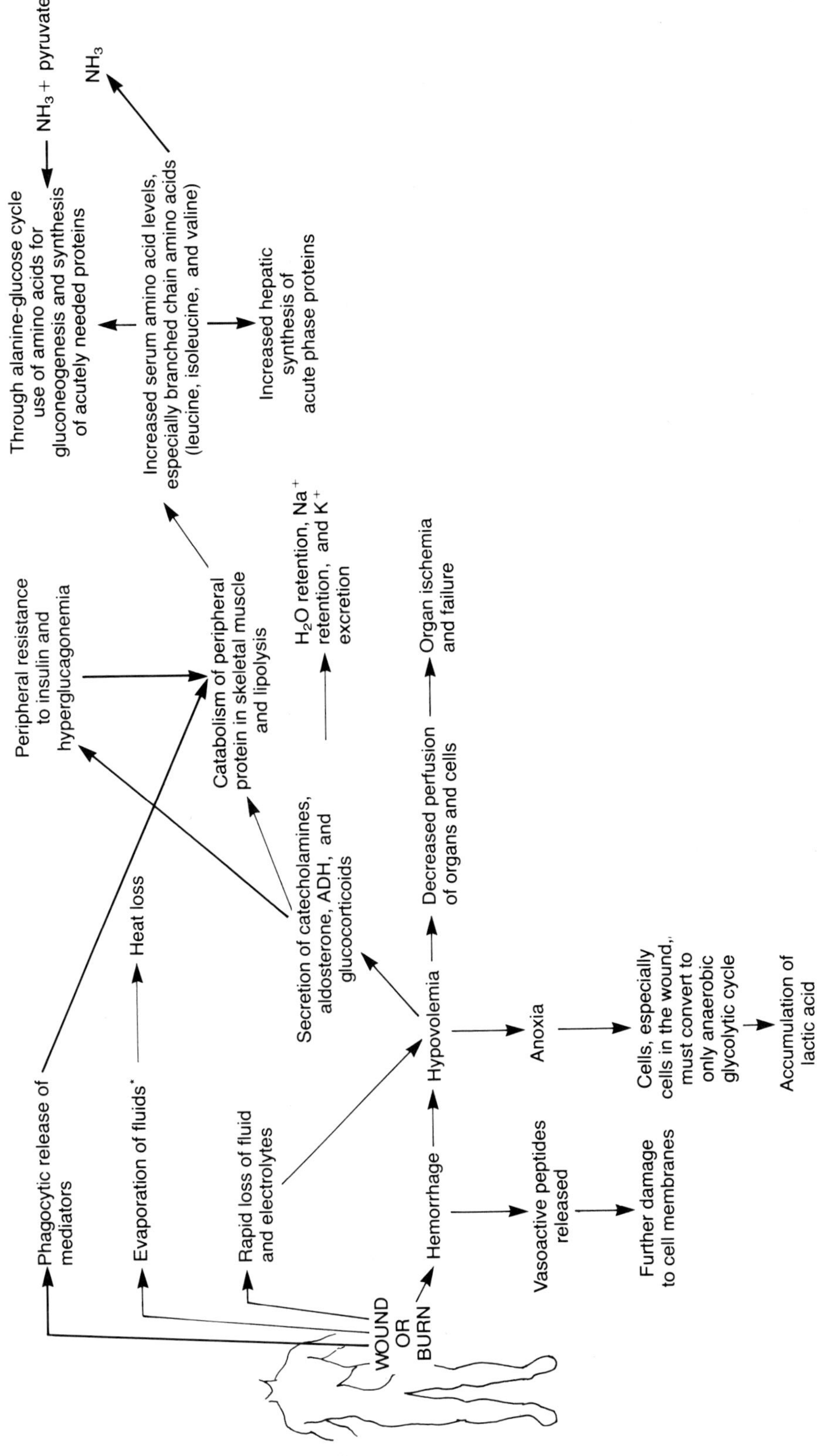

*Mainly occurs in the patient with extensive burns

FIGURE 29–3. *Physiologic and metabolic changes immediately after an injury or burn. The extent of these changes depends on the severity of the trauma.*

in the United States. This type of physiologic stress is characterized by pain and shock and frequently hypovolemia as a result of blood loss from severe wounds. Although the stress response to this type of injury is similar to that seen in other forms of physiologic stress, it is frequently more intense and often continues for a longer period. Severe functional imbalance and loss of fluids and electrolytes may take place (Fig. 29–3).

Protein catabolism characteristic of the stress response is amplified by losses of protein-rich fluids from open wounds. Healing of multiple fractures often involves prolonged immobilization, which contributes to the loss of calcium as well as to further loss of protein. With immobilization, body weight may increase dramatically 10 to 20% above earlier levels.

Nutritional Care

Replacement of losses and promotion of healing are the aims of nutritional care. During the first 24 to 48 hours after the injury, it is necessary to maintain blood volume and electrolyte balance, and aggressive nutritional support is not important. After this time, the diet should be appropriate to resist infection, promote wound healing, regain muscular strength, and prevent weight loss. Adequate protein and calories should be supplied to meet the patient's estimated needs.

When the injury involves bone fracture, intakes of calcium and vitamin D require special attention. Evidence suggests that calcium intakes in excess of the recommended daily allowance (RDA) may be necessary to achieve optimal bone health and healing. Excessive intakes of protein may also increase calcium requirements.

If the patient is unable to eat an adequate amount at meals, high-protein, high-calorie beverages can be served between meals. Tube feeding is necessary for comatose patients or for those unable to take food by the normal route. Gastrointestinal injury requires placement of the tube at a point below the injury so that food can still be absorbed.

A severe traumatic injury may cause gastrointestinal ileus. Jejunal and colonic ileus are short-lived, and early enteral tube feeding is usually possible. A gastric ileus usually lasts longer, and fat-containing formulas are poorly tolerated because they take longer to leave the stomach. Low-fat formulas can be used until the ileus resolves.

Parenteral nutrition is indicated if adequate nutrition by the gastrointestinal route is impossible. It may be given as either peripheral vein supplementation or central vein total nutrition, as discussed in Chapter 30.

HEAD INJURY

Major injury to the brain is unique because of the brain's central role in metabolic control. Severe head injury has been compared with the severe burn in its intensity (Chiolero et al, 1989; Clifton et al, 1984; Fruin et al, 1986). The more severe the head injury, the greater will be the release of catecholamines (norepinephrine and epinephrine) and cortisol and the greater will be the hypermetabolic response. There is even a slight hypermetabolism for as much as 1 year after the injury (Haider et al, 1975).

Hypermetabolism of the brain-injured patient may be a response to treatment with exogenous steroids, but several studies have shown that even patients who do not have steroid treatment exhibit the high metabolic rate (Robertson et al, 1985; Young et al, 1985). Nevertheless, steroids greatly increase the nitrogen loss in the case of the head-injured patient during the first 6 days after the injury (Greenblatt et al, 1989). After this time, the nitrogen balance becomes equal in the brain-injured patients, whether they are treated with steroids or not (Robertson et al, 1985).

It is also suggested that the IL-1 released into the intracerebroventricular space after brain injury possesses enhanced biologic activity compared with its release intravenously or intraperitoneally (Ott et al, 1987).

EXTENSIVE BURNS

Extensive burns result in severe trauma. Energy requirements can increase as much as 100% above resting expenditures, depending on the extent of the injury. This hypermetabolism is accompanied by exaggerated

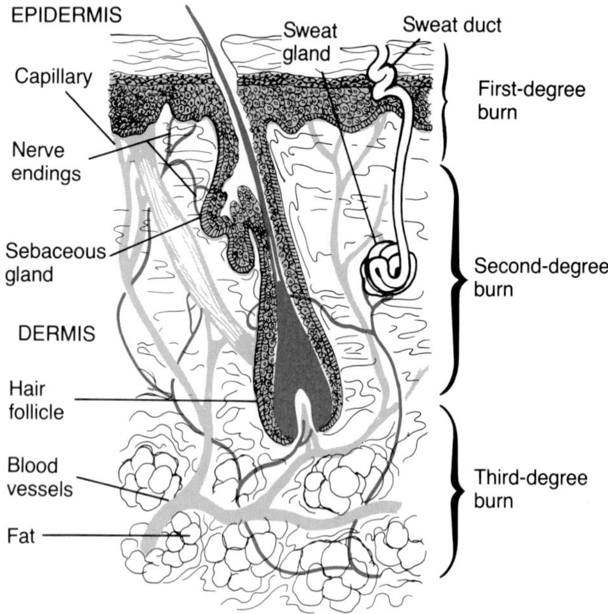

FIGURE 29–4. *Burn depth. (Modified from Luckmann J and Sorensen KC: Medical-Surgical Nursing, 3rd ed. Philadelphia, WB Saunders, 1987, p 1616.)*

protein catabolism and by increased urinary nitrogen excretion, with further protein loss through wound exudate (Fig. 29–4). Burn patients are particularly susceptible to infection, which markedly increases requirements for both energy and protein. Because patients with major burns usually develop ileus (loss of intestinal peristalsis or lack of effective coordinated peristalsis) and are anorexic, their nutritional support becomes a real challenge.

Fluid and Electrolyte Replacement

Because of extensive fluid and electrolyte losses through the wound, the first 24 to 48 hours of treatment are devoted to their replacement. A variety of formulas have been developed to calculate the volume of resuscitation fluid needed. Most agree that half of the calculated volume for the first 24 hours be given during the first 8 hours, because this is the period of the greatest intravascular loss.

The volume of fluid needed is based on the age and weight of the patient and on the extent of the burn. Variations of the Lund and Browder chart (Herndon et al, 1985; Lund and Browder, 1944) can be used to determine the percentage of total body surface area (TBSA) burned. Composition of the resuscitation fluid is controversial. Solutions containing water, electrolytes, and albumin have all been advocated in varying proportions.

General appearance, clear sensorium, and adequate urinary output help to determine if resuscitation has been sufficient. Once resuscitation is complete, ample fluids must be given to cover both maintenance requirements and evaporative losses that continue through open wounds. Provision of adequate fluids and electrolytes as early as possible after injury is paramount for maintaining circulatory volume and for preventing acute renal failure.

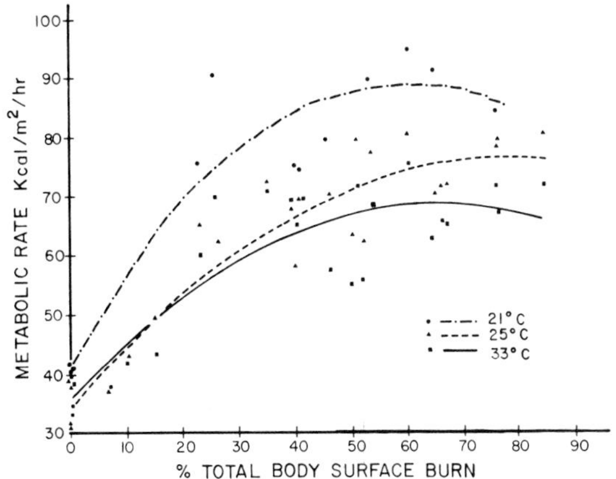

FIGURE 29–5. *Relationship between metabolic rate and burn size at three ambient temperatures. Resting metabolic rate is minimized in a thermal neutral environment. Cooling accelerates metabolic rate and increases energy requirements. (From Rombeau JL and Caldwell MD: Parenteral Nutrition, Vol. 2. Philadelphia, WB Saunders, 1986, p 249.)*

Wound Management

Wound management depends on the depth and extent of the burn. The current trend is for early excision and grafting. Metabolic needs are reduced slightly by the practice of covering wounds as early as possible to reduce evaporative and nitrogen losses and to prevent infection.

Nutritional Care

Along with early wound coverage and infection control, nutritional support is recognized as being one of the most significant aspects of care of the burned patient. Wound healing can take place only in an anabolic state. Feeding should be initiated soon after resuscitation is complete. Some burn centers advocate the introduction of nutritional support shortly after the patient's admission to the hospital, before complete resuscitation has been achieved (McArdle et al, 1984; Saito et al, 1987). By the fifth to seventh day after injury, patients should be able to consistently meet their estimated energy and protein needs. Table 29–3 summarizes the goals of nutritional care for burned patients.

Energy

The increased energy needs of the burn patient vary according to the size of the burn (see Fig. 29–5). Various formulas have been developed for estimating energy needs, of which the following is one of the simplest and easiest to use (Curreri, 1979):

kcal needed per day =
25 kcal × kg usual body weight
+ 40 kcal × % TBSA burned
(using a maximum of a 50% burn)

TBSA = total body surface area

TABLE 29–3. Nutritional Care Goals for Burned Patients

1. Minimizing metabolic response by:
   - Controlling environmental temperature
   - Maintaining fluid and electrolyte balance
   - Controlling pain and anxiety
   - Covering wounds early
   - Preventing infection
2. Meeting nutritional needs by:
   - Providing adequate calories to prevent weight loss of greater than 10% of usual body weight
   - Providing protein adequate for positive nitrogen balance and maintenance or repletion of visceral protein stores
   - Providing vitamin and mineral supplementation as indicated
3. Preventing Curling's ulcer by:
   - Providing antacids or continuous enteral feedings

Some formulas do not establish an upper limit to the number of kilocalories required. When these formulas are used, it should be noted that the maximum caloric load that the body can handle is approximately 100% above resting metabolic expenditure (2 × REE) (Cunningham et al, 1989).

Additional kilocalories may be required to meet the needs of fever, sepsis, multiple trauma, stress of surgery, or promotion of weight gain in the severely underweight patient. Weight maintenance should be the goal for overweight patients until the healing process is complete. The energy requirement for the obese burned person is probably more than calculated when IBW is used but less than calculated when actual body weight is used (Feurer et al, 1981).

An accurate formula for calculating the nutritional needs of the pediatric burn patient remains to be developed. Because basic requirements depend on the stage of growth and development, it is difficult to provide a formula to cover all age groups. Furthermore, the extent of increase required above basic needs is controversial. Some authors feel that because burned children are less active, their nutritional requirements are met as specified by the RDA (Young et al, 1981). Other proposals include a 50% increase above the RDA (Klein et al, 1978) or twice the calculated basal metabolic expenditure (Molnar et al, 1983).

Protein

Protein recommendations for burned patients are not well defined (Snelling et al, 1982). A common recommendation is for 1 gram of nitrogen per 100 to 150 kcal of intake. Others suggest protein levels at 20 to 25% of the total calories or 2 to 3 g/kg of body weight (Molnar et al, 1983; Stinnett et al, 1982). Patients with burns over 30% of the body surface area generally require more protein, with kilocalorie : nitrogen ratios closer to 100 : 1.

Although protein recommendations for children are even less clear, it is generally agreed that protein needs are increased above the RDA. Calorie to nitrogen ratios between 150 : 1 and 100 : 1 with protein providing 20 to 25% of kilocalories are recommended (Alexander et al, 1980). The ability of pediatric burn patients to tolerate protein depends on their renal function and fluid balance.

Whether it is protein in general or specific amino acids that are required in increased amounts is the subject of current study. It has been suggested that BCAA or their keto derivatives should be increased (Aussel et al, 1986), but this has not been confirmed. It may be that arginine is useful in the burn patient as it seems to result in less wound infection (Gottschich, 1990).

ASSESSMENT OF PROTEIN ADEQUACY. The adequacy of protein and energy intake is best evaluated by following wound healing, graft-take, and basic nutritional assessment parameters. Wound healing or graft-take may be delayed if weight loss exceeds 10% of the usual weight. An exact evaluation of weight loss may be difficult to obtain, because of fluid shifts or edema or because of differences in the weights of dressings or splints. However, weight change trends can be identified.

Nitrogen balance may give a rough estimate of protein needs but cannot be considered to be accurate without accounting for wound losses. One formula suggests using 0.2 grams of protein per % of full thickness burn per day to account for wound losses (Soroff et al, 1961). Nitrogen excretion should begin to decrease as wounds heal or are covered; however, serum albumin usually remains depressed until major burns are healed. Proteins with shorter half-lives, such as prealbumin, transferrin, and retinol-binding protein, show promise for helping to assess the protein status of burn patients.

Carbohydrate

Even though carbohydrate is recommended as the chief energy source in burn patients, there appears to be a maximum glucose load of 7 mg/kg/min above which glucose is not oxidized but rather is converted to fat (Wolfe, 1985). This state of lipogenesis causes increased O_2 consumption and CO_2 production.

Lipid

The use of lipid in nutritional support of burn patients is controversial, because although lipid is a concentrated source of calories, high levels of lipid may have deleterious effects on immunologic responses and may cause increased susceptibility to infections (Gottschlich et al, 1990). Composition of the lipid is probably important because diets high in omega-3 fatty acids may result in improved immune response and in tube feeding tolerance (Alexander et al, 1986). A reasonable approach is to begin by limiting lipid to 15% of nonprotein calories with attention to indicators of immune function, feeding tolerance, and serum triglycerides if higher amounts are used (Gottschlich et al, 1990; Ireton-Jones and Baxter, 1991).

Vitamins

It is generally agreed that vitamin needs are increased for burn patients but that exact requirements have not been established. Supplements may be needed for patients on oral intakes; however, most patients on tube feeding or TPN receive vitamins in excess of the RDA because of high-calorie needs. Vitamin C is involved in collagen synthesis and may be required in increased amounts for wound healing. It has also been recommended that vitamin A be provided in amounts above the RDA (Gottschlich and Warden, 1990).

Minerals

Electrolyte imbalances involving serum sodium or potassium are usually corrected by adjusting fluid therapy. Hyponatremia may be seen in patients whose evaporative losses are reduced drastically by the application of dressings or grafts without appropriate change in maintenance fluids or in those who are treated with silver nitrate soaks that tend to draw sodium from the wound. Restricting the oral consumption of free water and sodium-free fluids may help to correct hyponatremia. A slightly elevated serum potassium may indicate inadequate hydration.

Depression of serum calcium levels may be seen in patients with burns involving greater than 30% of TBSA. Calcium losses may be exaggerated if the patient is immobile or being treated with silver nitrate soaks. Early ambulation and exercise should help to decrease these losses. Administration of calcium supplements may be necessary to treat symptomatic hypocalcemia.

A depressed serum zinc level has been reported in burn patients, but it is unclear whether this is representative of total body zinc levels. Zinc supplementation may not be warranted for every patient; however, it has been suggested for treating post-burn anorexia and impaired wound healing and for those receiving total parenteral support for an extended period (Bell and Wyatt, 1986).

Hypophosphatemia has also been identified in patients with extensive burns. This occurs most commonly in patients receiving large volumes of resuscitation fluid along with parenteral infusion of glucose solutions and large amounts of antacids for stress ulcer therapy. Serum levels need to be monitored and appropriate phosphate supplementation provided, usually parenterally. Magnesium levels may also require attention because significant magnesium can be lost from the wound in patients with major burns. Supplemental magnesium may be required.

The anemia initially seen following a burn is usually unrelated to iron deficiency and is treated by giving packed red blood cells.

Methods of Nutritional Support

Methods of nutritional support need to be determined on an individual basis. Most patients with burns over less than 20% of their bodies are able to meet their needs on a regular diet. Patients with extensive burns, severely exaggerated nutritional needs, or poor appetites usually require tube feeding or TPN. Although most patients with burns covering more than 40% of TBSA cannot meet their estimated energy and protein needs with oral intakes alone, the appropriate method of support needs to be individually assessed for each patient.

Enteral feeding is usually preferred, but parenteral nutrition may be necessary with early excision and grafting to avoid the frequent interruptions in enteral nutritional support required because of anesthesia. TPN may be the method of choice for patients with persistent ileus who are not tolerating tube feeding or who have a high risk of aspiration. However, it may be that ileus can be avoided by early enteral feeding (McArdle et al, 1984). Central lines for TPN can be maintained through burn wounds with careful monitoring.

Ancillary Measures

Physical therapy helps to prevent contractures and may facilitate the incorporation of nitrogen into muscle (Legaspi, 1989). Provision of a warm environment minimizes heat loss and the expenditure of energy to maintain body temperature (see Fig. 29–5). Individual heat shields are often used above the patients' beds to maintain the environmental temperature near 30° C. Minimizing fear and pain with reassurance from the staff and adequate pain medication also helps to decrease catecholamine stimulation, which increases energy requirements.

Antacids should be given to patients with major burns to prevent formation of Curling's ulcer in the gastric or duodenal mucosa.

SURGERY

Nutritional Assessment

Emergency situations offer little opportunity for nutritional assessment or preparatory nutritional care. However, a nutritional assessment should be made in elective cases, particularly those involving recent previous surgery, malabsorption, prolonged immobilization, chronic alcoholism, or bizarre eating habits.

Illness requiring surgery may cause anorexia or restriction of food intake for days or weeks, predisposing to nutritional depletion and weight loss. In some cases, vomiting, diarrhea, and bleeding contribute to marked losses of sodium, chloride, potassium, and iron. When long periods of malabsorption are involved, the patient may also be depleted in protein, vitamins, and other minerals. Preoperative diagnostic procedures requiring that the patient fast or receive only clear liquids may promote nutritional inadequacies that are particularly detrimental to the already depleted or underweight patient.

Preoperative Nutritional Care

A well-nourished patient will usually tolerate major surgery better than a severely malnourished patient, and malnutrition appears to be associated with a high incidence of operative complications and death (Dempsey et al, 1988). A chemically defined or elemental liquid diet with minimal residue can be used preoperatively for patients at nutritional risk. Except for patients who are unable to take food enterally, there is no conclusive evidence that perioperative nutritional support (other than in the form of oral intake) is effective in reducing operative complications and deaths, even though it does improve nutritional status (Detsky et al, 1987). A large multicenter study of surgical patients in Veterans Administration hospitals is presently underway to help answer this question (Veterans Administration . . . , 1988).

Patients determined to need preoperative repletion will require energy and protein at levels 30 to 50% above maintenance level. Providing energy and protein much beyond these levels has not been beneficial. A depleted patient can be expected to gain a maximum of 50 to 100 mg/day of lean tissue.

Overweight patients may be required to lose weight before elective surgery. In this event, special attention should be given to the rate and composition of weight loss, because losses of lean body mass exceeding 10% over a short period may delay operative wound healing.

Operative risk appears to be associated with the status of protein metabolism rather than with the achievement of full repletion, which could take months. Patients who demonstrate positive nitrogen balance and improved visceral protein or immune status are thought to have fewer operative complications. Individual response to repletion is variable; it has been suggested therefore that nutritional status be evaluated every 7 days in order to determine readiness for surgery.

It is important that the stomach be empty of food at the time of the operation to avoid the danger of vomitus aspiration during the induction of anesthesia or upon awakening. In elective cases, no food is allowed by mouth for at least 6 hours before surgery. In emergency cases, it is advisable to perform gastric lavage to remove stomach contents before starting anesthesia.

Prior to abdominal surgery, the colon should be free of residue to prevent postoperative infection. Colonic bacteria are reduced when less food residue is present. Low-fiber foods or a liquid diet are commonly given for 2 to 3 days preceding surgery, and the patient receives an enema a few hours before going to the operating room.

Surgery should not be performed on a dehydrated patient. If oral fluids are not tolerated or there is insufficient time for oral administration, fluids can be given parenterally.

Postoperative Nutritional Care

Nutritional care following surgery should be individualized and should be related to the type of surgery performed. Although some surgeons may be very specific about postoperative diet orders, a number of general principles are applicable to all patients who have undergone surgery.

Introduction of Food

Oral feeding is often delayed for the first 24 to 48 hours following surgery to await the return of bowel tones. However, evidence suggests that the small intestine regains motility within hours and the stomach begins to empty at 24 hours after surgery, thus bowel tones may not be a good measure of return of bowel function (Moss, 1985). The "norm" of postoperative catabolism due to malnutrition may thus be an avoidable complication if patients are fed within 24 hours of surgery using the appropriate enteral feeding tubes (Moss, 1985). Infusion of an elemental diet by needle-catheter jejunostomy into the small bowel, distal to the operative procedures, is useful in the critically ill patient in whom oral feeding is not possible for 5 days or more (see Chapter 30).

The introduction of solid food depends on the condition of the gastrointestinal tract. A general practice has been to progress from clear liquids to full liquids and finally to solid foods over a period of several meals. However, there is no physiologic reason why solid foods should not be introduced once the gastrointestinal tract is functioning and a few liquids are being tolerated.

Energy and Protein

The extent to which energy expenditure increases above the BEE varies with the nature and extent of surgery. For the elective uncomplicated surgical patient, the energy requirement is the BEE × 1.4 or 1.5 depending on whether the patient is in bed. However, if the surgery was preceded by multiple fractures or trauma, the energy requirement can be the BEE × (1.65 − 1.8). See Table 29-1 for the increased energy requirements of stressful clinical situations surrounding surgery, such as infection.

Depletion of body protein is largely responsible for postoperative weakness and slow recovery. It causes edema, inhibits wound healing, makes the body more vulnerable to infection, renders the liver more liable to toxic damage, impedes regeneration of hemoglobin, prevents resumption of normal gastrointestinal activity, and delays the return of muscular strength. Table 29-2 presents methods for calculating protein requirements.

Many patients will be able to meet their energy and protein needs with the standard hospital diet. Patients with small appetites, drastically increased nutritional needs, or poorly functioning gastrointestinal tracts may require supplemental oral liquids, tube feeding, or parenteral support. See Chapter 30 for discussion of alternative routes of nutritional care.

Vitamins and Minerals

Vitamin supplements are not required after minor surgery in a well-nourished individual. Fasting for long periods before or after surgery, as well as the stress of major surgery, particularly after a long debilitating illness, are circumstances that justify therapeutic doses of vitamins, sometimes in amounts two and three times the RDA.

Wound healing is improved with the administration of zinc to patients with low serum zinc levels. Although its specific role in wound healing is unclear, this mineral appears to be required for amino acid metabolism and synthesis of collagen precursors. The role of zinc is discussed more fully in Chapter 7.

Fluids

Blood, fluids, and electrolytes are lost during surgery and further loss can occur through vomiting and drainage. To prevent dehydration and shock during the immediate postoperative period, fluid and electrolyte balance should be maintained by intravenous, subcutaneous, or rectal infusion. The patient at this time may experience difficulty with the intake of large quantities of water by mouth. In some cases, oral fluids can be given immediately after recovery from anesthesia.

CITED REFERENCES

Alexander JW et al: Beneficial effects of aggressive protein feeding in severely burned children. Ann Surg 192:505, 1980.

Alexander JW et al: The importance of lipid type in the diet after burn injury. Ann Surg 204:1, 1986.

Alvarez OM and Gilbreath RL: Thiamine influence on collagen during the granulation of skin wounds. J Surg Res 32:24, 1982.

A.S.P.E.N. Board of Directors: Guidelines for use of total parenteral nutrition in the hospitalized adult patient. J Parenter Enteral Nutr 10:441, 1986.

Aussel C et al: Plasma branched-chain keto acids in burn patients. Am J Clin Nutr 44:825, 1986.

Bell SJ and Wyatt J: Nutrition guidelines for burned patients. J Am Diet Assoc 86:648, 1986.

Berdanier CD: The many faces of stress. Nutr Today 22(2):12, 1987.

Blackburn GL: In search of the "preferred fuel" (Editorial). Nutr Clin Prac 4:3, 1989.

Bower RH et al: Branched chain amino acid-enriched solutions in the septic patient: A randomized, prospective trial. Ann Surg 203:13, 1986.

Bynoe RP et al: Nutrition support in trauma patients. Nutr Clin Prac 3:137, 1988.

Chandra RK (ed): Nutrition and Immunology: Contemporary Issues in Clinical Nutrition, Vol 11. New York, Alan R Liss, 1988.

Chiolero R et al: Hormonal and metabolic changes following severe head injury or noncranial injury. J Parenter Enteral Nutr 13:5, 1989.

Clifton GL et al: The metabolic response to severe head injury. J Neurosurg 60:687, 1984.

Cunningham JJ et al: Measured and predicted calorie requirements of adults during recovery from severe burn trauma. Am J Clin Nutr 49:404, 1989.

Curreri PW: Nutritional replacement modalities. J Trauma 19:904, 1979.

Dempsey DT, Mullen JL, and Buzby GP: The link between nutritional status and clinical outcome: Can nutritional intervention modify it? Am J Clin Nutr 47(Suppl 2):352, 1988.

Detsky AS et al: Perioperative Parenteral Nutrition: A Meta-analysis. Ann Intern Med 107:195, 1987.

Feurer I et al: Resting energy expenditure in morbid obesity (Abstract No. 28). J Parenter Enteral Nutr 5:562, 1981.

Fruin AH, Taylor C, and Pettis MS: Caloric requirements in patients with severe head injuries. Surg Neurol 25:25, 1986.

Gottschlich MM et al: Differential effects of three enteral dietary regimens on selected outcome variables in burn patients. J Parenter Enteral Nutr 14:225, 1990.

Gottschlich MM and Warden GD: Vitamin supplementation in the patient with burns. J Burn Care Rehabil 11:275, 1990.

Greenblatt SH et al: Catabolic effect of dexamethasone in patients with major head injuries. J Parenter Enteral Nutr 13:372, 1989.

Grieg PD et al: Parenteral nutrition in septic patients: Effect of increasing nitrogen intake. Am J Clin Nutr 46:1040, 1987.

Haider W et al: Metabolic changes in the course of severe acute brain damage. Eur J Intens Care Med 1:19, 1975.

Herndon DN et al: Treatment of burns in children. Pediatr Clin North Am 32:1311, 1985.

Ireton-Jones CS and Baxter CR: Nutrition for adult burn patients: A review. Nutr Clin Prac 6:3, 1991.

Keenan RA et al: An altered response by peripheral leukocytes to synthesize or release leukocyte endogenous mediator in critically ill, protein malnourished patients. J Lab Clin Med 100:844, 1982.

Klein CL et al: Increased rates of whole body protein synthesis and breakdown in children recovering from burns. Ann Surg 187:383, 1978.

Legaspi A: Adjunctive therapy for nutritional support in hospitalized patients. Nutr Clin Prac 4:95, 1989.

Loggie BW and Hinchey EJ: Effect of iron administration on the outcome of bacterial peritonitis. Surg Forum 35:111, 1984.

Long CL et al: Metabolic response to injury and illness: Estimation of energy and protein needs from indirect calorimetry and nitrogen balance. J Parenter Enteral Nutr 3:452, 1979.

Lund CL and Browder NC: The estimation of areas of burns. Surg Gynecol Obstet 79:352, 1944.

McArdle AH et al: Early enteral feeding of patients with major burns: Prevention of catabolism. Ann Plast Surg 13:396, 1984.

Molnar JA, Wolfe RR, and Burke JF: Burns: Metabolism and nutritional therapy in thermal injury. *In* Schneider HA, Anderson CE, and Coursin DB (eds): Nutritional Support of Medical Practice, 2nd ed. Philadelphia, Harper & Row, 1983.

Moore EE and Jones TN: Benefits of immediate jejunostomy feeding after major abdominal trauma — a prospective, randomized study. J Trauma 26:874, 1986.

Moss G: Early enteral feeding after abdominal surgery. *In* Deitel M (ed): Nutrition in Clinical Surgery, 2nd ed. Baltimore, MD, Williams & Wilkins, 1985.

Ott L, Young B, and McClain C: The metabolic response to brain injury. J Parenter Enteral Nutr 11:488, 1987.

Pomposelli JJ, Flores EA, and Bistrian BR: Role of biochemical mediators in clinical nutrition and surgical metabolism. J Parenter Enteral Nutr 12:212, 1988.

Robertson CS, Clifton GL, and Goodman JC: Steroid administration and nitrogen excretion in the head-injured patient. J Neurosurg 63:714, 1985.

Saito H et al: The effect of route administration on the nutritional state, catabolic hormone secretion and gut mucosal integrity after burn injury. J Parenter Enteral Nutr 11:1, 1987.

Snelling CFT et al: Amino acid metabolism in burn patients. Surgery 91:474, 1982.

Soroff HS, Pearson E, and Artz CP: An estimation of the nitrogen requirements for equilibrium in burn patients. Surg Gynecol Obstet 112:159, 1961.

Souba WW and Wilmore DW: Diet and nutrition in the care of the patient with surgery, trauma and sepsis. *In* Shils ME and Young VR (eds): Modern Nutrition in Health and Disease, 7th ed. Philadelphia, Lea & Febiger, 1988.

Spitzer JJ et al: Alterations in lipid and carbohydrate metabolism in sepsis. J Parenter Enteral Nutr 12(6)(Suppl):53s, 1988.

Stinnett JD et al: Plasma and skeletal muscle amino acids following severe burn injury in patients and experimental animals. Ann Surg 195:75, 1982.

Thiamin and wound repair. Nutr Rev 40:316, 1982.

Veterans Administration cooperative trial of perioperative total parenteral nutrition in malnourished surgical patients: Background, rationale and study protocol. Am J Clin Nutr 47(Suppl 2):351–391, 1988.

Wolfe RR: Glucose metabolism in burn injury: A review. J Burn Care Rehabil 6:408, 1985.

Young B et al: The metabolic and nutritional sequela of the non-steroid treated injury patient. Neurosurgery 17:784, 1985.

Young VR, Motil KJ, and Burke JF: Energy and protein metabolism in relation to requirements of the burned pediatric patient. *In* Suskind RM (ed): Textbook of Pediatric Nutrition. New York, Raven Press, 1981.

ADDITIONAL REFERENCES

Starvation

Cahill GF: Starvation in man. N Engl J Med 282:668, 1970.

Metabolic Stress Response

Fleck A: The acute phase response: Implications for nutrition and recovery. Nutrition 4:109, 1988.

Jensen TG: Determination of nutritional status in critical care. J Am Diet Assoc 84:1345, 1984.

Burns

Boosalis MG et al: Serum copper and ceruloplasmin levels and urinary copper excretion in thermal injury. Am J Clin Nutr 44:899, 1986.

Boosalis MG et al: Serum zinc response in thermal injury. J Am Coll Nutr 7:69, 1988.

Cunningham JJ, Harris LJ, and Briggs SE: Nutritional support of the severely burned infant. Nutrition in Clinical Practice 3:69, 1988.

Gottschlich MM: Acute thermal injury. *In* Lang CE (ed): Nutritional Support in Critical Care. Rockville, MD, Aspen Publishers, 1987.

King N and Goodwin CW: Use of vitamin supplements for burned patients: A national survey. J Am Diet Assoc 84:923, 1984.

Sutherland AB and Batchelor ADR: Nitrogen balance in burned children. *In* Wilkinson AW (ed): International Congress on Research in Burns. Edinburgh, Churchill Livingstone, 1966, pp 147–157.

Wachtel TL: Nutritional support of the burn patient. *In* Boswick JA Jr (ed): The Art and Science of Burn Care. Rockville, MD, Aspen Publishers, 1987.

Bed Rest

Rubin M: The physiology of bed rest. Am J Nurs 88:50, 1988.

Trauma

Cerra FB et al: Enteral nutrition in hypermetabolic surgical patients. Crit Care Med 17:619, 1989.

Hurst JM, Koetting CA, and Lang CE: Multiple trauma. *In* Lang CE (ed): Nutritional Support in Critical Care, Rockville, MD, Aspen Publishers, 1987.

Popp M and Brennan M: Metabolic response to trauma and infection. *In* Fischer JE (ed): Surgical Nutrition. Boston, Little, Brown, 1983.

Sepsis

Endres S et al: The effect of dietary supplementation with n-3 polyunsaturated fatty acids on the synthesis of interleukin-1 and tumor necrosis factor by mononuclear cells. N Engl J Med 320:265, 1989.

Hasselgren P-O and Fischer JE: Nutritional support in sepsis. *In* Lang CE (ed): Nutritional Support in Critical Care. Rockville, MD, Aspen Publishers, 1987.

Hoffman-Goetz L: Lymphokines and monokines in protein-energy malnutrition. *In* Chandra RK (ed): Nutrition and Immunology: Contemporary Issues in Clinical Nutrition, Vol 11. New York, Alan R Liss, 1988.

Keusch GT and Farthing MJG: Nutrition and infection. Ann Rev Nutr 6:131, 1986.

Nelson KM and Long CL: Physiological basis for nutrition in sepsis. Nutr Clin Prac 4:6, 1989.

Shizgal HM and Martin MF: Caloric requirement of the critically ill septic patient. Crit Care Med 16:312, 1988.

Surgery

Cerra FB et al: Enteral nutrition in hypermetabolic surgical patients. Crit Care Med 17:619, 1989.

Delany HM: Nutritional support following major surgery (Editorial). Nutrition 4:478, 1988.

Fletcher JP and Little JM: The effect of nutritional support on nitrogen balance following major surgery. Nutrition 4:447, 1988.

Grimes CJC, Younathan MT, and Lee WC: The effect of preoperative total parenteral nutrition on surgery outcomes. J Am Diet Assoc 87:1202, 1987.

Health and Public Policy Committee, American College of Physicians: Perioperative parenteral nutrition: Position paper. Ann Intern Med 107:252, 1987.

Smith RC and Hartemick R: Improvement of nutritional measures during preoperative parenteral nutrition in patients selected by the Prognostic Nutritional Index: A randomized controlled trial. J Parenter Enteral Nutr 12:587, 1988.

CHAPTER 30

METHODS OF NUTRITIONAL SUPPORT

CHAPTER OUTLINE

- Enteral Feeding
- Parenteral Nutrition
- Transitional Feeding
- Enteral or Parenteral Tube Feeding at Home
- Psychosocial Aspects of Alternative Forms of Nutritional Support

KEY TERMS

ADMIXTURES OR "THREE-IN-ONE MIXTURES"—referring to a parenteral nutrition mixture in which all three nutrients—amino acids, lipid, and glucose—are included in the same container

CYCLIC TOTAL PARENTERAL NUTRITION—administration of total parenteral nutrition solution for 12 to 18 consecutive hours, usually at night, followed by a 6- to 12-hour period of no TPN

DEFINED FORMULA DIET (sometimes called ELEMENTAL DIET)—a nutritionally adequate liquid diet designed for easy digestion and absorption, which leaves minimal residue in the bowel; administered either orally or enterally

ENTERAL NUTRITION—the delivery of nutrients directly into the stomach, duodenum, or jejunum

NASOENTERIC TUBE—a tube inserted through the nasal passage into the stomach, duodenum, or jejunum

NEEDLE CATHETER JEJUNOSTOMY (NCJ)—a feeding tube using a small-bore needle and tube that is usually inserted into the jejunum at the time of surgery

NUTRITIONAL RECOVERY SYNDROME—a syndrome marked by clinical signs (especially hypophosphatemia and hypokalemia), indicative of overly aggressive refeeding of patients who have been without food for a period of time

PARENTERAL NUTRITION (PN)—the delivery of nutrients directly into the circulation; can be either peripheral or central, total or supplemental

PERCUTANEOUS ENDOSCOPIC GASTROSTOMY (PEG)—a feeding tube whose insertion into the stomach involves using an endoscope and pulling the tube through a small incision in the abdominal wall

PERIPHERAL PARENTERAL NUTRITION (PPN)—delivery of nutrients into a peripheral vein

POLYMERIC—when referring to nutrients, the form in which the nutrient appears before digestion into its smaller parts

TOTAL PARENTERAL NUTRITION (TPN) also called CENTRAL PARENTERAL NUTRITION (CPN)—delivery of nutrients into a large central vein, usually the superior vena cava

TRANSITIONAL FEEDING—nutritional support during the time when the patient is moved from one form of feeding to another

ENTERAL FEEDING

Oral Feeding

The preferable and most palatable method of meeting the increased demands of catabolism and recovery is provision of abundant, nutritious, and frequent meals and supplements given orally. (See Table 18–6, which gives suggestions for increasing energy intake with whole foods.)

Nutritional Supplements

When a sufficient quantity of food is not eaten at meals, calories and protein can be supplemented with between-meal puddings or drinks. Some supplements are concentrated and contain additional vitamins and minerals, whereas others are commonly used foods; not all are nutritionally adequate. The choice of a nutritional supplement will depend on the nutritional requirements and tolerance of the patient as well as the cost, composition, palatability, availability, and the shelf life of the supplement, as well as the staff available for preparation. The composition and indications for oral use of available nutritional supplements are given in Table 30–1.

Supplements can be formulated using fluid or powdered milk, powdered whole eggs, and powdered egg albumin as concentrated protein sources. Milk is used frequently because it is one of the few liquid sources of a complete protein. Eight ounces of whole milk provide 160 kilocalories and 8 grams of protein of high biologic value; one tablespoon of powdered skim milk provides 15 kilocalories and 1.5 grams of protein. Protein content of the diet can be augmented at low cost by the addition of casein and lactalbumin. Milk-free or lactose-free formulas can be used as nutritional supplements in the presence of lactose intolerance or milk allergy (see Appendix Table 33).

Nutritionally Complete Formulas

Liquid feedings meeting nutritional requirements are used in the care of patients unable to take solid food. Ideally these feedings are given orally, but part or all of the intake is usually given enterally by tube.

Enteral Tube Feeding

Patients with conditions that prevent oral intake, such as oral surgery, gastrointestinal surgery, dysphagia, unconsciousness, anorexia, or esophageal obstruction require liquid feeding through a tube. Others who for various reasons are unable to obtain adequate nourish-

TABLE 30–1. Situations Requiring Artificial Feeding Techniques

Physiologic Problem	Recommended Feeding	Clinical Situation or Disorder
Inability to ingest food	Liquid feedings: whole food or milk-based formula Route of administration: Tube Nasogastric Gastrostomy Jejunostomy Oral	Carcinoma of esophagus or stomach Dental or oral surgery Inflammatory disease of esophagus Coma
Inability to digest food	Chemically defined diet Route of administration: Oral Tube	Pancreatitis Biliary tract disease
Decreased ability or inability to absorb food	Chemically defined diet Route of administration: Oral Tube Peripheral vein nutritional support Total parenteral nutrition	Radiation therapy Sprue Inflammatory bowel disease Short bowel syndrome
Inability to handle colonic residue	Chemically defined diet Route of administration: Oral Tube Peripheral vein nutritional support Total parenteral nutrition	Inflammatory bowel disease Presurgical preparation Ileostomy, colostomy Draining fistula
Inability to meet nutritional requirements fully with normal foods	Liquid feeding Oral supplement Tube feeding Peripheral vein nutritional support Central vein nutritional supplementation	Major surgery Burns Trauma Extended fever Anorexia of chronic illness Anorexia nervosa

ment through oral intake alone, require additional feedings supplied enterally (see Table 30–1).

Indications and Advantages

Enteral tube feeding is the proper choice over parenteral feeding whenever the digestive and absorptive capacities of the gastrointestinal tract are still functional. The cost is considerably less (one sixth) and fewer technical, metabolic, and infectious complications are involved. Enteral feeding usually requires less patient monitoring (although initial problems with formula intolerance may necessitate more attention), and normal immunologic and physiologic gastrointestinal functions are maintained (Bynoe et al, 1988). However, to be solely maintained by enteral feeding does require at least 2 and preferably 3 ft (60 to 100 cm) of functioning small bowel (Ryan and Beshlian, 1987).

Tube Type and Position

The placement and type of tube used for feeding is determined by the patient's condition and particularly the status of his or her gastrointestinal tract. Placement may be nasoenteric or through an ostomy into the stomach, jejunum, or duodenum. Because no surgery is required, *nasoenteric* tubes are placed more easily and cost less than an ostomy. The tube can remain in place or be reinserted with each feeding. *Transpyloric placement* of the tube is indicated when there is risk of aspiration, as in patients with gastroesophageal reflux, delayed gastric emptying, intractable vomiting, or coma. A tube *enterostomy* is used when the esophagus is blocked, facial trauma is present, or when the tube must remain in for a month or more and patient appearance and convenience are factors (Fig. 30–1).

A recent innovation is the *percutaneous endoscopic gastrostomy (PEG)*, whose insertion does not require general anesthesia, takes less time, and therefore makes the procedure less expensive than other gastrostomies. The procedure is performed at the bedside, or in the endoscopy suite, using an endoscope and pulling the tube through a small incision in the abdominal wall.

A *jejunostomy* is recommended if aspiration is a problem, when major abdominal surgery is contemplated and postoperative nutritional support is necessary, or in the presence of esophageal, gastric, pancreatic, or hepatobiliary complications. Because the small bowel recovers normal peristalsis rapidly after surgery, a jejunostomy allows earlier infusion of enteral feedings than is possible with the oral gastric route (Moore and Jones, 1986).

The *needle catheter jejunostomy (NCJ)* inserted at the time of surgery is especially useful in postoperative nutritional management. The Witzel jejunostomy using a red rubber tubing sutured into the jejunum at the time of surgery is also used.

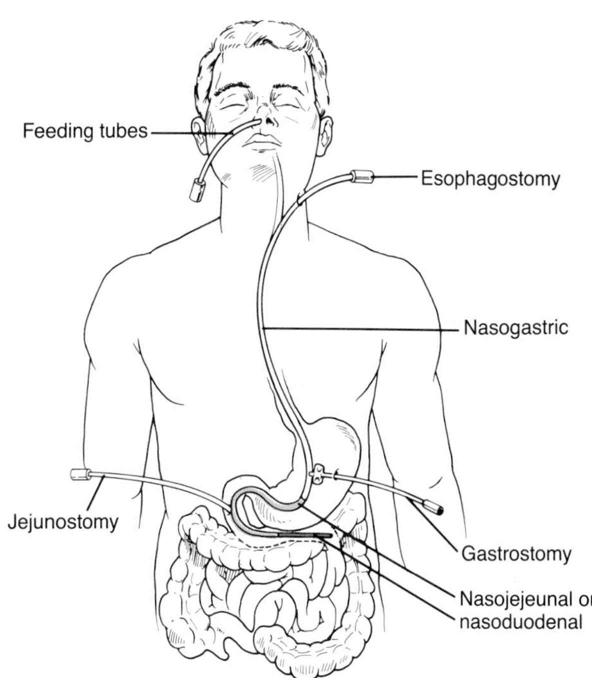

FIGURE 30–1. *Diagram of the placement of enteral feeding tubes.*

A small tube (No. 8 French) is more comfortable for a nasoenteric feeding and most formulas will pass through a tube of this size, especially when it is used in conjunction with a mechanical pump. A small tube also has less tendency to diminish competence of the lower esophageal sphincter and possibly lead to gastroesophageal reflux. A blenderized formula requires a large tube (No. 16 French) of the type usually reserved for ostomy feedings.

Composition

Commercial formulas suitable for tube feedings are described in Appendix Table 33. Commercial products save time in preparation, are less likely to be contaminated, and are of a known composition; however, they are not quite as flexible in meeting patient needs as tube feedings prepared especially for the individual. Their limitations can be overcome by the preparation of individualized feedings combining modular components. *Modular formulas* are prepared from the components or "modules"—carbohydrate, protein, fat, water, vitamins, and minerals (see Appendix Table 33). Preparing a formula from modules is useful in patients with hepatic or renal failure or fluid restrictions. However, it is usually more expensive due to the labor and training costs of preparation.

Feedings may also be made from a mixture of the foods served in the normal diet, or from food or supplement combinations planned to meet specific therapeutic needs. These should be finely homogenized, strained, and diluted to a consistency that will ensure passage through the tube. Formulas made from whole foods have the advantage of including naturally present trace minerals and vitamins that may not be added to a commercial formula diet. Disadvantages of such a formula are a thick consistency that requires a larger feeding tube for administration, the longer labor time required for preparation, and a higher potential for contamination. Table 30–2 presents a typical formula made from strained infant foods. Use of strained infant foods is recommended because of their predictable nutrient content and consistency. Parameters for evaluation of a feeding formula are osmolality; nutrient and energy density; the type of protein, carbohydrate, and fat; the vitamin and mineral composition; the fiber content; the viscosity; and the amount of feeding necessary to meet the Recommended Dietary Allowances (RDA) (Table 30–3).

OSMOLALITY. Many tube feedings are hyperosmolar with respect to body osmolality. If given too rapidly, they will cause water to be drawn into the gastrointestinal tract. Slow initial administration with gradually increasing amounts is usually better tolerated. Diluting the formula and gradually increasing it to the normal concentration will also enhance tolerance. This should take 2 days in the case of gastric feedings and 4 to 5 days with jejunal or duodenal feedings. See Appendix Table 33 for the osmolality of feeding formulas. Products with osmolalities of 500 mOsm/kg can generally be fed full strength right away.

ENERGY. Feedings usually provide 1 to 1.2 kcal/ml when mixed full strength according to directions. Some high-calorie formulas contain up to 2 kcal/ml. These calorically dense formulas are useful for patients with increased energy requirements who also have fluid restrictions or decreased ability to handle large volumes of liquid. However, they may not provide enough water; thus, hydration must be monitored.

TABLE 30–2. Designing a Home-Blenderized Tube Feeding*

Using the following ingredients, the dietitian can prescribe the proper amounts for a tube feeding that meets the nutritional needs of the patient. The usual daily intake of the blenderized feeding would be 1,800 to 2,500 ml.

_______ jar of strained meat (3½ oz jar)†
_______ jar of strained vegetables (4½ oz jar)†
_______ jar of strained fruits (4½ oz jar)†
_______ cup of dried skim milk powder
_______ T vegetable oil
_______ T corn syrup
_______ cups water
_______ cups whole milk
_______ other

* Adapted from The American Dietetic Association: Home Enteral/Parenteral Nutrition Therapy: A Practitioner's Guide. ©1986, The American Dietetic Association. Used by permission.
† The selection of strained infant foods should be varied daily.

TABLE 30–3. Factors to Consider in Choosing a Feeding Formula

Integrity of the patient's gastrointestinal system.
The type of protein, fat, carbohydrate, and fiber in the formula as related to the patient's digestive and absorptive capacity.
Caloric and protein density (i.e., kcal/ml, g protein/ml, and kcal : nitrogen ratio).
Ability of the formula, taken in the amounts tolerated, to meet the patient's nutritional requirements.
Sodium, potassium, and phosphorus content of the formula, especially for patients with renal, hepatic, or cardiac dysfunction.
Viscosity of formula as related to type of tube-feeding equipment.
Cost of formula (i.e., per g protein, per kcal, per ml).

PROTEIN. The protein content of formulas varies from 4 to 26% of kilocalories. Most contain 14 to 16% of the kilocalories as protein, and the "high-nitrogen" products may contain 18 to 26% of the kilocalories from protein. The number of kilocalories provided per gram of nitrogen can range from 100 to 300. Protein may be supplied in the intact form of whole proteins, also called *polymeric,* or hydrolyzed into peptide fragments or free amino acids. The protein source can be casein (milk protein), puréed beef, egg albumin, skim milk powder, soy protein, hydrolyzed soy, hydrolyzed casein, or amino acids. Formulas that contain the whole protein are more palatable than those containing hydrolyzed protein or amino acids, and they are also cheaper. The hydrolyzed forms of protein are a good source of peptides for a patient with maldigestion, malabsorption, or allergy who needs protein in an easily digested form. Small peptides are more rapidly absorbed than free amino acids and are preferable in many ways (Brinson et al, 1989). Whole proteins are preferable for individuals with a healthy intestine because they offer greater trophic stimulus to the bowel, are more efficiently assimilated than hydrolyzed proteins, and have fewer side effects (Kerzner, 1988).

Formula proteins are also being modified to better meet the requirements posed by specific problems. For example, trauma patients are being treated with formulas higher in branched-chain amino acids (see Chapter 29). Glutamine may also be a preferential fuel for the gut mucosa during stress, as it appears to enhance cell mass and height of the mucosal villi (Smith, 1988; Souba, 1988). The presence of this amino acid may make enteral feeding preferable over parenteral feeding in maintaining gastrointestinal integrity. Some enteral formulas now contain glutamine.

LIPID. The fat in most commercial formulas is in the form of corn, soy, or safflower oil, in amounts ranging from 1 to 43% of kilocalories. A few products contain *medium-chain triglycerides (MCT)* and are used when fat malabsorption is involved. An alternate in such cases is the use of a fat-free formula, with the fat intake increased gradually in amounts of 10 g/l each day. When limiting the fat in enteral feeding, it is important to provide essential fatty acid at the level of 1 to 2% of total energy intake.

Fat is an important component of a feeding because it increases kilocalories without increasing osmolality and it also contributes to a feeling of satiety. Fat metabolism requires less CO_2 production, which may be of significance for the patient on a ventilator; formulas for patients with respiratory disease contain a higher percentage of calories from fat (see Chapter 34).

The type of fat in formulas used in critical care is receiving attention because of its potential role in gut and immune function. *Long-chain triglycerides (LCT)* exert a hypertrophic stimulus on the gut mucosa (Kerzner, 1988). By entering the portal system, MCT can bypass lipase and bile salt digestion and should therefore be used when gastrointestinal function is compromised by chylous effusions, lymphangiectasia, or abetalipoproteinemia. However, unlike LCT, MCT do not have a hypertrophic stimulus on the gut mucosa (Kerzner, 1988). They supply only 8.3 kcal/g and appear to increase metabolic rate and energy requirements.

CARBOHYDRATE. The many possible sources of carbohydrate in a liquid feeding range from puréed fruits and vegetables to corn syrup solids, oligosaccharides (maltodextrin and partial hydrolysates of cornstarch), glucose, fructose, sucrose, and lactose. The carbohydrate source considerably affects the palatability of the formula, and the amount affects its osmolarity. The digestive and absorptive capacity of the bowel determines whether monosaccharides or more complex oligosaccharides can be used.

Because lactase deficiency occurs frequently as a result of genetic disease or stress, many formulas eliminate lactose as a carbohydrate source.

FIBER. Fiber in the form of soy polysaccharide is added to some formulas for the purpose of preventing diarrhea or decreasing the constipation that can complicate enteral formula feeding. The dietary fiber content is similar to that in a whole-foods diet, ranging from 6 to 14 g/l. The fiber maintains normal bowel function, but some patients report increased flatulence during the adaptation period. The short-chain fatty acid content of the fiber source may also be beneficial in maintaining the colonic mucosa, where these fatty acids are the preferential fuel of the mucosal cells.

VITAMINS AND MINERALS. Most commercially available liquid diets are fortified with vitamins and minerals to meet the RDA for healthy individuals. Unfortunately the vitamin and mineral requirements needed to fulfill the RDA of stressed individuals are not known. The adequacy of formulas prepared from whole foods depends upon the choice of foods; therefore, the use of a multivitamin and mineral supplement is advised. Additional vitamins may be necessary in cases of vitamin deficiency, drug-nutrient interactions, or excessively high requirements. In some circumstances, replacement of lost electrolytes may also be required. Patients who are not taking a formula full strength or are not taking the recommended amount will not meet their requirements for vitamins and minerals. Appendix Table 33 indicates the amount of formula needed to provide the RDA for these nutrients.

DEFINED FORMULA DIETS. These formulas are designed for easy digestion and absorption. Because they leave minimal residue in the bowel, stool passage is halted or markedly reduced. They contain known quantities of purified substances, but the substances are not truly elements and the name *elemental diet,* although widely used, is erroneous. It is true, however, that the protein and carbohydrate used in these diets are in simpler forms than those found in other formulas. Carbohydrate is present in the form of glucose or dextrins (disaccharides and oligosaccharides). Protein is in the form of amino acids, dipeptides, or tripeptides, all of which appear to be equally well absorbed (Brinson et al, 1989; Grimble, 1987). Any fat is present either in very small amounts, in the form of MCT, or as monoglycerides or diglycerides (see Appendix Table 33).

Defined formulas are especially suited for cases of steatorrhea and malabsorption caused by disease, short-bowel syndrome, radiation, or antibiotic damage to the intestinal tract. These formulas can also be made using modular components as listed in Appendix Table 33. All of the products are supplemented with vitamins and minerals to meet the RDA.

When formulas are fed nasoduodenally or through a jejunostomy, a defined formula is not necessarily required. The choice of feeding is based on the feeding tube size and the viscosity of the formula. A small feeding tube such as in a needle catheter jejunostomy requires a less viscous and therefore a defined formula feeding. An open-ended red rubber catheter (Witzel technique) can accommodate a more viscous formula; thus a polymeric formula could be used.

Defined formula products can be administered orally or through a tube. Because they contain peptides and amino acids, they are less palatable when taken by mouth. However, if they are to be taken orally they should be offered to the patient well chilled, "on the rocks," masked with flavor supplements, and with a positive attitude.

Administration

RATE AND STRENGTH. Continuous drip via gravity or enteral pump is probably the most common method of administration. Continuous drip feeding with a pump is the preferred method for the hospitalized patient. Bolus feedings are often used for home patients to allow greater degree of mobility. They are also frequently used in nursing homes where pumps are often not available.

The gastrointestinal tract can adapt to a hyperosmolar formula when it is fed in a manner that allows for a slow increase of the osmolarity. Cramping and diarrhea may occur initially as water is drawn into the intestinal tract. Patients who are debilitated or who have hypoalbuminemia, gastrointestinal disorders, or short-bowel syndrome, or those whose gastrointestinal tracts have been without food for a long period of time are more likely to be intolerant of the hyperosmolar formula and require special attention.

Continuous Drip Feeding. Giving not more than 40 to 60 ml/hr for 18 to 24 hours (20 to 40 ml/hr for pediatric patients) in the first 8 to 12 hours enables gradual development of tolerance to the osmolarity of the formula (Andrassy, 1988). The rate is then increased approximately 25 ml every 8 to 12 hours. The final rate is 50 to 100 ml/hr for 18 to 24 hours. Isotonic formulas (300 mOsm/kg of water) may be started at full strength. Hypertonic (500+ mOsm/kg of water) formula should be started at no more than one-half strength. Monitoring is especially important when the feeding is being given into the duodenum or jejunum of a gastrointestinal tract that has been without nutritional support for 2 weeks or more. In the event of intolerance to the formula, concentration can be reduced to one half and gradually increased to full strength as tolerated. The rate may also be decreased and then gradually increased to meet the patient's needs. Rate and strength should not be increased at the same time.

Formula given by pump or continuous drip should not be allowed to hang more than 4 to 8 hours, and new formula should not be added to old formula. Unused formula should be kept refrigerated but should not be used after 24 hours.

Bolus Feeding. The patient's total daily formula needs should be divided into six regular daytime feedings of 250 to 350 ml (usually 3 hours apart). Isotonic formulas can be started at full strength, whereas hypertonic formulas should be started at one-half strength the first day. The feeding should be given over at least 15 minutes and followed by 25 to 60 ml of water. The additional water after feeding is important to prevent hypertonic dehydration from solute overload. The water is also used for careful rinsing of the tube because the protein in the feeding tends to coagulate when it comes in contact with gastric HCl and can then clog the tube.

If by the fifth day the tolerated volume of formula still is not sufficient to meet the patient's nutritional requirements, a more calorically dense formula should be considered.

Fluid Needs. Fluid needs are not always met with the amount of enteral formula tolerated and the water used to flush the tube after feedings. This is often the case with calorically dense formulas (1.5 kcal/ml or greater) where the free water content of the formula may be as low as 60% of the formula amount. Most adults require 1 ml of water/kcal or 35 ml/kg usual body weight, whereas children require 70 to 100 ml/kg and infants require 150 ml/kg. Most enteral formulas contain 80 to 85% water.

POSITION. A bolus tube feeding can be administered when the patient is standing, sitting, or lying in bed with the head and thorax elevated at least 30 degrees from the horizontal. Maintaining these positions during feeding and for at least 30 minutes afterward decreases risk of aspiration of formula into the lungs. This also applies to nasogastric continuous drip feeding. With a nasoduodenal or jejunostomy feeding, this is not necessary.

With bolus feeding, the tube should be properly positioned in the stomach and not in the duodenum or jejunum unless it is supposed to be there. The gastric contents should be suctioned out and returned to the stomach before a new feeding is administered to make sure that only minimal residue remains from the previous feeding. Excessive residue may indicate an obstruction or digestive problem that should be resolved before feeding is continued. Sources vary on the acceptable amount of residue in adults; a maximum of 100 to 150 ml has been proposed (Breach and Saldanha, 1988a, 1988b, and 1988c).

MONITORING. The *actual* formula intake of the patient and any signs of hypertonic dehydration or inadequate feeding should be recorded. The actual parenteral intake of any patient should be closely monitored to see if nutritional requirements are being met. One study showed that on a given day, less than half of tube-fed patients received 100% of their energy intake. The most common reasons for loss of feeding time were: (1) tube falling out, (2) gastrointestinal intolerance, (3) medical procedures that required discontinuation of feeding, and (4) feeding tube position difficulties (Abernathy, 1989).

Assessment of hydration is particularly important in comatose, weak, very ill, or frightened patients who are unable to communicate their feelings of thirst. Tracheostomy patients who are unable to express their thirst are typical of those who may become dehydrated from a tube feeding. Renal or cardiovascular disease that causes malfunction of the water elimination and retention mechanism is also likely to cause dehydration. If insensible water loss is great as a result of fever or fistula drainage, or if the formula is high in protein or electrolytes, the water intake of a tube-fed patient should be increased. Table 30-4 provides a list of factors that should be monitored routinely for the tube-fed patient.

ALBUMIN. Albumin can be clinically useful in maintaining oncotic pressure and thus allowing tolerance of enteral feeding when more costly parenteral feeding would otherwise be required. Colloid oncotic pressure promotes movement of water from the interstitial space back into the capillaries. Over 20 years ago it was shown that serum albumin level correlated with decreased absorption and increased fluid retention in the bowel (Moss, 1967). Some other studies have shown that serum albumin levels, usually 2.5 mg/dl or less, appear to correlate with intolerance of enteral feeding (Brinson et al, 1987; Ford et al, 1987). However, other studies have shown no correlation.

Albumin administration is expensive and serum albumin levels often are not maintained. Thus, at this time, albumin administration does not appear to be justified as a method for improving tolerance of an enteral nutrition formula.

Problems and Solutions

Diarrhea is the most common complication of enteral tube feeding (Table 30-5). It can be caused by many circumstances including lactose intolerance, formula hyperosmolality, too rapid infusion rate, bacterial contamination of the formula, concomitant drug therapy, altered gastrointestinal flora, hypoalbuminemia, or gastrointestinal tract impairment due to shock, ischemia, or hypoxia. If diarrhea continues even after the measures stated in Table 30-5 are taken, the addition of soy polysaccharide fiber, pectin in the form of applesauce, or powdered pectin may help to bring the diarrhea under control. Switching to a fiber-containing formula may also help. Kaopectate or Lomotil (antidiarrheal agents) can be added to the feeding just before administration. After the patient has become stabilized on the tube feeding, constipation may develop because of the low-fiber content of the formula and the large amounts of casein used in some formulas. Methylcellulose and other forms of fiber can be added to the formula; however, these supplements increase the viscosity of the tube feeding and interfere with its passage through the tube. If the constipation remains unresolved, stool softeners or cathartics may be necessary.

Some medications cause clogging of the feeding tube because of incompatibility with the feeding formula. Feeding tubes should always be flushed with water after they have been used for drug administration. Coca Cola and cranberry juice have been used to flush feeding tubes; however, cranberry juice is not as effective as Coca Cola or warm water (Metheny et al, 1988).

The goal of tube feeding is to promote anabolism or at least nitrogen balance. If this is not achieved, it usually means that the patient is not receiving adequate nutritional support. This may be the result of intolerance or resistance. It may also reflect lack of knowledge or inattention on the part of the hospital staff and failure to deliver all of the nutritional support ordered. Daily use of the nutritional index as discussed in Chapter 24, particularly for protein and energy, is a valuable guide. Patients who are being tube fed need a great deal of encouragement to help them adjust to the situation.

TABLE 30-4. Monitoring the Enterally Tube-Fed Patient

Weight (at least 3 times/week)
Signs of edema (daily)
Signs of dehydration (daily)
Fluid intake and output (daily)
Calorie, protein, fat, carbohydrate, vitamin, and mineral intake (at least 2 times/week)
Nitrogen balance (24-hr urine urea nitrogen) (weekly)
Gastric residuals (every 4 hours)
Stool output and consistency (daily)
Urine glucose (every 6 hours until maximum feeding rate established, then daily for diabetics)
Serum electrolytes, blood urea nitrogen (BUN), creatinine, and blood count (2-3 times weekly)
Chemistry profile including serum total protein, albumin, prealbumin, calcium, magnesium, phosphorus, and liver function tests (weekly)

PARENTERAL NUTRITION

The administration of nutrients of varying strengths directly into the circulation is called *parenteral nutrition (PN).* This method of feeding is appropriate only when the gastrointestinal tract cannot be used. When necessary, however, PN can be lifesaving.

The two major types of PN solutions are (1) isotonic or slightly hypertonic solutions given by peripheral vein *(peripheral parenteral nutrition [PPN]),* usually as adjunct nutritional therapy, and (2) hypertonic solutions given by central vein *(central parenteral nutrition [CPN]),* which often provide total nutrition support. CPN is often referred to as *total parenteral nutrition (TPN)* even though it may or may not be providing total nutrition. It has also been called hyperalimentation (HA), or intravenous hyperalimentation

TABLE 30–5. Complications of Enteral Tube Feeding

Problem	Signs	Possible Reasons	Solutions
Gastrointestinal			
Profuse diarrhea	More than 3 liquid stools/day	Gastric hypersecretion Lactose intolerance Formula hyperosmolality Too rapid infusion rate Bolus feeding Bacterial contamination of formula Concomitant drug therapy (antibiotics, magnesium-based acids) Altered GI flora* Malabsorption Impaction Hypoalbuminemia	Add cellulose bulking agent Change to lactose-free formula Change to continuous drip feeding Take more care to prevent bacterial contamination of formula Medication to control diarrhea Reduce osmolality of formula Give albumin in IV line†
Inadequate gastric emptying	Large volumes of gastric residuals	Nonfunctioning GI tract Too rapid infusion rate Formula too high in fat Hypoalbuminemia—delayed gastric emptying	Reduce rate of infusion Reposition feeding tube, possibly into duodenum Hold feedings for 2–8 hr, then resume at reduced rate Medication to increase gastric emptying
Nausea or vomiting	Expulsion of gastric contents	Nonfunctioning GI tract	Reduce rate of infusion Reposition feeding tube, possibly into duodenum Hold feedings for 2–8 hr, then resume at reduced rate Medication to increase gastric emptying
GI bleeding	Coffee-ground aspirates or blood in residuals	Non–tube feeding problem	Change to parenteral feeding
Mechanical			
Transnasal tube lodged or obstructed	Inability to aspirate gastric residual More than 12 hr of feeding not received	Inadequate flushing of feeding tube Too small a bore in feeding tube Incompatibility of formula with concomitant drug therapy	More frequent flushing of tube, especially before and after medication administration Flush feeding tube with Coca Cola, cranberry juice, or solution of pancreatic enzyme tablets mixed with water Change to continuous infusion
Aspiration pneumonia	Evidence of formula in airways	Inadequate elevation of head during feeding Improper placement of feeding tube Improper gastric emptying due to high-fat formula or hypoalbuminemia Incompetent lower esophageal sphincter due to large feeding catheter	Change feeding tube placement to the duodenum Frequent gastric residual checks Change to formula with lower fat content Change to smaller, softer feeding tube
Metabolic			
Hyperkalemia	Serum potassium >5.5 mEq/l	Formula with excessive potassium Potassium retention due to anabolism Secondary to metabolic acidosis Secondary to renal insufficiency	Substitute enteral formula with less potassium
Prerenal azotemia	Hypernatremic dehydration; serum osmolality >300 mOsm/kg	Secondary to free water loss or inadequate intake Formula with too high a protein concentration	Increase free water intake Decrease protein content of formula
Hyponatremia	Low serum sodium	Fluid retention secondary to hepatic, renal, or cardiac dysfunction Inappropriate antidiuretic hormone production in head-injured patients	Restrict free water intake Choose formula with greater nutrient density
Macronutrient or micronutrient deficiencies	Abnormal lab tests	Secondary to feeding problems and inadequate intake Secondary to increased requirements	Supplement enteral feeding Correct feeding problems to permit adequate intake
Hyperglycemia	Osmotic diuresis Elevated blood glucose	Too rapid infusion rate Infection History of diabetes	Slow formula infusion rate Change to formula with less sugar and more fiber

* GI = gastrointestinal.
† IV = intravenous.

(IVH), although both are misnomers because the formulas are usually designed to meet desirable rather than excessive nutrient requirements.

The decision to use central versus peripheral PN is based upon energy requirements, the length of time PN will be needed, status of the peripheral veins, and whether the patient requires nutritional rehabilitation. Table 30–6 gives the indications for the two types of PN.

Peripheral Parenteral Nutrition

The oldest regimen of intravenous nutritional therapy is administration of a 5% glucose solution intravenously, which provides 50 g glucose/l. This is equivalent to about 100 to 150 g glucose/day, or 400 to 600 kcal. This clinical practice, which has been widely used in the past, is of little benefit except for maintenance of fluid balance. It is appropriate only for patients who will soon resume eating, as in the "clean" surgical patient who is expected to regain complete oral nourishment within 3 to 5 days postoperatively.

When short-term nutritional support is necessary, it can be provided peripherally as a mixture of 5 to 10% glucose, a 3.5 to 5% amino acid solution, and a 10 to 20% lipid emulsion. Total fat intake should not exceed 2.5 g/kg/day. Vitamins, minerals, and electrolytes are added as necessary, based on requirements and concurrent oral or enteral intake. The osmolarity of the PPN solution is the limiting factor and should usually be no greater than 600 mOsm/l. This means that large amounts of the solution are needed to meet nutritional requirements. Because total nutritional requirements are often unmet by this method, it is appropriate only as short-term (5 to 7 days) support for a mildly malnourished patient. The usual energy intake by this method is 700 to 1,800 kcal/day. Fluid balance, weight, lipid clearance, and electrolytes should be monitored. In addition, the PPN patient must be observed for signs of peripheral vein intolerance such as phlebitis or infiltration at the catheter site. Inasmuch as PPN solutions are nearly iso-osmolar, it is not necessary to start infusions slowly or taper off their administration (Clinical Insight, p. 516).

PPN is also useful as a supplement to oral feeding in the patient who, because of gastrointestinal problems, cannot meet nutritional requirements completely by the oral or enteral route.

TABLE 30–6. Indications for Using Peripheral Versus Central Vein Feedings*

Peripheral Vein Feedings

1. Enteral intake interrupted, but enteral feeding expected to resume within 5–7 days
2. Supplementation to enteral feedings or as transitional phase until enteral feedings meet needs
3. Mild to moderate malnutrition, necessitating intervention in order to prevent further depletion
4. Normal or mildly elevated metabolic rate
5. No organ failure necessitating fluid restriction

Central Vein Feedings

1. Unable to tolerate enteral intake for greater than 7 days
2. Moderately to severely elevated metabolic rate
3. Moderate to severe malnutrition, not correctable with enteral feedings
4. Cardiac, renal, or hepatic failure, or other conditions necessitating fluid restriction
5. Limited access to peripheral veins
6. Able to access central vein

* Adapted from Young LS: Principles of parenteral nutrition: Indications, administration and monitoring. *In* Krey SH and Murray RL: Dynamics of Nutrition Support. Assessment, Implementation, Evaluation. Norwalk, CT, Appleton-Century-Crofts, 1986, Table 17–2, p 379.

Central or Total Parenteral Nutrition

TPN is a method of providing complete nutritional support in which the gastrointestinal tract is bypassed by introducing assimilable nutrients into a central vein, usually the superior vena cava. Because the central vein is able to tolerate a hyperosmolar solution, nutritional support can be provided in a form that will meet all nutritional needs. This is in contrast to PPN, where total nutritional requirements rarely can be met.

Indications for Use

This method of feeding is used for individuals who are debilitated and malnourished, with a weight loss of 10% of body weight or more, and who are unable to obtain adequate nutrition enterally or with PPN. Patients with short-bowel syndrome, bowel fistulas or obstruction, inflammatory bowel disease, or hypermetabolic states in which the gastrointestinal tract is completely or partially unusable benefit from this form of nutritional support. It is useful for patients with cancer who are malnourished but who still have a chance of responding to oncologic treatment if they can be nutritionally rehabilitated. TPN can meet the high energy and protein needs of burned patients whose gastrointestinal tracts may be unusable because of multiple surgeries, sepsis-induced ileus, or organ failure. It is also useful in the treatment of neonatal abnormalities, anorexia, or extreme cachexia; in some pulmonary diseases involving danger of food aspiration; and in acute hepatic and renal failure when the composition of the amino acid intake must be manipulated (see Chapters 28 and 35).

Unlike PPN, which at most provides 1,800 kcal/day, TPN can supply enough energy for anabolism — up to 4,000 kcal/day if necessary. This is possible because the solution is administered through a Hickman or Broviac-type catheter inserted into the superior vena cava, where the hypertonic solution can be rapidly diluted by the large, fast-flowing volume of blood. If such a concentrated solution were introduced into a peripheral

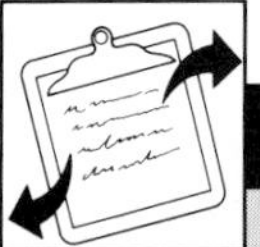

CLINICAL INSIGHT: Calculation of the Osmolarity of a Parenteral Nutrition Solution

1. Multiply the grams of dextrose per liter by 5.
   Example: 50 grams of dextrose × 5 = 250 mOsm/l
2. Multiply the grams of protein per liter by 10.
   Example: 30 grams of protein × 10 = 300 mOsm/l
3. Fat is isotonic, does not contribute to osmolarity.
4. Electrolytes would further add to osmolarity.
   Total osmolarity = 250 + 300 = 550 mOsm/l

vein, phlebitis would develop in 4 to 8 hours. The central catheter should only be used for the nutrient solution and not for blood products or medications. If it is a double-lumen or triple-lumen catheter, one lumen should be reserved for the nutrient solution. This minimizes the risk of contaminating the feeding system.

Nutritional Requirements and Formula Composition

ENERGY. A typical TPN solution at the usual strength is a concentrated liquid providing 1 kcal/ml, or 1,000 kcal and approximately 42 grams of protein per liter of solution. The kilocalorie : nitrogen ratio is usually around 150 : 1, which is appropriate for protein synthesis and anabolism. If the patient is under severe stress, a kilocalorie : nitrogen ratio of 100 : 1 may be necessary (see Chapter 29). However, the formula can be designed with great flexibility to meet individual needs.

PROTEIN. Protein in TPN formulas is provided by crystalline amino acids. Standard solutions contain 5.5, 8.5, and 10% amino acids. Five hundred milliliters of the 8.5% amino acid solution is usually mixed with 500 ml of a 50% dextrose solution to provide 1 liter of solution. Because amino acid intake should be used for body maintenance and not for energy, often the energy from protein is not counted as a part of the total energy requirement.

Commonly used solutions are Freamine, Travasol, and Aminosyn. Inasmuch as the usual TPN solution contains 25 to 50 g protein/l, most patients require at least 2 to 3 l/day in order to meet their protein requirements (1 to 2 g protein/kg ideal body weight [IBW]/day). Infants usually require at least 2 g protein/kg IBW. (Requirements for neonates are discussed in Chapter 11.) The composition of amino acids can be adjusted with reference to the metabolic state. For example, solutions containing only essential amino acids (e.g., Nephramine) can be used in renal failure. Solutions high in branched-chain amino acids are available for patients with trauma, stress (Freamine HBC), or hepatic failure (Heptamine).

Carbohydrate. Carbohydrate in TPN is usually in the form of a 50% dextrose (D50) solution, which is a much higher osmolality than the usual 5% glucose solution administered in peripheral intravenous therapy. This amounts to 500 ml of the dextrose solution per liter of TPN, with a concentration of 25% in the final TPN solution. This provides 250 grams of glucose or 850 kcal/l (250 grams of glucose × 3.4 kcal/g of glucose = 850 kcal). To this may or may not be added the calories provided by the protein in the mixture (42.5 g of protein × 4 kcal/g = 170 kcal), resulting in a final solution containing 1,020 kcal/l, or about 1 kcal/ml. For patients requiring more concentrated carbohydrate energy sources because of large energy requirements or fluid restrictions, D70 (350 g/glucose/500 ml) is available. However, it has been reported that high glucose loads can increase minute ventilation, carbon dioxide production, the respiratory quotient (RQ), and oxygen consumption. Lipid does not have the same effect and has been shown to be useful in patients with impaired ventilatory function (see Chapter 34).

LIPID. The role of lipids in PN originally was merely as a source of essential fatty acids. At least 2 to 4% of the total energy should be provided as lipid emulsion to meet these essential fatty acid requirements. However, currently lipids are included as a major energy source in TPN. It is usual to provide 25 to 35% of the calories as fat, with higher levels in patients with respiratory distress, but not exceeding 60% of total calories. The presence of fat as a major energy source with glucose helps to prevent TPN-induced changes in hepatic function tests, cholestasis, and fatty liver.

Lipid emulsions for intravenous use can be of three kinds. The first type consists of either soybean oil, safflower oil, or a mixture of these two, and provides LCT in which a large fraction of the fatty acids consists of linoleic acid. The second type consists of fully saturated MCT that can be given separately or as a mixture with LCT. The third type, not yet commercially available, is a "structured" emulsion made up of a rearranged triacylglycerol (triglyceride) containing both medium and long-chain fatty acids (Heird et al, 1986; Mascioli et al, 1988). At present the ideal mixture of MCT and LCT is not known (Further Reading, p. 517).

Short-chain triglycerides (SCT) are also being considered as an alternative energy source as they are

FURTHER READING: Advantages of MCT or MCFA or an MCT/LCT Mixture Over LCT or LCFA

1. MCT or a mixture of MCT and LCT is oxidized and cleared more rapidly than LCT. MCT constitute a more immediate energy source and are not re-esterified and stored in the liver.
2. Oxidation of MCFA is independent of the carnitine acyl transferase system.
3. MCT stimulate ketogenesis and possibly increase the energy supply.
4. Oxidation of MCT is greater than that of LCT in the hyperinsulinemia related to catabolic stress (Bach et al, 1988), and there is no hypertriglyceridemia as seen with LCT.
5. MCT may have a greater protein-sparing effect than LCT (Bach et al, 1988).
6. MCT do not compromise host defense by interfering with the functioning of the reticuloendothelial system and other aspects of the immune system.

The single disadvantage of MCT over LCT emulsions is an increase of 9% in oxygen consumption and energy expenditure (Mascioli et al, 1987). Also, because MCT promote ketogenesis they have limited use in patients with diabetes and other conditions associated with acidosis.

LCFA = long-chain fatty acids; LCT = long-chain triglycerides; MCFA = medium-chain fatty acids; MCT = medium-chain triglycerides.

water-soluble and seem to incorporate all the advantages of MCT. In addition they appear to be a primary energy source for the gut epithelium and may have a special place in enteral nutrition (Campos and Meguid, 1988). However, toxic effects such as central nervous system changes and induction of coma have been reported.

Four lipid emulsions are currently available: Intralipid (soybean oil, Kabi-Vitrum Labs), Liposyn II (safflower and soybean oils, Abbott Labs), Travamulsion (soybean oil, Travenol Laboratories), and Soyacal (soybean oil, Alpha Therapeutic). Lipid emulsions are available in 10 or 20% concentrations, providing 1.1 kcal/ml (550 kcal/500 ml bottle) and 2.2 kcal/ml (1,010 kcal/500 ml bottle), respectively. Although theoretically 60% of the daily energy requirement could be provided as fat, as in the case of respiratory distress, a practical goal is 45%; 2.5 g fat/kg can be given daily. Most patients receive 25 to 35% of their calories from fat.

Lipid emulsions are usually administered separately from the rest of the TPN mixture of glucose, amino acids, vitamins, and minerals. If a Y-catheter is used, both can be infused at the same time, but 2 pumps are required. TPN *admixtures* or *three-in-one mixtures* that combine all three nutrients are available and widely used because of their convenience. However, questions of stability and compatibility still exist, and these solutions are not as flexible in meeting patient needs. In addition there is the problem of larger size lipid molecules clogging the filter usually used for the glucose–amino acid solution.

Lipid emulsions must be administered carefully in patients with hyperlipidemia, pancreatitis, severe liver damage, pulmonary disease, blood coagulation disorders, or anemia. Tolerance should be assessed in all patients by giving a 10% emulsion at 1 ml/min or 20% at 5 ml/min for 15 to 30 minutes and watching for adverse reactions such as dyspnea, cyanosis, allergic reactions to the egg phospholipids used in the lipid emulsions, nausea, vomiting, headache, fever, or chest or back pain. After the first bottle has run, the patient should be checked for tolerance with a serum triglyceride level. The infusion should not exceed 125 ml/hr and the solution should not be allowed to hang more than 24 hours. If the concentration of serum triglycerides at 6 hours after completion of infusion is 300 mg/dl or more, the rate and/or concentration of lipid should be decreased, and the use of fat emulsions should be limited to provide for essential fatty acid requirements only (Roesner and Grant, 1987). If there are no adverse reactions, the rate may be increased to 80 to 100 ml/hr for a 10% emulsion and 60 ml/hr for a 20% emulsion. Patients who do not tolerate even the amount of lipids required to prevent essential fatty acid deficiency have been treated with cutaneous application of oils. However, the usefulness of this procedure is questionable (Shapiro and Rosen, 1989).

ELECTROLYTES. Electrolytes must be added to the solution to promote efficient tissue synthesis. The potassium requirement may be increased at the onset of anabolism, when glucose and potassium move into the cells. Sodium and chloride are also important. Without adequate phosphorus, dangerous hypophosphatemia can develop in the presence of high-energy feedings. Calcium is necessary to balance the phosphate infusion. Table 30–7 lists the suggested electrolyte and major mineral concentrations in parenteral nutrition.

VITAMINS. The precise vitamin requirements for patients receiving TPN are still not known, although

TABLE 30–7. Electrolyte Requirements During Total Parenteral Nutrition*

Ion	Units	Infants and Young Children (per kg/day)	Adults (per day)
Sodium†	mEq	3–5	60 and up
Potassium†	mEq	3–5	60 and up
Magnesium†	mEq	0.3–0.5	12–20 or higher
Calcium	mEq	1–2	10–25‡
Phosphorus§	mg	15–30	450 and up

* Adapted from Shils ME: Enteral (tube) and parenteral nutrition support. *In* Shils ME and Young VR (eds): Modern Nutrition in Health and Disease, 7th ed. Philadelphia, Lea & Febiger, 1988, Table 54–8, p 1052.

† For patients with normal cardiovascular, renal, and intestinal function. The higher ranges are suggested for children with rapid growth rate and for adults with large gastrointestinal losses and adequate renal functions. In such patients, periodic evaluation of serum, stool, and urine levels is indicated.

‡ The higher calcium intakes are indicated for children with rapid growth and adults with conditions predisposing to prior bone demineralization and chronic acidosis.

§ As inorganic phosphate. Increased amounts are indicated when initiating total parenteral nutrition with large amounts of glucose to counteract resulting hypophosphatemia.

knowledge in the area is rapidly accumulating. Table 30–8 presents the most recent vitamin recommendations for children and adults on TPN. It is important to note that these guidelines are appropriate for parenteral administration of vitamins to patients in nonstressed normal metabolic states, and should be adapted to meet the needs of particular disease states (American Medical Association, 1975; Multivitamin preparations for parenteral use, 1979). For example, the need for ascorbic acid is higher in patients with burns or severe trauma than the 100 mg recommended (see Chapter 29). Requirements for specific vitamins are affected by the nutritional composition of parenteral solutions as well as by the influence of infection and other disease states, problems whose specific needs as yet remain unresolved.

Some products formulated for use with TPN contain the usual multiple vitamin preparation with the addition of biotin, folic acid, and vitamin B_{12}, but still may not be adequate for all patients. It may be preferable to formulate vitamin combinations according to individual needs. To prevent excessive excretion of the water-soluble vitamins, the daily dosage of the multiple vitamin preparation should be administered over several hours as part of the intravenous feeding schedule. It is usually added to the glucose–amino acid mixture and is easily identified in the TPN solution because it turns it yellow.

Requirements for fat-soluble vitamins are not as clearly understood. Normal serum vitamin A levels can be maintained using 1,500 to 2,000 IU/day, an amount less than the RDA. However, although the recommendation for vitamin E in Table 30–8 is 10 IU (0.67 mg d,1-alpha-tocopherol), it has been suggested that as much as 50 mg may be needed (Greig et al, 1982).

Vitamin K in the amounts normally provided by gut bacteria should be adequate for TPN patients. However, if there are changes in the gut flora due to antibiotic administration or to the TPN feeding, additional vitamin K may be necessary. Ten milligrams of the water-soluble form (Synkavite) weekly in the TPN solution is adequate.

The need for vitamin D in TPN is not well established, even though 200 IU are recommended. Aggravation of a syndrome of skeletal calcium loss with a histologic picture of increased bone osteoid with re-

TABLE 30–8. Recommendations for Vitamin Intakes During Parenteral Nutrition*

Formulations for Infants and Children Under 11 Years†

Vitamins	*AAP‡ Minimum/100 kcal Orally*	*Multivitamin Formulation§ for Intravenous Use*
A (retinol) (IU)	250.0	2,300.0‖
D (IU)	40.0	400.0¶
E (α-tocopherol) (IU)	0.3	7.0
K_1 (phylloquinone) (mg)		0.2
Ascorbic acid (mg)	8.0	80.0
Folacin (μg)	4.0	140.0
Niacin (mg)	0.25	17.0
Riboflavin (mg)	0.06	1.4
Thiamin (mg)	0.025	1.2
B_6 (pyridoxine) (mg)	0.035	1.0
B_{12} (cyanocobalamin) (μg)	0.15	1.0
Pantothenic acid (mg)	0.3	5.0**
Biotin (μg)		20.0**

Children Age 11 Years and Older, and Adults†

Vitamins	*Multivitamin Formulation for Intravenous Use*
A (IU)	3,300.0
D (IU)	200.0
E (IU)	10.0
Ascorbic acid (mg)	100.0
Folacin (μg)	400.0
Niacin (mg)	40.0
Riboflavin (mg)	3.6
Thiamin (mg)	3.0
B_6 (pyridoxine) (mg)	4.0
B_{12} (cyanocobalamin) (μg)	5.0
Pantothenic acid (mg)	15.0
Biotin (μg)	60.0

* Adapted from Multivitamin preparations for parenteral use. A statement by the Nutrition Advisory Group. J Parenter Enteral Nutr 3:258, 1979.

† Adapted from Guidelines for Multivitamin Preparations for Parenteral Use. Chicago, AMA, 1975.

‡ AAP = American Academy of Pediatrics.

§ MVI-pediatric meets these guidelines.

‖ 700 μg of retinol.

¶ As ergocalciferol or cholecalciferol.

** RDA not established; amount = 20 times the amount in 100 kcal of human milk.

duced calcification has been reported at vitamin D levels of 250 IU/day (Shike et al, 1981). On the other hand, it has been suggested that a single weekly intake of 100 IU is appropriate (Greig et al, 1982).

TRACE MINERALS. Trace mineral needs during TPN are not clarified with precision, but their need is well appreciated. This has been demonstrated for several elements in extended follow-up of patients for whom TPN is the sole source of nutrition. For example, chromium deficiency has been identified as the reason for the development of unexplained hyperglycemia in long-term TPN patients (Jeejeebhoy et al, 1977). At least one pharmaceutical company has formulated a trace mineral preparation containing zinc, copper, chromium, and manganese that can be added to the TPN solution. Other formulations containing single minerals such as selenium and molybdenum are also available. In administering trace elements intravenously, special care must be taken to avoid toxic complications and to consider the amounts of these elements that are already present in the TPN solutions as contaminants. Table 30–9 lists the recommended amounts of trace elements in TPN solution.

Administration

Insertion of the TPN catheter into the superior vena cava is a surgical technique performed under sterile conditions with local anesthesia (Fig. 30–2). Once placement of the tube has been confirmed with a chest x-ray, administration of TPN can begin. Because the TPN solution is hyperosmolar and a very concentrated source of glucose, it must be administered slowly at first.

Usually 1 liter is given in 24 hours, using a constant

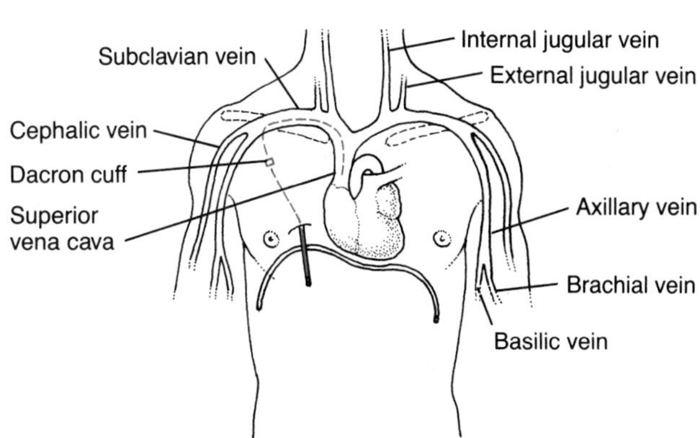

FIGURE 30–2. *Venous access sites from which the superior vena cava may be cannulated.*

drip infusion or a volumetric infusion pump. The rate of TPN should be increased gradually to allow for adjustment of endogenous insulin production and to avoid hypoglycemia and hyperglycemic episodes, especially in those with diabetes, metabolic stress, or sepsis. Another reason for gradual rate increases is to avoid overwhelming the system with a large increase in fluid intake, especially in cardiac and pulmonary patients. If the TPN solution is temporarily unavailable, D10W or D20W can be given until it can be obtained. Blood glucose, urine glucose, and electrolyte levels should be closely monitored. The rate of administration is gradually increased, usually over 2 to 3 days, until the full requirement is being given. Four liters per day of TPN formula is the maximum that most patients can tolerate.

The solution should be administered at a steady rate. If the administration falls behind, the rate should be corrected. Any attempt to "catch up" will result in an excessive glucose load. When TPN is no longer needed,

TABLE 30–9. Recommendations for Daily Trace Elements During Total Parenteral Nutrition*

	Child (μg/kg)†	Stable Adult	Adult in Acute Catabolic State‡	Stable Adult With Intestinal Losses‡
Zinc	300§ 100‖	2.5–4.0 mg	Additional 2.0 mg	Add 12.2 mg/l of small-bowel fluid losses and 17.1 mg/kg of stool or ileostomy output
Copper	20	0.5–1.5 mg	—	—
Chromium	0.14–0.2	10–15 μg	—	20 μg
Manganese	2–10	0.15–0.8 mg	—	—

* Adapted from Shils ME: Enteral (tube) and parenteral nutrition support. *In* Shils ME and Young VR (eds): Modern Nutrition in Health and Disease, 7th ed. Philadelphia, Lea & Febiger, 1988, p 1053, and Shils ME et al: Guidelines for essential trace element preparations for parenteral use: A statement by an expert panel. JAMA 241:2051, 1979.

† Limited data available for infants weighing less than 1,500 g.

‡ Frequent monitoring of blood levels in these patients is essential to guide proper dosage.

§ For premature infants up to 3 kg of body weight; thereafter, recommendations for full-term infants apply.

‖ For full-term infants and children up to 5 years old. Thereafter, the recommendations for adults apply up to a maximum of 4 mg/day.

it is a subject of debate as to whether the rate of TPN administration should be gradually tapered over a period of 2 hours or abruptly stopped. After abrupt cessation, some patients may experience a rebound hypoglycemia; others may not. Those at higher risk of hypoglycemia are patients with diabetes, metabolic stress, and sepsis. Most stabilized TPN patients do not have hypoglycemia with abrupt cessation of TPN (Rohde and Braun, 1986).

Cyclic TPN is a technique often used for those receiving long-term TPN. It involves "cycling" the TPN so that the person is fed for 12 to 18 hours, usually at night, and then fasts in the remaining hours of the day. It has the advantages of (1) providing freedom and a more normal life during the day and (2) preventing hepatotoxicity, common in long-term patients fed continuously (Bennett and Rosen, 1990).

Some patients receiving TPN still feel hungry and if possible, can take some food orally. If complete bowel rest is required, however, the patient should not be given anything by mouth, not even water, but sometimes can suck on ice chips.

TPN should be given in amounts to allow a daily weight gain of ¼ to ½ lb (0.1 to 0.2 kg), the limit for the amount of body tissue that can be synthesized in 24 hours. A weight gain greater than this indicates fluid retention. This is commonly seen initially in malnourished patients who are given TPN with nonprotein calories as glucose only; it is not seen with systems that use lipid. Once ideal weight is achieved, it should be maintained by adjustment of the TPN intake.

CARE OF THE CATHETER SITE. Catheter site care requires special attention because it is an easy entrance for microorganisms into a major vein. In addition, the TPN solution is a perfect medium for fungal and bacterial growth. Patients receiving TPN are often immunologically compromised due to underlying medical conditions, therapies, or their depleted state.

The dressings around the site should be changed every 48 to 72 hours and the tubing from the catheter to the TPN bottle changed every 24 to 72 hours. The whole catheter is not removed until it is no longer needed or until there is indication of an infection at the tip where it enters the vein. However, burn patients may need their TPN catheters changed weekly, especially if the catheter was introduced through burned tissue. With proper care, infectious complications are infrequent. Signs of catheter sepsis are fever, chills, tachycardia, and glucose intolerance. Onset of hyperglycemia in a previously stable patient usually indicates the beginning of an infection.

TABLE 30–10. Monitoring the Parenterally Fed Patient*

Variables to Be Monitored	Suggested Frequency†	
	Initial Period	*Later Period*
Growth Variables		
Weight	Daily	Daily
Length (infants only)	Weekly	Weekly
Head circumference (infants only)	Weekly	Weekly
Metabolic Variables		
Blood		
Serum electrolytes (Na^+, K^+, Cl^-)	Daily	3/week
Blood urea nitrogen	3/week	
Plasma total calcium or ionized Ca^{2+} and inorganic phosphorus	3/week	2/week
Blood glucose	Daily	3/week
Plasma transaminases	3/week	2/week
Plasma total protein and fractions	2/week	Weekly
Blood acid-base status	Daily	3/week
Hemoglobin	Weekly	Weekly
Prothrombin time	Weekly	Weekly
Ammonia	2/week	Weekly
Magnesium	2/week	Weekly
Zinc	Weekly	Weekly
Copper	Weekly	Weekly
Triglycerides	Weekly	Weekly
Urine		
Glucose and ketones	4–6/day	2/day
Specific gravity or osmolarity	2–4/day	Daily
Urinary urea nitrogen	Weekly	Weekly
General Measurements		
Volume of infusate	Daily	Daily
Oral intake (if any)	Daily	Daily
Urinary output	Daily	Daily
Prevention and Detection of Infection		
Clinical observations (activity, temperature, etc.)	Daily	Daily
WBC‡ count and differential	As indicated	As indicated
Cultures	As indicated	As indicated

* Adapted from Winters RW and Wilmore DW: Evaluation of the patient. *In* White PL, Nagy ME, and Fletcher DC (eds): Total Parenteral Nutrition. Acton, MA, Publishing Sciences Group, 1974; Grant JP: Handbook of Total Parenteral Nutrition. Philadelphia, WB Saunders, 1980.

† *Initial period* refers to that period in which a full glucose intake is being achieved; *later period* implies that the patient has achieved a steady metabolic state. In the presence of metabolic instability, the more intensive monitoring outlined under *initial period* should be followed.

‡ WBC = white blood cell.

Monitoring

Table 30–10 lists the clinical factors that should be monitored in the patient receiving TPN. Monitoring of blood and urine glucose concentrations, urinary output, blood urea nitrogen (BUN), and electrolyte levels show whether the patient is metabolically stable. If insulin response is not sufficient, insulin may need to be added. Four liters per day of TPN formula is the maximum that most patients can tolerate. As in the case with enterally tube-fed patients, the actual administration of parenteral feeding should be closely monitored. Often prescribed volume does not match the given amount because of decreased feeding time due to patient ambulation and bathing, frequent tests or treatments away from bedside, intravenous administration of medications, and inappropriate infusion rates (Lenssen, 1989).

Exercise

Exercise and physical therapy are an important part of total treatment if possible and allow efficient use of the nutritional support being provided. Skeletal muscle protein synthesis is enhanced if the muscles are exercised. For example, in states of protein depletion the heart muscle is spared until the end, apparently because it receives constant exercise.

Complications

Although TPN appears to be the answer to many clinical nutritional problems, it is not without risk. Some of the complications are listed in Table 30–11. The risk of TPN should always be balanced against the benefit and compared with risks and benefits of enteral nutrition.

TABLE 30–11. Complications of Total Parenteral Nutrition

Subclavian Catheterization
Pneumothorax
Hemothorax
Hydrothorax
Tension pneumothorax
Subcutaneous emphysema
Brachial plexus injury
Subclavian artery injury
Subclavian hematoma
Central vein thrombophlebitis
Arteriovenous fistula
Thoracic duct injury
Hydromediastinum
Air embolism
Catheter fragment embolism
Catheter misplacement
Cardiac perforation; tamponade
Endocarditis

Infection and Sepsis
Catheter entrance site
    Contamination during insertion
    Long-term catheter placement
Catheter seeding from blood-borne or distant infection
Solution contamination

Mechanical Problems

Metabolic Complications
Dehydration from osmotic diuresis
Hyperosmolar, nonketotic, hyperglycemic coma
Rebound hypoglycemia on sudden cessation of treatment
Hypomagnesemia
Hypocalcemia
Hypercalcemia
Hyperphosphatemia and hypophosphatemia
Hyperchloremic metabolic acidosis
Uremia
Hyperammonemia
Electrolyte imbalance
Trace mineral deficiencies
Essential fatty acid deficiency
Hyperlipidemia

TRANSITIONAL FEEDING

Nutritional support during the time when the patient is moved from one form of feeding to another is called *transitional feeding.* Transition can be from parenteral nutrition to enteral tube feeding or oral intake, from enteral tube feeding to oral formula or food, or a combination of these.

Nutritional Recovery Syndrome

Nutritional recovery syndrome is marked by clinical signs, most importantly *hypophosphatemia,* which is seen in the overly aggressive refeeding of patients who have been without food or malnourished for a period of time (Table 30–12). The hypophosphatemia is due to the shift of phosphorus from the plasma to the intracellular compartment as it is used for adenosine triphosphate synthesis. The hypophosphatemia has severe metabolic, neuromuscular, and hematologic effects. Patients undergoing refeeding should have their serum phosphates monitored and phosphate replacement therapy such as phospho-soda or IV potassium phosphate given (Postoperative hypophosphatemia, 1989). A similar situation also exists for potassium—hypokalemia can occur as potassium moves into cells with the glucose during refeeding.

The state of starvation also appears to result in a decrease in the intestinal enzymes sucrase and lactase. Upon refeeding, the activity of these enzymes increases; however, lactase increases at a much slower rate than sucrase, so that the sugar lactose is poorly tolerated in the beginning (Knudsen et al, 1968).

Refeeding the malnourished patient disrupts the adaptive state of starvation and therefore must proceed slowly with close patient monitoring. It appears that the ideal early feedings are moderate in carbohydrate, low in sodium, lactose-free, and supplemented with phosphorus and potassium (Havala, 1990).

Parenteral to Enteral Tube Feeding

In the initial phase of moving from parenteral to enteral tube feeding, the parenteral support is continued at the prevailing rate. This allows for maintenance of adequate nutrient and fluid intake as tolerance of en-

TABLE 30–12. Refeeding Syndrome

Hyperglycemia
Hyperosmolar, hyperglycemic nonketotic coma
Rebound hypoglycemia
Dehydration
Congestive heart failure
Hypercapnia
Hypophosphatemia
    Increased risk in: alcoholics
        those with renal insufficiency
        diabetics
Hypokalemia
Hyperkalemia
Magnesium deficiency
    Increased risk in: alcoholics
        those with malabsorption
Hypocalcemia
Hypoalbuminemia

teral feeding is assessed. Continuous drip or pumped enteral tube feeding is usually started at 40 to 60 ml/hr and increased by 25 ml/hr every 8 to 24 hours. The rate or concentration of parenteral support is decreased in proportion to the amount (based on nutrient intake) of enteral nutrition support that is tolerated. This transition usually takes 2 to 3 days, but more time may be needed for patients who have received nothing enterally or orally for 2 weeks or more. These patients, and others with malabsorption, may require enteral feeding at half strength, with the initial rate reduced to 30 ml/hour.

Symptoms of gastrointestinal intolerance are nausea, vomiting, distention, diarrhea, cramping, and the presence of large amounts of residual feeding. If any of these are present, the enteral feeding should be (1) maintained temporarily at the prevailing level, (2) reduced in concentration or in the rate of infusion, (3) replaced with another formula, or (4) discontinued with a return to full parenteral nutrition support.

If formula feedings are not tolerated, it may be useful to start again with a protein feeding module diluted to an isomolar level. These amino acid solutions or protein modules will stimulate gut hypertrophy and function and allow for tolerance of a more complete formula (Wade, 1986).

Bolus or meal feedings by syringe are not appropriate during early stages of transition from parenteral to enteral tube feeding because the volume loads (150 to 350 ml) may not be tolerated.

Parenteral to Oral Formula or Foods

In moving from parenteral to oral intake, it is again important to maintain parenteral support during the time when oral intake is started and gradually increased. Tolerance must be monitored, and adequate intake must be maintained. Small volumes (30 to 60 ml/hr) are sipped for 20 to 30 minutes. This is increased by 30 to 60 ml/hr each day, and the time between feedings is gradually expanded. At first the formula may need to be diluted to ¼ or ½ strength. Once the required volume is tolerated, the concentration of the formula can be increased to normal. Simultaneous increases in volume and concentration should be avoided.

The transition from PN to oral formula intake is harder to manage than PN to enteral tube feeding. Difficulties involve the patient's subjective tolerance of the taste of the formula, the less controlled rate of consumption, and the necessity for oral consumption of the large volume needed (sometimes as much as 3 liters) to provide for daily fluid and nutrient requirements (Wade, 1986).

When it is anticipated that transition from PN to oral feeding will progress rapidly, foods may be introduced initially in place of a formula. Simple liquid foods such as a clear liquid diet are recommended first foods. However, even these may need to be diluted at first because of their high osmolalities (Table 30–13). At first, patients with limited gastrointestinal tolerance should receive hyposmolar or mildly hyperosmolar liquids (up to 400 mOsm/kg) (Bell et al, 1987). The complexity of the foods can be increased based upon the individual's tolerance. Volumes begin at 30 to 60 ml/hr and are increased gradually to ad libitum consumption within 48 hours. During the next 3 days, food consistency and complexity are increased and foods provided

TABLE 30–13. Osmolalities of Beverages*

Beverage	Dilutions	mOsm/kg
Juice		
Prune	1:3	1,076
Cranberry	1:3	836
Pineapple	—†	772
Apple	—	705
Tomato	—	619
Grapefruit	—	618
Orange	—	601
V-8	—	578
Low-calorie cranberry	—	287
Broth		
Low-sodium, low-fat chicken	—	452
Regular chicken	—	389
Water Ice		
Cherry‡	1:3	1,064
Jello		
Cherry	1:4	735
Low calorie	—	57
Soft drinks		
Cola	—	714
Ginger ale	—	565
Diet ginger ale	—	53
Diet cola	—	43
Coffee/tea — 1 cup		
Coffee with 1 tsp sugar	—	128
Coffee with artificial sweetener	—	114
Tea with 1 tsp sugar	—	106
Tea with artificial sweetener	—	84
Coffee	—	83
Tea	—	8
Milk		
Ice cream	—	1,150
Carnation Instant Breakfast with skim milk and Lactaid	—	727
Carnation Instant Breakfast with whole milk and Lactaid	—	723
Eggnog	—	695
Carnation Instant Breakfast with whole milk	—	653
Carnation Instant Breakfast with skim milk	—	617
Whole milk with Lactaid	—	413
Skim milk with Lactaid	—	375
Skim milk	—	280
Whole milk	—	277

* Adapted from Bell SJ et al: Osmolality of beverages commonly provided on clear and full liquid menu. Nutr Clin Prac 2:241, 1987.

† Dash indicates no dilution.

‡ Like a popsicle.

often (6 to 8 times per day) in small amounts (1 to 2 oz) with only two to five items at each meal. Nutrient-dense foods are emphasized until adequate oral intake is established. When adequate oral intake, based upon intake calculations, is maintained for 3 to 4 days, the IV line can be discontinued.

Overzealous dietary progression can lead to problems of intolerance (see Table 30–12). On the other hand, the anorexic patient with a functioning gastrointestinal tract needs to be encouraged and supported by creativity on the part of the clinical nutritionist and hospital staff.

Enteral to Oral Formula or Foods

A common problem in transition from enteral tube feeding to oral feeding is poor appetite and satiety as long as enteral feeding is available. Cyclic feeding during the night or a specified portion of the day provides the nutrient and fluid requirements not met by oral intake. Detachment from the continuous infusion during the remaining time allows for more activity and opportunity for oral intake. Infusion of the feeding for 8 to 20 hr/day rather than continuously is the goal for those preparing for an oral diet or who are on home tube-feeding programs. The length of the cycle will depend on the patient's ability to tolerate large fluid volumes at an increased rate and the amount of the oral intake.

ENTERAL OR PARENTERAL TUBE FEEDING AT HOME

When a patient is basically well except for the need for long-term or continuous nutritional therapy, discharge from the hospital to a nursing home, long-term care facility, or home is a routine occurrence. In fact, even some critically ill or terminally ill patients are discharged to the home setting (Table 30–14). Patients can be maintained indefinitely with enteral or parenteral feeding either as a supplement to oral intake or as the sole method of intake. Some have been maintained for several decades with enteral feeding and almost 2 decades with parenteral feeding. Many children maintained all of their lives with enteral or parenteral nutrition therapy grow and mature normally.

Most effective in educating the patient and family as well as providing for ongoing support, is a home nutrition therapy team usually consisting of a physician, dietitian, nurse, pharmacist, and sometimes social worker and rehabilitative therapist. There are now commercial companies that provide this home care in addition to providing the feeding formula and supplies to the home. Monitoring and following protocol for formula preparation and infection control are just as important at home as they are in the hospital (McCrae, 1989; McCrae and Hall, 1989; Rohde and Braun, 1986).

TABLE 30–14. Concerns in the Selection of Patients for Home Nutrition Support*

Social/Psychologic
Patient motivation
Potential improvement in the patient's life
Financial
Third-party insurance reimbursement
Patient's or family's ability to handle the financial situation
Educational
Patient's or caretaker's ability to learn the protocol for administration
Ability to comply with the standards for safety
Medical
Benefit of long-term nutrition support to the patient's condition
Nutritional
Benefit of the long-term nutrition support to the patient's nutritional status
Physical
Patient's or caretaker's physical limitations that influence the ability to administer nutrition support safely

* Adapted from Porcelli KA and Krey SH: Home enteral nutrition. *In* Krey SH and Murray RL (eds): Dynamics of Nutritional Support. Assessment, Implementation and Evaluation. Norwalk, CT, Appleton-Century-Crofts, 1986.

Home enteral or parenteral nutrition is usually administered in the evening hours when the patient is at home or asleep, so that life during the day can be as normal as possible. However, some patients who require infusion for longer periods of time in order to maintain their nutritional intake can wear portable feeding bags and pumps that do not restrict them.

The ability of nutrition support to maintain life past the point where the quality of that life is not acceptable to the patient leads to the ethical issue of when life support should be discontinued. Standards for its initiation and termination have been determined, but the decision remains a complex, controversial, and an individual one (American Dietetic Association, 1987; American Society for Parenteral and Enteral Nutrition, 1989).

PSYCHOSOCIAL ASPECTS OF ALTERNATIVE FORMS OF NUTRITIONAL SUPPORT

Several psychologic and social issues surround nutritional support, and the longer the period of anticipated support, the greater is their scope (Gulledge et al, 1987). Patients' feelings of loss of control and independence can be combined with frustration and anger at having a tube extending from the body, possible surgical scarring, and possible chronic underweight. Sexual dysfunction and loss of libido may result.

An individual's lifestyle usually changes dramatically as social activities may need to be scheduled around feeding times or avoided because of the inability to partake of a meal. The patient who may have been independent and a care-giver is now a care-receiver and may be unable to return to work, which affects family roles and income. The home may have to be rearranged to accommodate the equipment, supplies, and solutions necessary for home nutrition support.

Reactions to these many changes are variable and normal. A response should be considered abnormal only if it persists beyond a reasonable length of time or becomes debilitating. The home health nurse or dietitian can be very useful in assessing the patient's ability to cope, providing psychologic support, or encouraging further counseling.

CITED REFERENCES

Abernathy GB et al: Efficacy of tube feeding in supplying energy requirements of hospitalized patients. J Parenter Enteral Nutr 13:387, 1989.

American Dietetic Association: Position of the American Dietetic Association: Issues in feeding the terminally ill. J Am Diet Assoc 87:78, 1987.

American Medical Association, Nutrition Advisory Group: Statement on guidelines for multivitamin preparations for parenteral use. Chicago, AMA, 1975.

American Society for Parenteral and Enteral Nutrition: Standards for nutrition support for residents of long-term care facilities. Nutr Clin Prac 4:148, 1989.

Andrassy RJ: Enteral feeding: Complications and monitoring. *In* Enteral Feeding: Scientific Basis and Clinical Applications. Columbus, OH, Ross Laboratories, 1988.

Bach AC, Storck D, and Meraihi A: Medium-chain triglyceride-based fat emulsions: An alternative energy supply in stress and sepsis. J Parenter Enteral Nutr 12(Suppl):82s, 1988.

Bell SJ et al: Osmolality of beverages commonly provided on clear and full liquid menu. Nutr Clin Prac 2:241, 1987.

Bennett KM and Rosen GH: Cyclic total parenteral nutrition. Nutr Clin Prac 5:163, 1990.

Breach CL and Saldanha LG: Tube feeding complications. Part I: Gastrointestinal. Nutr Suppl Serv 8(2):15, 1988a.

Breach CL and Saldanha LG: Tube feeding complications. Part II: Mechanical. Nutr Suppl Serv 8(5):28, 1988b.

Breach CL and Saldanha LG: Tube feeding complications. Part III: Metabolic. Nutr Suppl Serv 8(6):16, 1988c.

Brinson RR, Anderson WM, and Singh M: Hypoalbuminemia-associated diarrhea in critically ill patients, J Crit Illness 2(7):9, 1987.

Brinson RR, Hanumanthu SK, and Pitts WM: A reappraisal of the peptide-based enteral formulas: Clinical applications. Nutr Clin Prac 4:211, 1989.

Bynoe RP et al: Nutrition support in trauma patients. Nutr Clin Prac 3:137, 1988.

Campos ACL and Meguid MM: Invited comment: Short-chain fatty acids: Present prospect—Future alternative? J Parenter Enteral Nutr 12(Suppl):98S, 1988.

Foley EF et al: Albumin supplementation in the critically ill. Arch Surg 125:739, 1990.

Ford EG, Jennings LM, and Andrassy RJ: Serum albumin (oncotic pressure) correlates with enteral feeding tolerance in the pediatric surgical patient. J Pediatr Surg 22:597, 1987.

Greig PD, Baker JP, and Jeejeebhoy KN: Metabolic effects of total parenteral nutrition. Annu Rev Nutr 2:179, 1982.

Grimble G: Effect of peptide chain length on absorption of egg protein hydrolysates in the normal human jejunum. Gastroenterology 92:136, 1987.

Gulledge AD et al: Psychosocial issues of home parenteral and enteral nutrition. Nutr Clin Prac 2:183, 1987.

Harak T and Shronts E: Managing the complications associated with refeeding. Nutr Clin Prac 5:23, 1990.

Havala T and Shronts E: Managing the complications associated with refeeding. Nutr Clin Prac 5:23, 1990.

Heird WC, Grundy SM, and Van Hubbard S: Structured lipids and their use in clinical nutrition. Am J Clin Nutr 43:320, 1986.

Hunter AMB: Ethical issues in nutritional support. *In* Skipper A (ed): Dietitian's Handbook of Enteral and Parenteral Nutrition. Rockville, MD, Aspen Publishers, 1989.

Jeejeebhoy KN et al: Chromium deficiency, glucose intolerance, and neuropathy reversed by chromium supplementation in a patient receiving long-term parenteral nutrition. Am J Clin Nutr 30:531, 1977.

Kerzner B: Determinants of optimal nitrogen, fat and carbohydrate sources for enteral feeding. *In* Enteral Feeding: Scientific Basis and Clinical Applications. Columbus, OH, Ross Laboratories, 1988.

Knudsen K et al: Effect of fasting and refeeding on the histology of the human intestine. Gastroenterology 55:46, 1968.

Lenssen P: Monitoring and complications of parenteral nutrition. *In* Skipper A (ed): Dietitian's Handbook of Enteral and Parenteral Nutrition. Rockville, MD, Aspen Publishers, 1989.

Mascioli EA et al: Medium chain triglycerides and structured lipids as unique nonglucose energy sources in hyperalimentation. Lipids 22:421, 1987.

Mascioli EA et al: Novel triglycerides for special medical purposes. J Parenter Enteral Nutr 12(Suppl):127S, 1988.

McCrae JAD: Home parenteral nutrition. *In* Skipper A (ed): Dietitian's Handbook of Enteral and Parenteral Nutrition. Rockville, MD, Aspen Publishers, 1989.

McCrae JAD and Hall NH: Current practices for home enteral nutrition. J Am Diet Assoc 89:233, 1989.

Metheny N, Eisenberg P, and McSweeney M: Effect of feeding tube properties and three irrigants on clogging rates. Nurs Res 37:165, 1988.

Moore EE and Jones TN: Benefits of immediate jejunostomy feeding after major abdominal trauma—a prospective, randomized study. J Trauma 26:874, 1986.

Moss G: Postoperative metabolism: The role of plasma albumin in the enteral absorption of water and electrolytes. Pacific Med Surg 75:355, 1967.

Multivitamin preparations for parenteral use. A statement by the Nutrition Advisory Group. J Parenter Enteral Nutr 3:258, 1979.

Postoperative hypophosphatemia: A multifactorial problem. Nutr Rev 47:111, 1989.

Roesner M and Grant JP: Intravenous lipid emulsions. Nutr Clin Prac 2:96, 1987.

Rohde CL and Braun TM: Home Enteral/Parenteral Nutrition Therapy. Chicago, American Dietetic Association, 1986.

Ryan JA and Beshlian K: Nutritional significance of the small intestine. *In* Lang CE (ed): Nutritional Support in Critical Care. Rockville, MD, Aspen Publishers, 1987.

Shapiro M and Rosen GH: Topical oil applications in essential fatty acid deficiency. Nutr Clin Prac 4:140, 1989.

Shike M et al: A possible role of vitamin D in the genesis of parenteral nutrition-induced metabolic bone disease. Ann Intern Med 95:560, 1981.

Smith RJ et al: Glutamine nutrition and the gastrointestinal tract. *In* The Gastrointestinal Response to Injury, Starvation, and Enteral Nutrition, Report of the 8th Ross Conference on Medical Research. Columbus, OH, Ross Laboratories, 1988.

Souba WW et al: Gut glutamine metabolism. J Parenter Enteral Nutr 14(Suppl):45s, 1990.

Wade J: Parenteral and enteral transition techniques. *In* Krey SH and Murray RL (eds): Dynamics of Nutritional Support. Assessment, Implementation, and Evaluation. Norwalk, CT, Appleton-Century-Crofts, 1986.

Wayman L: The effect of acute discontinuation of TPN. Ann Surg 204:524, 1986.

ADDITIONAL REFERENCES

Albumin supplementation during TPN. Nutr MD 16(2):3, 1990.

Andrassy RJ: Role of albumin in enhancing gastrointestinal function. Nutr MD 14(6):1, 1988.

Burns PE, McCall L, and Wirsching R: Physical compatibility of

enteral formulas with various common medications. J Am Diet Assoc 88:1094, 1988.
Ferraro RT and Albu J: Nutrition support of the critically ill obese patient (Editorial). Nutr Clin Prac 4:125, 1989.
Fleming CR and Berkner S (eds): Home Parenteral Nutrition: A Handbook for Patients. Philadelphia, JB Lippincott, 1989.
Lo CW and Walker WA: Changes in the gastrointestinal tract during enteral or parenteral feeding. Nutr Rev 47:193, 1989.
Mc Mahon M et al: Parenteral nutrition in patients with diabetes mellitus: Theoretical and practical considerations. J Parenter Enteral Nutr 13:545, 1989.
Mobarhan S: The role of albumin in nutritional support. J Am Coll Nutr 7:445, 1988.
Moss G: The role of albumin in nutritional support. J Am Coll Nutr 7:441, 1988.
Patterson ML: Enteral feeding in the hypoalbuminemic patient. J Parenter Enteral Nutr 14:362, 1990.
Rombeau JL and Caldwell MD: Clinical Nutrition: Enteral and Tube Feeding, 2nd ed. Philadelphia, WB Saunders, 1990.
Rombeau JL et al (eds): Atlas of Nutritional Support Techniques. Boston, Little, Brown & Co, 1989.
Seaton TB et al: Thermic effect of medium-chain and long-chain triglycerides in man. Am J Clin Nutr 44:630, 1986.
Skeie B et al: The beneficial effects of fat on ventilation and pulmonary function. Nutrition 3:149, 1987.
Skipper A (ed): Dietitian's Handbook of Enteral and Parenteral Nutrition. Rockville, MD, Aspen Publishers, 1989.
Steinbrook R and Lo B: Artificial feeding—Solid ground, not a slippery slope. N Engl J Med 318:286, 1988.
The ethics of artificial feeding (Letter). N Engl J Med 319:306, 1988.

CHAPTER 31

NUTRITIONAL CARE IN DIABETES MELLITUS AND REACTIVE HYPOGLYCEMIA

KEY TERMS

CONTINUOUS SUBCUTANEOUS INSULIN INFUSION—continuous delivery of insulin by means of indwelling catheter and a programmed pump worn outside the body

DIABETIC GASTROPARESIS—paralysis of the stomach caused by diabetes-induced visceral autonomic neuropathy

DIABETIC KETOACIDOSIS—acidosis accompanied by the accumulation of ketone bodies in the body tissues and fluids; caused by a lack or inadequacy of insulin

FASTING HYPOGLYCEMIA—abnormally low blood glucose concentration 6 hours or more after a meal

GESTATIONAL DIABETES MELLITUS—glucose intolerance with onset during pregnancy

GLUCOSE TOLERANCE FACTOR—a biologically active complex of chromium and nicotinic acid that appears to facilitate the reaction of insulin with receptor sites on cells

GLYCOSYLATED HEMOGLOBIN—hemoglobin A with a hexose attached to the N-terminal of the beta-chain

HONEYMOON PERIOD—the period after diagnosis in the patient with insulin-dependent diabetes mellitus when the insulin requirements diminish or disappear temporarily

HYPEROSMOLAR, HYPERGLYCEMIC NONKETOTIC COMA—diabetic coma in which the level of ketone bodies is normal; usually seen in untreated NIDDM

HYPOGLYCEMIA—plasma glucose usually of 50 mg/dl or less, which results in symptoms caused by compensatory sympathetic nervous system activity

INSULIN-DEPENDENT DIABETES MELLITUS OR TYPE 1—diabetes usually occurring in childhood and characterized by abrupt onset of symptoms—insulinopenia, dependence on exogenous insulin to sustain life, and a tendency to develop ketoacidosis

MACROVASCULAR DISEASE—coronary heart disease, cerebrovascular disease, and peripheral vascular disease

MATURITY ONSET DIABETES OF YOUTH—a subtype of non–insulin-dependent diabetes mellitus that appears before age 20

MICROVASCULAR DISEASE—disease of the smaller blood vessels with an internal diameter of 100 μm or less

NON–INSULIN-DEPENDENT DIABETES MELLITUS—diabetes characterized by a gradual onset with minimal or no symptoms of metabolic disturbance and no requirement for exogenous insulin to prevent ketonuria and ketoacidosis

ORAL HYPOGLYCEMIC AGENTS—medications that act to regulate blood glucose by improving the action or secretion of endogenous insulin

POLYOL PATHWAY—the non-insulin dependent pathway by which glucose is converted to sorbitol and fructose in tissues, such as the lens, peripheral nerve cells, and kidney cells

REACTIVE POSTPRANDIAL HYPOGLYCEMIA—abnormally low concentration of blood glucose within 2 to 5 hours after eating

DIABETES MELLITUS

Diabetes mellitus is an ancient disease. The Greek word *diabetes* means "to flow through a siphon." *Mellitus,* meaning "honeyed," was added many centuries later to describe the sweet taste of the urine.

Diabetes affects about 6 million Americans and may be undetected in another 4 to 5 million. It is estimated that about 7% of the adult population has diabetes, half of which is undiagnosed (Hadden and Harris, 1987). Diabetes is the most common cause of blindness in this country and is responsible for 25% of all new end-stage renal disease each year. The rate of heart disease is 2 to 3 times as high as in nondiabetics, and life expectancy is only two thirds of that of the general population (Harris and Hamman, 1985).

Classification

The clinical syndrome of diabetes is characterized by an impaired ability to metabolize carbohydrates and fats, resulting in an increased concentration of glucose (hyperglycemia) and lipids (hyperlipidemia) in the circulating blood and eventually leading to premature vascular degeneration. The abnormal metabolism is the result of inadequate insulin secretion or ineffectiveness of the available insulin.

Insulin-dependent diabetes mellitus (IDDM), also called Type I or juvenile-onset diabetes, most commonly appears in youth and young adults but can occur at any age. The symptoms appear abruptly and require insulin for control. IDDM accounts for only 5 to 10% of all diabetes in this country, and incidence rates have been stable since 1965 (Harris and Hamman 1985).

Non-insulin-dependent diabetes mellitus (NIDDM), also called Type II or adult-onset diabetes, usually appears in middle age. This type is much more common, afflicting about 90 to 95% of all persons who have diabetes. Although the two types of diabetes appear to be different in etiology and pathophysiology, the manifestations of hyperglycemia and hyperlipidemia and their potentially damaging effects are similar (Table 31-1).

A *maturity-onset diabetes of youth (MODY)* is a type of NIDDM that appears before age 20. *Type III diabetes* is another subtype, seen only in black youth, in which the initial clinical course imitates the acute insulin deficiency of IDDM, but insulin dependency is transient and the eventual course is NIDDM. This atypical form accounts for at least 10% of all cases of youth-onset diabetes in black Americans in the southeastern United States (Winter et al, 1987).

Normal and Pathologic Physiology

Hormonal and Biochemical Relationships

GLUCOSE METABOLISM. Blood glucose levels are maintained by glucose from dietary carbohydrate and from liver glycogen. As glucose enters the blood stream, it is rapidly delivered to the cells, where it may be (1) utilized for energy (cellular oxidation), (2) converted to glycogen for storage in the liver or muscle (glycogenesis), or (3) converted to fat for storage in adipose tissue (lipogenesis).

Transport of glucose to the interior of most cells is dependent upon the presence of insulin attached to receptor sites on the cell membranes. In the absence of sufficient insulin or in the presence of reduced insulin effectiveness, glucose cannot cross the cell membrane and accumulates in the blood, leading to hyperglycemia and glycosuria. Exceptions are the brain, liver, lens of the eye, red blood cells, and renal medulla, in which

TABLE 31-1. Differences Between Insulin-Dependent Diabetes Mellitus and Non-Insulin-Dependent Diabetes Mellitus

Features	Insulin-Dependent	Non-Insulin-Dependent
Age at onset	Usually under 40	Usually over 40
Proportion of all diabetics	Less than 10%	Greater than 90%
Seasonal trend	Fall and winter	None
Family history of diabetes	Uncommon	Common
Appearance of symptoms	Acute or subacute	Slow
Metabolic ketoacidosis	Frequent	Rare
Obesity at onset	Uncommon	Common
Beta cells	Decreased	Variable
Insulin	Decreased or absent	Variable
Insulin receptors	Normal	Low or normal
Inflammatory cells in islets	Present initially	Absent
HLA association	Yes	No
Antibodies to islet cells	Yes	No
Clinical remission	Short-lived after treatment started	May be prolonged (if weight loss successful)
Primary immediate objective of dietary management	Synchronization of food intake and insulin injectons	Weight reduction

glucose is able to diffuse across the cell membrane without the intervention of insulin.

Insulin promotes fatty acid synthesis in the liver. It also promotes subsequent fat storage by stimulating activity of the enzyme lipoprotein lipase, one of whose functions is to facilitate uptake of triglyceride by adipose tissue. In the absence of insulin or effective insulin activity, lipolysis is promoted and free fatty acids, triglycerides, cholesterol, and phospholipids increase in the blood.

Insulin promotes the transport of amino acids through the cell membrane in a carrier transport system similar to that for glucose. It promotes protein synthesis in muscle tissue and the liver. In the absence of sufficient insulin, amino acids are deaminated and the non-nitrogenous portion used to synthesize glucose or fatty acids.

PANCREATIC SECRETIONS. Insulin, glucagon, and somatostatin are hormones secreted by adjacent cells in the pancreatic islets of Langerhans. Insulin lowers blood glucose; glucagon, along with epinephrine, cortisol, and growth hormone, raises blood glucose. Somatostatin inhibits the secretion of both insulin and glucagon, and also inhibits the release of growth hormone. It may also function to control the rate of absorption of nutrients into the circulation.

CELLULAR RECEPTOR SITES. NIDDM is characterized by insulin resistance at the cellular level in both hepatic and muscle tissue. The number of insulin-binding receptors on the surface of the cell membrane decreases as the basal insulin level increases. Basal insulin levels are typically increased in NIDDM. Any intervention, such as diet, that reduces the basal insulin level will increase the number of receptors and improve the action of insulin. However, there is also a postreceptor defect in the cell that explains some of the insulin resistance.

Degenerative Complications

Degenerative complications are the cause of most diabetes morbidity and mortality. Whether normalizing blood glucose levels can postpone and minimize the onset of retinopathy, neuropathy, renal disease, and severe atherosclerosis is not entirely clear. The Diabetes Control and Complications Trial (DCCT), a 10-year multicenter clinical trial initiated in 1982 by the National Institute of Arthritis, Diabetes and Digestive and Kidney Diseases has been designed to provide an answer to this question (Diabetes Control and Complications Trial Research Group, 1987).

VASCULAR DISEASE. The increased life expectancy of persons with diabetes, made possible by the availability of insulin and oral hypoglycemic agents, has been accompanied by a steady increase in the incidence of vascular complications.

Macrovascular disease (coronary heart disease, cerebrovascular disease, and peripheral vascular disease) is not specific to diabetes, but it generally develops at an earlier age and is the major cause of death in patients with this disease. A common consequence of peripheral vascular disease is reduced circulation, particularly to the legs and feet. Other complaints are coldness and fatigue in these areas. Wounds and infections can be dangerous because of poor healing due to the poor blood supply, and gangrene can develop. In addition, there is reduced pain sensation and impairment of inflammatory response to injury, so that the person with diabetes may not have the usual pain and redness in response to injury. Table 31-2 lists some of the degenerative complications of diabetes.

Microvascular disease occurs in tissues where glucose transport into the cell does not depend on insulin. When the extracellular glucose level is high, cellular glucose concentration rises and glucose is converted to sorbitol and fructose by the *polyol pathway.* Sorbitol and fructose cannot leave the cell easily, and as their cellular concentration increases, they promote osmotic accumulation of water with subsequent swelling and cellular dysfunction, especially in the lens of the eye. In the peripheral nerve cells and possibly other tissues, sorbitol and fructose accumulation reduces the cellular concentration of myo-inositol, another sugar alcohol. Dietary myo-inositol has improved nerve conduction in some patients, but its use is not yet an accepted general

TABLE 31-2. Degenerative Complications of Diabetes Mellitus*

- Ophthalmologic
  - Retinopathy (most frequent complication of insulin-dependent diabetes mellitus)
  - Glaucoma
  - Cataract
- Macrovascular
  - Coronary artery disease
  - Cerebrovascular disease
  - Peripheral vascular disease
    - Gangrene
  - Hypertension
- Nephropathy
  - Renal failure (Kimmelstiel-Wilson disease)
- Neuropathy
  - Polyneuropathy
  - Autonomic neuropathy
    - Gastroparesis
    - Impotence
- Infections
- Osteopenia
- Pancreatic exocrine insufficiency
  (mild, usually clinically insignificant)

* Adapted from Molitch ME: Complications of diabetes mellitus. *In Handbook of Diabetes Nutritional Management* by MA Powers, p. 31, with permission of Aspen Publishers, Inc., © 1987.

practice (Green et al, 1987a). Aldose reductase inhibitors, medications that inhibit the polyol pathway, may be useful in the future in preventing the hyperglycemia-induced complications of diabetes.

Hyperglycemia leads to the excessive accumulation of glycosylation end products on glycoproteins in the blood vessel walls. The resulting dysfunction may be a cause of some diabetic complications; for example, the thickening of capillary basement membranes that results in the dysfunction of the retina, renal glomerulus, and nerve Schwann cells (Brownlee et al, 1988).

INFECTIONS. Hyperglycemia damages components of the immune system, with the result that the person with diabetes is highly susceptible to infections that typically destroy the glucose-insulin homeostasis and put the diabetes "out of control." The combination of infection, slow wound healing, and impaired circulation to the extremities imposes extreme risk for injuries of the feet to become unmanageable.

Etiology

Insulin-Dependent Diabetes Mellitus

IDDM is a disorder that appears to result from immunologically mediated destruction of pancreatic beta cells in genetically susceptible individuals. A virus-invaded beta cell may become identified as a foreign substance leading to an immune response, or a virus may provoke a lymphocytic infiltration of pancreatic islets that progresses to destruction of beta cells and the sudden appearance of symptoms. Antibodies to islet cells are present in most newly diagnosed IDDM patients, and may be detected up to 11 years before the clinical onset of the disease (Srikanta et al, 1983). A variety of viruses, including mumps, rubella, and measles, may be involved.

Non – Insulin-Dependent Diabetes Mellitus

NIDDM is also genetically determined, and is expressed with age and the influence of environmental factors. The hereditary mechanism is more predominant in NIDDM and does not appear to involve the immune response (Further Reading, p. 532).

AGE. Glucose tolerance declines with age. In the population examined in the NHANES II, males aged 65 to 74 years were 10 times as likely to have diabetes as males aged 25 to 34 years (19% and 1.9%, respectively) and older females were 11 times more likely to have diabetes than younger females (16.5% and 1.5%, respectively) (Yetley and Johnson, 1987).

Several theories have been proposed to explain the hyperglycemia that occurs with aging, such as decreased insulin synthesis, insulin receptor changes, or changes in body composition. The higher glucose standards of "impaired glucose tolerance" (Table 31 – 3) are used to diagnose excessive and problematic glucose intolerance in the elderly.

OBESITY. The prevalence of diabetes is almost 3 times as high in the obese as in the nonobese (Yetley and Johnson, 1987). Hyperinsulinism is also seen, and it is thought that insulin resistance develops from an increase in adipose tissue mass. It also appears that android (upper body) obesity is more frequently associated with abnormal glucose tolerance than gynoid (lower body) obesity (Kawahara and Amemiya, 1989) (see p. 318 in Chapter 18). Weight reduction in the obese with NIDDM usually ameliorates insulin resistance and the severity of the disease.

STRESS. Physiologic and mental stress may decrease glucose tolerance and can precipitate diabetes in persons whose tolerance is already impaired.

The stress of infectious disease or the trauma of injury, surgery, or myocardial infarction can precipitate diabetes in a person with impaired glucose tolerance. The physiologic stress of pregnancy may decrease glucose tolerance. Mental stress may aggravate the disease by causing the release of catecholamines, which decreases glucose tolerance.

DRUGS. Diuretics such as furosemide and glucocorticoids can impair glucose tolerance or aggravate existing diabetes.

TRACE MINERALS. Zinc has been shown to enhance the action of insulin in promoting uptake of glucose by adipose tissue. Chromium occurs with nicotinic acid and amino acids in a *glucose tolerance factor (GTF),* which is required for normal carbohydrate and lipid metabolism and appears to facilitate insulin binding with receptors. A chromium deficiency, often seen with advancing age, may account for impaired glucose tolerance seen in some elderly persons (Anderson and Kozlovsky, 1985).

Clinical Findings

Blood Glucose Levels

Diagnosis of diabetes mellitus is usually made by measuring a fasting plasma glucose (FPG), sometimes combined with a postprandial plasma glucose or with an oral glucose tolerance test (OGTT).

STANDARDS FOR BLOOD GLUCOSE. FPG is elevated in all but the mildest cases of diabetes. The normal plasma glucose level is 70 to 115 mg/dl; a diagnosis of diabetes

TABLE 31-3. Classification of Diabetes Mellitus*

Classification	Diagnostic Criteria†
Insulin-dependent diabetes mellitus (IDDM) or Type I (formerly called juvenile-onset diabetes mellitus)	1. Classic symptoms of diabetes such as polyuria, polydipsia, ketonuria, and rapid weight loss together with random plasma glucose (PG) > 200 mg/dl 2. Fasting plasma glucose (FPG) ≥ 140 mg/dl 3. FPG < 140 mg/dl but sustained elevated plasma glucose during the oral glucose tolerance test (OGTT) on more than one occasion; both the 2-hr sample and some other sample taken between administration of the glucose and 2 hr later must be ≥200 mg/dl
Non-insulin-dependent diabetes mellitus (NIDDM) or Type II (formerly called adult-onset diabetes mellitus)	1. Classic symptoms as described above 2. FPG ≥ 140 mg/dl 3. FPG < 140 mg/dl but sustained elevated plasma glucose on OGTT as described above
Diabetes mellitus associated with certain conditions or syndromes (formerly called secondary diabetes mellitus)	1. Diagnosis of diabetes (as described above) and the presence of the associated condition or syndrome
Impaired glucose tolerance (formerly called chemical, latent or subclinical diabetes mellitus)—affects many elderly individuals	1. FPG < 140 mg/dl 2. PG 2 hr after glucose administration in an OGTT must be between 140 and 200 mg/dl 3. PG between ½ and 1½ hr after the glucose administration in OGTT must be ≥200 mg/dl
Gestational diabetes—glucose intolerance has its onset or recognition during pregnancy; associated with increased perinatal complications	1. Two or more of the following values during the OGTT must be met or exceeded: FPG = 105 mg/dl 1-hr PG = 190 mg/dl 2-hr PG = 165 mg/dl 3-hr PG = 145 mg/dl

* From National Diabetes Data Group: Classification and diagnosis of diabetes mellitus and other categories of glucose intolerance. Diabetes 28:1039, 1979.

† Based on venous plasma or serum samples. Whole blood or capillary blood values are about 10-15% lower than plasma values; 120 mg/dl is the upper limit for a fasting value on whole blood; 140 mg/dl is the upper limit for a fasting value on plasma or serum.

is made if on two separate occasions the FPG is greater than 140 mg/dl (capillary or whole blood—120 mg/dl). The 2-hour postprandial plasma glucose, which is elevated in the presence of diabetes, indicates how well glucose is handled after a meal. An elevated postprandial, but not fasting, glucose is classified as *impaired glucose tolerance (IGT)*. The OGTT indicates the ability to utilize a specific amount of glucose over time. Diagnostic criteria for diabetes and impaired glucose tolerance are shown in Table 31-3.

Oral Glucose Tolerance Test. The OGTT is controversial because it often is improperly standardized. However, a properly performed OGTT can be clinically useful in diagnosing patients with fasting normoglycemia. When administered correctly, a standard glucose load (1 g/kg body weight in adults with a maximum of 100 grams, and 1.75 g/kg body weight for children) is given as a glucose drink. Plasma glucose is measured before the glucose preparation is given, and again ½ hour, 1 hour, 2 hours, 3 hours, and possibly 4 and 5 hours after the glucose preparation has been taken. Urinary glucose is frequently measured at the same time.

The patient should be instructed to follow a diet unrestricted in carbohydrate (at least 150 g/day) for 3 days prior to the test. The OGTT is diagnostic of diabetes when two of the plasma glucose measurements between the time of glucose administration and 2 hours later are greater than 200 mg/dl.

Symptoms

Symptoms of uncontrolled diabetes reflect the consequences of cellular glucose deprivation and the efforts of the kidney to reduce elevated blood glucose levels. These include increased appetite (polyphagia), increased urination (polyuria), increased thirst (polydipsia), loss of weight, and failing strength. Failure to balance excessive urinary output with increased fluid intake leads to dehydration, electrolyte imbalance, and possibly ketoacidosis. These symptoms are seen classically in IDDM; however, less than 50% of cases of NIDDM present in this manner.

Reduced tissue healing ability leads to degenerative changes, especially in advanced cases. Pruritus vulvae, skin infections or irritation, and visual disturbances are frequently present and are often precipitating factors leading to the diagnosis of NIDDM.

Management

Philosophy of Management

The present philosophy of diabetes management is to maintain blood glucose levels as close to normal as possible without causing hypoglycemia. With the avail-

FURTHER READING: Diabetes in the Pima Indians

The incidence of diabetes in some American Indians has been recorded as the highest in the world. Studies conducted in the 1960s on Pima Indians living in the desert of central Arizona found that NIDDM occurred with a frequency 11 to 15 times that of the general population and 19 times that of a group of predominantly white adults in Rochester, Minnesota (Knowler, 1978).

Complications of NIDDM as seen among the Pimas follow the typical pattern; however, the disease does present some unique characteristics. Although of the "maturity onset" type, it commonly develops during adolescence, from age 15 and older. Although hypoglycemia is common, it is usually asymptomatic and acidosis is infrequent. Incidence plateaus around 40 years of age (Sievers, 1966; Savage, 1979).

Along with the strong genetic predisposition to NIDDM, the Pimas share with other southwestern desert tribes an extremely high incidence of obesity, possibly reflecting the presence of a "thrifty gene" that favors fat storage in anticipation of the food shortages that once were common. Obesity is widespread in adolescents and affects most adults over 35 years of age.

Diabetes may have been triggered in this susceptible population by departure from a traditional diet based on foods high in starch of a variety that is slowly digested and absorbed. Prior to 1930, the Pima diet consisted principally of wild and cultivated legumes, mesquite, and corn, supplemented with seeds, fish, and cacti (Brand, 1990).

However, the only correlation to date established between dietary factors and the risk of NIDDM is through the relation of obesity to the disease.

ability of self-monitoring of blood glucose (SMBG) and multiple daily insulin injections, it has become possible to achieve euglycemia. Nutritional management is receiving increased attention, particularly with NIDDM patients.

Insulin

Since their introduction in 1922, commercial insulin preparations have been the cornerstone of IDDM treatment. The NIDDM patient produces insulin and may in fact have hyperinsulinemia, but the insulin is not effective because of aberrations in the insulin receptor sites and a decrease in their number. As a result, these patients may require exogenous insulin in order to achieve euglycemia. However, in comparison with patients with IDDM, they are not ketosis-prone and therefore may be called *insulin requiring* rather than *insulin dependent.*

TYPES OF COMMERCIAL INSULIN. The several types of commercial insulin can be divided into three general categories: (1) short-acting (regular), (2) intermediate-acting (NPH and lente), and (3) long-acting (ultralente) insulin. Insulins available in the United States are summarized in Table 31–4. Until 1984, all insulin was extracted from animal pancreases. Now it can be made to duplicate human insulin (Humulin), either using recombinant DNA or by a process that modifies pork insulin. Humulin is nonallergenic, and its absorption is faster and its duration of action is less (Sotsky and Shamoon, 1986).

DOSAGES. All insulin is sold in a standard potency of U-100 (100 units/ml). A single unit (U) of insulin provides for the use of 1.5 to 3 grams of glucose.

The type, dosage, and frequency of insulin administration is individualized, depending upon the patient's stage of growth, physical state, activity, eating habits, and psychologic stability. It may be a single dose, or a mixture of insulins in one injection, or a regimen of two or three injections during a 24-hour period. It may be given as a continuous subcutaneous insulin infusion (CSII) with small additional amounts before meals and snacks. A balance must be maintained among insulin, dietary glucose, and activity level.

The average child needs 0.6 U/kg of insulin per 24-hour period, whereas the adolescent may require 1 to 2 U/kg/day. Moderately active adults usually need 0.6 U/kg/day but may require 1 U/kg/day when ill or under stress. Insulin dosages significantly greater than this may represent "overinsulinization." The insulin-requiring NIDDM patient usually begins with 10 to 15 U/day. Insulin dosage is adjusted as needed based upon blood glucose monitoring.

TABLE 31–4. Types and Actions of Insulin

Insulin	Onset (hr)	Peak (hr)	Usual Effective Duration (hr)	Usual Maximum Duration (hr)
Animal				
Regular	0.5–2.0	3–4	4–6	6–8
NPH	4–6	8–14	16–20	20–24
Lente	4–6	8–14	16–20	20–24
Ultralente	8–14	Minimal	24–36	24–36
Human				
Regular	0.5–1.0	2–3	3–6	4–6
NPH	2–4	4–10	10–16	14–18
Lente	3–4	4–12	12–18	16–20
Ultralente	6–10	?	18–20	20–30

* From American Diabetes Association: Physician's Guide to Insulin-Dependent (Type I) Diabetes: Diagnosis and Treatment. Alexandria, VA, American Diabetes Association, 1988, Table 6.

Insulin administration must be continued during the period when the pancreas is unable to function adequately. Very often, improvement occurs in the patient with IDDM for a short time after insulin has been started. This clinical remission, or *honeymoon phase,* may last for a period of weeks or up to 1 year but is only temporary. During the remission, insulin is either reduced or omitted. The NIDDM patient who requires insulin at first may, after sufficient weight loss, be able to control hyperglycemia by diet alone or by diet plus one of the oral hypoglycemic agents.

INJECTION SITES

Administration. Insulin is best injected in the area between fat and muscle where the skin is loose (Fig. 31-1). It should be injected into the same area of the body for the injection at a particular time of the day. For example, the morning injection in the arm and the evening injection in the legs. The injection site should be rotated within the injection area (see Fig. 31-1).

Continuous subcutaneous insulin infusion delivers insulin by means of a pump worn outside the body. It is programmed to give an approximation of basal insulin levels (often as a slow-acting insulin), with additional increments of regular insulin just before meals or snacks. Blood glucose must be checked several times per day and the insulin infusion adjusted accordingly.

Two other methods of insulin administration are available. The *jet injector,* still relatively expensive, forces insulin under pressure through the skin. The *button infuser* is a needle with a resealable cap that remains in the abdomen for 2 to 3 days. It is good for those taking multiple daily injections; however, it is also expensive.

Insulin Allergy. Local cutaneous reactions can develop to the insulin being used, especially to beef insulins, or to the alcohol used for cleansing or sterilization. Changing the type of insulin does not help; desensitization is the only effective treatment (Pulini, 1985). Small but gradually increasing amounts of insulin are given at frequent intervals.

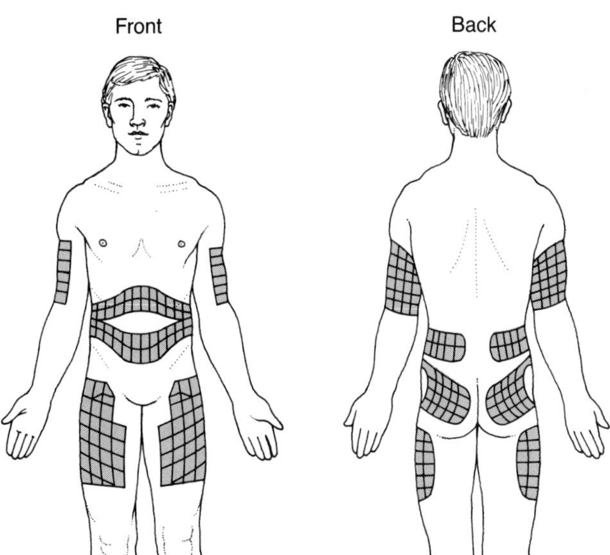

FIGURE 31-1. *Sites for insulin injection. Insulin injected into abdomen is absorbed 30% faster than from any other site.*

Insulin Antibodies. Occasionally antibodies develop to injected insulin. An immune reaction occurs, and insulin becomes ineffective. Dosages must be greatly increased, sometimes up to several hundred units per day depending on the degree of resistance. Usually insulin sensitivity returns and the dosage can be reduced. Common causes of insulin resistance are physiologic stresses such as pregnancy, infection, obesity, or an endocrine disorder.

Insulin Resistance. Insulin resistance is defined as the situation in which there is a need for large doses of insulin—at least 200 U for more than 2 days—but without the presence of antibodies. This can develop in the presence of Cushing's syndrome, acromegaly, hemochromatosis, and acanthosis nigricans. Patients with insulin resistance are candidates for U-500, a more concentrated insulin available by special order.

Lipodystrophy. Repeated insulin injections at the same site may lead to development of either lipoatrophy (loss of subcutaneous fat) or lipohypertrophy (overgrowth of subcutaneous fat). Lipoatrophy is treated by using a purer insulin at the same site; lipohypertrophy is treated by avoiding the area for injections. Proper rotation of injection sites should be emphasized in both situations.

SOMOGYI PHENOMENON. The occurrence of rebound hyperglycemia after a period of hypoglycemia before meals or during the night is called the *Somogyi phenomenon.* This effect is caused by the release of counter-regulatory hormones, particularly epinephrine, which acts to raise blood glucose (Perriello et al, 1988). Waning of insulin action and excess eating that may occur in order to overcome hypoglycemic symptoms can add to the hyperglycemia (Cryer and Gerich, 1985). As a consequence, insulin dosages can be mistakenly increased with a worsening of the situation. The blood glucose must be tested several times during the day and night, and when the presence of hypoglycemia is documented, the evening insulin dosage should be decreased or the evening snack increased.

DAWN PHENOMENON. Early morning hyperglycemia, thought to be caused by a surge of growth hormone released during sleep, is known as the *dawn phenomenon.* It also appears in persons without diabetes, but is compounded in those with diabetes by the fact that the evening insulin dosage may also be waning at that time (4:00 A.M. to 7:00 A.M.). A 3:00 A.M. blood test will discriminate between the Somogyi and dawn phenomena.

A low blood glucose at that time (70 mg/dl or less) is indicative of the Somogyi phenomenon and a normal value identifies the dawn phenomenon. The latter is treated by adjusting the evening dosage of insulin to provide additional coverage between 4:00 A.M. to 7:00 A.M.

WEIGHT GAIN. Weight gain is common after intensive insulin therapy, probably because utilization of energy improves when glycosuria is decreased. This should be anticipated so that management can be modified accordingly (Diabetes Control and Complications Trial Research Group, 1988). Instead of adjusting insulin, these patients may be better counseled to adjust the diet based on SMBG.

Oral Hypoglycemic Agents

Patients with NIDDM who do not respond appropriately to dietary measures are usually treated with *oral hypoglycemic agents (OHA).*

TYPES. The OHA commonly in use in the United States are the sulfonylureas listed in Table 31–5. Glyburide and glipizide are newer and more potent drugs with fewer side effects and are safer for patients with renal disease. OHA lower the blood glucose level and reduce glycosuria by (1) stimulating the pancreatic beta cells to secrete insulin, (2) enhancing insulin sensitivity of the receptor cell, and (3) inhibiting glucose formation from liver glycogen. However, these compounds are effective only in those who have beta cells that are able to respond to the stimulus.

RISKS. Users of oral hypoglycemic agents are at risk of hypoglycemia but this response is not common. In 1970, the University Group Diabetes Program reported increased cardiovascular disease and death in some patients taking tolbutamide. However, these findings were not confirmed in subsequent studies.

TABLE 31–5. Oral Hypoglycemic Agents*

Agent	Equivalent Doses (mg)	Doses per Day	Onset (hr)	Duration (hr)
First Generation				
Tolbutamide (Orinase)	1000	2–3	1	6–12
Acetohexamide (Dymelor)	500	1–2	1	12–24
Tolazamide (Tolinase)	250	1–2	4–6	10–16
Chlorpropamide (Diabinese)	250	1	1	Up to 60
Second Generation				
Glyburide (Diabeta, Micronase)	5	1–2	2–4	24
Glipizide† (Glucotrol)	5	1–2	1–1.5	10–24

* Adapted from Samowich AS: Medications and Delivery Methods. *In* Powers MA: Handbook of Diabetes Nutritional Management. Rockville, MD, Aspen Publications, 1987, p. 70; adapted from Drug Facts and Comparisons, 1987 Edition (p. 376) with permission of Facts and Comparisons Division, JB Lippincott Company, 1986.

† Take 30 minutes before a meal to maximize effect.

INTERACTION WITH ALCOHOL AND OTHER DRUGS. Alcohol can potentiate the hypoglycemic effect of sulfonylureas. Aspirin, phenylbutazone, sulfonamides, and monoamine oxidase inhibitors may have a similar effect, but not to the degree exerted by alcohol. Corticosteroids have a hyperglycemic effect, as do oral contraceptives and thiazide diuretics. Hypoglycemia appears more commonly with chlorpropamide (Diabinese) and glyburide (Micronase, DiaBeta). This hypoglycemia may last 24 to 48 hours and may be very severe.

Monitoring

SELF-MONITORING OF BLOOD GLUCOSE (SMBG). SMBG using a finger prick of capillary blood with glucose-oxidase reagent strips (e.g., Dextrostix, Chemstrip), read visually or from a reflectance meter (glucometer), has been a major factor in improving glycemic control. When carefully done, either test will give results within 10 to 15% of glucose concentrations measured by standard laboratory methods. Readings before meals and 1 to 2 hours afterward permit adjustment of daily insulin dosage, exercise, and diet in accordance with the observed effect on blood glucose. An appropriate premeal or fasting blood glucose in NIDDM should be 115 mg/dl to 140 mg/dl; equivalent postprandial (1 to 2 hours after a meal) values are between 140 mg/dl and 175 mg/dl. Patients with IDDM have wider fluctuations and target ranges should be established individually (Rifkin, 1983).

URINE MONITORING. Urine glucose concentrations are only crude assessments of diabetes management. However, urinary testing for ketones is important, especially if blood glucose is greater than 240 mg/dl. Urine specimens are checked before breakfast, lunch, dinner, and bedtime. Ketone measurements are even more important during illness when their use is recommended in addition to SMBG.

GLYCOSYLATED HEMOGLOBIN. *Glycosylated hemoglobin* (HbA_1 or HbA_{1c}) is produced when hemoglobin reacts with high concentrations of serum glucose. Because it increases with continued glucose exposure for the life of the red blood cell, it affords an assessment of long-term (60 to 120 days) blood glucose control. However, it is not helpful in adjusting daily insulin doses.

Measurements are either of HbA_1 or of a subgroup, HbA_{1c}, that reflects most closely the increases in blood glucose; thus, recommended values will vary depending upon the technique used. The normal ranges for glycosylated hemoglobin are 4 to 6% for HbA_{1c} and 5 to 8% for HbA_1 (American Diabetes Association, 1988).

Food and Activity Records. When combined with SMBG, food and activity records kept by the patient can provide valuable information on the effect of meals, food choices, and exercise on the level of blood glucose. They are useful in identifying problem eating times, problem foods, and situations that trigger overeating in the obese.

Blood Lipids. Because the person with diabetes is at risk for hyperlipidemia, lipid levels should be assessed every 2 to 3 years. Measurements should be made of triglycerides, total cholesterol, high-density lipoprotein-cholesterol (HDL-C), and low-density lipoprotein-cholesterol (LDL-C) (see Chapter 20).

Renal Function Tests. Renal function tests on a regular basis are important to identify renal insufficiency as early as possible and to monitor its progress. Detection at an early stage is through protein excretion tests; elevation of blood urea nitrogen (BUN) and serum creatinine occurs at a late phase of renal insufficiency.

Nutritional Management

Although there is some controversy regarding the principles of nutritional care, authorities do agree that in addition to achieving and maintaining optimal body weight and nutritional status, the diabetic diet should maintain plasma glucose as near the normal physiologic range as possible, with the goal of preventing or delaying the development and progression of cardiovascular, renal, retinal, neurologic, and other complications of diabetes insofar as these are related to metabolic control.

To achieve these goals in the person with IDDM, it is important to consider the timing of meals, composition of the diet, energy content of the diet, and physical activity. Insofar as possible, the insulin should be adjusted to fit a preferred eating plan rather than adjusting the diet to fit the insulin dosage. Timing of meals is not as important with NIDDM unless insulin is being used.

Dietary Components

Energy. Effective determinations of appropriate energy intake are made by (1) monitoring weight and adjusting energy intake accordingly, (2) mimicking the present energy intake if weight is appropriate, or (3) calculating energy intake as follows:

1. Using the Harris-Benedict formula in Table 2-5 or the nomogram in Figure 2-1, determine the basal energy expenditure (BEE) for 24 hours based upon age, sex, and size. In the individual at ideal body weight this is about

$$1 \text{ kcal/kg/hr} \times 24 \text{ hr}$$

2. Add an activity increment as a percentage of the BEE as follows: sedentary, 20%; light, 30%; and active, 50 to 75%.
3. Add an additional 10% of this total for the thermal effect of food (TEF). The sum is the total energy requirement. A rough estimation for the sum of these three factors is 10 to 12 kcal/lb of present weight for the sedentary person, 13 to 15 kcal/lb for the active person, and 16 to 20 kcal/lb for the very active individual. Calculations for the obese person are performed using the desirable body weight (DBW) rather than the present weight.
4. Another method for determining the energy level for the obese person who needs to reduce weight is to subtract 500 to 750 kcal from the total daily energy requirement based on present weight. The very sedentary obese may need to subtract as much as 1,000 kcal/day. The energy deficit can also be increased by the addition of daily exercise. In some situations, the obese person with diabetes may follow a modified fast with a calorie level of 400 to 600 kcal/day (see Chapter 18). Once the appropriate weight is reached, maintenance can be maintained by adjusting the energy level of the diet. No matter how it is constructed, a regimen for achieving weight loss is more important for the obese patient than alterations in the macronutrient composition of the diet.
5. The energy needs for children range between 36 and 45 kcal/lb, with a gradual decline in energy needs per pound as age increases. Adolescent boys need 20 to 36 kcal/lb and girls need 15 to 20 kcal/lb depending upon activity.

Protein. The protein requirement is determined in the same manner as for the person without diabetes and, depending on age, may vary from 0.75 to 2.2 g/kg ideal body weight (0.4 to 1 g/lb). Children require between 1 and 1.2 g/kg, whereas infants require 1.6 to 2.2 g/kg. This usually means a protein intake of 12 to 20% of total energy. Pregnant and lactating women have additional needs as do individuals with catabolic stress.

Current research addresses the differing insulin response to carbohydrate- and protein-containing meals depending on the source of protein. This makes sense in light of the fact that some amino acids promote insulin secretion and others promote glucagon secretion. Other new research suggests that a protein intake at the Recommended Dietary Allowance (0.75 g/kg), which is lower than most Americans consume, may delay the progression of diabetic renal disease (Kaysen et al, 1986). Protein intakes in the range of 40 to 60 g/day have been accompanied by improved kidney function in patients with nephrosis (Carlson, 1987) (see Chapter 35). In children, this would be equivalent to 12 to 15% of energy from protein.

Carbohydrate. Estimation of the amount and type of carbohydrate in the diet is guided by the patient's blood glucose response, lipid levels, and individual eating patterns. Carbohydrates provide 45 to 50% of the total energy in the diet of most Americans, but may be increased up to 55 to 60% in the diabetic diet.

It appears that the insulin-dependent person is able to metabolize diets of varying carbohydrate content without serious impact on blood glucose control. A high-carbohydrate diet also lowers blood glucose and enhances glycemia control in NIDDM. However, in some patients with NIDDM, high-carbohydrate diets reduce serum HDL-C and increase triglyceride levels (American Diabetes Association, 1987a). It may be that providing part of the energy in the form of monounsaturated fats rather than as complex carbohydrates may result in a better lipid profile (Garg et al, 1988).

Small amounts of sucrose and other refined sugars (up to 5% of the energy contributed by carbohydrate) are acceptable if the patient is in metabolic control and is managing his weight. Often these small amounts of sucrose can mean the difference between noncompliance and diabetic control.

Glycemic Response. The availability of SMBG has made it possible to evaluate the glycemic response to individual foods and combinations of foods. Results suggest that the rate of carbohydrate digestion, absorption, and metabolism may be as important as the actual amount consumed. This rate is dependent upon the form of food (e.g., mashed or whole, boiled, or raw); cooking (e.g., home-cooked or canned, especially in reference to beans); processing (e.g., the high-gluten flour in pasta versus the regular flour in bread); presence of antinutrients (phytates, tannins, and lectins as found in beans); amount and type of fiber content (e.g., soluble versus insoluble); and the combination of nutrients in the meal (carbohydrate alone or carbohydrate with fat). All starches (complex carbohydrates) in equal amounts do not produce the same rise in blood glucose, and sugars (simple carbohydrates) do not necessarily cause a greater rise in blood glucose than starches (Jenkins, 1984 and 1988). Even the addition of salt to a meal increases the glycemic response (Thorburn et al, 1986).

A "glycemic index" has been established for many foods, based on the rise in blood glucose following their ingestion compared with a standard defined as the rise in blood glucose after the ingestion of either white bread or glucose (Jenkins, 1984). Table 31-6, which gives the glycemic range for some common foods, includes some surprises. For example, the glycemic response to cornflakes is almost equal to glucose, while that for ice cream is less than half that of cornflakes. Responses to sugars are variable. Dextrose produces higher blood glucose concentrations than sucrose, and fructose results in relatively flat blood glucose response curves compared with either sucrose or dextrose (Bohannon et al, 1980; Crapo et al, 1982). Legumes produce the flattest glycemic responses and even flatten the glycemic response to the meal taken after their ingestion (Wolever et al, 1988).

TABLE 31-6. Glycemic Index for Selected Foods*

Food	Mean GI†‡
White bread	100
Whole-grain bread	100 ± 2
Spaghetti, white, boiled 5 min	45
Spaghetti, wholegrain, boiled 15 min	61
Rice, brown	81
Rice, white, boiled 15 min	79 ± 5
Sweet corn	80 ± 4
All bran cereal	74 ± 1
Cornflakes	115 ± 4
Muesli	96
Shredded wheat	97
Oatmeal cookies	78
Potato, mashed	100
Potato, russet, baked	128
Potato, sweet	70
Beans, baked, canned	60
Beans, kidney	45 ± 11
Beans, soy, canned	22
Peanuts	15
Green peas, frozen	65
Apple	53
Banana	84 ± 7
Orange juice	67
Fructose	31 ± 2
Honey	126
Sucrose	89 ± 2
Potato chips	77
Corn chips	99
Ice cream	52
Skim milk	46

* From Jenkins DJA, Wolever TMS and Jenkins AL: Starchy foods and glycemic index. Diabetes Care 11:149, 1988. Copyright 1988 by American Diabetes Association, Inc. Modified by permission.

† These values are the mean values from several studies of diabetic, both insulin- and non-insulin-dependent, and nondiabetic subjects.

‡ Mean Glycemic Index (GI) of foods adjusted so that GI of white bread = 100.

In view of the many factors that affect glycemic response and the small number of foods tested to date, it is not yet possible to say which foods or combinations of foods will have the best effect on glycemia control. Future research may lead to development of a glycemic index (GI) system that can be used in diabetic education. Currently it appears that the glycemic response to a meal containing either high- or low-GI foods is not extremely different (Fig. 31-2), and the exchange list system is equally accurate in predicting the glycemic outcome (Laine et al, 1987). It is essential to remember that the composition of the entire diet is important.

Fiber. Soluble dietary fiber, found primarily in fruits, vegetables, barley, and especially oats and legumes, has been shown to improve control of blood glucose, possibly by slowing gastric emptying and increasing intes-

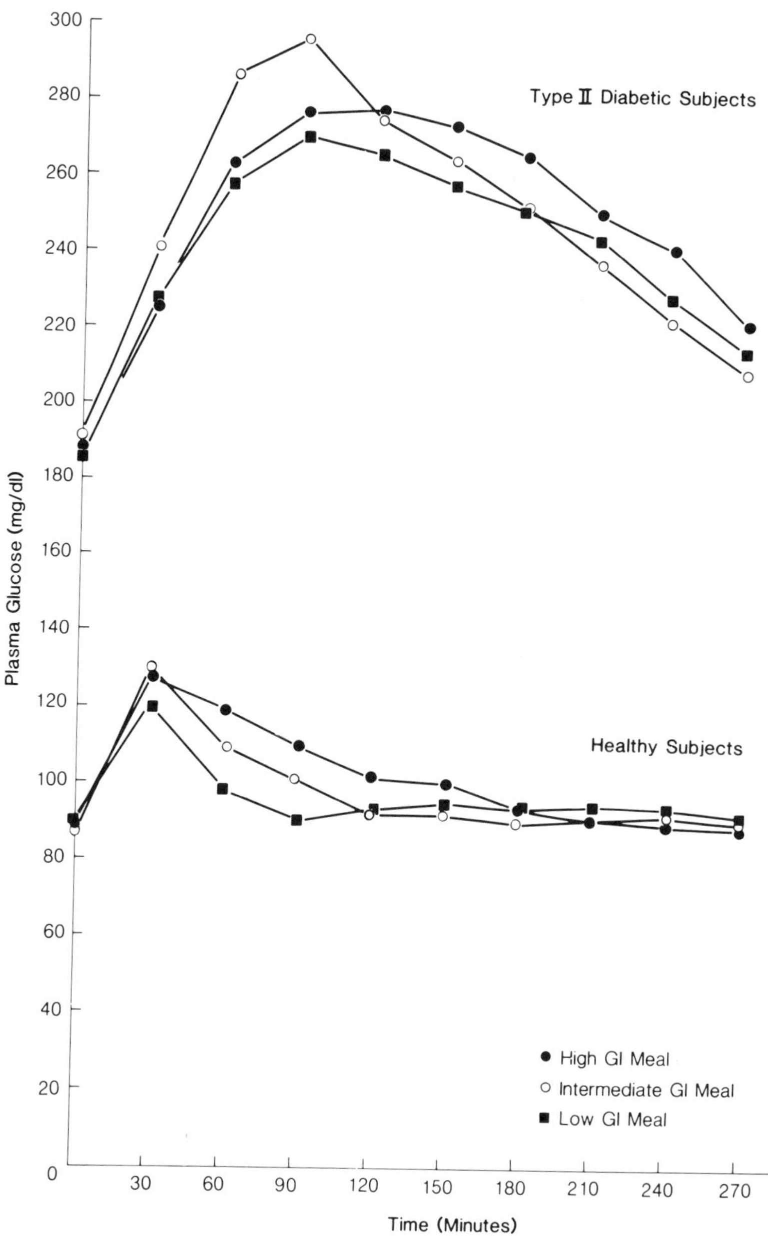

FIGURE 31–2. *Mean plasma glucose concentrations before and after ingestion of high, intermediate, and low glycemic index (GI) test meals in type II diabetic and healthy subjects. (From Laine DC, Thomas W, Levitt MD, et al: Comparison of the predictive capabilities of diabetic exchange lists and glycemic index of foods. Diabetes Care 10:387–394, 1987; with permission.)*

tinal transit time, thereby slowing glucose absorption (see Chapter 3).

Supplements of soluble fiber added to diabetic diets have shown the same positive results (Aro et al, 1981). However, guar gum and other highly purified supplements can have unpleasant side effects (Anderson et al, 1987). As the fiber in the diet is increased, patients may complain of increased flatulence, eructation, and stool frequency. These complaints can be minimized by starting with small portions of high-fiber foods and increasing them gradually.

When patients are started on high-fiber diets, insulin requirements and blood glucose should be closely monitored and insulin dosage reduced as necessary. Studies suggest that long-term use of high-fiber diets will not affect mineral absorption (Anderson et al, 1980; Rattan et al, 1981). However, high-risk groups such as postmenopausal women, children, or the elderly may require supplements of calcium or trace minerals (American Diabetes Association, 1987a).

The amount of dietary fiber recommended for the diabetic diet is about 40 g, or 25 g/1,000 kcal, composed of approximately equal amounts of soluble and insoluble fiber (see Chapter 3 and Table 3–5). As the average American consumes 13 to 19 grams of fiber/day, this would require doubling the usual intake. Fiber intake can be calculated using the average values for the exchange lists in Table 31–7, or Appendix Table 2. Any increase in dietary fiber should be accompanied by a corresponding increase in water.

TABLE 31–7. American Diabetes Association–American Dietetic Association Exchange List Calculation Guide*

Exchange Group	Carbohydrate (g)	Protein (g)	Fat (g)	Calories	Fiber (g)
Starch/bread					
Whole-grain bread, cereals, crackers	15	3	tr†	80	2
Starchy vegetables and legumes	15	3	tr†	80	3–4
Bran cereals	15	3	tr†	80	3–8
Others	15	3	tr†	80	0–1
Meat					
Lean	—	7	3	55	0
Medium-fat	—	7	5	75	0
High-fat	—	7	8	100	0
Vegetable					
Raw	5	2	—	25	3
Cooked, canned, frozen cooked	5	2	—	25	2
Fruit					
Fresh, frozen, canned	15	—	—	60	2
Dried	15	—	—	60	3
Juices	15	—	—	60	0
Milk					
Skim	12	8	tr†	90	0
Low-fat	12	8	5	120	0
Whole	12	8	10	150	0
Fat	—	—	5	45	0
Nuts and seeds	—	—	5	45	1

* From American Diabetes Association and American Dietetic Association: Exchange Lists for Meal Planning, 1986, and Powers MA (ed): Nutrition Guide for Professionals. Diabetes Education and Meal Planning, Chicago, American Diabetes Association, Inc. and American Dietetic Association, 1988.

† One gram of fat can be used for calculation purposes.

Fat. To balance the energy requirement, the remaining energy in the diet is supplied by fats. As a preventive measure against atherosclerosis and coronary heart disease, it is recommended that fat be restricted to less than 30% of calories, and made up of approximately one third each polyunsaturated, saturated, and monounsaturated fat. Cholesterol should total less than 300 mg/day. In some hyperlipidemic patients, further reduction of saturated fat to 7% of total energy intake and dietary cholesterol to 200 mg/day may be necessary (see Step 1 and Step 2 diets of the National Cholesterol Education Program, Chapter 20).

Reduction of hyperglycemia can lower serum triglycerides, raise HDL-C, and lower LDL-C and very low-density lipoprotein cholesterol (VLDL-C). Persons with diabetes who continue to show increased VLDL-triglyceride and VLDL-C concentrations after the first reduction of fat to 30% of kilocalories are not likely to benefit from further fat restriction (American Diabetes Association, 1987a).

Minerals and Vitamins. Mineral and vitamin supplements are not necessary when the diet is adequate and the glycosuria controlled. A possible exception is chromium, a component of the GTF. This organic complex of chromium, nicotinic acid, and amino acids is required for normal carbohydrate and lipid metabolism. Some studies have shown increased glucose tolerance, decreased insulin levels, increased insulin receptors and binding, and even cholesterol lowering after chromium supplementation (Anderson, 1983; Offenbacher and Pi-Sunyer, 1980). However, it is not yet possible to identify those who might benefit from higher levels of chromium, and at present supplementation is still on an experimental basis. The most likely candidates are elderly patients with NIDDM. Chromium supplementation should be used cautiously, with an upper limit of 200 μg/day. Two to 3 months of supplementation may be required to see results (Anderson, 1988). Some studies suggest that chromium supplementation cannot be effective unless there is adequate nicotinic acid present that may also be deficient (Urberg and Zemel, 1987).

Good food sources of chromium are brewer's yeast, oysters, potatoes and apples with skins, liver, wheat germ, cheese, and egg yolks.

Alcohol. Even though the metabolism of alcohol is not dependent upon insulin, its use is discouraged except in limited amounts. As a concentrated energy source providing 7 kcal/g, it is inappropriate for those who need to lose weight. It increases serum triglycerides, an undesirable circumstance in the patient who may already have hypertriglyceridemia. Also, it can induce hypoglycemia in some patients taking sulfonylureas. Alcohol dehydrogenase, which is involved in alcohol metabolism, inhibits gluconeogenesis, and thus alcohol can produce hypoglycemia in the fasting state even without sulfonylurea medication.

IMPLEMENTING THE DIET. The type and amount of insulin, the time of insulin administration, and the timing, type, and amount of daily activity and exercise determine the optimal amount and timing of food intake throughout the day.

Relation of Diet and Insulin Use

Using No Insulin. When no insulin is prescribed, the intake of food is spread evenly throughout the day according to the patient's preference, activity, and eating pattern. SMBG will help determine the ideal spacing of meals to maximize endogenous insulin production. Many find small meals interspersed with snacks more effective than three meals. Others find that spacing meals 4 to 5 hours apart allows time for the insulin to lower blood glucose. Strict daily consistency of meal times is not usually necessary. It becomes more important when the patient is taking an oral hypoglycemic agent.

Regular Insulin. When regular, short-acting insulin is given before meals, the amount is adjusted to match the usual meal or snack size. The patient should eat within ½ hour after regular insulin is taken.

Intermediate-Acting Insulin (NPH, Lente). The action of these insulins is intermediate in duration and intensity. When they are given before breakfast, a late afternoon nourishment (3:00 to 4:00 P.M.) is frequently required to counteract a hypoglycemic tendency, since these insulins have peak activity 8 to 12 hours after injection. A bedtime feeding is often necessary, especially if there is a second predinner NPH injection.

Long-Acting Insulin (Ultralente). The maximum availability of glucose from foods should coincide with the maximum availability of insulin. Thus, when Ultralente, with a prolonged activity of approximately 36 hours, is administered, an evening feeding (bedtime) is usually required to prevent hypoglycemia during the night or early morning.

Continuous Subcutaneous Insulin Infusion. Meal timing can be more flexible for patients using CSII (the "pump"). An additional bolus of regular insulin can be administered to cover the increased insulin needs of a meal or a snack. The amount of insulin to be administered continuously throughout the day and prior to a meal is based on frequent tests of SMBG correlated with food intake and exercise. Nutrition education to prevent weight gain while liberalizing the diet is an important feature of nutritional follow-up.

Planning the Diet. In planning the diabetic diet, the patient's current dietary pattern should be followed as much as possible. A diet history will define the present energy intake and distribution of protein, fat, and carbohydrate. Gradual modification of current eating patterns is often the most effective way of attaining a goal. For example, if the patient is eating the equivalent of 8 fat servings/day, reduction to 5 would be an improvement even though 3 would be ideal. Any changes are dictated by the total energy requirement, the recommended content of protein, fat, and carbohydrate, and the timing of meals to promote glucose control. The optimal eating plan may only be reached over several months of change, when a more realistic pattern between present eating habits and the optimal will develop.

The effective nutrition counselor will individualize the eating plan to the patient. This means not only including foods that the patient likes, but also individualizing the method by which the patient learns to manage eating in relation to diabetes. The practitioner should feel free to use any one of the plans mentioned later, or even a combination of two or more to meet the educational needs of the individual. An excellent resource for deciding upon the teaching method is *Meal Planning Approaches in the Nutrition Management of the Person with Diabetes* (Diabetes Care and Education Practice Group, 1987).

Meal Planning with Exchange Lists. The most widely used procedure for calculating a diabetic diet and planning appropriate meals was published in 1950 as a joint effort of the American Diabetes Association, the United States Public Health Service, and the American Dietetic Association. Foods were organized into six groups or "exchanges" on the basis of their protein, fat, and carbohydrate content. In 1976, this system was updated to provide for reductions in fat and cholesterol. In 1986, the system was further modified to emphasize reduced sodium and increased fiber in addition to the fat modifications. Foods have so far not been grouped with regard to fiber content or glycemic index. Table 31–7 summarizes the exchange lists. Table 31–8 is a useful worksheet for assessing present intake. Table 31–9 presents the steps in designing an exchange meal plan. The exchange lists are shown in Table 31–10, and Table 31–11 shows how these are translated into an eating pattern. Table 31–12 illustrates a sample menu.

Other Planning Systems. Other systems for planning meals for the diabetic are discussed in Table 31–13.

Special Foods. With the exception of a reduced amount of simple sugars and foods prepared with sugars, the person with diabetes can eat the same variety of foods as the rest of the family. Although special "diabetic" foods are not needed, foods lower in fat such as reduced-calorie mayonnaise, salad dressings, and margarines can be very useful.

Sweeteners. Fructose elicits a lower plasma glucose and insulin response than either dextrose or sucrose, and is therefore an acceptable sweetener for well-controlled diabetic patients (Bohannon et al, 1980). It is a nutritive sweetener however, so its caloric contribution to the diet must be considered (1 T of fructose, 15 grams, can be counted as 1 fruit serving). However, because fructose is 1½ times as sweet, substitution for sucrose ultimately reduces the total carbohydrate intake. 30 g/day can usually be used without loss of glucose control (Grigoresco et al, 1988; Birchwood and Jenkins, 1988).

The sweeteners sorbitol, mannitol, and xylitol are the alcohols of sucrose, mannose, and xylose, respectively. They are absorbed more slowly than sucrose; however, they are eventually metabolized to glucose and therefore must be considered in the diet calculation. In large amounts, they tend to cause diarrhea; 50 to 60 g/day is acceptable (Olefsky and Crapo, 1980).

Aspartame, marketed under the label of Nutrasweet, was approved for use by the Food and Drug Administration (FDA) in 1981 after rigorous testing. It is made from aspartic acid and phenylalanine and is therefore not appropriate for use by persons with phenylketonuria. Because it is made of amino acids, it is technically a nutritive sweetener; however because of its intense sweetness (180 to 220 times that of sucrose), it is used in only minute amounts and its nutritive value is negligible. Because it loses its sweetness when heated, aspartame is effective only in foods that do not require cooking or baking. The acceptable daily intake (ADI) is 50

Text continued on pg. 545

TABLE 31–8. Worksheet for Evaluation of Meal Plan*

Food Group	Breakfast	Snack	Lunch	Snack	Dinner	Snack	Total Servings/ Day	CHO (g)	Protein (g)	Fat† (g)	Kilo-calories
	Meal/Snack/Time										
Starch/Bread								15	3	1	80
Meats/ Substitutes									7	5	75
Vegetables								5	2		25
Fruits								15			60
Milk								12	8	1	90
Fats										5	45
							Total				
							Calories	×4 =	×4 =	×9 =	Total =
							Per cent calories				

* From Powers MA (ed): Nutrition Guide for Professionals. Diabetes Education and Meal Planning, p. 31. © 1988, American Diabetes Association, Inc., and The American Dietetic Association. Used by permission.

† Calculations are based on medium-fat meats and skim/very low fat milk. If diet consists predominantly of low-fat meats, use the factor 3 g instead of 5 g fat; if predominantly high-fat meats, use 8 g fat. If low-fat (2%) milk is used, use 5 g fat; if whole milk is used, use 8 g fat.

TABLE 31–9. Designing an Exchange Meal Plan*

Step 1: Assessment of Desirable Body Weight and Energy Requirements.

Step 2: Assessment of Current Food Intake with Exchange System Using the Worksheet in Table 31–8.

Categorize usual food intake into exchange amounts and divide the exchanges among meals and snacks, staying as close as possible to the patient's present eating pattern.

Fill in the grams of protein, fat, and carbohydrate according to the total number of exchanges per day.

Total the grams of carbohydrate, protein, and fat and the calories for the day and determine the percentages of calories provided by protein, fat, and carbohydrate.

Evaluate appropriateness of present food intake by considering:
- energy intake versus energy requirements
- percentage of calories from protein, fat, and carbohydrate
- timing and size of snacks and meals
- integration of insulin therapy into meal plan for those using insulin
- distribution of food to promote maximal use of endogenous insulin in patients with non–insulin-dependent diabetes mellitus

Determine necessary changes based on the evaluation and discuss which changes the patient is willing to make.

Adjust insulin regimen to conform as closely as possible to individual's eating patterns and lifestyle.

Step 3: Distribution of Meals and Snacks

Distribute meals and snacks based on lifestyle and activity patterns.

With consistent food intake from day to day, insulin therapy can be adjusted.

Self-monitoring of blood glucose (SMBG) gives feedback on appropriateness of food distribution, activity, and insulin therapy.

Step 4: Calculation of Meal Plan for Initial Education

Meal plan can be designed with the changes the patient is willing to make.

Use information from Table 31–8 and adjust.

Step 5: Followup and Continuing Education

After 2 to 3 weeks on initial plan, its effectiveness should be assessed based on SMBG, weight, food records and acceptance by patient.

Adjustments that patient agrees to can be made.

* Adapted from Powers MA (ed): Nutrition Guide for Professionals. Diabetes Education and Meal Planning. © 1988, American Diabetes Association, Inc., and The American Dietetic Association. Adapted by permission.

TABLE 31–10. Exchange Lists for Diabetes Nutrition Management

Starch/Bread List

Each item in this list contains approximately 15 g carbohydrate, 3 g protein, a trace of fat, and 80 kcal. Whole-grain products average about 2 g fiber per serving. Some foods are higher in fiber.

Starch exchanges can be chosen from any of the items on this list. The general rule for starch foods not on this list is that:
½ cup of cereal, grain, or pasta is one serving.
1 oz of a bread product is one serving.

Cereals/Grains/Pasta

*Bran cereals, concentrated	⅓ cup
*Bran cereals, flaked (such as Bran Buds, All Bran)	½ cup
Bulgur (cooked)	½ cup
Cooked cereals	½ cup
Cornmeal (dry)	2½ T
Grape-nuts	3 T
Grits (cooked)	½ cup
Other ready-to-eat unsweetened cereals	¾ cup
Pasta (cooked)	½ cup
Puffed cereal	1½ cup
Rice, white or brown (cooked)	⅓ cup
Shredded wheat	½ cup
*Wheat germ	3 T

Dried Beans/Peas/Lentils

*Beans and peas (cooked) (such as kidney, white, split, blackeye)	⅓ cup
*Lentils (cooked)	⅓ cup
*Baked beans	¼ cup

Starchy Vegetables

*Corn	½ cup
*Corn on cob, 6-in long	1
*Lima beans	½ cup
*Peas, green (canned or frozen)	½ cup
*Plantain	½ cup
Potato, baked	1 small (3 oz)
Potato, mashed	½ cup
Squash, winter (acorn, butternut)	¾ cup
Yam, sweet potato, plain	⅓ cup

Bread

Bagel	½ (1 oz)
Bread sticks, crisp, 4-in long × ½ in	2 (⅔ oz)
Croutons, low-fat	1 cup
English muffin	½
Frankfurter or hamburger bun	½ (1 oz)
Pita, 6-in across	½
Plain roll, small	1 (1 oz)
Raisin, unfrosted	1 slice (1 oz)
*Rye, pumpernickel	1 slice (1 oz)
Tortilla, 6-in across	1
White (including French, Italian)	1 slice (1 oz)
Whole wheat	1 slice (1 oz)
Taco shell, 6-in across	2
Waffle, 4½-in square	1
Whole wheat crackers, fat added (such as Triscuits)	4–6 (1 oz)

Crackers/Snacks

Animal crackers	8
Graham crackers, 2½-in square	3
Matzoth	¾ oz
Melba toast	5 slices
Oyster crackers	24
Popcorn (popped, no fat added)	3 cups
Pretzels	¾ oz
Rye crisp, 2-in × 3½-in	4
Saltine-type crackers	6
Whole wheat crackers, no fat added (crisp breads, such as Finn, Kavli, Wasa)	2–4 slices (¾ oz)

Starch Foods Prepared with Fat
(Count as 1 starch/bread serving, plus 1 fat serving)

Biscuit, 2½-in across	1
Chow mein noodles	½ cup
Corn bread, 2-in cube	1 (2 oz)
Cracker, round butter type	6
French fried potatoes, 2-in to 3½-in long	10 (1½ oz)
Muffin, plain, small	1
Pancake, 4-in across	2
Stuffing, bread (prepared)	¼ cup

* Foods with 3 or more grams of fiber per serving.

Meat List

Each serving of meat and substitutes on this list contains about 7 g protein. The amounts of fat and number of calories vary, depending on the kind of meat or substitute chosen. The list is divided into three parts based on the amount of fat and calories: lean meat, medium-fat meat, and high-fat meat. One ounce (one meat exchange) of each of these includes:

	Carbohydrate (g)	Protein (g)	Fat (g)	Calories
Lean	0	7	3	55
Medium-fat	0	7	5	75
High-Fat	0	7	8	100

Lean Meat and Substitutes
(One exchange is equal to any one of the following items.)

Beef:	USDA Good or Choice grades of lean beef, such as round, sirloin, and flank steak; tenderloin; and chipped beef†	1 oz
Pork:	Lean pork, such as fresh ham; canned, cured or boiled ham;† Canadian bacon,† tenderloin.	1 oz
Veal:	All cuts are lean except for veal cutlets (ground or cubed). Examples of lean veal are chops and roasts.	1 oz

Medium-Fat Meat and Substitutes
(One exchange is equal to any one of the following items.)

Beef:	Most beef products fall into this category. Examples are: all ground beef, roast (rib, chuck, rump), steak (cubed, Porterhouse, T-bone), and meatloaf.	1 oz
Pork:	Most pork products fall into this category. Examples are: chops, loin roast, Boston butt, cutlets.	1 oz
Lamb:	Most lamb products fall into this category. Examples are: chops, leg, and roast.	1 oz
Veal:	Cutlet (ground or cubed, unbreaded)	1 oz

Table continued on following page

TABLE 31–10. Exchange Lists for Diabetes Nutrition Management *Continued*

Meat List *Continued*

Lean Meat and Substitutes *Continued*

Poultry:	Chicken, turkey, Cornish hen (without skin)	1 oz
Fish:	All fresh and frozen fish	1 oz
	Crab, lobster, scallops, shrimp, clams (fresh or canned in water†)	2 oz
	Oysters	6 medium
	Tuna† (canned in water)	¼ cup
	Herring (uncreamed or smoked)	1 oz
	Sardines (canned)	2 medium
Wild Game:	Venison, rabbit, squirrel	1 oz
	Pheasant, duck, goose (without skin)	1 oz
Cheese:	Any cottage cheese	¼ cup
	Grated Parmesan	2 T
	Diet cheeses† (with less than 55 kcal/oz)	1 oz
Other:	95% fat-free luncheon meat	1 oz
	Egg whites	3 whites
	Egg substitutes with less than 55 kcal per ¼ cup	¼ cup

Medium-Fat Meat and Substitutes *Continued*

Poultry:	Chicken (with skin), domestic duck or goose (well-drained of fat), ground turkey	1 oz
Fish:	Tuna† (canned in oil and drained)	¼ cup
	Salmon† (canned)	¼ cup
Cheese:	Skim or part-skim milk cheeses, such as:	
	Ricotta	¼ cup
	Mozzarella	1 oz
	Diet cheeses† (with 56–80 kcal/oz)	1 oz
Other:	86% fat-free luncheon meat†	1 oz
	Egg (high in cholesterol, limit to 3 per week)	1
	Egg substitutes with 56–80 kcal per ¼ cup	¼ cup
	Tofu (2½ in × 2¾ in × 1 in)	4 oz
	Liver, heart, kidney, sweetbreads (high in cholesterol)	1 oz

High-Fat Meat and Substitutes

Remember, these items are high in saturated fat, cholesterol, and calories, and should be used only three (3) times per week. (One exchange is equal to any one of the following items.)

Beef:	Most USDA Prime cuts of beef, such as ribs, corned beef†	1 oz
Pork:	Spareribs, ground pork, pork sausage† (patty or link)	1 oz
Lamb:	Patties (ground lamb)	1 oz
Fish:	Any fried fish product	1 oz
Cheese:	All regular cheeses,† such as American, Blue, Cheddar, Monterey, Swiss	1 oz
Other:	Luncheon meat,† such as bologna, salami, pimento loaf	1 oz
	Sausage,† such as Polish, Italian	1 oz
	Knockwurst, smoked	1 oz
	Bratwurst†	1 oz
	Frankfurter† (turkey or chicken)	1 frank (10/lb)
	Peanut butter (contains unsaturated fat)	1 T

Count as one high-fat meat plus one fat exchange:

Frankfurter† (beef, pork, or combination)	1 frank (10/lb)

† Foods with 400 mg or more of sodium per exchange.

Vegetable List

Each vegetable serving on this list contains about 5 g carbohydrate, 2 g protein, and 25 kcal. Vegetables contain 2–3 grams of dietary fiber. Vegetables are a good source of vitamins and minerals. Fresh and frozen vegetables have more vitamins and less added salt.
Unless otherwise noted, the serving size for vegetables (one vegetable exchange) is:
½ cup of cooked vegetables or vegetable juice.
1 cup of raw vegetables.

Artichoke (½ medium)	Cabbage, cooked	Mushrooms, cooked	Spinach, cooked
Asparagus	Carrots	Okra	Summer squash (crookneck)
Beans (green, wax, Italian)	Cauliflower	Onions	Tomato (one large)
Bean sprouts	Eggplant	Pea pods	Tomato/vegetable juice†
Beets	Greens (collard, mustard, turnip)	Peppers (green)	Turnips
Broccoli	Kohlrabi	Rutabaga	Water chestnuts
Brussels sprouts	Leeks	Sauerkraut†	Zucchini, cooked

Starchy vegetables such as corn, peas, and potatoes are found on the Starch/Bread List.
† 400 mg or more sodium per exchange

TABLE 31–10. Exchange Lists for Diabetes Nutrition Management *Continued*

Fruit List

Each item on this list contains about 15 g carbohydrate, and 60 kcal. Fresh, frozen, and dry fruits have about 2 g fiber per serving. Fruit juices contain very little dietary fiber.

The carbohydrate and calorie content for a fruit serving are based on the usual serving of the most commonly eaten fruits. Use fresh fruits or fruits frozen or canned without sugar added. Whole fruit is more filling than fruit juice and may be a better choice for those who are trying to lose weight. Unless otherwise noted, the serving size for one fruit serving is:

½ cup of fresh fruit or fruit juice.
¼ cup of dried fruit.

Fresh, Frozen, and Unsweetened Canned Fruit

Apple (raw, 2-in across)	1 apple
Applesauce (unsweetened)	½ cup
Apricots (medium, raw) or	4 apricots
Apricots (canned)	½ cup, or 4 halves
Banana (9-in long)	½ banana
*Blackberries (raw)	¾ cup
*Blueberries (raw)	¾ cup
Cantaloupe (5-in across)	⅓ melon
(cubes)	1 cup
Cherries (large, raw)	12 cherries
Cherries (canned)	½ cup
Figs (raw, 2-in across)	2 figs
Fruit cocktail (canned)	½ cup
Grapefruit (medium)	½ grapefruit
Grapefruit (segments)	¾ cup
Grapes (small)	15 grapes
Honeydew melon (medium)	⅛ melon
(cubes)	1 cup
Kiwi (large)	1 kiwi
Mandarin oranges	¾ cup
Mango (small)	½ mango
*Nectarine (1½-in across)	1 nectarine
Orange (2½-in across)	1 orange
Papaya	1 cup
Peach (2¾-in across)	1 peach, or ¾ cup
Peaches (canned)	½ cup, or 2 halves
Pear	½ large, or 1 small
Pears (canned)	½ cup or 2 halves
Persimmon (medium, native)	2 persimmons
Pineapple (raw)	¾ cup
Pineapple (canned)	⅓ cup
Plum (raw, 2-in across)	2 plums
*Pomegranate	½ pomegranate
*Raspberries (raw)	1 cup
*Strawberries (raw, whole)	1¼ cup
Tangerine (2½-in across)	2 tangerines
Watermelon (cubes)	1¼ cup

Dried Fruit

*Apples	4 rings
*Apricots	7 halves
Dates	2½ medium
*Figs	1½
*Prunes	3 medium
Raisins	2 T

Fruit Juice

Apple juice/cider	½ cup
Cranberry juice cocktail	⅓ cup
Grapefruit juice	½ cup
Grape juice	⅓ cup
Orange juice	½ cup
Pineapple juice	½ cup
Prune juice	⅓ cup

* 3 or more grams of fiber per serving

Milk List

Each serving of milk or milk products on this list contains about 12 g carbohydrate and 8 g protein. The amount of fat in milk is measured in percent (%) of butterfat. The calories vary, depending on the kind of milk chosen. The list is divided into three parts based on the amount of fat and calories: skim/very low fat milk, low-fat milk, and whole milk. One serving (one milk exchange) of each of these includes:

	Carbohydrate (g)	*Protein (g)*	*Fat (g)*	*Calories*
Skim/Very low fat	12	8	trace	90
Low fat	12	8	5	120
Whole	12	8	8	150

Skim and Very Low Fat Milk

Skim milk	1 cup
½% milk	1 cup
1% milk	1 cup
Low-fat buttermilk	1 cup
Evaporated skim milk	½ cup
Dry nonfat milk	⅓ cup
Plain nonfat yogurt	8 oz

Low-Fat Milk

2% milk	1 cup fluid
Plain low-fat yogurt (with added nonfat milk solids)	8 oz

Whole Milk

The whole milk group has much more fat per serving than the skim and low-fat groups. Whole milk has more than 3¼% butterfat. Try to limit choices from the whole milk group as much as possible.

Whole milk	1 cup
Evaporated whole milk	½ cup
Whole plain yogurt	8 oz

Table continued on following page

TABLE 31–10. Exchange Lists for Diabetes Nutrition Management *Continued*

Fat List

Each serving on the fat list contains about 5 g fat and 45 kcal. The foods on the fat list contain mostly fat, although some items may also contain a small amount of protein. All fats are high in calories and should be carefully measured. Everyone should modify fat intake by eating unsaturated fats instead of saturated fats. The sodium content of these foods varies widely. Check the label for sodium information.

Unsaturated Fats		*Saturated Fats*	
Avocado	⅛ medium	Butter	1 tsp
Margarine	1 tsp	ǂBacon	1 slice
ǂMargarine, diet	1 T	Chitterlings	½ oz
Mayonnaise	1 tsp	Coconut, shredded	2 T
ǂMayonnaise, reduced-calorie	1 T	Coffee whitener, liquid	2 T
Nuts and Seeds:		Coffee whitener, powder	4 tsp
Almonds, dry roasted	6 whole	Cream (light, coffee, table)	2 T
Cashews, dry roasted	1 T	Cream, sour	2 T
Pecans	2 whole	Cream (heavy, whipping)	1 T
Peanuts	20 small or 10 large	Cream cheese	1 T
		ǂSalt pork	¼ oz
Walnuts	2 whole		
Other nuts	1 T		
Seeds, pine nuts, sunflower (without shells)	1 T		
Pumpkin seeds	2 tsp		
Oil (corn, cottonseed, safflower, soybean, sunflower, olive, peanut)	1 tsp		
ǂOlives	10 small or 5 large		
Salad dressing, mayonnaise-type	2 tsp		
Salad dressing, mayonnaise-type, reduced-calorie	1 T		
ǂSalad dressing (all varieties)	1 T		
†Salad dressing, reduced-calorie	2 T		
(Two tablespoons of low-calorie salad dressing is a free food.)			

ǂ If more than 2 servings eaten, these foods have 400 mg or more sodium.

Free Foods

A free food is any food or drink that contains less than 20 kcal/serving, and can be taken in unlimited amounts. Two or three servings per day of those items that have a specific serving size can be eaten.

Drinks
Bouillon† or broth without fat
Bouillon, low sodium
Carbonated drinks, sugar-free
Carbonated water
Club soda
Cocoa powder, unsweetened (1 T)
Coffee/Tea
Drink mixes, sugar free
Tonic water, sugar-free

Nonstick pan spray

Fruit
Cranberries, unsweetened (½ cup)
Rhubarb, unsweetened (½ cup)

Vegetables (raw, 1 cup)
Cabbage*
Celery*
Chinese cabbage*
Cucumber
Green onion
Hot peppers
Mushrooms
Radishes
Zucchini*

Salad greens
Endive
Escarole
Lettuce
Romaine*
Spinach*

Sweet substitutes
Candy, hard, sugar-free
Gelatin, sugar-free
Gum, sugar-free
Jam/Jelly, sugar-free (2 tsp)
Pancake syrup, sugar free (1–2 T)
Sugar substitutes (saccharin, aspartame)
Whipped topping (2 T)

Condiments
Catsup (1 T)
Horseradish
Mustard
Pickles†, dill, unsweetened
Salad dressing, low-calorie (2 T)
Taco sauce (1 T)
Vinegar

Seasonings can be very helpful in making food taste better. Be careful of how much sodium is used. Read the label, and choose those seasonings that do not contain sodium or salt.

Basil (fresh)
Celery seeds
Cinnamon
Chili powder
Chives
Curry
Dill
Flavoring extracts (vanilla, almond, walnut, peppermint, butter, lemon, etc.)
Garlic
Garlic powder
Herbs
Hot pepper sauce
Lemon
Lemon juice
Lemon pepper
Lime
Lime juice
Mint
Onion powder
Oregano
Paprika
Pepper
Pimento
Spices
Soy sauce†
Soy sauce, low sodium ("lite")
Wine, used in cooking (¼ cup)
Worcestershire sauce

* 3 g or more of fiber per serving.
† 400 mg or more of sodium per serving.

TABLE 31–10. Exchange Lists for Diabetes Nutrition Management *Continued*

Combination Foods

These combination foods do not fit into only one exchange list. It can be quite hard to tell what is in a certain casserole dish or baked food item. This is a list of average values of some typical combination foods.

Food	*Amount*	*Exchanges*
Casseroles, homemade	1 cup (8 oz)	2 starch, 2 medium-fat meat, 1 fat
Cheese pizza,† thin crust	¼ of 15 oz or ¼ of 10 in	2 starch, 1 medium-fat meat, 1 fat
Chili with beans*† (commercial)	1 cup (8 oz)	2 starch, 2 medium-fat meat, 2 fat
Chow mein*† (without noodles or rice)	2 cups (16 oz)	1 starch, 2 vegetable, 2 lean meat
Macaroni and cheese†	1 cup (8 oz)	2 starch, 1 medium-fat meat, 2 fat
Soup		
Bean*†	1 cup (8 oz)	1 starch, 1 vegetable, 1 lean meat
Chunky, all varieties†	10¾ oz can	1 starch, 1 vegetable, 1 medium-fat meat
Cream† (made with water)	1 cup (8 oz)	1 starch, 1 fat
Vegetable† or broth†	1 cup (8 oz)	1 starch
Spaghetti and meatballs† (canned)	1 cup (8 oz)	2 starch, 1 medium-fat meat, 1 fat
Sugar-free pudding (made with skim milk)	½ cup	1 starch
If beans are used as a meat substitute:		
Dried beans,* peas,* lentils*	1 cup (cooked)	2 starch, 1 lean meat

Foods for Occasional Use

Moderate amounts of some foods can be used in the meal plan, in spite of their sugar or fat content, as long as blood glucose control is maintained. The following list includes average exchange values for some of these foods. Because they are concentrated sources of carbohydrate, the portion sizes are very small.

Food	*Amount*	*Exchanges*
Angel food cake	1/12 cake	2 starch
Cake, no icing	1/12 cake, or a 3-in square	2 starch, 2 fat
Cookies	2 small (1¾-in across)	1 starch, 1 fat
Frozen fruit yogurt	⅓ cup	1 starch
Gingersnaps	3	1 starch
Granola	¼ cup	1 starch, 1 fat
Granola bars	1 small	1 starch, 1 fat
Ice cream, any flavor	½ cup	1 starch, 2 fat
Ice milk, any flavor	½ cup	1 starch, 1 fat
Sherbet, any flavor	¼ cup	1 starch
Snack chips,‡ all varieties	1 oz	1 starch, 2 fat
Vanilla wafers	6 small	1 starch, 1 fat

* 3 or more g fiber per serving.
† 400 mg or more of sodium per exchange
‡ If more than one or two servings are eaten, these foods have 400 mg or more of sodium.

mg/kg body weight/day in the United States and 40 mg/kg/day in Canada. (One 12-oz can of diet drink contains about 200 mg of aspartame and a packet of Equal contains 35 mg of aspartame, equivalent in sweetness to 2 tsp of sucrose.)

Acesulfame, approved by the FDA in 1988, is the newest artificial sweetener (FDA . . . , 1989). Unlike saccharin and aspartame, it does not break down at high temperatures and can be used in baked products. It has no aftertaste. However a packet of Sweet One contains 1 g of glucose as a carrier, which could be a problem for someone using many packets.

Non-Nutritive Sweeteners. A variety of non-nutritive sweeteners has been developed to replace sugars. The oldest of these is *saccharin,* which was discovered in 1879 and which is 300 times as sweet as sugar. In early 1977, the FDA proposed banning the use of saccharin on the basis of Canadian studies that reported development of bladder tumors in rats fed large doses of this sweetener. Subsequent studies have not demonstrated a health risk to humans from use in normal dietary amounts (American Medical Association, 1985). It is still available as a nonprescription drug. The Joint Food and Agriculture Organization/World Health Organization (FAO/WHO) Committee on Food Additives recommends an ADI of saccharin at 2.5 mg/kg/day, which for a 70 kg person would be about 175 mg/day. In the United States, a recommendation for the upper limit of safe intake established at 1,000 mg/day for adults and 500 mg/day for children has been accepted

TABLE 31–11. 1,500-Kilocalorie Meal Plan with Snacks for Person with Non–Insulin-Dependent Diabetes Mellitus*

	Meal/Snack/Time										
Food Group	*Breakfast 7:30*	*Snack*	*Lunch 11:30*	*Snack 3:00*	*Dinner 6:30*	*Snack 10:30*	Total Servings/ Day	CHO (g)	Protein (g)	Fat† (g)	Kilo-calories
Starch/Bread	2		2	1 or 1 fruit	1	1	7	15 105	3 21	1 7	80 560
Meats/ Substitutes			2		3		5		7 35	5 25	75 375
Vegetables			0–1		2		2	5 10	2 4		25 50
Fruits	1		1		1		3	15 45			60 180
Milk	½		1			½	2	12 24	8 16	1 2	90 180
Fats	1		1		1	0–1	3			5 15	45 135
							Total	184	76	49	
							Calories	×4 = 736	×4 = 304	×9 = 441	Total = 1481
							Per cent calories	50%	20%	30%	

* From Powers MA (ed): Nutrition Guide for Professionals. Diabetes Education and Meal Planning. Chicago, American Diabetes Association and American Dietetic Association, 1988, p. 34.

† Calculations are based on medium-fat meats and skim/very low fat milk. If diet consists predominantly of low-fat meats, use the factor 3 g instead of 5 g fat; if predominantly high-fat meats, use 8 g fat. If low-fat (2%) milk is used, use 5 g fat; if whole milk is used, use 8 g fat.

TABLE 31–12. Sample Menu for 1,500-Kilocalorie Meal Plan

Breakfast—7:30 A.M.	
2 starch/bread	½ cup raisin bran cereal ½ bagel
1 fruit	⅓ 5-in cantaloupe
½ milk	½ cup skim milk
1 fat	1 T cream cheese
Lunch—11:30 A.M.	
2 starch/bread	2 slices whole-wheat bread
2 meat/substitutes	2 oz lite cheese
1 fruit	1 small apple
1 milk	1 cup skim milk
1 fat	1 tsp mayonnaise
Snack—3:00 P.M.	
1 starch/bread or fruit	¾ oz pretzels
Dinner—6:30 P.M.	
1 starch/bread	1 small baked potato
3 meat/substitutes	3 oz baked chicken breast
2 vegetables	½ cup broccoli spears ½ small tomato ¼ cup fresh mushrooms
1 fruit	¾ cup mandarin oranges
1 fat	1 T sour cream 1½ tsp low-cal salad dressing
Snack—10:30 P.M.	
1 starch/bread	3 graham cracker squares
½ milk	½ cup skim milk

by the American Diabetes Association (American Diabetes Association, 1987b; Saccharin and its Salts, 1977). One teaspoon of powdered saccharin contains 14 to 20 mg of saccharin.

The use of *cyclamate,* a popular sweetener without the aftertaste of saccharin, was banned in 1971. Although further testing failed to support research leading to the ban, applications of the manufacturer to return cyclamates to the market have been denied. The WHO recommendation for cyclamate ADI is 2.5 mg/kg body weight.

Other sweeteners are in the developmental stage.

Fat Substitutes. Two fat substitutes have been approved for dietary use by the FDA; others are pending. *Sucrose polyester (Olestra)* is not absorbed and metabolized and is therefore calorie-free. It replaces part of the fat in cooking oil, commercial snacks, and fast foods. *Simplesse* is a fat substitute made from egg white and whey that has the "mouth feel" of fat. For more discussion of these products, see New Directions, page 50.

Labeling. Labeling information on packaged foods frequently provides information on the carbohydrate, protein, fat, and kilocalorie content that can be used to incorporate one or more servings into an exchange system meal plan or a calorie-counting approach. Many

TABLE 31–13. Summary of Meal Planning Approaches*

Low Structure, Simple Approaches

Dietary Guidelines for Americans: General guidelines for the public, which will define an appropriate diet for the diabetic. Is not quantity controlled.

Kentucky Personal Guidelines: Designed by the Kentucky Diabetes Foundation to assist diabetics in choosing appropriate foods for glycemia and lipid control. Not quantity controlled.

Healthy Food Choices: Provides guidelines for diabetics for choosing foods appropriate for glycemia and lipid control—emphasis on complex carbohydrate, high-fiber, and low-fat foods. Concise with simplified exchange list.

Low Structure, Complex Approaches

Calorie Counting; Total Available Glucose (TAG); Point System: These methods of counting, either calories or grams of glucose available in the food, or carbohydrate equivalents provide quantity control.

High Structure, Simple Approaches

Food Choice Plan: Based on the person's stated plan of how he or she would like to eat for the week with the dietitian's input on amounts and preparation.

Individual Menus: Specific menus based on the person's preferences but without much flexibility. For those with limited interest or limited reading skills.

High Structure, Complex Approaches

ADA Exchange Lists: Provides guidelines for meal timing and composition for glycemia and lipid control with emphasis on low-fat foods.

High-Carbohydrate, High-Fiber *(HCF) Exchange Lists:* Provides guidelines for meal timing and composition for glycemia and lipid control with emphasis on low-fat, high-fiber, complex carbohydrate foods, especially beans and bran.

* Adapted from Diabetes Care and Education Practice Group: Meal Planning Approaches in the Nutrition Management of the Person with Diabetes. Chicago, American Dietetic Association, 1987.

food companies will provide the exchange values for their products upon request.

The shopper should remember that the term *dietetic* does not necessarily mean that a food is appropriate for someone with diabetes. For example, *dietetic* might describe a food that could be used on a low-sodium diet but, because of a high-fat or high-sugar content, would not be appropriate for a diabetic diet (Table 16–7). (Labeling information is discussed in Chapter 16.)

Alcohol. An occasional alcoholic beverage can be included in the diet by exchanging the kilocalories from alcohol for the kilocalories in fat. An average drink, 12 oz of regular or light beer, 4 oz of wine, or 1½ oz of distilled beverage, is an "alcohol equivalent" and can be substituted for 2 fat exchanges in the diet of the patient with NIDDM. Alcohol intake should not exceed 1 to 2 alcohol equivalents 1 to 2 times per week.

Alcohol should be mixed with sugar-free mixers whenever possible, and very sweet wines should be avoided. Alcohol should not be taken on an empty stomach in order to avoid the potential hypoglycemic effect. The person with IDDM diabetes whose weight is normal does not usually have to adjust his or her meal plan for the occasional drink of alcohol. Up to 2 alcohol equivalents can be consumed in addition to the regular meal plan.

Exercise. Regular exercise is an important part of diabetic management. Exercise appears to blunt the rise in blood glucose following carbohydrate ingestion and may increase insulin sensitivity for 2 to 3 days afterward (National Institutes of Health, 1987). However, for patients with IDDM, it also introduces management problems. The increase in hepatic glucose production in response to exercise enhances hyperglycemia and accelerates ketone production in poorly controlled diabetics (blood glucose of 250 to 300 mg/dl). Those in poor control should be brought into good control before beginning exercise.

On the other hand, hypoglycemia can be precipitated in diabetics who are in good control. Insulin production in normal individuals decreases during exercise to allow for glucose production by the liver to maintain blood glucose levels and match the glucose uptake by the exercising muscles. The diabetic taking exogenous insulin cannot make this adjustment. Hypoglycemia can be prevented by increasing the food intake before exercise, or adjusting insulin to accommodate the effects of exercise, or by both. After strenuous or prolonged exercise, hypoglycemia can occur for up to 24 hours while muscles take up blood glucose to replenish glycogen stores. During this time insulin dosage may need to be lowered.

Sometimes exercise results in hyperglycemia afterwards, the result of excess glucose production to meet glucose requirements during exercise. SMBG is important to determine the need for increased insulin or reduced food intake.

Retinopathy, nephropathy, or neuropathy can be worsened by strenuous exercise, especially that which increases blood pressure, involves abrupt changes in head motion, and has significant potential for joint or bone injury (Franz, 1987).

In NIDDM, exercise can enhance peripheral glucose utilization due to the glucose uptake by muscle and an apparent increased insulin sensitivity (Bogardus et al, 1984).

The following are guidelines for safe exercise:

1. SMBG is essential so that hyperglycemia and hypoglycemia can be prevented as much as possible, especially in those with IDDM. Ideally, exercise should take place at the same time every day; however, this is not usually possible, so SMBG is even more important. Depending on the blood glucose level, the amount of food taken before exercise is adjusted. If blood glucose is between 180 and 200 mg/dl, no additional food is needed prior to exercise unless the activity will be strenuous and lasts longer than 1 hour. In that case, 15 grams of carbohydrate (1 fruit or bread/starch exchange) is recommended. If the blood glucose is 100 to 180 mg/dl, then 15 grams of carbohydrate should be taken, and if the exercise will last longer than 1 hour, 25 to 50 grams

of carbohydrate should be taken along with some protein (e.g., ½ sandwich and 1 cup milk) (Franz, 1987). If blood glucose is less than 100 mg/dl and the exercise is of short duration (less than ½ hour) and of moderate intensity, 10 to 15 grams of carbohydrate is recommended. If the exercise is of moderate duration and intensity, 25 to 50 grams of carbohydrate is recommended; if the exercise is strenuous or of long duration, 50 grams or more of carbohydrate is recommended.

Persons with NIDDM are not likely to become hypoglycemic with exercise. Those taking OHA or insulin may need food before exercise, but usually their glucose levels are more stable than those of the patient with IDDM.

2. Exercisers should be in good control before beginning exercise. If not, exercise should be postponed until blood glucose is less than 300 mg/dl and preferably less than 250 mg/dl.
3. In order to prevent hypoglycemia, exercise should not be undertaken when insulin activity is at its peak. If this is not possible, food intake should be increased before and possibly during and after exercise.
4. Exercise can accelerate the absorption of insulin from an exercised injection site if it is done within 40 minutes after an injection of regular insulin, or within 2½ hours after an injection of intermediate-acting insulin. If exercise must begin soon after an insulin injection, then the insulin should be given in an unexercised part of the body.
5. Exercisers should increase their fluid intake. This is often overlooked in the attention to carbohydrate intake and the prevention of hypoglycemia. A fluid replacement mixture of one part juice and one part water (5 to 10% carbohydrate) provides the best ratio for absorption (see Chapter 19).

Special Situations

EMERGENCIES

Illness. Diabetes can get out of control very quickly during febrile illness. Insulin requirements usually increase, probably due to increased glucagon levels. Blood glucose should be monitored frequently and the urine tested for ketones. The presence of ketones indicates the potential for ketoacidosis and a physician should be called.

Sometimes a diabetic patient may become too ill to eat. It is important in this situation that the patient with IDDM continue to take insulin and if possible, carbohydrate should be given at the rate of 50 to 75 grams every 6 to 8 hours to prevent ketosis. The intake may be in the form of simple carbohydrate such as juices and even sugar-containing drinks, as listed in Table 31-14. At times a liquid diet is useful to replace uneaten carbohydrate (Appendix Table 33). If necessary, the protein and fat allowances may be sacrificed and the amounts limited to provide maximum comfort for the patient. If blood glucose is 240 mg/dl or higher, some of the carbohydrate can be omitted. Consumption of adequate fluids is very important.

Hypoglycemia. Insulin reactions are the result of an imbalance of blood glucose and insulin or oral hypoglycemic agents leading to hypoglycemia (blood glucose less than 70 mg/dl). Early symptoms include sweating, impatience, double vision, hunger, pallor, trembling, palpitation, headache, faintness and an "all gone" feeling. Although fleeting, these reactions can be relieved by the immediate consumption of a rapidly assimilated carbohydrate such as fruit juice, candy, or sugar (see Table 31-15). Reactions may be caused by an unusual amount of exercise, a delay in eating, the omission of a meal or of the prescribed amount of food, by an error resulting in the administration of an excessive amount of insulin, or by a decreased need for insulin as may occur after changing to a high-complex carbohydrate, high-fiber diet, or after weight loss. Diabetics taking insulin are advised to carry some candy or rapidly absorbed carbohydrate for the hypoglycemic emergency.

Reactions from regular unmodified insulin given before breakfast often occur before lunch (between 3 and 6 hours after injection). Reactions from intermediate-acting insulins (NPH, Lente) are more likely to occur in the afternoon before the evening meal, and reactions from Ultralente occur later. Patients receiving two injections with some NPH in the afternoon may have reactions in the evening or at night.

SMBG should be done before and after treating hypoglycemia so that overzealous treatment and resulting hyperglycemia can be avoided. If blood glucose is less than 70 mg/dl, the patient should take 15 g of carbohydrate, wait 15 minutes (the "15/15 rule") and retest the blood glucose. If it is still less than 70 mg/dl, another 15 g of glucose should be taken, followed by a retest 15 minutes later. The sequence should be repeated until blood glucose reaches at least 70 mg/dl (Powers et al, 1987).

Subcutaneous injections of glucagon may also be used in the treatment of hypoglycemic reactions because glucagon stimulates glycogenolysis, causing the liver to release glucose rapidly into the blood stream.

A more serious type of insulin reaction is one that develops slowly as the result of an excessive and continuous overdosage of insulin. Not only is blood glucose lowered but glycogen reserves are also depleted, leading eventually to central nervous system involvement. Gastric stasis often is present. Oral glucose is inadequate in this circumstance, and intravenous glucose or glucagon should be given immediately.

Occasionally hypoglycemia can occur in the patient taking oral hypoglycemic agents, most commonly with

TABLE 31–14. Foods or Glucose Sources Equivalent to 15 g Carbohydrate*

Food/Glucose Source	Amount	Carbohydrate Glucose (g)†	Total (g)	Kilocalories
Gelatin, regular, prepared	½ cup	6.0	17	71
Hard candy (Life Savers), flavored	5	0‡	15	50
Honey	1 T	7.1	17.3	64
Juice, apple	½ cup	3.1	14.5	58
Juice, orange	½ cup	6.6	12.8	54
Milk, skim	1 cup	0	12	86
Raisins	2T	5.6	14.2	54
Soft drinks, regular				
Cola	½ cup	5	12.8	50
Ginger ale	¾ cup	5.6	15.9	62
Sugar, granulated†	4 t	0	15.5	61
Sugar, ½-in cubes†	6	0	14.5	57
Syrup, corn	1 T	4.4	15	44
Thirst quencher (Gatorade)	1 cup	5.8	15.2	60
Glucose tablets	3	15	15	60
Glutose, 80 g bottle	½	16	16	64
Insta Glucose, 31 g tube	½	6.4	12.5	50
Insulin Reaction Gel, 25-g packets	1½	15	17	69

* From Powers MA (ed): Nutrition Guide for Professionals. Diabetes Education and Meal Planning. Chicago, American Diabetes Association and American Dietetic Association, 1988, p. 43.

† Values from Matthews RH, Pehrsson PR, Farhat-Sabet M: Sugar content of selected foods: individual and total foods. USDA/HNIS/Home Economics Research Rep no 48, 1987. This is the amount of glucose found in food before digestion and metabolism. For example, common table sugar is the disaccharide sucrose. Sucrose consists of the 2 monosaccharides glucose and fructose *joined* by a glycosidic linkage. Consequently, digestion and metabolism need to occur before glucose in sucrose is available.

‡ Glucose is known to be present, but there is a lack of reliable data.

chlorpropamide (Diabinese) and glyburide (Micronase and DiaBeta). These reactions can be very severe and require attention to blood glucose levels for several hours.

Diabetic Ketoacidosis. Uncontrolled diabetes can lead to ketosis followed by ketoacidosis and coma. Ketoacidosis can occur in the presence of an insulin lack caused by omission of prescribed insulin, or an insulin deficiency relative to the levels of the counter-regulatory hormones glucagon, epinephrine, cortisol, and growth hormone. These hormones can be increased during times of stress such as infection, illness, injury, surgery, or severe emotional upset. The resultant hyperglycemia, glycosuria, and osmotic load provoke sodium and water losses, leading to dehydration and further hyperglycemia.

Fatty acids are mobilized at a rate that cannot be handled by the Krebs cycle. The resulting incomplete oxidation of fatty acids results in the production of acetone, beta-hydroxybutyric acid, and acetoacetic acid (ketone bodies) that accumulate in the blood and depress the pH to hazardous levels. The reserve of bicarbonate buffers is depleted and subsequent respiratory compensation raises the blood pH. Coma is the result of brain response to the abnormal acid levels.

The warning symptoms of *coma* are thirst and dry mouth, flushed face, progressive drowsiness, nausea, vomiting, abdominal pain, cold and dry skin, characteristic acid breath (ketoacidosis), deep sighing (Kussmaul breathing), headache, dizziness, pain in the back and legs, and extreme weakness. The urine will contain large amounts of sugar.

It is probable that enough insulin is still available in NIDDM to inhibit excessive fat mobilization and excessive production of ketones by the liver and development of ketonemia. However, in these patients a hyperosmolar, hyperglycemic, nonketotic coma is sometimes seen. It has an insidious onset and frequently develops in adults with undiagnosed or mild diabetes who experience a precipitating stress such as an infection, injury, acute pancreatitis, myocardial infarction, septicemia, or gastroenteritis. The resulting hyperglycemia, 600 to 3,000 mg/dl, leads to hyperosmolarity and osmotic diuresis. The inevitable consequence is severe dehydration and hypovolemia, leading to compromised renal blood flow, thromboembolic complications, and eventually cerebral dehydration and coma.

Treatment. Speed in treatment is essential; diabetic coma may prove fatal if not treated promptly and efficiently. The treatment consists of (1) insulin, (2) electrolytes, and (3) fluids. Regular insulin is given intravenously as a low-dose constant infusion or as an hourly intramuscular injection. In severe ketoacidosis, fluids and electrolytes are replaced with normal saline and sometimes bicarbonate given intravenously. As hyperglycemia and glycosuria diminish, 5% glucose is added. The patient should not be fed orally for 24 hours because a flare-up of autonomic neuropathy could lead to emesis and aspiration. Potassium and possibly phosphate are also given, preferably monitored by electrocardiogram. Urinary output must be adequate.

RENAL DISEASE. Persistent proteinuria (microalbuminuria) of more than 1 g/day indicates the early stage of diabetic nephropathy. This usually occurs about 2 decades after diabetes is diagnosed. The renal deterioration progresses and a period of uremia (nitrogenous wastes accumulating in the blood) lasts from 1 to 3 years, followed in another 2 or 3 years by kidney failure (Levine, 1987). See Chapter 35 for further discussion of diabetic renal disease and management of renal failure.

GASTROPARESIS. Diabetic gastroparesis results from an alteration of the activity of the stomach and is thought to be related to visceral autonomic neuropathy. Stomach emptying of fluids is normal, but the emptying of solids is markedly delayed. Symptoms include bouts of nausea, vomiting, bloating, and abdominal pain after eating. Attacks of gastric stasis may contribute to brittle diabetes marked by diabetic ketoacidosis or severe insulin reactions, poor nutritional intake, and resultant malnutrition and death.

The treatment involves synchronizing insulin activity with food intake and emptying from the stomach, providing adequate energy, and ameliorating the psychological burden of constant abdominal distress. Nutrient-dense liquid supplements may be necessary to meet energy needs, and medication such as metoclopramide is used to improve gastric emptying. Jejunostomy tube feeding may be necessary if the patient does not respond to other measures.

Autonomic neuropathy affecting intestinal peristalsis may manifest as uncontrollable diarrhea, especially nocturnal. Medication and the usual dietary recommendations for diarrhea management may help.

SURGERY. The person with diabetes does not have increased surgical risk over the nondiabetic; however, risk of complications is increased. Preoperative care involves hydration and control of hyperglycemia. Patients on OHA should continue them until the day of surgery, with the exception of chlorpropamide (Diabinese), which should be discontinued a day earlier because of its longer half-life. During this time, blood glucose can be managed by the addition of regular insulin to the intravenous fluids that usually also provide dextrose. The diabetic requires close monitoring during surgery.

Fluid and dextrose are provided postoperatively to achieve adequate vascular volume as well as to provide substrate until adequate oral intake is achieved. Insulin requirements, which may have greatly increased during surgery, gradually diminish to preoperative levels. Blood glucose should be checked every 4 to 6 hours to determine the amount of regular insulin to provide. Urine acetone should also be checked to monitor for impending ketosis. Sharp increases in blood glucose can signal postoperative complications such as infection.

If a liquid diet is necessary either preoperatively or postoperatively, the choice should be one with a carbohydrate, protein, and fat calorie distribution of 50%, 20%, and 30%, respectively. The carbohydrate should be mainly complex, as in soy products. If feeding is via a tube enterally, injections of insulin will be necessary with dosage and timing dependent upon blood glucose and urine acetone done every 6 hours. The patient who must receive parenteral nutrition benefits from a lipid-containing solution because glucose intolerance is lessened, as are insulin requirements. Blood glucose should be maintained in the 150 to 200 mg/dl range. The best method for providing insulin is to add it to the nutrient formula. If it is provided through an additional insulin drip, there is the danger of hypoglycemia if the insulin drip continues, and for some reason administration of the nutrient formula is stopped. Both blood glucose and acetone should be measured every 4 hours.

When the patient begins to eat normally, it is important that energy intake remain constant; uneaten food may need to be replaced with liquid forms of carbohydrate. The total available glucose is determined, and a replacement is offered.

DIABETES IN THE ELDERLY

It has been argued that different glucose tolerance standards should be used in diagnosing true cases of NIDDM in the elderly inasmuch as there is a "natural" glucose intolerance, especially postprandial glucose intolerance, that occurs with aging. However, with the increasing evidence for the risks of atherosclerosis and other vascular damage, and the definition of IGT in the diagnostic criteria for diabetes (see Table 31–3), more aggressive treatment is being recommended for the elderly with IGT. In most cases, this means reducing plasma glucose levels through weight reduction and increased exercise.

Nutritional management of the elderly is the same as with younger diabetics except for special attention to appropriate methods of education, interest in eating, ability to exercise, and perhaps special mineral requirements. A chromium deficiency often present in the elderly may be a cause for glucose intolerance.

Insulin injections can be hazardous for the nearly blind, forgetful, frightened, and unconfident elderly patient, and the necessity for outside supervision or chronic institutionalization can mark the end of independence. Hypoglycemia because of failure to eat or overdosage of insulin, is always a danger. Care of the elderly diabetic calls for special empathy and concern.

DIABETES IN PREGNANCY

The Pregnant Woman with Diabetes. Pregnancy imposes additional stress on the woman with diabetes. Even well-controlled cases may become unbalanced and require modifications in both diet and insulin. However, the incidence of fetal morbidity and mortality is steadily decreasing with improvement in mothers' glucose control, and statistics for the pregnant woman with diabetes are approaching those of normal pregnancy (Mills et al, 1988). The ultimate goal is preconceptional control of blood glucose.

Infants born to women with diabetes are, as a rule, larger than those of nondiabetics. Hyperglycemia in the mother causes high levels of glucose to cross the placenta and supernormal levels of the fetus' own insulin stimulate accelerated growth. The increased secretion of insulin results in a tendency for these infants to become hypoglycemic shortly after birth.

Management. Successful pregnancy depends upon adequate dietary and insulin management to meet the growth needs of the fetus, prevent depletion of the mother's nutritional stores, and provide optimal glucose and insulin levels for fetal development. The demands of pregnancy may impose a need for insulin in a diabetic gravid woman whose condition was previously controlled by diet alone.

Insulin requirements usually increase, and multiple injections of regular insulin throughout the day are often a necessity by the end of the second trimester. Frequent changes in the diet and the insulin dosage may be necessary.

Individualized, expert care is needed for nutritional management. Many pregnant women with diabetes are hospitalized for a few days shortly after learning of a pregnancy in order to regain diabetic control and be administered renal function tests and provided with patient education. The major dietary goal is to avoid large fluctuations in blood glucose during the day. The range of normal blood glucose values is lower during pregnancy: fasting and premeal, 60 to 90 mg/dl; peak postprandial, 120 to 140 mg/dl (Rifkin, 1983; Powers et al, 1987).

Gestational Diabetes Mellitus. Diabetes may exist only during the stress of pregnancy and resolve itself after delivery. The etiology of "gestational diabetes" is not completely understood, but it often can be controlled by diet alone. In normal pregnancy, maternal insulin does not cross the placenta, but the effect of gradually increasing placental secretion of hormones such as estrogen and progesterone is to blunt the efficacy of a given amount of insulin and to stimulate increased secretion of maternal insulin. In women unable to increase their insulin secretion, gestational diabetes mellitus (GDM) results. Evidence suggests that the large offspring of mothers with GDM may experience increased risk of obesity and impaired glucose tolerance in later years due to the altered metabolic milieu (Green et al, 1987b).

The parameters for diagnosing gestational diabetes are shown in Table 31–3. All pregnant women should be screened for fasting blood glucose at 24 to 28 weeks. If the FBG is greater than 105 mg/dl, the oral glucose tolerance test should be given. Two or more of the following venous plasma concentrations must be met or exceeded for a positive diagnosis: fasting, 105 mg/dl; 1 hr, 190 mg/dl; 2 hr, 165 mg/dl; 3 hr, 145 mg/dl (Diabetes Care and Education Practice Group, 1987). As soon as diagnosis is made, the patient should be given a meal plan providing approximately 30 to 32 kcal/kg ideal prepregnant weight during the first trimester and about 38 kcal/kg during the last two trimesters. In the obese woman, this may be less than the energy intake to maintain weight and may need to be adjusted upward to prevent ketonemia. There is no definitive answer to the question of optimal energy requirements for the obese pregnant woman with diabetes. The distribution of protein, carbohydrate, and fat is similar to that for the nonpregnant diabetic except that there needs to be special attention given to the need for 30 g additional protein so that the percentage of calories from protein may be higher.

During lactation, the energy requirements for the woman with diabetes are the same (38 kcal/kg ideal prepregnant body weight). During the postpartum time, it is also important to make plans with the mother for reducing to her ideal weight, especially in the case of the obese GDM mother. Preliminary evidence suggests that diet and exercise appropriate for diabetic management and follow-up can delay onset of overt diabetes in later years (Stowers et al, 1985).

CHILDREN WITH DIABETES

The peak incidence for the age of onset of IDDM in children is 8 to 15 years of age (Cruickshanks et al, 1985). This is when children are normally working toward independence, are being influenced by peers more than by parents, are learning the physical capabilities of their bodies, and are exploring and testing the environment. Learning at this time that he or she has diabetes and must be dependent on insulin and schedules can be devastating and, at the least, troublesome for the child and the family. It takes coordinated team effort, empathy, and continuous attention by the health care providers to help the new diabetic make the transition to a lifestyle appropriate for diabetes management.

Insulin Therapy. Some time after beginning insulin therapy, it is not uncommon for juvenile patients to experience a period of remission when they do not need as much, or in rare cases, any insulin. This "honeymoon period" may last for months or years; however, this period is always temporary, and the child and parents should be so informed. This temporary remission is not well understood, but it appears to be a final effort by the pancreas to secrete insulin and control the level of blood glucose. The period seems to last longer in children who are diagnosed and treated early.

After the remission period, insulin requirements increase and then remain fairly stable except for a 25 to 30% increase during the accelerated growth and the insulin resistance of adolescence (Yki-Jarvinen and Koivisto, 1986). Requirements also increase after a hypoglycemic attack and during an infection. Energy requirements lessen with approaching adulthood, and it is important to reduce insulin dosage and energy intake accordingly.

Nutritional Care. The general pattern of the diet for a child with diabetes is the same as that suggested for the adult except that snacks in the mid-afternoon and evening are almost always included. Energy and protein requirements are higher to allow for growth and development. (Recommended allowances for energy, protein, vitamins, and minerals for normal children are listed in Table 16–1.) Food intake, exercise, and insulin distribution should be adjusted to avoid insulin reactions and, insofar as practical, glycosuria. The diet is adjusted to provide 12 to 20% of the calories from protein, 25 to 35% from fat, and 50 to 60% from carbohydrate. The distribution of the carbohydrates and calories throughout the day must be relatively uniform to maintain a high degree of control and to prevent hypoglycemia.

Counseling Children With Diabetes. The interpretation of diets for children with diabetes should be flexible, especially if the child and family are conscientious about glucose monitoring. An eating plan that fits into the familiar dietary pattern of the family is usually more acceptable. Approaching the child and family with the idea that the eating plan will be based on what the child is already eating, and that the calorie level will be determined from the present intake, makes the diet seem more acceptable. This can be done only with an extensive interview and dietary history and with sympathetic listening on the part of the dietetic practitioner.

Children are capable students and learn quickly how to plan their own diets once they have accepted their disease and are ready to learn. By 5 to 6 years of age, most children can select the appropriate foods for their eating plan; by 9 to 10 years of age, they are capable of self-injection; and by approximately 11 years of age, they are able to do SMBG independently.

Patient and Family Education

Persons with diabetes should know how to plan their own diets, adjust exercise and insulin when necessary, and monitor serum glucose. Changes in eating habits and dietary pattern are not easy, particularly when weight reduction is necessary, and frequent adjustments are necessary until an acceptable pattern evolves.

It is important to recognize when patients are ready to learn. Diet is frequently the least important focus of attention in new patients. They are likely to be more concerned about giving themselves insulin injections, and education regarding their eating practices may have to wait until a more appropriate time.

Dietary patterns and timing and spacing of meals should be planned to conform as closely as possible with individual lifestyles and customary eating habits. Standardized diet sheets are never appropriate, and education techniques should be individualized to match learning patterns.

At each follow-up visit, the interview should begin with a determination of the dietary pattern the patient is now following. If there has been a change in weight, or blood tests have not been acceptable, well-informed persons with diabetes usually know the reason. They often need assistance in adjusting to changing conditions in their lives.

REACTIVE HYPOGLYCEMIA (POSTPRANDIAL SYNDROME)

Hypoglycemia is a symptom of disordered carbohydrate metabolism. It is usually defined by a plasma glucose level below 50 mg/dl (blood glucose of 40 mg/dl or less) after a meal or glucose load, accompanied by typical symptoms of adrenergic neural activation. Accurate diagnosis of hypoglycemia should include measurement of plasma glucose at the time of symptoms (Palardy et al, 1989). The mixed meal tolerance test entails measurement of plasma or blood glucose at specific times after consumption of a meal containing 75 grams of carbohydrate combined with fat and protein that would be present in a normal meal.

The typical symptoms of sweating, weakness, hunger, tachycardia, and "inward trembling" are produced by a compensatory increase in sympathetic nervous system activity as the body attempts to increase hepatic glycogenolysis to offset the falling blood glucose level. Other nonspecific symptoms are headache, blurred vision, mental confusion, incoherent speech, bizarre behavior, or convulsions, which usually result from a slow and severe decline in blood glucose.

Fasting hypoglycemia is characterized by the development of hypoglycemic symptoms 6 or more hours after a meal. Although fasting hypoglycemia occurs rarely, there are several possible causes, some of which are hypersecretion of insulin due to an insulinoma (tumor of the pancreatic islet beta cells), other endocrine tumors, hypothyroidism, overadministration of insulin or sulfonylureas, and liver damage. The treatment for this type of hypoglycemia is to correct the underlying medical problem or treat the symptoms with diazoxide, which decreases secretion of insulin and elevates blood glucose.

Hypoglycemia in the "fed" state, or *reactive postprandial hypoglycemia,* occurs 2 to 5 hours after the intake of food, especially of carbohydrates. Sensitive individuals are those with impaired glucose tolerance due to a delayed but excessive insulin response to glucose, or those with alimentary hypoglycemia resulting from dumping syndrome (see p. 446 in Chapter 26). In the opinion of some authorities, the former represents one of the earliest manifestations of the diabetic state. It is characterized by a delay in insulin secretion, with the peak response occurring between 90 and 180 minutes after a meal as opposed to a normal peak occurring between 30 and 60 minutes postprandially. The liver has already started taking up glucose at this time, so that maximal levels of serum glucose and serum insulin do not coincide. Thus, the late-arriving insulin causes an excessively large drop in serum glucose between 180 and 270 minutes after food intake, and hypoglycemia and symptoms result. The symptoms are relieved with carbohydrate intake.

The work-up for the patient who has hypoglycemic symptoms should include a dietary history to identify the content of the diet and the timing of symptoms. In addition, it should be determined how the symptoms are relieved and what triggers them. Symptoms of true hypoglycemia should be relieved by carbohydrate intake. An oral glucose tolerance test may or may not be useful in the diagnosis.

Management

Surgery is the preferred treatment when a tumor is established as the cause of fasting hypoglycemia. Some patients refuse to have an operation, and others with mild symptoms, may prefer to try medical regimens including diet. The basic principles of the dietary treatment for hypoglycemia focus upon slowing the quick absorption and utilization of carbohydrates, which stimulate the islet cells of the pancreas to secrete insulin and move glucose from the blood. Because the glucose available after the absorption and metabolism of complex carbohydrate, fiber, and protein is released into the blood stream evenly and more slowly causing less stimulation of insulin secretion, a diet rich in these components is recommended.

The diet for hypoglycemia is calculated in a procedure similar to that used to plan the diabetic diet, and the Exchange Lists given in Table 31 – 10 can be used. A diet divided into five or six meals, with some protein and fiber in each meal in order to provide a less rapidly available source of glucose and slow down glucose absorption, helps to maintain blood glucose at a normal level.

The energy content of the diet is based upon the patient's normal requirements. A moderate protein content of 70 to 130 g (12 to 20% of calories) is average, and a moderate carbohydrate content of 40 to 55% of calories is the usual range. The balance of kilocalories is allotted to fats. Concentrated sweets are avoided. Fruits, vegetables, breads, cereals, and potatoes should provide the carbohydrate in the diet. Because alcohol can potentiate hypoglycemia by blocking gluconeogenesis, it should be omitted or restricted to one drink per day. Caffeine should also be omitted, as it affects blood glucose levels through epinephrine stimulation.

CITED REFERENCES

American Diabetes Association: Nutritional recommendations and principles for individuals with diabetes mellitus: 1986. Diabetes Care 10:126, 1987a.

American Diabetes Association: Physician's Guide to Insulin-Dependent (Type I) Diabetes: Diagnosis and Treatment. Alexandria, VA, American Diabetes Association, 1988, p 18.

American Diabetes Association: Position statement: Use of noncaloric sweeteners. Diabetes Care 10:526, 1987b.

American Medical Association: Saccharin: Review of safety issues. JAMA 254:2622, 1985.

Anderson RA: Selenium, chromium, and manganese. B. Chromium. *In* Shils ME and Young VR (eds): Modern Nutrition in Health and Disease. Philadelphia, Lea & Febiger, 1988, p 268.

Anderson RA and Kozlovsky AS: Chromium intake, absorption and excretion of subjects consuming self-selected diets. Am J Clin Nutr 41:1177, 1985.

Anderson RA et al: Chromium supplementation of human subjects: Effects on glucose, insulin and lipid variables. Metabolism 32:894, 1983.

Anderson JW et al: Dietary fiber and diabetes: A comprehensive review and practical application. J Am Diet Assoc 87:1189, 1987.

Anderson JW et al: Mineral and vitamin status on high-fiber diets: Long-term studies of diabetic patients. Diabetes Care 3:38, 1980.

Aro A et al: Improved diabetic control and hypocholesterolemic effect induced by long term dietary supplementation with guar gum in type II (non-insulin-dependent) diabetes. Diabetologia 21:29, 1981.

Birchwood BA and Jenkins AL: Fructose and sorbitol in the management of diabetes mellitus. J Can Diet Assoc 49:153, 1988.

Bogardus C et al: Effects of physical training and diet therapy on carbohydrate metabolism in patients with glucose intolerance and non-insulin dependent diabetes. Diabetes 33:311, 1984.

Bohannon NV, Karam JH, and Forsham PH: Endocrine response to sugar ingestion in man. J Am Diet Assoc 76:555, 1980.

Brand JC et al: Plasma glucose and insulin responses to traditional Pima Indian meals. Am J Clin Nutr 51:416, 1990.

Brownlee M, Cerami A, and Vlassara H: Advanced glycosylation end products in tissue and the biochemical basis of diabetic complications. N Engl J Med 318:1315, 1988.

Carlson SK: Protein. *In* Powers MA: Handbook of Diabetes Nutritional Management. Rockville, MD, Aspen Publishers, 1987.

Crapo PA, Scarlett JA, and Kolterman OG: Comparison of the metabolic responses to fructose and sucrose sweetened foods. Am J Clin Nutr 36:256, 1982.

Cruickshanks KJ et al: The epidemiology of insulin-dependent diabetes mellitus: Etiology and prognosis. *In* Ahmed PI and Ahmed N (eds): Coping with Juvenile Diabetes. Springfield, IL, Charles C Thomas, 1985.

Cryer PE and Gerich JE: Glucose counterregulation, hypoglycemia, and intensive insulin therapy in diabetes mellitus. N Engl J Med 313:232, 1985.

Diabetes Care and Education Practice Group, American Dietetic Association: Meal Planning Approaches in the Nutrition Management of the Person with Diabetes. Chicago, The American Dietetic Association, 1987.

Diabetes Control and Complications Trial Research Group: Diabetes Control and Complications Trial (DCCT): Results of feasibility study. Diabetes Care 10:1, 1987.

Diabetes Control and Complications Trial Research Group: Weight gain associated with intensive therapy in diabetes control and complications trial. Diabetes Care 11:567, 1988.

FDA OKs new sweetener. Nutr MD 15(3):4, 1989.

Franz M: Exercise and diabetes mellitus. *In* Powers MA: Handbook of Diabetes Nutritional Management. Rockville, MD, Aspen Publications, 1987.

Garg A et al: Comparison of a high-carbohydrate diet with a high-monounsaturated-fat diet in patients with non-insulin-dependent diabetes mellitus. N Engl J Med 319:862, 1988.

Green DA, Lattimer SA, and Sima AAF: Sorbitol, phosphoinositides, and sodium-potassium-ATPase in the pathogenesis of diabetic complications. N Engl J Med 316:599, 1987a.

Green OC et al: Fuel-mediated teratogenesis: Prospective correlations between anthropometric development in childhood and antepartum maternal metabolism. Clin Res 35:657A, 1987b.

Grigoresco C et al: Lack of detectable deleterious effects on metabolic control of daily fructose ingestion for 2 mo in NIDDM patients. Diabetes Care 11:546, 1988.

Hadden WC and Harris MI, National Center for Health Statistics: The prevalence of diagnosed diabetes, undiagnosed diabetes and impaired glucose tolerance in adults 20–74 years of age, United States, 1976–80. Vital and Health Statistics, Series 11, No 237. DHHS Publ No (PHS) 87-1687. Washington, DC, Government Printing Office, February 1987.

Harris M and Hamman R (eds): Diabetes in America. NIH Publication No 85-1468, 1985.

Jenkins DJA: Starchy foods and glycemic index. Diabetes Care 11:149, 1988.

Jenkins DJA et al: The glycemic response to carbohydrate foods. Lancet 2:388, 1984.

Kawahara R and Amemiya T: Obesity and diabetes mellitus. Asian Med J 32:379, 1989.

Kaysen GA et al: Effect of dietary protein on a albumin homeostasis in nephrotic patients. Kidney Internat 29:572, 1986.

Knowler WC et al: Diabetes incidence and prevalence in Pima Indians: A 19-fold greater incidence than in Rochester, Minnesota. Am J Epidemiol 108:497, 1978.

Laine DC et al: Comparison of predictive capabilities of diabetic exchange lists and glycemic index of foods. Diabetes Care 10:387, 1987.

Levine SE: Renal failure: Diabetic nephropathy. *In* Powers MA: Handbook of Diabetes Nutritional Management. Rockville, MD, Aspen Publications, 1987, p. 378.

Mills JL et al: Incidence of spontaneous abortion among normal women and insulin-dependent diabetic women whose pregnancies were identified within 21 days of conception. N Engl J Med 319:1617, 1988.

Offenbacher EG and Pi-Sunyer FX: Beneficial effect of chromium rich brewer's yeast on glucose tolerance and blood lipids in elderly subjects. Diabetes 29:919, 1980.

Olefsky JM and Crapo PA: Fructose, xylitol and sorbitol. Diabetes Care 3:390, 1980.

Palardy J et al: Blood glucose measurements during symptomatic episodes in patients with suspected postprandial hypoglycemia. N Engl J Med 321:1421, 1989.

Perriello G et al: The effect of asymptomatic nocturnal hypoglycemia on glycemic control in diabetes mellitus. N Engl J Med 319:1233, 1988.

Powers MA, Metzger BE, and Freinkel N: Pregnancy and Diabetes. *In* Powers MA: Handbook of Diabetes Nutritional Management. Rockville, MD, Aspen Publications, 1987, pp. 332–351.

Pulini M: Insulin allergy in clinical practice. Pract Diabetology 4:1, 1985.

Rattan J et al: A high-fiber diet does not cause mineral and nutrient deficiencies. J Clin Gastroenterol 3:389, 1981.

Rifkin H (ed): Physician's Guide to Type II Diabetes (NIDDM): Diagnosis and Treatment. Alexandria, VA, American Diabetes Association, 1983.

Saccharin and its salts. Federal Register, April 15:19,996, 1977.

Savage PJ et al: High prevalence of diabetes in young Pima Indians: Evidence of phenotypic variation in a genetically isolated population. Diabetes 28:937, 1979.

Sievers ML: Disease patterns among Southwestern Indians. Pub Health Rep 81:1075, 1966.

Sotsky M and Shamoon H: Human insulin: A second revolution? Clin Diabetes 4:2, 1986.

Srikanta S et al: Islet-cell antibodies and beta-cell function in monozygotic triplets and twins initially discordant for Type I diabetes mellitus. N Engl J Med 30:322, 1983.

Stowers JM, Sutherland HW, and Kerridge DF: Long-range implications for the mother. Diabetes 34(Suppl 2):106, 1985.

Thorburn AW et al: Salt and glycaemic response. Br Med J 292:1697, 1986.

Urberg M and Zemel MB: Evidence for synergism between chromium and nicotinic acid in the control of glucose tolerance in elderly humans. Metabolism 36:896, 1987.

Winter WE et al: Maturity-onset diabetes of youth in Black Americans. N Engl J Med 316:285, 1987.

Wolever TMS et al: Second-meal effect: Low-glycemic-index foods eaten at dinner improve subsequent breakfast glycemic response. Am J Clin Nutr 48:1041, 1988.

Yetley E and Johnson C: Nutritional applications of the Health and Nutrition Examination Surveys (HANES). Annu Rev Nutr 7:441, 1987.

Yki-Jarvinen H and Koivisto VA: Natural course of insulin resistance in Type I diabetes. N Engl J Med 315:224, 1986.

ADDITIONAL REFERENCES

American Diabetes Association: Consensus Statement. Role of cardiovascular risk factors in prevention and treatment of macrovascular disease in diabetes. Diabetes Care 12:573, 1989.

Anderson RA: Chromium in human health and disease. Nutr MD, 14(3):1, 1988.

Andreni D, Marks V, and Lefebvre PJ: Hypoglycemia. New York, Raven Press, 1987.

Aspartame and headache. Nutrition Research Newsletter 7:82, 1988.

Beebe CA and Rubenstein AH: Classification, diagnosis and treatment of diabetes. *In* Powers MA: Handbook of Diabetes Nutritional Management. Rockville, MD, Aspen Publishers, 1987.

Beebe C: Self-blood glucose monitoring: An adjunct to dietary and insulin management of the patient with diabetes. J Am Diet Assoc 87:61, 1987.

Bernstein RK: Meaningful screening test for reactive hypoglycemia. Diabetes Care 10:792, 1988.

Chromium and nicotinic acid in glucose tolerance. Nutr MD 14(3):1, 1988.

Cooper PL, Wahlqvist ML, and Simpson RW: Sucrose versus saccharin as an added sweetener in non-insulin-dependent diabetes: Short- and medium-term metabolic effects. Diabetic Med 5:676, 1988.

Crapo PA: Use of alternative sweeteners in the diabetic diet, Diabetes Care 11:174, 1988.

Crapo PA, Kilterman OG, and Olefsky JM: Effects of oral fructose in normal, diabetic and impaired glucose tolerance subjects. Diabetes Care 3:575, 1980.

Crapo PA et al: Postprandial hormonal responses to different types of complex carbohydrate in individuals with impaired glucose tolerance. Am J Clin Nutr 33:1723, 1980.

Cryer PE et al: Hypoglycemia in IDDM, Diabetes 38:1193, 1989.

deFronzo RA, Sherwin RS, and Kraemer N: Effect of physical training on insulin action in obesity. Diabetes 36:1379, 1987.

Diabetes Care and Education Practice Group: Meal Planning Approaches in the Nutrition Management of the Person with Diabetes. Chicago, The American Dietetic Association, 1987.

Gavin JR: Diabetes and exercise. Am J Nurs 88:178, 1988.

Gerich JE: Oral hypoglycemic agents. N Engl J Med 321:1231, 1989.

Glauber H et al: Adverse metabolic effect of omega-3 fatty acids in non-insulin-dependent diabetes mellitus. Ann Intern Med 108:663, 1988.

Hansen BC: Dietary considerations for obese diabetic subjects. Diabetes Care 11:183, 1988.

Hollenbeck CB, Coulston AM, and Reaven GM: Comparison of plasma glucose and insulin responses to mixed meals of high-, intermediate-, and low-glycemic potential. Diabetes Care 11:323, 1988.

Jenkins DJA et al: Glycemic index of foods: A physiological basis for carbohydrate exchange. Am J Clin Nutr 34:362, 1981.

Karjalainen J et al: A comparison of childhood and adult Type I diabetes mellitus. N Engl J Med 320:881, 1989.

Kissebah A and Schectman G: Polyunsaturated and saturated fat, cholesterol and fatty acid supplementation. Diabetes Care 10:129, 1988.

Kovar MG, Harris MI, and Hadden WC: The scope of diabetes in the United States population. Am J Public Health 77:1549, 1987.

Leon AS et al: Safety of long-term large doses of aspartame. Arch Intern Med 149:2318, 1989.

Malik RL et al: Adjustment of caloric intake based on self-monitoring in noninsulin-dependent diabetes mellitus: Development and feasibility. J Am Diet Assoc 89:960, 1989.

Mitchell TH et al: Hyperglycemia after intense exercise in IDDM subjects during continuous subcutaneous insulin infusion. Diabetes Care 11:311, 1988.

Molitch ME: Complications of diabetes mellitus. *In* Powers MA: Handbook of Diabetes Nutritional Management. Rockville, MD, Aspen Publishing, 1987.

Morley JE et al: Diabetes mellitus in elderly patients. Is it different? Am J Med 83:533, 1987.

National Institutes of Health: Consensus development conference on diet and exercise in non-insulin-dependent diabetes mellitus. Diabetes Care 10:639, 1987.

Nelson RL: Hypoglycemia: Fact or Fiction? Mayo Clin Proc 60:844, 1985.

Nompleggi D et al: Overview of gastrointestinal disorders due to diabetes mellitus: Emphasis on nutritional support. J Parenter Enteral Nutr 13:84, 1989.

Powers MA (ed): Nutrition Guide for Professionals. Diabetes Education and Meal Planning. Chicago, American Diabetes Association and American Dietetic Association, 1988.

Ramsay RC et al: Progression of diabetic retinopathy after pancreas transplantation for insulin-dependent diabetes mellitus. N Engl J Med 318:208, 1988.

Samowich AS: Medications and delivery methods. *In* Powers MA: Handbook of Diabetes Nutritional Management. Rockville, MD, Aspen Publications, 1987.

Simpson RW et al: Macronutrients have different metabolic effects in nondiabetics and diabetics. Am J Clin Nutr 42:449, 1985.

Sweeteners in Diabetes. Proceedings of a Conference. Diabetes Care 12(Suppl 1):47–82, 1989.

Tordjman KM et al: Failure of nocturnal hypoglycemia to cause fasting hyperglycemia in patients with insulin-dependent diabetes mellitus. N Engl J Med 317:1552, 1987.

US Dept of Health and Human Services and US Dept of Agriculture: Nutrition Monitoring in the United States. A Progress Report from the Joint Nutrition Monitoring Evaluation Committee. DHHS Publ No (PHS) 86-1255. US Public Health Service. Washington, DC, US Government Printing Office, 1986.

Vinik AI and Jenkins DJA: Dietary fiber in management of diabetes. Diabetes Care 11:160, 1988.

Weinstock RS and Levine RA: The role of dietary fiber in the management of diabetes mellitus. Nutrition 4:187, 1988.

Wing RR et al: Calorie counting compared to exchange system diets in the treatment of overweight patients with Type II diabetes. Addict Behav 11:163, 1986.

Wurtman RJ: Aspartame: Possible effect on seizure susceptibility. Lancet 2:1060, 1985.

Wylie-Rosett J: Evaluation of protein in dietary management of diabetes mellitus. Diabetes Care 11:143, 1988.

CHAPTER 32

NUTRITIONAL CARE IN ANEMIA

CHAPTER OUTLINE

Nutritional Anemias
Other Anemias
Iron Overload

KEY TERMS

ANEMIA—a deficiency in the size or number of red blood cells or in the amount of hemoglobin they contain that limits the exchange of oxygen and carbon dioxide between the blood and the tissue cells

FERRITIN—an iron-apoferritin complex; one of the chief iron storage forms

HEMATOCRIT—the volume percentage of erythrocytes in the blood

HEME—the nonprotein, iron protoporphyrin constituent of hemoglobin

HEME IRON—the form in which iron occurs in meat, fish, and poultry

HEMOCHROMATOSIS—a genetically determined form of iron overload that results in progressive hepatic damage

HEMOGLOBIN—a conjugated protein containing four heme groups and globin; the oxygen-carrying pigment of the erythrocytes

HEMOLYTIC ANEMIA—anemia caused by shortened survival of mature red blood cells

HYPOCHROMIC—deficient hemoglobin content of red blood cells

INTRINSIC FACTOR—a glycoprotein secreted by the gastric glands necessary for the absorption of vitamin B_{12}

MACROCYTIC ANEMIA—anemia characterized by larger than normal red blood cells, increased mean corpuscular volume and mean corpuscular hemoglobin

MEGALOBLASTIC ANEMIA—anemia characterized by the presence of large, immature, abnormal red blood cell progenitors in the bone marrow; characteristic of a folic acid or vitamin B_{12} deficiency

MICROCYTIC ANEMIA—anemia characterized by smaller than normal erythrocytes and less circulating hemoglobin; usually caused by a deficiency of iron

NONHEME IRON—iron that is not a part of the heme complex and that is present in foods such as eggs, grains, vegetables, and fruits; also present in small amounts in meat, fish, and poultry

PERNICIOUS ANEMIA—a macrocytic, megaloblastic anemia caused by a deficiency of vitamin B_{12}

PROTOPORPHYRIN—an iron-containing portion of the respiratory pigments which, when combined with protein, forms hemoglobin or myoglobin

TOTAL IRON BINDING CAPACITY—the capacity of transferrin to take on or become saturated with iron

TRANSFERRIN SATURATION—a gauge of iron supply to the tissues; a measure of the amount of iron bound to transferrin, the globulin that binds and transports iron

Anemia is a condition in which a deficiency in the size or number of erythrocytes or in the amount of hemoglobin they contain limits the exchange of oxygen and carbon dioxide between the blood and the tissue cells. The anemias are classified on the basis of cell size and hemoglobin content as macrocytic, hypochromic-microcytic, and normochromic normocytic (Table 32–1). Most are caused by a lack of nutrients required for normal erythrocyte synthesis, principally iron, vitamin B_{12}, and folic acid. Others result from a variety of conditions, such as hemorrhage, genetic abnormalities, chronic disease states, or drug toxicity.

NUTRITIONAL ANEMIAS

The anemias that result from an inadequate intake of iron, protein, certain vitamins (B_{12}, folic acid, pyridoxine, and ascorbic acid), copper, and other heavy metals are frequently called nutritional anemias. The most common nutritional anemias in the United States are expressions of iron or folic acid deficiency.

Iron Deficiency Anemia

Iron deficiency anemia is characterized by the production of small (microcytic) erythrocytes and a diminished level of circulating hemoglobin. This is actually the last stage of iron deficiency, and it represents the endpoint of a long period of iron deprivation.

Etiology

The three primary causes of iron deficiency anemia are (1) chronic blood loss, such as from a bleeding peptic ulcer, hemorrhoids, parasites, or malignancy; (2) faulty iron intake or absorption, resulting from an iron-poor diet or chronic gastrointestinal disturbances, such as diarrhea, achlorhydria, or intestinal disease; and (3) increased iron requirement of expanded blood volume as seen in infancy, adolescence, and pregnancy. With few exceptions, iron deficiency anemia in male adults is the result of blood loss. Large losses of menstrual blood can cause iron deficiency in women, many of whom are unaware that their menses are unusually heavy.

TABLE 32–1. Morphological Classification of Anemia*

Morphologic Type of Anemia†	Underlying Abnormality	Clinical Syndromes	Treatment
Macrocytic (MCV > 94, MCHC > 31)			
Megaloblastic	Vitamin B_{12} deficiency	Pernicious anemia	Vitamin B_{12}
	Folic acid deficiency	Nutritional megaloblastic anemias, sprue, and other malabsorption syndromes	Folic acid
	Inherited disorders of DNA synthesis	Orotic aciduria	According to nature of disorder
	Drug-induced disorders of DNA synthesis	Chemotherapeutic agents, anticonvulsants, oral contraceptives	Stop offending drug and administer folic acid
Nonmegaloblastic	Accelerated erythropoiesis	Hemolytic anemia	Treatment of underlying disease
	Increased membrane surface area		
	Obscure		
Hypochromic-microcytic (MCV < 80, MCHC < 31)			
	Iron deficiency	Chronic loss of blood, inadequate diet, impaired absorption, increased demands	Ferrous sulfate and correction of underlying cause
	Disorders of globin synthesis	Thalassemia	Nonspecific
	Disorders of porphyrin and heme synthesis	Pyridoxine-responsive anemia	Pyridoxine
	Other disorders of iron metabolism		
Normochromic-normocytic (MCV 82–92, MCHC > 30)			
	Recent blood loss	Various	Transfusion, iron
			Correct underlying condition
	Overexpansion of plasma volume	Pregnancy	Restore homeostasis
		Overhydration	
	Hemolytic diseases		According to nature of disorder
	Hypoplastic bone marrow	Aplastic anemia	Transfusions
		Pure red blood cell aplasia	Androgens
	Infiltrated bone marrow	Leukemia, multiple myeloma, myelofibrosis	Chemotherapy
	Endocrine abnormality	Hypothyroidism, adrenal insufficiency	Treatment of underlying disease
	Chronic disorders		Treatment of underlying disease
	Renal disease	Renal disease	Treatment of underlying disease
	Liver disease	Cirrhosis	Treatment of underlying disease

* Adapted from Wintrobe MM et al: Clinical Hematology, 8th ed. Philadelphia, Lea & Febiger, 1981.
† MCV (mean corpuscular volume) = volume of one red blood cell expressed in femtoliters (fl); MCHC (mean corpuscular hemoglobin concentration) = concentration of hemoglobin expressed in grams per deciliter (dl).

The development of iron deficiency is characterized by three stages: (1) iron stores depletion, (2) deficient erythropoiesis, and (3) anemia. In the early stage, the storage forms of iron (*ferritin* and *hemosiderin*) are depleted. Subsequent depletion of iron in the plasma protein transport vehicle (*transferrin*) is reflected in the measure of total iron-binding capacity (TIBC). At this point, the rate of absorption from gastrointestinal mucosal cells is greatly enhanced. Depletion of iron-containing enzymes in the tissues may also occur.

When plasma iron content falls below 60 μg/dl and the percentage saturation of transferrin falls below 15%, the iron supply to the bone marrow is inadequate for making red blood cells (RBC). The falling level of hemoglobin results in production of erythrocytes that are smaller (*microcytic*) and contain less hemoglobin (*hypochromic*).

Clinical Findings

Because anemia is the last manifestation of a chronic iron deficiency of long standing, the symptoms reflect a malfunction of a variety of body systems. Inadequate muscle function is reflected in decreased work performance and exercise tolerance. Neurologic involvement is manifested in behavioral changes—fatigue, anorexia, and pica, especially pagophagia (ice eating). Abnormal cognitive development in children suggests the presence of iron deficiency before it has developed into overt anemia (Pollitt et al, 1986). Growth abnormalities, epithelial disorders, and reduction in gastric acidity are common. A possible sign of early iron deficiency is a reduction in immunocompetence, particularly defects in cell-mediated immunity and the phagocytic activity of neutrophils that might lead to an increased propensity for infection (Dallman, 1987).

As iron deficiency anemia becomes more severe, defects develop in the structure and function of the epithelial tissues, especially of the tongue, nails, mouth, and stomach. Skin color may appear pale, and the inside of the lower eyelid will be light pink instead of red. Fingernails become thin and flat, and eventually koilonychia (spoon-shaped nails) develops as shown in Figure 32-1. Mouth changes include atrophy of the lingual papillae, burning, and redness and, in severe cases, a completely smooth, waxy, and glistening appearance to the tongue (glossitis). Angular stomatitis may also develop as well as a form of dysphagia (difficulty in swallowing). Gastritis occurs frequently and may result in achlorhydria. Progressive, untreated anemia results in cardiovascular and respiratory changes that can eventually result in cardiac failure.

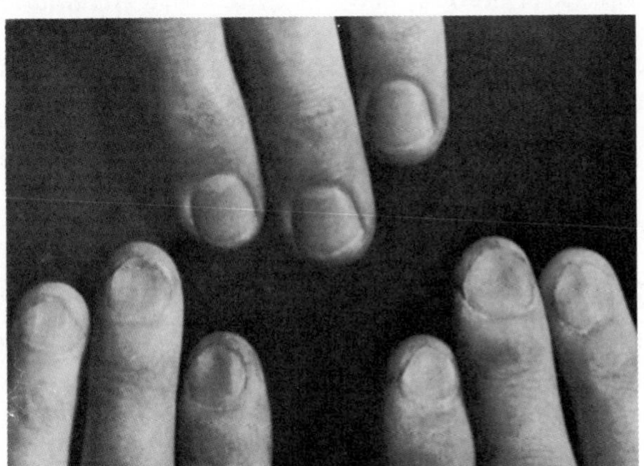

FIGURE 32-1. *Fingernails of an iron-deficient adult (below) compared with those of a normal subject. (From Rosenbaum E and Leonard JW: Nutritional iron deficiency anemia in an adult male. Ann Intern Med 60:683, 1964, p 684.)*

Some behavioral symptoms of iron deficiency seem to respond to iron therapy before the anemia is cured, suggesting they may be the result of tissue depletion of iron-containing enzymes rather than of a decreased level of hemoglobin.

Diagnosis

The progressive degrees of iron deficiency can be evaluated by four different measurements. (1) Plasma ferritin provides a measure of iron stores. (2) Transferrin saturation is a gauge of iron supply to the tissues. It is calculated by dividing serum iron by TIBC; levels below 16% are considered inadequate for erythropoiesis. (3) The ratio of zinc protoporphyrin (erythrocyte protoporphyrin) to heme (ZnPP/heme) is a sensitive indicator of the iron supply to the developing RBC. When insufficient substrate iron is available to incorporate into porphyrin, zinc is then substituted. Although it can combine with globin and circulate, this zinc-containing molecule cannot bind oxygen. (4) Either the hemoglobin or hematocrit measurement indicates anemia. Most patients develop symptoms of anemia when hemoglobin is approximately 8 to 11 g/dl (Table 32-2).

The proper diagnosis of iron deficiency anemia must include more than one iron evaluation and preferably all of the four stated. It should also include an assessment of cell morphology. Serum or plasma ferritin is the most sensitive parameter of iron status. It falls only with true iron deficiency, whereas transferrin saturation (TS), ZnPP/heme ratio, and hemoglobin levels are affected by chronic infection as well as by other factors that may produce a condition that looks like iron deficiency anemia when in fact iron is adequate.

By itself hemoglobin concentration is unsuitable as a diagnostic tool of iron deficiency anemia, because (1) it is affected only late in the disease, (2) it does not indicate the type of anemia that exists, and (3) there is a wide variation in values in normal subjects. Using the data from the second National Health and Examina-

TABLE 32–2. Laboratory Values in Various Stages of Iron Deficiency*

Stage	Stainable Marrow Iron	Serum Ferritin (μg/l)	Serum Iron	TIBC†	Transferrin Saturation (%)	Erythrocyte Abnormalities	Hemoglobin
Normal	Present	>15	Normal	Normal	>16	None	Normal
Early depletion of iron stores	None	<15	Normal	Normal	>16	None	Normal
Early iron-deficient erythropoiesis	None	<15	Decreased	Normal	<16	Early anisocytosis	Normal
Late iron-deficient erythropoiesis	None	<15	Decreased	Increased	<16	Characteristic peripheral smear	Decreased

* From Beissner RS and Trowbridge AA: Clinical assessment of anemia. Postgrad Med 80:83, 1986.
† TIBC = total iron-binding capacity.

tion Survey (NHANES II), Dallman derived 95% reference ranges for hemoglobin concentration for black and white males and females of all ages (Dallman et al, 1984). A hemoglobin value below the 95% reference range for sex, age, and race could be indicative of iron deficiency anemia.

Treatment

Treatment should focus primarily on the underlying disease or situation leading to the anemia. This is often very difficult to determine. Repletion of iron stores, not merely alleviation of the anemia, should be the goal.

MEDICATION. The chief treatment for iron deficiency anemia consists of oral administration of inorganic iron in the ferrous form. At a dose of 30 mg, absorption of ferrous iron is three times greater than if the same amount were given in the ferric form. With larger doses, the difference is even more marked. The most widely used preparation is ferrous sulfate, and the dose is calculated in terms of the amount of elemental iron provided. Other salts absorbed to about the same degree are the ferrous forms of lactate, fumarate, glycine sulfate, glutamate, and gluconate.

Iron is best absorbed when the stomach is empty; however, under these conditions it tends to cause gastric irritation. Gastrointestinal side effects of nausea, epigastric discomfort and distention, heartburn, diarrhea, or constipation can be minimized by increasing the dose slowly over a few days until the required amount is reached and by giving the iron in at least three doses per day. Sustained-release iron preparations reduce gastrointestinal side effects by preventing rapid dissolution of iron, but at the same time they may allow the iron to bypass the jejunum, which is the most active site of iron absorption. Side effects are dose-related, and smaller dosages have been suggested with the expectation that the therapeutic program will take longer (Crosby, 1986).

Depending on the severity of the anemia and the tolerance of iron medication, daily dosage for adults should be 50 to 200 mg of elemental iron. The dosage for children should be 6 mg/kg of elemental iron. Ascorbic acid greatly increases iron absorption through its capacity to maintain iron in the reduced state. Absorption of 10 to 20 mg/day of iron permits an RBC production rate of about three times normal and, in the absence of blood loss, a hemoglobin concentration rise of 0.2 g/dl/day. Increased reticulocytosis is seen within 2 to 3 days after iron administration, but subjective improvement in mood and appetite may be seen even sooner. Hemoglobin level begins to increase by day 4. Iron therapy should be continued for several months, even after hemoglobin levels have been restored in order to allow for repletion of body iron reserves.

If iron supplementation fails to correct the anemia, it may be that (1) the patient is not taking the medication, most likely because of unpleasant side effects; (2) bleeding is continuing at a rate faster than the erythroid marrow can replace blood cells; or (3) the supplemental iron is not being absorbed, possibly as a result of malabsorption caused by idiopathic steatorrhea or celiac sprue. In these circumstances, parenteral administration of iron in the form of iron-dextran may be necessary. Although replenishment of stores by this route is faster, it is more expensive and is not as safe.

NUTRITIONAL CARE. In addition to medication, attention should be given to the amount of absorbable iron in food. Liver, kidney, beef, egg yolk, dried fruits, dried peas and beans, nuts, green leafy vegetables, molasses, whole-grain breads and cereals, and fortified cereals rank highest among foods in their iron content. (See Table 7–9 and Appendix Table 1 for a more complete list; see also Figure 32–2.)

It is estimated that 1.8 mg of iron must be absorbed daily to meet the needs of 80 to 90% of adult women and adolescent males and females. Because the content of iron in typical Western diets is 6 mg/1,000 kcal with surprising consistency, it is apparent that the bioavailability of the iron in the diet is of greater importance than the total dietary iron in correcting or preventing iron deficiency.

Bioavailability of Dietary Iron. Several factors influence the bioavailability of dietary iron. The rate of absorption depends on the iron status of the individual, as

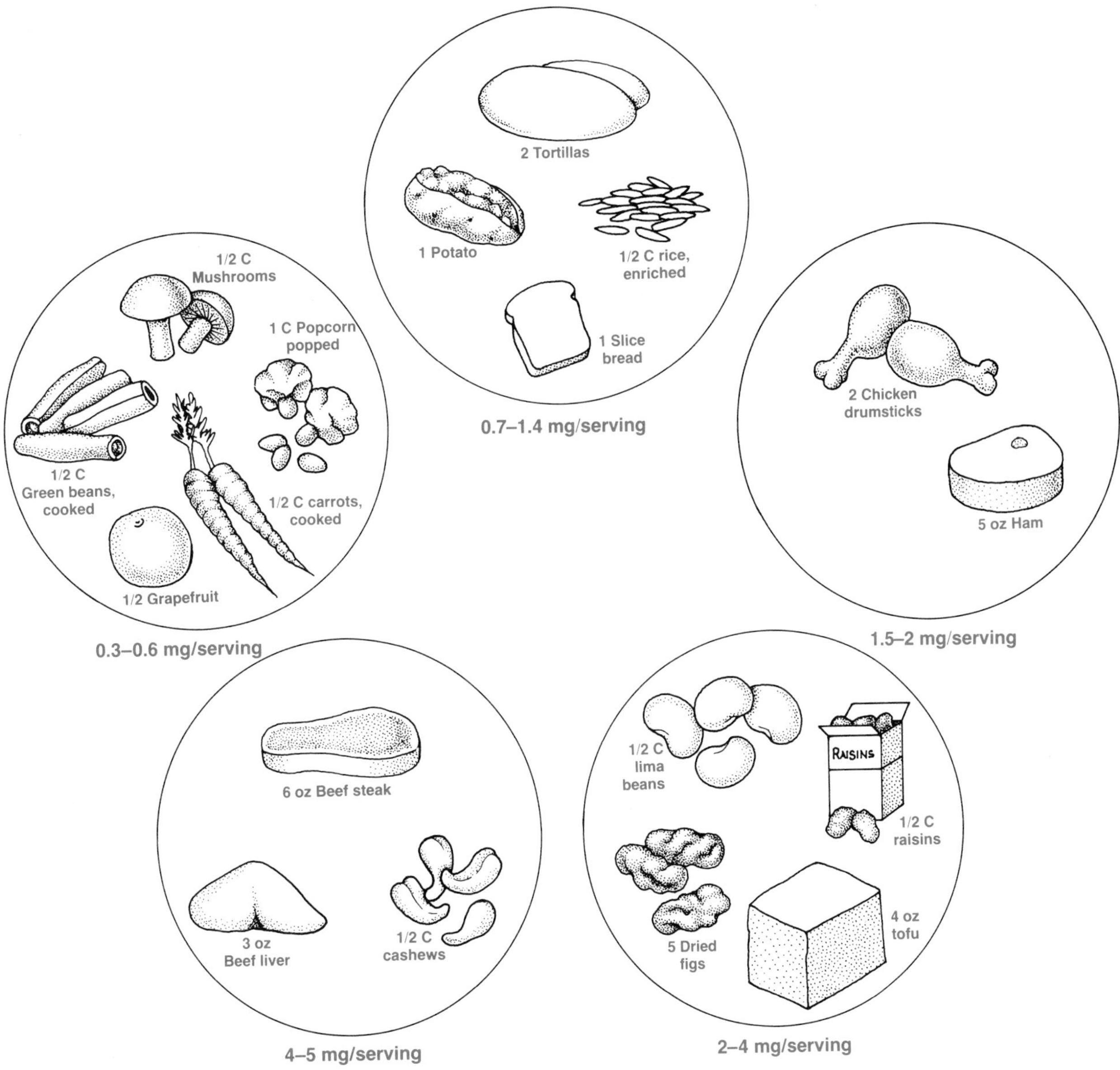
2 Tortillas
1 Potato
1/2 C rice, enriched
1 Slice bread
0.7–1.4 mg/serving
1/2 C Mushrooms
1 C Popcorn popped
1/2 C Green beans, cooked
1/2 C carrots, cooked
1/2 Grapefruit
0.3–0.6 mg/serving
2 Chicken drumsticks
5 oz Ham
1.5–2 mg/serving
6 oz Beef steak
3 oz Beef liver
1/2 C cashews
4–5 mg/serving
1/2 C lima beans
RAISINS
1/2 C raisins
5 Dried figs
4 oz tofu
2–4 mg/serving

FIGURE 32–2. *Iron content of selected foods.*

reflected in the level of iron stores. The lower the iron stores, the greater will be the rate of iron absorption. Absorption is also influenced by the form of iron in the diet. *Heme iron,* present in meat, fish, and poultry (MFP), is much better absorbed than is *nonheme iron,* which is also present in MFP as well as in eggs, grains, vegetables, and fruits. Absorption rate of nonheme iron can vary between 3 and 8% depending on the presence of dietary enhancing factors—specifically ascorbic acid and MFP. Ascorbic acid is not only a powerful reducing agent, but it also binds iron to form a readily absorbed complex. The mechanism by which MFP potentiates the absorption of nonheme iron in other foodstuffs is unknown. MFP digestion may lead to the release of amino acids and polypeptides in the upper small bowel, which then form soluble, absorbable complexes with nonheme iron (Monsen et al, 1978). To be effective, the enhancing substances must be consumed along with the nonheme iron. Ascorbic acid given 4 hours before a meal has no effect (Cook and Monsen, 1977). See Clinical Insight, page 562, for calculation of the amount of absorbable iron.

Iron absorption can be inhibited to a varying degree by a number of factors, including carbonates, oxalates, phosphates, and phytates (unleavened bread, unrefined cereals, and soybeans). Factors in vegetable fiber may inhibit nonheme iron absorption. When taken with meals, tea can reduce iron absorption by 50% through the formation of insoluble iron compounds with tannin (Rossander et al, 1979). Ethylenediaminetetra-acetic acid (EDTA), a food preservative, causes a 50% reduction in the absorption of nonheme iron. Iron

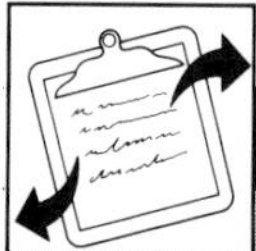

CLINICAL INSIGHT: Calculation of Absorbed Iron

The amount of iron absorbed from a meal includes both heme and nonheme iron and depends on the efficiency of absorption and the presence of enhancing factors.

Between 15 and 35% of *heme* iron is absorbed, depending on the level of body iron stores. Calculations are based on the assumption that iron stores are at the desirable level of 500 mg.

Between 3 and 8% of *nonheme* iron is absorbed, depending on the number of enhancing factors from meat, fish, and poultry (MFP) and from ascorbic acid. One mg of ascorbic acid is equivalent in enhancing power to approximately 1 g of cooked or raw MFP. The sum of the enhancing factors (Σ EF) is therefore determined by totaling the milligrams of ascorbic acid and the grams of MFP present in a meal. These sums have been mathematically summarized in Table A, in such a manner that when the total number of enhancing factors (Σ EF) is known, it is possible to determine the percentage of nonheme iron that will be absorbed.

The following examples demonstrate how the amount of absorbable iron can vary by as much as 300% between two meals, both of which contain the same amount of total iron.

Example Meal 1 (MFP-containing, high ascorbic acid)

Food	Total Iron (mg)	Heme Factor	Heme Iron (mg)	Nonheme Iron (mg)	Ascorbic Acid (mg)
Beef-vegetable stew					
Beef, lean, cooked, 3 oz (85 g)	2.7	0.4[1]	1.1	1.6	0
Potatoes, ½ cup	0.4			0.4	13
Carrots, 2 T	0.1			0.1	1
Onions, 2 T	0.1			0.1	2
Green pepper, raw, 2 slices	0.2			0.2	26
Breadstick, 2 medium	0.3			0.3	Trace
Margarine, 2 tsp	0			0	0
Peaches, canned, ½ cup	0.4			0.4	4
Gingerbread	1.0			1.0	Trace
Total	5.2		1.1	4.1	46
Ascorbic acid (46 mg)					
Meat, fish, poultry cooked (85 g)					
Σ Enhancing factors = 131	% Absorbable iron		23%[2]	8%[3]	
	Absorbable iron (mg)		0.25	0.33	
	Total absorbable iron (mg)		0.58		

[1] Although the proportions of heme and nonheme iron probably vary in different animal tissues, distributions of 40% heme iron and 60% nonheme iron are usually assumed.
[2] Percentage absorption of heme iron depends on individual iron stores. In this table, factors for heme iron are based on stores of 500 mg, which means that 23% of heme iron is estimated to be absorbed.
[3] From Table A.

Table A. Percentage of Nonheme Iron That Will Be Absorbed Based on the Sum of Enhancing Factors (Σ EF)* †

Σ EF	%	Σ EF	%	Σ EF	%	Σ EF	%	Σ EF	%
0	3.00	16	4.33	31	5.41	46	6.38	61	7.26
1	3.09	17	4.40	32	5.48	47	6.44	62	7.31
2	3.18	18	4.48	33	5.55	48	6.50	63	7.37
3	3.26	19	4.55	34	5.61	49	6.56	64	7.42
4	3.35	20	4.63	35	5.68	50	6.62	65	7.47
5	3.44	21	4.70	36	5.75	51	6.68	66	7.53
6	3.52	22	4.78	37	5.81	52	6.74	67	7.58
7	3.60	23	4.85	38	5.88	53	6.80	68	7.64
8	3.69	24	4.92	39	5.94	54	6.86	69	7.69
9	3.77	25	5.00	40	6.01	55	6.92	70	7.74
10	3.85	26	5.06	41	6.07	56	6.97	71	7.79
11	3.93	27	5.14	42	6.13	57	7.03	72	7.85
12	4.01	28	5.21	43	6.20	58	7.09	73	7.90
13	4.09	29	5.28	44	6.26	59	7.14	74	7.95
14	4.17	30	5.34	45	6.32	60	7.20	75	8.00
15	4.25								

For Σ EF < 75: $\% = 3 + 8.93 \log n \frac{EF + 100}{100}$; For Σ EF ≥ 75: % = 8

* Developed by Elaine Monsen, Ph.D., R.D., Professor, University of Washington, Seattle, Washington.
† Factors are based on 500 mg, the desirable level of iron stores. The amount of iron absorbed would be increased with lower stores.

Calculations:

The total iron in Meal 1 is 5.2 mg.

Absorbable heme iron:

Total heme iron = 40% of beef iron® (2.7 mg) = 1.1 mg.

Percentage of heme iron absorption = 23%®

Absorbable heme iron = 0.23 × 1.1 mg = 0.25 mg

Absorbable nonheme iron:

Total nonheme iron = 60% of beef iron® (2.7 × .6 = 1.6 mg) + nonheme iron in remaining foods = 2.5 mg

Σ EF = 1 EF/g MFP (85) + 1 EF/mg ascorbic acid (46) = 131

From Table A: Σ EF ≥ 75: % absorption = 8%

Absorbable nonheme iron = 0.08 × 4.1 mg = 0.33 mg

Total absorbable iron in Meal 1 = 0.25 mg heme iron + 0.33 mg nonheme iron = 0.58 mg

Example Meal 2 (Non-MFP, low ascorbic acid)

Food	Total Iron (mg)	Heme Factor	Heme Iron (mg)	Non-heme Iron (mg)	Ascorbic Acid (mg)
Beans, navy, cooked ½ cup	2.6			2.6	0
Rice, brown, cooked ½ cup	0.5			0.5	0
Cornbread, 1 piece	0.9			0.9	1
Margarine, 1 T	0			0	0
Apple slices, ½ cup	0.1			0.1	1
Walnuts, black, raw, 1 T	0.5			0.5	0
Almonds, raw, 1 tablespoon	0.4			0.4	Trace
Yogurt, skim milk, 1 cup	0.1			0.1	2
Total	5.1			5.1	4
Ascorbic acid (4 mg)					
Meat, fish, poultry, 0					
Σ Enhancing factors = 4	% Absorbable iron			3.35%	
	Absorbable iron (mg)			0.17	
	Total absorbable iron (mg)		0.12		

Calculations:

All of the iron in Meal 2 is nonheme iron (5.1 mg).

Σ EF = 4 (from 4 mg of ascorbic acid)

From Table A: percentage of nonheme iron absorbed when Σ EF = 4 is 3.35%.

Absorbable nonheme iron = 0.0335 × 5.1 mg = 0.17 mg

Total absorbable iron in Meal 2 = 0.17 mg

in egg yolk is poorly absorbed because of the presence of phosvitin.

Summary. In general, the following recommendations can be made: (1) improve food choices to increase amount of total dietary iron, (2) include a source of vitamin C at every meal, (3) include MFP at every meal if possible, (4) avoid drinking large amounts of tea or coffee with meals (both contain tannin), and (5) avoid high quantities of EDTA by checking food labels for its presence in foods. With children, this often means reducing milk consumption to no more than 3 cups per day and replacing it with iron-containing foods.

Anorexia, if present, must be considered when selecting food or planning the diet. Gastrointestinal side effects from concurrent iron medication should also be considered.

Megaloblastic Anemias

Megaloblastic anemias reflect a disturbed synthesis of DNA, which results in morphologic and functional changes in the erythrocytes, leukocytes, platelets, and their precursors in the blood and bone marrow. Megaloblastic anemia is usually caused by a deficiency of vitamin B_{12} or folic acid, both of which are essential to the synthesis of nucleoproteins. Hematologic changes are the same for both; however, the folic acid deficiency is the first to appear. Normal body folate stores are depleted within 2 to 4 months on a folate-deficient diet, whereas vitamin B_{12} stores are depleted only after several years.

Folic Acid Deficiency Anemia

Etiology. This anemia is present in tropical sprue, in some pregnant women, and in infants born to deficient mothers. Inadequate diets of long duration, faulty absorption and utilization of folic acid, and increased requirements due to growth are believed to be the most frequent causes (Table 32–3).

Clinical Findings. Because of their interrelated roles in protein synthesis, a deficiency of either vitamin B_{12} or folic acid will result in the same clinical sign — a megaloblastic anemia. Erythrocyte protein cannot be synthesized properly in the deficient state, and a large

TABLE 32–3. Pathogenetic Classification of the Causes of Megaloblastic Anemia*

Vitamin B_{12} Deficiency	**Folate Deficiency**
Dietary deficiency (rare)	Dietary deficiency
Lack of Castle's intrinsic factor	Increased requirements
Pernicious anemia	Cirrhosis
Congenital form	Pregnancy
Adult form	Infancy
Gastrectomy	Diseases associated with rapid cellular proliferation
Total	Congenital folate malabsorption
Partial	Drug-induced folate malabsorption
Ingestion of caustic materials	Anticonvulsants
Functionally abnormal intrinsic factor	Oral contraceptives
Biologic competition	Extensive intestinal resection, jejunal resection
Small-bowel bacterial overgrowth	**Combined Folate and Vitamin B_{12} Deficiency**
Small-bowel diverticulosis	Tropical sprue
Anastomoses and fistulae	Gluten-induced enteropathy
Blind loops and pouches	**Inherited Disorders of DNA Synthesis**
Strictures	Orotic aciduria
Scleroderma	Lesch-Nyhan syndrome
Achlorhydria	Thiamin-responsive megaloblastic anemia
Fish tapeworm disease	Deficiency of enzymes required for folate metabolism
Familial selective vitamin B_{12} malabsorption (Imerslund's syndrome)	Congenital megaloblastic anemia responsive to large doses of folate and vitamin B_{12}
Drug-induced vitamin B_{12} malabsorption	**Drug-Induced Disorders of DNA Synthesis**
Chronic disease of the pancreas	Folate antagonists (e.g., methotrexate)
Zollinger-Ellison syndrome	Purine antagonists (e.g., 6-mercaptopurine)
Diseases especially affecting the ileum	Pyrimidine antagonists (e.g., cytosine arabinoside)
Ileal resection and bypass	**Erythroleukemia**
Regional enteritis	

* Adapted from Wintrobe M M et al: Clinical Hematology, 8th ed. Philadelphia, Lea & Febiger, 1981.

(*macrocytic*) immature (*megaloblastic*) blood cell is the result. This state is also characterized by a decreased number of erythrocytes, leukocytes, and platelets.

Folate deficiency anemia is manifested by very low serum folate levels (less than 3 ng/ml) and RBC folate levels (less than 140 ng/ml). RBC folate is the superior measurement of folate nutriture because it reflects body folate status at the time when the RBC were formed. Serum levels of vitamin B_{12} are lowered moderately. To differentiate folate deficiency anemia from vitamin B_{12} deficiency anemia, both serum folate and B_{12} levels should be measured. The formiminoglutamic acid (FIGLU) urinary excretion test can also be used. Excretion of FIGLU is increased in folic acid deficiency and to a lesser extent in vitamin B_{12} deficiency (see Chapter 6).

The common clinical picture of folic acid deficiency is fatigue, dyspnea, sore tongue, diarrhea, irritability, forgetfulness, anorexia, glossitis, and weight loss.

TREATMENT. Before initiating treatment, it is important to make a proper diagnosis. Administration of folate in the presence of a vitamin B_{12} deficiency will correct the megaloblastic anemia, but it will not correct the vitamin B_{12} deficiency that will continue and cause progressive nerve disease.

To replenish folate stores, 1 mg of folate taken orally every day for 2 to 3 weeks is recommended. Maintaining repleted stores requires an intake of at least 50 to 100 μg of folic acid every day, either in food or in a supplement. (One cup of orange juice supplies between 50 and 100 μg folic acid.) When folate deficiency is complicated by conditions that suppress hematopoiesis, increase folate requirement, or reduce folate absorption, therapy should begin with 500 to 1,000 μg/day.

Symptomatic improvement, such as increased alertness, cooperativeness, and appetite may be apparent before the hematologic values revert to normal. After the anemia is corrected, the patient should be instructed about ways to include folate in the diet. Because folate is destroyed easily by heat, fruits and vegetables should be eaten fresh or with very little cooking.

Pernicious and Other Vitamin B_{12} Deficiency Anemias

ETIOLOGY. Pernicious anemia is a macrocytic megaloblastic anemia caused by a deficiency of vitamin B_{12}. Most commonly the vitamin deficiency is secondary to a lack of the *intrinsic factor* (*IF*), a glycoprotein in the gastric juice that is necessary for the absorption of dietary vitamin B_{12}. Very rarely, vitamin B_{12} deficiency anemia occurs in strict vegetarians, whose diet contains no vitamin B_{12} except for traces found in plants contaminated by microorganisms capable of synthesizing vitamin B_{12}. Other causes are shown in Table 32–3.

Methylfolate Trap. Deficiency of vitamin B_{12} can result in a deficiency of folic acid by causing the entrapment of folate as 5-methyltetrahydrofolate as shown in Figure 32–3. Without B_{12}, methyltetrahydrofolate is unable to release its methyl group to become tetrahydrofolate (THFA), the optimal substrate for folate polyglutamate synthesis in the cell. Thus other folate coenzymes cannot be synthesized and a folic acid deficiency results.

DIAGNOSIS. The most popular method for testing vitamin B_{12} absorption is by the Schilling urinary excretion test. After an oral dose of radioactive B_{12}, excretion of vitamin B_{12} is low in patients with pernicious anemia because the B_{12} was not absorbed. When the same test is repeated with IF also given orally, the urinary excretion becomes almost normal. A deficiency of vitamin B_{12} due to a malabsorption syndrome is reflected in decreased urinary excretion of B_{12} that remains unchanged on administration of IF.

CLINICAL FINDINGS. Pernicious anemia affects not only the blood but also the gastrointestinal tract and the peripheral and central nervous systems as well. This distinguishes it from folic acid deficiency anemia. The overt symptoms are caused by inadequate myelinization of the nerves and include paresthesia, especially numbness and tingling in the hands and feet, diminution of the senses of vibration and position, poor muscular coordination, poor memory, and hallucinations. If the deficiency continues long enough, the nervous system damage may be irreversible, even with treatment.

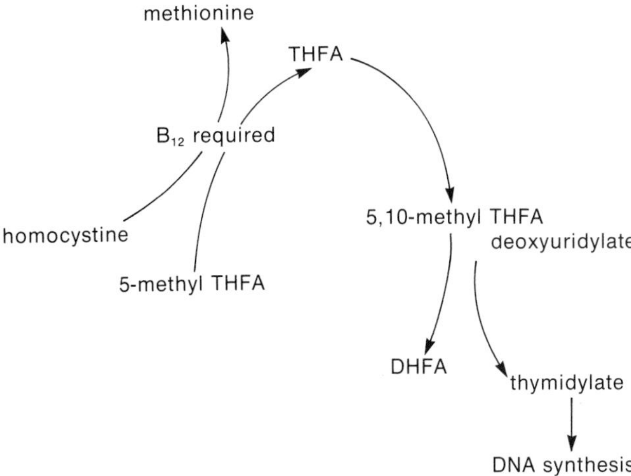

FIGURE 32–3. *Methylfolate trap. Deficiency of vitamin B_{12} can result in a deficiency of folic acid because folate is trapped in the form of 5-methyltetrahydrofolate (5-methyl THFA), which cannot be converted to tetrahydrofolate (THFA) by the vitamin B_{12}-dependent pathway.*

Vitamin B_{12} deficiency has been reported to impair the microbicidal activity of leukocytes, the cells involved in phagocytosis. The function of leukocytes in folic acid-deficient individuals is not impaired; therefore, vitamin B_{12} appears to have a specific role separate from that of folic acid in the production of the intermediates necessary for normal cell metabolism and function.

NUTRITIONAL CARE. Prior to 1926, pernicious anemia was an incurable disease, and a diagnosis meant death in a relatively short time. In 1926, Minot and Murphy reported the effectiveness of liver therapy, and active concentrates of liver suitable for oral use were soon developed. By 1936, relatively purified extracts of liver were available for intramuscular injection. In 1948, vitamin B_{12} was determined to be the active principle in liver and is now available for use either orally or parenterally. Treatment usually consists of intramuscular or subcutaneous injections of 50 to 100 μg/day of vitamin B_{12} for 1 to 2 weeks. After response, the frequency of administration is reduced until remission can be maintained indefinitely with monthly injections of 100 μg. Very large oral doses of B_{12} (1,000 μg) are also effective, even in the absence of intrinsic factor, because about 1% of B_{12} will be absorbed by diffusion. When a vitamin B_{12} deficiency is complicated by debilitating illness, such as infection, hepatic disease, uremia, coma, severe disorientation, or marked neurologic damage, initial dosages should be higher.

Response is evidenced by improved appetite, alertness, and cooperativeness followed by improved hematologic results, as seen by marked reticulocytosis within hours of an injection. Neurologic improvement may take 6 months or more. The shorter the duration of the B_{12} deficiency, the greater will be the neurologic response. Neurologic manifestations that have been present less than 3 months before treatment are usually reversible.

A high-protein diet (1.5 g/kg of body weight) is desirable both for liver function and blood regeneration. Because green leafy vegetables contain both iron and folic acid, the diet should contain increased amounts of these necessary components. Liver should be included frequently because it carries a good supply of iron, vitamin B_{12}, folic acid, and other important nutrients. Meats (especially beef and pork), eggs, milk, and milk products are particularly rich in vitamin B_{12}, although the cholesterol content should be considered.

Copper Deficiency Anemia

Copper and other heavy metals are essential for the proper formation of hemoglobin. *Ceruloplasmin*, a copper-containing protein, is required for normal mobilization of iron from its storage sites to the plasma. In the copper-deficient state iron cannot be released, leading to low serum iron and hemoglobin levels even in the presence of normal iron stores. Other consequences of copper deficiency suggest that copper proteins are needed for utilization of iron by the developing erythrocyte and for optimal functioning of the erythrocyte membrane.

The amounts of copper needed for normal hemoglobin synthesis are so minute that they are usually amply supplied by an adequate diet. Copper deficiency may occur in infants who are fed cow's milk or a copper-deficient infant formula. It is also seen in children or adults who have a malabsorption syndrome or who are receiving long-term total parenteral nutrition that does not supply copper.

Anemia of Protein-Energy Malnutrition (PEM)

Protein is essential for the proper production of hemoglobin and RBC. Because of the reduction in cell mass and thus oxygen requirements in PEM, fewer RBC are required to oxygenate the tissue. Since blood volume remains the same, this reduced number of RBC can look like an iron deficiency anemia with a low hemoglobin. In acute PEM, the loss of active tissue mass may be greater than the reduction of the number of RBC, leading to polycythemia. The body responds to this with suppression of RBC production, which is not a reflection of protein and amino acid deficiency but of an oversupply of RBC. Iron released from normal RBC destruction is not reused in RBC production and is stored so that often there will be adequate iron stores. Iron deficiency anemia can reappear with rehabilitation when there is a rapid expansion of RBC mass.

The anemia of PEM may be complicated by deficiencies of iron and other nutrients and by associated infections, parasitic infestation, and malabsorption. A diet lacking in protein is usually deficient in iron, folic acid, and less frequently, vitamin B_{12}.

Pyridoxine-Responsive Anemia

A *sideroblastic* anemia that responds to vitamin B_6 therapy has been reported. This is a severe microcytic, hypochromic anemia in the presence of high serum iron and tissue iron levels. Transferrin saturation is increased. Frequently, this condition is not due to a pyridoxine deficiency but is an inherited sex-linked anemia. The synthesis of heme appears to be impaired because of an inherited defect in the formation of D-aminolevulinic acid synthetase, an enzyme involved in heme synthesis. Pyridoxal-5-phosphate is necessary in this reaction. The iron that cannot be used for heme synthesis is stored in the mitochondria of immature RBC, called sideroblasts. These iron-laden mitochondria do not function normally, and the development and production of RBC becomes ineffective. The symptoms are those of anemia and iron overload. The neurologic and cutaneous manifestations of vitamin B_6 deficiency are not observed. The anemia responds to administration of pyridoxine.

Treatment consists of a therapeutic trial dose of pyridoxine of 50 to 200 mg/day, which is 25 to 100 times the RDA. If the anemia responds, pyridoxine therapy is continued for life. However, the anemia is only partially corrected; normal RBC morphology is never achieved. Patients respond to this treatment in varying degrees, and some may achieve normal hemoglobin levels.

Vitamin E-Responsive Hemolytic Anemia

A hemolytic anemia exists when defects in the membranes of RBC lead to oxidative damage and eventually to cell lysis. Vitamin E, an antioxidant, is involved in protecting the membrane against oxidative damage, and one of the few signs noted in vitamin E deficiency is hemolysis of RBC. Vitamin E-responsive hemolytic anemia in the newborn is discussed in Chapter 11.

OTHER ANEMIAS

Sickle Cell Anemia

Sickle cell anemia is an inherited hemolytic anemia in which defective hemoglobin causes the erythrocytes to be sickle-shaped. It occurs almost exclusively in black populations that trace their origins to areas of endemic malaria, and manifests itself clinically in persons homozygous for the gene. It is usually diagnosed toward the end of the first year of life. Degrees of severity depend on the amount of abnormal hemoglobin and on the number of erythrocytes with the characteristic odd shape.

Clinical Findings

In addition to the usual symptoms of anemia, sickle cell anemia is characterized by episodes of pain resulting from the occlusion of small blood vessels by the abnormally shaped erythrocytes. The occlusions frequently occur in the abdomen, causing acute, severe abdominal pain. The hemolytic anemia and vaso-occlusive disease result in impairment of liver function, hepatitis, jaundice, gallstones, and deteriorating renal function. Growth slows to below normal. Because of the constant hemolysis of erythrocytes, iron stores in the liver are increased. However, iron deficiency anemia and sickle cell anemia can coexist, and if so they are usually seen in children and pregnant women (Reed et al, 1987). It is suggested that iron deficiency, through reduction of the mean corpuscular hemoglobin (MCH) concentration, may actually be beneficial in sickle cell disease (Rao et al, 1983). Iron overload is a less common situation and is thought to be a problem only in patients who have received many transfusions.

Treatment

There is no specific treatment other than relief of pain during a crisis and possibly administration of an exchange transfusion. It is important that sickle cell anemia is not mistaken for iron deficiency anemia and treated with iron supplements.

Nutritional Care

Because iron stores are frequently in excess in the patient with sickle cell anemia, the diet should be low in iron. Iron-rich foods, such as liver, iron-fortified formula, and iron-fortified cereals are excluded. Factors, such as ascorbic acid, that enhance iron absorption should not be taken with meals. It is important to remember, however, that iron deficiency is present in some cases of sickle cell anemia, possibly owing to repeated phlebotomies, hematuria due to renal papillary necrosis, or other unknown mechanisms.

The diet should be high in folate (400 to 600 μg) because the increased production of erythrocytes needed to replace the cells being continuously destroyed also increases folic acid requirements. However, there is no proof that administration of folate supplements is effective in reducing the crises of sickle cell anemia (Reed et al, 1987).

The symptoms of sickle cell disease, such as delayed onset of puberty and hypogonadism in males, low body weight, defects in the immune system, impaired healing of chronic leg ulcers, and poor appetite, are similar to those seen with zinc deficiency. Decreased levels of zinc in plasma, erythrocytes, and hair, as well as decreased growth have been reported in patients with sickle cell anemia. Gains in height and weight in zinc-treated adolescents have also been reported (Prasad and Cossack, 1984). It has also been shown that zinc can increase the oxygen affinity of both normal and sickle-shaped erythrocytes. Thus zinc supplementation may be beneficial in the management of sickle cell disease, although the long-term effects are unknown. Because zinc competes with copper for binding sites on proteins, the use of high doses of zinc may precipitate a copper deficiency.

Decreased plasma and RBC levels of vitamin E (alpha-tocopherol) have been observed in sickle cell anemia. As there is some evidence that formation of irreversibly sickled cells is related to changes in the erythrocyte membrane rather than hemoglobin structure, it has been postulated that vitamin E has a protective effect against sickling by stabilizing the erythrocyte membrane against oxidative stress (Natta et al, 1980).

Sports Anemia

Heavy physical training can cause a transient anemia or "sports anemia," which is characterized by a significant decrease in RBC count, hemoglobin concentration, and packed cell volume, but the erythrocyte morphology remains normal. The cause is not clear, but reasons such as a hemodilution effect of expanded blood volume and increased rate of destruction of RBC due to intravascular hemolysis have been postulated. See Chapter 19.

IRON OVERLOAD

Iron Toxicity

An overdose of iron medication, seen occasionally in children who eat iron tablets because they think that the tablets are candy, can be fatal in doses of 3 to 10 grams. Iron can cause irritation of the mucosa with ulceration and bleeding, hypoxia, metabolic acidosis, alveolar and hepatic damage, and renal failure, and death can occur in 12 to 48 hours. Treatment is with intravenous desferrioxamine-B, which chelates with iron and leaves by way of the kidneys. Calcium disodium EDTA can also be used.

Hemochromatosis

Hemochromatosis is a genetically determined form of iron overload that is believed to affect as much as 0.5% of the population (Gordeuk et al, 1987). Men are particularly susceptible because they have no mechanisms for losing iron such as menstruation, pregnancy, or lactation. The source of excessive intake is usually the accidental incorporation of iron into the diet from environmental sources. In developing countries, solution of iron from cast-iron cooking vessels and contamination by iron-containing soils is common.

A chronic positive iron balance results in progressive hepatic damage, primarily involving the parenchymal cells. The classic case exhibits hepatomegaly, skin pigmentation, diabetes mellitus, and hypogonadism. Mortality from hemochromatosis is preventable if excess body iron is removed by phlebotomy therapy before hepatic cirrhosis develops. For heavily loaded patients, weekly phlebotomy for 2 to 3 years may be required to eliminate all excess iron.

Iron-Loading Anemias

Iron-loading anemias are a group of refractory disorders associated with ineffective erythropoiesis, in which massive iron overload may develop that is not accounted for by RBC transfusions. These refractory anemias include several thalassemias, a variety of sideroblastic anemias, and a number of anemias associated with blocks in the incorporation of iron into hemoglobin.

CITED REFERENCES

Cook JD and Monsen ER: Vitamin C, the common cold and iron absorption in man. Am J Clin Nutr 30:235, 1977.

Crosby WH: Overtreating the deficiency anemias. Arch Intern Med 146:779, 1986.

Dallman PR: Iron deficiency and the immune response. Am J Clin Nutr 46:329, 1987.

Dallman PR, Yip R, and Johnson C: Prevalence and causes of anemia in the United States, 1976—1980. Am J Clin Nutr 39:437, 1984.

Gordeuk VR, Bacon BR, and Brittenham GM: Iron overload: Causes and consequences. Annu Rev Nutr 7:485, 1987.

Monsen ER et al: Estimation of available dietary iron. Am J Clin Nutr 31:134, 1978.

Natta CL, Machlin LJ, and Brin M: A decrease in irreversibly sickled erythrocytes in sickle cell anemia patients given vitamin E. Am J Clin Nutr 33:968, 1980.

Pollitt E et al: Iron deficiency and behavioral development in infants and preschool children. Am J Clin Nutr 43:555, 1986.

Prasad AS and Cossack ZT: Zinc supplementation and growth in sickle cell disease. Ann Intern Med 100:367, 1984.

Rao KRP et al: Iron deficiency and sickle cell anemia. Arch Intern Med 143:1030, 1983.

Reed JD, Redding-Lallinger R, and Orringer EP: Nutrition and sickle cell disease. Am J Hematol 24:441, 1987.

Rossander L, Hallberg L, and Bjorn-Rasmussen E: Absorption of iron from breakfast meals. Am J Clin Nutr 32:2484, 1979.

ADDITIONAL REFERENCES

Beutler E: The common anemias: State of the art review. JAMA 259:2433, 1988.

Clinical assessment of mild iron-deficiency anemia. Nutr MD 13(3):3, 1987

Expert Scientific Working Group: Summary of a report on assessment of the iron nutritional status of the United States population. Am J Clin Nutr 42:1318, 1985.

Hallberg L, Brune M, and Rossander L: Iron absorption in man: Ascorbic acid and dose-dependent inhibition by phytate. Am J Clin Nutr 49:140, 1989.

Howe RB: Current concepts of anemia in elderly patients. Compr Ther 13(5):30, 1987.

Monsen ER: Iron nutrition and absorption: Dietary factors which impact iron bioavailability. J Am Diet Assoc 88:786, 1988.

Ratcliffe SD et al: Lead toxicity and iron deficiency in Utah migrant children. Am J Public Health 79:631, 1989.

Skikne BS and Cook JD: Screening test for iron overload. Am J Clin Nutr 46:840, 1987.

Soemantri AG, Pollitt E, and Kim I: Iron deficiency anemia and educational achievement. Am J Clin Nutr 42:1221, 1985.

Yip R and Dallman P: The roles of inflammation and iron deficiency as causes of anemia. Am J Clin Nutr 48:1295, 1988.

CHAPTER 33

NUTRITIONAL CARE IN CONGESTIVE HEART DISEASE

CHAPTER OUTLINE

KEY TERMS

CACHECTIC HEART—a soft, flabby heart characterized by loss of myocardial mass as the result of extreme malnutrition

CARDIAC CACHEXIA (CC)—a profound state of malnutrition characterized by loss of fat and muscle mass, especially in the temporal and supraclavicular region due to severe congestive heart failure

CONGESTIVE HEART FAILURE (CHF)—a clinical syndrome caused by heart disease, which is characterized by breathlessness, chest pain, and abnormal sodium and water retention

LOW SALT SYNDROME—a syndrome of hyponatremia, hypochloremia, and eventually azotemia as glomerular filtration rate falls as the result of salt depletion

MILD SODIUM RESTRICTION—restriction of dietary sodium to 2 to 3 grams (87 to 130 mEq) per day

MODERATE SODIUM RESTRICTION—restriction of dietary sodium to 1 gram (43 mEq) per day

NO ADDED SALT DIET—a diet containing 4 grams (174 mEq) of sodium

ORTHOPNEA—respiratory distress while in a recumbent position

SEVERE SODIUM RESTRICTION—restriction of dietary sodium to 250 mg (11 mEq) per day

STRICT SODIUM RESTRICTION—restriction of dietary sodium to 500 mg (22 mEq) per day

Some categories of heart disease such as congestive heart failure and cardiac cachexia are characterized by gradual failure of the heart to act as a pump. Nutritional care in these conditions is concerned primarily with the consequences of poor circulation throughout the body. Necessary dietary modifications differ considerably from those involved in treatment of the kinds of vascular disease involved in atherosclerosis and hypertension, which are discussed with respect to nutritional care in Chapters 20 and 21.

CONGESTIVE HEART FAILURE

Congestive heart failure (CHF) is the result of an extended process in which the heart gradually loses the capability for normal function (Fig. 33–1). For a time the organ is able to compensate for inefficiency and maintain almost normal circulation by enlarging and increasing the pulse rate (compensated heart disease). In decompensated heart disease, normal circulation is no longer possible. Shortness of breath (dyspnea) and chest pains occur with any activity. The reduced cardiac output results in complex changes in the renal, nervous, and endocrine management of blood pressure, leading to increased tubular resorption of sodium and finally to edema. Other organs such as the liver and brain are affected as blood flow to these organs declines (What . . . , 1988).

Heart disease becomes acute in the presence of infections resulting in endocarditis or carditis, in cardiac failure, after myocardial infarction, and after cardiac surgery. Diseases outside of the heart that cause an increased workload on the heart can cause a secondary CHF.

Cardiac Cachexia

Cardiac cachexia is an outcome of moderate to severe CHF characterized by a state of malnutrition of life-threatening severity. The underlying heart disease is usually valvular in etiology, with a predominant right ventricular component. Loss of both fat and muscle mass are obvious in the temporal and supraclavicular areas.

Although it is not understood why this condition is precipitated in some patients, a variety of factors are known to contribute to the malnourished state. (1) Anorexia can result from ascites, which causes pressure in the abdominal cavity with a constant feeling of fullness, as well as from the breathlessness and exhaustion that can accompany eating, the often unpalatable sodium-restricted diet, altered taste and smell sensations, possible digitalis toxicity, and depression. (2)

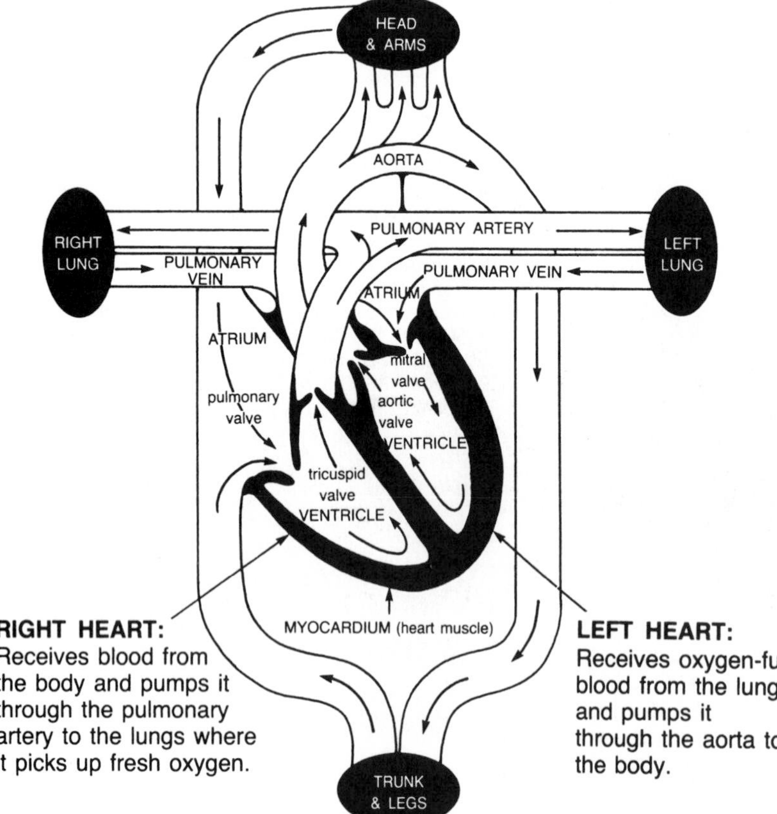

FIGURE 33–1. *The structure of the heart pump. (Redrawn from Katch FI and McArdle WD: Nutrition, Weight Control and Exercise, 3rd ed. Philadelphia, Lea & Febiger, 1988, p 83.)*

The basal metabolic rate can be elevated by cardiomegaly and by increased cardiac and pulmonary work. (3) Inadequate perfusion and tissue hypoxia impede the process of digestion and absorption by the abdominal organs and lead to malabsorption, especially of calcium and magnesium. (4) Diuretic use contributes to loss of zinc, magnesium, and potassium. Other sources of nutrient loss are the presence of protein-losing gastroenteropathy and extensive blood tests both of which can lead to marginal iron status (Table 33–1).

Eventually the cachexia is reflected in a loss of myocardial mass, hypotension, reduction of heart rate, basal metabolic rate and oxygen consumption, electrocardiogram (ECG) abnormalities, and finally heart failure. A *"cachetic heart"* can occur in any clinical situation of extreme malnutrition.

The cachectic patient who must undergo cardiac surgery is at high risk of increased morbidity and mortality, delayed wound healing, increased time for weaning from ventilatory support, and increased susceptibility to postoperative acute renal failure (Warnold and Lundholm, 1984). Nutritional support and rehabilitation should begin before surgery.

SYMPTOMS

Breathlessness is the most common symptom of CHF and may occur during various activities. As CHF worsens, *orthopnea,* or respiratory distress while recumbent, can develop. Other symptoms that reflect inadequate blood supply to the abdominal organs include anorexia, nausea, feeling of fullness, constipation, abdominal pain, malabsorption, enlarged liver, and liver tenderness. Decreased cranial blood supply can lead to mental confusion, memory loss, anxiety, insomnia, and headache. Cool extremities, sweating, and edema in the legs are common. As failure progresses, the amount of blood that the heart must pump increases. The myocardium is weakened by overstretching, and the heart eventually fails.

Table 33–1. Factors in the Development of Cardiac Cachexia

- Generalized cellular hypoxia
- Decreased energy intake
  - Anorexia due to gastric and hepatic congestion
  - Unpalatable diet and fluid restriction
  - Breathlessness and exhaustion while eating
  - Altered taste and smell sensations
  - Depression
- Decreased energy assimilation
  - Increased myocardial oxygen consumption
  - Increased work of breathing
  - Elevated basal metabolic rate
  - Fever
- Nutrient losses
  - Aggressive use of diuretics
  - Protein-losing enteropathy
  - Renal protein loss

TREATMENT

Treatment involves eliminating or minimizing the cause of CHF as much as possible, reducing the workload on the heart, and providing adequate nourishment. This is accomplished by providing oxygen, decreasing physical activity, using medication, and manipulating the diet. The goal of nutritional care is to provide adequate nourishment with as little work for the heart as possible and to prevent edema. Commonly used medications are furosemide (a diuretic), digitalis, and glycosides. Nonglycoside positive inotropic agents such as dopamine increase heart muscle contractility. Cardiac preload- and afterload-reducing agents such as nitroprusside dilate arterial and venous vessels.

Nutritional Care

Assessment

Assessing the patient with CHF with or without cardiac cachexia is complicated by the altered renal and fluid balance. Edema confounds weight changes and triceps skinfold measurements. A considerable loss of muscle mass can be disguised by increasing edema with little net change in body weight. In cardiac cachexia, however, the wasting is so extensive that it is usually reflected in a 10 to 15% loss in body weight. Because of the dilutional effect of excess extracellular fluid, the usual nutrition markers such as serum albumin, retinol-binding protein, or transferrin may be disproportionately low. Nutritional assessment thus depends primarily on a dietary history and the mid–upper arm circumference—the anthropometric measurement least affected by edema (Talamini, 1987).

Dietary Components

ENERGY. Well-compensated heart failure may not require any diet modification other than the achievement and maintenance of appropriate weight. Perhaps most common is the undernourished patient who may need anabolic nutritional support. The appropriate energy intake depends on the activity of the individual.

The energy needs of the patient in severe failure or with cardiac cachexia may be as much as 30 to 50% above basal. This requirement should be provided by an energy-dense diet that also needs to be controlled for fluid intake. Protein requirements may also be increased to 1.5 to 2 g/kg (Ansari, 1987). The calorie-to-nitrogen ratio should be 150:1.

The amount of carbohydrate in the diet may need manipulation, depending on the arterial Pco_2. (This is discussed further in Chapter 34.) It also depends on hyperglycemia, which is very common in patients with heart disease. Incidence of diabetes is increased in this population, and the hypoperfusion of the pancreas caused by the CHF may lead to an acute hyperinsulinemia and insulin resistance.

Nutritional support for the patient with cardiac cachexia may need to include enteral tube feeding. In this situation the feeding should begin slowly with constant attention to fluid and sodium balance by assessing for moist crackles (rales) in the lungs, edema in the extremities, and daily weight. Overly aggressive nutritional repletion can worsen CHF and can result in pulmonary edema. The nutritional formula should have a high calorie-to-volume ratio (2 kcal/ml) and a moderate to low sodium content (see Appendix Table 33). Patients with CHF who receive proper nutritional support can enter an anabolic state, although there may be initial weight loss due to mobilization and excretion of excess extracellular fluid (Heymsfield and Casper, 1989).

Parenteral nutrition becomes necessary when the patient cannot tolerate a tube of any kind compromising the airway, the gastrointestinal function is inadequate, or the infusion of feedings causes intra-abdominal pressure and increased work of breathing. Parenteral therapy must begin slowly because stress from the increased blood volume and basal metabolic rate can lead to worsened CHF. It is wise to begin with one half of the estimated requirements and to increase the amount gradually. Central venous pressure, pulse rate, arterial blood pressure, urine output, and serial x-rays for pulmonary status and cardiac silhouette are monitored as fluid volume is increased.

Enteral or parenteral therapy should begin early at the first sign of inadequate oral intake, as it takes longer to advance nutritional support and to reach adequate energy levels in the cardiac patient. Achievement of any nutritional rehabilitation requires at least 3 weeks.

SODIUM. Edema in decompensated heart disease results from the impaired cardiac function. Circulation to the kidneys is decreased, thus allowing sodium, and therefore fluid, to accumulate in the tissues. A sodium-restricted diet and diuretics are required to relieve the strain on the heart and prevent further damage and edema. Because sodium restriction enhances the sodium-depleting effects of diuretics, the use of sodium restriction in conjunction with diuretics will give the best results. The degree to which sodium and sometimes fluids are restricted depends on the needs of the individual. The maximal sodium load tolerated in the acute phase is usually 1 to 2 g/day. This is usually liberalized to 3 to 4 g/day when the patient improves or is discharged. In the rare situation requiring sodium levels of 500 mg/day or less, the restriction should only be instituted for short periods because these diets are unpalatable and potentially inadequate nutritionally. It would be more appropriate to maintain a higher level of sodium and to increase the use of diuretics.

Sodium-Restricted Diets. Sodium-restricted diets are usually prescribed at four levels as shown below. Clinical Insight, page 575, shows the conversion of milliequivalents to milligrams of sodium or salt.

4 grams (174 mEq) Sodium

Foods high in sodium are limited. Salt is allowed in cooking, but no salt is added to food after cooking. This is often referred to as a *no added salt* diet.

2 to 3 grams (87 to 130 mEq) Sodium—Mild Sodium Restriction

Foods high in sodium are omitted. A limited amount of salt is allowed in cooking, and no salt is added after cooking.

1 gram (43 mEq) Sodium—Moderate Sodium Restriction

Foods high in sodium are omitted. No salt is used in the preparation of food or at the table. Canned or processed foods containing salt are omitted. Frozen peas, lima beans, mixed vegetables, and corn are omitted because brine is used during the preparation for freezing. The use of regular bread and baked goods is limited. This diet may be difficult for most patients to follow at home.

500 mg (22 mEq) Sodium—Strict Sodium Restriction

Foods high in sodium are omitted. No salt is used in the preparation of food or at the table. Canned or processed foods containing salt are omitted. The frozen vegetables mentioned in the 1-gram sodium diet are omitted as well as the following vegetables that are naturally high in sodium: beets, beet greens, carrots, kale, spinach, celery, white turnips, rutabagas, mustard greens, chard, and dandelion greens. Low-sodium bread replaces regular bread. This diet is unpalatable and should be used only for short periods. It can be nutritionally deficient if not planned carefully.

250 mg (11 mEq) Sodium—Severe Sodium Restriction

Foods high in sodium are omitted. No salt is used in the preparation of food or at the table. Canned or processed foods containing salt are omitted. Low-sodium bread replaces regular bread, and the frozen and fresh vegetables naturally higher in sodium are omitted. Low-sodium milk replaces regular milk, and protein foods are limited. This is an extreme diet and is rarely used.

Designing a Sodium-Restricted Diet. In designing a sodium-restricted diet, the initial consideration is given to minimizing or eliminating the use of salt and highly salted foods. Table 33–2 lists foods that should not be used unless they are calculated into the diet. As the restriction becomes more severe, attention is given to foods prepared with salt or sodium-containing compounds, such as breads and cereals that contribute 30% of the sodium in the American diet. These are listed in Table 33–3. Finally, foods that naturally contain sodium —milk, meat, and vegetables—are considered. Table 33–4 lists the sodium content of food groups and

Table 33–2. Foods High in Sodium

1. Salt.
2. Monosodium glutamate (MSG).
3. Vegetable salts and flakes, such as onion, garlic, or celery salt.
4. Smoked, processed, or cured meats and fish, such as ham, bacon, corned beef, cold cuts, frankfurters, sausage, tongue, salt pork, chipped beef, pickled herring, and anchovies.
5. Meat extracts, bouillon cubes, and meat sauces.
6. Salted foods, such as potato chips, tortilla chips, corn chips, pretzels, salted nuts, popcorn, and crackers.
7. Prepared condiments, relishes, Worcestershire sauce, barbecue sauce, soy sauce, commercial salad dressings, catsup, pickles, mustard, and olives.
8. Prepackaged frozen foods (plain frozen vegetables, except for peas and other vegetables soaked in brine, and fruits are acceptable), packaged mixes for sauces, gravies, casseroles, and noodle, rice, or potato dishes.*
9. Canned soup unless made without salt.
10. Prepared flour mixes or packaged baking mixes.*
11. All canned meat and vegetable products unless prepared without salt.

* May be used in some circumstances, if calculated into the diet.

Table 33–3. Some Sodium-Containing Additives

Name	Foods Likely to Contain
Disodium phosphate	Cereals, cheeses, ice cream, bottled drinks
Monosodium glutamate	Accent (a flavor enhancer), meats, condiments, pickles, soups, candy, baked goods
Sodium alginate	Ice cream, chocolate milk
Sodium benzoate	Fruit juices
Sodium hydroxide	Pretzels, sour cream, cocoa products, canned peas
Sodium propionate	Breads
Sodium sulfite	Dried fruits, cut salad greens
Sodium pectinate	Syrups and toppings, ice cream, sherbet, salad dressings, jams and jellies
Sodium caseinate	Ice cream and other frozen products
Sodium bicarbonate	Baking powder, tomato soup, self-rising flour, sherbets, confections

the number of servings from each group to include at each level of sodium restriction. Table 33–5 presents the plan for a 2-gram sodium diet.

It is important to keep in mind the variety of ways in which the restriction can be implemented. For example, a patient may prefer to follow a 1-gram sodium diet, in which regular bread is limited and canned vegetables are omitted, in order to have 1/2 tsp of salt (1,150 mg of sodium) to use on his food throughout the day. This would bring the total intake to 2 g/day.

Experience has shown that patients eating a diet of low-sodium foods do not "make up" the sodium difference when allowed use of a salt shaker ad libitum. This supports the hypothesis that a substantial reduction in dietary sodium is possible if low-sodium foods are consumed in conjunction with ad libitum use of table salt and that acceptable dietary saltiness can be attained with less salt (Beauchamp et al, 1987).

Dietary Sources of Sodium. Dietary sources of sodium

Table 33–4. Sodium-Controlled Diets

Food Group	Serving Size	mg Na^+	mEq Na^+	Suggested Number of Servings for Diet				
				3 g	*2 g*	*1 g*	*500 mg*	*250m*
Milk, low sodium	8 oz	7	—				1	2
Milk, regular	8 oz	120	5	2	2	2	1	—
Buttermilk, salted	8 oz	280	13	—	—	—	—	—
Cottage cheese, regular	¼ cup	130	6	1	1	1	—	—
Cheese, regular	1 oz	200	9	1	—	—	—	—
Meat, fish, poultry, unsalted cheese	1 oz	25	1	6	6	6	5	4
Fresh shellfish	1 oz	50	2	1	1	—	—	—
Peanut butter, regular	1 T	80	3	1	1	—	—	—
Egg	1	70	3	Not restricted		1	1	—
Vegetables, cooked, fresh, frozen	½ cup	10	—			Not restricted		
Vegetables, naturally higher in sodium	½ cup	40	2		Not restricted		1	—
Vegetables, canned regular	½ cup	230	10	—	—	—	—	—
Vegetable juices, canned	½ cup	200	9	—	—	—	—	—
Fruits	½ cup	2	—			Not restricted		
Bread, regular	1 slice	150	7	4	4	1	—	—
Bread, low sodium	1 slice	5	—			Not restricted		
Quick bread, muffin	1 serving	300	14	1	—	—	—	—
Cereal, ready to eat, salted	1 cup	300	14	1	—	—	—	—
Cereal, unsalted	½ cup	5	—			Not restricted		
Butter or margarine, salted	1 tsp	50	2	3	3	2	—	—
Butter or margarine, unsalted	1 tsp	1	—			Not restricted		
Mayonnaise, regular	1½ tsp	50	2	1	1	1	1	1
Salad dressing, regular	1 T	350	16	1	—	—	—	—
Soup, regular	1 cup	900	42	—	—	—	—	—
Soup, low sodium	1 cup	25	1			Not restricted		
Desserts, regular	1 serving	300	14	1	—	—	—	—
Desserts, low sodium	1 serving	15	—			Not restricted		
Salt	1 tsp	2,300	10	¼ tsp	—	—	—	—

Table 33–5. 2-Gram Sodium Diet*

Food Category	Foods Recommended	Foods Excluded
Milk and milk products (limit to 16 oz/day)	Any milk—whole, low-fat, skim, chocolate, cocoa Yogurt Eggnog Substitute 8 oz of milk for one of the following: 4 oz evaporated milk 4 oz condensed milk ⅓ cup dry milk powder	Buttermilk, malted milk, and milkshake
Vegetables (2–4 servings/day)	Fresh, frozen, and low-sodium canned vegetables Low-sodium vegetable juices	Regular canned vegetables and vegetable juices Sauerkraut Pickled vegetables and others prepared in brine Frozen vegetables in sauce
Fruits (2 or more servings/day)	All fruits and fruit juices	None
Breads and cereals (4 or more servings/day)	Enriched white, wheat, rye, and pumpernickel bread Hard dinner rolls Cooked cereal without salt Dry low-sodium cereals Unsalted crackers and breadsticks Biscuits, muffins, cornbread, pancakes, and waffles made with low-sodium baking powder and without salt Low-sodium or homemade bread crumbs	Breads and rolls with salted tops Quick breads Instant hot cereals Dry cereals with added sodium Crackers with salted tops Pancakes, waffles, muffins, biscuits, and cornbread with salt, baking powder, self-rising flour, and instant mixes Regular bread crumbs or cracker crumbs
Potato or substitute	White or sweet potatoes Salt-free potato chips Enriched rice, barley, noodles, spaghetti, macaroni, and other pastas Homemade bread stuffing	Potato casserole mixes Salted potato chips and other snack chips Instant rice and pasta mixes Commercial casserole mixes Commercial stuffing
Meats or substitute (6 oz or more/day)	Any fresh or fresh-frozen meats: beef, lamb, pork, veal, and game Any fresh or fresh-frozen poultry: chicken, turkey, Cornish hen, and others Any fresh-water or fresh-frozen unbreaded fish and shellfish Low-sodium canned tuna, salmon, or sardines Eggs Low-sodium cheese Cream cheese Ricotta cheese Dry cottage cheese Low-sodium peanut butter Dried peas and beans	Any meat, fish, or poultry that is smoked, cured, salted, or canned: bacon, chipped beef, corned beef, cold cuts, ham, hot dogs, and sausages Sardines, anchovies, marinated herring, and pickled meats Regular canned tuna and salmon Pickled eggs Regular hard and processed cheese Cheese spreads Regular peanut butter Frozen dinner entrées
Fats	Unsalted butter or margarine Unsalted salad dressings Vegetable oils, shortening Mayonnaise-type salad dressing Light, heavy, and sour cream	Salted butter or margarine Regular salad dressings Bacon fat, salt pork Snack dips made with cheese, bacon, buttermilk, instant soup mixes, etc.
Soups	Low-sodium bouillon, broth, and consomme Low-sodium commercial canned or dehydrated soups Homemade soups made with allowed vegetables or milk	Regular bouillon, broth, or consomme Regular canned or dehydrated commercial soups
Sweets and desserts	Any sweets and desserts (desserts made from milk should be within milk allowance)	None
Beverages	All beverages (see milk allowance)	Commercially softened water Beverages and foods made with commercially softened water Sport drinks
Miscellaneous	Limit salt to ¼ to ½ tsp/day† Salt substitute with physician's approval Pepper, herbs, and spices Flavorings Vinegar and lemon or lime juice Salt-free seasoning mixes Following low-sodium condiments: catsup, chili sauce, mustard, and pickles Fresh-ground horseradish Tabasco sauce Low-sodium baking powder Following unsalted snacks: nuts, seeds, pretzels, and popcorn	Garlic salt, celery salt, onion salt, and seasoned salt Sea salt, rock salt, and kosher salt Any other seasoning containing salt and sodium compounds Monosodium glutamate (Accent) Regular catsup, chili sauce, mustard, pickles, relishes, olives, and horseradish Kitchen Bouquet, gravy, and sauce mixes Barbecue sauce, soy and teriyaki sauce, Worcestershire and steak sauce Salted snack items: nuts, seeds, pretzels, and popcorn All commercially prepared and convenience foods

* © 1988, The American Dietetic Association. Manual of Clinical Dietetics, 3rd ed. Used by permission.
† This is salt used in cooking. The amount allowed depends on the adherence to the rest of the diet.

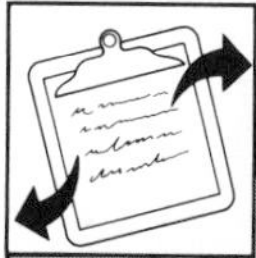

CLINICAL INSIGHT: Sodium and Salt Measurement Equivalents

Sodium chloride is approximately 40% (39.3%) sodium and 60% chloride. To convert a specified weight of sodium chloride to its sodium equivalent, multiply the weight by 0.393. Sodium is also measured in milliequivalents (mEq). To convert milligrams of sodium to mEq, divide by atomic weight of 23. To convert sodium to sodium chloride, multiply by 2.54. Millimoles (mmol) and milliequivalents (mEq) of sodium are the same. Examples:

1 tsp of salt = approximately 6 grams of sodium chloride = 6,096 mg NaCl

6,096 mg NaCl × 0.393 = 2,396 mg Na

2,396 mg Na/23 = 104 mEq Na

1 g Na = 1,000 mg/23 = 43 mEq

Sodium and Salt in Gram and Milliequivalent Measurements

mEq Na^+ (Approximate)	Mg Na^+	g NaCl (Approximate)
11	250	0.6
22	500	1.3
43	1,000	2.5
65	1,500	3.8
87	2,000	5.0
130	3,000	7.6
174	4,000	10.2
217	5,000	12.7

are (1) salt added to foods at the table, (2) foods to which salt or sodium compounds are added during their preparation or processing, (3) foods that naturally contain sodium, and (4) chemically softened water. It has been estimated that the average American consumes about 4 to 7 grams of sodium daily, one third of which comes from salt added to food in its preparation or at the table. This is much more than the minimum 250 mg (9 mEq) required by the human to maintain life.

The amount of sodium in drinking water is significant only in a diet containing 500 mg of sodium or less, and only if the concentration is greater than 40 parts per million (40 mg or 2 mEq/l). Sodium is likely to be high in "softened" water. Typical water softeners exchange sodium ions for calcium and other ions that cause water hardness. Distilled water may be necessary, or only the hot water should be softened.

The animal protein foods — milk, cheese, eggs, meat, poultry, and fish — are relatively high in sodium. Like human muscle cells, animal tissue cells are surrounded by sodium chloride-physiologic saline. Thus these foods must be used in measured amounts. Kosher meats and poultry are soaked in salt water for 1 hour after slaughter to remove the blood. Although the meat is washed thoroughly before cooking, the sodium content may be increased as much as four times to 90 to 115 mg/oz. Alternatives are the use of ammonium chloride in place of sodium chloride, or boiling the meat and discarding the broth before eating. Low-sodium kosher meats are also available.

Sodium Labeling. The term "salt-free" does not necessarily guarantee that a product is low in sodium. The food may have natural sodium or sodium-containing additives, such as those listed in Table 33-3. With the Nutrition Labeling and Education Act (NLEA) of 1990, the FDA revised regulations to require labeling of sodium content on more foods and to provide legal definitions for the terms "low sodium," "moderately low sodium," and "reduced sodium" (Table 33-6).

Non-Nutrient Sources of Sodium. Most *commercial salt substitutes* are mineral bases consisting of potassium chloride, calcium chloride, or ammonium chloride. Administration of a substitute containing large amounts of potassium to patients with renal insufficiency could conceivably be harmful. However, for patients requiring potassium supplementation because of diuretic therapy, the use of potassium chloride salt substitutes is an easy way to add potassium to the diet.

"Low-sodium" salt substitutes, which still contain half as much sodium as regular table salt, can be used only in a mildly sodium-restricted diet. Vegetized salts use powdered dehydrated vegetables as a base, in combination with a variety of additional ingredients. However, they may contain considerable quantities of sodium and should therefore not be used unless the sodium content is counted as part of the dietary total.

Table 33-6. Sodium and Salt Food Labeling

The following terms defined by the Nutrition Labeling and Education Act (NLEA), 1990, designate foods truly low in sodium and appropriate for a low-sodium diet:

Sodium free, no sodium: containing less than 5 mg per serving.
Very low sodium: containing 35 mg or less per serving.
Low sodium: containing 140 mg or less per serving.

The following terms designate foods lower in sodium than their usual counterparts. They may still be relatively high in sodium depending on amounts present in the foods before processing:

Reduced sodium: processed to reduce the usual level of sodium by 75%. Label must identify the comparison food.
Unsalted, no salt added; without added salt: processed without salt; may still contain sodium that is naturally present in the food. The food must resemble the usual salted food. The sodium content is declared as required.

Spices, herbs, and other seasonings can be used to improve the flavor of low-sodium foods. Most spices contain less than 0.05% sodium, and almost all are below 0.1%. Exceptions are allspice, celery seed, dehydrated celery flakes, whole mace, and dehydrated parsley flakes. Any of the herb or spice "salts," such as garlic salt, should also be avoided.

Nondietary Sources of Added Sodium. In addition to the sodium in food and water, incidental amounts may be ingested in the form of medicines and dentifrices. Barbiturates, sulfonamides, antibiotics and other drugs, cough medicines, stomach alkalizers, laxatives, tooth pastes and powders, and mouthwashes may contain large amounts of sodium. For example, some over-the-counter chewable antacid tablets can add between 1,200 and 7,000 mg of sodium daily when used as therapy for ulcer or gastrointestinal distress. Aspirin supplies about 50 mg of sodium per tablet. Most medicines contain less than 5 mg of sodium per dose; only those containing 80 to 120 mg/dose contribute substantially to sodium intake.

Low-Sodium or Low-Salt Syndrome. Severe sodium restriction is intended for the hospitalized patient whose sodium tolerance is unusually low. Care should be taken to avoid hyponatremia, hypochloremia, and eventually azotemia as the glomerular filtration rate falls. *Low-salt syndrome* can also result from adrenal insufficiency, marked vomiting, diarrhea, and burns. Symptoms of potential *low-sodium syndrome* or salt depletion are weakness, lassitude, anorexia, vomiting, abdominal cramps, aching skeletal muscles, and mental confusion.

POTASSIUM. Many diuretics deplete potassium, requiring the use of potassium supplements and the inclusion of high-potassium foods in the diet (see Appendix Table 1 or Table 35-7). Potassium depletion may lead to digitalis toxicity, which is characterized by anorexia, nausea and vomiting, abdominal discomfort, hallucinations, depression, drowsiness, and cardiac arrhythmias. In the depleted patient who begins receiving nutritional support the process of anabolism increases the uptake of potassium, which is another potential reason for increased potassium needs.

Salt substitutes are a source of potassium; most use potassium chloride instead of sodium chloride. They can provide between 500 to 2,000 mg (13 to 72 mEq) potassium per teaspoon—usually a welcome addition to the diet. However, in some cases (e.g., renal failure) excess potassium is not desirable; thus use of salt substitutes should always be approved by a physician.

FLUIDS. Fluid intake often needs to be controlled in CHF, but it depends on the individual. A fluid restriction of 1 to 1.5 l/day or less will reduce the need for diuretic therapy but may not be necessary if the patient complies with the low-sodium diet. Occasionally, foods with a high fluid content will need to be restricted. It is important to monitor fluid status through urine specific gravity, serum electrolyte measurements, and clinical signs of edema.

LIPIDS. Patients with atherosclerosis should follow a cholesterol-lowering diet after recovering from the acute phase of CHF.

CARDIAC SURGERY: POSTOPERATIVE NUTRITIONAL CARE

General Principles

Nutritional support of the cardiac patient undergoing surgery should begin before surgery, if at all possible. The failure of cardiac patients to tolerate surgery as well as adequately nourished controls may be due to poor nutritional status prior to surgery (Talamini, 1987).

Nutritional care should be in concert with the goals of minimizing myocardial work, pain, and discomfort; maintaining adequate myocardial oxygenation and normal extracellular volume; and avoiding significant cardiac arrhythmias.

In acute cardiac failure, such as after myocardial infarction, cardiac surgery, or carditis, the diet is reduced to the minimum. Food is given in soft or liquid form. Large-volume feedings should be avoided, because they potentially increase postprandial cardiac work and increase the chance of vomiting and aspiration in the event of cardiac emergencies. Five or six small meals are recommended.

Use of *caffeine* is controversial. Some data have shown that caffeine does not increase the occurrence or severity of ventricular cardiac work in postinfarction patients (Myers et al, 1987), nor does it increase ventricular or atrial arrhythmias (Graboys et al, 1989). However, many cardiologists prefer that their patients avoid the use of caffeine, theobromine, and other methylxanthines.

Constipation should be avoided because straining with bowel movements can predispose to vagal cardiac rhythm changes. Inclusion of high-fiber foods and stool softeners is useful. (See Chapter 27 for further discussion of constipation.)

The postsurgical patient with *hypertension* requires a 2- to 4-gram sodium diet, combined with a low-energy diet if weight reduction is necessary, and a cholesterol-lowering diet when appropriate. A 2-gram sodium diet is usually prescribed for the patient with CHF and hypertension. Potassium intake should be ample.

Hyperglycemia and *glucose intolerence* are observed in the perioperative and early postoperative period of cardiac surgery. This is in the presence of normal or elevated plasma insulin levels, indicating an impaired glucoregulatory effect of insulin. It is not known why this happens or how it can be prevented. However, blood glucose should be monitored closely in the postoperative period, and the patient should be nourished appropriately.

Cardiac cachexia is common in patients undergoing valvular surgery; thus, the main postoperative concern is getting the patient to eat. Usually after surgery, correction of the heart failure allows elimination of sodium and fluid restrictions; however, these may still be necessary in the immediate postoperative period.

Heart Transplant

The main nutritional concerns of the transplant patient are maintenance during the period of immunosuppression and dealing with the complications necessitated by the medications. (See the nutritional recommendations in Chapter 36 for patients with bone marrow transplants.) Some CHF requiring nutritional manipulation may also be present. If the patient was severely cachectic prior to surgery, active nutritional rehabilitation should be continued postsurgically.

CITED REFERENCES

Ansari A: Syndromes of cardiac cachexia and the cachectic heart: Current perspective. Prog Cardiovasc Dis 30:45, 1987.

Beauchamp GK et al: Failure to compensate decreased dietary sodium with increased table salt usage. JAMA 258:3275, 1987.

Graboys TB et al: The effect of caffeine on ventricular ectopic activity in patients with malignant ventricular arrhythmia. Arch Int Med 149:637, 1989.

Heymsfield SB and Casper K: Congestive heart failure: Clinical management by use of continued nasoenteric feeding. Am J Clin Nutr 50:539, 1989.

Myers MG et al: Caffeine as a possible cause of ventricular arrhythmias during the healing phase of acute myocardial infarction. Am J Cardiol 59:1024, 1987.

Talamini M: The cardiac patient. *In* Lang CE (ed): Nutritional Support in Critical Care. Rockville, MD, Aspen Publishers, 1987.

Warnold I and Lundholm D: Clinical significance of preoperative and nutritional status in 215 non-cancer patients. Ann Surg 199:299, 1984.

What causes oedema? Lancet 1:1028, 1988.

ADDITIONAL REFERENCES

Beauchamp GK et al: Modification of salt taste. Ann Intern Med 98:763, 1983.

Caffeine effects on heart rate and rhythm. Am J Nurs 88:1679, 1988.

Firth JD, Raine AEG, and Ledingham JGG: Raised venous pressure: A direct cause of renal sodium retention in oedema. Lancet 1:1033, 1988.

Harris P: Role of arterial pressure in oedema of heart disease. Lancet 1:1036, 1988.

Morganroth J and Moore EN (eds): Congestive Heart Failure, Developments in Cardiovascular Medicine. Boston, Martinus Nijhoff, 1987.

CHAPTER 34

NUTRITIONAL CARE IN PULMONARY DISEASE

Elizabeth Adams, M.S., R.D.

CHAPTER OUTLINE

Nutrition and the Respiratory System
Nutritional Care in Pulmonary Diseases

KEY TERMS

BRONCHOPULMONARY DYSPLASIA (BPD)—a chronic lung disease of infancy, commonly following respiratory distress syndrome and treatment with oxygen; characterized by bronchiolar metaplasia and interstitial fibrosis

CHRONIC BRONCHITIS—a chronic productive cough with inflammation of one or more of the bronchi and secondary changes in lung tissue

CHRONIC OBSTRUCTIVE PULMONARY DISEASE (COPD)—a process characterized by the presence of chronic bronchitis, emphysema, or both, leading to the development of airway obstruction

COR PULMONALE—a heart condition that may develop in patients with severe COPD, which is characterized by right ventricular failure due to increased pressure within the pulmonary arteries

CYSTIC FIBROSIS (CF)—an autosomal recessive disorder characterized by dysfunction of the exocrine glands and production of abnormally thick secretions that obstruct airway, pancreatic, and other ducts

EMPHYSEMA—a condition of the lung characterized by abnormal permanent enlargement of alveoli, accompanied by destruction of their walls without obvious fibrosis

ENZYME REPLACEMENT THERAPY (ERT)—use of exogenous pancreatic enzymes in order to simulate the normal digestive environment

MECONIUM ILEUS EQUIVALENT—intestinal obstruction from fecal impaction

RESPIRATORY DISTRESS SYNDROME (RDS)—a condition of the newborn, particularly the premature newborn, marked by dyspnea with cyanosis

Nutritional support is an integral part of care for the pulmonary patient. The malnutrition that often occurs in conjunction with pulmonary disease adversely affects lung structure and function, respiratory muscle strength and endurance, immune defense mechanisms, and control of breathing. At the same time, nutritional needs are often increased by lung disease. Good nutritional status has an important role in maintaining the integrity of the respiratory system and in allowing maximal participation in activities of daily living.

NUTRITION AND THE RESPIRATORY SYSTEM

Together, malnutrition and pulmonary disease can establish the cycle shown in Figure 34–1. As pulmonary function declines, nutritional status worsens, thus contributing to further decline in pulmonary function. The goal of medical and nutritional care is to break this cycle.

Impact of Malnutrition

The relationship between malnutrition and respiratory disease has long been recognized. During times of famine, respiratory infections are frequent complications of starvation. After 12 weeks of semistarvation, healthy volunteers exhibited impaired pulmonary function in the form of decreased vital capacity (lung volume), minute ventilation (volume exhaled/minute), and efficiency of ventilation (Keys et al, 1959). Subsequent research has documented the impact of malnutrition on components of the respiratory system.

The structure and function of the pulmonary parenchyma are altered by malnutrition. Lung tissue may be more susceptible to damage and the repair process disrupted in states of malnutrition. Increased compliance (distensibility) and decreased elasticity of the lung have been produced by malnutrition, and may impair lung function. Decreased levels of surfactant, a phospholipid that functions to decrease surface tension within the alveoli, contribute to the collapse of alveoli and to the subsequent increased work of breathing. Hypoproteinemia resulting from malnutrition contributes to the development of pulmonary edema. Low serum protein levels and decreased colloid osmotic pressure allow fluid to move into the interstitial space. Lastly, the oxygen-carrying capacity of the blood declines when hemoglobin levels are low, as they are likely to be in malnutrition.

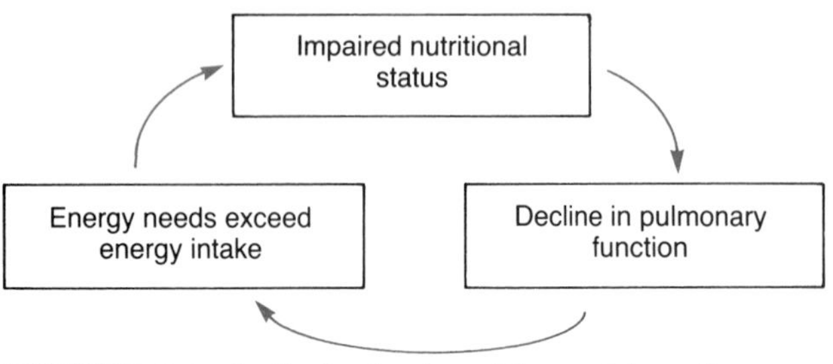

FIGURE 34–1. *Cycle of malnutrition and lung disease.*

With starvation, respiratory muscle mass, strength, endurance, and efficiency decline. Respiratory muscle mass is thought to decline in proportion to the decline in body weight, whereas respiratory muscle strength probably declines to a greater extent. Both respiratory muscle strength and function have been shown to improve with nutrition repletion (Efthimiou et al, 1988).

At the cellular level, low levels of energy substrates and of minerals and electrolytes (iron, magnesium, and potassium) also compromise respiratory muscle function (Bilbrey et al, 1973; Molloy et al, 1984; Rochester, 1986). Acute respiratory failure has been associated with hypophosphatemia (Aubier et al, 1985).

Acute malnutrition alters the control of breathing in healthy volunteers. The ventilatory response to hypoxia is decreased (Doekel et al, 1976; Zwillich et al, 1977). Depression of the hypoxic ventilatory drive with starvation may be most detrimental for patients with diseases such as cystic fibrosis or emphysema who may depend on the hypoxic ventilatory drive for adequate ventilation.

The association of malnutrition with impaired immunity places the malnourished patient with lung disease at risk for developing respiratory infections. The impact of malnutrition on other pulmonary defense mechanisms, such as pulmonary epithelium, cilia, and alveolar macrophages, is not well understood. Bacterial colonization patterns of the lower respiratory tract may be altered by changes in nutritional status (Niederman et al, 1986).

Impact of Lung Disease on Nutritional Status

Lung disease often adversely affects nutritional status, and patients with respiratory disease are at increased risk for malnutrition. Although energy needs can be increased substantially by lung disease, complications of the disease or its treatment can make adequate intake and retention of nutrients difficult. Factors that may limit intake are listed in Table 34–1. Required medications may alter absorption, utilization, intake, and retention of nutrients. Drug-nutrient interactions of medications commonly used in pulmonary disease, such as steroids, diuretics, antibiotics, and bronchodilators, are described in Chapter 25.

Infants, children, and adults with chronic lung disease expend about 25 to 50% more energy than if they did not have lung disease (Field et al, 1982; Yeh et al, 1989). This increase has been attributed mainly to the

TABLE 34–1. Adverse Effects of Lung Disease on Nutritional Status

Increased Energy Expenditure
Increased work of breathing
Chronic infection
Medical treatments (e.g., bronchodilators, chest physical therapy)
Reduced Intake
Fluid restriction
Shortness of breath
Decreased oxygen saturation when eating
Anorexia due to chronic disease
Gastrointestinal distress and vomiting
Additional Limitations
Difficulty in preparing food due to fatigue
Lack of financial resources
Impaired feeding skills (for infants and children)
Altered metabolism

increased work of breathing. However, infection, fever, and treatments such as the use of bronchodilators and chest physical therapy also contribute to increased energy expenditure. A 10% increase in resting energy expenditure associated with the use of albutamol, a bronchodilator, has been documented (Vaisman et al, 1987). A 35% increase in oxygen consumption has been associated with chest physical therapy for critically ill, mechanically ventilated patients (Weissman et al, 1984).

NUTRITIONAL CARE IN PULMONARY DISEASES

Bronchopulmonary Dysplasia

Bronchopulmonary dysplasia (BPD) is a chronic lung disease of infancy which occurs most frequently in premature infants following *respiratory distress syndrome* (RDS) in the neonatal period. Factors implicated in the etiology of BPD include prematurity, mechanical ventilation, supplemental oxygen, endotracheal intubation, patent ductus arteriosus (a congenital heart condition), and malnutrition. Infants with severe disease often require prolonged intensive medical care. They may remain medically fragile and require therapies such as mechanical ventilation, supplemental oxygen, or tube feedings long after discharge from the hospital.

Infants with BPD have special nutritional needs related to both their disease and their prematurity (see Chapter 11). BPD and its treatment affect growth, energy needs, nutrient metabolism, and the development of feeding skills. The goal of nutritional care is to promote linear growth and fluid balance, with adequate nutrient intake and development of feeding skills.

Nutritional Assessment

The growth of infants with BPD is followed closely as an indicator of medical and nutritional status. Because lung size is stature-dependent, linear growth is thought to be important for the growth of healthy lung tissue and for the resolution of the disease. Limited observations of growth patterns of infants with BPD suggest that these infants grow more slowly than other prematures initially, but they may catch up to their peers during the first 3 years of life (Vohr and Bell, 1982). Reasons for growth failure among infants with BPD are thought to include increased energy needs combined with inadequate dietary intake, chronic hypoxia, or emotional deprivation (Yeh et al, 1989).

The growth of infants with BPD should be evaluated and compared to other infants of the same post-conceptional age (see Chapter 11). The goal of care is to promote linear growth that parallels or advances on the growth channel for age, with weight proportional to length. Additional factors to be included in nutrition screening and assessment are listed in Table 34–2.

TABLE 34–2. Components of Nutritional Assessment for the Infant with Bronchopulmonary Dysplasia*

Historical Parameters	Medical Parameters	Nutritional Parameters
Birthweight	Respiratory status	Weight
Gestational age	Oxygen saturation	Length
Medical history	Use of medications	Head circumference
Nutritional history	Emesis	Hemoglobin and hematocrit
Previous growth pattern	Stool pattern	Serum electrolytes
	Urine output	Other biochemical tests as needed
	Urine specific gravity	(e.g., serum albumin, alkaline phosphatase, phosphorus)
Feeding History	**Environmental Parameters**	
Volume	Parent-child interaction	
Frequency of feedings	Home facilities	
Behavior during feedings	Community resources	
Formula composition	Economic resources	
Use of solids		
Feeding milestones		

* Adapted from Sirois LW: Nutritional assessment and management of the infant with bronchopulmonary dysplasia. Nutritional Support Services 4(5):62–66, 1984.

Nutritional Care

Increased energy needs are well recognized in infants with BPD. Although the reasons are not completely understood, increased work of breathing is thought to be an important factor. Resting energy expenditure for infants with BPD has been documented to be 25 to 50% greater than for age-matched controls. Infants with BPD who have growth failure may have energy needs 50% higher than those who are growing well (Kurzner et al, 1988). Energy needs also may vary over the course of the disease. In the acute phase, when infants are in controlled temperature environments, are fed parenterally, are inactive, and are not growing or are growing slowly, energy requirements may be 50 to 85 kcal/kg/day. In contrast, during the convalescent phase when infants are growing rapidly, are being fed orally, and are using additional energy for temperature regulation, activity, and the work of breathing, they may require 120 to 130 kcal/kg/day or more (Oh, 1986).

Meeting energy needs is a major challenge in the care of infants with BPD. Barriers to adequate intake include anorexia, fluid restriction, fatigue, poor coordination of breathing and swallowing, weakness of suck, and other feeding problems. To meet energy needs, calorically dense formulas, small frequent feedings, use of a soft nipple, and nasogastric or gastrostomy tube feedings may be needed. When calorically dense formulas are used (>20 to 24 kcal/oz), adequacy of fluid intake and urinary output should be monitored. Introduction of solids when developmentally appropriate can help infants to meet energy needs; some infants find it easier to take solids than liquids.

Protein intake should be within the advised range for infants of comparable postconceptional age. As the caloric density of the diet is increased by the addition of fat and carbohydrate, protein should continue to provide 7% or more of total calories. Lesser amounts can be inadequate for growth. Additions of fat or carbohydrate should be made to formula after it has been concentrated to 24 kcal/oz to keep protein at an acceptable level (Table 34-3; see also Table 11-13).

Fat provides essential fatty acids (EFA) and helps to meet energy demands when tolerance for fluid and carbon dioxide load is limited. Biochemical evidence of EFA deficiency has been documented within the first week of life for very low birthweight (VLBW) infants not receiving lipids (Farrell et al, 1988). Although the clinical importance of these alterations is not well understood, EFA deficiency may be linked to coagulation abnormalities or to altered fatty acid composition of pulmonary surfactant phospholipids (Adamkin, 1986).

Use of parenteral lipids for the neonate with RDS or BPD is an area of debate. Questions center around the relationship between oxygen diffusion and the rate of lipid administration as well as the physiologic impact of prostaglandin precursors (arachidonic and linoleic acids) on vascular tone and adequacy of oxygenation. Several investigators have evaluated the relationships between lipid infusion and hypoxemia, pulmonary vascular resistance, and clinical outcome of VLBW infants. Collectively, these studies highlight the need to exercise judgment in administration of parenteral lipids for infants with respiratory compromise (Brans et al, 1986; Lloyd and Boucek, 1986; Hammerman and Aramburo, 1988). For infants with RDS, administration of parenteral lipid emulsions at doses to prevent EFA deficiency (0.5 to 1 g/kg) may be started on the third day of life and slowly increased by 0.5 g/kg increments to 3 g/kg/day as tolerated. Lipids should be administered over 24 hours to prevent significant fluctuation of triglycerides, free fatty acids, and free fatty acid/albumin molar ratio. Triglyceride levels should remain at less than 150 mg/dl. Infants with pulmonary disease or at risk for pulmonary hypertension should be monitored closely as lipids are gradually advanced (see Chapter 11).

To maintain fluid balance, infants with BPD may require fluid restriction, sodium restriction, and long-term treatment with diuretics, all of which have nutritional implications. When fluid intake is restricted, the use of parenteral lipids or calorically dense enteral feedings helps to meet energy needs. For infants sensitive to sodium loads, formulas with lower sodium content can be selected (see Table 10-1). When evaluating sodium loads, the sodium content of medications should not be overlooked.

TABLE 34-3. Methods for Increasing the Energy Concentration of Infant Formulas

		Kcal/oz	% Cho	% Pro	% Fat
13 oz 13 oz	Formula concentrate Water	20	42	9	49
13 oz 11 oz	Formula concentrate Water	22	42	9	49
13 oz 9 oz	Concentrate Water	24	42	9	49
13 oz 9 oz 1¼ tsp ½ tsp	Concentrate Water White sugar* Vegetable oil (2.5 ml)	26	42	8	50
13 oz 9 oz 2½ tsp 1 tsp	Concentrate Water White sugar* Vegetable oil (5 ml)	28	42	8	50
13 oz 9 oz 3¾ tsp 1½ tsp	Concentrate Water White sugar* Vegetable oil (7.5 ml)	30	43	7	50

* In infants older than 1 year, light corn syrup (Karo syrup) can be substituted for sugar—1¼ tsp sugar = 1 tsp corn syrup. Polycose can also be used—1½ T polycose = 1 T corn syrup.

Furosemide, a diuretic, is associated with increased loss of minerals including chloride, potassium, and calcium. Additional chloride losses may occur for infants with chronic CO_2 retention and respiratory acidosis because of metabolic correction for the acidosis. Potassium and chloride levels should be monitored regularly and supplemented as needed to maintain normal levels. Deficiencies of chloride or potassium are associated with muscle weakness and impaired growth. Low levels of chloride have been described in infants dying with BPD (Perlman et al, 1986).

Chronic use of diuretics, combined with a history of total parenteral nutrition, limited volume of intake, and respiratory acidosis, as well as limited stores of calcium and phosphorus related to prematurity, may place infants with BPD at risk for poor bone mineralization (Greer, 1986). Calcium and phosphorus intake should be optimized as for other VLBW infants. Serial measurements of serum alkaline phosphatase and serum phosphorus are helpful in evaluating bone mineral status. Dual photon absorptiometry may be available in some centers for direct measurement of bone mineral content.

Other factors such as adequacy of oxygenation, gastroesophageal reflux, and feeding difficulties also affect the growth and nutritional status of infants with BPD. When oxygen saturation is low, there can be decreased growth (Groothuis and Rosenberg, 1987). Brief episodes of decreased oxygen saturation are thought to occur frequently in infants with BPD, especially during feeding (Garg et al, 1988). The impact of these episodes on growth and dietary intake is unknown. When growth is poor, low oxygen saturation should be evaluated as a contributing factor (Figure 34–2).

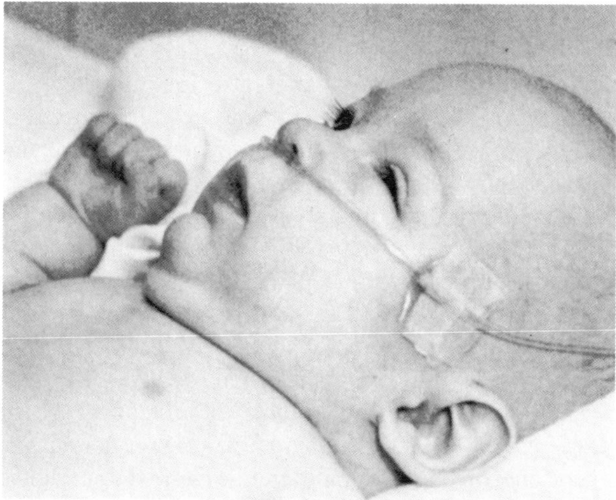

FIGURE 34–2. *Continuous low-flow oxygen therapy is used to supply adequate oxygen saturation for this 5-month-old infant with bronchopulmonary dysplasia. (From Foster RLR et al: Family-Centered Nursing Care of Children. Philadelphia, WB Saunders, 1989, p 1187.)*

Infants with BPD have a high incidence of gastroesophageal reflux. When uncontrolled it may worsen lung disease, and associated vomiting may result in inadequate retention of feedings. Treatment includes thickened feedings, prone positioning, medications, and surgical fundoplication in severe cases. To thicken formula, 1/2 to 1 tablespoon of infant cereal is added per ounce of formula, and then adjustments are made as needed.

Feeding difficulties occur frequently among infants with BPD. Infants may tire with breast-feeding or bottle-feeding and require small frequent feedings or supplementation by feeding tube. They may also have difficulty in tolerating the introduction of solids, especially as texture is increased. Risk factors for feeding difficulties are thought to include history of unpleasant oral experiences (e.g., intubation, frequent suctioning, or recurrent vomiting), history of nonoral feedings, delayed introduction of solids, or discomfort or choking associated with eating solids. Approaches that may be useful include creating a pleasant mealtime environment, the use of consistent and appropriate feeding techniques, oral stimulation during tube feedings, attention to the timing of the introduction of solids, oral desensitization techniques, gradual progression of texture and flavor changes, and behavior modification programs. Suggestions on how to meet nutritional needs in nonthreatening ways can reduce the stress associated with feeding as the child learns to eat. An interdisciplinary approach involving the primary care giver as a team member is recommended for management of feeding difficulties.

Cystic Fibrosis

Cystic fibrosis (CF) is a genetic disease that is inherited in an autosomal recessive pattern and occurs in approximately 1/2,000 live births in the white population. Although the incidence is lower among nonwhites, CF can occur in these populations as well. Since CF was first recognized 50 years ago, many advances have been made in diagnosis and treatment, and the life span of individuals with CF has increased dramatically. The median life span for patients with CF in the United States in 1987 was 28 years (Cystic Fibrosis Foundation, 1987).

The underlying lesion in CF is unknown but is thought to involve a disorder of electrolyte transport. The disease is characterized by dysfunction of the exocrine glands. This results in the production of abnormally thick secretions that may obstruct airway and pancreatic ducts, as well as ducts in many different organ systems. Manifestations of CF usually include pulmonary and gastrointestinal symptoms and elevated levels of sodium and chloride in the sweat, although other organ systems are also affected.

The most reliable test for diagnosis of CF is the *sweat test.* Elevated levels of sodium and chloride (> 60 mEq/l) in collected sweat samples are indicative of CF. Criteria for the diagnosis of CF include a positive result on a sweat test and the presence of chronic lung disease, failure to thrive and malabsorption, or a family history of CF.

CF can have a profound impact on the digestive system. Thick mucous plugs reduce the quantity of digestive enzymes released from the pancreas into the small intestine. The resultant enzyme insufficiency causes malabsorption of nutrients, including protein, fat, starch, vitamins, and minerals. Eighty-five per cent of all individuals with CF have pancreatic insufficiency (Durie and Forstner, 1989). Decreased bicarbonate secretion can further reduce digestive enzyme activity and impair digestion. Decreased bile acid reabsorption contributes further to fat malabsorption. The presence of excessive mucus may also interfere with nutrient absorption. Gastrointestinal complications include bulky, foul-smelling stools, cramping and intestinal obstruction, rectal prolapse, and liver involvement. As the disease progresses, damage to the pancreas can cause impaired glucose tolerance and development of diabetes mellitus. The prevalence of insulin-requiring diabetes is estimated to be 7% in the entire population with CF and up to 15% in the adult CF population. As many as 50% of adults with CF may demonstrate glucose intolerance (Finkelstein et al, 1988).

Nutritional Status

Individuals with CF are at high risk for malnutrition. Although nutritional needs are increased by CF and malabsorption, complications of the disease often make it difficult to meet these needs. Factors that interfere with adequate intake and retention of nutrients include shortness of breath, coughing and cough-induced vomiting, gastrointestinal discomfort, anorexia during episodes of infection, impaired sense of smell, and glucosuria. Growth retardation and difficulty in maintaining desired weight for height are common problems. Before diagnosis, infants with CF often demonstrate growth failure. With treatment, growth generally improves in childhood. For some patients, especially adolescent and adult females, growth rate and weight for height may then decline as lung disease progresses (Durie and Pencharz, 1989). Although it was previously thought that this growth pattern was unavoidable due to pulmonary disease or endocrine abnormalities, it now appears that energy deficit is a significant contributing factor. When energy intake is adequate, growth appropriate for age can usually be achieved. The long-term relationship between nutritional support, growth, and survival is not known; however, improved nutritional status on a long-term basis is suggested to be a contributing factor to increased survival (Corey et al, 1988).

Nutritional Requirements and Care

The goal of nutritional care is to control malabsorption, to provide adequate energy, protein, and other nutrients to promote optimal linear growth and maintenance of ideal weight for height, and to prevent nutritional deficiencies.

Enzyme replacement therapy is the first step taken to control malabsorption. Pancreatic enzymes are taken with meals and snacks to improve the digestion of starches, protein, and fat. Even when replacement enzymes are taken, digestion is often not complete. The most widely used enzyme preparations contain "beads" of enterically coated pancreatic enzymes. Coating around the beads protects the enzymes from destruction in the acidic stomach. As the beads pass into the less acidic small intestine, enzymes are released and are made available to aid digestion. The enzyme content of preparations varies widely. High lipase formulations introduced in the late 1980s were designed to reduce the number and size of capsules required. Agents such as histamine antagonists and bicarbonate, which reduce the acidity of the small intestine, can be used as adjunct therapies when enzymes have not been effective. The efficacy of these additional therapies in long-term weight gain has been debated, but some individuals may benefit from a trial. Nonenterically coated enzymes that are active immediately upon contact with food were used extensively before enterically coated preparations became available. These enzymes cause irritation when they come into contact with the skin. However, they may still be used in situations when enterically coated enzymes cannot be used effectively.

The quantity of enzymes to be taken with food depends on the degree of pancreatic insufficiency, the quantity of food eaten, the fat and protein content of food consumed, and the type of enzymes used. Enzyme dosage is adjusted empirically to control gastrointestinal symptoms, including steatorrhea, and to promote growth appropriate for age. For infants or children unable to swallow enzyme capsules, the capsules can be opened and the beads can be mixed with a soft food such as applesauce. *Beads should not be mixed with foods that have a pH greater than 6.0 such as milk, custard, ice cream, or many other dairy products because the enteric coating will be destroyed.* To retain benefits of enteric coating, beads should not be chewed or crushed. If gastrointestinal symptoms cannot be controlled, dosage of enzymes, patient adherence, and enzyme type should be re-evaluated. Fecal fat or nitrogen balance studies may help to evaluate the adequacy of enzyme supplementation.

Inadequate enzyme use and fluid intake contribute to the development of *meconium ileus equivalent,* which is intestinal obstruction from fecal impaction. Treatment for meconium ileus equivalent includes adequate enzymes and fluids, high-fiber diet, exercise, bulk laxatives, and stool softeners.

ENERGY REQUIREMENTS. The amount of energy required by the patient with CF depends on the severity of lung disease, presence of infection, control of malabsorption, rate of growth, and physical activity level. Increase in energy needs may also be related to the basic defect of CF. Energy intakes of 120 to 150% of the recommended daily allowance (RDA) for age and gender are often recommended. Patients may tire of the need to keep energy intake high, and conflicts around eating may develop within the family.

PROTEIN AND FAT REQUIREMENTS. Protein needs are increased due to malabsorption. However, when energy needs are adequately supplied, individuals with CF are generally able to meet their protein needs by following a typical North American diet of at least 15 to 20% of total calories as protein. The protein intake should meet the RDA for age, weight, and gender when energy intake is adequate.

Fat intake should be encouraged and should provide 35 to 40% or more of total kilocalories, as tolerated. Dietary fat helps to provide required energy and essential fatty acids, limits the volume of food required to meet energy demands, and improves palatability of the diet. In the past, low-fat diets were recommended to patients with CF for control of steatorrhea, but with improved enzyme preparations and recognition of the difficulty in providing adequate energy using a low-fat diet, increased fat intake is widely recommended. Tolerance for fat and for specific high-fat foods in the diet varies for each individual. Extra enzymes can be taken with high-fat foods, such as pizza or French fries, to help with digestion. Indications of fat intolerance include an increase in the number of stools, greasy stools, or abdominal cramping. Among patients with CF who have pancreatic insufficiency and who are treated with enzymes to control malabsorption, clinical signs of EFA deficiency are rare, although blood and tissue lipid levels are likely to be abnormal (Farrell et al, 1985).

VITAMIN AND MINERAL REQUIREMENTS. Water-soluble vitamins, with the exception of vitamin B_{12}, are well absorbed in CF and needs can usually be met by diet. Vitamin B_{12} absorption is normalized with pancreatic enzyme supplementation. Because of fat malabsorption in pancreatic insufficiency, the fat-soluble vitamins may be poorly absorbed. Low serum concentrations of vitamin A and increased hepatic stores have been documented in CF, suggesting impaired mobilization/transport of the vitamin from the liver (Farrell and Hubbard, 1983). Decreased levels of vitamin D metabolites have been documented in subjects with CF. This is one of several factors that may be related to the decreased bone mineral content, which has been described in populations with CF (Mischler et al, 1979; Reiter et al, 1985). Low vitamin E levels have been associated with hemolytic anemia and abnormal neurologic findings in infants at diagnosis (Cynamon et al, 1988; Dolan, 1976). Individuals with CF are thought to be at increased risk for vitamin K deficiency due to long-term use of antibiotics, liver disease, as well as malabsorption. Although most patients maintain normal prothrombin times without supplementation, decreased biologic activity of vitamin K has been reported.

Sodium requirements are increased in CF due to increased losses in sweat. When sodium intake is inadequate, lethargy, vomiting, and dehydration may occur. Adequate salt is provided in the diet of most children and adults following a typical North American diet, including dairy products and processed foods. However, supplemental salt is required under some conditions. Infants require extra salt due to the low-sodium content of breast milk, formula, and infant foods, and ⅛ to ¼ tsp/day is usually adequate for needs. Children and adults need additional salt during periods of fever, hot weather, or physical exertion. Other minerals are not routinely supplemented in CF, although mineral status should be evaluated on an individual basis. Decreased bone mineralization, low iron stores, and low magnesium levels have all been described in CF (Ater et al, 1983; Green et al, 1985). Plasma zinc levels may be low in cases of moderate to severe malnutrition (Durie and Pencharz, 1989). Specific protocols for supplementation of vitamins and minerals vary, but one example is shown in Table 34–4.

DIET MODIFICATION. Diet modification is the first approach used to meet increased energy needs. Energy and protein intake can be increased by increasing the food portions at meals, by adding extra snacks, and by selecting foods of high-caloric density (Table 34–5; see also Table 30–1). Special nutrition supplements including fortified beverages and puddings, and carbohydrate supplements can help some individuals to meet nutritional needs (Appendix Table 33).

Night-time supplementation by feeding tube is an alternative available for those who are unable to meet nutritional needs by the oral route. Formulas are provided by continuous infusion through a nasogastric, gastrostomy, or jejunostomy tube while the patient sleeps. Elemental and nonelemental formulas with enzymes have both been used effectively. Enzyme powder can be added directly to the formula, or capsules can be taken by mouth when the feeding is started and again

TABLE 34–4. Vitamin and Mineral Supplementation in Cystic Fibrosis*

Nutrient	Quantity
Vitamin A	1–2 times the RDA/day†
Vitamin D	1–2 times the RDA/day†
Vitamin E	
Infants	25–50 IU/day‡
Children ≤ 10	100 IU/day
Children > 10	200 IU/day
Vitamin K	
Infants (<1 year)	2.5–5.0 mg weekly
Children and adults with long-term antibiotic therapy or liver disease	2.5–5.0 mg twice weekly
Sodium	
Infants	¼ tsp salt daily
Children and adults at times of vigorous exercise, heat stress, or profuse diarrhea	250 mg–2 g, 2–3 times per day

* Adapted from Adams EJ: Nutritional care in cystic fibrosis. Nutrition News Vol 51, No 3, 1988. Courtesy of National Dairy Council®.
† Vitamins A and D can be provided by 1 to 2 multivitamins daily.
‡ Vitamin E is provided in a water-soluble form.

once or twice during the night. Intensive supplementation has been associated with improved growth rate, slowed decline in pulmonary function, decreased incidence of respiratory infection, and improved sense of well-being (O'Laughlin et al, 1986; Shepherd et al, 1988). Although the short-term benefits of supplementation have been well documented, nutritional status is likely to deteriorate when supplementation is stopped. The long-term impact of intensive supplementation on disease course has not been determined. Factors that should be considered in the decision to proceed with night-time supplementation include nutritional and medical status, risks associated with tube feeding such as aspiration, and psychosocial and financial impact.

The immunologic and psychosocial benefits of breast-feeding are well established and are potentially very important for infants with CF and their families. For the infant with pancreatic insufficiency, enzymes are required with breast-milk feedings. Enzyme beads can be added to a small amount of baby food or can be placed directly in the infant's mouth by finger. Supplementation with high-calorie formula may be necessary to meet energy and protein needs if growth has been inadequate. For formula-fed infants, standard formulas at 20 to 27 kcal/oz with supplemental enzymes are usually adequate. Protein hydrolysate formulas with medium-chain triglycerides may also be used (Farrell et al, 1987).

TABLE 34–5. Suggestions for Increasing Energy Intake*

Include foods of high-energy density.
Include snacks regularly, especially before bedtime. Serve snacks at least 2 hours before the next meal.
Keep foods readily accessible for snacking.
Soft foods and beverages may be easier to eat when there is shortness of breath.
If lack of appetite is a problem, cold, low-fat foods will leave the stomach most quickly.
To enhance appetite, pay attention to appearance, texture, and aroma of foods offered.
Simplify food preparation by using convenience foods or preprepared foods.
Identify financial and food resources in the community to help meet needs.
Encourage companionship at meals.

* Adapted from Adams EJ: Nutrition care in cystic fibrosis. Nutrition News Vol 51, No 3, 1988. Courtesy of National Dairy Council®.

Chronic Obstructive Pulmonary Disease

Chronic obstructive pulmonary disease (COPD) is a process characterized by the presence of chronic bronchitis, emphysema, or both, leading to the development of airway obstruction. Clinically, *chronic bronchitis* is defined by a chronic productive cough that is present for more than half the time for 2 years. *Emphysema* is a condition of the lung characterized by abnormal permanent enlargement of alveoli, accompanied by destruction of their walls without obvious fibrosis (Fig. 34–3).

Cor pulmonale is a heart condition that may develop in patients with severe COPD. It is characterized by enlargement of the right ventricle and by right ventricular failure due to increased pressure within the pulmonary arteries. Vasoconstriction caused by chronic hypoxemia is a major factor in the development of *cor pulmonale.* Loss of pulmonary vascular bed due to emphysema, transmission of increased intrathoracic pressures, and increased blood volume may also contribute to the development of this condition. Treat-

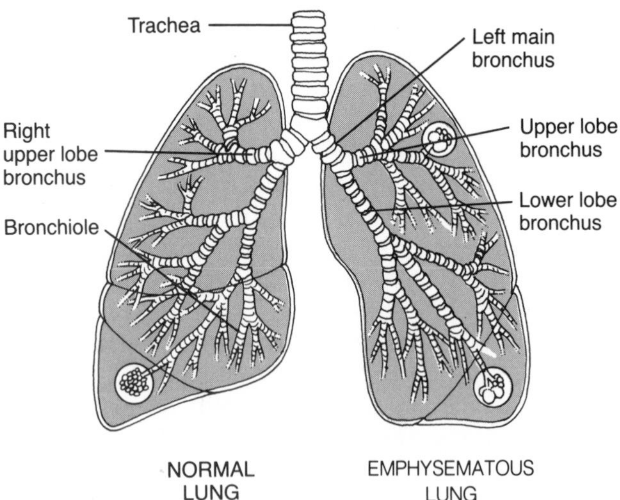

FIGURE 34–3. *Comparison of normal with emphysematous lung tissue. Increased energy expenditure, decreased energy intake, and impaired oxygenation are involved in nutritional wasting in COPD.*

ment of ventricular failure includes adequate oxygen therapy and the use of diuretics for control of edema.

Data from the National Health Interview Survey provide estimates that 10 million Americans have COPD (7.5 million with chronic bronchitis and 2.5 million with emphysema). COPD and related conditions represented the fifth leading cause of death in the United States in 1984. The prevalence, incidence, and mortality rate for COPD increase with age and are higher in males than in females. Cigarette smoking is the most important risk factor (Research Trends, page 588).

Nutritional Status

Epidemiologic studies indicate that malnourished patients with COPD have a worse prognosis than those who are well nourished. No large studies have been done to establish prevalence of malnutrition in COPD; however, clinical observations and surveys of small groups of affected patients confirm that weight loss is common. Nutritional depletion, characterized by low body weight and triceps skinfold measurements, has been shown to relate to the degree of airflow obstruction, diffusing capacity, CO_2 retention, respiratory and limb muscle strength, as well as altered muscle function (Efthimiou et al, 1988). Patients with emphysema may be at greater nutritional risk than those with chronic bronchitis. Historically, the patient with emphysema has been characterized as thin and wasted, and the patient with chronic bronchitis is described as overweight.

The cause for nutritional wasting in COPD is not completely understood, but is thought to involve a combination of increased energy expenditure, decreased energy intake, and impaired oxygenation as described in Table 34–1. Evidence of low weight for height despite reported caloric intakes of 156 to 162% of resting energy expenditure (REE) supports observations of increased oxygen consumption in this population (Keim et al, 1986).

Nutritional Care

The focus of nutritional care for patients with COPD is the maintenance of an acceptable weight for height as well as management of drug-nutrient interactions and fluid balance. Components of nutrition screening and assessment are listed in Table 34–6. History of recent weight loss or body weight less than 90% of ideal body weight (IBW) are considered to be significant, and identify patients in need of further evaluation. For patients with cor pulmonale and fluid retention, weight maintenance or gain may occur despite wasting of lean body mass. The concentration of biochemical indicators of nutritional status, such as serum proteins, hemoglobin, and electrolytes, are depressed by hemodilution in patients retaining fluid. Some patients with cor pulmonale and fluid retention require sodium and fluid restriction, whereas others are well controlled by diuretics alone (see Chapter 33).

Energy requirements vary for each patient but may be near 150% of REE calculated by the Harris-Benedict method (see Table 2–5). Factors listed in Table 34–1 can make it difficult for patients to meet increased energy needs. Suggestions to enhance appetite and promote dietary intake are included in Tables 30–1 and 34–5. When abdominal bloating is a problem, limitation of foods associated with gas formation can be helpful. These foods may include apples, beer, cabbage, cauliflower, legumes, melons, nuts, onions, and sauerkraut (see Chapter 27). Exercise, adequate fluids, and dietary fiber also enhance gastrointestinal motility. Patients with disease-related physical limitations may be helped by assistance with shopping and meal preparation, suggestions for simplified meal preparation, or participation in congregate meal programs. Linkage with community resources may also be necessary.

Enteral nutritional supplementation by mouth or by feeding tube can be used to increase total caloric intake for some patients with COPD. Supplementation for 3 months with a high-calorie liquid supplement has effectively increased total energy intake and has resulted in significant increases in weight, triceps skinfold, midarm circumference, and respiratory muscle

TABLE 34–6. Components of Nutrition Assessment for Adults with Chronic Obstructive Pulmonary Disease

Historical Parameters	Medical Parameters	Nutritional Parameters	Diet History	Environmental Parameters
Medical history Nutritional history Usual weight	Respiratory status Oxygen saturation Dental status Senses of smell and taste Gastrointestinal function	Weight Height Skinfold measurements Hemoglobin and hematocrit Serum electrolytes Serum proteins Additional biochemical tests as needed (e.g., immunologic testing, creatinine height index, nitrogen balance)	Usual home diet Use of supplements Where meals are eaten Social companionship with meals	Home facilities Physical abilities Financial resources

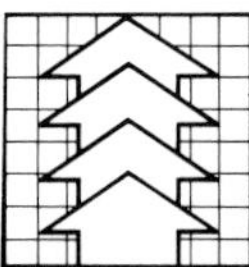

NEW DIRECTIONS: Cigarette Smoking, Vitamin C Status, and Pulmonary Disease

It is well known that smoking is a major contributor to the development of chronic respiratory lung disease. Cellular inflammation caused by cigarette smoke leads to the release of free radicals, which in turn cause direct injury to the lungs. It is suggested that vitamin C and other micronutrients reduce the release and destructive activity of free radicals by acting as cofactors for antioxidative enzymes. Other factors such as the ability of vitamin C to accelerate histamine metabolism may also be important.

Also well established is the fact that smoking reduces serum levels of vitamin C. Two studies using data from the NHANES II survey have explored this area.

One study investigated the relationship of dietary intake and serum levels of several nutrients to bronchitis and pulmonary wheezing. Of these, vitamin C showed the strongest negative correlation with these common symptoms of lung disease. The relationship was independent of current smoking status, suggesting a positive effect of vitamin C nutriture on lung health that is unrelated to prevention of the damage sustained from smoking (Schwartz and Weiss, 1990).

A second study explored the effect of smoking on dietary intakes and serum levels of vitamin C. Not unexpected was the finding that serum levels of vitamin C were negatively related to the amount of smoking, with the highest levels occurring in persons who had never smoked or who had quit smoking at least 1 year previously. A somewhat surprising finding was that smoking decreased the intake of vitamin C–rich foods in an amount proportional to the level of smoking. Serum vitamin C levels were influenced more by the effect of smoking than by the intake of the vitamin, suggesting that lowered levels represent a response to two different mechanisms (Schectman et al, 1989).

Many of the subjects in the second study were using dietary supplements. Unsupplemented smokers were approximately 11 times more at risk of marginal hypovitaminosis C than smokers who took vitamin C supplements. Raising serum vitamin C levels of unsupplemented smokers to those of nonsmokers required approximately 130 mg/day. The authors suggested that although the optimal solution would be to quit smoking, the next approach might be supplementation with this amount, which is well under the level of vitamin C supplementation that provokes undesirable response.

strength (Efthimiou et al, 1988). However, when supplementation is inadequate for weight gain, improvement in respiratory muscle strength does not usually occur (Lewis et al, 1987).

Acute Respiratory Failure

Nutritional support has a critical role for the patient recovering from acute respiratory failure who requires mechanical ventilation. Respiratory muscle weakness is a central factor in failure to wean from mechanical ventilation, and nutritional status is linked closely to respiratory muscle strength and endurance. Retrospective studies suggest that patients who respond to nutritional support with an increase in protein synthesis are more likely to wean from mechanical ventilation.

Nutritional Status

Nutritional needs vary widely within this group of patients, depending on the underlying disease process and on prior nutritional status. Collectively, patients with acute respiratory failure are likely to present in poor nutritional condition and to be at high risk for nutritional depletion during hospitalization.

Nutritional Care

The goal of nutritional support for the patient with acute respiratory failure is to meet energy and nutrient needs, preserve lean body mass, and maintain fluid balance without exceeding the capacity of the respiratory system to clear carbon dioxide. Weight is the most useful screening parameter. Weight less than 90% IBW or history of loss of 10% IBW are significant findings. Triceps skinfold measurements have limited value when patients are followed only for a short time. Other indicators of protein-energy status may be useful as described for the patient with COPD (see Table 34–6).

Energy requirements depend on the underlying conditions and on the respiratory effort required. Energy needs can be estimated by indirect calorimetry, which measures oxygen consumption and carbon dioxide production (see Chapter 2). However, these measurements may be affected significantly by routine procedures in critical care, and may be unreliable for patients receiving high concentrations of oxygen (Pingleton, 1988). When indirect calorimetry is not available or is impractical, the Harris-Benedict equation can be used to estimate resting energy expenditure for age, gender, and size, and additional energy requirements associated with specific conditions can be added to the REE (see Table 2–5). Afebrile, mechanically ventilated patients with COPD have been documented to require an additional 29 to 34% of calories beyond REE (Harmon et al, 1986). Although energy requirements for patients recovering from conditions such as adult respiratory distress syndrome have not been quantified, needs of nonseptic patients rarely exceed 150% of the calculated REE (Pingleton, 1988).

Diet composition should be planned to meet protein

and energy needs while minimizing CO_2 production. Dietary regimens that include fat and are associated with lower respiratory quotients (RQ) are of theoretical benefit to minimize the quantity of CO_2 that must be cleared by the lungs (see Chapter 2). Increased CO_2 loads associated with carbohydrate metabolism may be a critical problem during weaning from mechanical ventilation (Dark et al, 1985). For parenterally nourished patients with respiratory failure, recommended energy intakes provide 1.0 to 1.2 times energy expenditure for weight maintenance and 1.4 to 1.6 times energy expenditure for repletion, with 50% of the nonprotein calories provided as lipid (Askanazi et al, 1982).

Routes of Nutritional Support

Most patients who are not intubated or who have tracheostomies will be able to meet all or some of their nutritional needs by mouth. Patients who are intubated require non-oral nutritional support. The enteral route is preferred if the gastrointestinal tract is functioning (see Chapter 30). Of special concern for the mechanically ventilated patient is the potential risk of aspiration. Feeding procedures that may help to minimize aspiration include the use of a continuous feeding method, tube placement in the duodenum, chest elevation, frequent evaluation for residuals, and endotracheal tube cuff inflation.

When enteral feeding is not possible, parenteral nutritional support is required. Concerns have been raised about the use of lipids for critically ill patients requiring mechanical ventilation because of potential adverse effects on gas exchange and pulmonary vascular tone (Hageman and Hunt, 1986). Administration of intravenous lipids to healthy volunteers and critically ill ventilator-dependent patients without adverse effects on gas exchange has been documented (Jarnberg et al, 1981). However, the potential impact of the lipid may vary with underlying conditions. Therefore, lipids should be administered slowly, and respiratory status should be monitored carefully as the dose is gradually advanced.

CITED REFERENCES

Adamkin DH: Total parenteral nutrition in hyaline membrane disease. *In* Lebenthal E: Total Parenteral Nutrition: Indications, Utilization, Complications and Pathophysiological Considerations. New York, Raven Press, 1986.

Askanazi J et al: Nutrition and the respiratory system. Crit Care Med 10:163, 1982.

Ater JL et al: Relative anemia and iron deficiency in cystic fibrosis. Pediatrics 71:810, 1983.

Aubier M et al: Effect of hypophosphatemia on diaphragmatic contractility in patients with acute respiratory failure. N Engl J Med 313:420, 1985.

Bilbrey GL et al: Skeletal muscle resting membrane potential in potassium deficiency. J Clin Invest 52:3011, 1973.

Brans YW et al: Fat emulsion tolerance in very low birth weight neonates: Effect on diffusion of oxygen in the lungs and blood pH. Pediatrics 78:79, 1986.

Corey M et al: A comparison of survival, growth and pulmonary function in patients with cystic fibrosis in Boston and Toronto. J Clin Epidemiol 41:588, 1988.

Cynamon HA et al: Effect of vitamin E deficiency on neurologic function in patients with cystic fibrosis. J Pediatr 113:637, 1988.

Cystic Fibrosis Foundation: Patient Registry Data, 1987.

Dark DS, Pingleton SK, and Kerby GR: Hypercapnia during weaning: A complication of nutritional support. Chest 88:141, 1985.

Doekel RC et al: Clinical semistarvation: Depression of hypoxic ventilatory response. N Engl J Med 295:358, 1976.

Dolan TF: Hemolytic anemia and edema as the initial signs in infants with cystic fibrosis. Clin Pediatr 15:597, 1976.

Durie PR and Forstner CG: Pathophysiology of the exocrine pancreas in cystic fibrosis. J R Soc Med 82:2, 1989.

Durie PR and Pencharz PB: A rational approach to the nutritional care of patients with cystic fibrosis. J R Soc Med 82:11, 1989.

Efthimiou J et al: The effect of supplementary oral nutrition in poorly nourished patients with chronic obstructive pulmonary disease. Am Rev Respir Dis 137:1075, 1988.

Farrell PM and Hubbard VS: Nutrition in cystic fibrosis: Vitamins, fatty acids and minerals. *In* Lloyd-Still JD: Textbook of Cystic Fibrosis. Boston, John Wright-PSG, 1983.

Farrell PM, Mischler EH, and Sondel SA: Predigested formula for infants with cystic fibrosis. J Am Diet Assoc 87:1353, 1987.

Farrell PM et al: Essential fatty acid deficiency in premature infants. Am J Clin Nutr 48:220, 1988.

Farrell PM et al: Fatty acid abnormalities in cystic fibrosis. Pediatr Res 19:104, 1985.

Field S, Kelly SM, and Macklem PT: The oxygen cost of breathing in patients with cardiorespiratory distress. Am Rev Respir Dis 128:9, 1982.

Finkelstein SM et al: Diabetes mellitus associated with cystic fibrosis. J Pediatr 112:373, 1988.

Garg M et al: Clinically unsuspected hypoxia during sleep and feeding in infants with bronchopulmonary dysplasia. Pediatrics 81:635, 1988.

Green CG, Doershuk CF, and Stern RC: Symptomatic hypomagnesemia in cystic fibrosis. J Pediatr 107:425, 1985.

Greer FR: Bronchopulmonary dysplasia and the rickets of prematurity. *In* Bronchopulmonary Dysplasia and Related Chronic Respiratory Disorders, Report of the Ninetieth Ross Conference on Pediatric Research, Ross Laboratories, Columbus, OH, 1986.

Groothuis JR and Rosenberg AA: Home oxygen promotes weight gain in infants with bronchopulmonary dysplasia. Am J Dis Child 141:992, 1987.

Hageman JR and Hunt CE: Fat emulsions and lung function. Clin Chest Med 7:68, 1986.

Hammerman C and Aramburo MJ: Decreased lipid intake reduces morbidity in sick premature neonates. J Pediatr 113:1083, 1988.

Harmon GS, Whitman RA, and Pingleton SK: Energy requirements in mechanically ventilated COPD patients. Am Rev Respir Dis 133:A203, 1986.

Jarnberg PO, Lindholm J, and Eklund J: Lipid infusion in critically ill patients: Acute effects on hemodynamics and pulmonary gas exchange. Crit Care Med 9:27, 1981.

Keim NL et al: Dietary evaluation of outpatients with chronic obstructive pulmonary disease. J Am Diet Assoc 86:902, 1986.

Keys A et al: The Biology of Human Starvation. Minneapolis, The University of Minnesota Press, 1959.

Kurzner SI et al: Growth failure in infants with bronchopulmonary dysplasia: Nutrition and elevated resting metabolic expenditure. Pediatrics 81:379, 1988.

Lewis MI, Belman MJ, and Dorr-Uyemura L: Nutritional supplementation in ambulatory patients with chronic obstructive pulmonary disease. Am Rev Respir Dis 135:1062, 1987.

Lloyd TR and Boucek MM: Effect of intralipid on the neonatal pulmonary bed: An echographic study. J Pediatr 108:130, 1986.

Mischler EH et al: Demineralization in cystic fibrosis. Am J Dis Child 133:632, 1979.

Molloy DW et al: Hypomagnesemia and respiratory muscle power. Am Rev Respir Dis 129:497, 1984.

Niederman MS et al: Malnutrition affects patterns of tracheobronchial colonization by gram-negative bacteria in mechanically ventilated patients. Am Rev Respir Dis 133:204A, 1986.

Oh, W: Nutritional management of infants with bronchopulmonary dysplasia. Bronchopulmonary dysplasia and related chronic respiratory disorders. *In* Report of the Ninetieth Ross Conference on Pediatric Research, Ross Laboratories, Columbus, OH, 1986.

O'Laughlin W et al: Nutritional rehabilitation of malnourished patients with cystic fibrosis. Am J Clin Nutr 43:732, 1986.

Perlman JM et al: Is chloride depletion an important contributing cause of death in infants with bronchopulmonary dysplasia? Pediatrics 77:212, 1986.

Pingleton SK: Nutritional support in the mechanically ventilated patient. Clin Chest Med 9:101, 1988.

Reiter EO et al: Vitamin D metabolites in adolescents and young adults with cystic fibrosis: Effects of sun and season. J Pediatr 106:21, 1985.

Rochester DF: Respiratory effects of respiratory muscle weakness and atrophy. Am Rev Respir Dis 134:1083, 1986.

Schectman G et al: The influence of smoking on vitamin C status in adults. Am J Public Health 79:158, 1989.

Schwartz J and Weiss ST: Dietary factors and their relation to respiratory symptoms: The Second National Health and Nutrition Examination Survey. Am J Epidemiol 132:67, 1990.

Shepherd RW et al: Increased energy expenditure in young children with cystic fibrosis. Lancet 1:1300, 1988.

Vaisman N et al: Effect of salbutamol on resting energy expenditure in patients with cystic fibrosis. J Pediatr 111:137, 1987.

Vohr BR and Bell EF: Infants with bronchopulmonary dysplasia: Growth pattern and neurologic and developmental outcome. Am J Dis Child 136:443, 1982.

Weissman C et al: Effect of routine intensive care interactions on metabolic rate. Chest 86:815, 1984.

Yeh TF et al: Metabolic rate and energy balance in infants with bronchopulmonary dysplasia. J Pediatr 114:448, 1989.

Zwillich CW, Sahn SA and Weil JV: Effects of hypermetabolism on ventilation and chemosensitivity. J Clin Invest 60:900, 1977.

ADDITIONAL REFERENCES

Arora NS and Rochester DF: Respiratory muscle strength and maximal voluntary ventilation in undernourished patients. Am Rev Respir Dis 126:5, 1982.

Chalmers DM et al: The influence of long-term cimetidine as an adjuvant to pancreatic enzyme therapy in cystic fibrosis. Acta Paediatr Scand 74:114, 1985.

Edelman NH, Rucker RB, and Peavy HH: NIH Workshop Summary: Nutrition and the respiratory system. Am Rev Respir Dis 134:347, 1986.

Elpern EH, Jacobs ER, and Bone RC: Incidence of aspiration in tracheally intubated adults. Heart Lung 16:527, 1987.

Frank L and Sosenko IRS: Undernutrition as a major contributing factor in the pathogenesis of bronchopulmonary dysplasia. Am Rev Respir Dis 138:725, 1988.

Handen BL, Mandell R, and Russo DC: Feeding induction in children who refuse to eat. Am J Dis Child 140:52, 1986.

Katz DP and Askanazi J: Nutrition and pulmonary function. Nutr MD 16(2):1, 1990.

Knowles MR and Fernald GW: Diabetes and cystic fibrosis: New questions emerging from increased longevity. J Pediatr 112:419, 1988.

Rothkopf MM et al: Nutritional support in respiratory failure. Nutr Clin Prac 4:166, 1989.

Rubenstein S, Moss R, and Lewiston N: Constipation and meconium ileus equivalent in patients with cystic fibrosis. Pediatrics 78:473, 1986.

Soutter VL et al: Chronic undernutrition/growth retardation in cystic fibrosis. Clin Gastroenterol 15:131, 1986.

CHAPTER 35

NUTRITIONAL CARE IN RENAL DISEASE

Charles J. Pruchno, M.D., Katy E. Wilkens, M.S., R.D., and Kris W. Schroeder, R.D., C.D.

CHAPTER OUTLINE

KEY TERMS

ACUTE GLOMERULONEPHRITIDES—a group of diseases characterized by inflammation of the capillary loops of the glomerulus

AZOTEMIA—the accumulation in the blood of abnormal quantities of urea, uric acid, creatinine, and other nitrogenous wastes

CONTINUOUS ARTERIOVENOUS HEMOFILTRATION (CAVH)—a method of acute renal failure management in which an ultrafiltration membrane, powered by the patient's own blood, produces an ultrafiltrate that can then be replaced by parenteral nutrition fluids

DIALYSATE—the solution used in dialysis to remove waste products and excess fluids from the blood; similar to plasma but without waste products

END-STAGE RENAL DISEASE—a disease characterized by the kidney's inability to excrete waste products, maintain fluid and electrolyte balance, and produce hormones

ERYTHROPOIETIN—a hormone secreted chiefly by the kidney in the adult and by the liver in the fetus, which acts on stem cells of the bone marrow to stimulate red blood cell production

GLOMERULAR FILTRATION RATE (GFR)—the quantity of glomerular filtrate formed per unit time in all nephrons of both kidneys

HEMODIALYSIS—a method of clearing waste products from the blood in which blood passes by the semipermeable membrane of the artificial kidney and waste products are removed by diffusion

ISCHEMIC ACUTE TUBULAR NECROSIS—extensive kidney tissue destruction that is the result of a prolonged episode of blood deprivation

METASTATIC CALCIFICATION—the deposition of calcium in tissues as a result of abnormalities in calcium and phosphate levels in the blood and fluids

NEPHRITIC SYNDROME—the syndrome of hematuria, hypertension, and mild loss of renal function that results from acute inflammation of the capillary loops of the glomerulus

NEPHROLITHIASIS—a condition marked by the presence of renal calculi

NEPHROTIC SYNDROME—a condition resulting from loss of the glomerular barrier to protein and is characterized by massive edema and proteinuria, hypoalbuminemia, hypercholesterolemia, hypercoagulability, and abnormal bone metabolism

OLIGURIC—the condition of having urinary volumes of less than 500 ml/day

OSTEITIS FIBROSA CYSTICA—inflammation of the bone with fibrous degeneration and formation of cysts secondary to parathyroid gland hyperfunction

PERITONEAL DIALYSIS—a method of removal of waste products from the blood in which diffusion carries waste products from the blood through the semipermeable peritoneal membrane and into the dialysate

RENAL FAILURE—the inability of a kidney to excrete the daily load of wastes

RENAL OSTEODYSTROPHY—metabolic bone disease as a complication of end-stage renal disease

RENIN-ANGIOTENSIN MECHANISM—a major control of blood pressure involving kidney-secreted renin that acts in the plasma to form angiotensin I, which is converted to angiotensin II, a powerful vasoconstrictor and potent stimulus of aldosterone secretion by the adrenal gland

SOLUTE LOAD—the end waste products of metabolism

UREMIA—clinical syndrome of malaise, weakness, nausea and vomiting, muscle cramps, itching, metallic mouth taste, and often neurologic impairment, which is brought about by an unacceptable level of nitrogenous wastes in the blood

PHYSIOLOGY AND FUNCTION OF THE KIDNEYS

The main function of the kidney is to maintain homeostatic balance with respect to fluids, electrolytes, and organic solutes. The normal kidney has the ability to perform this function over a wide range of dietary fluctuations in sodium, water, and various solutes. This task is accomplished by the continuous filtration of blood and by alterations (secretion and reabsorption) in this filtered fluid. The kidney receives 20% of cardiac output, which allows the filtering of approximately 1,600 l/day of blood. Approximately 180 liters of fluid (ultrafiltrate) are produced in filtering this blood, and through active processes of reabsorbing certain components and secreting others, the composition of this fluid is changed into the 1.5 liters of urine excreted in an average day.

Each kidney consists of approximately 1 million functioning units called nephrons (Fig. 35–1). The *nephron* consists of a *glomerulus* connected to a series of *tubules,* which can be broken into functionally different segments: the proximal convoluted tubule, loop of Henle, distal tubule, and collecting duct. Each nephron functions independently in producing a contribution to the final urine, although all are under similar control and are thus coordinated. Nevertheless, when one segment of a nephron is destroyed, that complete nephron is no longer functional.

The glomerulus is a spherically shaped mass of capillaries surrounded by a membrane, *Bowman's capsule.* The function of the glomerulus is to produce the large amount of ultrafiltrate, which the ensuing segments of the nephron will then modify. The ultrafiltrate produced in the glomerulus is very similar in composition to blood. Owing to the barrier function of the glomerulus, it lacks blood cells as well as molecules of molecular weight greater than 6,500, most notably protein. The production of ultrafiltrate is mainly a passive one, relying on the perfusion pressure generated by the heart and supplied by the renal artery.

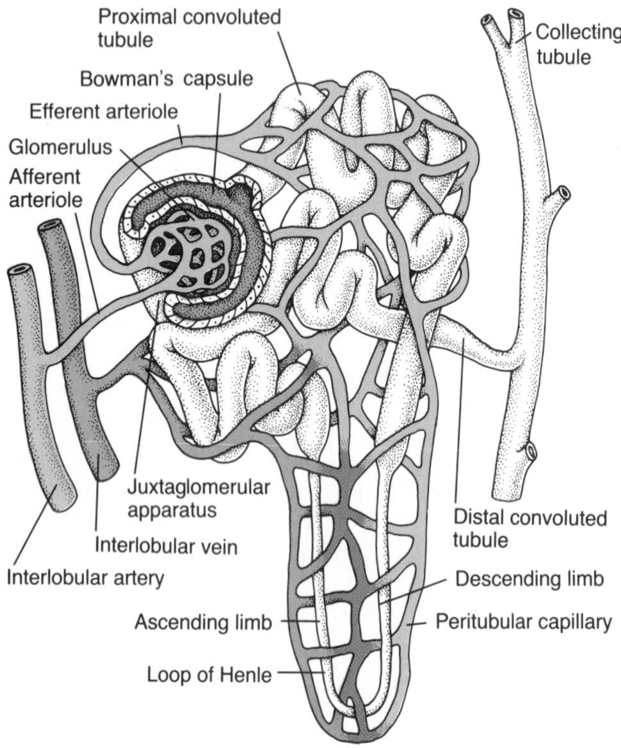

FIGURE 35–1. *The nephron.*

The tubules function to reabsorb the vast majority of components that compose the ultrafiltrate. Much of this process is active and requires a large expenditure of energy in the form of adenosine triphosphate (ATP). Due to a unique structure, differences in permeabilities between the various segments, and the response to hormonal control, the tubule is able to produce a final urine with a wide range of variability in concentration of sodium, potassium, other electrolytes, osmolality, pH, and volume.

Ultimately, the final urine produced is funneled into common collecting tubules and into the renal pelvis. The renal pelvis narrows into a single ureter per kidney, and each ureter carries urine into the bladder, where it is allowed to accumulate prior to elimination.

Although the homeostatic mechanisms are interrelated to a large extent, occasional demands are placed on the kidney to regulate one substance while sacrificing tight control of others. In this regard, the control of circulating blood volume predominates over the control of all other parameters. Thus sodium, the most important molecule in determining the body's circulating volume, is regulated at the expense of all other substances. A gain or loss of 1% of circulating volume will be reflected in marked changes in urine as well as in serum composition of potassium, bicarbonate, and water.

The kidney has almost unlimited ability to regulate water homeostasis. Owing to its ability to form a large concentration gradient between its inner medulla and outer cortex, the kidney can excrete urine as dilute as 50 mOsm or as concentrated as 1,200 mOsm. Given a daily fixed solute load of about 600 mOsm (the solute load representing the end waste products of normal metabolism), the kidney can get rid of as little as 500 ml of concentrated urine or as much as 12 liters. Control of water excretion is regulated by *antidiuretic hormone (ADH),* a small peptide hormone secreted by the posterior pituitary. An excess of relative body water, indicated by a fall in osmolality, leads to a prompt shut-off of all ADH secretion. Likewise, a small rise in osmolality brings about marked ADH secretion and retention of water. However, the need to conserve sodium sometimes leads to a sacrifice of the homeostatic control of water for the sake of volume.

The minimum urinary volume capable of eliminating a relatively fixed 600 mOsm of solute is 500 ml, assuming that the kidney is capable of maximum concentration. Urinary volumes of less than 500 ml/day are called *oliguric;* it is impossible for such a urine volume to eliminate all of the daily waste.

The majority of the solute load consists of nitrogenous wastes, largely the end product of protein metabolism. Urea predominates in amounts depending on the protein content of the diet; uric acid, creatinine, and ammonia are present in small amounts. If these normal waste products are not eliminated appropriately, they collect in abnormal quantities in the blood, a condition described as *azotemia.* The ability of the kidney to adequately eliminate nitrogenous waste products is defined as *renal function; renal failure* is the consequence of inability to excrete the daily load of these wastes.

The kidney also performs functions unrelated to excretion. One of these involves the *renin-angiotensin mechanism,* a major control of blood pressure (Fig. 35–2). Decreased blood volume causes cells of the glomerulus (the *juxtaglomerular apparatus*) to react by secreting *renin,* a proteolytic enzyme. Renin acts in the plasma to form *angiotensin I,* which is converted to *angiotensin II,* a powerful vasoconstrictor and a potent stimulus of aldosterone secretion by the adrenal gland. As a consequence, sodium is reabsorbed, and blood pressure is returned to normal.

The kidney also produces *erythropoietin,* a critical determinant of erythroid activity in the bone marrow. A deficiency of erythropoietin is a factor in the severe anemia present in chronic renal disease.

Maintenance of *calcium-phosphorus homeostasis* involves the complex interactions of parathyroid hormone (PTH), calcitonin, vitamin D, and three effector organs, the gut, kidney, and bone. The role of the kidney includes the production of the active form of vitamin D—$1,25(OH)_2D_3$—as well as the elimination of both calcium and phosphorus. Active vitamin D promotes efficient absorption of calcium by the gut and is one of the substances necessary for bone remodeling and maintenance (see Chapter 22).

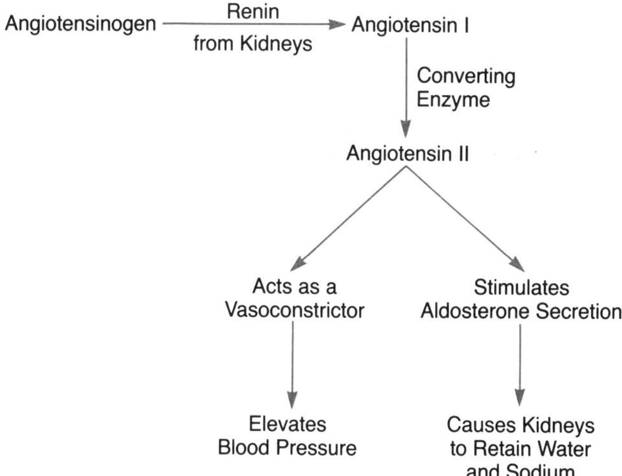

FIGURE 35–2. *Renin-angiotensin mechanism.*

DISEASES OF THE KIDNEY

The manifestations of renal disease are a direct consequence of the portion of the nephron most affected. These include: (1) nephrotic syndrome, (2) nephritic syndrome, (3) acute renal failure (ARF), (4) tubular defects, (5) renal stones, and finally (6) end-stage renal disease (ESRD). Objectives of nutritional care depend on the abnormality to be treated.

Glomerular Diseases

The functions of the glomerulus that are important with respect to disease include the production of an adequate ultrafiltrate and prevention of certain substances from entering this ultrafiltrate.

Nephrotic Syndrome

Nephrotic syndrome describes a heterogeneous group of diseases whose common manifestations derive from a loss of the glomerular barrier to protein. Large protein losses in the urine lead to hypoalbuminemia with consequent edema, hypercholesterolemia, hypercoagulability, and abnormal bone metabolism.

More than 95% of cases seen with this syndrome are accounted for by three systemic diseases (diabetes mellitus, systemic lupus erythematosus [SLE], and amyloidosis) and four diseases primarily of the kidney (minimal change disease, membranous nephropathy, focal glomerulosclerosis, and membranoproliferative glomerulonephritis). Although renal function can deteriorate during the course of these diseases, it is not a consistent feature.

NUTRITIONAL CARE. The primary objective of the diet treatment in nephrotic syndrome is the replacement of albumin and other protein lost from the plasma into the urine. Patients with an established severe protein deficiency who continue to lose protein may require an extended time of carefully supervised nutritional care.

The diet should provide sufficient protein and energy to maintain a positive nitrogen balance and to produce an increase in plasma albumin concentration and disappearance of edema. The dietary protein level for patients with nephrotic syndrome remains controversial. Historically, these patients received diets high in protein (up to as much as 1.5 g/kg/day) in an attempt to increase serum albumin and to prevent protein malnutrition. However, studies have shown that a reduction of protein intake to as low as 0.6 mg/kg/day can decrease proteinuria without adversely affecting serum albumin (Kaysen, 1986). To allow for optimal protein use, 80% of the protein should be from sources of high biologic value (HBV), and energy intake should be 35 to 50 kcal/kg/day for adults and 100 to 150 kcal/kg/day for children.

Edema, the most clinically apparent manifestation of this group of diseases, indicates a state of total body sodium overload. Yet, due to the low oncotic pressure in the circulating blood volume that results from hypoalbuminemia, the volume of circulating blood is actually reduced. Attempts to limit sodium intake more than modestly, and attempts to eliminate large amounts of extra sodium with diuretics, can result in marked hypotension, exacerbation of the coagulopathy, and deterioration of renal function. Control of edema in this group of diseases should therefore not be complete, should rely to some extent on elastic full-length support hose, and should entail only modest sodium restriction — approximately 3 g/day of sodium.

The important consequence of hypercholesterolemia lies in the potential for inducing cardiovascular disease. Although a satisfactory answer is not apparent, it is believed that patients with longstanding nephrotic syndrome are at increased risk (Bernard, 1988). Many pediatric patients with frequently relapsing or resistant nephrotic syndrome are at particular risk for premature atherosclerosis. Certain lipid-lowering agents, when combined with a cholesterol-lowering diet, can reduce total cholesterol, low-density lipoprotein (LDL) cholesterol, and triglycerides in patients with nephrotic syndrome (see Chapter 20).

Nephritic Syndrome

Nephritic syndrome describes the clinical manifestations of a group of diseases characterized by inflammation of the capillary loops of the glomerulus. These diseases, also referred to as *acute glomerulonephritides,* are sudden in onset, last a short time, and proceed to either complete recovery, development of chronic nephrotic syndrome (as already discussed), or ESRD.

The primary manifestation of these diseases is hematuria (blood in the urine), a consequence of the capillary inflammation that damages the glomerular barrier to blood cells. The syndrome is also characterized by hypertension and by mild loss of renal function. The most common presentation follows a streptococcal infection and is usually, although not always, self-limiting. Other causes include primary kidney diseases, such as IgA nephropathy and hereditary nephritis, as well as secondary diseases, such as SLE, vasculitides, and glomerulonephritis associated with endocarditis, abscesses, or infected ventriculoperitoneal shunts.

NUTRITIONAL CARE. The treatment of acute glomerulonephritis attempts to maintain good nutritional status while allowing time for the disease to resolve spontaneously. In cases in which an underlying disease is responsible, treatment of that disease predominates and largely determines patient outcome. There is no reason to restrict protein or potassium intake unless significant uremia or hyperkalemia develops. When hypertension is present, it is related mainly to extracellular volume excess and should be treated with sodium restriction.

Diseases of the Tubules and Interstitium

To a great extent, the functions of the kidney tubules make them susceptible to injury. The enormous energy requirements and expenditures of the tubules in performing work of active secretion and reabsorption leave this part of the kidney particularly vulnerable to ischemic injuries. High local concentrations of many toxic drugs can destroy or damage various segments of the tubules. Finally, the high-solute concentration generated in the medullary interstitium exposes it to the damage of oxidants, precipitation of calcium-phosphate product (extraosseous calcification), and favors the sickling of red blood cells in sickle cell anemia.

Acute Renal Failure

ARF is characterized by a sudden reduction in *glomerular filtration rate (GFR)* and an alteration in the ability of the kidney to excrete the daily production of metabolic waste. It can occur either in association with a reduction in urine output (*oliguria,* strictly defined as production of less than 500 ml in 24 hours) or with normal urine flow. ARF typically occurs in previously healthy kidneys. Its duration varies from a few days to several weeks. The causes of ARF are numerous, and often several occur simultaneously (Table 35–1).

TABLE 35–1. Some Causes of Acute Renal Failure

- Prerenal
  - Severe dehydration
  - Circulatory collapse
- Intrinsic
  - Acute tubular necrosis
    - Trauma, surgery
    - Septicemia
  - Nephrotoxicity
    - Antibiotics, contrast agents, and other drugs
  - Vascular disorders
    - Bilateral renal infarction
  - Acute glomerulonephritis of any cause
    - Poststreptococcal infection
    - Systemic lupus erythematosus
- Postrenal-Obstruction
  - Benign prostatic hypertrophy
  - Carcinoma of the bladder or prostate
  - Ureterovesical stricture

These causes are generally classified into three categories: (1) inadequate renal perfusion *(prerenal)*, (2) diseases within the renal parenchyma *(intrinsic)*, and (3) obstruction *(postrenal)*. Generally, if careful attention is directed at diagnosing and correcting the prerenal and obstructive causes, ARF is short-lived and requires no particular nutritional intervention.

Intrinsic ARF can result from toxic drug exposure, a local allergic reaction to drugs, rapidly progressive glomerulonephritis, or a prolonged episode of ischemia leading to *ischemic acute tubular necrosis*. Of these, the latter is the most devastating. Typically, patients develop this illness as a complication of sustained shock due to an overwhelming infection, severe trauma, surgical accidents, or cardiogenic shock.

The clinical course and outcome depend mainly on the underlying cause. Patients with ARF that is caused by drug toxicity generally recover fully after they stop taking the drug. On the other hand, the mortality associated with ischemic acute tubular necrosis due to shock is approximately 70%. Typically, these patients are highly catabolic, and extensive tissue destruction occurs in the early stages. Hemodialysis is used to reduce the acidosis, correct the uremia, and control hyperkalemia.

If recovery is to occur, it generally takes place within 2 to 3 weeks of the time when the underlying insults have been corrected. The recovery (diuretic) phase is characterized first by an increase in urine output and later by a return of waste elimination. During this period, dialysis may still be required, and careful attention must be paid to fluid and electrolyte balance and to appropriate replacement.

NUTRITIONAL CARE. Nutritional care in ARF is particularly important, because the patient not only has uremia, metabolic acidosis, and fluid and electrolyte imbalance, but usually also suffers from physiologic stress (e.g., infection or tissue destruction) that increases protein needs. The problem of balancing protein and energy needs with treatment of acidosis and excessive nitrogenous waste is complicated and delicate.

In the early stages of ARF, the patient is often moribund and is unable to eat. It has been clearly shown that early attention to nutritional status, often in the form of total parenteral nutrition (TPN) and early dialysis, have a positive impact on patient survival (Bartlett et al, 1986; Cerra, 1987).

Replacement of renal function during ARF can be carried out as standard hemodialysis, peritoneal dialysis, or *continuous arteriovenous hemofiltration (CAVH)*. CAVH uses a small ultrafiltration membrane powered by the patient's own blood to produce an ultrafiltrate that can be replaced by parenteral nutrition fluids (Feinstein, 1988; Kaplan, 1988). This allows parenteral feeding without fluid overload.

Protein. At the onset of ARF, when few patients can tolerate oral feedings because of vomiting and diarrhea, intravenous (IV) preparations have been used to reduce protein catabolism. Giving carbohydrate alone (e.g., 100 grams over a 24-hour period) only reduces protein breakdown by 50%. The preferred treatment is parenteral administration of glucose and an essential amino acid solution, such as Nephramine (McGaw Labs), Aminosyn-RF (Abbott Labs), or Aminess (Clintec) (Feinstein and Massry, 1988). This reduces the protein catabolism and urea production to a minimum until the patient can tolerate oral feeding.

Considerations regarding the amount of protein that should be given to the patient with ARF must balance the extraordinary catabolic needs of a patient in intensive care with the inability to excrete the fluid, electrolytes, and solute that this treatment requires. A large protein load necessitates frequent dialysis, often in a patient who is not hemodynamically stable, and the patient is therefore at high risk for dialysis complications. This issue is therefore quite controversial. Some authorities recommend protein intakes as low as 0.3 g/kg body weight during the initial phase of ARF; however, protein intakes from 0.5 g/kg to 1.5 g/kg have been advocated by others (Brenner and Lazarus, 1988). As the patient's overall medical status stabilizes and improves, metabolic requirements decrease, and dialysis becomes less hazardous. During this stable period prior to the return of renal function, it is generally agreed that a daily intake of 0.8 to 1.0 g/kg of ideal body weight (IBW) should be given.

Energy. Energy needs are high (approximately 50 kcal/kg IBW/day) in order to provide positive nitrogen balance under stress situations. Alternative fuel sources that will prevent the use of protein for energy production must come from a high intake of carbohydrate and fat. For patients receiving TPN, high concentrations of both carbohydrate and lipid can be administered to fulfill these needs.

In addition to the usual dietary sources of refined sweets and fats, special high-calorie, low-protein, and low-electrolyte formulas have been developed to augment the diet. Some of these supplements are Controlyte (Doyle), Polycose (Ross), Cal-Power (General Mills), and Hycal (Beecham) (see Appendix Table 33). The liquid products contain 70 to 85 kcal/oz, and the powders contain approximately 140 kcal/oz. Special recipes that are low in protein and electrolytes and extremely high in calories have been developed, and several cookbooks are listed at the end of this chapter.

Fluid and Sodium Balance. During the early (often oliguric) phase of ARF, meticulous attention to fluid status is essential. Ideally, fluid and electrolyte intake should balance net body output. With negligible urine output, significant contributions to total body output include emesis and diarrhea, body cavity drains, and

TABLE 35–2. Sample Calculation of Fluid Requirements in Acute Renal Failure

Measured urine output of previous 24 hr	−200 ml
Insensible water loss in 24 hr	−1,000 ml
(Varies with room temperature, room humidity and body temperature)	
Water loss in vomitus	−100 ml
Total water loss in 24 hr	−1,300 ml
Water produced by metabolism in 24 hr (provided catabolism and weight loss are not occurring)	−500 ml
Water requirements for 24 hr	800 ml
Water in usual diet in 24 hr	500 ml
Additional fluid intake needed in 24 hr	300 ml

skin and respiratory losses. If fever is present, skin losses can be excessive, whereas if the patient is on humidified air, almost no respiratory losses occur. Table 35–2 provides an example of the calculations of water requirements. Due to the numerous IV drugs as well as blood and blood products necessitated by the underlying disease, the challenge in managing patients at this point invariably becomes how to cut fluid intake as much as possible while providing adequate protein and energy.

Sodium is restricted depending on the level of urinary excretion. In the oliguric phase when the sodium output is very low, an attempt is made to keep intake low as well, perhaps as low as 20 to 40 mEq. However, it is often impossible to limit sodium, due to the requirement for many IV solutions (including IV antibiotics, pressors, and TPN). The administration of these solutions in electrolyte-free water, in the face of oliguria, leads quickly to water intoxication (hyponatremia). For this reason, all fluid above the daily calculated water loss should be presented in a balanced salt solution.

Potassium Balance. The majority of potassium excretion and the control of potassium balance are normal functions of the kidney. When renal function is impaired, potassium balance should be scrutinized carefully. In addition to dietary sources, all body tissues contain large amounts of potassium, thus tissue destruction can lead to tremendous overload. For this reason, potassium intake must be restricted as much as possible (30 to 50 mEq/day).

The primary mechanism of potassium removal during ARF is dialysis. Control of serum potassium levels between dialysis administrations relies mainly on IV infusions of glucose, insulin, and bicarbonate, all of which serve to drive potassium into cells.

Exchange resins, such as Kayexalate, which exchange K^+ for Na^+ in the gastrointestinal (GI) tract, can be used to treat high K^+ concentrations, but for many reasons these resins are less than ideal. The treatment is unpleasant, regardless of whether it is given orally or by retention enema. In addition, because it can gel in the GI tract causing obstruction, it must therefore be given with sorbitol, which is a nonabsorbable sugar that induces diarrhea. Administration requires a functioning GI tract, both with respect to absorption and motility, which is often not the case in the critically ill patient. Finally, the exchanged sodium leads to volume overload, which must also be controlled mainly by dialysis during renal failure. Table 35–3 summarizes nutritional care during ARF.

Other Tubular or Interstitial Diseases

A wide variety of diseases or disorders of the tubules and interstitium exist. They share common manifestations and can be considered together with respect to dietary management.

Chronic interstitial nephritis can occur as a result of analgesic abuse, sickle cell disease, diabetes mellitus, or vesicouretero reflux and manifests primarily as an inability to concentrate the urine and mild renal insufficiency. A hereditary disorder of the interstitium, *medullary cystic disease,* also presents this picture. Dietary management consists of adequate fluid intake, which can require several liters of extra fluid. This is generally quite well tolerated by the patient, except when intercurrent illness occurs.

Fanconi syndrome is characterized by an inability to reabsorb the proper amount of glucose, amino acids, phosphate, and bicarbonate in the proximal tubule, leading to excretion of these substances in the urine. Adults with this syndrome present with acidosis, hypokalemia, polyuria, or osteomalacia, whereas children present with polyuria, growth retardation rickets, or vomiting. A specific treatment is usually not available, and dietary treatment is therefore the main form of management. Replacement therapy usually consists of large volumes of water, as well as dietary supplements of bicarbonate, potassium, phosphate, calcium, and vitamin D.

Other tubular defects, generally affecting reabsorption of only a single solute, are treated with replace-

TABLE 35–3. Nutritional Care During Acute Renal Failure

Nutrient	Amount
Protein	0.5 g/kg IBW, increasing as GFR returns to normal. 80% should be HBV protein.
Energy	45–55 kcal/kg body weight.
Potassium	30–50 mEq/day in oliguric phase (depending on urinary output, dialysis and serum K^+ level); replace losses in diuretic phase.
Sodium	20–40 mEq/day in oliguric phase (depending on urinary output, edema, dialysis and serum Na^+ level); replace losses in diuretic phase.
Fluid	Replace output from the previous day (vomitus, diarrhea, urine) plus 500 ml.

GFR = glomerular filtration rate; HBV = high biologic value; IBW = ideal body weight.

ment of that particular solute. *Renal tubular acidosis* (RTA), a defect in tubular handling of bicarbonate, can either be caused by a proximal tubular defect (type 2) or by a defect in the distal tubule (type 1). The proximal lesion can be associated with other proximal defects, such as in the Fanconi syndrome, and has very little clinical significance by itself, whereas distal RTA leads to severe osteomalacia, kidney stones, and often nephrocalcinosis (calcification of the kidney). Distal RTA is treated with small amounts of bicarbonate, 70 to 100 mEq/day, with complete resolution of disease manifestations. *Isolate proximal RTA* in the adult is a benign disease, which is often made worse with bicarbonate treatment and should therefore not be treated.

Nephrolithiasis (Kidney Stones)

Kidney stones are formed when the concentration of components in the urine reaches a level in which crystallization is possible. They generally are composed of calcium salts, uric acid, cystine, or struvite (triple salt of ammonium, magnesium, and phosphate). Although, the clinical manifestations of these stones is similar, their pathogenesis and treatment differ. Several long-term follow-up studies suggest that most patients who pass a single stone will have stone recurrence (Williams et al, 1963). For this reason, most authors suggest stone analysis as well as metabolic evaluation after the first or second stone (Coe, 1981; Pak et al, 1981). Analysis of stone type is not as important as identifying and treating the underlying metabolic abnormality. Regardless of the type of stone or its cause, the encouragement of large volumes of oral fluid intake (1.5–2 l/day) to produce at least 2 l/day of urine is an essential component of effective prophylactic treatment (Office of Medical Applications . . . , 1988). The goal of rigorous hydration is to keep the urine dilute, preventing the crystallization of stone-forming minerals.

Calcium Oxalate and Calcium Phosphate Stones

Calcium oxalate and *calcium phosphate stones* account for the majority (75%) of stones and are most common in middle-aged men. Calcium oxalate stones occur most frequently. Their causes are multiple, including hyperparathyroidism, hyperuricosuria, idiopathic hypercalciuria, hypercitraturia, distal RTA, and hyperoxaluria. The primary treatment involves correction of the specific defect. This includes the removal of parathyroid adenoma for hyperparathyroidism, protein reduction, and medication with allopurinol for hyperuricosuria, protein restriction for hypercalciuria, and medication with bicarbonate and potassium for RTA.

Overproduction *hyperoxaluria* is treated with pyridoxine; however, it is not uniformly effective (Larsson and Tiselins, 1987). Another form results from gut overabsorption of oxalate, commonly seen in small intestinal diseases such as Crohn's disease, celiac sprue, intestinal bypass surgery or pancreatic insufficiency, or with excessive intakes of vitamin C (which is metabolized to oxalate). Treatment of this disorder requires adequate calcium intake (which binds oxalate) as well as a low-oxalate (40 to 50 mg) diet (Table 35–4).

Hypercalciuria (more than 200 mg of calcium in a 24-hour urine collection) may be the single most important condition underlying calcium stone formation (Zerwekh, 1987). This condition can be either *absorptive* (increased intestinal absorption of calcium), *renal* (impaired renal tubular absorption of calcium; a renal "leaker"), or *resorptive* (excessive resorption of calcium from bone due to primary hyperparathyroidism; treated with surgery). Whether the absorptive and renal conditions are two different types or simply manifestations of the same defect of $1,25(OH)_2D_3$ production is controversial (Coe, 1984; Pak et al, 1980).

If the treatment is to be effective, the type of hypercalciuria must be determined. The only situation in which a low-calcium diet is appropriate is in a subtype of the absorptive form, in which the hypercalciuria occurs only with an extremely high calcium intake (2,000 mg/day or more) (Pak et al, 1980). In this situation, dietary calcium should be limited to the RDA of 800 to 1,200 mg/day. This level is usually achieved by limiting the amount of fluid milk to 16 oz/day or less; however, dietary counseling is required to identify all sources of calcium in the patient's diet. This strikes a compromise between the possible risk of osteoporosis from inadequate calcium and the possibility of stone formation (Erickson, 1987). Cellulose phosphate is sometimes used to decrease intestinal calcium absorption. However, it also increases oxalate absorption and decreases magnesium absorption. Diets of these patients should therefore be low in oxalate and should be supplemented with magnesium.

In all other forms of hypercalciuria, a low-calcium diet is not indicated. In fact, a low-calcium diet could be detrimental in renal hypercalciuria (Wainer et al, 1987).

Patients with idiopathic hypercalciuria have been treated effectively with ample fluid intake and thiazide diuretics, which decrease urinary calcium. Maximal effectiveness of thiazides is accomplished by mildly restricting sodium intake to 4 to 5 g/day. Dramatic drops in urine calcium have been reported with more severe dietary sodium restriction (Goldfarb, 1988) (see Chapter 33).

Hyperuricosuria usually leads to the formation of calcium oxalate rather than to uric acid stones. Uric acid crystals may form a nidus on which calcium oxalate precipitates. Uric acid also encourages calcium oxalate growth by binding calcium oxalate inhibitors.

TABLE 35–4. Approximate Oxalate Content of Selected Foods*†

Foods	Little or No Oxalate (<2 mg/Serving)	Moderate Oxalate (2–10 mg/Serving)	High Oxalate Foods (>10 mg/Serving)
Beverages	Beer, bottled Carbonated cola (limit to 12 oz/day) Distilled alcohol Lemonade or limeade without peel Wine: red, rose, white	Coffee (limit to 8 oz/day)	Draft beer Ovaltine and other beverage mixes Tea Cocoa
Milk	Buttermilk Whole, low-fat, or skim milk Yogurt with allowed fruit		
Meat and substitutes	Eggs Cheese Beef, lamb, or pork Poultry Fish and shellfish	Sardines	Baked beans canned in tomato sauce Peanut butter Tofu
Vegetables	Avocado Brussels sprouts Cauliflower Cabbage Mushrooms Onions Peas, green, fresh, or frozen Potatoes, white Radishes	Asparagus Broccoli Carrots Corn: Sweet, white Sweet, yellow Cucumber, peeled Green peas, canned Lettuce Lima beans Parsnips Tomato, 1 small or juice (4 oz) Turnips	Beans: green, wax, dried Beets: tops, roots, greens Celery Chives Collards Dandelion greens Eggplant Escarole Kale Leeks Mustard greens Okra Parsley Peppers, green Pokeweed Potatoes, sweet Rutabagas Spinach Summer squash Swiss chard Watercress
Fruits/juices	Apple juice Avocado Banana Cherries, bing Grapefruit, fruit and juice Grapes, green Mangoes Melons: Cantaloupe Casaba Honeydew Watermelon Nectarines Peaches Pineapple juice Plums, green or yellow	Apple Apricots Black currants Cherries, red, sour Cranberry juice (4 oz) Grape juice (4 oz) Orange, fruit and juice (4 oz) Peaches Pears Pineapple Plums, purple Prunes	Blackberries Blueberries Currants, red Dewberries Fruit cocktail Grapes, purple Gooseberries Lemon peel Lime peel Orange peel Raspberries Rhubarb Strawberries Tangerine Juices made from the above fruits
Bread/starches	Breakfast cereals Macaroni Noodles Rice Spaghetti Bread	Cornbread Sponge cake Spaghetti, canned in tomato sauce	Fruit cake Grits, white corn Soybean crackers Wheat germ
Fats and oils	Bacon Mayonnaise Salad dressing Vegetable oils Butter, margarine		Nuts: Peanuts, almonds, pecans, cashews, walnuts

TABLE 35-4. Approximate Oxalate Content of Selected Foods*† *Continued*

Foods	Little or No Oxalate (<2 mg/Serving)	Moderate Oxalate (2-10 mg/Serving)	High Oxalate Foods (>10 mg/Serving)
Miscellaneous	Coconut Jelly or preserves (made with allowed fruits) Lemon, lime juice Salt, pepper (limit to 1 tsp/day) Soups with allowed ingredients Sugar	Chicken noodle soup, dehydrated	Chocolate, cocoa Vegetable soup Tomato soup Marmalade

* From Pemberton CM et al: Mayo Clinic Diet Manual. 6th ed. Philadelphia, BC Decker, 1988, pp 253-254.

† Considerable variation in the oxalate content of a single type of food exists. Factors such as growing conditions, age of the plant, bioavailability, and gastrointestinal abnormalities all affect individual absorption of oxalate. Therefore, the foods have been categorized into low, moderate, and high oxalate groups, rather than giving an exact value. The data available on the oxalate content of foods are limited and variable.

Hyperuricosuria is treated by limiting protein intake to the level of the RDA.

Uric Acid Stones

Uric acid stones are associated with gout and malignant disease as well as some GI diseases characterized by diarrhea. Drugs such as aspirin or probenecid can increase uric acid excretion and thus can lead to stone formation. The most important factor involved in forming uric acid stones appears to be the production of an acid urine (Coe and Favus, 1986). For this reason, the cornerstone of management of uric acid stones, in addition to fluid ingestion, involves raising the normally slightly acidic urine pH to within the range of 6.0 to 6.5. This can be accomplished with a high-alkaline ash diet, supplemented with citrate or bicarbonate (Clinical Insight, page 600). Protein may be decreased to the RDA if hyperuricosuria is extreme.

Cystinine Stones

Cystinine stones, caused by a rare hereditary disorder of amino acid transport, represent a rare and exceedingly difficult management problem. Treatment consists of extremely high oral intakes of fluid (>4 l/day). The patient should be encouraged to get up during the night to drink. In addition, an alkaline ash diet and alkaline therapy are needed to raise the urinary pH to 7.5. If these measures alone do not control stone formation, the addition of penicillamine has been beneficial but has significant risks for serious systemic side effects. Cystinine stones usually cause relentless, progressive renal destruction.

Struvite Stones

Struvite stones, containing ammonium, magnesium, and phosphate, are usually seen in women. They are formed when the urinary tract is infected with urease-splitting organisms. These organisms, most commonly *Proteus* or *Klebsiella,* produce high concentrations of ammonium upon cleavage of urea. Large stones typically lodge in the renal pelvis, forming staghorn calculi (Fig. 35-3). Recurrent pyelonephritis and progressive renal failure usually develop with eventual obstruction. Treatment consists of long-term effective antibiotics as well as surgical or ultrasonic removal of stones. Dietary management has no significant role in this form of stone disease.

PROGRESSIVE NATURE OF RENAL DISEASE

A wide range of kidney lesions are characterized by a slow steady decline in renal function. A number of the diseases discussed earlier lead to renal failure in some patients, whereas other patients have a benign course without loss of renal function. The factors involved in

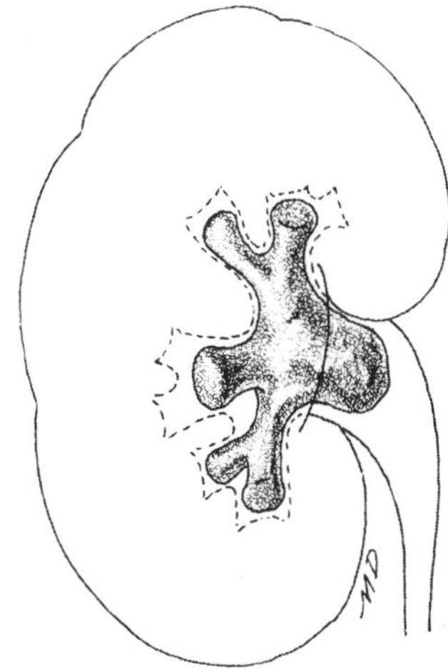

FIGURE 35-3. *Staghorn calculus. (From Luckmann J and Sorensen KC: Medical-Surgical Nursing, 3rd ed. Philadelphia, WB Saunders, 1987, p 1209.)*

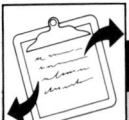

CLINICAL INSIGHT: "Acid Ash" and "Alkaline Ash" Diets

Dietary intake influences the acidity or alkalinity of the urine (Sherman and Gettler, 1912). The acid-forming potential is contributed by chloride, phosphorus, and sulfur (anions) and the base-forming potential by sodium, potassium, calcium, and magnesium (cations). In general, fruits and vegetables contribute alkaline "ash" to the urine, except in the case of prunes, plums, and cranberries. These fruits contain benzoic and quinic acids that are excreted in the urine as hippuric acid. However, the effectiveness of these foods, particularly cranberry juice, as urine acidifiers is poorly established (Soloway and Smith, 1988).

High-protein foods (meat, fish, poultry, eggs, and cheese), and breads and cereals are the primary contributors of acid "ash." Milk contributes to both categories. However, because factors of digestion, absorption, use of salt or medications, hormonal status, and homeostatic mechanisms all affect renal excretion and urine production, urine pH cannot be predicted by calculation of intake. Such information can be obtained only by direct measurement of the urine (Dwyer et al, 1985).

The following food lists serve as a guide to influencing urine pH. They are usually used to supplement the effect of medication in altering urine pH; therefore, it may be sufficient to avoid excessive use of particular foods rather than to avoid them completely.

Potentially Acid or Acid-Ash Foods*	
Meat	Meat, fish, fowl, shellfish, eggs, all types of cheese, peanut butter, peanuts
Fat	Bacon, nuts (Brazil nuts, filberts, walnuts)
Starch	All types of bread (especially whole wheat), cereal, crackers, macaroni, spaghetti, noodles, rice
Vegetable	Corn, lentils
Fruit	Cranberries, plums, prunes
Desserts	Plain cakes, cookies
Potentially Basic or Alkaline-Ash Foods	
Milk	Milk and milk products, cream, buttermilk
Fat	Nuts (almonds, chestnuts, coconut)
Vegetables	All types (except corn, lentils), especially beets, beet greens, Swiss chard, dandelion greens, kale, mustard greens, spinach, turnip greens
Fruit	All types (except cranberries, prunes, plums)
Sweets	Molasses
Neutral Foods	
Fats	Butter, margarine, cooking fats, oils
Sweets	Plain candies, sugar, syrup, honey
Starch	Arrowroot, corn, tapioca
Beverages	Coffee, tea

* Adapted from Pemberton CM et al: Mayo Clinic Diet Manual, 6th ed. Toronto, BC Decker, 1988, p 256.

producing a benign disease in one patient and renal failure in another patient are not clear. However, it has been recognized in all kidney diseases that once approximately three quarters of kidney function has been lost, regardless of the underlying disease, progressive further loss of kidney function ensues. This is true even in diseases in which the underlying cause has been eliminated completely, such as in vesicoureteral reflux, cortical necrosis of pregnancy, or analgesic abuse. The nature of this progressive loss of function has been the subject of an enormous amount of basic and clinical research during the past decade and has also been the subject of several excellent reviews (Brenner, 1983; Klahr et al, 1988).

It is currently believed that in response to a decreasing GFR, the kidney undergoes a series of adaptations in order to prevent this decrease. Although in the short term this leads to improvement in filtration rate, in the long term it leads to an accelerated loss of nephrons and to progressive renal insufficiency. The nature of these adaptations involves a change in the hemodynamic characteristics of the remaining glomeruli, specifically leading to increased glomerular pressure. Factors that increase glomerular pressure tend to accelerate this process, whereas factors that decrease glomerular pressure tend to alleviate it.

The role of dietary protein has been championed as a factor that increases glomerular pressure and thus leads to accelerated loss of renal function (Brenner and Lazarus, 1988). Numerous studies in experimental models of moderate renal insufficiency demonstrate a significant decline in this process upon protein restriction. Clinical studies appear to corroborate the experimental models, demonstrating a role for protein restriction in the management of patients with mild to moderate renal insufficiency, for the purpose of preserving renal function (Evanoff et al, 1987; Giordano, 1981; Ihle et al, 1989; Maschio et al, 1982). Whereas it must be pointed out that these clinical studies are small, often retrospective, and uncontrolled, the bulk of scientific evidence favors such a role. A large multicenter trial, Modification of Diet in Renal Disease, is underway to determine the role of both protein and phosphorous restriction (Klahr, 1989).

Most studies have demonstrated a beneficial effect using dietary protein intakes of 0.4 to 0.6 g/kg IBW or have supplemented lower protein intakes with essential amino acids or ketoacids. At least 75% of the protein intake in such a diet should be HBV protein to ensure that the essential amino acid requirements are met. It must be pointed out that systemic hypertension, another factor that mitigates the progressive loss of renal function, must be well controlled in order to see benefits from protein restriction.

Long before evidence regarding the role of protein restriction in halting the progression of renal failure was known, this dietary maneuver was carried out in order to decrease the amount of nitrogenous waste produced. It has long been demonstrated that this maneuver decreases the symptoms of uremia. Prior to the age of dialysis, this was paramount in the management of patients with renal failure (Addis, 1948).

The potential benefits of protein restriction in the patient with moderate renal insufficiency must be weighed against the potential hazards of such treatment, namely protein malnutrition. Much controversy still remains, based mainly on this consideration (Jamison, 1983). If protein restriction is elected, careful monitoring, including urea generation rate, and anthropomorphic studies should be carried out periodically.

END-STAGE RENAL DISEASE

ESRD can result from a wide variety of different kidney diseases. Currently, 90% of patients reaching ESRD had either (1) diabetes mellitus, (2) glomerulonephritis, or (3) hypertension. With ESRD comes a myriad of problems related to the kidney's inability to excrete waste products, maintain fluid and electrolyte balance, and produce hormones. As renal failure slowly progresses, a point is reached at which the level of circulating waste products leads to symptoms of uremia.

Uremia is defined as the clinical syndrome of malaise, weakness, nausea and vomiting, muscle cramps and itching, metallic taste in the mouth, and often neurologic impairment that is brought about by an unacceptable level of nitrogenous wastes. The manifestations are somewhat nonspecific and vary from one patient to another. There is no reliable laboratory parameter that corresponds directly with the beginning of symptoms. However, as a rule of thumb a blood urea nitrogen (BUN) above 100 and a creatinine of 10 to 12 are usually quite close to this threshold.

Medical Treatment

Treatment of ESRD requires either transplantation or dialysis.

Transplantation

Transplantation involves the surgical implantation of a kidney from a living related donor or from a cadaver. Rejection of the foreign tissue is a major complication. Currently, patients awaiting transplantation by far outnumber the number of donated kidneys available.

NUTRITIONAL CARE. The nutritional care of the adult patient who has received a transplanted kidney is based mainly on the metabolic effects of the required immunosuppressive therapy. Corticosteroids are associated with accelerated protein catabolism, hyperlipidemia, sodium retention, weight gain, glucose intolerance, and inhibition of normal calcium, phosphorus, and vitamin D metabolism. Cyclosporine therapy is associated with hyperkalemia, hypertension, and hyperlipidemia. The doses of these medications used after transplantation are decreased over time until a "maintenance level" is reached.

During the first month after transplantation, and during high-dose steroid therapy used for acute rejection episodes, a high-protein diet (1.5 to 2 g/kg body weight) with an energy intake of 30 to 35 kcal/kg is recommended to prevent negative nitrogen balance. A moderate sodium restriction (80 to 100 mEq) during this period minimizes fluid retention and helps to control blood pressure. After this time, protein intake can be decreased to 1 g/kg, and calorie intake should be at a level sufficient to achieve and maintain an appropriate weight for height. Sodium intakes are individualized based on fluid retention and blood pressure.

In patients exhibiting glucose intolerance, limitation of simple carbohydrates is appropriate. Hyperkalemia, commonly associated with cyclosporine therapy, warrants dietary potassium restriction, although this is usually only temporary. Following transplantation, many patients exhibit hypophosphatemia and mild hypercalcemia (due to bone resorption) associated with persistent hyperparathyroidism and the effects of steroids on calcium, phosphorus, and vitamin D metabolism. The diet should contain adequate amounts of calcium and phosphorus (1,200 mg of each daily), and serum levels should be monitored periodically. Supplemental phosphorus may be necessary to correct hypophosphatemia.

The majority of transplant recipients have elevated serum triglycerides or cholesterol, or both. The etiology of this hyperlipidemia is multifactorial, and it is unclear whether treatment should be given and if so what treatment (Morris, 1988). Intervention consists of calorie restriction for those who are overweight, limiting cholesterol intake to less than 300 mg/day, limiting total fat (see Chapter 20) and simple carbohydrates and maintaining a regular moderate exercise regimen (Hunsicker, 1988).

Dialysis

Dialysis can be accomplished either by hemodialysis or by peritoneal dialysis. The most common method is *hemodialysis*, in which blood passes by the semipermeable membrane of the artificial kidney and waste products are removed by diffusion.

Hemodialysis. Hemodialysis requires a permanent access to the blood stream through a fistula created by surgery to connect an artery and a vein. Fistulas are often made near the wrist, causing the forearm veins to become greatly enlarged. Large needles are inserted into the fistula prior to each dialysis and are removed when dialysis is complete (Fig. 35–4).

The dialysis fluid is similar to that of normal plasma. Waste products and electrolytes move by osmosis from the blood into the dialysate and are removed. Hemodialysis usually requires 4 to 6 hours three times per week. Dietary protein needs are about 1 g/kg to make up for some losses through dialysate (see Table 35–5).

Peritoneal Dialysis. *Peritoneal dialysis* makes use of the semipermeable membrane of the peritoneum. A catheter is surgically implanted in the abdomen and into the peritoneal cavity, as shown in Figure 35–5. Dialysate containing a high-dextrose concentration is instilled into the peritoneum, where diffusion carries waste products from the blood through the peritoneal membrane and into the dialysate. This fluid is then withdrawn and discarded, and new solution is added.

Peritoneal dialysis is a less efficient method of removing waste products from the blood. Treatments usually last longer than hemodialysis, about 10 to 12 hr/day, three times per week. Patients with peritoneal dialysis have higher protein needs (about 1.2 to 1.5 g/kg of protein) because of greater protein losses.

Continuous ambulatory peritoneal dialysis (CAPD) is similar to peritoneal dialysis, except that the dialysate is left in the peritoneum and is exchanged manually so that no machine is required. Exchanges of dialysis fluid are done four to five times daily, making it a 24-hour treatment. Protein losses are similar to those from regular peritoneal dialysis. Advantages of this form of treatment are avoidance of large fluctuations in blood chemistry and the ability of the patient to achieve a somewhat more normal lifestyle.

Patients with CAPD are on more liberal fluid, sodium, and potassium allowances because the therapy is continuous and more of these products are removed. The loss of sodium can be as much as 6 g/day, thus these patients may need higher sodium intakes as shown in Table 35–5. Complications associated with CAPD include peritonitis, hypotension requiring additional fluid and sodium replacement, and weight gain. The weight gain is experienced by most patients with CAPD as a result of absorbing 600 to 800 calories/day from the glucose dialysate. This may be desirable in

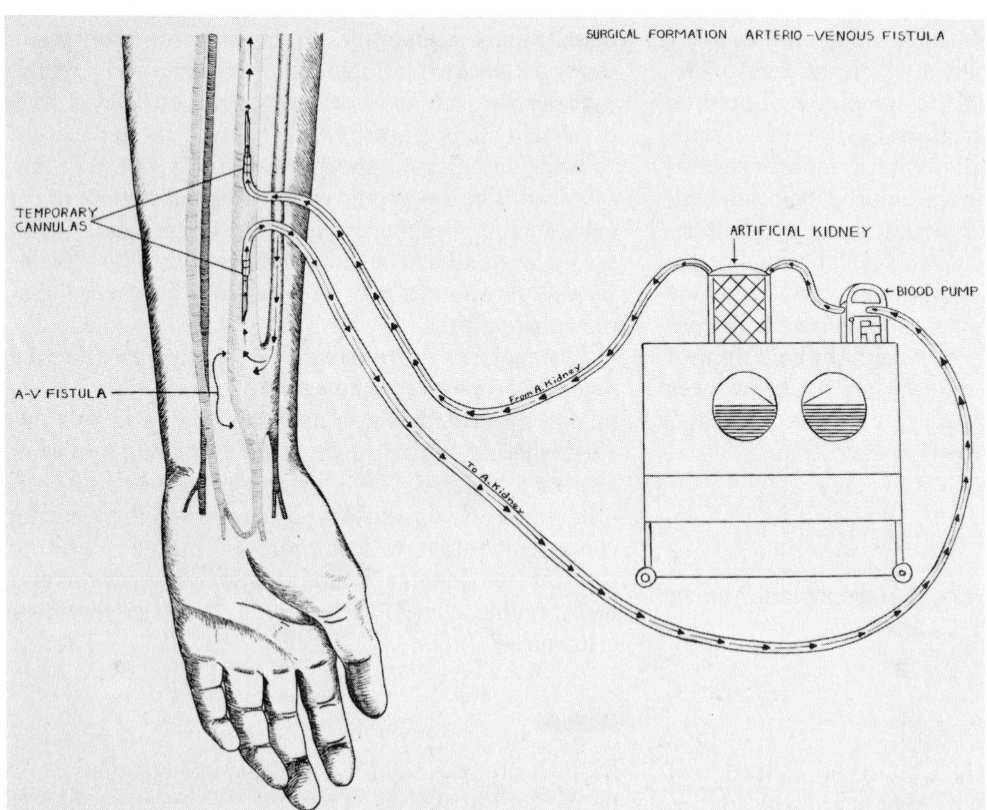

FIGURE 35–4. *Arteriovenous fistula with temporary cannulas in place and blood circulating to and from the artificial kidney.* Arrows *show the direction of blood flow. (Photograph courtesy of Northwest Kidney Center, Seattle, Washington.)*

TABLE 35–5. Nutrient Requirements for Adults with Renal Disease Based on Type of Therapy

Therapy	Energy	Protein	Fluid	Sodium	Potassium	Phosphorus
Impaired renal function (predialysis)	40–50 kcal/kg IBW*	0.6 g/kg IBW	Ad libitum	Variable, 2–3 g/day	Variable, usually ad lib. or increased to cover losses with diuretics	1–1.2 g/day
Hemodialysis	35 kcal/kg IBW	1 gm/kg IBW (1.2–1.5 g/kg for repletion)	750 ml/day + urine output	2–3 g/day	2–3 g/day	1–1.2 g/day
Intermittent peritoneal dialysis (IPD)	30 kcal/kg IBW (40–50 kcal/kg for repletion)	1.2 g/kg IBW (1.5 g/kg for repletion)	750 ml/day + urine output	2–3 g/day	2–3 g/day	1–1.2 g/day
Continuous ambulatory peritoneal dialysis (CAPD)	25 kcal/kg IBW (40–50 kcal/kg for repletion)	1.2 g/kg IBW (1.5 g/kg for repletion)	Ad libitum (minimum of 2,000 ml/day + urine output)	6–8 g/day	3–4 g/day	1.5–2 g/day
Diabetic on hemodialysis, IPD, or CAPD	35 kcal/kg IBW (40–50 kcal/kg for repletion)	1.5 g/kg IBW	Same as for hemodialysis, IPD, or CAPD. Monitor thirst, blood sugar, and weight changes		Same as for hemodialysis, IPD, or CAPD. (Increased blood sugar may cause increased potassium)	1–1.2 g/day (Often liberalized due to other restrictions)
Transplant 4 to 6 weeks after transplant	30–35 kcal/kg IBW	1.5–2 g/kg IBW	Ad libitum	Variable	Variable; may require restriction with cyclosporine-induced hyperkalemia	1.2 g/day Calcium 1.2 g/day
6 weeks or longer after transplant Carbohydrate—limit simple carbohydrate Fat less than 35% of calories Cholesterol no more than 400 mg/day Polyunsaturated/saturated fat ratio of greater than 1.0.	To achieve/maintain IBW	1 g/kg IBW	Ad libitum	Variable	Variable	Calcium 1.2 g/day

* IBW = ideal body weight.

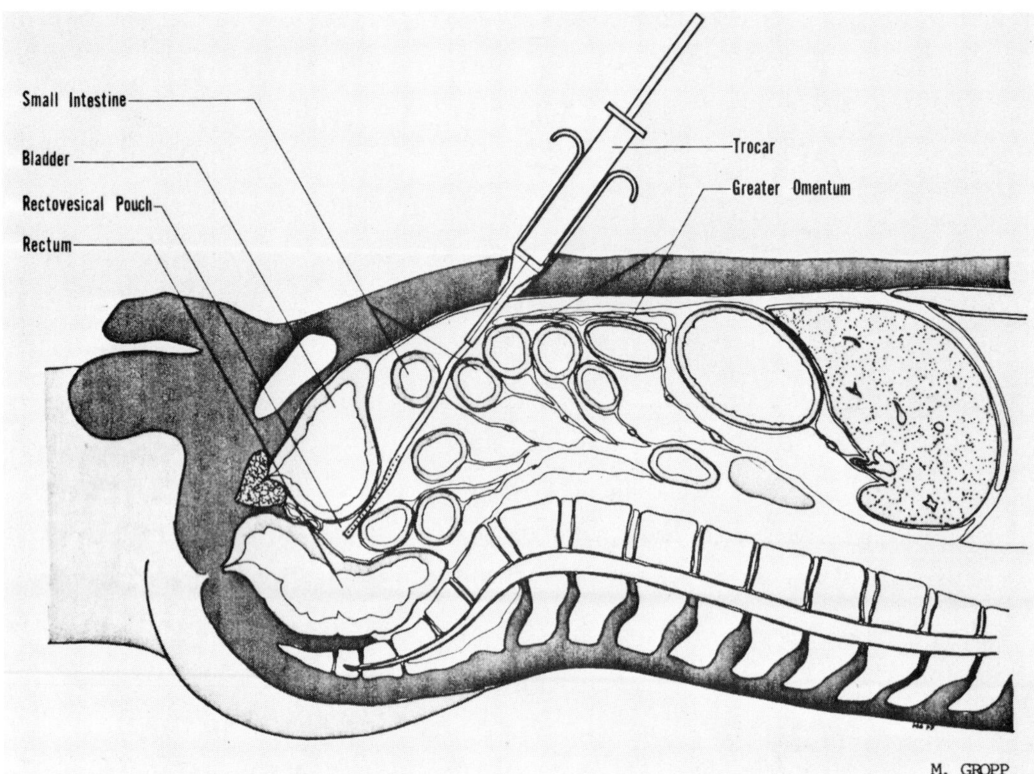

FIGURE 35–5. *Catheter position for peritoneal dialysis. (Adapted from Shapter RK and Yonkman FK: The kidneys, ureters, and urinary bladder. CIBA 1973.)*

patients who are underweight, but eventually dietary intake may have to be modified to account for energy absorbed from dialysate.

Psychologic Support

Patients with renal failure must deal not only with conflicting feelings about being dependent on artificial means of elimination, but also with changes in the quality of their lives and the necessity for adapting to a chronic, progressive illness. Control becomes a central issue, as they must devote large quantities of time to dialysis, follow fairly strict dietary limitations (Fig. 35–6), and often take several medications. Those who work with renal dialysis patients must be especially empathetic to their feelings of thirst, anorexia when faced with eating, and taste changes due to uremia.

Nutritional Care

The goals of nutritional care in the management of ESRD are:

1. To prevent deficiency and maintain good nutritional status (and growth, in the case of children) through adequate protein, energy, vitamin, and mineral intake.
2. To control edema and electrolyte imbalance by controlling sodium, potassium, and fluid intake.
3. To prevent or retard the development of renal osteodystrophy by controlling calcium, phosphorus, and vitamin D intake.
4. To enable the patient to eat a palatable attractive diet that fits his or her lifestyle as much as possible.

Even with the development of dialysis methods and transplantation techniques, nutritional care remains essential to enhance dialysis, maintain optimal nutritional status, and prevent complications.

Because treatment is on an outpatient basis or dialysis is done at home, patients with ESRD assume responsibility for their diet. Most patients know their diets very well, having been instructed by a dietitian prior to each hospital discharge. However, the patient facing long-term compliance with a difficult diet regimen is assisted by periodic professional counseling. Monitoring the patient's long-term nutritional status is an important role of the dietitian. Table 35–6 presents a guide for teaching patients about their blood values and control of their disease.

Fluid and Sodium Balance

The ability of the kidney to handle sodium and water in ESRD changes must be assessed frequently through measurement of urinary sodium excretion, blood pressure, presence of edema, serum sodium level, and dietary intake. The diet and fluid intake are then modified accordingly.

Although sodium is retained by most patients with ESRD, it may be lost by others. Examples of diseases with a salt-losing tendency are polycystic disease of the kidney, chronic obstructive uropathy, chronic pyelonephritis, and analgesic nephropathy. To prevent hypotension, hypovolemia, cramps, and further deterioration of renal function, extra sodium may be required. Measurement of urinary sodium in patients receiving a known amount of sodium should be made several times to assess the extent of losses.

The diet should be matched to the urinary sodium and fluid excretion. Usually, this is 130 mEq (3 grams) or higher of sodium per day, which is the amount in a normal diet without added salt. Needs for extra sodium

RENAL DIET

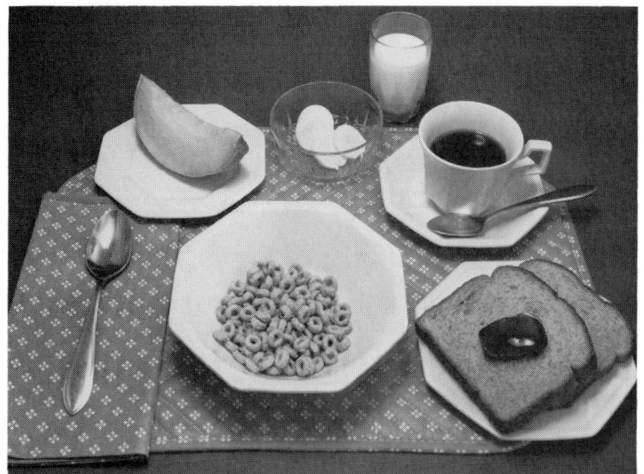

BREAKFAST

Slice of cantaloupe
¾ c dry cereal
2 slices whole-wheat toast
1 tsp jelly
1 hardboiled egg
5 oz coffee
2 tsp sugar
½ c nondairy creamer

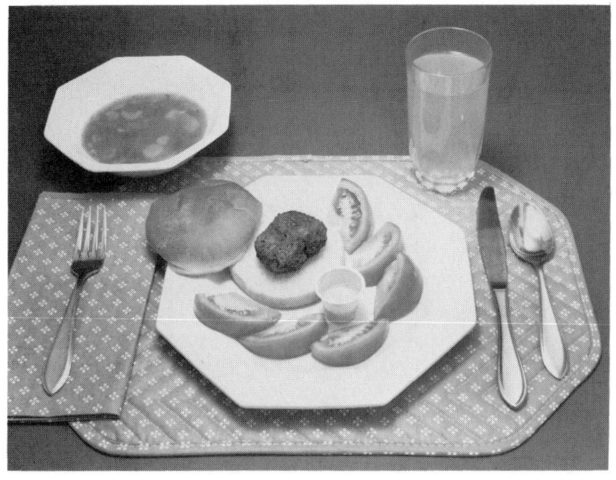

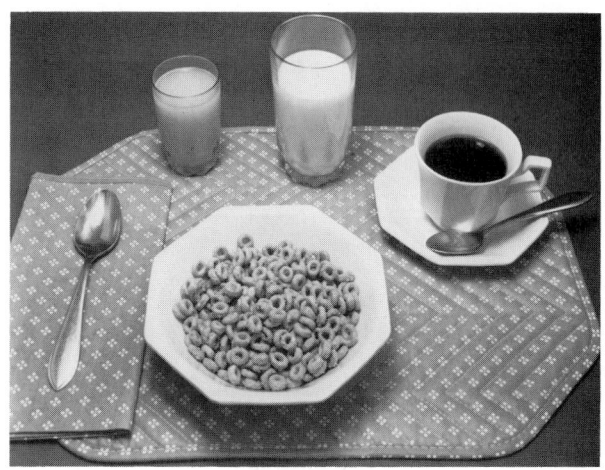

LUNCH

⅔ c low-sodium vegetable soup
2 oz lean hamburger on bun
1 medium-sliced tomato
1 tsp salt-free thousand island dressing
8 oz glass lemonade

STANDARD AMERICAN DIET

BREAKFAST

1½ c Cheerios
¾ c orange juice
1 c 2% milk
5 oz coffee

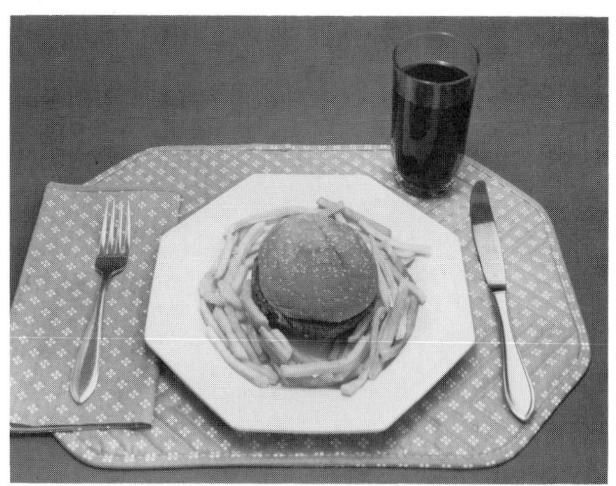

LUNCH

1 quarter-pound cheeseburger, lettuce, tomatoes
French fries
8 oz diet soda

FIGURE 35–6. *A typical menu for a renal diet compared to a menu typical of a US diet.*

RENAL DIET

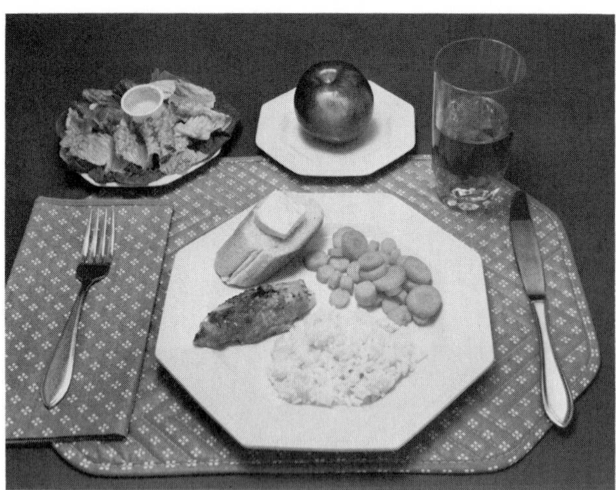

DINNER

2 oz broiled chicken
½ c white rice
½ c carrots
1 slice French bread
3 tsp margarine
1 c green salad
1 tsp vinegar and oil dressing
1 baked apple, 4 tsp sugar
1 c ginger ale

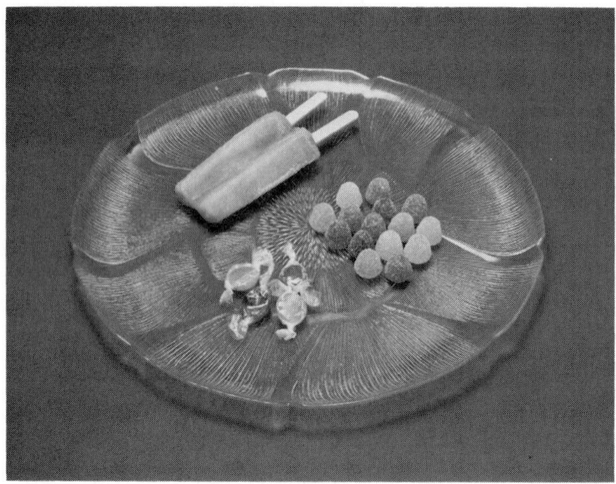

SNACKS

4 pieces hard candy
15 gum drops
1 3-oz popsicle

STANDARD AMERICAN DIET

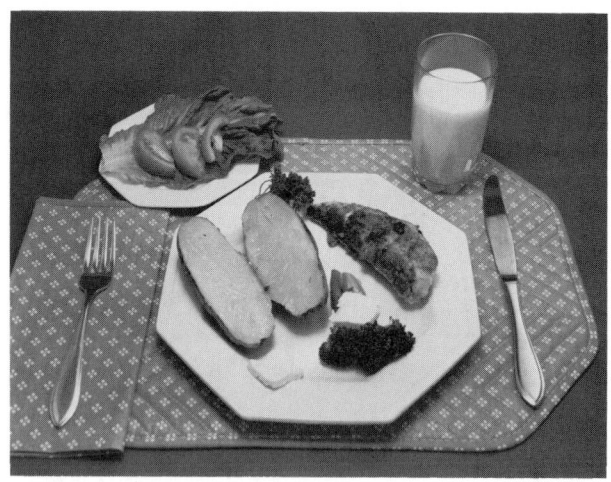

DINNER

1 baked potato, 1 tsp margarine
1 broiled chicken breast (4 oz after cooking)
1½ c 2% milk
½ c broccoli, margarine
2 c salad (lettuce, tomatoes, 2 T creamy dressing)

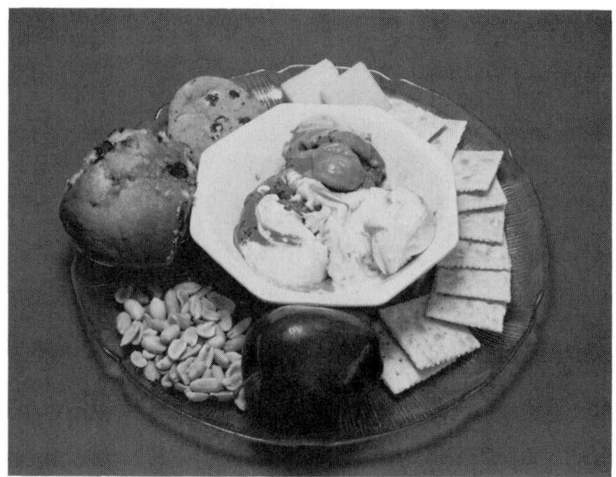

SNACKS

1 large blueberry muffin
Coffee
8 oz 2% milk
1 cookie
10 saltines
1 apple
2 oz cheese
1¼ c ice cream
¼ c peanuts

FIGURE 35–6 *Continued*

TABLE 35–6. Dialysis Patient's Guide to Blood Values*

This guide is to help in the understanding of lab reports. The normal values are for people with good kidney function. Acceptable values for dialysis patients are given in the next column. Blood values should fall within the range for dialysis patients. Many things affect blood values and diet is one of these. Understanding blood chemistry will help diet control.

Blood Test	Normal Values	Values for Dialysis Patients	Function	Diet Changes
Sodium	136–145 mEq/l	Same	Found in salt and many preserved foods. A diet high in sodium will make you thirsty. When you drink too much fluid, it may dilute the sodium and it will look low. If you eat too much sodium and do not drink water, it may be high. Always check your weight gains against your sodium value.	High: Eat less salt and salty foods. Make sure you are gaining about 1.5 kg between dialyses and are not dehydrated. Low: Probably drinking too much fluid. Limit weight gains to 1.5 kg between dialyses. Eat less salt and fewer salty foods.
Potassium	3.5–5.5 mEq/l	Same	Found in most high-protein foods, fruits, and vegetables. It affects muscle action, especially the heart. High levels can cause your heart to stop. Low levels can also cause symptoms, such as weakness.	High: Avoid foods with over 250 mg of potassium per serving and limit daily intake to 2,000 mg. Consult a dietitian. Low: Add one 250-mg potassium food per day and recheck blood level.
Chloride	97–108 mEq/l	Same	Usually associated with amount of sodium in the blood.	No dietary changes.
Total CO_2	23–30 mEq/l	Lower than normal	Total carbon dioxide is a measure of how acidic your blood is. Your kidneys normally keep this normal. When they fail, your blood becomes more acidic, and your CO_2 is lower.	No dietary changes.
Creatinine	0.7–1.5 mg/dl	10–15 mg/dl	A normal waste product of muscle breakdown. This value is controlled by dialysis. You have a higher amount because the artificial kidney is not working all the time like the normal kidney does.	No dietary changes; normal dialysis controls creatinine.
Glucose	60–125 mg/dl	Same (higher for diabetic)	This sugar in the blood is made from the food that you eat, especially the starches and sugars. The body uses glucose for energy. For diabetics: a high blood sugar can make you thirsty; be sure to follow diet.	You need a *minimum* of 4 servings of breads/starches or cereals and 2–3 servings of fruit to provide energy. For diabetics: Avoid concentrated sweets unless your blood sugar is low.
Calcium	8.5–10.5 mg/dl	8.5–11 mg/dl	Found in dairy products, meats, and green vegetables. It is used by the body to make bone and help muscle movement. It is closely related to phosphorus; vitamin D is needed for its absorption. Calcium and phosphorus are 2 minerals needed for strong bones. They have a "see-saw" relationship, thus when phosphorus is up, calcium is down. The ratio should be kept within normal for strong bones.	High: Eat fewer milk products. Check with a doctor if you are taking calcium supplement like Tums or vitamin D (DHT or Rocaltrol). Low: Increase calcium in diet (if phosphorus is normal) by adding more milk products. You may need a calcium supplement like Tums or vitamin D. Check with your doctor before taking.
Phosphorus	2.3–4.3 mg/dl	Same	Found in milk products, dried beans, peas, nuts, and meat. It is also used to build bones.	High: Limit milk and milk products to 1 serving per day. Take phosphate binders as prescribed. Low: Add 1 serving milk product or other high-phosphorus food per day.

Table continued on following page

TABLE 35–6. Dialysis Patient's Guide to Blood Values* *Continued*

This guide is to help in the understanding of lab reports. The normal values are for people with good kidney function. Acceptable values for dialysis patients are given in the next column. Blood values should fall within the range for dialysis patients. Many things affect blood values and diet is one of these. Understanding blood chemistry will help diet control.

Blood Test	Normal Values	Values for Dialysis Patients	Function	Diet Changes
BUN	4–22 mg/dl	Less than 100 mg/dl	Waste product of protein breakdown. Unlike creatinine, this is affected by the amount of protein in your diet. Dialysis removes urea nitrogen.	High: Limit intake of meat, fish, chicken, and dairy products to about 3 servings per day and contact the dietitian. Low: May be low if you are not eating and are losing weight. May also increase with loss of muscle. Contact the dietitian.
Uric acid	4.0–8.5 mg/dl	Same	A waste product of purine. A high level may be related to symptoms of gout. Purines are found in a variety of foods.	No dietary changes. Since purines are found in most foods, you would have to stop eating! If you have gout, your doctor can prescribe a medicine to lower it.
Alk Phos	30–115 IU/l	Same	Found in normal bone. Released from bone when calcium is being removed.	Keep calcium and phosphorus within normal range.
LDH SGOT	80–220 IU/l 0–41 IU/l	Same Same	Enzymes released when tissue is damaged. Increased in infection, heart problems, liver damage, and damage of any tissue.	No dietary changes.
Cholesterol	150–240 mg/dl	Often lower	Found in high-fat foods from animal sources (e.g., meat, milk, eggs). Your body can also make its own if there is not enough in your diet. Within normal levels, cholesterol is not harmful.	Usually no dietary changes are necessary.
Total protein Albumin	6.0–8.2 g/dl 3.5–5.0 g/dl	Same Same	Proteins make up all body cells. Albumin is a type of protein. Both are needed by the body. Protein is lost with dialysis. Peritoneal dialysis protein loss is much more than hemodialysis, so you need even more protein. If albumin is low, fluid will "leak" from blood vessels into tissue, causing edema. When fluid is in the tissue, it is more difficult to remove with dialysis.	Low: Increase intake of protein-rich foods: meat, fish, chicken, eggs. Ask your dietitian for high-protein recipes.
HCT	35–45%	Usually lower	This is the percentage of red blood cells in the blood. Red blood cells carry oxygen to the cells. Everyone's value is different; learn what is normal for you.	If hematocrit is dropping, check with your doctor.
Serum ferritin	15–200 μg/l (men) 12–150 μg/l (women)	Same Same	Ferritin is the form of iron stored in the liver. If iron stores are low, you cannot make new red blood cells.	Iron in food is not well enough absorbed. Ask your doctor about an iron supplement. Do not take iron with your phosphate binders.
Hepatitis B surface antigen (hepatitis)	Negative		A protein in your body if you have serum hepatitis, a liver disease.	No dietary changes.

* Developed by Linda Peterson, R.N., and Katy Wilkens, R.D., Northwest Kidney Center, Seattle, Washington.
Alk Phos = alkaline phosphatase; BUN = blood urea nitrogen; HCT = hematocrit; LDH = lactic dehydrogenase; SGOT = serum glutamic oxaloacetic transaminase.

can be met by adding salt or salty foods, such as bouillon (one cube contains 20 mEq of sodium). Patients with hypertension and edema may need to restrict intakes of sodium and fluids. Because solid foods in the average diet contribute approximately 500 to 800 ml of fluid, these foods will replace the 500 ml of net insensible water loss (insensible water loss of 1,000 ml offset by water of metabolism of 500 ml) as shown in Table 35–2. Additional fluid is given to replace urinary loss.

Fluid and sodium requirements can increase in the presence of perspiration, vomiting, or fever. Hypotension and the possibility of clotting at the shunt site must be avoided by scrupulous attention to fluid and sodium intake.

In the *anuric* (without urine) patient who is maintained with dialysis, sodium intake and fluid intake are regulated to allow for a weight gain from increased fluid in the vasculature of 4 to 5 lb (2 to 3 kg) between dialyses. This means a sodium intake of 130 mEq (3 grams) per day and a fluid intake of 1,000 ml/day plus the amount equal to the urine output. A 130-mEq sodium diet allows for light salting of foods during cooking but no additional salt at the table and no salted, smoked, or cured meat or fish; salted snack foods; bouillon and canned soups; or foods canned in brine. Chapter 33 gives the details of the 130-mEq (3 grams) sodium diet plan.

When educating about fluid balance, the health care provider must teach the patient how to deal with thirst without drinking. Sucking on a few ice chips, cold sliced fruit, or sour candies; using a spray mouth wash; or chewing "sports gum" containing citric acid may help to alleviate the dryness.

Patients must be taught to measure their fluid intake and urine output, examine their ankles for edema, weigh themselves regularly each morning, and record their weight. Occasionally (in about 15 to 20% of patients), hypertension is not alleviated even after meticulous attention is paid to fluid and water balance. In these cases, hypertension is usually perpetuated by a high level of renin secretion and requires medication for control.

Potassium

Potassium usually requires restriction, depending on the individual's body size, the 24-hour urinary potassium excretion, the serum K^+ level, and the frequency of dialysis. High intakes are not tolerated with less frequent dialysis. The daily intake of potassium for most Americans is 75 to 100 mEq (3 to 4 grams). This is usually reduced in ESRD to 40 to 65 mEq (1.5 to 2.5 grams) per day and is reduced for the anuric patient on dialysis to 51 mEq (2 grams). The potassium content of foods is listed in Appendix Table 1. The exchange lists in Table 35–7 show the potassium content for groups of food.

Protein

Dialysis is a drain on body protein, and the daily intake should be increased to compensate. Losses of 20 to 30 grams of protein can occur during a 24-hour peritoneal dialysis, with an average of 1 g/hr. Hourly losses in hemodialysis are similar. Patients receiving peritoneal dialysis three times per week or continuous ambulatory dialysis require a daily protein intake of at least 1.2 to 1.5 g/kg body weight. Those receiving hemodialysis three times per week should have 1 g/kg body weight. Protein requirements for patients on different types of dialysis are summarized in Table 35–5. Serum BUN and serum creatinine levels, uremic symptoms, and

TABLE 35–7. Exchange Lists for Diets Controlled for Protein, Sodium and Potassium

Food	Protein (g)	Kcal	Sodium (mEq)		Potassium (mEq)
			Unsalted	*Salted*	
Meat and meat substitutes	7	75	1.0	3.0	2.5
Milk and milk products	4	Varies	2.5	2.5	4.0
Starches	3	70	0.5	8.0	1.5
Starchy vegetables	3	70	0.5	8.0	Varies
Vegetables					
Moderate potassium	2	20	0.5	12.0	4.0
Higher potassium	2	20	0.5	12.0	7.0
Fruit					
Low potassium	0.5	60	—	—	2.0
Moderate potassium	0.5	60	—	—	4.0
High potassium	0.5	60	—	—	7.0
Low-protein products	0.2	100	0.5	0.5	—
Fats and oils	—	35	—	2	—
CHO supplements	—	100	—	—	—
Beverages	—	Varies	—	—	Varies

Table continued on following page

TABLE 35–7. Exchange Lists for Diets Controlled for Protein, Sodium and Potassium *Continued*

Meat and Meat Substitutes

Each exchange contains approximately 7 g protein and 2.5 mEq potassium. The sodium content varies. Portion sizes refer to cooked weights.

Unsalted: 1 mEq sodium	
1 oz	Beef, lamb, pork, or veal
1 oz	Poultry
1 oz	Fish: any fresh or frozen
¼ cup	Salmon or tuna, fresh or unsalted, waterpacked
1 oz	Unsalted cheese
2 Tbsp	Unsalted peanut butter* (limit to 1 serving daily)
Salted: 3 mEq sodium	
1	Egg (no salt added)
¼ cup	Egg substitute (no salt added)
1 oz	Lightly salted meat, fish, poultry (¼ tsp salt per pound)
1 oz	Liver, heart, kidneys
2 oz (⅓ cup)	Clams, crab, lobster
3 oz (6 medium)	Oysters
2 oz (5 medium)	Shrimp
1 oz	Swiss cheese†
High sodium: 8 mEq sodium	
¼ cup	Cottage cheese†
1 oz	Cheese†: brick, cheddar, colby, mozzarella
2 Tbsp	Regular peanut butter* (limit to 1 serving per day)

* Contains 6 mEq potassium and is low biologic value protein
† Contains 1 mEq potassium

Milk and Milk Products

Each exchange contains approximately 4 g protein, 2.5 mEq sodium, and 4 mEq potassium.

½ cup	Skim, 2%, or whole milk
½ cup	Half and half
¼ cup	Evaporated milk
2 Tbsp	Nonfat dry milk (before adding liquid)
⅔ cup	Whipping cream, light
¾ cup	Whipping cream, heavy
½ cup	Yogurt (plain)

Desserts (made with milk)

The following milk products contain additional carbohydrate. Omit one-half serving of carbohydrate supplement in addition to one serving of milk for diabetic patients.

⅓ cup	Custard
½ cup	Pudding
¼ cup	Bread pudding
¾ cup	Ice cream*
⅔ cup	Ice milk*
½ cup	Frozen yogurt dessert*
½ cup	Yogurt (flavored)
½ cup	Chocolate milk*

* These foods to be included in fluid allowance

Starch

Each exchange contains approximately 3 g of protein and 1.5 mEq of potassium unless otherwise specified. Sodium content is indicated.

Unsalted: less than 1 mEq sodium (average 0.5 mEq)	
Bread	
1 slice	Unsalted bread
1	Tortilla, 6-in diameter
Cereal	
¾ cup	Corn flakes, unsalted
1½ cups	Puffed wheat or rice, unsalted, unsweetened

TABLE 35–7. Exchange Lists for Diets Controlled for Protein, Sodium and Potassium *Continued*

***Starch** Continued*	
***Unsalted** Continued*	
1 biscuit	Shredded wheat, unsalted
½ cup	Cooked cereal, no salt
½ cup	Grits (cooked, no salt)
½ cup	Barley
1 Tbsp	Wheat germ (2 mEq potassium)
Rice and Pasta	
⅓ cup	Rice (brown or white), cooked (no salt)
½ cup	Pasta, spaghetti, noodles, macaroni (cooked, no salt)
Other Bread Products	
2½ Tbsp	Cornmeal, dry
3 Tbsp	Flour
1½ cups	Popcorn (popped, no salt)
Crackers	
6	Saltines, unsalted, 2½-in square
Salted: 5 to 10 mEq sodium (average 8 mEq)	
Bread: 1.5 mEq potassium	
½	Bagel or English muffin
1 slice	Bread: white (including French or Italian), whole wheat, rye, raisin
4	Breadsticks (unsalted tops)
½	Hamburger bun
1	Plain roll
Bread: 3 to 5 mEq potassium	
½	English muffin
1 slice	Pumpernickle bread
Cereal: 1.5 mEq potassium	
¾ cup	Cereals, ready to eat, unsweetened
½ cup	Cereals, cooked (with ⅛ tsp of salt)
½ cup	Barley, cooked (with ⅛ tsp of salt)
3 Tbsp	Grapenuts
½ cup	Grits, cooked (with ⅛ tsp of salt)
½ cup	Barley, cooked (with ⅛ tsp of salt)
Cereal: 5 to 10 mEq potassium	
½ cup	Bran cereals, flakes, chex, etc.
⅓ cup	Bran cereals, All Bran, Bran Buds
Crackers: 1.5 mEq potassium	
10	Animal crackers
3	Arrowroot
3	Graham crackers, 2½-in square
¾	Matzo, 4 in by 6 in
5	Melba toast, 2 in by 3¾ in
3	Rye wafers, 2 in by 3½ in
6	Round butter or whole wheat crackers (low sodium)
6	Saltines, unsalted tops, 2½-in square
Rice and Pasta	
⅓ cup	Rice (brown or white), cooked (with ⅛ tsp of salt)
½ cup	Pasta, spaghetti, noodles, macaroni (cooked with ⅛ tsp of salt)
Other Bread Products	
1 square	Cornbread, 2 in by 2 in by 1 in*
1 small	Croissant†
½ cup	Chow mein noodles*
½ cup	Croutons
¼ cup (4 Tbsp)	Dried bread crumbs
2	Pancakes from mix, 4-in diameter*
1	Pita bread, 6-in diameter
1 small	Plain muffin, biscuit, 2-in diameter*
¾ oz (25 sticks)	Pretzels, unsalted
2	Taco shells, 6-in diameter*
1	Tortilla, 6-in diameter
1	Waffle, 5-in diameter*

* These foods contain one additional fat exchange
† These foods contain two additional fat exchanges

Table continued on following page

TABLE 35–7. Exchange Lists for Diets Controlled for Protein, Sodium and Potassium *Continued*

Starchy Vegetables

***Unsalted:* Prepared without salt (less than 1 mEq sodium)**
***Salted:* Prepared with ⅛ tsp of salt per serving (approximately 8 mEq sodium)**

3 to 5 mEq potassium

⅓ cup	Corn
1 small ear	Corn on the cob, 3½ in
¼ cup	Sweet potato or yam, canned
½ small	Sweet potato, baked
⅓ cup	Lima beans
10 (1½ oz)	French fried potatoes, 2 to 3½ in long

5 to 10 mEq potassium

½ cup	Mashed potato
1 small	Potato, peeled and boiled

10 to 15 mEq potassium

⅔ cup	Parsnips
1 small	Potato, baked
¾ cup	Squash, acorn, butternut, or winter
1 cup	Pumpkin

Vegetables

Each exchange equals approximately 2 g protein. Unsalted vegetables are prepared without salt (less than 1 mEq sodium). Salted vegetables are canned with added salt or prepared with ⅛ tsp salt per serving (approximately 12 mEq sodium).
One serving of vegetable equals ½ cup cooked or 1 cup raw vegetables unless otherwise specified. There are no "free" vegetables.

Moderate Potassium—3 to 5 mEq potassium (average 4 mEq)

Alfalfa sprouts	Escarole	Radishes
Asparagus	Green pepper	Rhubarb
Bamboo shoots	Green string beans	Rutabaga
Bean sprouts	Kale	Summer squash
Beets	Lettuce	Turnip
Cauliflower	Mustard greens	Water chestnuts
Chicory	Okra	Watercress
Chinese cabbage	Onion	Yellow string beans
Eggplant	Peas, green (¼ cup)	Zucchini
Endive	Pea pods or snow peas	

Higher Potassium—5 to 10 mEq potassium (average 7 mEq)

Artichokes	Chard	Spinach
Beet greens	Collards	Tomatoes
Broccoli	Cucumber	Tomato juice, unsalted
Brussels sprouts	Dandelion greens	Turnip greens
Cabbage	Kohlrabi	Vegetable juice cocktail, unsalted
Carrots	Mushrooms	
Celery	Parsley	

Fruit

Each exchange contains 0.5 to 1 g protein, trace of sodium, and averages of 2, 4, or 7 mEq potassium.

Low potassium—less than 3 mEq potassium (average 2 mEq)

1 small	Apple, fresh, 2-in diameter	⅓ cup	Cranberry juice cocktail
½ cup	Apple juice or cider	1¼ cup	Cranberry juice cocktail (low calorie)
½ cup	Applesauce		
¾ cup	Blueberries		
1¼ cup	Cranberries		

Moderate Potassium—3 to 5 mEq potassium (average 4 mEq)

1 cup	Raspberries	½ cup	Canned peaches
12	Cherries, fresh	2 halves	Dried peaches
½ cup	Canned cherries	½ cup	Peach nectar

TABLE 35–7. Exchange Lists for Diets Controlled for Protein, Sodium and Potassium *Continued*

Fruit *Continued*

Moderate Potassium *Continued*

2 large	Dates	1 small	Pear, fresh
2 medium	Fig, fresh	1 half	Pear, dried
1 medium	Fig, dried	½ cup	Pear, canned
1½	Canned figs	½ cup	Pear, nectar
½ cup	Fruit cocktail	2 medium	Persimmon, native
½ medium	Grapefruit, fresh	¾ cup	Pineapple, fresh
½ cup	Grapefruit juice	⅓ cup	Pineapple, canned
¾ cup	Grapefruit sections	½ cup	Pineapple juice
15 small	Grapes, fresh	2	Plum, fresh, 2 in
⅓ cup	Grape juice	3 or ½ cup	Plums, canned
5 medium	Kumquats	2 Tbsp	Raisins
½ small	Mango	1 cup	Rhubarb
1 medium	Peach, fresh		

High potassium—5 to 10 mEq potassium (average 7 mEq)

4 medium	Apricots, fresh	1¼ cup	Watermelon
½ cup or 4 halves	Canned apricots	½	Nectarine, 3 in
7 halves	Dried apricots	1 small	Orange, fresh, 2½
½ cup	Apricot nectar	¾ cup	Orange sections
½	Banana, 9 in	½ cup	Orange juice
¾ cup	Blackberries	1 cup	Papaya
1¼ cup	Strawberries	3 medium	Passion fruit
		½ medium	Pomegranate
1 medium	Guava	1 medium	Prickly pear
1 large	Kiwi fruit	3 medium	Prunes
1 cup	Lemon juice*	⅓ cup	Prune juice
¼ small or 1 cup	Cataloupe, 6 in	1 medium	Tangelo
		2 medium	Tangerine, fresh
⅛ medium or 1 cup	Honeydew	½ cup	Tangerine juice

* Up to 2 Tbsp of lemon juice may be used per day without considering this as a part of the fruit group.

Low-Protein Products

Each exchange contains 0.2 g protein, 0.5 mEq sodium, trace potassium, and 100 kilocalories.

1 slice (1½ oz)	Low-protein bread
2 slices	Low-protein rusks
½ cup, cooked (¼ cup dry)	Low-protein macaroni, ring macaroni, or noodles
½ cup, prepared	Low-protein gelatin (negligible protein, 1 mEq sodium, 2 mEq potassium, 85 kilocalories)
2	Low-protein cookies (0.2 g protein, 2 mEq sodium, 1 mEq potassium, 1 fat serving, and 140 kilocalories

Fats and Oils

Each exchange contains negligible amounts of protein and a trace of potassium. Sodium varies.

Unsalted: trace of sodium

1 tsp	Margarine, unsalted
1 tsp	Butter, unsalted
1 tsp	Mayonnaise, low sodium
1 tsp	Oil
1 tsp	Shortening
2 Tbsp	Gravy (meat drippings with fat thickened with cornstarch), unsalted

Salted: 2 mEq sodium

1 tsp	Margarine
1 tsp	Butter
1 tsp	Mayonnaise
2 Tbsp	Nondairy creamer
2 Tbsp	Sour cream (limit to one serving per day)

Table continued on following page

TABLE 35–7. Exchange Lists for Diets Controlled for Protein, Sodium and Potassium *Continued*

Carbohydrate Supplements

Each exchange contains negligible amounts of protein, sodium, and potassium and 100 kilocalories.

Sugar and syrups	
2 Tbsp	Sugar
2 Tbsp	Honey
2 Tbsp	Jelly or jam
2 Tbsp	Syrup
Candy	
3 large	Fondant or sugar mints
3 large	Gumdrops
6 pieces	Hard candy, unfilled
20	Jelly beans
1 medium	Lollipop, unfilled
Fruit desserts	
¼ cup	Cranberry sauce or relish
½ cup	Fruit ice (sherbert made without milk) (contains 80 ml fluid)
1 twin bar	Popsicle (2½ oz bar contains 75 ml fluid)
Flavored beverages	
1 cup (8 oz)	Carbonated, fruit flavored Kool Aid, artificially flavored lemonade
Flour products	
¼ cup	Cornstarch or tapioca (may be used to thicken sauces and gravies)
Other carbohydrate supplements	
¼ cup	Polycose powder or liquid (contains 2 mEq sodium, use as suggested)

Beverages

One cup (8 oz) of the following beverages contains only a trace of protein and sodium.

Trace potassium	*1 mEq potassium*	*2 mEq potassium*	*4 mEq potassium*
Cola	Limeade	Coffee, instant	Coffee, brewed
Ginger ale		Coffee, decaffeinated, instant, and freeze dried	
Kool Aid		Lemonade, from frozen concentrate	
Root beer		Tea	
Seven-up			

12 oz of beer contain 1.5 mEq sodium and 3 mEq potassium
4 oz of wine contain a trace of sodium and 3 mEq potassium

* From Pemberton CM et al: Mayo Clinic Diet Manual, 6th ed. Philadelphia, BC Decker, 1988, p. 235.

weight should be monitored, and the diet should be adjusted accordingly.

Most patients find it difficult if not impossible to consume adequate calories and still have a palatable diet. In addition, the uremia itself causes some taste aberrations, notably to red meats, sometimes making it difficult to achieve the high HBV/low biological value (LBV) protein ratio. Clinical Insight, page 615, gives an example of foods that will provide 75% of the protein as HBV protein.

Table 35–7 contains the exchange lists quantified for controlled intakes of protein, sodium, potassium, and calories. A sample menu is given in Table 35–8.

Although the exchange lists may simplify calculation of the diet, some patients may prefer to learn the actual protein, potassium, and sodium content of foods and adjust their intake accordingly. Sodium, potassium, and protein values of foods are given in Appendix Table 1.

TUBE FEEDING. Patients with ESRD who require enteral tube feeding may be given a product such as Amin-Aid (McGaw), which contains only the essential amino acids plus histidine in the amount required and which, when mixed with water, provides amino acids, carbohydrate, and a few electrolytes (see Appendix

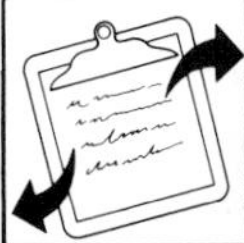

CLINICAL INSIGHT: Protein Calculation for a Dialysis Patient

A 60-kg anuric female receiving hemodialysis three times per week should be eating 60 g/day of protein. If 75% of this protein is to be HBV protein, then 46 grams of protein should be in the form of eggs, meat, fish, poultry, milk, or cheese. A possible combination of these foods that would contribute 46 grams of HBV protein would be:

Food	Protein (g)
1 egg	7
2 oz chicken	14
3 oz beef	21
½ cup milk	4
Total	46

The remaining 14 grams is obtained from LBV protein sources: breads and cereals, vegetables, potatoes, pasta, and milk-free desserts. A combination of foods that would provide 14 grams of LBV protein is:

Food	Protein (g)
3 slices bread	6
¾ cup cereal	3
½ cup mashed potato	2
½ cup carrots	1
½ cup peas	1
½ cup orange juice	0.5
1 small apple	0.5
Total	14

Table 33). A side effect of this formulation may be diarrhea due to the high osmotic effect of these solutions. Electrodialyzed whey (lactalbumin treated to remove the electrolytes) combined with glucose and water provides HBV protein with adequate calories and few electrolytes. However, unless the patient is experiencing severe shifts in electrolytes or requires a very large volume, most standard house tube feedings can be tailored to meet requirements. As soon as possible, the patient should be encouraged to eat a moderate-protein, high-calorie diet with controlled sodium and potassium intake.

Energy

Energy intake must be adequate to spare protein for tissue protein synthesis and to prevent its metabolism for energy. Depending on the patient's nutritional status and degree of stress, between 35 and 50 kcal/kg body weight should be provided.

Calcium, Phosphorus, and Vitamin D

A major complication of ESRD is metabolic bone disease or *renal osteodystrophy*. The disease is essentially of three types: *osteomalacia*, or bone demineralization;

TABLE 35–8. Sample Menu for Renal Diet Prescription

60 g protein
2 g sodium (87 mEq)
2 g potassium (51 mEq)
1,000 mg phosphorus

Breakfast	Lunch	Dinner
Slice of cantaloupe (⅛)	Low-sodium vegetable soup (⅔ cup)	Broiled chicken (2 oz)
Dry cereal (¾ cup)	Lean hamburger patty (2 oz)	White rice (½ cup)
Whole-wheat toast (2 slices)	Hamburger bun (whole)	Carrot coins (½ cup)
Margarine (2 tsp)	Sliced tomato (1 medium)	Hard dinner roll (1)
Jelly (1 T)	Salt-free Thousand Island dressing (1 T)	Margarine (3 tsp)
Hard boiled egg (1)	Lemonade (8 oz)	Lettuce and cucumber salad (1 cup)
Coffee (5 oz)		Vinegar + oil dressing (1 T)
Sugar (2 t)		Baked apple w/4 tsp sugar (1)
Nondairy creamer (½ cup)		Ginger ale (1 cup)

Snack Throughout Day

Hard candy (4 pieces)
Gum drops (15)
Popsicle (3 oz)

osteitis fibrosa cystica, caused by hyperparathyroidism; and *metastatic calcification* of joints and soft tissues.

As the GFR decreases, phosphorus, whose level is controlled by renal excretion, is retained in the plasma. Serum calcium level declines for several reasons. Decreased 1,25$(OH)_2D_3$, brought about by decreased ability of the kidney to convert the inactive form, appears to be most important. In addition, the calcium-phosphate product, which increases as phosphate increases, leads to extraosseus calcifications throughout the body and brings about a decreased calcium level. The low calcium level triggers several mechanisms by which the healthy body increases calcium to normal. These include the release of PTH from the parathyroid glands as well as increased synthesis of the active form of vitamin D by the kidney. This in turn acts on the gut to increase absorption of both calcium and phosphate and, in concert with PTH, acts to increase bone resorption, thus liberating both calcium and phosphate. PTH also acts on the kidney to increase secretion of phosphate while retaining extra calcium. With decreased ability to produce 1,25$(OH)_2D_3$, the patient with failing kidneys cannot increase gut absorption of calcium and must therefore rely on the effects of PTH to keep calcium levels up and phosphate down through bone resorption, and to increase renal elimination of phosphate. The dependence of calcium-phosphate control on increasing levels of PTH thus leads to a characteristic hyperplastic demineralized bone disease, *osteitis fibrosa cystica.* The disease is characterized by dull aching bone pain.

Even though the serum calcium level is elevated in response to PTH, the serum phosphate concentration remains high as the GFR falls lower. If the product of the serum calcium level (milligrams per 100 ml) multiplied by the serum phosphate level (milligrams per 100 ml) is greater than 70, *metastatic calcification* is imminent. Clinical management aims to keep the product below 70 by preventing transient elevations in serum phosphate concentration.

In essence, calcium and phosphorus intake must be controlled to as great a degree as possible in order to avoid aggravation of the delicate situation posed by hyperparathyroidism, phosphate retention, and hypocalcemia in renal failure. In practical terms, calcium intake is kept high and phosphorus intake is kept low. This is a problem as far as food is concerned, because most of the high-calcium foods (milk and milk products) are also high in phosphorus. Consequently, methods other than dietary must be relied on.

Calcium is increased by giving calcium supplements in the form of calcium carbonate (e.g., Tums), lactate, or gluconate along with the 300 to 500 mg of calcium provided in the diet. Calcium is added to the dialysate bath so that a smaller amount of serum calcium is drawn off during dialysis. Starting calcium supplementation early is more likely to prevent hyperparathyroidism (Slatopolsky, 1986).

Phosphate intake is lowered by restricting dietary sources to 1,200 mg or less (see Table 35–9) and by using phosphate-binding resins such as Basaljel or Amphojel. These aluminum hydroxide products (also used as antacids) bind with phosphate and prevent its absorption from the gut. Taken by themselves the resins may be distasteful, thus recipes for cookies and other products that incorporate the aluminum hydroxide products have been developed. Several potential risks of aluminum-containing phosphate binders must be considered (Andress, 1986; Coburn and Norris,

TABLE 35–9. Common Foods High in Phosphorus*

	Milligrams of Phosphorus Per Exchange†
Milk Group	
Yogurt (plain)	165
Pudding	130
Milk (including chocolate and evaporated)	125
Half and Half	115
Ice cream	100
Custard	100
Meat and Meat Substitutes	
Cheese (processed)	215
Cheese (Swiss)	175
Cheese (cheddar, mozzarella)	145
Liver	130
Fish (salmon, bass, mackerel)	120
Lentils, ½ cup	120
Egg	90
Cottage cheese	70
Starch	
Cereal (100% bran)	400
Cereal (All Bran, Bran Buds, granola-type)	265
Cereal (Bran Chex, bran flakes)	150
Waffle (frozen)	135
Cooked cereal (instant)	135
Biscuit (from mix)	130
Cake, white (from mix)	115
Wheat germ	80
Bread (whole wheat)	70
Lima Beans	60
Vegetables	
Mushrooms	80
Peas	50
Fats and Oils	
Nondairy creamer	50
Carbohydrate Supplements	
Cola beverage	30

* From Pemberton CM et al: Mayo Clinic Diet Manual 6th ed. Philadelphia, BC Decker, 1988, p. 242.

† As listed in the Exchange Lists for Protein, Sodium, and Potassium Control, Table 35–7.

1986). Aluminum is absorbed from the gut and is deposited throughout the body, most importantly in brain and bone. Long-term administration of high doses of aluminum can lead to a neurologic syndrome referred to as *dialysis dementia.* Aluminum deposits in bone can halt the mineralization process and lead to osteomalacia. For this reason, no more than 1,200 mg of aluminum three times daily (total of 3,600 mg) should be administered. Calcium carbonate or calcium acetate (Phos-Ex) are being substituted for aluminum hydroxide as preferred phosphate binders with aluminum gels reserved for patients needing them (Mactier, 1987).

Severe constipation leading to intestinal impaction is another potential risk of excessive consumption of phosphate binders. Occasionally, this may lead to perforation of the intestine with resultant peritonitis and death. Constipation is often the reason why patients will not take the prescribed aluminum hydroxide gels. Suggestions for using bran or other high-fiber foods and regular light exercise may contribute to patient compliance. Giving phosphate binders with food increases their efficiency and thus less may be required (Schiller et al, 1989).

As with calcium supplementation, the early initiation of phosphate reduction therapies is advantageous in order to delay hyperparathyroidism and bone disease. Unfortunately, most patients are asymptomatic during the early phase of hyperparathyroidism and are not attentive about following a modified diet and taking the calcium supplements and phosphate binders. However, they should be encouraged to do so.

Because of potential *hypermagnesemia,* which can exacerbate the already existent bone disease, magnesium-containing antacids such as Maalox, Gelusil, or Mylanta should not be used.

Vitamin D is given only when the hypocalcemia of renal failure is severe or causing osteomalacia. Because so little vitamin D is changed into its active form in the patient with ESRD, large amounts (10,000 to 30,000 IU/day) must be given. The dangers inherent in the use of these large doses of vitamin D are hypercalcemia and hypomagnesemia from overdosage and metastatic calcification from combined hypercalcemia and hyperphosphatemia. Phosphate binders are even more important when a vitamin D sterol is used (Coburn and Salusky, 1989).

Because of this, the routine drug of choice is $1,25(OH)_2D_3$, which is available as calcitriol (Rocaltrol, Roche Labs). Analogues such as $1\text{-a},(OH)D_3$ and $1\text{-a},25(OH)_2D_3$ (DHT, Roxane Labs), which have similar configurations, have been produced, and are also available.

Hemodialysis or peritoneal dialysis does not alleviate osteodystrophy. However, it can reduce the progression of the disease because the infused calcium results in decreased PTH secretion. Patients must still be responsible for following a low-phosphorous diet and for taking calcium or aluminum to bind phosphate.

Fluoride

High levels of fluoride in the serum of the uremic patient appear to aggravate the existing bone disease, possibly by enhancing bone demineralization. Increased serum fluoride levels in dialyzed uremic patients have been reported and may possibly be attributed to the fluoride content of the dialysate bath. It is recommended that water from fluoridated supplies be deionized before using it in dialysis (Rao and Friedman, 1975).

Iron

The hypoproliferative, normochromic, normocytic anemia of chronic renal failure usually stabilizes with dialysis; however, it manifests itself in complaints of fatigue. It is caused by both an inability of the kidney to produce *erythropoietin (EPO),* a hormone that stimulates the bone marrow to produce red blood cells, as well as an increased destruction of red blood cells secondary to the circulating uremic waste products. It is typically characterized by normal or increased iron stores that cannot be used effectively. Treatment with iron supplementation, therefore, is only required when special circumstances of iron deficiency exist, such as after a significant GI bleed. Anabolic steroids are sometimes used to help stimulate erythropoiesis.

A synthetic form of EPO, *recombinant human erythropoietin (rHuEPO),* has been approved by the FDA. Clinical trials have demonstrated a dramatic effect in correction of anemia, as well as in restoration of a general sense of well being (Eschbach et al, 1987). Accompanying the rise in hematocrit is often an increased need for iron, sometimes requiring supplementation. The main side effect of rHuEPO administration has been improved appetite, occasionally leading to problems with potassium control. The drug is available commercially and is routinely used.

Blood transfusion is not recommended for most patients with ESRD because of (1) its depression of erythropoiesis in the bone marrow, (2) the possibility of overexpansion of the blood volume, (3) the risk of hepatitis, and (4) hemochromatosis and hemosiderosis due to increased iron stores and administration of parenteral iron.

Serum ferritin is an accurate indicator of iron overload. Patients who have received excess transfusions and who are storing extra iron may have serum ferritin levels of 800 to 5,000 ng/ml. (A normal level is 68 ng/ml for women and 150 ng/ml for men.)

Vitamins

One of the several causes for vitamin deficiency in uremia is the decreased intake due to the restriction of dietary phosphorus and potassium. Water-soluble vitamins are usually abundant in high-potassium foods such as citrus fruits and vegetables, and high-phosphorus foods, such as meat and milk. Diets for patients on dialysis tend to be low in folacin, niacin, riboflavin, and vitamin B_6 ascorbic acid is marginal. With frequent episodes of anorexia or illness, the vitamin intake is decreased even further.

Altered metabolism and excretory function as well as drug administration also may alter vitamin levels. Little is known about GI absorption in uremia, but it may be significantly decreased. It is possible that uremic toxins interfere with the activity of some vitamins; for example, the phosphorylation of pyridoxine (vitamin B_6) and its analogues may be inhibited.

Water-soluble vitamins are also lost during dialysis. In general, ascorbic acid and most of the B-complex vitamins are dialyzable. Because vitamin B_{12} is protein-bound, losses during dialysis are minimal. Fat-soluble vitamins do not require supplementation in renal disease.

A few vitamin supplements are now available that fit the needs of the uremic patient or of the patient receiving dialysis (Nephrocaps, Fleming and Co.; Tabron, Park-Davis). A supplement of vitamin B complex and vitamin C is often used. Additional supplements of folic acid and pyridoxine may also be given.

Carbohydrate

Glucose intolerance with both hyperglycemia and hypoglycemia is frequently observed in patients with ESRD. It seems to reflect a delayed and erratic action of insulin due to tissue resistance to insulin action or to an insulin antagonism by the products of uremia. In any case, this glucose intolerance rarely requires administration of insulin and never requires control of the carbohydrate in the diet. If there are problems with hypoglycemia, the addition of dextrose to the dialysate usually alleviates the problem.

Lipid

Atherosclerotic cardiovascular disease is the most frequent cause of death among patients maintained on long-term hemodialysis. This appears to be a function of both underlying disease (e.g., diabetes mellitus, hypertension, nephrotic syndrome) as well as a lipid abnormality common among patients with ESRD. Typically, the patient with ESRD has an elevated triglyceride level with or without an increase in cholesterol. The lipid abnormality likely represents both increased synthesis of very low density lipoprotein (VLDL) (Reaven et al, 1980) as well as decreased clearance (Henck and Ritz, 1980).

Treatment of hyperlipidemia with diet or pharmacologic agents remains controversial. Epidemiologic evidence demonstrating increased incidence of atherosclerotic coronary disease (Lindner et al, 1974), is balanced by studies demonstrating that patients with clearly defined clinical evidence of atherosclerosis at the initiation of dialysis are at no increased risk above age-matched cohorts (Rostand et al, 1982).

Whereas routine treatment appears unwarranted, a good case can be made for dietary and pharmacologic treatment of patients with ESRD with underlying lipid disorders and evidence of accelerated atherosclerosis. The new generation of lipid-lowering drugs, including lovostatin, may have a significant impact on future management.

Improvement of the plasma lipid profile in ESRD may also result from supplementation with the amino acid carnitine. Since the kidney is a major site of carnitine synthesis, dialysis patients typically have abnormal carnitine metabolism and low plasma-free carnitine levels. Presently research is investigating the effectiveness of carnitine supplementation to increase free and acyl carnitine levels in these patients. So far carnitine supplementation has been associated with improved muscle function and less cramping, fewer hypotensive episodes and less protein catabolism. However it is still considered experimental therapy (Bellinghieri, 1983; Vacha, 1983).

Parenteral Nutrition

When a patient with ESRD becomes too ill to maintain an adequate oral intake, and when tube feeding is not advisable due to GI complications, parenteral nutrition should be considered (see Chapter 30).

Parenteral nutrition in ESRD is similar to parenteral nutrition used for other malnourished patients. Use of essential amino acid solutions, such as Nephramine, are usually recommended in cases of acute renal failure or when a patient is not receiving dialysis treatment. Patients receiving dialysis therapy tolerate routine amino acid solutions, such as Freeamine (McGaw), Travasol 8.5 (Clintec), and Aminosyn (Abbott Labs).

Vitamins and Minerals

Most researchers agree that vitamin needs for ESRD are different from normal requirements during parenteral nutrition but do not agree on their recommendations for individual nutrients. It is generally accepted that folate, pyridoxine, and biotin should be supplemented and that vitamin A should not be provided parenterally unless retinol-binding protein is monitored, because it is elevated in patients with renal failure (Table 35–10).

Little information is available relating to trace mineral supplementation in renal failure. Because most trace minerals, including zinc, chromium, and magnesium, are excreted in the urine, a close monitoring of these minerals in the serum seems to be appropriate.

Hypophosphatemia is a potential complication of parenteral nutrition in ESRD, which may be more commonly seen due to routine ingestion of phosphate-binding antacids. If adequate protein and calories are provided and the patient becomes anabolic, the phosphate binder regime may need to be altered to prevent hypophosphatemia and potential respiratory arrest.

Intradialytic Parenteral Nutrition

Malnourished patients with chronic renal failure who are on hemodialysis have a unique potential for parenteral nutrition due to the requirements of the dialysis therapy itself. Because direct access to the blood must be made at every treatment, parenteral nutrition may be administered without additional invasive procedures or surgery.

Typically, *intradialytic parenteral nutrition* is administered through a connection to the venous side of the extracorporeal circuit during dialysis (Olsham et al, 1987). Due to the high blood flow rate achieved through use of the surgically created fistula and the high blood pump speeds attained, hypertonic glucose and protein can be administered without danger of phlebitis. Lipids may also be administered (Tables 35–11, 35–12; 35–13).

TABLE 35–10. Guidelines for Daily Parenteral Vitamin Supplementation in Total Parenteral Nutrition for Patients with Renal Failure*

Vitamin	Silberman	Kopple
A, as retinol (IU)	3,300	0
E, tocopherol (IU)	10	10
K, (mg)		7.5
Niacin (mg)	40	20
Thiamin HCl (mg)	3	2
Riboflavin (mg)	3.6	2
Pantothenic acid (mg)	15	10
Pyridoxine (mg)	5	10
Ascorbic acid (mg)	100	100
Biotin (mg)	60	200
Folic acid (mg)	1	2
B_{12} (μg)	5	3

* From Kouba, J.: Vitamin and Electrolytes in Patients with Renal Failure Requiring Total Parenteral Nutrition. Dietitians in Critical Care, p 5, December 1985, American Dietetic Association, Chicago.

These are general guidelines and may need more specific evaluation and adjustment in patients in severe stress or with gastrointestinal losses from diarrhea, ostomies, fistula drainage, etc.

TABLE 35–11. Regimen for Parenteral Nutrition by Peripheral Vein for Dialysis Patients

Infusion	Quantity	Calories (kcal)	Volume (ml)
10% Glucose	50 g glucose	170	500
10% Amino acids	40–50 g protein	160	500
10% Lipid emulsion	50 g fat	550	500
Total		880	1,500*

Monitor serum glucose, sodium, potassium, bicarbonate, phosphate, triglycerides

* Additional volume may include insulin and vitamins.

Developed by Katy Wilkens, R.D., Northwest Kidney Center, Seattle, Washington.

COMPLICATIONS. Complications are similar to those encountered in TPN with the exception of *postdialysis hypoglycemia* due to the abrupt ending of the glucose supply. To avoid this problem, glucose administration is typically tapered up and down during the first and last half hour of the 3- to 4-hour treatment. Additionally, some patients may benefit from a snack of complex carbohydrate toward the end of the treatment (Foulkes, 1988).

Amino acid losses through the dialysate average about 10%, or about 2 grams per treatment. Vitamins and trace minerals are typically not administered with these solutions, because patients are able to tolerate oral vitamin preparations and have some oral intake.

Other potential methods of nutritional support include the use of a hemodialysis dialysate solution containing amino acids and the use of peritoneal dialysate solution containing amino acids as well as dextrose. These methods are currently experimental.

End-Stage Renal Disease in Patients With Diabetes

Since renal failure is a complication of diabetes, approximately 35% of all new patients starting dialysis are diabetic. Because of the need to control blood sugar, these patients require even more specialized diet therapy. The diabetic diet (as discussed in Chapter 31) can

TABLE 35–12. Regimen for Intermittent Parenteral Nutrition Administered During Hemodialysis Therapy*

Infusion	Quantity	Calories (kcal)	Volume (ml)
70% Glucose	350 g glucose	1,160	500
10% Amino acids	25 g protein	100	250
20% Lipid emulsion	50 g fat	550	250
Totals		1,810	1,000†

* Developed by Katy Wilkens, R.D., Northwest Kidney Center, Seattle, Washington.

† Additional volume may include insulin and vitamins.

TABLE 35–13. Regimen for Total Parenteral Nutrition by Subclavian Vein for Dialysis Patients

Infusion	Quantity	Calories (kcal)	Volume (ml)
70% Glucose	700 g glucose	2,380	1,000
10% Amino acids	40–50 g protein	160–200	500
20% Lipid emulsion	100 g fat	1,100	500
Total		3,640–3,680	2,000*

Monitor serum glucose, sodium potassium, bicarbonate, phosphate, triglycerides

* Additional volume may include insulin and vitamins.

Developed by Katy Wilkens, R.D., Northwest Kidney Center, Seattle, Washington.

be modified for the patient on dialysis (American Dietetic Association, 1991).

In the presence of hyperglycemia, most diabetics experience thirst, and fluid overload becomes a serious problem. Increased osmolarity due to high levels of glucose may cause water and potassium to be pulled out of cells with resultant hyperkalemia.

In addition, the diabetic patient on dialysis often has other complications, such as retinopathy, neuropathy, gastroparesis, and amputation, all of which can place the diabetic at high nutritional risk.

End-Stage Renal Disease in Children

Renal failure may occur in children at any age, from the newborn infant through the adolescent. As with all children, the major concern is to promote normal growth and development. Without aggressive monitoring and encouragement, the child rarely meets his or her nutritional needs. If the renal disease is present from birth, nutritional support needs to begin immediately to avoid losing the growth potential of the first few months of life.

Growth in children with ESRD is usually retarded. Although no specific therapy ensures normal growth, factors capable of responding to therapy include metabolic acidosis, electrolyte depletion, osteodystrophy, chronic infection, and protein-calorie malnutrition. Energy and protein needs for children with chronic renal disease are at least equivalent to the RDA for normal children of the same height and age. If nutritional status is poor, energy needs may be greater to promote weight gain and linear growth. Parenteral nutrition or feeding by tube may be necessary in the presence of poor intake, particularly in the critical growth period of the first 2 years of life (Abitbol, 1984). Table 35–14 presents the nutritional requirements of children with renal failure.

Control of calcium and phosphorus balance is especially important to maintain good growth. The goal is to restrict phosphorus intake while promoting calcium absorption with the aid of 1,25-$(OH)_2D_3$. This helps to prevent renal osteodystrophy, which can cause severe growth retardation during the rapid growth of childhood. Use of calcium carbonate formulations to supplement the dietary intake enhances calcium intake while binding excess phosphorus. Aluminum-containing preparations are used only in cases of extreme hyperphosphatemia and only on a short-term basis. Aluminum is very toxic, especially in infancy.

Persistent metabolic acidosis is often associated with growth failure in infancy. In chronic acidosis, the titration of acid by the bone causes calcium loss and contributes to bone demineralization. Bicarbonate may be added to the formula to counteract this effect.

Restriction of protein in pediatric diets is controversial. The so-called "protective" effect on kidney function must be weighed against the clearly negative effect of possible protein malnutrition on growth. The RDA for protein for age is usually the minimum to be given (see Table 16–1).

Each child's diet should be individualized to meet his or her food preferences, family eating patterns, and biochemical needs. This is often not an easy task. In addition, care must be taken not to place too much emphasis on the diet to avoid its becoming a manipulative tool and an attention-getting device.

Special encouragement, creativity, and attention are required to help the child with ESRD consume the necessary energy. When possible, CAPD appears to be a viable therapy of choice for children because it allows liberalization of the diet. The child is more likely to meet nutritional requirements with fewer dietary restrictions and therefore experience better growth.

New developments that may help with treatment of renal disease in children include the use of rHuEPO and *rDNA-produced growth hormone (rHGH).* Correction of anemia with the use of EPO may increase appetite, intake and feeling of well-being, and may lead to increased growth. But even with seemingly adequate nutritional support and rHuEPO, some children with ESRD still do not grow well (Powell et al, 1988). rHGH is currently under study to determine its effectiveness in promoting normal growth in children with ESRD (Koch et al, 1989).

HUMAN IMMUNODEFICIENCY VIRUS AND RENAL DISEASE

Exposure to human immunodeficiency virus (HIV) may occur in patients with renal disease. HIV infection with eventual development of acquired immunodeficiency syndrome (AIDS) may then occur.

Drugs often used in the treatment of patients with HIV may be nephrotoxic and cause reversible kidney disease. Sepsis, common in the patient with HIV, may

TABLE 35–14. Nutrient Requirements Based on Type of Therapy for Children with Renal Disease*

Therapy	Energy	Protein		Fluid	Sodium	Potassium	Phosphorus
		Creatinine Clearance	*Protein Requirement*				
Impaired renal function (predialysis)	Infant (under 1 yr): 120–150 kcal/kg	10–50	1.5 g/kg	35 ml/100 kcal + urine output	23–69 mg/kg/day (1–3 mEq/kg/day)	29–87 mg/kg/day (1–3 mEq/kg/day)	0.5–1 g/day
	Child: First 10 kg = 100 kcal/kg	<10	1 g/kg				
	Second 10 kg = 50 kcal/kg	<5	0.3–0.5 g/kg				
	Every kg thereafter: 20 kcal/kg						
		Weight of Child					
Hemodialysis	Same as above	10–20 kg 20–30 kg 30–40 kg 40+ kg	2 g/kg 1.5 g/kg 1.0–1.5 g/kg 1.0 g/kg	Same as above, plus losses from dialysis. Child's fluid gains should be about 5% of body weight.	57 mg/kg/day (2.5 mEq/kg/day)	Same as above	0.5–1 g/day
Intermittent peritoneal dialysis (IPD)	Same as above	10–20 kg 20–40 kg 40+ kg	2 g/kg 1.5 g/kg 1.0–1.5 g/kg	Same as above	Same as above	Same as above	0.5–1 g/day
Continuous ambulatory peritoneal dialysis (CAPD)	100–120 kcal/kg	10–20 kg 20–40 kg 40+ kg	2–3 g/kg 1.5–2 g/kg 1.0–1.5 g/kg	100–160 ml/kg/day + urine output	Same as above	Same as above	0.5–1 g/day
Transplant	Normal energy requirement for age. Tendency toward obesity due to steroids. Not more than 35% of total calories from fat. Low saturated fat.		2–3 g/kg	Ad libitum	Variable	Variable, usually ad libitum	Ad libitum Supplement if necessary. Calcium ad lib supplement if necessary. Vitamin D as necessary.

* Developed by Katy Wilkens, R.D., Northwest Kidney Center, Seattle, and Anne Hetrick, R.D., Shands Teaching Hospital, University of Florida, Gainesville.

also lead to renal failure. The prognosis of HIV patients who develop acute renal failure appears to be somewhat improved if they receive repetitive dialysis therapy (Rao and Friedman, 1987).

A specific form of *AIDS-associated renal disease* has been suggested, but its existence is controversial. Patients who develop this type of renal failure have a poor prognosis and less than 10% survive longer than 6 months after the initiation of dialysis (Humphreys and Schoenfeld, 1987).

The patient with ESRD with previously diagnosed renal disease who develops *positive HIV antibodies* has a somewhat better prognosis. Survival on dialysis treatment may range from 3 months to several years, with death resulting from other complications of renal failure or the development of AIDS.

Several cases of patients becoming infected with HIV as a result of *organ transplantation* from an HIV-positive donor, either living-related or cadaveric, have been reported. The Centers for Disease Control recommends that no person from a high-risk category should be considered as a donor for organ transplantation and that HIV testing should be performed on all donors.

Conversely, transplantation of a kidney to an HIV-positive patient may be contraindicated as the immunosuppressive drugs may shorten the time required to develop AIDS. The 2-year survival rate for asymptomatic HIV-positive patients who have had transplants has been reported to be significantly lower than for non–HIV-positive transplant recipients (AIDS Working Group, 1985).

Nutritional Care

Weight loss and malnutrition are common findings in patients with AIDS, apparently due to malabsorption, altered metabolism, and altered organ function (see Chapter 37). Problems with nutritional treatment in such patients are compounded by restrictions on sodium, potassium, and fluid. As in any patient with renal disease who has malnutrition, all restrictions not absolutely necessary for the patient's immediate well-being are usually omitted. The emphasis is on provision of adequate oral intake tolerated by the patient.

Parenteral nutrition, either total or intermittent, may be used as an adjunctive treatment in these patients, although some centers have reported little success (Ricco-Pena, 1988). Open communication with these terminally ill patients is required among the patient, family, and health-care team to provide the patient with adequate but not heroic treatment.

CITED REFERENCES

Abitbol CL: Effects of amino acid addition during hemodialysis of children. J Parenter Enter Nutr 8:25, 1984.

Addis T: Glomerular Nephritis: Diagnosis and Treatment. New York, MacMillan, 1948, p 222–314.

AIDS Working Group: HTLV-III infection in kidney transplant recipients. Lancet 2:1361, 1985.

Andress DL: Aluminum-associated bone disease in chronic renal failure: High prevalence in the long-term dialysis population. J Bone Miner Res 1:391, 1986.

Bartlett R et al: Continuous arteriovenous hemofiltration: Improved survival in surgical acute renal failure? Surgery 100:400, 1986.

Bellinghieri G, et al: Correlation between increased serum and tissue L-Carnitine levels and improved muscle symptoms in hemodialyzed patients. Am. J Clin Nutr 38:523, 1983

Bernard DB: Extrarenal complications of the nephrotic syndrome. Kidney Int 33:1184, 1988.

Brenner BM: Hemodynamically mediated glomerular injury and the progressive nature of kidney disease. Kidney Int 23:647, 1983.

Brenner BM and Lazarus JM (eds): Acute Renal Failure, 2nd ed. New York, Churchill-Livingstone, 1988.

Cerra F: Hypermetabolism, organ failure and metabolic support. Surgery 101:1, 1987.

Coburn JW and Norris KC: Diagnosis of aluminum-related bone disease and treatment of aluminum toxicity with desferoxamine. Semin Nephrol 4:12, 1986.

Coburn JW and Salusky IB: Control of serum phosphorous in uremia. N Engl J Med 320:1140, 1989.

Coe FL: Nephrolithiasis: Causes, classification and management. Hosp Pract 16(4):33, 1981.

Coe FL: Treatment of hypercalciuria (Editorial). N Engl J Med 311:116, 1984.

Coe FL and Favus MJ: Disorders of stone formation. *In* Brenner BM and Rector FC (eds): The Kidney, 3rd ed. Philadelphia, WB Saunders, 1986.

Dwyer J et al: Acid/alkaline ash diets: Time for assessment and change. J Am Diet Assoc 85:841, 1985.

Erickson SB: Idiopathic nephrolithiasis. *In* Rous SN (ed): Stone Disease: Diagnosis and Management. Orlando, FL, Harcourt Brace Jovanovich, 1987.

Eschbach J et al: Correction of the anemia of end-stage renal disease with recombinant human erythropoietin. N Engl J Med 316:73, 1987.

Evanoff GV et al: Effect of dietary protein restriction on the progression of diabetic nephropathy. Arch Intern Med 147:492, 1987.

Feinstein EI: Total parenteral nutrition support of patients with acute renal failure. Nutr Clin Prac 3:9, 1988.

Feinstein E and Massry S: Nutritional therapy in acute renal failure. *In* Mitch W and Klahr S: Nutrition and the Kidney. Boston, Little, Brown, 1988.

Fine, RN et al: Accelerated growth following recombinant human growth hormone therapy, (Abstract), Am. Soc. Nephrol., 20th Annual Meeting, 1987.

Foulkes C: Nutritional evaluation of patients on maintenance dialysis therapy. Am Nephrol Nurses Assoc J 15(1):13, 1988.

Giordano C: Early diet to slow the course of chronic renal failure. *In* Zurukzoglu W and Papadimetrious M (eds): Eighth International Congress of Nephrology, June, 1981. Basel, S Karger, 1981.

Goldfarb S: Dietary factors in the pathogenesis and prophylaxis of calcium nephrolithiasis. Kidney Int 34:544, 1988.

Henck C-C and Ritz E: Hyperlipoproteinemia in renal insufficiency. Nephron 25:1, 1980.

Humphreys MH and Schoenfeld PY: AIDS and renal disease. Kidney 20:7, 1987.

Hunsicker LG: Nutritional requirements of renal transplant patients. *In* Mitch WE and Klahr S (eds): Nutrition and the Kidney. Boston, Little, Brown, 1988.

Ihle BU et al: The effect of protein restriction on the progression of renal inefficiency. N Engl J Med 321:1773, 1989.

Jamison RL: Dietary protein, glomerular hyperemia and progressive renal failure. Ann Intern Med 99:849, 1983.

Kaplan A: Continuous arteriovenous hemofiltration: Coming of age. Dial Transplant 17:252, 1988.

Kaysen G: Effect of dietary protein intake on albumin homeostasis in nephrotic patients. Kidney Int 29:572, 1986.

Klahr S: The modification of diet in renal disease study. N Engl J Med 320:864, 1989.

Klahr S, Schreiner G, and Ichikawa I: The progression of renal disease. N Engl J Med 318:1657, 1988.
Koch VH et al: Accelerated growth after recombinant human growth hormone treatment of children with chronic renal failure. J Pediatr 113:365, 1989.
Larsson L and Tiselius H-G: Hyperoxaluria. Miner Electrolyte Metab 13:242, 1987.
Lindner A et al: Accelerated atherosclerosis in prolonged maintenance hemodialysis. N Engl J Med 290:697, 1974.
Mactier RA: Control of hyperphosphatemia in dialysis patients: Comparison of aluminum hydroxide, calcium carbonate and magnesium trisilicate. Dialy Transplant Nephrol 11:599, 1987.
Maschio G et al: Effects of dietary protein and phosphorus restriction in the progression of early renal failure. Kidney Int 22:371, 1982.
Morris P: Renal transplantation indications, outcome, complications and results. *In* Schrier RW and Gottschalk CW (eds): Diseases of the Kidney, 4th ed. Boston, Little, Brown, 1988.
Office of Medical Applications and Research, National Institutes of Health: Consensus conference: Prevention and treatment of kidney stones. JAMA 260:977, 1988.
Olsham AR, Bruce J, and Schwartz A: Intradialytic parenteral nutrition administration during outpatient hemodialysis. Dialy Transplant 16:495, 1987.
Pak CYC et al: Ambulatory evaluation of nephrolithiasis: Classification, clinical presentation and diagnostic criteria. Am J Med 69:19, 1980.
Pak CYC et al: Is selective therapy of recurrent nephrolithiasis possible? Am J Med 71:615, 1981.
Pemberton CM et al: Mayo Clinic Diet Manual, 6th ed. Toronto, BC Decker, 1988.
Powell DR, Resenfeld RG, and Hintz RI: Effects of growth hormone therapy and malnutrition on the growth of rats with renal failure. Pediatr Nephrol 2:425, 1988.
Rao TKS and Friedman EA: Fluoride and bone disease in uremia. Kidney Int 7:125, 1975.
Rao T and Friedman E: The types of renal disease in the acquired immunodeficiency syndrome. N Engl J Med 316:1062, 1987.
Reaven GM, Swenson RS, and Sanfelippo ML: An inquiry into the mechanism of hypertriglyceridemia in patients with chronic renal failure. Am J Clin Nutr 33:1476, 1980.
Ricco-Pena G: AIDS and nutritional support in a health maintenance organization setting. Nutr Suppl Serv 8(8):14, 1988.
Rostand St G, Kirk KA, and Rutsby EA: Relationship of coronary risk factors to hemodialysis-associated ischemic heart disease. Kidney Int 22:304, 1982.
Schiller LR et al: Effect of the time of administration of calcium acetate on phosphorous binding. N Engl J Med 320:1110, 1989.
Sherman HC and Gettler AO: The balance of acid forming and base forming elements in foods and its relation to ammonia metabolism. J Biol Chem 11:323, 1912.
Slatopolsky E: Calcium carbonate as a phosphate binder in patients with chronic renal failure undergoing dialysis. N Engl J Med 315:157, 1986.
Soloway MS and Smith RA: Cranberry juice as a urine acidifier. JAMA 260:1465, 1988.
Vacha GM, Giorcelli G, Siliprandi N: Favorable effects of L-carnitine treatment on hypertryglyceridemia in hemodialysis patients. Am J Clin Nutr 38:523, 1983.
Wainer L, Resnick VA, and Resnick MI: Nutritional aspects of stone disease. *In* Pak CYC: Renal Stone Disease. Pathogenesis, Prevention and Treatment. Boston, Martinus Nijhoff, 1987.
Williams RC et al: Long-term survey of 538 patients with upper urinary tract stones. Br J Urol 35:416, 1963.
Zerwekh JE: Pathogenesis of hypercalciuria. *In* Pak CYC (ed): Renal Stone Disease. Pathogenesis, Prevention and Treatment. Boston, Martinus Nijhoff, 1987.

ADDITIONAL REFERENCES

A Healthy Food Guide for Patients with Diabetes and Kidney Disease. Chicago, The American Dietetic Association, in press.
Appel GB et al: The hyperlipidemia of the nephrotic syndrome. Relation to plasma albumin concentration, oncotic pressure, and viscosity. N Engl J Med 312:1544, 1985.
Barsotti G: Effects on renal function of a low nitrogen diet supplemented with essential amino acids and ketoanalogues and of hemodialysis and free protein supply in patients with chronic renal failure. Nephron 27:113, 1981.
Cranberries and urinary infections. Nutr MD 8(8):3, 1982.
Furst P: Principles of essential amino acid therapy in uremia. Am J Clin Nutr 31:1744, 1978.
Gillet D, Stover J, and Spizozzi NS (eds): A Clinical Guide to Nutrition Care in End-Stage Renal Disease. Chicago, American Dietetic Association, 1987.
Giovanetti S and Maggiore Q: A low-nitrogen diet with proteins of high biological value for severe uraemia. Lancet 1:1000, 1964.
Goldstein DJ: Nutrition for acute renal failure patients on continuous hemofiltration. Nutr Clin Prac 3:238, 1988.
Kaysen GA and Martinez CA: Nutritional management of the proteinuric patient. Nutr MD 15(12):1, 1989.
Kopple JD: Nutrition, diet and the kidney. *In* Shils ME and Young VR (eds): Modern Nutrition in Health and Disease, 7th ed. Philadelphia, Lea & Febiger, 1988, pp 1230–1268.
Ljunghall S, Fellstrom B, and Johansson G: Prevention of renal stones by a high fluid intake? Eur Urol 14:381, 1988.
Mault JR and Bartlett RH: Energy balance and survival in patients with acute renal failure. *In* Kramer P (ed): Arteriovenous Hemofiltration: A Kidney Replacement Therapy for the Intensive Care Unit. Berlin, Springer-Verlag, 1985, pp. 154–159.
Mitch WE and Klahr S: Nutrition and the Kidney. Boston, Little, Brown, 1988.
Robertson WG: Diet and calcium stones. Miner Electrolyte Metab 13:228, 1987.
Rosenberg ME: Nutrition and transplantation. Kidney 18:19, 1986.
Stover J and Nelson P: Nutritional recommendations for infants, children and adolescents with ESRD. *In* Gillit D, Stover J, and Spinozzi NS (eds): A Clinical Guide to Nutrition Care in End-Stage Renal Disease. Chicago, IL, The American Dietetic Association, 1987.
Task Force on Nutritional Management of Children with Chronic Renal Failure: Nutritional Management of Children with Chronic Renal Failure. Elk Grove Village, IL, American Academy of Pediatrics, 1986.
Walser M: 1988 Herman Award Lecture: Effect of ketoanalogues in chronic renal failure and other disorders. Am J Clin Nutr 49:17, 1989.
Wilkens K (ed): Suggested Guidelines for Nutrition Care of Renal Patients. Chicago, IL, American Dietetic Association, 1986.
Ziegler VS, Sucher KP, and Downes NJ: Southeast Asian renal exchange list. J Am Diet Assoc 89:85, 1989.

CHAPTER 36

NUTRITIONAL CARE IN NEOPLASTIC DISEASE*

Carrie L. Cheney, Ph.D., R.D., and Saundra N. Aker, R.D.

CHAPTER OUTLINE

KEY TERMS

CANCER CACHEXIA—the weak, malnourished, and emaciated condition that results from cancer

GLUTATHIONE PEROXIDASE—a selenium-containing enzyme that catalyzes the oxidation of glutathione

GRAFT-VERSUS-HOST DISEASE (GVHD)—a disease caused by the immune response of histoincompatible, immunocompetent donor cells against the tissues of an immunoincompetent host

INITIATION—the initial stage of tumorigenesis involving transformation of cellular DNA

OLIGOPHAGY—eating only a few foods

PROMOTION—the stage of tumorigenesis in which initiated cells are activated by a promoting agent to multiply and form a discrete tumor

TUMOR NECROSIS FACTOR (CACHECTIN)—a hormone-like protein that releases fat and reduces the concentration of enzymes required for the production and storage of fat; induces a state of anorexia

VENO-OCCLUSIVE DISEASE (VOD)—symptomatic occlusion of the small hepatic venules caused by hepatotoxins and radiation; may resolve after removal of the offending agent or may progress to portal hypertension and liver failure

XEROSTOMIA—mouth dryness

* *This work was supported by grants CA18029 and DK38516, National Cancer Institute and Clinical Nutrition Research Unit, DHHS.*

The study of diet and nutrition as it relates to cancer addresses both the causes and the consequences of cancer. Tumorigenesis or carcinogenesis is thought to be a multistage process, involving initiation, promotion, and tumor progression. The simplistic model of tumorigenesis conceives of two qualitatively different stages, initiation and promotion. *Initiation* involves a transformation of the cell that is produced by the interaction of chemicals, radiation, or viruses with cellular deoxyribonucleic acid (DNA). The transformation occurs rapidly, but the resultant cell remains dormant for a variable period until activated by a promoting agent. During *promotion,* initiated cells multiply to form a discrete tumor.

Although the exact mechanisms are unknown, nutrition may modify the carcinogenic process at any stage, including carcinogen metabolism, cellular and host defenses, cell differentiation, and tumor growth. Nutrition itself is also adversely affected, both by the tumor and by the medical treatment given, posing special problems for nutritional care.

NUTRITION IN THE ETIOLOGY OF CANCER

If the estimate that 80 to 90% of cancer is related to environmental factors is correct, including an estimated 35% related to diet, then the majority of human cancer may be potentially preventable. The strong influence of environmental factors is readily seen in studies of migration between cultures, which in many types of cancer are marked by changes in the pattern of occurrence to resemble that of the new country. For example, in Japan, mortality from breast and colon cancer is low and mortality from stomach cancer is high, whereas the reverse is seen in the United States. After two or three generations, the cancer pattern of Japanese immigrants is the same as that of their new home. The change coincides with differences in environmental exposure, lifestyle, and diet (see New Directions, p. 390).

Studies evaluating the role of diet in the etiology of cancer tend to produce conflicting results. When one major component of the diet is altered, other changes take place simultaneously. For example, decreasing animal protein also decreases animal fat and cholesterol. This makes the interpretation of research findings difficult because the effects cannot be clearly associated with a single factor. Many tumors have a long latency period, and the diet at the time of initiation or promotion, not at the time of diagnosis, may be important. Some prospective epidemiologic studies attempt to circumvent this difficulty by measuring diet at one point in time and by following the same subjects for several years (New Directions, p. 628). Diets contain both inhibitors and enhancers of carcinogenesis. Furthermore, the effects of a nutrient can vary depending on the type of cancer.

The National Cancer Institute and the Committee on Diet, Nutrition, and Cancer of the National Research Council have both made recommendations for dietary practices that may contribute to cancer prevention. These recommendations are discussed in Chapter 16.

Energy

In animal studies, chronic restriction of food inhibits the growth of most experimentally induced tumors and the occurrence of many spontaneous tumors. The degree of effect depends mainly on the extent and timing of caloric restriction and the tumor type. Underfeeding is most effective when maintained during both initiation and promotion; if limited to one phase, caloric restriction during the promotion phase is more effective in inhibiting tumor growth (Kritchevsky and Klurfeld, 1986).

It is not known how energy restriction inhibits tumor growth. According to one theory, mitotic activity is inhibited by the limited amount of carbohydrate and carbohydrate intermediates available for energy production. Other theories postulate that changes in hormones or host immunity produced by energy restriction inhibit tumorigenesis by complex mechanisms yet to be clarified.

Energy excess is more difficult to relate to cancer incidence. In the animal model, obesity per se is associated with more rapid tumor formation, but its role in susceptibility to cancer is interrelated with a number of dietary factors. Genetically determined body weight–related factors are also involved (Wolff, 1987). Excess weight is associated with increased cancer mortality in men and women. Increased incidence in obese women of estrogen-related tumors, such as breast and endometrial cancers, may be related to increased estrogen production, primarily in adipose tissue, which leads to increased exposure of estrogen-sensitive tissues (Hershcopf and Bradlow, 1987). Some studies implicating caloric expenditure and exercise suggest the need for further study of exercise, diet, obesity, and hormones with respect to cancer risk (Pariza and Boutwell, 1987).

Lipid

Some experimental and epidemiologic data show a link between some neoplasms and the amount of fat in the diet. Geographic variations in the incidence and mortality of cancers of the breast, colon, and prostate suggest that high-fat intake is related to higher risk of these cancers. Mortality from breast cancer varies internationally by per capita dietary fat consumption (Carroll and Khor, 1975) as shown in Figure 36–1. Because dietary fat intake is correlated with intake of other nutrients and dietary components, it is difficult to distinguish between the effects of dietary fats and protein, total calories, or fiber. A complex interaction of fat with these or other dietary components may account for inconsistent results of epidemiologic and experimental investigations (Kolonel, 1987). Other lipid constituents may also be important.

Fats are thought to affect the promotion stage of carcinogenesis. Some bile acids have been shown to act as tumor promotors; in the ionized state, both bile acids and fatty acids can be toxic to colonic epithelium (Carroll et al, 1986). Some experimental and clinical data support this hypothesis, although much remains to be clarified.

It is possible that the composition of the fat may also have a role in carcinogenesis. High intake of total fat increases the risk of breast cancer in animals, provided that a threshold requirement for unsaturated fatty acids is met (Rohan and Bain, 1987). The degree of desaturation of the fatty acid appears to be important. Some experimental data show that tumor incidence is enhanced by feeding lipids containing higher amounts of linoleic and linolenic acids. Linoleic acid is a precursor for prostaglandins and related compounds, and its effect on tumorigenesis may involve this mechanism. Research is underway to delineate the mechanisms involved. The long-chain ω-3 polyunsaturated fatty acids do not appear to enhance tumor incidence, and studies show that olive oil, which is high in monounsaturated fatty acids, is associated with lower cancer incidence in both experimental models and epidemiologic observations (Weisburger, 1986).

Increased dietary cholesterol has been associated with increased risk of cancer, especially colon and breast cancer (McMichael et al, 1984). Blood cholesterol levels have been related inversely to risk of colon cancer in many, but not all, epidemiologic studies. However, it does not seem that deliberate lowering of blood cholesterol levels by drugs or by diet alters the risk of cancer. A plausible explanation may be differing cholesterol dynamics in susceptible individuals. It is possible that the hypocholesterolemic individual consuming a relatively high-fat diet may produce greater amounts of bile acids and may thus excrete more fecal acids and neutral steroids (Broitman, 1986). Increased excretion of bile acids in turn may enhance colonic mucosal proliferation rate, increasing the susceptibility of the mucosa to carcinogens in the lumen.

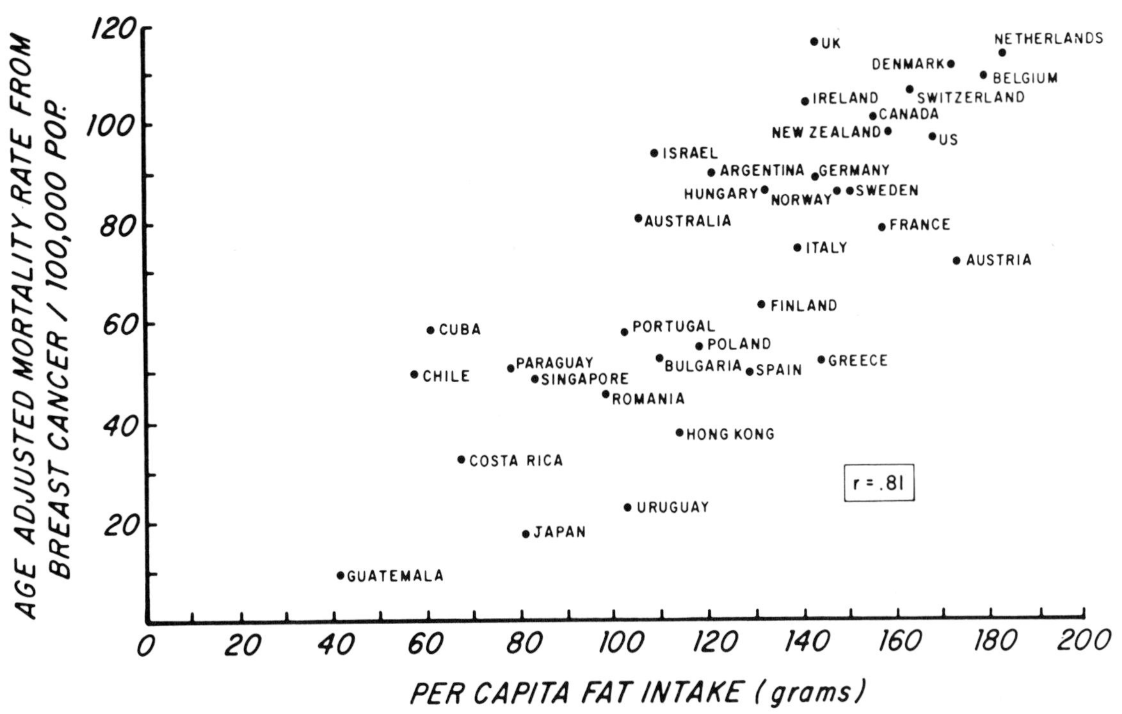

FIGURE 36–1. *Correlation between age-specific breast cancer mortality rates (>55 yr) and per capita fat intake. Data are from Food Balance 1979–81 Average, FAO, UN, Rome, 1984 and from Kurihara M, Aoki K, and Tominaga S: Cancer Mortality Statistics in the World. Nagoya, Japan University of Nagoya Press, 1984. (Redrawn from Wynder EL, Rose DP, and Cohen LA: Diet and breast cancer in causation and therapy. Cancer 58:1804, 1986.)*

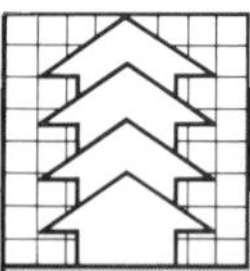

NEW DIRECTIONS: Intervention Trials in the Study of Cancer

Diet and cancer are increasingly linked in the public mind, and indeed the recommendations of the Surgeon General, the National Cancer Institute, and the US Dietary Guidelines reflect this association. However, the supporting evidence continues to be primarily circumstantial, and the desirability of recommending dietary changes for the population remains controversial among some members of the scientific community.

The most compelling evidence is derived from epidemiologic data comparing food intakes with cancer incidence in the 21 countries that maintain good cancer registration, and from migrant data that show dramatic changes in incidence of certain types of cancer as people change residence from one country to another. The strongest evidence relates total intake of dietary fat with cancers of the breast, colon, and prostate. Acceptance of this relationship is hindered by a lack of hard data, as well as of a plausible hypothesis to explain the mechanism by which fat intake causes, or more probably, promotes, these cancers. Unfortunately the kind of intervention trials that would be required to establish positive evidence involve the use of large numbers of subjects over a long period and are very expensive.

An example of the difficulty involved is the Women's Health Trial that was designed to define the relationship between dietary fat and breast cancer (Prentice et al, 1988). The proposed study involved a sample of 32,000 women aged 45 to 69 years with a cost estimated at 90 million dollars over a 10-year period. A feasibility phase conducted in 1984 to 1985 in three cities successfully demonstrated that women in this age group were able to successfully reduce their total fat intake from approximately 38% to 20% of total calories. However, before the trial moved into the final phase, a scientific review panel questioned the power of the trial to provide a convincing test of the hypothesis. The panel considered that the possibility of several confounding variables, particularly the effects of dietary fat and energy intake, would require an increase in sample size that would elevate the anticipated price tag to unacceptable levels. Although the trial was cancelled, other test options are currently under investigation.

Protein

Understanding the role of protein in tumor development is complicated by the fact that most diets high in protein are also high in meat and fat and low in fiber. The effect of protein on experimental carcinogenesis depends on the tissue of origin and the type of tumor, as well as on the type of protein and the caloric adequacy of the diet. In general, tumorigenesis is suppressed by diets containing levels of protein below that required for optimal growth, while it is enhanced by protein levels two to three times the amount that is required (Visek, 1986). The effects may be due to specific amino acids, a general effect of protein, or, in the case of low-protein diets, depressed food intake. Epidemiologic data are limited and conflicting. Increased meat intake has been associated with increased risk of colorectal and breast cancers in some studies, but not in others.

Because certain amino acid deficiencies inhibit some tumors, the feeding of amino acid–deficient diets or amino acid antagonists has been proposed as an adjunct to cancer therapy (Harper, 1986). Unfortunately, results are equivocal; restriction of protein or amino acid intake is effective on some tumors but is ineffective or has the opposite effect on others. The difference in response is likely to be due to differences in metabolism of individual amino acids or carcinogens, degree of amino acid pool depletion, or effects of depletion on the immune system, enzyme activities, or tumor cell metabolism.

Fiber

In recent years, much attention has been focused on the possible protective role of fiber in the prevention of cancer of the colon and rectum. This interest has arisen from the observation of low incidence of colon cancer among black Africans who consume a diet high in unabsorbable fiber. Subsequent epidemiologic studies have been inconclusive, in part because of limited knowledge of fiber components. Fiber is a generic term referring to a number of substances differing in chemical structure, physical properties, and physiologic effects (see Chapter 3). Most studies of the relationship between fiber and cancer have measured fiber-rich foods or total dietary crude fiber rather than fiber components.

Documenting the intake of fiber and its influence on other dietary components is also difficult. The intake of dietary fiber influences the intake of meat, fat, and refined carbohydrates. The physiologic effects of the fiber-rich food may, in turn, be the factors to consider in fiber's protective effect.

The quantity and type of dietary fiber affect intestinal microflora, bile salt metabolism, fecal bulk, and transit time, any or all of which may be involved in bowel carcinogenesis. Fiber may also protect by limiting energy intake and by enhancing fecal energy loss (Kritchevsky, 1986).

Metabolic studies have measured fecal characteristics and constituents against dietary fiber intakes in an attempt to provide evidence for these mechanisms. The experimental results are conflicting. Studies in animals demonstrate a protective effect with wheat bran and cellulose, but dietary pectin, corn bran, undegraded carageenan, agar, and hydrophilic mucilloid have an opposite effect (Jacobs, 1986). Human studies are also inconclusive. Dietary fiber increases fecal bulk, which may reduce cancer risk by decreasing the concentration of potential carcinogens such as bile acids in the stool, and thus limiting their contact with the colonic mucosa (Kritchevsky, 1986; Weisberger, 1986). Additional support for a protective mechanism comes from a 4-year nutritional intervention trial in patients with familial adenomatous polyposis, a premalignant condition. Patients who received daily grain-fiber supplements had fewer new polyps develop during the study period than patients who did not receive fiber supplements or who received vitamin C or E supplements (DeCosse et al, 1989). Some reports suggest that physical activity and bowel motility also have a role in the risk of colorectal cancer (Vena et al, 1987).

Vitamin A

Vitamin A (*retinol*), its analogues (*13-cis-retinoic acid, all-trans-retinoic acid*), and its precursors (the *carotenoids*) have all been suggested as possible inhibitors of carcinogenesis. Supplemental retinoids inhibit chemical carcinogenesis in the skin, mammary gland, esophagus, respiratory tract, pancreas, and urinary bladder of experimental animals (Moon and Mehta, 1986). Furthermore, the incidence of chemically induced tumors is greater in animals maintained on a vitamin A–deficient diet than in those fed adequate diets. Other experiments indicate that retinoids can reverse premalignant changes in the epithelium. Proposed mechanisms of action include influencing gene expression and cellular differentiation, and enhancing both humoral and cell-mediated immunity, possibly even stimulating specific antitumor immunity (Olson, 1986). Unfortunately, effective doses are large, and the potential for toxicity may prevent use in humans.

Beta-carotene is not toxic and may be protective in a mechanism independent of its role as a vitamin A precursor. As a protective antioxidant, it is able to trap toxic organic free radicals and single oxygen molecules. Limited animal data suggest that beta-carotene supplementation reduces the incidence of chemically induced tumors (Temple and Basu, 1987).

Studies of blood retinol levels and retinol intake and the risk of cancer in humans have not consistently detected an association (Hennekens et al, 1986). Evidence for the protective effect of high intake and high blood levels of beta-carotene is seen more consistently from studies of lung cancer and is found somewhat less consistently in studies of other sites (Connett et al, 1989; Paganini-Hill et al, 1987; Wald et al, 1988; Ziegler et al, 1984). The difficulty in assessing the role of dietary beta-carotene is that some other component of the carotene-rich vegetables and fruits may be responsible for the decreased risk of cancer (Wald et al, 1988). Moreover, a diet higher in vegetables and fruits is generally also higher in fiber and lower in fat, and these factors may be influential as well.

Vitamin C

The antioxidant properties of ascorbic acid may influence tumorigenesis. In the animal model, ascorbic acid inhibits the formation of carcinogenic nitrosamines. It is not known whether this reaction exists in humans; however, epidemiologic studies suggest that increased intake of fruits and vegetables rich in ascorbic acid is protective against cancer, particularly in the stomach and esophagus (Glatthaar et al, 1986).

Ascorbic acid deficiency among cancer patients has been described by several investigators, suggesting the therapeutic use of ascorbic acid. The reasons for low leukocyte ascorbate concentrations are unknown. Several mechanisms besides low dietary intake have been postulated, including the accumulation of the vitamin in tumors, and increased requirements for host resistance and cell-mediated immune function (Glatthaar et al, 1986). Clinical studies of the effect of supplemental ascorbic acid on the prognosis of cancer patients have yielded conflicting results. The two most carefully conducted randomized trials have shown no therapeutic benefit (Creagan et al, 1979; Moertel et al, 1985).

Vitamin E

Vitamin E has received attention because its function as an intracellular antioxidant may protect against carcinogen-induced chromosomal damage. A protective effect of vitamin E has not been consistently observed in animal studies. Epidemiologic data show an inverse relationship between serum vitamin E levels and subsequent development of cancer (Knekt, 1988; Kneckt et al, 1988), but conflicting results have been reported by others (Russell et al, 1988). The effect of vitamin E may be modified by selenium status in a synergistic relationship (Knekt, 1988), supporting the proposed interaction between vitamin E and selenium as antioxidants protecting against intracellular lipid peroxidation. Peroxidative cell damage is increased by high intakes of polyunsaturated fatty acids in animals, and the relationship between vitamin E and cancer in humans could depend on lipid intake or other dietary factors.

Calcium and Vitamin D

An inverse association between colon cancer incidence and per capita calcium intake has been observed in the United States and in other countries (McKeown-Eyssen and Bright-See, 1984). Although few in number, the epidemiologic studies have shown that milk or dietary calcium is associated with lower risk of disease (Wargovich, 1988). The mechanism proposed is that ionic calcium in the intestinal lumen binds with fats and bile acids to form calcium soaps, reducing the exposure of the bowel epithelium to potentially toxic substances. Calcium may also be involved in the regulation of epithelial proliferation in the bowel (Lipkin and Newmark, 1985).

Dietary vitamin D has also been associated with lower risk of colon cancer (Garland et al, 1985). Because vitamin D facilitates transport of calcium out of the intestinal lumen, a systemic protective mechanism for calcium is implied. Alternatively, vitamin D may have an independent effect, possibly by a role in cell proliferation and differentiation (DeLuca and Ostrem, 1986).

Selenium

Selenium supplementation inhibits the incidence and total number of tumors in a number of experimental models (Ip, 1986). Selenium is a component of glutathione peroxidase, an enzyme that protects against oxidative tissue damage. Available data suggest that chemopreventive effect is not mediated by the function of this enzyme or by the inhibition of lipid peroxidation (Medina, 1986). Instead, selenium may modulate carcinogenesis by inhibiting DNA synthesis and by enhancing host immune response.

Descriptive geographic studies have shown an inverse relationship between cancer mortality rates and selenium availability. Studies of cancer patients have generally shown that they have lower serum selenium levels than noncancer controls; however, most studies have a number of methodologic problems, and the low serum levels may have been a result of the disease (Clark, 1985). Prospective studies measuring serum selenium before diagnosis of cancer have recently reported that individuals with low serum selenium levels have an increased risk of cancer (Nomura et al, 1987; Virtamo et al, 1987), although conflicting results have also been reported.

Zinc

Experimental zinc deficiency increases the incidence of tumors induced by nitrosamines, although the mechanism is unknown (Barch and Iannaccone, 1986). Epidemiologic studies have shown an association between dietary zinc deficiency and increased incidence of esophageal cancer (Van Rensberg, 1981). Dietary zinc deficiency is uncommon except in areas of the world where zinc is relatively lacking in the soil and thus in the food supply, and the minimal intake is combined with high dietary phytate intake.

Alcohol

Several epidemiologic studies suggest that alcohol has a causal role in carcinogenesis, especially for cancers of the mouth, pharynx, larynx, and esophagus. Alcohol appears to have a greater effect on those tissues directly exposed to it during its consumption and to act synergistically with tobacco. In carcinogenesis, alcohol could act directly as a cell toxin or as a vehicle for cocarcinogens. Alternatively, alcohol could act indirectly by depressing the immune response, altering the metabolism of epithelial cells, enhancing absorption of carcinogens, or increasing the susceptibility to carcinogens (Rogers and Conner, 1986). The malnutrition associated with alcoholism is also likely to be important in the increased risk for certain cancers in the alcoholic individual.

Coffee

Coffee intake has been investigated as a possible risk factor for a variety of cancers. Although laboratory data indicate that the methylxanthine component (e.g., caffeine, theophylline, theobromine) is not carcinogenic, mortality from pancreatic cancer varies internationally with per capita coffee consumption (Binstock et al, 1983). However, the majority of evidence does not support a causal role for coffee in pancreatic cancer (Hiatt et al, 1988). Studies of other cancers suggest that neither cancer mortality rate nor the total cancer incidence is adversely related to coffee drinking (Jacobsen et al, 1986; LeGrady, 1987).

Artificial Sweeteners

The use of artificial sweeteners has been investigated primarily in relation to bladder cancer, mainly because of experimental evidence showing that large doses of saccharin produce tumors of the urinary tract and promote the action of carcinogens in the bladder of rats. Further studies defining the dose-response relationship for bladder tumor risk in the rat have led to the conclusion that the present level of exposure of humans presents an insignificant cancer risk (Newberne and Conner, 1986). Several epidemiologic studies suggest that the use of saccharin does not increase the risk of bladder cancer. It should be recognized, however, that detection of a weak carcinogenic effect is difficult and that there may be an effect of heavy use in certain individuals (Morrison and Buring, 1980).

The artificial sweetener *cyclamate* was removed from use because of presumed toxic effects of its principal metabolite. Subsequent reviews by the Federal Drug Administration (FDA) Cancer Assessment Committee and the National Academy of Sciences concluded that cyclamate is not carcinogenic (National Academy of Sciences, 1985). Cyclamate is used in many countries, and approval by the FDA for its use in the United States is pending.

Aspartame has not been carcinogenic in experimental studies; clinical studies have shown no ill effect in humans consuming large doses (Newberne and Conner, 1986). Epidemiologic data are not available because its approval for use is relatively recent.

Preservatives

Butylated hydroxytoluene (BHT) and *butylated hydroxyanisol (BHA)* are antioxidants widely used as preservatives. Studies conducted by FDA and the National Cancer Institute indicated no carcinogenic activity of either compound. Recent work, however, has found that BHA and BHT cause proliferative lesions in the stomachs of rats given large doses (Newberne and Conner, 1986), and further evaluation is in progress. Conversely, BHT appears to protect experimental animals from the effects of a number of carcinogens (Fukiyama and Hsieh, 1985).

Nitrates, Nitrites, and Nitrosamines

Nitrates and nitrites have received attention because of their relationship with nitrosamines, which are potent carcinogens in various species. *Nitrate* can be readily reduced to *nitrite*, which in turn can interact with dietary substrates such as amines and amides to produce *N-nitroso compounds,* or *nitrosamines* and *nitrosamides*. This conversion, known as *N*-nitrosation, has been demonstrated to occur in saliva as well as in the stomach, colon, and bladder. It is not known, however, whether *N*-nitrosation is a cause of any human cancer. Gastric cancer is not common, and incidence has decreased steadily during the past 50 years.

Nitrates are present in a variety of foods, but the main dietary sources are vegetables and drinking water. Sodium and potassium nitrates are used in the processes of salting, pickling, and curing foods. Nitrosamines are present in tobacco and tobacco smoke.

Epidemiologic studies implicate an interplay of dietary factors in the development of cancer in the gastric mucosa (Howson et al, 1986; Weisberger, 1986). Available evidence suggests that the mucosa may be damaged by a diet rich in salt, thus increasing vulnerability to a carcinogen derived from a diet rich in nitrate/nitrites. It also appears that both disease initiation and progression may be inhibited by consumption of fresh vegetables, especially those that contain vitamin C, which has been shown to inhibit nitrosamine formation. The *N*-nitrosation reaction is also inhibited by tocopherol (Mirvish, 1986), although the significance of this is unknown.

Method of Food Preparation

Cooking methods can cause contamination of the food by carcinogens, especially *polycyclic aromatic hydrocarbons* (e.g., benzo(a)pyrene) and *heterocyclic aromatic amines* (Miller and Miller, 1986). These toxic substances are formed during combustion of carbon fuel and pyrolysis of protein, which commonly occurs during charcoal broiling, frying, and smoking of meats. Several investigators have found mutagenic activity in foods after frying and charcoal broiling. Furthermore, mutagenic activity has been demonstrated in the urine of human subjects after eating fried meats (Baker et al, 1982). Epidemiologic studies have indicated an increased risk of stomach and esophageal cancers with the frequent intake of smoked and fried foods (Howson et al, 1986; Yu et al, 1988).

NUTRITIONAL EFFECTS OF CANCER

The adverse nutritional effects of cancer can be severe and may be compounded by effects of the therapeutic regimens and the psychologic impact of cancer. The result is often a profound state of depletion. Recent data suggesting an association between minor weight loss and a shortened duration of survival (Fearon and Carter, 1988) imply a very subtle relationship between nutritional status and the outcome of malignant disease.

Cachexia

Malnutrition is a major cause of morbidity and mortality in cancer patients, in whom it is usually seen as a syndrome known as *cancer cachexia* (Fig. 36–2). A number of factors predispose the patient to the development of cachexia; however, the malignancy itself is responsible for initiating the syndrome, and its reversal is achieved only by control of the disease (Kern and Norton, 1988). Cancer cachexia presents clinically with anorexia, weight loss, anemia, diminished reflexes, asthenia, and emaciation. It appears to be a complex metabolic problem unique to malignant disease and involves aberrations in substrate metabolism, water, electrolyte and acid-base balance, vitamin metabolism, enzyme systems, and immune and endocrine functions.

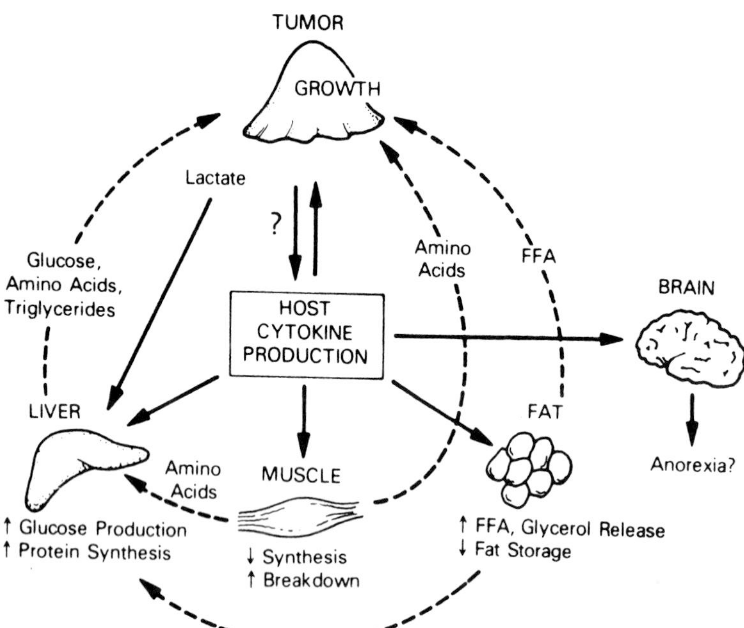

FIGURE 36–2. *The mechanism of cachexia in patients with cancer. (From Rombeau JL and Caldwell MD: Enteral and Tube Feeding, 2nd ed. Philadelphia, WB Saunders, 1990, p 273.)*

Energy Metabolism

Weight loss results from a negative energy balance, although whether the wasting is due to a reduction in energy intake or to an increase in expenditure is unclear. Experimental and clinical evidence indicate that both mechanisms occur (Fearon and Carter, 1988).

Energy intake has been repeatedly shown to be voluntarily reduced in tumor-bearing animals. Similar reductions have been reported in patients with various malignancies and stages of disease. However, the severity of the weight loss does not directly correlate with nutrient consumption; decreased intake cannot entirely explain the progressive weight loss (Fearon et al, 1988).

The normal response to decreased food intake, or semistarvation is lowered basal metabolic rate (BMR). However, patients with cancer and tumor-bearing animals exhibit the opposite response. Significantly increased BMR and total energy expenditure have been seen in cancer patients compared with age, sex, and activity matched controls (Schersten et al, 1980). The mechanism for this increase is unknown; it does not appear to be a result of tumor growth alone but to host metabolic alterations as well. Rates of protein synthesis and degradation may be changed in patients with cancer; however, these alterations do not necessarily result in a measurable increase in BMR. The assumption that energy expended in elevation of whole body protein turnover causes weight loss in cancer patients may be an oversimplification (Fearon et al, 1988).

Substrate Metabolism

Energy metabolism is intimately related to carbohydrate, protein, and lipid metabolism, all of which are altered by tumor growth. The tumor exerts a consistent demand for glucose. The neoplastic cell exhibits a characteristically high rate of anaerobic metabolism yielding lactate as the end product. This expanded lactic acid pool requires an increased rate of host gluconeogenesis via the Cori cycle activity, which is increased in some cancer patients but not in others (Fearon and Carter, 1988). Thus, it is unclear whether the weight loss of cancer patients is due primarily to reduced food intake, increased energy expenditure, or a combination of the two. Moreover, the mechanism of any proposed elevation of energy expenditure is not established.

Alterations are seen in protein metabolism and appear to be directed toward providing adequate amino acids for tumor growth. Most notable is the loss of skeletal muscle protein, which is due to both a decrease in the rate of synthesis and an increase in the rate of muscle protein degradation (Kern and Norton, 1988). Likewise, the rate of serum albumin synthesis diminishes and in some cases the rate of its degradation increases, accounting in part for the hypoalbuminemia characteristic of cachectic cancer patients.

Recent work has focused on the macrophage-produced monokine *cachectin/tumor necrosis factor (TNF)* as a possible mediator of cancer cachexia. Cachectin/TNF or other host-derived cytokines have been implicated as signal molecules in cachexia, based on similar metabolic derangements produced by these cytokines in other chronic wasting illnesses (Kern and Norton, 1988).

Lipid metabolism is altered, as evidenced by inappropriate mobilization of free fatty acids from adipose tissues and subsequent depletion of total body fat. Disorders may also be seen in the form of decreased lipid clearance from serum and elevated plasma-free fatty acid levels (Kern and Norton, 1988). Supporting evidence suggests that the tumor produces lipolytic substances that are directly responsible for increased fat mobilization (Thompson et al, 1986).

Other Metabolic Abnormalities

Fluid and electrolyte imbalances are seen in patients with advanced cancer, the most frequent being hyponatremia. Hypoalbuminemia and hypocalcemia are also often seen. Severe imbalances in fluid and electrolyte status may be present in patients with cancers that promote excessive diarrhea or vomiting, and similar consequences result from hormone-secreting tumors that impair renal function.

Radioisotope tracer studies have shown advanced cancer patients to be overhydrated (Cohn et al, 1981). Because body weight is used as an index of nutritional status, this overhydration may be misleading. Therefore, other indices of nutritional status should be used in conjunction with body weight.

Vitamin and mineral metabolism is altered in malignant disease. Serum levels of ascorbic acid, thiamin, folate, vitamin A, iron, and zinc are often depressed, whereas serum copper is increased (Dickerson, 1981). The significance of these changes remains speculative.

The activities of several enzyme systems are affected, as are certain endocrine functions, and the nature of the alterations varies by tumor type. Host immunologic function is impaired, apparently the result of both the neoplasm and the progressive malnutrition.

In addition to the cancer-induced metabolic effects, the mass of the tumor may anatomically alter the normal physiology of specific organ systems.

Sensory Changes

Alterations in taste and smell sensations are common and contribute to the anorexia frequently seen in cancer patients. The recognition threshold for sweet is increased and for bitter is often lowered, whereas thresholds for sour and salt tend to increase, although there is considerable variation among reported studies (Trant et al, 1982). Lowered taste threshold for bitter may lead to total meat aversion. The sensation abnormalities do not consistently correlate with the extent of tumor involvement, tumor response to therapy, or food preferences and intake.

NUTRITIONAL EFFECTS OF CANCER THERAPY

Antitumor therapy may involve chemotherapy, radiation, surgery, or immunotherapy or may be a multimodal combination of these. Certain hematologic malignancies are treated by bone marrow transplantation. Each of these therapeutic programs contributes to the nutrient alterations in the cancer patient by reducing food intake, decreasing absorption, or altering metabolism.

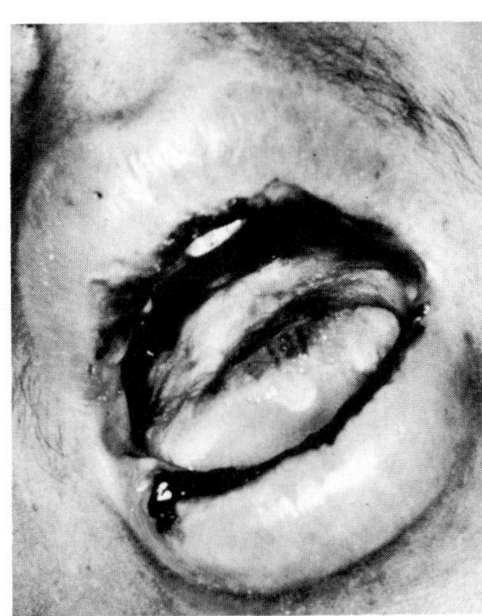

FIGURE 36–3. *Severe oral mucositis following marrow transplantation. Patient has also had high dose cyclophosphamide and whole body radiation. (From Peterson DE and Sonis ST [eds]: Oral Complications of Cancer Therapy. The Hague, Martinus Nijhoff Publishing, 1983, p 128.)*

Chemotherapy

The action of chemotherapeutic agents is not limited to malignant tissue but affects normal cells as well. As a result, major organ toxicities are seen, and dietary intake and nutritional status are adversely affected. Food intake is inhibited by *mucositis* (Fig. 36–3), cheilosis, glossitis, stomatitis, and esophagitis caused by many drugs. Table 36–1 summarizes the side effects of many drugs. Nausea and vomiting occur with almost all anti-

TABLE 36–1. Common Problems Associated with Oncologic Medications*

Anorexia, nausea, and vomiting can be caused by:
  Nitrogen mustard, imidazole, carboxamide, *cis*-platinum, hexamethylmelamine, streptozotocin, adriamycin, cyclophosphamide, bleomycin, asparaginase, carmustine, dactyinomycin, doxorubicin, methotrexate, and procarbazine
Mucositis can be caused by:
  5-fluorouracil, methotrexate, vinblastine, bleomycin, antinomycin D, adriamycin, dactinomycin, doxorubicin, and hydroxyurea
Constipation can be caused by:
  Vincristine and vinblastine
Fluid retention can be caused by:
  Hormonal therapy
Liver toxicity can be caused by:
  Methotrexate, mithramycin, and asparaginase
Reaction to monoamine oxidase inhibitors can be caused by:
  Procarbazine

* From Kouba J: Nutritional care of the individual with cancer. Nutr Clin Prac 3:176, 1988.

neoplastic drugs. Taste abnormalities lead to anorexia and *oligophagy* (eating few foods). Diarrhea may be induced, or there may be constipation or *adynamic ileus* (inhibition of bowel motility). Symptoms of gastrointestinal toxicity are usually not long-lasting; however, some combination chemotherapeutic programs have severe and prolonged gastrointestinal effects. Some agents, especially corticosteroids, cause tissue breakdown and promote excessive urinary loss of protein, potassium, and calcium. The intestinal mucosa and digestive processes are affected, altering digestion and absorption to some degree. Protein, energy, and vitamin metabolism may be impaired, although the consequences of this are not known. Total lymphocyte count is depressed and does not accurately reflect nutritional status following antineoplastic agent administration.

Radiation Therapy

The effects of radiation vary according to the region irradiated. Radiation to the head and neck causes a variety of food ingestion problems, including sore throat, mucositis, *xerostomia* (*mouth dryness*), severe dental and gum destruction, and altered taste and smell (Schubert and Izutsu, 1987). Anorexia is common, and weight loss is a major problem. Radiation to the thorax induces esophagitis with accompanying dysphagia. Esophageal stricture leading to obstruction can occur. Radiation to the abdomen may produce acute gastritis or enteritis with nausea, vomiting, diarrhea, and anorexia; severe gastrointestinal damage is accompanied by malabsorption of glucose, lactose, fats, and electrolytes. *Radiation enteritis* can develop into a chronic form, with symptoms of ulceration or obstruction intensifying the risk of malnutrition. Total body irradiation may cause all of the aforementioned acute symptoms to some extent. As with chemotherapy, radiation depresses immune function, thus limiting the applicability of this as a nutrition assessment indicator.

Radiochemotherapy

When radiation is used concurrently with chemotherapy, the combined toxic effects of the two treatments may simply be additive. However, in some cases the severity is even greater than the sum of individual toxicities (Schubert and Izutsu, 1987).

Immunotherapy

Biologic agents are natural products made in quantities through cloning and genetic engineering. Used directly as cytotoxic agents or indirectly as stimulators of the patient's own natural defenses, biological agents can kill tumor cells. *Monoclonal antibodies* have produced complete or partial remission in patients with lymphoma, gastrointestinal cancer, and neuroblastoma. Alpha-interferon is used to treat hairy cell leukemia. Clinical trials are in progress with TNF, colony stimulating factors, and interleukin-2 (IL-2).

Marrow Transplantation

Marrow transplantation is performed for the treatment of certain hematologic malignancies, such as leukemia, lymphoma, and occasionally solid tumors. The preparative regimen includes cytotoxic chemotherapy and total body irradiation to suppress immunologic reactivity and to eradicate malignant cells. This is followed by intravenous infusion of bone marrow from a suitable donor. Acute toxic reactions, such as nausea, vomiting, and diarrhea, diminish 24 to 48 hours after the administration of preconditioning therapy. Delayed effects during the first 2 months after the transplant include mucositis, stomatitis, esophagitis, salivary and taste alterations, and gut damage. Patients typically have little or no oral intake during the first 30 days post transplant and require support by way of enteral or parenteral nutrition.

Graft-versus-host disease (GVHD) is a major complication in which donor marrow cells react against the tissues of the "foreign" host. The functions of several target organs (skin, liver, gut, lymphoid cells) are disrupted, and susceptibility to infection is increased. GVHD of the intestinal tract is usually manifested within the first 70 days post transplant and may be resolved or may go on to a chronic form requiring long-term treatment and dietary management. GVHD of the liver, evidenced by icterus and abnormal liver function tests, frequently accompanies gastrointestinal GVHD and further complicates nutritional management.

The symptoms of gastrointestinal GVHD are severe. The volumes of secretory diarrhea often exceed 3 l/day, and total gut rest is indicated until diarrhea is reduced to less than 500 ml/day (McDonald et al, 1986). Initial oral feedings begin with beverages that are iso-osmotic, low-fat, and lactose-free because of the loss of intestinal enzymes due to intestinal villi and mucosa alterations. As those are tolerated, solids of the same nature are introduced individually. Dietary restrictions are progressively reduced as foods are gradually introduced in the absence of increasing symptoms.

Veno-occlusive disease (VOD) of the liver is characterized by chemotherapy induced damage to the hepatic venules. It can develop 1 to 3 weeks post transplant, resulting in symptoms of hepatomegaly, ascites, jaundice, renal failure, and encephalopathy and presents a difficult clinical nutritional management situation (McDonald et al, 1985). Other complications of marrow transplantation include pulmonary disease and multiple organ failure. The side effects of cancer therapy that may cause nutritional problems are summarized in Table 36–2.

NUTRITIONAL CARE OF THE PATIENT WITH CANCER

General Nutritional Care

A common secondary diagnosis in patients with advanced neoplastic disease is protein-energy malnutrition. Weight loss and altered nutritional status have been associated with decreased survival, reduced tolerance to therapy, and increased postoperative morbidity (Chlebowski, 1985; Silberman, 1985). Even small amounts of weight loss prior to therapy (less than 5% of body weight) may worsen prognosis significantly (DeWys et al, 1980). Because of this, the importance of early nutritional assessment and intervention as a preventive measure seems clear.

Although the detrimental effect of malnutrition on survival is evident, the favorable influence of nutritional intervention is not clear. Nutritional repletion is usually achieved by aggressive modes of support using enteral intubation or parenteral alimentation, which can successfully replenish lean body mass, visceral protein stores, and immunocompetence. Except in one study of marrow transplant patients supported with total parenteral nutrition (TPN) (Weisdorf et al, 1987), the beneficial effect of nutritional intervention on survival has not been demonstrated (Koretz, 1984). A review of the studies of parenteral nutrition (PN) given to adequately nourished patients undergoing chemotherapy has led the American College of Physicians to conclude that it has no benefit to such patients and should not be used routinely, although it may be beneficial to malnourished patients (American College of Physicians, 1989). Further study is needed to clarify if subgroups of patients or conditions of treatments exist for which PN is beneficial.

Of concern is the possibility that nutritional support will preferentially benefit the tumor. In tumor-bearing animals, nutritional repletion stimulates tumor growth while improving host nutritional status. Tumor stimulation has not been observed in cancer patients, although further study is warranted (Torosian and Daly, 1986). Thus the controversy regarding the merits of nutritional support for cancer patients remains. Nevertheless, the adverse effects of malnutrition are clear. Nutritional support does serve as prevention and therapy for malnutrition, and in this function plays an important role in care of the cancer patient (Buss, 1987).

TABLE 36–2. Side Effects of Cancer Therapy That May Cause Nutritional Problems

Radiation Treatment
Nausea, vomiting, and general loss of appetite
Taste and smell changes
Dental problems
Mucositis and xerostomia
Esophageal stricture from radiation to the thorax
Diarrhea and malabsorption from bowel damage
Depressed immune function
Chemotherapy Treatment
Taste abnormalities
Mucositis, cheilosis, glossitis, stomatitis, and esophagitis
Diarrhea and malabsorption from gastrointestinal toxicity
Nausea, vomiting, and anorexia
Anemias
Depressed immune function
Immunotherapy
Fever
Nausea and vomiting
Immune stimulation including reversal of neutropenia
Weight loss
Marrow Transplantation
Mucositis, stomatitis, and esophagitis
Taste and salivary changes
Diarrhea and malabsorption from bowel damage
Acute and chronic graft-versus-host disease
Veno-occlusive disease
Pulmonary disease
Renal disease

Goals of Nutritional Care

The overall goals of the nutritional care of the cancer patient are to (1) prevent or correct nutritional deficiencies, and (2) to minimize weight loss. The emphasis is on prevention. Unfortunately, nutritional consultation is often considered only after the patient becomes severely depleted. The initial health care plan should include an assessment to determine the risk of nutritional depletion with supportive care planned (see Chapter 17).

Strategies for modifying nutrient intake depend on the specific feeding problem and on the extent of depletion. The oral route is the preferred mode of feeding but may be resisted by the patient who has nausea, altered taste sensations, and dysphagia. Eating is encouraged by modifying the food and its presentation. Patients who have altered taste acuity may benefit from increased use of flavorings and seasonings during food preparation. Meat aversion requires eliminating red meats, which are stronger in flavor, or emphasizing alternate protein sources. Dysphagia due to lesions in the oral and esophageal tissues can be lessened with foods that are soft and liquid and at moderate or room temperature. Artificial saliva preparations and saliva stimulants are useful in cases of diminished salivation, as are foods with high-moisture content. Patients with intestinal damage may require dietary modifications in lactose, fat, and fiber content as well as in texture. Commercial nutritional supplements can be included in many dietary plans. Guidelines for oral feedings are presented in Table 36–3. Management of diarrhea and steatorrhea is discussed in Chapter 27.

Timing of Food Presentation

The timing of food presentation deserves consideration. Cancer patients complain of decreased ability to eat as the day progresses (the morning being the best time for eating). This symptom may be due to sluggish digestion and gastric emptying as a result of decreased production of digestive secretions, gastrointestinal mucosal atrophy, and gastric muscle atrophy. Frequent small feedings with particular emphasis on feedings given in the morning are suggested.

The timing of meals or snacks relative to gastrointestinal toxic therapy may have a bearing on subsequent learned food aversions, which develop when specific foods are associated with unpleasant symptoms such as nausea and vomiting and psychologic stimuli such as anxiety (Dolgin and Katz, 1988; Padilla, 1986). The effect may not be limited to new food items but may also involve foods in the patient's usual diet eaten before treatment.

Enteral Tube Feeding

Efforts to encourage oral intake sometimes fail or are inappropriate, and more aggressive feeding methods are required. If the gut is functional, enteral tube feeding is utilized. The nasogastric route is most often used, although tubes may be inserted elsewhere in the intestinal tract when necessary (see Chapter 30). The selection of the enteral solution is determined by several factors, including the functional capacity of the gut, the intubation site, the patient's metabolic status, and the cost and convenience considerations, especially if used at home. Appendix Table 33 describes available enteral preparations. Blenderized formulas (see Table 30–3) may be used with large-diameter tubes and have the advantage of lower cost, but these formulas are not suitable for the more common small-diameter feeding tubes. Commercial milk-based or soy-based formulas serve most needs. Defined formula diets can be utilized in patients with decreased digestive capacity. Patients with radiation enteritis or existing malnutrition may have multiple malabsorption problems and benefit from soy-based (lactose-free), low-residue, and low-fat formulas.

TABLE 36–3. Guidelines for Oral Feeding During Antitumor Therapy*

Problem	Diet	Supplements and Aids	Poorly Tolerated Foods
Acute gastrointestinal toxicity	Clear, cold liquids Light, low-fat foods.	None	Milk products; cream soups; fried foods; sandwiches; sweet desserts.
Stomatitis, esophagitis	Liquid and soft diet Broth based soups; fruit ades; carbonated beverages; melons. Alter texture and temperature.	Glucose polymers; mild-flavored supplements; frequent oral hygiene; frequent saline rinses.	Juices, especially citrus; bananas; crisp or raw foods; meats; spicy entrees; textured or granular foods; coarse bread products; extremely hot or cold foods.
Viscous mucous production, xerostomia (mouth dryness)	Liquid diet. Tea with lemon; juices; fruit ades; popsicles; carbonated beverages; broth-based soups; thinned hot cereal.	Glucose polymers; artificial saliva; frequent saline rinses and oral hygiene.	Thick nectars and liquids; thick cream soups; thick hot cereals; bread products; gelatin; oily foods.
Decreased salivation	Regular diet with high-moisture foods. Gravies; sauces; casseroles; chicken; fish; beverages with foods; citric acid-containing foods; sherbet; melons; vegetables with sauces.	Artifical saliva; glucose polymers; saliva stimulants, such as sugarless lemon drops and gum; frequent saline rinses.	Dry foods; bread products; meats; crackers; bananas; excessively hot foods; alcohol.
Mouth blindness (hypogeusia)	Regular diet with strongly flavored foods. Spicy foods with emphasis on aroma and texture.	Flavored supplements; frequent saline rinses.	Bland foods; plain meats; unsalted foods.
Taste alterations (dysgeusia)	Regular diet with many cold foods. Milk products. Emphasis on experimentation.	Fruit-flavored supplements.	Red meats; chocolate; coffee; tea.
Early satiety	High-calorie diet with calorically dense foods. Meat; fish; poultry; eggs; whole milk; cheese; cream soups; ice cream; whole-milk yogurt; creamed vegetables; rich desserts.	Calorically dense supplements; glucose polymers.	Low or nonfat milk products; broth soups; green salads; steamed, plain vegetables; low-calorie beverages.

* Adapted from Aker SN and Lenssen P: A Guide to Good Nutrition During and After Chemotherapy and Radiation, 3rd ed. Seattle, WA, Fred Hutchison Cancer Research Center, 1988.

Parenteral Nutrition

If the gastrointestinal tract is not functioning or enteral support is not feasible, intravenous alimentation, or PN, must be considered. This mode of feeding involves the administration of concentrated nutrient solutions via infusion into a larger-diameter vein, usually the subclavian vein. PN support may be partial, to supplement a limited oral intake, or it may be the only source of nutrient intake, in which case it is referred to as TPN.

The ideal parenteral formula for cancer patients has not been determined (Mahaffey and Copeland, 1987). Energy and protein are usually given as glucose and a mixture of amino acids. Energy is 35 to 55 kcal/kg, and protein intake should be 1.2 to 2 g/kg. Intravenous fat may be given to prevent essential fatty acid deficiency and to provide a balance of substrates to lessen possible deleterious effects on various organs, such as the liver or lungs. Electrolytes are added to the solution, as are certain trace metals and vitamins. Details regarding the nutrient composition and administration are given in Chapter 30.

The frequency and severity of complications of TPN in the cancer patient are no greater than those in the noncancer patient. Occasional complications include catheter-related infections, venous thrombosis, and fluid overload. Mild to moderate elevations in tests of liver function have been reported (Lindmark et al, 1986). Intense monitoring and specialized care are required. The use of TPN on an outpatient basis is successful in selected cases if the patient and family are cooperative and are instructed in its use (see Chapter 30).

Patient Cooperation

Regardless of which mode of feeding is utilized, nutritional goals should be specific, achievable, and limited in scope to encourage patient cooperation. The goals need to be directed toward a visible means of feedback, such as body weight or some other meaningful index. Instruction of the patient and family members regarding expected problems and their possible solution should be initiated early in the cancer therapy course, and should be ongoing in conjunction with follow-up nutritional assessment.

Pediatric Patient

Like the adult cancer patient, the child with cancer can suffer adverse nutritional consequences as a result of both the malignancy and the treatment. Overt malnutrition has been found in a high percentage of children at the time of diagnosis, indicating substantial metabolic and symptomatic effects of the tumor. The effects of antitumor therapy are similar to those described previously for cancer patients in general. Treatment commonly is multimodal, and the complications of radiation may be enhanced by combination with chemotherapy. In addition, the nutrient requirements per kilogram of body weight of a child are greater. Thus, the child with cancer is at high risk for protein-energy malnutrition, and its impact is reflected in tolerance to treatment, incidence of complications, response to therapy, and survival.

The psychologic impacts of fear, unpleasant hospital routines, unfamiliar foods, learned food aversions, and pain require creative efforts to minimize their effects. Nutritional supplements given orally can be useful, although their acceptance is often a problem, and the child should be offered a selection from which to choose. Because feeding by nasogastric tube is not usually an acceptable alternative in young children, efforts to promote eating by serving familiar foods and by encouraging parental involvement are vital.

If these efforts are not successful, or if the gastrointestinal tract is not functioning adequately, PN is an alternative. PN is also indicated for children who present at the beginning of therapy in a malnourished state.

Additionally, prophylactic use of TPN and bowel rest for patients at risk for enteritis might minimize intestinal trauma (Copeland et al, 1980). The efficacy of its routine use in all children at risk, however, has not been supported (Donaldson, 1982).

The nutritional requirements of pediatric cancer patients are similar to those of normal growing children with an adjustment for activity level. The pediatric cancer patient often is not bedridden and is as active as his or her healthy peers. Factors that may alter nutrient requirements in cancer include the impact of the malignancy on host metabolism, the catabolic effects of antineoplastic therapy, and physiologic stress such as surgery, fever, malabsorption, and infection. Fluid requirements are increased during cytoreductive therapy, fever, diarrhea, or high-output renal failure. Micronutrients may require supplementation during periods of poor intake, stress, or malabsorption. The best long-term indicator of adequate nutrient intake is growth (Sherry et al, 1987).

The long-term nutritional effects of cancer and its treatment in children are not well documented. Deficiencies in energy and protein can be expected to adversely affect growth, although the impact may be temporary and compensation may occur after cessation of successful tumor therapy. A survey of children with acute lymphocytic leukemia reported a delay in linear growth rate during the period of treatment followed by resumption of normal or even accelerated growth after completion of therapy (Verzosa et al, 1976). On the other hand, the treatment may have effects on growth independent of nutritional deprivation. Pastore and co-workers observed a high frequency of neurologic and musculoskeletal sequelae after therapy in infancy (Pastore et al, 1982). In older children, kyphoscoliosis was a common late effect of radiotherapy. With the increase in survival rates for several childhood cancers, further studies of the long-term effects are needed.

Terminal Cancer Patient

The use of aggressive nutritional support techniques can prolong life. It has questionable benefit, however, for patients who have failed antitumor therapy and have no meaningful expectations of a positive outcome (Ota et al, 1986). Extending the life of a terminal cancer patient usually represents an extension of suffering and financial burden. More appropriate priorities are suggestions for oral feedings as tolerated and the provision of emotional support. The pleasurable aspects of eating should be emphasized, without concern for quantity or nutrient content.

Marrow Transplant Patient

The marrow transplantation procedure presents severe nutritional consequences and requires prompt, aggressive nutritional intervention (Lenssen and Aker, 1985). During the preparatory phase, the patient has nausea, vomiting, and diarrhea caused by the chemoradiation conditioning therapy, and antiemetics may be helpful. Food intake may remain low for upwards of 4 to 5 weeks post transplant.

Following marrow transplantation, the delayed onset complications include varying degrees of mucositis, xerostomia, and dysgeusia (Schubert and Izutsu, 1987). Bland liquids and soft solids are best tolerated. Salivary stimulants and substitutes are beneficial for temporary relief of dry mouth; liquids and foods with sauces and gravies are suggested. Changes in taste acuity persist for 30 to 50 days post transplant (Barale et al, 1982). Strong flavored or spicy foods are better accepted if mucositis is absent. Nausea, vomiting, and diarrhea may occur with the administration of antibiotics and may increase the existing complications.

Because oral intake is virtually nonexistent for an extended period and the function of the gastrointestinal tract is compromised, TPN must be instituted. TPN is begun after the final dose of chemotherapy before the marrow transplant. A significant improvement in disease-free survival has been shown in marrow transplant patients receiving TPN compared with patients receiving no TPN (Weisdorf et al, 1987). The adequacy of TPN is determined on a daily basis by monitoring serum electrolyte and glucose levels, weight change, and chemical status. The administration of optimal levels of TPN is complicated by its frequent interruption for the infusion of antibiotics, blood products, and drugs, necessitating more concentrated nutrient solutions, increased flow rates, and the use of double and triple lumen catheters (Aker et al, 1982).

Patient Rehabilitation

Concern for the patient with cancer should continue until the patient has returned to a useful life. Patients need to be encouraged to care for themselves and to maintain their own nutritional intake. Many patients live at home or in temporary apartments during the later phases of treatment; thus much of their food preparation is independent of the treatment center. The clinic dietitian-nutritionist can help to guide food selections. Patient support groups can be formed for mutual encouragement. Several books with high-calorie and high-protein recipes and suggestions for making foods palatable are available, and could be used by patients to help maintain their dietary intake at home.

Unproven Dietary Treatments

The role of diet and nutrition in cancer causation and treatment is the focus of current scientific research. At the same time, several unorthodox, unproven therapies involving dietary modifications are increasingly used for cancer treatment and, in some cases, prevention. Among the current popular methods are metabolic therapy, dietary treatments, and megavitamins.

Metabolic therapy is possibly the most frequently used unorthodox treatment and is based on the theory that healing is inhibited by toxins and waste materials in the body and a lack of essential nutrients (Cassileth et al, 1984). Therapy regimens generally include colonic cleansing, special diets, and vitamin and mineral supplements. The major medical complications of these regimens result from the colonic irrigation, which is usually given in the form of enemas using coffee, wheatgrass, or other substances. Electrolyte imbalance, toxic colitis, bowel necrosis, and sepsis caused by colonic irrigation have been reported (Markman, 1985). The dietary component of metabolic therapy appears to be less restrictive than other regimens and thus causes fewer severe problems (Cassileth and Brown, 1988). Most regimens recommend restriction of animal products, refined flours and sugars, and foods that are processed or contain artificial ingredients. Some metabolic regimens include the administration of amygdalin (Laetrile), a toxic drug shown to be ineffective as a cancer treatment (Moertel et al, 1982).

Dietary treatments for cancer generally involve diet alone and are based on the "you are what you eat" principle. A number of diet therapies exist, consisting of specific foods prepared and consumed in a specified manner. Perhaps the most frequently used of these is the *macrobiotic diet* (Cassileth et al, 1984). This actually consists of several diets ranging in restriction from severe, consisting exclusively of cereals, to moderate, including increasing amounts of vegetables, fruits, and soups. The typical diet emphasizes whole-grain cereals and rice and contains small amounts of vegetables, fruits, and soybean products. Although the range of intakes varies, macrobiotic diets are generally low in energy, fat, and protein. They are also likely to provide inadequate amounts of micronutrients, particularly vitamin D, ascorbic acid, folic acid, vitamin B_{12}, riboflavin, calcium, and iron. Clinical cases of malnutrition and growth failure have been reported among individuals following macrobiotic diets (Bowman et al, 1984). Patients with cancer frequently have medical and nutritional complications that may be exacerbated by the nutrient deficits of such diets.

Megavitamin therapy is characterized by the use of large doses of one or more vitamins and is another of the most frequently practiced unproven therapies (Read et al, 1990). The treatment is based on the belief that the body's ability to destroy the tumor is enhanced by large doses of certain vitamins, such as vitamin A or ascorbic acid. Although it is true that studies with animals have sometimes shown a positive effect of micronutrients on tumor growth, the findings are not consistent and are difficult to interpret. Evidence from clinical trials with cancer patients indicates that large doses of ascorbic acid are not effective and in some cases are harmful (Moertel et al, 1985). Studies of the effects of retinoids and other micronutrients and human cancer are in progress.

CITED REFERENCES

Aker SN et al: Nutritional support in marrow graft recipients with single versus double lumen right atrial catheters. Exp Hematol 10:732, 1982.

American College of Physicians: Parenteral nutrition in patients receiving cancer chemotherapy. Ann Intern Med 110:734, 1989.

Baker R et al: Detection of mutagenic activity in human urine following fried pork or bacon meals. Cancer Lett 16:81, 1982.

Barale KV, Aker SN, and Martinsen CS: Primary taste thresholds in children with leukemia undergoing marrow transplantation. J Parenter Enter Nutr 6:287, 1982.

Barch DH and Iannaccone PM: Role of zinc deficiency in carcinogenesis. Adv Exp Med Biol 206:517, 1986.

Binstock M et al: Coffee and pancreatic cancer: An analysis of international mortality data. Am J Epidemiol 118:630, 1983.

Bowman BB et al: Macrobiotic diets for cancer treatment and prevention. J Clin Oncol 2:702, 1984.

Broitman SA: Dietary cholesterol, serum cholesterol, and colon cancer: A review. Adv Exp Med Biol 206:137, 1986.

Buss CL: Nutritional support of cancer patients. Prim Care 14:317, 1987.

Carroll KK and Khor HT: Dietary fat in relation to tumorigenesis. Prog Biochem Pharmacol 10:308, 1975.

Carroll KK et al: Fat and cancer. Cancer 58:1818, 1986.

Cassileth BR and Brown H: Unorthodox cancer medicine. Cancer 38:176, 1988.

Cassileth BR et al: Contemporary unorthodox treatments in cancer medicine. Ann Intern Med 101:105, 1984.

Chlebowski RT: Critical evaluation of the role of nutritional support with chemotherapy. Cancer 55:268, 1985.

Clark LC: The epidemiology of selenium and cancer. Fed Proc 44:2584, 1985.

Cohn SE et al: Compartmental body composition of cancer patients by measurement of total body nitrogen, potassium and water. Metabolism 30:222, 1981.

Connett JE et al: Relationship between carotenoids and cancer: The Multiple Risk Factor Intervention Trial (MRFIT) Study. Cancer 64:126, 1989.

Copeland EM, Daly JM, and Dudrick SJ: Intravenous hyperalimentation, bowel rest, and cancer. Crit Care Man 8:21, 1980.

Creagan ET et al: Failure of high dose vitamin C (ascorbic acid) therapy to benefit patients with advanced cancer. N Engl J Med 301:687, 1979.

DeCosse JJ, Miller HH, and Lesser ML: Effect of wheat fiber and vitamins C and E on rectal polyps in patients with familial adenomatous polypsis. J Natl Cancer Inst 81:1290, 1989.

DeLuca HF and Ostrem V: The relationship between the vitamin D system and cancer. Adv Exp Med Biol 206:413, 1986.

DeWys WD et al: Prognostic effect of weight loss prior to chemotherapy in patients. Am J Med 60:491, 1980.

Dickerson JWT: Nutrition and the patient with cancer. Proc Nutr Soc 40:31, 1981.

Dolgin MJ and Katz ER: Conditioned aversions in pediatric cancer patients receiving chemotherapy. J Dev Behav Pediatr 9:82, 1988.

Donaldson SS: Effects of therapy on nutritional status of the pediatric cancer patient. Cancer Res 42(Suppl):729s, 1982.

Fearon KCH and Carter DC: Cancer cachexia. Ann Surg 208:1, 1988.

Fearon KCH et al: Influence of whole body protein turnover rate on resting energy expenditure in patients with cancer. Cancer Res 48:2590, 1988.

Fukiyama MY and Hsieh DPH: Effect of butylated hydroxytoluene pretreatment on excretion, tissue distribution and DNA binding of carbon labelled aflatoxin B_1 in the rat. Food Chem Toxicol 23:567, 1985.

Garland C et al: Dietary vitamin D and calcium and risk of colorectal cancer: A 19-year prospective study in men. Lancet 1:307, 1985.

Glatthaar BE, Hornig DH, and Moser U: The role of ascorbic acid in carcinogenesis. Adv Exp Med Biol 206:357, 1986.

Harper AE: Proteins and amino acids: Effects of deficiencies and specific amino acids. Adv Exp Med Biol 206:153, 1986.

Hennekens CH, Mayrent SL, and Willett W: Vitamin A, carotenoids and retinoids. Cancer 58:1837, 1986.

Hershcopf RJ and Bradlow HL: Obesity, diet, endogenous estrogens, and the risk of hormone-sensitive cancer. Am J Clin Nutr 45:283, 1987.

Hiatt RA, Klatsky AL, and Armstrong MA: Pancreatic cancer, blood glucose and beverage consumption. Int J Cancer 41:794, 1988.

Howson CP, Hiyama T, and Wynder EL: The decline in gastric cancer: Epidemiology of an unplanned triumph. Epidemiol Rev 8:1, 1986.

Ip C: The chemopreventive role of selenium in carcinogenesis. Adv Exp Med Biol 206:431, 1986.

Jacobs LR: Modification of experimental colon carcinogenesis by dietary fibers. Adv Exp Med Biol 206:105, 1986.

Jacobsen BK et al: Coffee drinking, mortality, and cancer incidence: Results from a Norwegian prospective study. J Natl Cancer Inst 76:823, 1986.

Kern KA and Norton JA: Cancer cachexia. J Parenter Enter Nutr 12:286, 1988.

Knekt P: Serum vitamin E level and risk of female cancers. Int J Epidemiol 17:281, 1988.

Knekt P et al: Serum vitamin E and risk of cancer among Finnish men during a 10-year followup. Am J Epidemiol 127:28, 1988.

Kolonel LN: Fat and colon cancer: How firm is the epidemiologic evidence? Am J Clin Nutr 45:336, 1987.

Koretz RL: Parenteral nutrition: Is it oncologically logical? J Clin Oncol 2:534, 1984.

Kritchevsky D: Diet, nutrition and cancer: The role of fiber. Cancer 58:1830, 1986.

Kritchevsky D and Klurfeld DM: Influence of caloric intake on experimental carcinogenesis: A review. Adv Exp Med Biol 206:55, 1986.

LeGrady D et al: Coffee consumption and mortality in the Chicago Western Electric Company study. Am J Epidemiol 126:803, 1987.
Lenssen P and Aker SN (eds): Nutritional Assessment and Management During Marrow Transplantation: A Resource Manual. Seattle, Fred Hutchinson Cancer Research Center, 1985.
Lindmark L et al: Thermic effect and substrate oxidation in response to intravenous nutrition in cancer patients who lose weight. Ann Surg 204:628, 1986.
Lipkin M and Newmark H: Effect of added dietary calcium on colonic epithelial-cell proliferation in subjects at high risk for familial colonic cancer. N Engl J Med 313:1381, 1985.
Mahaffey SM and Copeland EM: Total parenteral nutrition in the cancer patient. Adv Surg 20:47, 1987.
Markman M: Medical complications of "alternative" cancer therapy. N Engl J Med 312:1640, 1985.
McDonald GB et al: Intestinal and hepatic complications of human bone marrow transplantation (Parts I and II). Gastroenterol 90:460 and 770, 1986.
McDonald GB et al: The clinical course of 53 patients with venocclusive disease of the liver after marrow transplantation. Transplantation 39:603, 1985.
McKeown-Eyssen GE and Bright-See E: Dietary factors in colon cancer: International relationships. Nutr Cancer 6:160, 1984.
McMichael AJ et al: Dietary and endogenous cholesterol and human cancer. Epidemiol Rev 6:192, 1984.
Medina D: Mechanisms of selenium inhibition of tumorigenesis. Adv Exp Med Biol 206:465, 1986.
Miller EC and Miller JA: Carcinogens and mutagens that may occur in foods. Cancer 58:1795, 1986.
Mirvish SS: Effects of vitamins C and E on *N*-nitroso compound formation, carcinogenesis and cancer. Cancer 58:184, 1986.
Moertel CG et al: A clinical trial of amygdalin (Laetrile) in the treatment of human cancer. N Engl J Med 306:201, 1982.
Moertel CG et al: High-dose vitamin C versus placebo in the treatment of patients with advanced cancer who have had no prior chemotherapy: A randomized double-blind comparison. N Engl J Med 312:137, 1985.
Moon RC and Mehta RG: Anticarcinogenic effects of retinoids in animals. Adv Exp Med Biol 206:399, 1986.
Morrison AS and Buring JE: Artificial sweetners and cancer of the lower urinary tract. N Engl J Med 302:537, 1980.
National Academy of Sciences: Report on Cyclamates. Washington, DC, National Academy Press, 1985.
Newberne PM and Conner MW: Food additives and contaminants: An update. Cancer 58:1851, 1986.
Nomura A et al: Serum selenium and the risk of cancer by specific sites: Case-control analysis of prospective data. J Nat Can Inst 79:103, 1987.
Olson JA: Some thoughts on the relationship between vitamin A and cancer. Adv Exp Med Biol 206:379, 1986.
Ota DM, Kleman G, and Diamond K: Practical considerations in the nutritional management of the cancer patient. Curr Probl Cancer Treat 7:345, 1986.
Padilla GV: Psychological aspects of nutrition and cancer. Surg Clin North Am 66:1121, 1986.
Paganini-Hill A et al: Vitamin A, beta-carotene and the risk of cancer: A prospective study. J Natl Cancer Inst 79:443, 1987.
Pariza MW and Boutwell RK: Historical perspective: Calories and energy expenditure in carcinogenesis. Am J Clin Nutr 45:151, 1987.
Pastore G et al: Late effects of treatment of cancer in infancy. Med Pediatr Oncol 10:369, 1982.
Prentice RL et al: Aspects of the rationale for the Women's Health Trial. J Natl Cancer Inst 80:802, 1988.
Read MH et al: Supplementation practices of a group of patients with cancer. J Am Diet Assoc 90:278, 1990.
Rogers AE and Conner MW: Alcohol and cancer. Adv Exp Med Biol 206:473, 1986.
Rohan TE and Bain CJ: Diet in the etiology of breast cancer. Epidemiol Rev 9:120, 1987.
Russell MJ, Thomas BS, and Bulbrook RD: A prospective study of the relationship between serum vitamins A and E and risk of breast cancer. Br J Cancer 57:213, 1988.
Schersten T et al: Energy metabolism in cancer. Acta Chir Scand 498(Suppl):130, 1980.
Schubert MM and Izutsu KT: Iatrogenic causes of salivary gland dysfunction. J Dent Res 66:680, 1987.
Sherry MEG, Aker SN, and Cheney CL: Nutrition assessment and management of the pediatric cancer patient. Top Clin Nutr 2:38, 1987.
Silberman H: The role of preoperative parenteral nutrition in cancer patients. Cancer 55:254, 1985.
Temple NJ and Basu TK: Protective effect of beta-carotene against colon tumors in mice. J Natl Cancer Inst 78:1211, 1987.
Thompson MP et al: Modified lipoprotein lipase activities, rates of lipogenesis, and lipolysis as factors leading to lipid depletion in C57BL mice bearing the preputial gland tumor, ESR-586. Ann Surg 204:637, 1986.
Torosian MH and Daly JM: Nutritional support in the cancer-bearing host: Effects on host and tumor. Cancer 58:1915, 1986.
Trant AS, Serin J, and Douglass HO: Is taste related to anorexia in cancer patients. Am J Clin Nutr 36:45, 1982.
Van Rensberg SJ: Epidemiological and dietary evidence for a specific nutritional predisposition to esophageal cancer. J Natl Cancer Inst 62:243, 1981.
Vena JE et al: Occupational exercise and risk of cancer. Am J Clin Nutr 45:318, 1987.
Verzosa MS et al: Five years after central nervous system irradiation of children with leukemia. Int J Radiat Oncol Biol Phys 1:209, 1976.
Virtamo J et al: Serum selenium and risk of cancer: A prospective follow-up of nine years. Cancer 60:145, 1987.
Visek WJ: Dietary protein and experimental carcinogenesis. Adv Esp Med Biol 206:163, 1986.
Wald NJ et al: Serum beta-carotene and subsequent risk of cancer: Results from BUPA study. Br J Cancer 57:428, 1988.
Wargovich MJ: Calcium and colon cancer. J Am Coll Nutr 7:295, 1988.
Weisberger JH: Role of fat, fiber, nitrate and food additives in carcinogenesis: A critical evaluation and recommendations. Nutr Cancer 8:47, 1986.
Weisdorf SA et al: Positive effect of prophylactic total parenteral nutrition on long-term outcome of bone marrow transplantation. Transplantation 43:833, 1987.
Wolff GL: Body weight and cancer. Am J Clin Nutr 45:168, 1987.
Yu MC et al: Tobacco, alcohol, diet, occupation, and carcinoma of the esophagus. Cancer Res 48:3843, 1988.
Ziegler RG et al: Dietary carotene and vitamin A and risk of lung cancer among white men in New Jersey. J Natl Cancer Inst 73:1429, 1984.

ADDITIONAL REFERENCES

Etiology

Alcohol consumption and breast cancer. Nutr Rev 46:9, 1988.
Aoki K et al: Smoking, alcohol drinking and serum carotenoid levels. Jpn J Cancer Res 78:1049, 1987.
Breast cancer and fat intake. Cancer 61:181, 1988.
de Waard F and Trichopoulos D: A unifying concept of the aetiology of breast cancer. Int J Cancer 41:666, 1988.
Diet and Cancer. Nutr Res Newsletter 7(7):73, 1988.
Eid A and Berry EM: The relationship between dietary fat, adipose tissue composition and neoplasms of the breast. Nutr Cancer 11:173, 1988.
Greenwald P, Lanza E, and Eddy GA: Dietary fiber in the reduction of colon cancer risk. J Am Diet Assoc 87:1178, 1987.
Harris RE and Wynder EL: Breast cancer and alcohol consumption: A study in weak associations. JAMA 259:2867, 1988.
Irwin M: Diet and cancer—what are the links? Am J Nurs 87:1086, 1987.
Jensen H and Madsen JL: Diet and cancer: Review of the literature. Acta Med Scand 223:293, 1988.
Katsouyanni K et al: Risk of breast cancer among Greek women in relation to nutrient intake. Cancer 61:181, 1988.
Kolonel LN, Yoshizawa CN, and Hankin JH: Diet and prostatic cancer: A case-control study in Hawaii. Am J Epidemiol 127:999, 1988.
Lippman SM and Meyskens FL: Vitamin A derivatives in the pre-

vention and treatment of human cancer. J Am Coll Nutr 7:269, 1988.
Pariza MW: Dietary fat, calorie restriction, ad libitum feeding and cancer risk. Nutr Rev 45:1, 1987.
Pastorino U et al: Vitamin A and female lung cancer: A case-controlled study on plasma and diet. Nutr Cancer 10:171, 1987.
Poirier LA: Stages in carcinogenesis: Alteration by diet. Am J Clin Nutr 45:185, 1987.
Rosen M, Nystrom L, and Wall S: Diet and cancer mortality in the counties of Sweden. Am J Epidemiol 127:42, 1988.
Wald NJ et al: Serum vitamin E and subsequent risk of cancer. Br J Cancer 56(1):69, 1987.
Wynder EL: Amount and type of fat/fiber in nutritional carcinogenesis. Prev Med 16:451, 1987.

Nutritional Care

Aker SN and Lenssen P: A Guide to Good Nutrition During and After Chemotherapy and Radiation, 3rd ed. Seattle, Fred Hutchinson Cancer Research Center, 1988.
Block AS: Nutrition Management of the Cancer Patient. Rockville, MD, Aspen Publishers, 1990.
Bozzetti F: Effects of artificial nutrition on the nutritional status of cancer patients. J Parenter Enter Nutr 13:406, 1989.
Copeland EM and Souba WW: Nutritional considerations in treatment of the cancer patient. Nutr Clin Prac 3:173, 1988.
Enck RE and Hogan CM: Management of nausea and vomiting. Am J Hospice Care 4:17, 1987.
Fearon KCH et al: Cancer cachexia: influence of systemic ketosis on substrate levels and nitrogen metabolism. Am J Clin Nutr 47:42, 1988.
Heber D: Malnutrition in cancer. Nutr MD 15(7):1, 1989.
Heimburger DC et al: Improvement in bronchial squamous metaplasia in smokers treated with folate and vitamin B_{12}: Report of preliminary randomized, double-blind intervention trial. JAMA 259:1525, 1988.
Lenssen P and Aker SA: Nutritional Assessment and Management During Marrow Transplantation: A Resource Manual. Seattle, Fred Hutchinson Cancer Research Center, 1985.
Lundholm KG and Drott C: Optimal nutritional indexes in cancer patients. J Parenter Enter Nutr 11(Suppl 5):135S, 1987.
Souba J: Nutritional care of the individual with cancer. Nutr Clin Prac 3:175, 1988.
Souba WW and Copeland EM: Parenteral nutrition and metabolic observations in cancer. Nutr Clin Prac 3:183, 1988.
Van der Merwe CR, Booyens J, and Katzeff IE: Oral gamma-linolenic acid in 21 patients with untreatable malignancy: An ongoing pilot open clinical trial. Br J Clin Prac 41(9):907, 1987.
White WS et al: Ultraviolet light-induced reductions in plasma carotenoid levels. Am J Clin Nutr 47:879, 1988.
Yetiv JZ: Popular Nutritional Practices: A Scientific Appraisal. Toledo, OH, Popular Medicine Press, 1986.
Zerwekh JV: Should fluid and nutritional support be withheld from terminally ill patients? Another opinion. Am J Hospice Care 4:37, 1987.

CHAPTER 37

NUTRITIONAL CARE IN AIDS

Barbara Eldridge, R.D., C.D., Carolyn Neary, R.D., M.S., C.D., and Sharon Furrer, R.D., M.S.

CHAPTER OUTLINE

KEY TERMS

ACUTE HUMAN IMMUNODEFICIENCY VIRUS (HIV) INFECTION—infection with human immunodeficiency virus with symptoms similar to a viral infection: fever, sore throat, arthralgias, and rash

AIDS ENTEROPATHY—changes in small and large bowel thought to be due to direct HIV infection and with no other identifiable pathogen; manifests as chronic diarrhea and possibly malabsorption

CONSTITUTIONAL DISEASE (AIDS WASTING SYNDROME)—disease characterized by lymphadenopathy and persistent fever, chronic or intermittent fatigue and malaise, and diarrhea of unknown etiology and weight loss

HIV-ASSOCIATED NEPHROPATHY—a syndrome of progressive renal failure with HIV infection

HIV ENCEPHALOPATHY (AIDS DEMENTIA)—degenerative disease of the brain due to infection with HIV

HIV POSITIVE—showing evidence of antibody to HIV and thus previous infection with HIV

KAPOSI'S SARCOMA—a malignant neoplastic vascular proliferation that is characterized by the development of bluish-red cutaneous nodules usually on the lower extremities and that appears in a particularly virulent form in immunocompromised individuals, particularly in those with AIDS

LYMPHADENOPATHY—disease of the lymph nodes characterized by enlarged lymph glands at two or more extrainguinal sites

OPPORTUNISTIC INFECTION—infection by an organism that does not ordinarily cause disease but that, under certain circumstances such as impaired immune response, becomes pathogenic

The acquired immunodeficiency syndrome (AIDS) was first described by the Centers for Disease Control (CDC) in 1981. Since then, more than 99,000 cases of persons diagnosed with AIDS have been reported in the United States. Of the cases reported, 61% have been homosexual or bisexual men and 20% have been intravenous drug users. Others affected include heterosexual contacts, hemophiliacs and other recipients of multiple blood transfusions, and infants born to mothers with AIDS (Centers for Disease Control, 1989). It is projected that by the year 1992 there will be a cumulative total of 365,000 reported cases of AIDS and human immunodeficiency virus (HIV) infection, of which 80,000 will be added in that year alone (AIDS Prevention Project, 1988a and b) (New Directions, p. 647).

ETIOLOGY AND CLASSIFICATION

AIDS is caused by the HIV, which invades the genetic core of T_4 lymphocyte cells (Bowen et al, 1985). Destruction of T lymphocyte function results in immune deficiency and consequent vulnerability to life-threatening neoplasms and opportunistic infections (Weller, 1985). The virus can also invade the brain, leading to HIV encephalopathy (Holland and Tross, 1985).

The virus can be transmitted via the blood and semen by intimate sexual contact, shared contaminated needles, injection of contaminated blood products, and across the placenta from the mother to the baby (Health and Public Policy Committee . . . , 1986). It is not transmitted in saliva or by casual contact. The virus is also found in breast milk, and

TABLE 37–1. Classification of Patients Diagnosed with Human Immunodeficiency Virus (HIV)*

Group I *Acute Infection:* Patients with transient signs and symptoms of HIV infection.

Group II *Asymptomatic Infection:* Patients without previous signs or symptoms leading to classification in group III or IV.

Group III *Persistent Generalized Lymphadenopathy:* Patients with palpable lymphadenopathy at two or more extrainguinal sites persisting for more than 3 months.

Group IV *Other Disease:* Patients designated to one or more subgroups below, whether they are minimally symptomatic or severely ill.

- A. **Constitutional disease:** HIV wasting syndrome; disabling weakness; or fevers
- B. **Neurologic disease:** HIV encephalopathy; peripheral neuropathy; or myelopathy
- C1. **Infectious diseases diagnostic of AIDS**
  1. *Pneumocystis carinii* pneumonia
  2. Cryptosporiodiosis
  3. Toxoplasmosis
  4. Extraintestinal strongyloidiasis‡
  5. Isosporiasis
  6. Candidiasis (esophageal, bronchial, pulmonary)
  7. Cryptococcosis (extrapulmonary)
  8. Histoplasmosis (disseminated)
  9. *Mycobacterium avium* or *M. kansasii* (disseminated)
  10. Cytomegalovirus infection (invasive)
  11. Herpes simplex virus (chronic mucocutaneous or disseminated)
  12. Progressive multifocal leukoencephalopathy
- C2. **Other secondary infectious diseases**
  1. Oral hairy leukoplakia‡
  2. Multidermatomal herpes zoster‡
  3. Recurrent *Salmonella* bacteremia
  4. Nocardiosis‡
  5. Tuberculosis
  6. Oral candidiasis‡
- D. **Secondary cancers**
  1. Kaposi's sarcoma
  2. Non-Hodgkin's lymphoma
  3. Primary lymphoma of the brain
- E. **Other HIV conditions**
  1. Idiopathic thrombocytopenia‡
  2. Coccidioidomycosis
  3. Chronic lymphoid interstitial pneumonia in children
  4. Serious recurrent or multiple pyogenic bacterial infections in children
  5. Any other disease or clinical finding not listed above that may be attributed to HIV‡

"Class IV non-AIDS"†

* From Centers for Disease Control: Classification system for human lymphotropic virus type III/lymphadenopathy-associated virus infections. MMWR 35:334, 1986; Washington State, Seattle-King County: AIDS. Quarterly AIDS surveillance report; 3rd quarter, 1987.

† Group IV is divided into 5 categories. Most of the group IV diseases fit the CDC case definition for AIDS. Diseases that do not fit the CDC case definition are indicated with a double dagger (‡) and are called "class IV non-AIDS."

although the risk of breast milk transmission is unknown, most researchers recommend that HIV-positive mothers should be discouraged from breast-feeding (Life Sciences Research Office, FASEB, 1990).

The time period between the initial infection with the HIV virus and the development of AIDS varies among individuals. The mean viral incubation period is thought to be 14 years (AIDS Prevention Project, 1988a and b). Whether all HIV-infected persons eventually develop AIDS is uncertain at this time. The CDC classification system described in Table 37-1 distinguishes between HIV infection and AIDS.

MANIFESTATIONS OF HIV INFECTION

The acute phase of the *initial HIV infection* may last for 2 weeks, with symptoms similar to a viral infection: fever, sore throat, arthralgias, and rash. Persistent generalized lymphadenopathy, characterized by enlarged lymph glands at two or more extrainguinal sites, may be present. In some cases, clinical manifestations may not be present. Seroconversion occurs within 8 weeks after infection, and individuals with and without symptoms will test positive for HIV at this time (Carey, 1988).

Constitutional disease, also known as *AIDS wasting syndrome,* is diagnostic of AIDS in the HIV-positive individual for whom no other cause of the symptoms has been identified (Centers for Disease Control, 1987). Common constitutional signs of HIV infection include persistent fever often with night sweats, chronic or intermittent fatigue and malaise, and diarrhea of unknown etiology. Involuntary weight loss of 10 to 15% is common.

Opportunistic Infections

Opportunistic infections from bacteria, fungi, protozoa, or viruses are common. They are often the cause of diarrhea, malabsorption, fever, and weight loss as well as many other symptoms. Common infections and their manifestations are summarized in Table 37-2.

Malignancies

Kaposi's sarcoma (KS), a malignancy of the endothelial cells, manifests as purple nodules that may be painless or may be accompanied by a burning sensation when present in the gastrointestinal tract. The skin, mucous membranes, lymph nodes, or bowels are common sites (Gelb and Miller, 1986) (Fig. 37-1). Lesions in the mouth and esophagus may result in dysphagia and odynophagia and may be associated with nausea and vomiting (Garcia et al, 1987). KS in the bowel may cause ulceration. *B cell lymphomas* may occur as lym-

TABLE 37-2. Problems and Symptoms Associated with AIDS-Related Infections*

AIDS-Related Infections	Common Physical Problems and Symptoms
Candida albicans (Fungi)	
Oral (thrush)	Loss of appetite, white plaques, mouth discomfort, change in taste
Pharyngeal	Dysphagia, sore throat
Esophageal	Substantial burning-type pain, difficulty in swallowing
Proctal	Rectal pain, weeping lesions (without plaques), pruritus
Cryptococcus neoformans (Fungi)	
Meningitis Pneumonia (occasionally)	Fever, severe headache, obtundation, stiff neck, change in mental status, untoward side effects related to antibiotics
Cryptosporidium enteritis (Protozoa) Infection of large and small bowels	Severe watery diarrhea (up to 15-20 l/day), weakness, electrolyte imbalance, abdominal cramping, fever, nausea, vomiting
Cytomegalovirus (virus) (CMV)	Blindness or visual loss (retinitis), fever, fatigue/severe malaise, weight loss, facial edema (secondary to adrenalitis), enteritis, or colitis
Herpes simplex (virus)	Weeping skin lesions (oral, perirectal), rectal bleeding, rectal discharge, pain
Herpes zoster (shingles) (virus)	Vesicular skin lesions along dermatomes, pain
Mycobacterium avium-intracellulare (bacteria) (MAI)	Fever, severe weight loss/cachexia, abdominal pain, diarrhea, malabsorption, antibiotic side effects
Pneumocystis carinii pneumonia (PCP) (Protozoa)	Fever, chills, night sweats, cough with or without sputum production, shortness of breath, antibiotic side effects, weight loss, weakness
Progressive multifocal leukoencephalopathy	Progressive weakness and dementia, speech problems, forgetfulness, perceptual problems, visual problems, incontinence

* Adapted from Martin J, Hughes A, and Franks P: AIDS Home Care and Hospice Manual, 2nd ed. San Francisco, Visiting Nurses and Hospice of San Francisco, 1990.

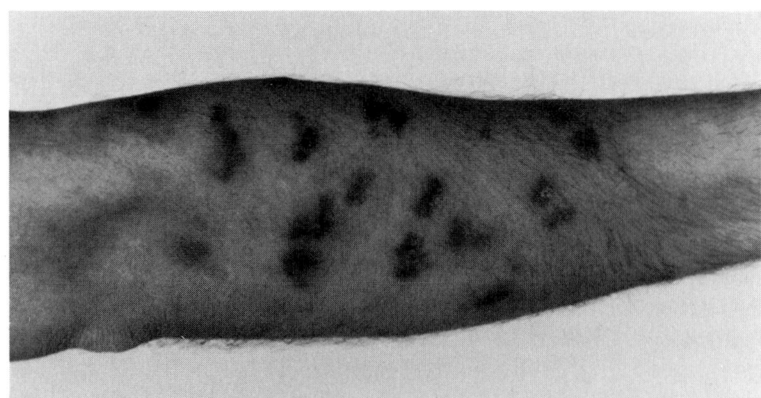

FIGURE 37–1. *Nodular lesions of Kaposi's sarcoma. (From Kelley WN et al: Textbook of Rheumatology, 3rd ed. Philadelphia, WB Saunders, 1989, p 1376.)*

phomas of the small bowel or brain or as increasing lymphadenopathy. Lymphomas respond poorly to therapy. Other malignancies reported with increased frequency in homosexual men are squamous cell carcinoma of the tongue and cloacogenic carcinoma of the colon. However, it is unknown if these are related to HIV (Carey, 1988).

Neurologic Disease

HIV encephalopathy, also known as *AIDS dementia,* appears to be associated with HIV infection of the central nervous system and is unrelated to and often precedes infection with opportunistic organisms or central nervous system neoplasms (Navia and Price, 1987). Symptoms of the initial phase include forgetfulness and concentration difficulties. Myelopathy with loss of balance, muscular leg weakness, and peripheral neuropathy with numbness or painful dysthesias may also develop as the disease progresses.

Other Affected Organ Systems

Nutritionally pertinent organs affected by the disease or its treatment include the liver, kidney, gastrointestinal tract (GI), and pancreas. Liver function may be compromised by infection with cytomegalovirus (Fig. 37–2), cryptosporidia, mycobacteria, and hepatitis B or by hepatic malignancies such as KS or lymphoma (Lefkowitch, 1986).

A syndrome of progressive renal failure, identified as *HIV-associated nephropathy,* has been reported (Sreepada Rao, 1988). Proteinuria may also result from repeated infections, volume depletion, or nephrotoxic drugs (Pardo et al, 1984) (see Chapter 35).

Chronic diarrhea may persist in the absence of identifiable enteric pathogens and may be the result of what is known as *AIDS enteropathy,* thought possibly to be the direct result of HIV infection (Gillin et al, 1985). Histologic findings in patients with AIDS show changes in the small and large bowel, including villous atrophy and infiltration of the lamina propria with chronic inflammatory cells. Diarrhea may be accompanied by steatorrhea or D-xylose malabsorption (Dworkin et al, 1985).

RELATIONSHIP BETWEEN MALNUTRITION AND AIDS

For the individual with AIDS, nutritional status can be compromised by decreased oral intake due to anorexia, nausea, vomiting, dyspnea, fatigue, neurologic disease, and disorders of the mouth and esophagus. When the GI tract is affected, nutrient absorption may be decreased due to malabsorption. At the same time, energy and protein needs may be increased by fevers and infection. Lipid metabolism and transport may also be affected by infection, causing lean body wasting.

Protein-energy malnutrition (PEM) is a common complication of AIDS, although the exact prevalence is

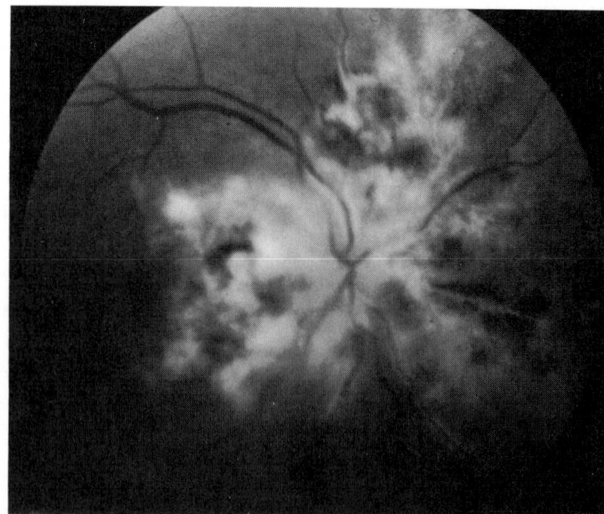

FIGURE 37–2. *Cytomegalovirus retinitis in an individual with AIDS. (From Kelley WN et al: Textbook of Rheumatology, 3rd ed. Philadelphia, WB Saunders, 1989, p 1376.)*

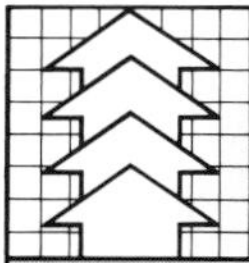

NEW DIRECTIONS: The Changing Face of AIDS

When AIDS was first identified about 10 years ago it was seen almost exclusively in the homosexual male population. However, the incidence of the disease is changing.

People of color (African American, native American, Hispanic, Asian/Pacific Islanders) now constitute 45% of the AIDS population and 78% of the pediatric cases. AIDS is also increasing in the heterosexual population among intravenous drug users and bisexual individuals. The World Health Organization estimates that there are 3 to 4 million females worldwide infected with HIV virus, and most of these are in the childbearing age. By the year 2000, 10 million children could be born to HIV-infected women.

To date there have been 167,830 diagnosed cases of AIDS and 106,361 deaths. By the end of 1993 it is estimated that there will be 390,000 to 480,000 cumulative diagnosed AIDS cases and 285,000 to 340,000 cumulative deaths from AIDS.

A 24-hour telephone recording of AIDS statistics, reported monthly, can be obtained from the Centers for Disease Control (CDC) as follows: ethnic/age categories, (404) 330-3020; gender/transmission categories, (404) 330-3021; and top 10 cities/states, (404) 330-3022.

unknown. Weight loss, body cell mass depletion, decreased skinfold thickness and mid-arm circumference, decreased iron-binding capacity, and hypoalbuminemia are frequently reported (Collins, 1988; Kotler et al, 1985; Malnutrition . . . , 1989; O'Sullivan et al, 1985). Deficiencies of zinc (Fabris, 1988; Falutz, 1988) have also been documented in patients with AIDS.

Immune changes in PEM are similar to those seen in AIDS (Gray, 1983; Jain and Chandra, 1984). Both conditions are marked by multiple opportunistic infections of viral, bacterial, parasitic, and fungal origin. KS and B cell lymphomas have been reported in individuals in Central and East Africa, where PEM is common.

It is hypothesized that malnutrition may contribute to the frequency and severity of infection seen in AIDS by further compromising immune function (Chlebowski, 1985). Deficiencies of protein, calories, copper, zinc, selenium, iron, essential fatty acids, pyridoxine, folate, and vitamins A, C, and E all interfere with immune function (Chandra, 1983). Severe weight loss can also result in organ damage, which may increase risk for fatal outcome of infections. Depletion of body cell mass in AIDS, independent of the underlying cause, has been shown to correlate with the timing of death in AIDS. Body weight at two thirds of ideal weight also appears to have a similar relationship to death (Kotler et al, 1989).

Although it is known that nutritional repletion in malnourished patients will reverse immunodeficiency in PEM, the effect of such repletion or maintenance of optimal nutritional status on the progression of AIDS is unknown. Therefore, the general goals of nutrition intervention are to preserve optimal somatic and visceral protein status, prevent nutrient deficiencies or excesses known to compromise immune function, minimize nutrition-related complications that interfere with either intake or absorption of nutrients, and enhance the quality of life.

NUTRITIONAL ASSESSMENT

The diet should be evaluated for adequacy of nutrient intake, especially nutrients involved in immune function. Because many of those infected with HIV are drug abusers, their eating habits prior to infection may have been erratic and nutritionally inadequate. Individuals should be asked about their use of nontraditional diet therapies that may be potentially harmful.

Psychosocial conditions should also be assessed. Fear, anxiety, depression, or social isolation can all affect appetite and nutrient intake. Illness or ostracism often leads to a lack of employment and to a subsequent loss of social contacts as well as income.

Monitoring anthropometric measurements over time is feasible, because many patients will have multiple clinic visits and hospitalizations. To estimate fat and skeletal protein stores, arm fat area and arm muscle area should be compared with reference data (see Chapter 17). For individuals who maintain a thin body, it may be more valid to assess weight change by using preillness weight rather than standard ideal body weight (Garcia et al, 1987). The percentage of weight change is a reliable measure of severity of weight loss and thus malnutrition.

Laboratory values such as serum albumin, prealbumin, retinol-binding protein, transferrin, and total iron-binding capacity can be used to monitor changes in visceral protein status. Total lymphocyte count and delayed hypersensitivity skin testing should not be used, since these immune functions are impaired and therefore are not indicative of nutritional status (Collins, 1988).

Many drugs used in the treatment of infections and cancers of AIDS have side effects with nutritional ramifications, and this should be included in the assessment (Table 37-3).

TABLE 37–3. Medications with Nutrition-Related Side Effects

Drugs	Use	Possible Gastrointestinal Interaction
Bactrim (trimethoprimsulfamethoxazole)	*Pneumocystis carinii pneumonia* (PCP)	•Nausea •Vomiting •Glossitis/stomatitis •Hyponatremia
Pentamidine isethionate	PCP	•Alterations in taste •Hypoglycemia and hyperglycemia •Nausea •Vomiting •Hypocalcemia
Dapsone	With sulfamethoxazole for PCP	•Anorexia •Nausea •Vomiting
Pyrimethamine	With sulfadiazine for toxoplasmosis	•Megaloblastic anemia •Vomiting •Anorexia •Tongue tenderness
Acyclovir (Zovirax)	*Herpes simplex* *Herpes zoster*	•Occasional nausea •Occasional vomiting
AZT (zidovudine Retravir)	Inhibits HIV replication	•Nausea •Vomiting •Taste alterations
DHPG	*Cytomegalovirus* (CMV)	•Diarrhea (rarely) •Vomiting (rarely) •Gastric ulceration and gastrointestinal perforation (rarely)
Amphotericin-B	Cryptococcal infection Histoplasmosis Candidiasis	•Anorexia •Vomiting •Hypokalemia •Hypomagnesemia •Metallic taste
Ketoconazole	Candidiasis Histoplasmosis	•Needs acidic stomach for absorption

NUTRITIONAL INTERVENTION

Nutrients

Energy

Energy and protein needs vary depending on the progression of the disease and the development of complications that will impair nutrient intake and utilization. No studies are as yet available to establish energy requirements for patients with AIDS. The Harris and Benedict equation can be used to determine basal energy expenditure (BEE) and multiplied by a stress factor to allow for maintenance and anabolism (see Table 29–2). Adjustment must also be made for the presence of fever. Energy requirements increase by 13% and protein requirements by 10% for every degree Celsius above normal (Hyman and Kaufman, 1989).

A general range for estimating energy needs is the BEE multiplied by 1.3 to 1.7. A realistic goal for oral intake is between 2,200 and 2,800 kcal.

Protein

Protein requirements may be estimated as 1 to 1.2 g/kg body weight for maintenance, with a calorie-to-nitrogen ratio of at least 150 : 1 to promote anabolism (Ota et al, 1986). However, protein may need to be restricted for patients with AIDS who develop renal or liver disease. Dietary intervention for these patients is the same as for noninfected persons (see Chapters 28 and 35).

Fat

Fat tolerance varies. When malabsorption as manifested by diarrhea is suspected, a low-fat diet and MCT oil may be useful (Resler, 1988).

Fluid

Fluid needs are the same as those of well individuals, except in the presence of severe diarrhea, nausea and vomiting, night sweats, and prolonged fever. In these conditions fluid needs are above normal, and losses should be replaced.

Vitamins and Minerals

Except for one study advocating the use of zinc supplementation (Fabris et al, 1988), which has been disputed (Falutz et al, 1988), there are few studies documenting vitamin and mineral needs of persons infected with the

AIDS virus. Early malabsorption of vitamin B_{12} may occur, even in patients who have no symptoms of malabsorption (Harriman et al, 1989). A Schilling test to measure vitamin B_{12} absorption may be useful in assessment. A vitamin and mineral supplement providing 100% of the RDA is recommended for individuals with diarrhea or malabsorption or for those who are consuming an inadequate diet (Taber Pike, 1987).

Megadoses of vitamins and minerals should be avoided, because excesses of these nutrients have been shown to be immunosuppressive (Beisel et al, 1981).

Nutritional Complications

Unless they were pre-existing, nutritional complications are not seen in the individual who is asymptomatic at the time of diagnosis. The treatment plan for this type of patient is therefore focused on the prevention of nutrition deficiencies and on attention to nutrition education (Task Force . . . , 1989).

As the disease progresses and signs and symptoms of HIV infection and AIDS appear, nutritional complications develop. The most common are weight loss, anorexia, fatigue, fever, dehydration, nausea, and vomiting. Treatments for these complications are the same as for patients with other chronic debilitating diseases. Treatment options for diarrhea and malnutrition, disorders of the oral cavity and esophagus, and neurologic dysfunction are more unique to AIDS.

Diarrhea and Malabsorption

Diarrhea and malabsorption are the major nutritional problems seen in persons who are HIV positive or who have developed AIDS (Smith et al, 1988). It is often the most difficult problem to resolve. Abnormal D-xylose absorption and steatorrhea are common. Malabsorption of fat, monosaccharides, disaccharides, nitrogen, vitamin B_{12}, folate, minerals, and trace elements occurs in patients with intestinal infections of the small bowel. When the large bowel is infected, malabsorption of fluids and electrolytes is seen.

The cause of diarrhea can be multifactorial. Organisms infecting the GI tract, KS, AIDS enteropathy (which is theoretically caused by direct HIV infection of the small bowel), hypoalbuminemia, malnutrition, and medications can all be involved (Brinson, 1985; Gelb and Miller, 1986; Smith et al, 1988). Intervention is based on a thorough diagnostic evaluation to identify the cause of the diarrhea.

Diarrhea resulting from KS, *Candidiasis, Herpes simplex, Salmonella,* and *Giardia lambia* infections can be treated. However, a type of severe secretory diarrhea (10 to 30 stools per day, 10- to 15-liter output) resulting in rapid weight loss is caused by treatment-resistant organisms (*Cytomegalovirus, Mycobacteria, Avium intracellularae, Cryptosporidium,* or *Isoporabelli*). As dietary intervention will not be effective in this case, parenteral nutritional support should be considered (Domaldo and Natividad, 1986; Resler, 1988; Smith et al, 1988). Chronic diarrhea of unknown etiology is referred to as AIDS enteropathy (Kotler et al, 1984). Table 37–4 describes nutritional interventions for treatable diarrhea, diarrhea resistant to treatment, and diarrhea resulting from AIDS enteropathy.

Patients with hypoalbuminemia-induced diarrhea may adequately absorb a chemically defined enteral formula despite mucosal changes induced by depressed serum albumin levels (Brinson, 1985). Some practitioners give albumin parenterally to restore albumin status and to improve intestinal absorption (see Chapter 30).

Disorders of the Oral Cavity and Esophagus

Oral candidiasis is common in persons with AIDS. Symptoms include soreness of the mouth and tongue, often described as a "burnt" feeling, and pain or difficulty with swallowing. Dysgeusia may also be present secondary to medications, nutrient deficiencies, candidiasis, xerostomia, or excessive mucus production. KS or herpes in the oropharyngeal or oroesophageal area can also inhibit normal chewing and swallowing and limit nutritional intake. Patients with extensive or chronic lesions may require alternative nutrition support, such as enteral or parenteral nutrition. Table 37–5 lists suggestions for improving the intake of the patient with AIDS who has a painful mouth.

TABLE 37–4. Nutrition Intervention for Diarrhea

Treatable Diarrhea

Maintain adequate nutritional intake for bowel regeneration.
Enhance absorption by using elemental diets.
Total bowel rest if indicated using total parenteral nutrition (TPN).
Infection and symptom control with antibiotics and antidiarrheals.

Diarrhea Resistant to Treatment

Promote patient comfort.
Maintain adequate hydration.
Try fiber-containing supplements.
Antidiarrheals or antispasmotics may be helpful.
TPN may be indicated for bowel rest, but is questionable in the setting of an untreatable gastrointestinal tract infection and may not outweigh the cost and risk of infection (Resler, 1988).

Diarrhea Resulting from AIDS Enteropathy

Diet modifications:
- Low lactose.
- Low fat if steatorrhea is present; try MCT oil.
- Increase fluid.
- Try bulking agents.
- Avoid caffeinated beverages.
- Incorporate small, frequent meals into meal plans.
- An elemental diet may enhance absorption.

Consider lactobacillus replacement if patient is on long-term antibiotic therapy.
Recommend a multivitamin/mineral supplement.
Gradually reintroduce suspect foods, one at a time, and check for tolerance.

TABLE 37–5. Diet Modification for Painful Eating

Use soft, moist, nonirritating foods, such as eggs, casseroles, cream soups, puddings, ice cream, yogurt, baked fish, ground meats, and cooked fruits.
Avoid spicy or acidic foods, such as citrus fruits, tomatoes, and red or black pepper.
Experiment with temperatures of foods. Avoid very hot or very cold foods; cool or room temperature is usually most acceptable.
Include nutrient-dense and energy-dense foods to maximize oral intake.
If xerostomia is present, use foods that are moist or served with a sauce or gravy. Serve liquids at mealtime and encourage fluids between meals.
Emphasis on good oral hygiene is vital. Encourage flossing and regular brushing with a soft toothbrush, along with baking soda or salt water rinses every 2 to 3 hours. Use a prescribed medication if oral or esophageal candidiasis is present.

Neurologic Disorders

Central nervous system manifestations of AIDS, ranging from psychomotor impairment to severe dementia, can significantly affect the ability to maintain adequate nutrition. Decreased sensory perception when chewing and swallowing can increase the risk of aspiration. In helping the patient to obtain an adequate nutritional intake, it is important to work closely with occupational and physical therapists, the speech pathologist, the nursing staff, and others involved in overall patient care.

Other Significant Nutritional Complications

Pentamidine, used in the treatment of *Pneumocystis carinii* pneumonia, can cause pancreatic damage with consequent hypoglycemia or hyperglycemia. Insulin-dependent diabetes mellitus (IDDM) may result. Nutritional management is the same as for individuals with IDDM (see Chapter 31).

Renal failure in AIDS is managed in the same manner as for others with renal disease (see Chapter 35). Weight maintenance in these individuals may be especially challenging, because accelerated wasting has been reported in individuals with HIV nephropathy (Sreepada Rao, 1988).

Fluid and sodium restriction may be necessary for patients with AIDS who have decreased liver function.

HIV infection via saliva has not been documented; therefore, special precautions for food service for HIV-infected individuals are unnecessary. Additionally, the virus does not survive long outside the body (Conte, 1986). As with any other patient population, precautions (e.g., wearing gloves) should be followed when handling dishes exposed to blood, feces, urine, or emesis (Resler, 1988). Usual dishwashing procedures will provide adequate decontamination (Conte, 1986).

UNPROVEN NUTRITIONAL THERAPIES

Persons with AIDS often become frustrated with the lack of definitive medical therapies for fighting and curing the disease. In their search for answers, some turn to unproven nutritional therapies. These regimens of diet or vitamin and mineral supplementation often can be costly, ineffective, and even harmful (Dwyer et al, 1988; Taber Pike, 1987 and 1988). Education should be started at the time of HIV diagnosis to instill and reinforce the basics of sensible nutritional practices and to point out accurate sources of nutrition information (Resler, 1988). Table 37–6 summarizes

TABLE 37–6. Unproven Nutritional Therapies*

Regimen	Description	Comment
Homeostatic macrobiotic diet	Based on the Zen Buddhist philosophy of the proper balance between yin and yang foods. The standard diet usually includes: 50–60% whole-grain cereals 20–25% vegetables 5–10% sea vegetables and beans 5% miso or tamari broth soup Emphasis on fluid restriction	Diet can be deficient in calories, complete protein, iron, calcium, vitamin D, vitamin B_{12}, folic acid, riboflavin, and ascorbic acid.
Anti-infective yeast-free diet	Claimed rationale is to prevent opportunistic yeast infections that can further weaken the immune system by eliminating foods containing yeast and foods that have high concentrations of simple sugars.	Diet claims are undemonstrated and are questioned by the American College of Allergy and Immunology Practice Standards Committee.
Megadoses of vitamins and minerals	High doses of vitamins A, C, E, B_{12} and selenium and zinc are advocated to strengthen and "revitalize" the immune system.	Recommendations are unproven, and toxicities can result from chronic and excessive intakes.
Anti-viral AL-721 and homemade formulas	"AL" or "active lipid" in the ratio 7:2:1, made from soy or egg yolk lecithin, can be given orally or by injection. Some studies report that this regimen can reduce or inhibit HIV replication.	AL-721 is approved for use in clinical trials by the FDA. Home formulas or generic substitutions are not approved, and may be impure.

* Data from Taber Pike, 1988; Dwyer, 1988; Bowman, 1984; Crook, 1986; Connolly, 1986; Sarin, 1985.

popular yet unproven nutritional therapies to which patients with AIDS are frequently attracted.

CITED REFERENCES

AIDS Prevention Project: AIDS — Quarterly AIDS Surveillance Report, 2nd quarter. Seattle, WA, Washington State Seattle-King County, 1988a.

AIDS Prevention Project: AIDS — Quarterly AIDS Surveillance Report, 3rd quarter. Seattle, WA, Washington State Seattle-King County, 1988b.

Beisel WR et al: Single-nutrient effects on immunological function. JAMA 245:53, 1981.

Bowen DL, Lane HC, and Fauci AS: Immunopathogenesis of the acquired immune deficiency syndrome. Ann Intern Med 103:704, 1985.

Bowman BB et al: Macrobiotic diets for cancer treatment and prevention — Review article. J Clin Oncol 2:702, 1984.

Brinson RR: Hypoalbuminemia, diarrhea, and the acquired immunodeficiency syndrome. Ann Intern Med 102:413, 1985.

Carey JT: The Clinical Spectrum of AIDS. *In* Blanchet KD (ed): AIDS, A Health Care Management Response. Rockville, MD, Aspen Publishers, 1988.

Centers for Disease Control: Revision of the CDC surveillance case definition for acquired immunodeficiency syndrome. MMWR 36(Suppl):3, 1989.

Centers for Disease Control: Classification system for human-lymphotropic virus type III/lymphadenopathy-associated virus infections. MMWR 35:334, 1986.

Centers for Disease Control: HIV/AIDS Surveillance Report, 2nd quarter, 1989.

Chandra RK: Nutrition, immunity and infection: Present knowledge and future directions. Lancet 1:688, 1983.

Chlebowski RT: Significance of altered nutritional status in acquired immunodeficiency syndrome (AIDS). Nutr Cancer 7:85, 1985.

Collins CL: Nutrition care in AIDS. Dietetic Currents, 15(3):1, 1988.

Connolly P: The *Candida albicans* Yeast Free Cookbook. New Canaan, CT, Keats Publishing, 1986.

Conte JE: Infection with human immunodeficiency virus in the hospital: Epidemiology, infection control, and biosafety considerations. Ann Intern Med 105:730, 1986.

Crook WG: The Yeast Connection. New York, Random House, 1986, pp 67–124.

Domaldo TL and Natividad LS: Nutritional management of patient with AIDS and *Cryptosporidium* infection. Nutr Support Serv 6(4):30, 1986.

Dworkin B et al: Gastrointestinal manifestations of the acquired immunodeficiency syndrome: A review of 22 cases. Am J Gastroenterol 80:774, 1985.

Dwyer JT et al: Unproven nutrition therapies for AIDS: What is the evidence? Nutr Today 23(2):25, 1988.

Fabris N et al: AIDS, zinc deficiency and thymic hormone failure. JAMA 259:839, 1988.

Falutz J, Tsoukas C, and Gold P: Zinc as a cofactor in human immunodeficiency virus — induced immunosuppression. JAMA 259:2850, 1988.

Garcia ME, Collins CL, and Mansell PWA: The acquired immune deficiency syndrome: Nutritional complications and assessment of body weight status. Nutr Clin Prac 2:108, 1987.

Gelb A and Miller S: AIDS and gastroenterology. Am J Gastroenterol 81:619, 1986.

Gillin JS et al: Malabsorption and mucosal abnormalities of the small intestine in the acquired immunodeficiency syndrome. Ann Intern Med 102:619, 1985.

Gray RH: Similarities between AIDS and PCM. Am J Publ Hlth 73:1332, 1983.

Harriman GR et al: Vitamin B_{12} malabsorption in patients with acquired immunodeficiency syndrome. Arch Intern Med 149:2039, 1989.

Health and Public Policy Committee, American College of Physicians, and The Infectious Diseases Society of America: Position paper: Acquired immunodeficiency syndrome. Ann Intern Med 104:575, 1986.

Holland JC and Tross S: The psychosocial and neuropsychiatric sequelae of the acquired immune deficiency syndrome and related disorders. Ann Intern Med 103:760, 1985.

Hughes A, Martin J, and Franks P: AIDS home care and hospice manual: AIDS home care and hospice program, San Francisco, Visiting Nurses Association of San Francisco, 1987.

Hyman C and Kaufman S: Nutritional impact of acquired immune deficiency syndrome: A unique counseling opportunity. J Am Diet Assoc 89:520, 1989.

Jain VK and Chandra RK: Does nutritional deficiency predispose to acquired immune deficiency syndrome? Nutr Res 4:537, 1984.

Kotler DP et al: Enteropathy associated with the acquired immunodeficiency syndrome. Ann Intern Med 101:421, 1984.

Kotler DP et al: Magnitude of body cell mass depletion and the timing of death from wasting in AIDS. Am J Clin Nutr 50:444, 1989.

Kotler DP, Wang J, and Pierson RN: Body composition studies in patients with the acquired immunodeficiency syndrome. Am J Clin Nutr 42:1255, 1985.

Lefkowitch JH: AIDS and the liver. Endocrin Rev 6:43, 1986.

Life Sciences Research Office, FASEB: Nutritional Therapy and Nutrition Education in the Care and Management of AIDS Patients, Tentative Report, Task Order #7, Washington, DC, Center for Food Safety and Nutrition, FDA, DHHS, 1990.

Malnutrition and weight loss in patients with AIDS. Nutr Rev 47:354, 1989.

Navia BA and Price RW: The acquired immunodeficiency syndrome dementia complex as the presenting or sole manifestation of human immunodeficiency virus. Arch Neurol 44:65, 1987.

O'Sullivan P, Linke RA, and Dalton S: Evaluation of body weight and nutritional status among AIDS patients. J Am Diet Assoc 85:1483, 1985.

Ota DM, Kleman G, and Dramond K: Practical considerations in nutritional management of the cancer patient. Curr Probl Cancer 10:353, 1986.

Pardo V et al: Glomerular lesions in the acquired immunodeficiency syndrome. Ann Intern Med 101:429, 1984.

Resler SS: Nutrition care of AIDS patients. J Am Diet Assoc 88:828, 1988.

Sarin PS et al: Effects of a novel compound (AL-721) on HTVL-111 infectivity in vitro. N Engl J Med 313:1289, 1985.

Smith D et al: Intestinal infections in patients with acquired immune deficiency syndrome. Ann Intern Med 108:328, 1988.

Sreepada Rao TK: Renal complications in patients with AIDS. J Crit Illness 3(3):55, 1988.

Taber Pike J: Nutrition Support. *In* Lewis A (ed): Nursing Care of Persons with AIDS/ARC. Rockville, MD, Aspen Publishers, 1987.

Taber Pike J: Alternative therapies — Where is the evidence? AIDS Patient Care 2(1):31, 1988.

Task Force on Nutrition Support in AIDS: Guidelines on nutritional support in AIDS. Nutrition 5(1):39, 1989.

Weller IVD: AIDS and the gut. Scand J Gastroenterol 114:77, 1985.

ADDITIONAL REFERENCES

Beach RS: Malnutrition in patients with HIV infection and AIDS. Nutr MD 15(8):1, 1989.

Breastfeeding and HIV transmission. Nutr MD 15(8):3, 1989.

Centers for Disease Control: Recommendations for preventing transmission of infection with human T-lymphotrophic virus type III/lymphadenopathy-associated virus in the workplace. MMWR 34:682, 1985.

Chandra RK (ed): Nutrition and Immunology, Contemporary Issues in Clinical Nutrition, Vol 11. New York, Alan R Liss, 1988.

Chelluri L and Jastremski MS: Incidence of malnutrition in patients with acquired immunodeficiency syndrome. Nutr Clin Prac 4:16, 1989.

Collins C and Garcia ME: Position of the American Dietetic Association: Nutrition intervention in the treatment of human immunodeficiency virus infection. J Am Diet Assoc 89:834, 1989.

De Brwyne, LK: Nutrition and AIDS. Nutr Clin 6(3):1, 1991.

DeVita VT, Heilman S, and Rosenberg SA: AIDS: Etiology, Diagno-

sis, Treatment and Prevention, 2nd ed. Philadelphia, JB Lippincott, 1988.
Diet for the AIDS patient. Nutr MD 15(8):7, 1989.
Hardy AM et al: The economic impact of the first 10,000 cases of the acquired immunodeficiency syndrome in the United States. JAMA 255:209, 1986.
Hyman C and Kaufman S: Nutritional impact of acquired immune deficiency syndrome: A unique counseling opportunity. J Am Diet Assoc 89:520, 1989.
Logan S et al: Breastfeeding and HIV infection. Lancet 1:1346, 1988.
Nutrition and Acquired Immunodeficiency Syndrome (AIDS): A review of the current literature. Norwich Eaton Pharmaceuticals, Wang Associates, 1988.
Nutrition and HIV infection: A review and evaluation of the extant knowledge of the relationship between nutrition and HIV infection. Nutr Clin Prac 6(3:Suppl), 1991.
O'Sullivan J: AIDS overview. Dietitians in Nutrition Support 9(6):14, 1988.
Rubin RH: Acquired immune deficiency syndrome. *In* Rubenstein E and Federman DD (eds): Scientific American Medicine. New York, Scientific American, 1987.
Shoemaker JD, Millard MC, and Johnson PB: Zinc in human immunodeficiency virus infection. JAMA 260:1881, 1987.
Singer P et al: Nutrition, the gastrointestinal tract and the acquired immune deficiency syndrome: Facts and perspectives. Clin Nutr 8:281, 1989.
Smith EJ and Larson E: AIDS and breast milk (Letter). J Obstet Gynecol Neonat Nursing 17:160, 1988.
Task Force Recommendations: Nutrition support of the AIDS patient. Nutr MD 15(8):3, 1989.
Task Force on Nutrition Support in AIDS: AIDS survey reveals need for greater nutrition support. Nutr Clin Prac 3:211, 1988.
Task Force on Nutrition Support in AIDS: Guidelines for nutrition support in AIDS. Nutr Today 24(4):27, 1989.
Tilkian SM, Lefevre G, and Coyle C: Altered folate metabolism in early HIV infection. JAMA 259:3128, 1988.

CHAPTER 38

NUTRITIONAL CARE IN FOOD ALLERGY AND FOOD INTOLERANCE

Elizabeth J. Adams, M.S., R.D.

CHAPTER OUTLINE

KEY TERMS

ANAPHYLAXIS—an acute, often severe, and sometimes fatal immune response that may affect any body system

CELL-MEDIATED IMMUNITY—immunity mediated by T lymphocytes either through the release of lymphokines or by direct cytotoxicity

ELIMINATION DIET—an eating plan in which individual foods suspected of causing intolerance or allergic reactions are omitted for a period of time in order to determine if there is an improvement in the individual's condition

FOOD ALLERGY—an adverse reaction to a food that is mediated by an immunologic mechanism; occurs consistently after consumption of that food and causes functional changes in target organs; food hypersensitivity

FOOD AND SYMPTOM DIARY—a record of food and drink consumed and symptoms experienced

FOOD HYPERSENSITIVITY—food allergy

FOOD INTOLERANCE—an adverse reaction to a food caused by toxic, pharmacologic, metabolic, or idiosyncratic reactions to the food or chemical substances in the food

HUMORAL IMMUNITY—immunity mediated by antibodies produced by B lymphocytes

IgE-MEDIATED ALLERGIC REACTION (IMMEDIATE HYPERSENSITIVITY)—IgE antibody–mediated hypersensitivity occurring within minutes after a sensitized individual is exposed to an antigen

RADIOALLERGOSORBENT TEST (RAST)—a test that measures specific IgE antibodies in serum; used as an alternative to skin tests

ROTATION DIET—an eating plan in which several foods known to cause allergic reactions or which are not tolerated, are eaten on separate days and then only every fourth or fifth day for each food

SENSITIZATION—exposure to an antigen or allergen that results in the development of hypersensitivity

SKIN TEST—a test in which an antigen is applied to the skin in order to observe the histamine response of the patient

Adverse reactions to foods, caused by many mechanisms and eliciting many different symptoms, are estimated to affect 15% of the American population. When immunologic mechanisms are the cause, these adverse reactions are called *food allergies.* Adverse reactions to foods caused by toxic, pharmacologic, metabolic, or idiosyncratic reactions to chemical substances are called *food intolerances* (American Academy of Allergy and Immunology, 1984). These nonallergenic reactions are thought to be much more common than food allergies.

DEFINITION

Much confusion surrounds the definition of food allergy. In popular literature, the term is frequently used to include any sensitivity to a food or substance that causes a reaction (Baker and Baker, 1987). In this text, *food allergy* refers to adverse responses to food that are mediated by immunologic mechanisms, occur consistently after consumption of a particular food, and cause functional changes in target organs (Taylor, 1986). The term *food hypersensitivity* may also be used to refer to these immunologically-mediated adverse reactions (Sampson, 1988).

Because the criteria for diagnosis of food allergy have not been clearly defined or universally accepted, estimates for the prevalence of food allergy vary widely. The Asthma and Allergy Foundation of America estimates that 0.8 to 1.8% of the American population is affected by food allergy (American Academy of Allergy and Immunology, 1984). Prevalence is thought to be highest in infancy, decreasing in childhood, and much lower in adulthood. Estimates of prevalence in the pediatric population range from 0.3 to 20% (Butkus and Mahan, 1986). In a well-controlled survey, reproducible adverse reactions to foods were reported in 8% of the children studied (Bock, 1987).

Food allergy is observed with greater frequency in at-risk populations; about 24% of children and adults with hay fever and asthma report some type of food allergies (American Academy of Allergy and Immunology, 1984).

IMMUNOLOGIC BASIS

Antigen Exclusion

In order for an allergic reaction to a food to occur, proteins or other large molecules from the food (antigens/allergens) must be absorbed from the gastrointestinal tract, interact with the immune system, and produce a response. Under normal conditions, the gastrointestinal tract and the immune system provide a barrier that prevents the absorption of most intact proteins. When this barrier fails, allergic sensitization may occur and re-exposure produces an allergic reaction. Some simple chemical substances (small molecules) can become allergens by combining with larger proteins.

Immune System

The immune system functions to clear the body of foreign substances (or antigens), such as viruses, bacteria, blood cells, and tissue cells. Normally, when antigens interact with cells of the immune system, they are cleared from the body without an adverse reaction. Three types of cells respond to antigens presented: *B lymphocytes, T lymphocytes,* and *macrophages.* The lymphocytes arise from the bone marrow and are the basis for the functioning of the two branches of the immune system, the humoral pathway and the cell-mediated pathway (Fig. 38–1).

The *humoral pathway* involves *antibodies* (immunoglobulins) and has an important role in food allergy. Antigen-specific antibodies are produced by the B lymphocytes (B cells) in response to the antigen presented. The union of an antigen and its antibody causes the production of chemical mediators or direct cellular damage that cause symptoms. Five classes of antibodies have been identified. *IgG, IgM,* and *IgD* antibodies protect the body against bacteria and viruses. Secretory *IgA* antibodies in breast milk provide local intestinal protection for infants against viruses and bacteria (Lawrence, 1985). *IgA* antibodies present in saliva and intestinal secretions block the absorption of antigens. *IgE* antibodies not only function to help eliminate

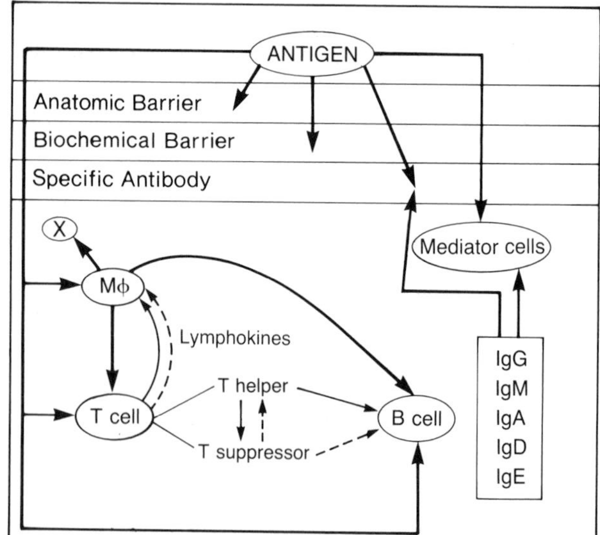

FIGURE 38–1. *The immune system's response to an antigen. (Mϕ = macrophage; X = excluded antigen.) (Redrawn from Bierman CW and Furukawa CT: Food allergy. Pediatr Rev 3(7):212, 1982. Reproduced by permission of Pediatrics.)*

parasites from the body but also are responsible for classic allergic reactions.

Cellular immunity involves the action of T lymphocytes (T cells). When antigens stimulate T cell growth, the T cells produce *lymphokines* and *cytokines*, substances that regulate the activities of other cells or cause direct cellular damage to target cells, resulting in the destruction of antigens. Cellular immunity has an important role in resistance to viruses, fungi, tumor cells, and other foreign cells. Allergic reactions such as contact dermatitis and the tuberculin reaction are also mediated by T cells. The role of cellular immunity in food allergy is unclear.

Tissue macrophages, derived from monocytes present in the blood, also have important roles in the recognition and clearance of antigens. Through the process of phagocytosis, the macrophage engulfs and destroys antigens. B cells, T cells, and macrophages are all thought to interact (see Fig. 38–1).

Allergic Reactions

Allergic reactions are unusual responses of the immune system and represent altered reactivity to an antigen. Antigens involved in allergic reactions are called *allergens.* Allergic reactions have been classified into four types: types I, II, and III, which are antibody dependent, and type IV, which is T cell dependent (Table 38–1).

Immediate hypersensitivity (*type I*), which involves IgE, is the most common allergic reaction and has the most clearly understood mechanism. The combination of an allergen with allergen-specific IgE fixed to tissue mast cells or circulating basophils causes the release of chemical mediators, including histamine, serotonin, kinins, and others. When released, these mediators can cause itching, contraction of smooth muscle, vasodilation, mucus secretion, and attraction of inflammatory cells. IgE-mediated allergic reactions are thought to have an important role in food allergy. Manifestations are most often systemic or involve the skin, gastrointestinal tract, or respiratory system (Table 38–2 and Fig. 38–2).

The contribution of non–IgE-mediated immunologic reactions to food allergy is unclear. Circulating food-specific antibodies (IgG, IgA, and IgM) occur commonly. Their clinical importance is unknown (American Academy of Allergy and Immunology, 1984; Kniker, 1987), although they may be part of normal mechanisms for clearing absorbed food antigens from the circulation. It has also been postulated that *antigen-antibody complexes* (*type III reaction*) may have a role in several food-related inflammatory diseases. These include celiac disease, various forms of colitis, enteritis with bleeding, malabsorptive disorders, ulceration, and chronic pneumonitis (Heiner syndrome). *Cell-mediated hypersensitivity* (*type IV reaction*) may have a role in celiac disease, protein-losing enteropathies, eosinophilic gastroenteritis, and inflammatory bowel disorders such as ulcerative colitis (Kniker, 1987).

TABLE 38–1. Types of Allergic Reactions*

Reaction/Classification	Mechanism	Comments
Type I		
Immediate hypersensitivity, anaphylactic IgE-mediated, or reaginic reaction	Allergen binds with sensitized IgE antibody on mast cell (specialized granular cells in the intestines, skin, and respiratory tract) or basophils (similar cells in blood). This results in release of mediators (histamine eosinophilic chemotactic factor, bradykinin, and so forth). IgG has also been identified as being involved in this type of reaction.	Includes hay fever, anaphylaxis, most food allergies. Symptoms occur within seconds or up to 2 hours. Symptoms of food reactions may include laryngeal edema, vomiting, diarrhea, eczema, itching, bronchospasm, and shock.
Type II		
Cytotoxic	IgG antibody reacts with cell membrane or antigen associated with cell membrane.	Results from transfusion of incompatible blood types. No food reactions have been demonstrated.
Type III		
Antigen-antibody complex Arthus reaction	Antigen and antibodies (IgG and IgM) form a complex called "precipitating antibody." The antigen–antibody complex is an Arthus reaction when it occurs in soft tissues like blood vessels, lungs, or kidneys, and is serum sickness when the complex circulates. Activation of complement also occurs in some cases.	Occurs in some food reactions; milk precipitins have been found in lungs of some children with chronic respiratory infection, and in GI tract in those with gastroenteropathies. Reactions usually take 6 hours or more to appear and may take several days to be clinically apparent.
Type IV		
Delayed or cell-mediated hypersensitivity	T cells interact directly with antigen.	Usual mechanism of graft rejection. Possibly involved in some food allergies, such as protein-losing enteropathies and celiac disease.

* Adapted from Butkus SN and Mahan LK: Food allergies: Immunological reactions to foods. © The American Dietetic Association. Reprinted by permission from Journal of the American Dietetic Association, Vol 86, p 601, 1986.

TABLE 38–2. Symptoms of Food Allergy

Gastrointestinal
Abdominal pain
Nausea
Vomiting
Diarrhea
Gastrointestinal bleeding
Protein-losing enteropathy
Oral and pharyngeal pruritus
Cutaneous
Urticaria
Eczema
Angioedema
Erythema
Itching
Respiratory
Rhinitis
Asthma
Cough
Milk-induced syndrome with respiratory disease (Heiner's syndrome)
Systemic
Anaphylaxis
Controversial or Unproven
Behavioral conditions
Tension-fatigue syndrome
Attention deficit hyperactivity disorder
Otitis media
Psychiatric disorders
Neurologic disorders
Musculoskeletal disorders
Migraine headache

SYMPTOMS

A wide range of symptoms have been attributed to food allergy (see Table 38–2). Gastrointestinal symptoms occur most frequently, followed by symptoms of the skin and respiratory system (Bock, 1986). Gastrointestinal symptoms have been reported in 70% of children studied; cutaneous symptoms have been reported in 24%, and respiratory symptoms have been found in 6% (Minford et al, 1982). Although the distribution of symptoms reported varies with the population evaluated, respiratory symptoms are thought to be the least common and occur most often in association with other symptoms (Bock, 1986; Novembre et al, 1988).

Anaphylaxis is an acute, often severe, and sometimes fatal immune response that usually occurs with a clear-cut temporal relationship after exposure to the antigen. Anaphylaxis may affect any body system. The most dangerous allergic reaction is systemic anaphylaxis, which can include abdominal pain, nausea, cyanosis, a drop in blood pressure, angioedema, chest pain, urticaria, diarrhea, shock, and death.

The role of food allergy in behavioral, psychologic, neurologic, and musculoskeletal disorders remains largely unproven. Behavioral symptoms such as hyperactivity and the tension fatigue syndrome, often anecdotally described, have not been reproduced in controlled challenge studies (Bock, 1986). Symptoms such as irritability and fussiness have been observed only in conjunction with gastrointestinal, skin, or respiratory symptoms (Bock, 1986 and 1987). A relationship between food allergy and migraine headaches has been suggested by preliminary studies (Egger et al, 1983; Mansfield et al, 1985). In children with migraine headaches and epilepsy, avoidance of specific foods has been prescribed to decrease seizure activity (Egger et al, 1989). However, the available data are too limited to establish food allergy as an important cause for migraine headaches or seizures. Similarly, exacerbation of rheumatoid arthritis symptoms by foods has been documented (Panaush, 1986a and b), but evidence for a relationship between food allergy and rheumatoid arthritis from controlled studies is limited at this time. A relationship between food allergy and otitis media in children has been proposed (Marshall et al, 1984), but

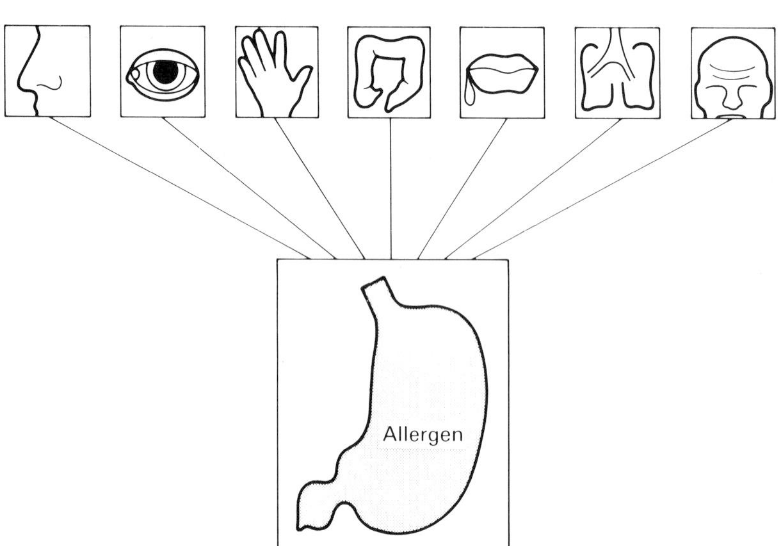

FIGURE 38–2. *Scheme of food allergy "target organs." (From Brostoff J and Challacombe SJ: Food Allergy and Intolerance. London, Baillière Tindall, 1987.)*

further evaluation is needed. However, when rheumatoid arthritis, otitis media, migraine headaches, and migraine headaches associated with untractable epilepsy do not respond to other treatments, evaluation of food allergy may be warranted.

The onset of symptoms after a food is eaten may be *immediate* (*less than 2 hours*), *intermediate* (*2 to 24 hours*), or *delayed* (*more than 24 hours*). Most documented allergic reactions to foods occur within 2 hours of ingestion (Bock, 1986) (Fig. 38–3). Symptoms displayed vary with the amount of antigen (allergen) ingested and absorbed, the types of reactions that occur, and the sensitivity of the target organ.

COMMON FOOD ALLERGENS

Many foods have been implicated in food allergy; however, relatively few foods have been documented to cause adverse reactions. The most common food allergens are commonly eaten foods with high-protein content, especially of plant or marine origin (Taylor et al, 1987). In children the foods most commonly documented to cause reactions are cow's milk, soy, peanut, egg, wheat, and fish (Bock, 1987; Eggleston, 1987; Marshall et al, 1984; Sampson, 1988). However, food allergy may develop to any food included in the diet (Bock, 1987). Positive reactions following ingestion of corn, rice, rye, nuts, shrimp, chicken, turkey, pork, beef, bananas, squash, and potatoes have also been reported (Bock, 1986 and 1987; Sampson, 1988). Although frequently described, allergic reactions to chocolate and strawberry have not been documented (Bock, 1986). Reactions to shellfish, peanuts, nuts, and grains have been described in the adult population (Atkins et al, 1985; Bernstein et al, 1982).

The antigens in food are often large proteins (mw 10,000 to 70,000 daltons). Individual foods contain many different proteins, of which only a few may be highly allergenic. For example, cow's milk contains more than 20 different proteins, of which beta-lactoglobulin, casein, and alpha-lactalbumin are among the most allergenic. *Cross-reactivity* between antigens may occur, especially between foods within the same biologic family. For example, an infant who is allergic to cow's milk may be allergic to goat's milk. A child who is allergic to ragweed pollen may not tolerate watermelon. However, allergy to one food or pollen does not necessarily mean that there will be allergy to all related foods. In children, clinically significant cross-reactivity between legumes, such as peanut and soybean, is rare (Bernhisel-Broadbent and Sampson, 1989). Adverse reactions to each food must be documented.

Although many allergens are unaffected by denaturation caused by heat and acid, the allergenicity of some proteins can be altered by heating (Aas, 1984). Antigens of some foods are removed by processing. For example, individuals sensitive to soybeans, cottonseed, peanuts, or corn usually tolerate soy, cottonseed, peanut, or corn oil, respectively (American Academy of Allergy and Immunology, 1984; Bush et al, 1984; Taylor et al, 1981 and 1985). However, caution is advised for those with a history of severe anaphylactic reactions (American Academy of Allergy and Immunology, 1984).

RISK FACTORS FOR THE DEVELOPMENT OF FOOD ALLERGY

The risk of developing food allergy depends on heredity, exposure to the food (antigen), gastrointestinal permeability, and environmental factors. *Heredity* is thought to have a major role in the development of

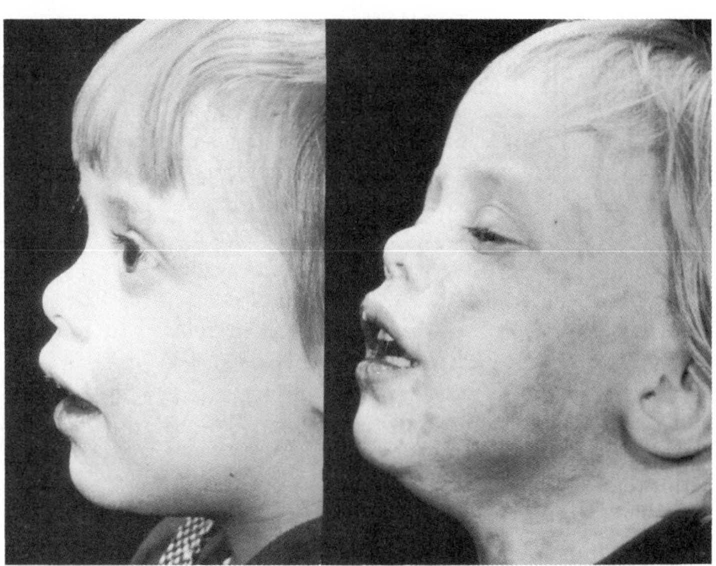

FIGURE 38–3. *Contact urticaria from egg white. This 3-year-old boy, with atopic eczema, was photographed before, and 15 minutes after, the application of raw egg white to his cheek. (From Brostoff J and Challacombe SJ: Food Allergy and Intolerance. London, Baillière Tindall, 1987.)*

allergy. *Atopy,* the tendency to develop IgE-mediated reactions, appears to be familial. A child's risk of being atopic is estimated to be from 47 to 100% when both parents are atopic and 13% when neither parent is atopic (Hamburger et al, 1983; Ziegler et al, 1989).

Antigen exposure is a prerequisite for development of food allergy. After the initial exposure to an antigen and sensitization of the immune cells, allergic reactions may occur. Infants may become sensitized to an antigen in breast milk, in which case allergic reactions may occur the first time an infant eats the antigen in food (Ziegler et al, 1989). Susceptibility to food allergy also depends on *gastrointestinal permeability,* which allows antigen penetration. Gastrointestinal permeability is thought to be greatest in early infancy and to decline with intestinal maturation. Other conditions such as gastrointestinal disease, malnutrition, prematurity, and immunodeficiency states may also be associated with increased permeability and the risk of developing food allergy.

The *amount of antigen presented* and *environmental factors* can also influence the development of food allergy. The effects of foods and other antigens are additive. Some foods may be tolerated only when they are eaten in small quantities. Clinical symptoms of food allergy may increase when inhalant allergies are exacerbated by seasonal or environmental changes. Common inhalant allergens include house dust, mites, feathers, animal dander, pollens, molds, and grain dust. Similarly, the effects of antigens that cross-react may be additive. Other environmental factors, such as tobacco smoke, stress, exercise, and cold, may enhance the clinical symptoms of food allergy. *Exercise-induced anaphylaxis* related to the ingestion of certain foods has been reported in adults (Kidd et al, 1983). This suggests interaction between nonspecific irritants and allergy in precipitating a reaction.

FOOD INTOLERANCES

Food intolerances are adverse reactions to foods caused by nonimmunologic mechanisms, including toxic, pharmacologic, metabolic, or idiosyncratic reactions (American Academy of Allergy and Immunology, 1984) (Table 38–3). Symptoms caused by food intolerances include gastrointestinal, cutaneous, and respiratory disorders and are often the same as those related to food allergy. Therefore, food intolerances must be considered in the differential diagnosis of food allergy. Although symptoms of food intolerance may be similar to symptoms of food allergy, treatment required may differ depending on the mechanism involved. Allergy skin testing is not useful in the diagnosis and treatment of these conditions.

Food Additives

Food additives, such as preservatives, flavor enhancers, and coloring agents, have historically been linked to adverse reactions. Additives implicated include tartrazine (FD&C No 5), azo dyes and other coloring agents, benzoic acid, sodium nitrates, butylated hydroxyanisole (BHA), butylated hydroxytoluene (BHT), and sulfites (Ortolani et al, 1988) (see Table 38–3).

Overall, adverse reactions to coloring agents and the preservatives benzoic acid, sodium nitrate, BHA, and BHT appear to be rare, even in the groups thought to be at greatest risk. Early reports suggested that intrinsic asthmatics and aspirin-sensitive asthmatics were the most likely to react to food additives (Weber et al, 1979). However, more recent controlled studies reveal that challenge with tartrazine, azo dyes, and benzoic acid elicited symptoms of asthma in up to 21% of the intrinsic asthmatics studied, whereas BHA and BHT challenge elicited no response (Stevenson et al, 1986; Weber et al, 1979). Similarly, in populations with chronic urticaria, challenge with tartrazine, sodium nitrate, and benzoate has been linked to urticaria in only 1 to 4% of those evaluated (Ortolani et al, 1988; Stevenson et al, 1986).

Adverse reactions to monosodium glutamate (MSG) have been reported to include headache, nausea, flushing, abdominal pain, and asthma and may occur from 1 to 14 hours after ingestion (Allen and Baker, 1980; Allen et al, 1983). Restaurant meals prepared without the use of MSG can be requested.

The association of food additives, dyes, and sugars with behavioral symptoms such as hyperactivity has been reported in the popular literature (Baker and Baker, 1987). These relationships have not been supported by most controlled challenge studies, however (American Academy of Allergy and Immunology; Mahan et al, 1985) (see Chapter 12). In contrast, improved behavior of preschool boys with attention deficit disorder and hyperactivity has been reported when receiving additive-free and caffeine-free diets that are low in sugar, although the effects may have been related to a reduction of caloric intake in the treatment diet (Kaplan et al, 1989). Alternatively, it is possible that some food additives were related to behavioral changes in a subset of this population. Although avoidance diets cannot be recommended for the routine management of hyperactivity, when families choose to pursue an additive-free diet in conjunction with recommended therapy, advice on implementing an adequate and safe diet should be provided.

Sulfites

Adverse reactions to sulfites in foods have been well documented (Brenner and Stevens, 1976; Bush et al, 1986; Taylor et al, 1988; Towns and Mellis, 1984). Sul-

TABLE 38–3. Representative Nonimmunologic Reactions to Food*

Cause	Associated Foods	Symptoms Described
Gastrointestinal Disorders		
Enzyme deficiency		
Lactase	Foods containing lactose and milk	Bloating, flatulence, diarrhea, abdominal pain
Glucose-6-phosphate dehydrogenase	Fava or broad beans	Hemolytic anemia
Disease Cystic fibrosis Gallbladder disease Enteropathies	Symptoms may be precipitated by many foods, especially high-fat foods or certain proteins	Bloating, loose stools, abdominal pain
Inborn Errors of Metabolism		
Phenylketonuria	Foods containing phenylalanine	Elevated serum phenylalanine levels, mental retardation
Galactosemia	Foods containing lactose or galactose	Vomiting, lethargy, failure to thrive
Psychologic Reactions	Symptoms may be precipitated by any food	Wide variety; any system may be involved
Reactions to Pharmacologic Agents in Foods		
Vasoactive amines		
Phenylethylamine	Chocolate, aged cheese, red wine	Migraine headaches
Tyramine	Cheddar cheese, French cheeses, brewer's yeast, Chianti wine, canned fish	Migraine headaches, cutaneous erythema, urticaria and hypertensive crisis in patients on monoamine oxidase inhibitors
Histamine	Fermented cheeses, fermented foods (e.g., sauerkraut, pork sausages, canned tuna, anchovies, sardines)	Erythema, headaches, decreased blood pressure
Histamine-releasing agents	Shellfish, chocolate, strawberries, tomatoes, peanuts, pork, wine, pineapple	Urticaria, eczema, pruritus

Cause	Associated Foods	Symptoms Described
Reactions to Food Additives		
Tartrazine or FD&C Yellow No. 5	Yellow or yellow-orange colored foods, soft drinks, medicine	Hives, rash, asthma
Benzoic acid or sodium benzoate	Soft drinks and some cheeses, salt-free margarines, and processed potato products	Hives, rash, asthma
Sulfites Sodium sulfite Potassium sulfite Sodium metabisulfite Potassium metabisulfite Sodium bisulfite Potassium bisulfite Sulfur dioxide	Shrimp, many processed foods—avocado, instant potatoes, dried fruits, vegetables, acidic juices, wine, beer	Acute asthma and anaphylaxis, loss of consciousness
Monosodium glutamate	Chinese and Japanese dishes	"Chinese restaurant syndrome"—headache, tenseness in face, sweating, chest pain, and dizziness
Reactions to Microorganism Contamination of Foods		
Proteus causes histidine to break down to histamine-like substance	Unrefrigerated scombroid fish (tuna, bonita, mackerel); heat stable toxin	Scombroid fish poisoning—itching, rash, vomiting, diarrhea
Gonyaulax catenella (red tide)	Mussels, clams that ingest organism that produces soxitoxin. Heat stable	Paralytic shellfish poisoning—progressive numbness from head to arms; frequently fatal

* From Butkus SN and Mahan LK: Food allergies: Immunological reactions to foods. © The American Dietetic Association. Reprinted by permission from Journal of the American Dietetic Association, vol 86, p 601, 1986.

fiting agents are added to many foods and beverages to prevent browning, to control microbial growth and spoilage, to modify texture, and to bleach certain foods. Sulfites are also used as antioxidants in pharmaceuticals. Although the prevalence of sulfite sensitivity in the general population is unknown, adverse reactions among nonasthmatics are rare (Bush et al, 1986; Simon, 1989). Sulfite sensitivity is most likely to occur in the asthmatic population. The prevalence of sulfite sensitivity among asthmatics is estimated at 3.9%, whereas the prevalence among steroid-dependent asthmatics has been estimated at 8.4% (Bush et al, 1986).

The diagnosis of sulfite sensitivity requires controlled provocative challenge with sulfites. Guidelines for challenge have been outlined (Taylor et al, 1988; Simon, 1989). Most adverse reactions occur with doses of 20 to 50 mg of sulfite given in solution (Simon, 1989). Reactions to sulfites present in foods may differ, however. Sulfite-sensitive asthmatics may not react after the ingestion of all sulfite-containing foods. The occurrence of reactions depends on the nature of the food, the level of residual sulfite, the sensitivity of the individual, and perhaps on the form of residual sulfite and the mechanism of the sulfite-induced reaction (Taylor et al, 1988).

Management of sulfite sensitivity requires avoidance of sulfite-containing foods. Foods containing high levels of sulfites are listed in Table 38–3. Since 1986, Food and Drug Administration (FDA) regulations have banned the use of sulfites on fresh fruits and vegetables other than potatoes that are served in the raw form (Further Reading, p. 664). Current regulations of the FDA and of the Bureau of Alcohol, Tobacco, and Firearms also require labeling of packaged foods that contain sulfites added as a preservative and alcoholic beverages containing 10 ppm or more of sulfite (Food and Drug Administration, 1988).

Carbohydrate Intolerance

Lactase deficiency is the most common enzyme deficiency on a world-wide basis (see Further Reading, p. 468). Individuals with a deficiency of the intestinal enzyme *lactase* have decreased ability to digest lactose, which is the sugar in milk. Symptoms after ingestion of lactose include abdominal cramping, flatulence, and diarrhea. Because the symptoms are similar, lactose intolerance is often confused with allergy to cow's milk. Deficiencies of lactase and other carbohydrate-digesting enzymes are discussed further in Chapter 27.

Gastrointestinal symptoms after ingestion of fruit juice are commonly reported in infants and children. These symptoms may be related to carbohydrate intolerance rather than to food allergy. Carbohydrate malabsorption has been documented following ingestion of pear, apple, and grape juices. A brief restriction of fruit juices may be useful in the evaluation of infants and children with chronic nonspecific diarrhea (Hyams et al, 1988).

DIAGNOSIS

No simple test can be used to diagnose food allergy. Diagnosis requires identification of the suspected food, proof that the food causes an adverse response, and verification of immunologic involvement. Nonallergic mechanisms must be ruled out. The omission of foods from the diet on the basis of improper diagnosis can threaten nutritional status.

A *history* is the first tool used in diagnosis. Information gathered includes a description of symptoms, time from ingestion of food to onset of symptoms, a description of the most recent reactions, a list of suspected foods, and an estimate of the quantity of food required to produce a reaction. Because food allergy may be linked to the introduction of new foods, early feeding history should be explored. Family history of allergy should also be reviewed.

Physical examination includes measurement of weight and height (and head circumference for the infant). Measurements are plotted on a growth chart and are evaluated in relationship to earlier measurements. Decreased weight for height may be related to malabsorption and food allergy. Therefore, patterns of growth and their relationship to the onset of symptoms should be explored. Clinical signs of malnutrition should be assessed, including the evaluation of fat and muscle stores (see Chapter 17). Evidence of chronic conditions, such as eczema, rhinitis, and asthma, are also evaluated.

A *food and symptom diary* is kept for 1 to 2 weeks (Fig. 38–4). Information recorded includes the type of food, the time and amount eaten, the time of appearance of symptoms, and the medications taken. Medications may alter the symptoms observed. The food and symptom diary helps to document symptoms and may suggest a relationship to diet that is not apparent from recall. This record also serves as a baseline for future intervention.

Biochemical testing serves to rule out nonallergenic causes for symptoms. A complete blood count and differential; tests of stool for reducing substances, ova, and parasite or occult blood; and a sweat chloride test for the exclusion of cystic fibrosis are examples of tests that may be useful.

Immunologic testing cannot be used to diagnose food allergy but can help to identify suspected foods and to confirm an immunologic mechanism. Positive immunologic test results must be confirmed by an adverse reaction when the food is eaten (Bock et al, 1977). Reli-

Name ______________

	DAY 1 DATE ___	DAY 2 DATE ___	DAY 3 DATE ___	DAY 4 DATE ___	DAY 5 DATE ___	DAY 6 DATE ___	DAY 7 DATE ___
SYMPTOMS							
B R E A K F A S T							
SNACK SUPPLEMENTS							
SYMPTOMS							
L U N C H							
SNACK SUPPLEMENTS							
SYMPTOMS							
D I N N E R							
SNACK							
SYMPTOMS							
MEDICATION							

FIGURE 38–4. *Food and symptom diary.*

able immunologic tests include the skin-prick test, the radioallergosorbent extract test (RAST), and the enzyme-linked immunosorbent assay (ELISA) (Table 38–4). A large weal (>3 mm) in reaction to a skin test is most likely to predict a positive result on a food challenge and can be useful for children over 3 years of age. For children less than 3 years old, the skin test is reserved to confirm immunologic mechanisms after symptoms have been confirmed by a positive result on a food challenge or when the history of the reaction is impressive (Bock, 1987). Most adverse reactions to foods in children under 3 years of age are not associated with a positive result on a skin test (Bock, 1987). RAST and ELISA are as reliable as the skin-prick test but are more costly; they may be useful for people who have had anaphylaxis or who have skin diseases such as widespread atopic dermatitis (American Academy of Allergy and Immunology, 1984).

Unreliable tests include cytotoxic testing, sublingual testing, provocative and neutralization testing, and kinesiologic testing (American Academy of Allergy, 1981; David, 1987) (see Table 38–4).

Food elimination is the next step in diagnosis. Suspected foods are omitted from the diet for 2 weeks or until symptoms clear. If symptoms do not clear and food allergy is still suspected, more restrictive diets can be implemented to omit cow's milk, eggs, wheat, and other common allergens. Examples of elimination diets are provided in Table 38–5. Elimination diets for infants depend on their developmental readiness for solids. Extensive elimination diets for infants may include casein hydrolysate formula (e.g., Nutramigen), rice cereal, and other solids including carrots, squash, sweet potatoes, chicken, lamb, peaches, pears, apricots, and tapioca (American Academy of Allergy and Immunology, 1984). Hypoallergenic elemental formulas such as Tolerex can be used for children (American Academy of Pediatrics, 1985) and adults in extreme cases, if symptoms have not cleared on an elimination diet. If symptoms persist, causes other than the foods eliminated should be investigated.

A food record is kept during the elimination phase. This record is used to ensure that all forms of suspected foods have been eliminated from the diet. This food record is also used to evaluate the nutritional adequacy of the diet. If a limited diet continues for several weeks, vitamin or mineral supplementation may be necessary.

If there has been a positive result on a skin test and symptoms improve unequivocally with the elimination of one or two foods, those foods can be eliminated from the diet empirically until it is appropriate to rechallenge. However, if symptoms improve only with elimination of multiple foods, food challenge is needed.

The *food challenge* is made after symptoms have cleared. Foods are reintroduced (challenged) one at a time while the person is carefully observed for the recurrence of symptoms. The initial challenge is made with 20 mg to 2 grams of dried food or 1/2 teaspoon to 1 tablespoon of fresh food, depending on the history reported. The quantity of food offered is then increased in a stepwise fashion until a reaction is observed or the quantity reaches 8 to 10 grams of dried food or a standard portion of fresh food. Reactions have been observed in children after consumption of 20 mg to 8 grams of dried food (Bock, 1986) and in adults after consumption of 5 to 100 grams of fresh food (Atkins et al, 1985). Although most allergic reactions occur within 2 hours of the challenge, non–IgE-mediated reactions may occur more than 24 hours after challenge, and

TABLE 38–4. Diagnostic Tests

Type of Test	Description	Comments
Skin Scratch, prick, or puncture	A drop of antigen is placed on skin, which is then scratched or punctured	Most sensitive test but overdiagnoses food allergy; should be followed by food challenge
Radioallergosorbent extract (RAST)	Serum mixed with food on paper disk and then washed with radioactively labeled IgE	No more accurate than skin test but more costly; may be useful for people who have had anaphylaxis or who have skin disease
Enzyme-linked immunosorbent assay (ELISA)	Much like RAST, except no radioactive material used	Same as RAST
Cytotoxic	Allergen mixed with whole blood or serum leukocyte suspension; lysed leukocytes are counted	Unreliable
Sublingual	Drops of allergen extract placed under the tongue and symptoms are recorded	Unreliable
Provocative and neutralization	Subcutaneous injection of extract elicits symptoms followed by weaker or stronger injection to neutralize symptoms	Unreliable
Kinesiologic	Arm extended and foods to be tested placed in hand; test is positive if arm moves more easily after food has been placed in hand	Unreliable

TABLE 38–5. Two Stages of Elimination Diets

	Elimination Diet 1—*Milk-, Egg-, and Wheat-Free*	
	Allowed	*Avoid*
Animal protein sources	Lamb, chicken, turkey, beef, pork	Cow's milk, chicken eggs
Vegetable protein sources	Soy milk, soy beans, other beans, lentils, peanuts	
Grains or alternate	White potato, sweet potato, yams, rice, tapioca, arrowroot, buckwheat, corn, barley, rye, millet, oats	Wheat
Vegetables	All vegetables	
Fruits	All fruits and juices	
Sweeteners	Cane or beet sugar, maple syrup, corn syrup	
Oils	Soy oil, corn oil, safflower oil, coconut oil, vegetable oil, olive oil, peanut oil, milk-free margarines	Butter and margarines that include milk
Other	Salt, all spices	
	Elimination Diet 2—*Minimal Elimination Diet*	
	Allowed	*Avoid*
Animal protein sources	Lamb	All other animal protein: meat, fish, poultry, eggs, and milk
Vegetable protein sources		Soy milk, soy beans, peas, other beans, lentils, peanuts, bean sprouts, all nuts
Grains or alternate starches	White potato, sweet potato, yams, rice, tapioca, buckwheat, arrowroot	Wheat, oats, corn, barley, millet, rye
Vegetables	All vegetables* except corn, peas, tomatoes	Corn, peas, tomatoes
Fruits	All fruits and juices* except citrus fruits, strawberries	Citrus fruits, strawberries
Sweeteners	Cane or beet sugar, maple syrup	Corn syrup, corn syrup solids
Oils	Safflower oil, coconut oil, olive oil, sesame oil	Butter, margarine, vegetable oils, soy oil, corn oil, peanut oil, nonspecific shortening, or fats of animal origin
Other	Salt, pepper, all spices,* vanilla or lemon extract, baking soda, cream of tartar	Chocolate, coffee, tea, colas and other soft drinks, alcoholic beverages Cornstarch, baking powder with cornstarch

* Suggest limiting number to five to minimize dietary variables.

reactions should continue to be monitored during this time.

Food challenges may precipitate anaphylactic reactions (David, 1984). To minimize risks to patients, all challenges that may cause an anaphylactic reaction should be carried out in a physician's office or hospital. The initial dose is increased in a stepwise fashion over 1 hour until a reaction is observed or a total of 8 to 10 grams of dried food has been consumed. The patient is then observed for an additional 2 hours before discharge. If there is a clear history of a life-threatening anaphylactic reaction after eating a specific food, it should not be challenged (Sampson, 1988).

A *double-blind food challenge* can be used when symptoms are subjective, when multiple food allergies have been suggested, or when psychosocial components are suspected. For the older child and adult who are able to swallow capsules, dried food is placed in opaque capsules. For the child who is not able to swallow capsules, the suspected food is concealed in a food or beverage known to be tolerated, such as applesauce, juice, or a specially prepared cookie. Capsules or masking foods are administered twice per challenge. On one occasion the individual receives the food being tested. On the other, a placebo is given. In a double-blind food challenge neither the person administering the challenge nor the person being challenged knows which has been offered. A *single-blind food challenge,* in which the person receiving the challenge does not know what has been offered, may be useful in similar situations and is easier to implement. Challenges carried out for research purposes should be double-blind (Bock, 1986; Sampson, 1988).

TREATMENT

Treatment of food allergy and of many food intolerances calls for eliminating the offending food from the diet. Each individual's sensitivity determines the degree to which foods must be omitted. Those who are very sensitive need to omit all forms of the offending food, whereas the less sensitive may tolerate small amounts (Butkus and Mahan, 1986). Families and individuals need suggestions on how to avoid foods, how to substitute for restricted foods in meal planning and preparation, and how to make nutritional replacements.

Restricted foods may be "hidden" in the diet in unfamiliar forms. To help in identification and avoidance of offending foods, allergy-specific lists describing

FURTHER READING: Is There Sulfite Present?

Approximately 5% of the estimated 9 million asthmatics in the United States are sensitive to sulfur-containing compounds that are frequently encountered in foods. In extreme cases, they may react with bronchospasms. Since 1985, four deaths (in restaurants) from this cause have been confirmed. Nonasthmatics may also be affected but react with lower-level symptoms.

Sulfur-containing compounds have for many years been added to a number of foods for the purpose of preventing oxidation, microbial infestation, and bleaching of colors. When sulfites in the final product exceed more than 10 parts per million, the label must carry the chemical name and purpose of the additive (e.g., "potassium bisulfate as a preservative"). Because sulfites destroy thiamin, they are not permitted in foods that are considered to be significant sources of this vitamin—primarily meats, some fish, and crab. (Information about foods in which added sulfites are "generally recognized as safe" can be found in the Code of Federal Regulations, 21 Food and Drugs, Parts 182 and 184.)

Sulfite-sensitive individuals can avoid offending foods by reading labels on packaged foods. However, such protection has not been available with respect to sulfite-treated foods that are served "fresh," such as salad bar ingredients and menu items that are delivered to restaurants in pre-prepared forms. (Sulfites preserve crispness of salad greens and the whiteness of peeled uncooked potatoes.) Although the institution packaging or containers of items such as raw French fries and hash browns may be properly labeled, this information does not usually reach the restaurant patron.

This potential hazard to asthmatics was addressed by the FDA in 1986 with the prohibition of sulfite use on fresh fruits and vegetables intended to be sold or served raw or presented to the consumer as "fresh." In February 1990, a similar ban was applied to potatoes. However, the latter ban was appealed on the basis of a legal technicality related to the FDA hearings, and in May of that year the regulation was overturned by a federal court. Alternatives are being explored by the FDA. At present, however, the safest way for the sensitive consumer to order potatoes at a restaurant is to order potatoes baked or otherwise cooked in their skins (Sulfite . . . , 1990; Information . . . , 1990).

foods to avoid, key words for ingredient identification, and acceptable substitutes are useful (Table 38–6). Caretakers need to read labels carefully before purchasing food.

When foods are removed from the diet, alternative nutrient sources must be provided. For example, when milk is omitted, other sources must provide calcium, vitamin D, protein, riboflavin, and energy. The nutritional adequacy of the diet should be monitored by ongoing evaluation of growth and nutritional status and by periodic evaluation of food records. Malnutrition has been documented in children consuming inadequate elimination diets (David et al, 1984; Silverman and Lecks, 1982). Vitamin and mineral supplementation may be needed, especially when multiple foods are omitted. Supplementation should not exceed 100% of the recommended dietary allowance (RDA) (see Chapter 16).

In long-term follow-up, the efficacy and patient acceptance of diets must be monitored. If symptoms persist or reappear, review of intake will determine if all forms of suspected foods have been omitted from the diet. If symptoms persist even with adherence to the diet, other causes should be investigated. Because food is an important part of an individual's culture, the social aspects of eating can make adherence difficult. Continued support from health care providers is needed to minimize the impact of diet changes on family and social life. Tips listed in Table 38–7 may help families and individuals to cope with food allergies.

Antigen load is sometimes limited by using the *rotation diet* for those with a large number of allergies. When a rotation diet is planned, allergenic foods or closely related foods are offered one at a time on 1 day of a 4- to 5-day cycle. In practice, these diets are rarely necessary and can be difficult to implement (American Academy of Allergy and Immunology, 1984).

Treatments with desensitization techniques or medications are not viable alternatives for management of food allergy. Although preliminary studies indicated that prophylactic use of sodium cromalyn may prevent symptoms of food allergy (Sogn, 1986), this role has not been confirmed (Burks and Sampson, 1988). Early studies suggested that ketotifen may block symptoms of food allergy, but further research is needed before its use can be recommended routinely (Molkhou and Dupont, 1987). The efficacy of desensitization shots and oral desensitization for food allergy is unproven and may place the patient at risk for anaphylaxis (Johnstone, 1972; Cohen et al, 1979).

NATURAL HISTORY

Food allergies that develop within the first 3 years of life tend to resolve with age, whereas those diagnosed after 3 years may be more persistent (Bock, 1987). In a prospective study of 480 children followed until 36 months of age, 80% of the initial complaints of adverse reactions to foods occurred during the first year of life (Bock, 1987). The majority of foods were returned to

TABLE 38–6. Food Selection for Allergy Diets

Foods likely to contain MILK . . .	Substitutes for MILK . . .
Milk	Soy milks
Buttermilk	Nut milks
Hot chocolate	Milk-free "shakes"
Many "nondairy" products	Some nondairy creamers
Many baked goods	Baked goods without milk—most French bread
Many baking mixes	
Granola	Bagels, saltines
Cheese	Soy cheese
Prepared meats (hot dogs, luncheon meats)	Kosher-prepared meats
Macaroni and cheese	Products labeled "parve" or pareve
Canned spaghetti	
Potatoes mashed with milk or butter	Foods prepared without milk or butter: potatoes, scrambled egg casseroles, etc.
Vegetables in cream, cheese, or butter sauces	
Many margarines	Milk-free margarines, salad dressings, sauces, and gravies
Many salad dressings	
Imitation sour cream	
Some gravies	
Ice cream	Milk-free sherbets, ices and sorbets
Some sherbets	
Yogurt	Frozen tofu desserts
Puddings	Cornstarch puddings with fruit juice
Milk chocolate	Jello

MILK may be listed on the label as . . .

Milk
Milk solids
Buttermilk solids
Curds
Whey solids
Whey
Casein
Lactalbumin
Caseinate
Cream
Sodium caseinate

Foods likely to contain EGG . . .	Substitutes for EGG . . .
Egg nog	
Root beers	
Many baked goods	Egg-free baked goods and specialty items
Pancakes, waffles, French toast	
Egg noodles	Pasta, rice, potatoes, egg-free egg substitutes
Eggs	
Most egg substitutes	
Many prepared meats (hot dogs, luncheon meats, imitation seafood)	Prepared meats and imitation seafood without egg products
Many batter-dipped foods	
Noodle soups	Soups without egg products
Mayonnaise	Imitation mayonnaise, sauces and salad dressings prepared without egg products
Hollandaise sauce	
Many salad dressings	
Tartar sauce	
Custards	Cornstarch, tapioca puddings prepared without eggs
Puddings	
Boiled frostings	Baked goods prepared without eggs
Meringues	
Macaroons	
Marshmallow products	
Fondants and other candies	

EGGS may be listed on the label as . . .

Albumin
Egg white
Egg white solids
Egg yolk
Yolks

Foods likely to contain WHEAT . . .	Substitutes for WHEAT . . .
Instant breakfast	
Postum	
Many baked goods	Breads and other wheat-free baked goods
Most baking mixes	
Pancakes, waffles	Wheat-free cereals, rice chex, cream of rice
Many cereals	
Many crackers	Rice cakes and crackers
	Rye crackers
Breaded foods	Cornmeal coating
Wheat tortillas	Corn tortillas
Pasta, noodles	Rice, corn pasta
Prepared meat products, hot dogs, luncheon meats	Meat products without wheat added
Gravies and sauces thickened with flour	Gravies and sauces thickened with cornstarch, potato starch, etc.
Cakes, cookies, pies, etc	Homemade baked goods made without wheat
Soy sauce	Worcestershire sauce
	Salt
Pretzels	Popcorn, corn chips
Beer, including nonalcoholic beer	

WHEAT may be listed on the label as . . .

Wheat
Flour
Wheat bran
Wheat germ
Wheat starch
Gluten
Graham flour
Enriched flour
Durum flour
Vegetable gums
Modified food starch
Vegetable starches
Malted cereal syrup
Hydrolyzed vegetable protein
Semolina

Foods likely to contain SOY . . .	Substitutes for SOY . . .
Soy formula	Casein hydrolysate formula
Soy milks	Milk or nut milks
Nondairy creamers	
Instant breakfast	Homemade breakfast shake
Many baked goods	Breads, cereals, and crackers made without soy products
Many baking mixes	
Many breakfast cereals	
Many crackers	
Imitation meats, bacon, and seafood	Meats and seafood
Meat filler products	Foods prepared without fillers or soy products
Tofu, miso, tempeh, soybean	
Canned spaghetti	
Packaged macaroni and cheese	
Breading mixes for poultry	
Tuna packed in oil*	Tuna packed in water
Peanut butter with added oil*	Peanut butter without added oils
Au gratin potato mixes	Potatoes without soy products
Soy bean oil*	Soy-free oils, margarines, and salad dressings
Soy margarines*	
Salad dressings*	
Spray shortenings*	
Many cakes, cookies	Cakes, cookies, and frostings prepared without soy products
Packaged frostings	
Chocolate chips and bars	
Canned puddings	
Soy and teriyaki sauces	Some Worcestershire sauces
Many snack foods: pretzels, chips, etc.*	Snack foods prepared without soy oil

* Tolerated by most people with soy allergy. Caution is advised for those with a history of anaphylaxis.
† Tolerated by most people with corn allergy. Caution is advised for those with history of anaphylaxis.

Table continued on following page

TABLE 38–6. Food Selection for Allergy Diets *Continued*

SOY may be listed on the label as . . .	
Soy	Vegetable starch
Soy flour	Vegetable gums
Soy protein	Soy bean oil*
Soy protein isolate	Vegetable shortening*
Hydrolyzed vegetable protein	Hydrogenated oils*

Foods likely to contain CORN . . .	**Substitutes for CORN . . .**
Carbonated beverages	Flavored seltzer
Many sweetened fruit drinks	Fruit juice
Instant breakfast	Homemade breakfast shake
Many bread products Many cereals Many crackers	Breads, crackers, and cereals made without corn products
Some baking and pancake mixes	
Corn tortillas	Wheat tortillas
Some processed meats	Processed meats made without corn products
Imitation seafood	
Imitation cheese	
Peanut butter with corn syrup added	Peanut butter without added sweeteners
Canned spaghetti and sauces Canned baked beans Canned soups Au gratin potato mixes	Foods without corn sweeteners or other corn products added
Corn oil†	Other oils
Corn oil margarine†	Soy-free margarines or butter
Salad dressings†	Homemade dressings made without corn oil
Sweetened canned fruit	Fresh fruit or packed in own juice
Corn syrup Pancake syrup	Sugar, pure maple syrup, or honey
Jellies and jams	Pure fruit spreads
Popsicles and ice creams	Frozen desserts without added corn sweeteners
Most baking powders	Featherweight baking powder
Cornstarch	Flour or potato starch
Condiments—sweet pickles	
Catsup and barbecue sauce	

CORN may be listed on the label as . . .
Corn
Cornstarch
Corn syrup
Corn oil†
Corn sweeteners
Corn syrup solids
High-fructose corn syrup
Maltodextrin
Vegetable oil†

* Tolerated by most people with soy allergy. Caution is advised for those with a history of anaphylaxis.
† Tolerated by most people with corn allergy. Caution is advised for those with history of anaphylaxis.

the diet within 9 months of the initial complaint, and all but 4 of the 37 confirmed or probable reactions resolved by 3 years of age. Allergies to cow's milk, soy, and egg are most likely to resolve with age (Bock, 1982). RAST or skin testing for IgE sensitization may remain positive even after the food can be eaten without symptoms (Bock, 1982; Eggleson, 1987).

Because symptoms of food allergy tend to resolve with age, foods should be reintroduced in a food challenge every 1 to 3 months to ensure that foods are not being restricted unnecessarily. After two to three positive open challenges, blinded challenges may be useful to overcome any bias that has developed (Bock, 1987).

Food allergies linked to severe reactions such as anaphylaxis may also resolve with age (Bock, 1985). Although these foods should not be challenged casually, challenge in controlled settings may be appropriate in some cases. Controlled challenge is preferable to accidental challenge in a setting where treatment is not available, and may help to reduce anxiety over possible adverse reactions. Challenges of foods that have caused severe reactions should only be carried out in settings where treatment for anaphylaxis is available, such as the intensive care unit, emergency room, or hospital outpatient clinic. An initial dose of one tenth of the amount thought to cause a reaction has been recommended (Bock, 1985). The dose is gradually increased

TABLE 38–7. Tips for Coping with Food Allergy

Substituting for foods: Substitute item for item at meals. If the family is eating ice cream, a frozen dessert may be a better accepted substitute than, for example, cookies.

Eating away from home: Bring "safe" foods along to make eating out easier. For breakfast, bring along soy milk if others will be having cereal with milk for breakfast.

Special occasions: Call the host family in advance and find out the menu planned. Offer to provide an acceptable dish that all can enjoy.

Grocery shopping: Be informed about what foods are acceptable and read labels carefully. Product ingredients change over time; continue to read the labels of "safe" foods. Shopping will take extra time.

Substitutions in cooking:
- *Milk:* Use herbal tea or fruit juice in recipes calling for milk. They add a spicy fragrance to cookies, cakes, puddings, and bread. Use soy or cashew milk for milk replacement. Combine 1 cup soy powder or ground cashews with 3 cups water in a large saucepan. Whisk until well dissolved. Bring to a boil over high heat, stirring constantly. Lower heat and simmer for 3 minutes. Serve hot or cold. Makes 3 cups.
- *Corn:* If a recipe calls for cornstarch, substitute equal amounts of arrowroot or potato starch or double the amount of whole wheat, soy, or barley flour. Most baking powders include cornstarch. Make corn-free baking powder by combining ¼ tsp baking soda with ½ tsp cream of tartar. This is equivalent to 1 tsp baking powder.
- *Egg:* In baking, achieve the emulsifying effect of one egg by combining 2 T whole-wheat flour, ½ tsp oil, ½ tsp baking powder, and 2 T milk, water, or fruit juice. Egg substitutes are also available.
- *Chocolate:* Use carob powder measure for measure when substituting for cocoa. As a substitute for one square of chocolate, use 3 T carob powder plus 2 T milk, water, butter, or margarine.
- *Wheat:* Wheat flour replacements and tips for cooking without wheat are listed in Table 27–10.

until a reaction occurs or a usual serving has been consumed under observation in a controlled setting. The amount tolerated under observation can then be offered at home.

There is some evidence in adults that complete avoidance of a proven food allergen can lead to tolerance of the food upon reintroduction 1 year later (Pastorello et al, 1989).

FOOD ALLERGY IN INFANCY

Cow's milk is the most common single allergen for infants (Bahna, 1987). Cow's milk allergy is thought to affect 3 to 5% of the infants fed cow's milk formula (Fig. 38–5). In a study involving three groups of infants based on their reactions to cow's milk, symptoms in 53% were characterized by pallor, vomiting, and diarrhea 45 minutes to 20 hours after ingestion of the food. Twenty-seven per cent had predominantly urticarial and angioedematous symptoms within 5 minutes of drinking milk and displayed positive skin test reactions to milk and elevated total and milk-specific IgE antibody levels. Twenty per cent of the infants displayed eczematous, bronchitic, or diarrheal symptoms, most of which developed more than 20 hours after beginning milk ingestion. These infants were the most difficult to identify clinically and had a history of chronic ill health and poor growth (Hill, 1986).

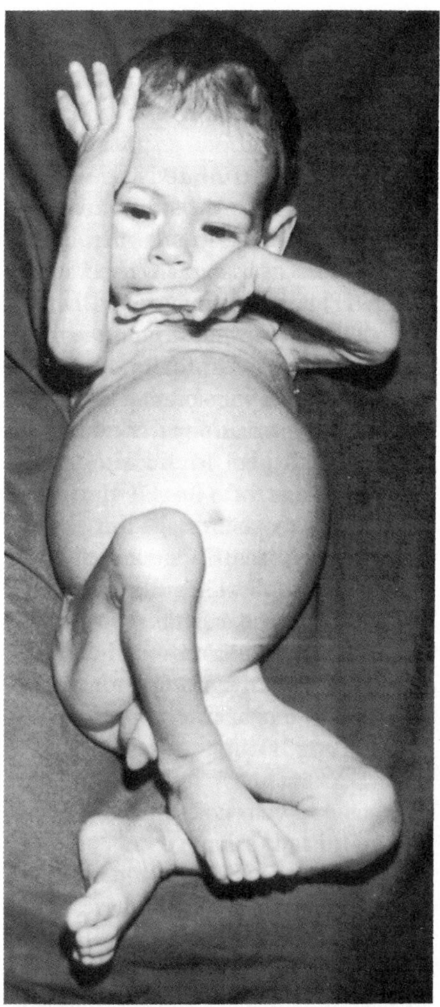

FIGURE 38–5. *Abdominal distention and muscular wasting in an infant due to cow's milk allergy. (From Brostoff J and Challacombe SJ: Food Allergy and Intolerance. London, Baillière Tindall, 1987.)*

Recommendations for Infant Feeding

Human milk is the preferred feeding for all infants. When use of human milk is not possible, soy protein or cow's milk protein hydrolysate formulas are alternatives to standard cow's milk formulas. Fifteen to 50% of infants allergic to cow's milk may also develop an allergy to soy (Sampson, 1991). Use of a protein hydrolysate formula instead of a soy formula when infants are showing clinical symptoms of allergic disease is recommended to reduce the likelihood of sensitization to soy protein (American Academy of Pediatrics, 1983). The American Academy of Pediatrics recommends the use of human milk or casein or whey protein hydrolysates with peptides of less than 1,200 molecular weight for infants with clinical symptoms of cow's milk or soy allergy. Commercially available casein protein hydrolysate formulas (Nutramigen and Pregestimil) that contain peptides of less than 1,200 molecular weight have been routinely used as feedings for infants allergic to cow's milk protein with adverse reactions rarely reported. However, available whey protein hydrolysate formulas (Good Start) contain larger peptides and may not be acceptable alternatives for the infant allergic to cow's milk protein (American Academy of Pediatrics, 1989).

The use of goat's milk as an alternative for cow's milk is not recommended because of the potential cross-reactivity with beta-lactoglobulin in cow's milk (American Academy of Allergy and Immunology, 1984). In addition, goat's milk is deficient in several nutrients and has a high renal solute load. Infants receiving goat's milk instead of infant formula would require supplements of iron, folacin, and vitamins A, C, and D. Goat's milk must be diluted to three-quarters strength and carbohydrate added to decrease the renal solute load.

Although uncommon, sensitivity to breast milk has been reported (Hamburger et al, 1983; Witington and Gibson, 1977). Allergens in the mother's diet, such as cow's milk or eggs, may pass into the breast milk and cause an allergic reaction in the infant. Foods in the mother's diet may also be associated with nonallergic reactions. Implicated foods have included caffeinated beverages, some herbal teas, cabbage, onions, turnips, garlic, radishes, rhubarb, spinach, and spices. Avoidance of the problem foods by the mother may alleviate her infant's symptoms.

Colic

The association between colic and food allergy remains controversial. Food intolerance and disturbed parent-child interaction have both been proposed as causes for infantile colic (Jakobsson and Lindberg, 1983; Lothe and Lindberg, 1989; Taubman, 1988). In some cases parental counseling on how to respond to infant crying has been more effective than diet change (Taubman, 1988). Symptoms of colic, sleeplessness, and irritability are rarely the result of an immune-mediated reaction to cow's milk protein (American Academy of Pediatrics, 1989). However, persistent colic may warrant trial of an elimination diet for the breast-feeding mother or of a casein hydrolysate formula for the infant receiving cow's milk or soy formula. The nutritional adequacy of the mother's diet should be monitored when foods are omitted from her diet, especially cow's milk. A calcium supplement with vitamin D can help to meet the RDA for calcium and vitamin D during lactation.

DIET AND PREVENTION OF ALLERGIC DISEASE

The role of early feeding in the development of food allergy and allergic disease remains an area of controversy. Breast feeding with maternal avoidance of allergens may delay the development of allergic disease in high-risk infants (Sampson, 1989). Reduced exposure to allergenic foods during infancy has been associated with lower prevalence of food allergy during the first year, but with no difference in prevalence of other allergic conditions at 2 years of age (Ziegler et al, 1989).

Because the optimal early feeding for infants at risk for developing allergy is still unknown, only conservative recommendations for feeding can be made. Exclusive breast-feeding for the first 6 months with protein hydrolysate formula supplements if necessary, and withholding of highly allergenic foods such as milk, egg, peanuts, and fish for the first 2 to 3 years of life in children at high risk for allergy have been recommended (Businco, 1983 and 1987; Sampson, 1989).

CITED REFERENCES

Aas K: Antigens in food. Nutr Rev 42:85, 1984.

Allen DH and Baker GJ: Chinese-restaurant asthma (Letter). N Engl J Med 305:1154, 1981.

Allen DH et al: Monosodium glutamate-induced asthma. J Allergy Clin Immunol 71:98, 1983.

American Academy of Pediatrics: Hypersensitivity to food. *In* Forbes GB and Woodruff CW (eds): Pediatric Nutrition Handbook. Elk Grove Village, IL, American Academy of Pediatrics, 1985.

American Academy of Allergy: Position statement: Controversial techniques. J Allergy Clin Immunol 67:333, 1981.

American Academy of Allergy and Immunology, Committee on Adverse Reactions to Foods, and National Institute of Allergy and Infectious Diseases: Adverse Reactions to Foods. NIH Publication No. (NIAID) 84-2442, July 1984.

American Academy of Pediatrics, Committee on Nutrition: Hypoallergenic infant formulas. Pediatrics 83:1068, 1989.

American Academy of Pediatrics, Committee on Nutrition: Soy protein formulas: Recommendations for use in infant feeding. Pediatrics 72:359, 1983.

Atkins FM et al: Evaluation of immediate adverse reactions to foods in adult patients. II: A detailed analysis of reaction patterns during oral food challenge. J Allergy Clin Immunol 75:356, 1985.

Bahna SL: Milk allergy in infancy. Ann Allergy 59:131, 1987.

Baker E and Baker E: The Unmedical Book: How to Conquer Disease, Lose Weight, Avoid Suffering and Save Money. Sagauche, CO, Drelwood Publications, 1987.

Bernhisel-Broadbent J and Sampson H: Cross-allergenicity in the legume botanical family in children with food hypersensitivity. J Allergy Clin Immunol 83:435, 1989.

Bernstein M, Day JH, and Welsh A: Double-blind food challenge in the diagnosis of food sensitivity in the adult. J Allergy Clin Immunol 70:205, 1982.

Bock SA: A critical evaluation of clinical trials in adverse reactions to foods in children. J Allergy Clin Immunol 78:165, 1986.

Bock SA: Prospective appraisal of complaints of adverse reactions to foods in children during the first 3 years of life. Pediatrics 79:683, 1987.

Bock SA: The natural history of food sensitivity. J Allergy Clin Immunol 69:173, 1982.

Bock SA: Natural history of severe reactions to foods in young children. J Pediatr 107:676, 1985.

Bock SA et al: Studies of hypersensitivity reactions to foods in infants and children. J Allergy Clin Immunol 62:327, 1978.

Bock SA et al: Proper use of skin tests with food extracts in diagnosis of hypersensitivity to food in children. Clin Allergy 7:375, 1977.

Brenner BM and Stevens JJ: Anaphylaxis after ingestion of sodium bisulfite. Ann Allergy 37:180, 1976.

Burks AW and Sampson HA: Double-blind placebo-controlled trial of oral cromolyn in children with atopic dermatitis and documented food hypersensitivity. J Allergy Clin Immunol 81:417, 1988.

Bush RK et al: A critical evaluation of clinical trials in reactions to sulfites. J Allergy Clin Immunol 78:191, 1986a.

Bush RK et al: Prevalence of sensitivity to sulfiting agents in asthmatic patients. Am J Med 81:816, 1986b.

Bush RK et al: Soybean oil is not allergenic to soybean sensitive individuals. J Allergy Clin Immunol 73:176, 1984.

Businco L et al: Prevention of atopic diseases in "at-risk newborns" by prolonged breastfeeding. Ann Allergy 51:296, 1983.

Businco L et al: Prevention of atopy: Results of a long-term (7 months to 8 years) follow-up. Ann Allergy 59:183, 1987.

Butkus SN and Mahan LK: Food allergies: Immunological reactions to foods. J Am Diet Assn 86:601, 1986.

Cohen SH et al: Acute allergic reaction after composite pollen ingestion. J Allergy Clin Immunol 64:270, 1979.

David TJ: Anaphylactic shock during elimination diets for severe atopic eczema. Arch Dis Child 59:983, 1984.

David TJ: Unorthodox allergy procedures. Arch Dis Child 62:1060, 1987.

David TJ, Waddington E, and Stanton RHJ: Nutritional hazards of elimination diets in children with atopic eczema. Arch Dis Child 59:323, 1984.

Egger J et al: Is migraine food allergy? Lancet 2:805, 1983.

Egger J et al: Oligoantigenic diet treatment of children with epilepsy and migraine. J Pediatr 114:51, 1989.

Eggleson PA: Prospective studies in the natural history of food allergy. Ann Allergy 59:179, 1987.

Food and Drug Administration: Information on Sulfites. March 1988.

Hamburger RN et al: Current status of the clinical and immunologic consequences of a prototype allergic disease prevention program. Ann Allergy 51:281, 1983.

Hill DJ et al: Manifestations of milk allergy in infancy: Clinical and immunologic findings. J Pediatr 109:270, 1986.
Hyams SJ et al: Carbohydrate malabsorption following fruit juice ingestion in young children. Pediatrics 82:64, 1988.
Information on foods containing sulfiting agents. Seattle District, WA, Food and Drug Administration, March 1990.
Jakobsson I and Lindberg T: Cow's milk proteins cause infantile colic in breast-fed infants: A double-blind crossover study. Pediatrics 71:268, 1983.
Johnstone DE: Uses and abuses of hyposensitization in children. Am J Dis Child 123:78, 1972.
Kaplan BJ et al: Dietary replacement in preschool-aged hyperactive boys. Pediatrics 83:7, 1989.
Kidd JM et al: Food-dependent exercise-induced anaphylaxis. J Allergy Clin Immunol 71:407, 1983.
Kniker WT: Immunologically-mediated reactions to food: State of the art. Ann Allergy 59:60, 1987.
Lawrence RA: Breastfeeding: A Guide for the Medical Profession, 2nd ed. St Louis, CV Mosby, 1985, p 234.
Lothe L and Lindberg T: Cow's milk whey protein elicits symptoms of infantile colic in colicky formula-fed infants: A double-blind crossover study. Pediatrics 83:262, 1989.
Mahan LK et al: Sugar allergy and children's behavior. J Allergy Clin Immunol 75:177, 1985.
Mansfield LE et al: Food allergy and adult migraine: Double-blind and mediator confirmation of allergic etiology. Ann Allergy 55:126, 1985.
Marshall SG, Bierman CW, and Shapiro GG: Otitis media with effusion in childhood. Ann Allergy 53:370, 1984.
Minford AMB, MacDonald A, and Littlewood JM: Food intolerance and food allergy in children: A review of 68 cases. Arch Dis Child 57:742, 1982.
Molkhou P and Dupont C: Ketotifen in prevention and therapy of food allergy. Ann Allergy 59:187, 1987.
Novembre E, de Martino M, and Vierucci A: Foods and respiratory allergy. J Allergy Clin Immunol 81:1059, 1988.
Ortolani C et al: Chemicals and drugs as triggers of food-associated disorder. Ann Allergy 60:358, 1988.
Panaush RS: Delayed reactions to foods, food allergy and rheumatic disease. Ann Allergy 56:500, 1986a.
Panaush RS: Food induced (allergic) arthritis. I: Inflammatory arthritis exacerbated by milk. Arthritis Rheum 29:220, 1986b.
Pastorello EA et al: Role of the elimination diet in adults with food allergy. J Allergy Clin Immunol 84:475, 1989.
Sampson HA: Food allergy. J Allergy Clin Immunol 84(6, pt. 2):1062, 1989.
Sampson HA: Immunologically-mediated food allergy: The importance of food challenge procedures. Ann Allergy 60:262, 1988.
Sampson HA et al: Safety of casein hydrolysate formula in children with cow's milk allergy. J Pediatr 118:520, 1991.
Silverman SH and Lecks HI: Protein-calorie deficiency and vitamin indiscretion in an atopic child who developed hypervitaminosis A. Clin Pediatr 21:172, 1982.
Simon RA: Sulfite challenge for the diagnosis of sensitivity. Allergy Proc 10:357, 1989.
Sogn D: Medications and their use in the treatment of adverse reactions to foods. J Allergy Clin Immunol 78:238, 1986.
Stevenson DD et al: Adverse reactions to tartrazine. J Allergy Clin Immunol 78:182, 1986.
Sulfite ban deemed null and void. Tufts University Diet and Nutr Lett 8(8), October 1990.
Taubman B: Parental counseling compared with elimination of cow's milk or soy milk protein for the treatment of infant colic syndrome: A randomized trial. Pediatrics 81:756, 1988.
Taylor SL: Food allergies and sensitivities. J Am Diet Assoc 86:599, 1986.
Taylor SL et al: Food allergens: Structure and immunologic properties. Ann Allergy 59:93, 1987.
Taylor SL et al: Peanut oil is not allergenic for peanut-sensitive individuals. J Allergy Clin Immunol 68:372, 1981.
Taylor SL et al: Sensitivity to sulfited foods among sulfite-sensitive subjects with asthma. J Allergy Clin Immunol 81:1159, 1988.
Towns SJ and Mellis CM: Role of acetyl salicylic acid and sodium metabisulfite in chronic childhood asthma. Pediatrics 73:631, 1984.
Weber RW et al: Incidence of bronchoconstriction due to aspirin, azo dyes, non-azo dyes, and preservatives in a population of perennial asthmatics. J Allergy Clin Immunol 64:32, 1979.
Ziegler RS et al: Effect of combined maternal and infant food-allergen avoidance on development of atopy in early infancy: A randomized study. J Allergy Clin Immunol 84:72, 1989.

ADDITIONAL REFERENCES

Allergy Information Association: The Food Allergy Cookbook (Diets Unlimited for Limited Diets). New York, NY, St. Martin's Press, 1983.
Bock SA: Food sensitivity: A critical review and practical approach. Am J Dis Child 134:973, 1980.
Ener-G Foods, Inc, P.O. Box 24723, Seattle, WA 98124. This company sells specialty foods for wheat-, corn-, soy-, and egg-free diets. Mail order is available.
Food allergy: Peanut anaphylaxis. Allergy Proc 10:249, 1989.
Frasier CA: Coping with Food Allergy. New York, NY, The New York Times Book Co, 1985.
Metcalfe DD: Diseases of food hypersensitivity. N Engl J Med 321:255, 1989.
Poysa L et al: Atopy in children with and without a family history of atopy. 1: Clinical manifestations with special reference to diet in infancy. Acta Paediatr Scand 78:896, 1989.
Roth J: The Allergic Gourmet. Chicago, IL, Contemporary Books, 1983.
Taylor SL: Food allergies. Food Technol 39:99, 1985.
Van Bever HP et al: Food and food additives in severe atopic dermatitis. Allergy 44:588, 1989.
Van Hooser B and Crawford LV: Allergy diets for infants and children. Comp Therapy 15(10):38, 1989.
Williams ML: Cooking Without: Recipes for the Allergic Child (And His Family). Blue Bell, PA, Tri Cor Inc, 1981.
Yoder ER: Allergy-Free Cooking. Reading, PA, Addison-Wesley, 1987.

CHAPTER 39

NUTRITIONAL CARE IN DISEASES OF THE NERVOUS SYSTEM

Carol Asbeck, M.S., R.D., L.D., and Berri L. Burns, R.D., L.D., B.S.

CHAPTER OUTLINE

KEY TERMS

ALZHEIMER'S DISEASE—primary degenerative dementia of presenile onset characterized by diffuse atrophy throughout the cerebral cortex and neurofibrillary tangles

AMYOTROPHIC LATERAL SCLEROSIS (ALS) OR LOU GEHRIG DISEASE—a progressive disease involving the degeneration of motor nerves throughout the body; may be bulbar, involving facial muscles, or spinal, involving the muscles of the neck, trunk, and limbs

APRAXIA—difficulty with perceptual motor planning; inability to perform certain purposeful movements

ATAXIA—loss of motor coordination

DRY BERIBERI—a nonedematous disease caused by a deficiency of thiamin in which there is flaccid paralysis, muscular atrophy, absence of reflexes, cardiac enlargement, and tachycardia

DYSARTHRIA—inability to produce intelligible words with proper articulation

DYSPHAGIA—difficulty in swallowing

EPILEPSY—intermittent derangement of the nervous system due to sudden, excessive, disorderly electrical discharge of cerebral neurons that causes convulsions

ESOPHAGEAL PHASE OF SWALLOWING—the final involuntary phase of swallowing during which the bolus continues through the esophagus into the stomach

FASCICULATIONS—coarse, involuntary twitching of a muscle group that is visible through the skin

GUILLAIN-BARRÉ SYNDROME—acute febrile neuritis

HEMIANOPSIA—defective vision or blindness in half of the visual field of one or both eyes

HEMIPARESIS—muscular weakness or partial paralysis affecting one side of the body

MIGRAINE—periodic vascular headache of marked severity, whose onset is usually temporal and unilateral and is preceded by constriction of the cranial arteries

MULTIPLE SCLEROSIS—a disease of the nervous tissue characterized by the destruction of the myelin sheath and its replacement with scar tissue

MYASTHENIA GRAVIS—a disorder of neuromuscular function due to the presence of antibodies to acetylcholine receptors at the neuromuscular junction

NEGLECT—inattention to a weakened or paralyzed side of the body

NEUROGENIC BLADDER—any condition of dysfunction of the urinary bladder caused by a lesion of the central or peripheral nervous system

NEUROPATHY—functional disturbances or pathologic changes in the peripheral nervous system; noninflammatory lesions in the peripheral nervous system

ORAL PHASE OF SWALLOWING—the phase in which the food is placed in the mouth, chewed, and collected into a bolus by the tongue and pressed backward against the hard palate

PARESTHESIA—abnormal tactile sensation

PARKINSON'S DISEASE—a slowly progressive disease characterized by mask-like facies, a characteristic tremor of resting muscles, a slowing of voluntary movements, a peculiar gait and posture, and weakness of muscles

PHARYNGEAL PHASE OF SWALLOWING—the second phase of swallowing during which the soft palate and larynx elevate to protect the airways and the pharynx constricts, thus allowing food to pass into the esophagus

STROKE—the result of complete ischemia in which the brain is deprived of blood and oxygen, and permanent damage, either focal or global, occurs

TRANSIENT ISCHEMIC ATTACK (TIA)—a brief attack (lasting from a few minutes to hours) of cerebral dysfunction of vascular origin with no persistent neurologic deficit

VALSALVA MANEUVER—forcible exhalation effort against a closed glottis; the resultant increase in intrathoracic pressure interferes with venous return to the heart

Neurologic disorders are often devastating for both the patient and the family. Independent function, particularly with respect to procurement of food or independent preparation of meals, often becomes impossible. The fulfillment of basic needs depends on the involvement of family and friends, or professional support such as that provided by home health aides.

Appropriate clinical care requires identification of problems and development of an overall care plan by an interdisciplinary team. The team usually includes a neurologist or neurosurgeon and/or a physiatrist (a medical doctor specializing in physical medicine and rehabilitation). Specific expertise is also provided by nurses, occupational and physical therapists, speech pathologists, social workers, and dietitians or nutritionists. In addition to clinical care, the team is also involved in the preparation and education for discharge to a nursing home, rehabilitation center, or home environment.

NEUROLOGIC DISEASES: FEEDING CONCERNS

Not all patients with neurologic diseases have the same feeding impairments; the region of the central nervous system (CNS) that is damaged determines the resultant disability (Table 39–1). An occupational therapist can perform a feeding evaluation and contribute to nutritional care planning and provide the patient with any needed adaptive equipment.

Dysphagia

Dysphagia, or difficulty in swallowing, is a common problem in the neurologic population. Initiation of the swallow begins voluntarily but is completed reflexively. The normal swallowing reflex causes food or fluid to pass from the mouth through the pharynx and esophagus into the stomach. This occurs by gravity and by muscular action.

During the first or *oral phase* of swallowing, the food is placed in the mouth, chewed if necessary, and collected by the tongue into a bolus. The tongue pushes the food to the rear of the oral cavity by gradually squeezing it backward against the hard palate (Fig. 39–1).

Increased intercranial pressure or cranial nerve damage can result in weakened or incoordinated tongue movements, leading to problems in completing the oral phase of swallowing. The patient may have difficulty forming a bolus and moving it through the oral cavity. Food can become pocketed in the sulcus area between the cheek and the teeth, especially if sensation is lost in the cheek (Fig. 39–2). Weakened lip muscles result in the inability to completely seal the lips, form a seal around a cup, or suck through a straw. Patients are embarrassed by drooling and may not want to eat in front of others.

The swallowing reflex is triggered at the beginning of the second or *pharyngeal phase* of swallowing. Four events must occur in rapid succession during this phase. The soft palate elevates to close off the nasal airway and to prevent nasal regurgitation. The larynx elevates, and the vocal cords close to protect the airway. The pharynx constricts while the cricopharyngeal sphincter relaxes, allowing the food to pass into the

TABLE 39–1. Common Disorders of Neurologic Diseases*

Site of the Brain	Impairment	Results
Cortical lesions of the parietal lobe (perception of sensory stimuli)	Sensory deficits	Fine regulation of muscle activities impossible if the patient is unable to perceive joint position, and motion and tension of contracting muscles
Lesions of the nondominant hemisphere	Hemi-inattention syndrome (neglect)	Patient neglects that side of the body
Optic tract lesions (usually of the middle cerebral artery or the artery near the internal capsule)	Visual field cuts	Patient reads one half of a page, eats from only one half of the plate, and so forth
Subcortically stored pattern of motor skills has been lost	Apraxia	Inability to perform a previously learned task (e.g., walking, rising from a chair), but paralysis, sensory loss, spasticity, and incoordination are not present
No identification with a particular brain disorder or a specifically located lesion	Language apraxia	Inability to produce meaningful speech, even though oral muscle function is intact and language production has not been affected
Lesion of Broca's area	Nonfluent aphasia	Thought and language formulation are intact, but the patient is unable to connect them into fluent speech production
Lesion of Wernicke's area	Fluent aphasia	Flow of speech and articulation seem normal, but language output makes little or no sense
Extensive brain damage	Global aphasia	Both expression and speech perception are severely impaired
Brain stem lesions Bilateral hemispheric lesions Cerebellar disorders	Dysarthria	Inability to produce intelligible words with proper articulation

* From Steinberg FU: Rehabilitating the older stroke patient: What's possible? Geriatrics 41:85, 1986.

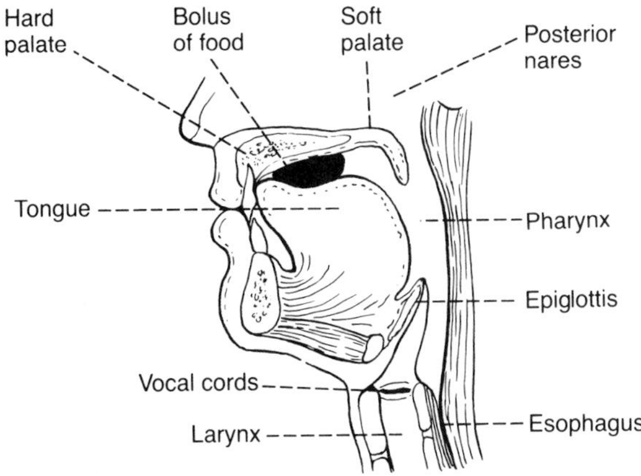

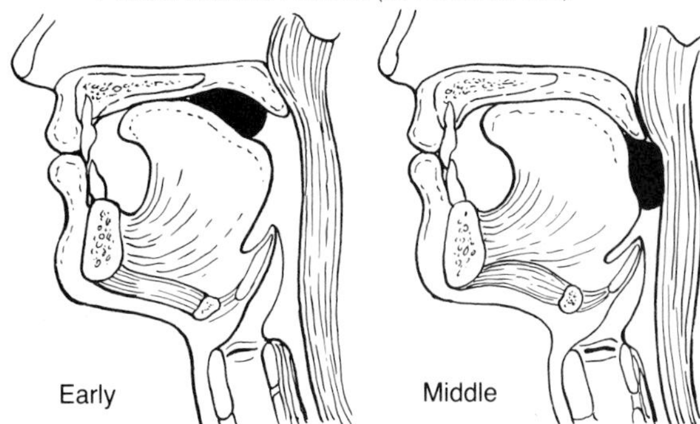

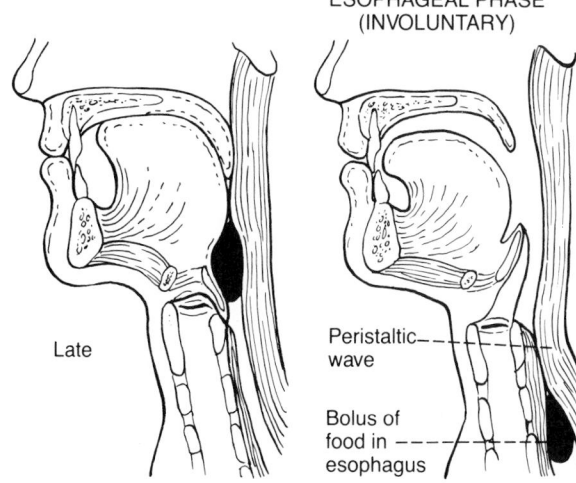

FIGURE 39–1. *Swallowing occurs in three phases: (1) Voluntary or oral phase. The tongue presses food against the hard palate, forcing it toward the pharynx. (2) Involuntary, pharyngeal phase. Early: wave of peristalsis forces a bolus between the tonsillar pillars. Middle: soft palate draws upward to close posterior nares and respirations cease momentarily. Late: vocal cords approximate and the larynx pulls upward, covering the airway and stretching the esophagus open. (3) Involuntary, esophageal phase. Relaxation of the upper esophageal (hypopharyngeal) sphincter allows the peristaltic wave to move the bolus down the esophagus. (From Luckmann J and Sorenson KC: Medical-Surgical Nursing, 3rd ed. Philadelphia, WB Saunders, 1987, p 1250.)*

esophagus. Breathing resumes at the end of the pharyngeal phase. Symptoms of incoordination during this phase include gagging, choking, and nasal regurgitation.

The final or *esophageal phase,* during which the bolus continues through the esophagus into the stomach, is completely involuntary. Any difficulties that occur during this phase are usually the result of a mechanical obstruction and are not due to neurologic disease.

Observation during meals allows the nurse or dietitian to screen informally for signs of dysphagia and bring them to the attention of the health care team. Symptoms include drooling, choking, coughing during or after meals, inability to suck from a straw, pocketing of food in the sulcus (of which the patient may not be aware), absent gag reflex, chronic upper respiratory infection, weight loss, or anorexia. Other signs are a gurgly voice quality or a moist cough after eating or drinking. A swallowing evaluation by a speech pathologist or occupational therapist is in order.

Dysphagia often leads to malnutrition because of inadequate intake. Modifications in diet should be individualized according to the type and extent of dysfunction. The dietitian can ensure that the diet remains as palatable and nutritionally adequate as possible (Table 39–2).

Nutritional Care

FLUIDS. Swallowing liquids of thin consistency requires the most coordination and control. They are easily aspirated into the lungs, which can be life threatening. If a patient has dysphagia with thin liquids, fluid requirements need to be met with solids and thick liquids. Liquids of all types can be thickened with nonfat

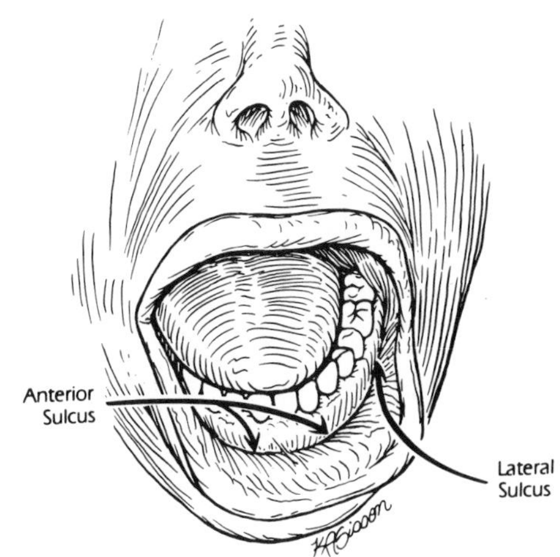

FIGURE 39–2. *If sensation is lost in the cheek, food can become lodged in the sulcus area between the cheek and the teeth. (From Logemann J: Evaluation and Treatment of Swallowing Disorders. San Diego, College-Hill Press, 1983, p 12.)*

TABLE 39–2. Guidelines for Feeding the Dysphagic Patient*

The following considerations are intended only as a starting point from which an individual's diet can be planned. Coordinated efforts between the dietitian and the swallowing therapist will determine the dietary prescription.

Neurologic Disorders

Condition	*Dietary Consideration*	*Rationale*
Slow/weak/uncoordinated swallow	Include highly seasoned, flavorful, aromatic foods. Add sugar, spices	Maximize stimulus for swallow
	Serve food at either very warm or at very cold temperatures	Maximize stimulus for swallow
	Include highly textured foods, such as diced cooked vegetables, diced canned fruit	Maximize stimulus for swallow
	Maintain semisolid consistencies that form a cohesive bolus. See examples	Need to avoid consistencies that will tend to fall apart in the pharynx
	Avoid sticky or bulky foods	Reduce risk of airway obstruction
	Caution with thin liquids (water, juices, milk, carbonated beverages) Try: Carbonated beverages (carbonation may stimulate reflex) Iced tart juices or crushed popsicles—banana and vanilla melt slowest (flavor and temperature may stimulate reflex) Medium or spoon-thick liquids may be substituted Thickening thin liquids with nonfat dry milk powder, fruit flakes, or commercial thickeners (Thick-It)	They are difficult to control, unpredictable, and may spill into pharynx prior to swallow reflex
	Small, frequent meals	Minimize fatigue; optimize food temperature and total nutrient intake
Weakened or poor oral-muscular control	Maintain semisolid consistencies that form a cohesive bolus	Requires less oral manipulation; purées are difficult to control
	Avoid slippery, sticky foods	
	Avoid thin liquids (see earlier description of thin liquids and recommendation)	See earlier rationale
	Small, frequent meals	Minimize fatigue, optimize total nutrient intake
Reduced oral sensation	Position food in most sensitive area	Maximize sensation
	Do not mix textures (e.g., vegetable soup)	Simplify swallow; minimize risk of aspirating thinner liquids
	Use colder temperatures	Maximize sensation; avoid potentially burning oral mucosa with liquids at too hot a temperature
	Use highly seasoned, flavorful foods	Maximize sensation
Crycopharyngeal dysfunction	Maintain liquid-puréed diet if no other contraindications are present	Liquids and purées pass into the esophagus more easily
Decreased laryngeal elevation	Limit diet to medium- and spoon-thick liquids, soft solids	Thin liquids easily penetrate the larynx
	Avoid sticky or bulky foods or food that will fall apart	Reduce the risk of airway obstruction
Decreased vocal cord closure	Avoid thin liquids	Easy, quick laryngeal penetration
	Avoid foods that will fall apart	Reduce risk of small pieces entering the larynx after the swallow

Mechanical Disorders

Condition	*Dietary Consideration*	*Rationale*
Stricture or partial obstruction of the pharynx or esophagus	Use semisolids or liquids	Solids may stick or lodge in the throat or esophagus
Partial glossectomy	Maintain semisolid consistencies that form a cohesive bolus	Reduce oral manipulation necessary
	Ensure very moist, well-lubricated foods. Add gravies, extra margarine, sauces	Aid oral manipulation
Base of tongue resection	Caution with thin liquids Maintain consistencies that form a cohesive bolus	Avoid quick, easy laryngeal penetration before the swallow. Reduce oral manipulation necessary
Total glossectomy	Very individual. May persistently aspirate all textures; may require nonoral feedings	
Floor of mouth resection	May require soft or semisolid textures	Difficulty chewing
	Maintain consistencies that form a cohesive bolus	Reduce oral manipulation necessary
Palate resection	Very individual. Mastication problems and nasal regurgitation dependent on the degree of resection and the adequacy of obturation	
Pharyngectomy	Use moist, well-lubricated foods	Aid bolus transport
	Caution with thin liquids	Avoid quick, easy laryngeal penetration
Supraglottic laryngectomy	Caution with thin liquids	Avoid quick, easy laryngeal penetration
	Maintain consistencies that form a cohesive bolus	Aid bolus transport
	Try superglottic swallow technique†	May reduce laryngeal penetration or clear material from larynx
Hemilaryngectomy; frontolateral laryngectomy	Generally can resume normal diet assuming that precautions are taken to protect airway	Airway protection usually intact if a vertical half of the larynx remains

Table continued on following page

TABLE 39–2. Guidelines for Feeding the Dysphagic Patient* *Continued*

Examples of Food Consistencies	
Solids	
Foods that form a cohesive bolus	**Foods that fall apart**
Egg dishes: soufflés, quiches	Dry, crumbly breads
Poached or scrambled eggs	Crackers
Egg, tuna, or meat salad	Thin, puréed foods: applesauce
Macaroni salad	Plain, chopped raw vegetables and fruits
Soft cheeses	Plain rice
Canned fruit	Cooked peas, corn
Macaroni or rice casseroles	Plain ground meats
Ground meats with gravy	Thin hot cereals
Moist, soft meat, or fish loaf	
Custard	**Sticky or bulky foods**
Cheesecake with sauce	Fresh white bread
Pudding	Peanut butter
Aspic	Plain mashed potatoes
Mousse	Bananas
Finger gelatin	Refried beans
Whipped gelatin	Bran cereals
Hot cereals	Chunks of plain meats
Vegetables in sauces	Raw vegetables or fruits
Liquids	
Thin liquids	
Apple juice	
Cranberry juice	
Orange juice	
Grape juice	
Broth	
Milk	
Chocolate milk	
Coffee	
Tea	
Water	
Soda	
Alcohol	
Ensure or Isocal	
Hot chocolate	
Medium-thick liquids	
Vegetable juice	
Blenderized or cream soups	
Ensure Plus or Sustacal HC	
Nectar	
Milkshakes, malts	
Eggnog	
Spoon-thick liquids	
Yogurt	
Puréed fruit	
Ice cream	
Sherbet	
Pudding	
Frozen shakes	
Popsicles	
Frozen juices	
Frozen sodas	

* Adapted from The American Dietetic Association: Manual of Clinical Dietetics. Chicago, The American Dietetic Association, 1988, p 195. Courtesy of Megan S. Veldee, M.S., RD, and Robert M. Miller, PhD. Seattle Veterans Administration Medical Center, Seattle, WA.

† Technique involving breath before swallow, consciously holding breath during swallow, forceful exhalation or gentle cough after swallow, and finally a reswallow to clear.

dry milk powder, cornstarch, fruit and vegetable flakes, and modular carbohydrate supplements. Commercial thickeners, such as Thick-It, designed for use with dysphagic individuals, are also available. Intermittent passage of an orogastric tube to administer water has been successful in some cases (Hillel and Miller, 1989).

When assessing fluid needs, the following equation is recommended (Segar, 1972):

$$(\text{Ideal body weight [kg]} - 20) \times 20 + 1{,}500 \text{ ml} = \text{fluid needs}$$

TEXTURES. In general, flavorful, very warm, or well-chilled foods with texture stimulate the swallow reflex better than bland, lukewarm foods. Sauces and gravies lubricate foods for ease in swallowing and can help to prevent fragmentation of foods in the oral cavity. Moist pastas, casseroles, and egg dishes are usually effective (Table 39–3). Patients should be warned not to wash food down with liquids.

Manipulation of textures as suggested by the swallowing therapist is necessary if the patient has difficulty with bolus formation. Small frequent feedings can help if fatigue or early satiety is a problem. Enteral feeding may be necessary if the risk of aspiration is high, or if the patient cannot eat enough to meet his or her needs. In the latter case, a tube feeding at night can bridge the gap between what the patient needs and what can be consumed orally. This allows the generation of a normal sensation of hunger and freedom from tube feeding during the day (Hynak-Hankinson et al, 1984; Logemann, 1983).

Other Self-Feeding Problems

The patient with neurologic disease may be unable to feed himself or herself due to limb weakness, poor body positioning, hemianopsia, neglect, apraxia, or confusion. The region of the CNS that is damaged determines the resultant disability (see Table 39–1).

If *limb weakness* or *paralysis* occurs on the dominant side of the body, incoordination results from a new reliance on the nondominant side. Eating with only one hand is difficult.

Hemiparesis causes the body to slump toward the affected side, increasing the risk of aspiration. The optimal position for feeding is to have both feet resting on the floor with the trunk nearly upright. If the patient must be in bed during mealtime, pillows can be used to bank and support the paretic side.

Hemianopsia is blindness (visual neglect) for one half of the field of vision (Fig. 39–3). The patient must learn to recognize that he or she no longer has a normal field of vision and to compensate by turning the head.

Neglect is inattention to a weakened or paralyzed side of the body. Neglect occurs only when the nondominant hemisphere (right) side of the brain is affected. The patient ignores the affected body part and his or her perception of the body's midline is shifted. Hemianopsia and neglect can occur together and impair the patient's function severely. For example, a patient may eat only half of the contents of a meal because he or she recognizes only half of it.

Another potential interference with self-feeding is *apraxia,* in which the patient has difficulty with perceptual motor planning. Even though the patient knows what needs to be done and has the physical ability to do it, he or she is unable to carry out an action and cannot follow directions. It may be possible to do the action after a demonstration, however, this may affect judgment and result in the performance of unsafe tasks, thus making it unsafe to leave the patient alone.

Confusion or *dementia* may prevent a patient from safely preparing meals or even remembering to eat regularly. Supervision, or even assistance with feeding, may be required.

TABLE 39–3. Diet for Easy Chewing and Swallowing

Type of Food	Foods Generally Included	Foods Commonly Excluded
Fluids	Thick juices,* sherbet,* sherbet shakes,* popsicles,* gelatin,* thin liquids thickened with Thick-It†	Water, thin juices, milk, coffee, tea
Bread and cereals	Bread, toast, cooked cereal, quick breads without nuts and raisins, pancakes, moist pastas, and casseroles	Crackers, dry rice, dry cereal flakes, crumbly bread, soft white bread
Dairy products	Butter, margarine, creamy or blenderized cottage cheese, soft cheeses, yogurt, thickened milk or dairy substitutes, and ice cream if tolerated	Dry cottage cheese, melted hot cheese
Eggs	Medium-cooked, poached, scrambled, soft omelet, custard	Runny eggs, thin eggnogs
Meat, fish, and poultry	Moist ground meat in casseroles, meatloaf, meatballs, ground meat with sauces and gravies, moist, tender fish without bones	Dry ground meats, chunky meats, dry fish, or fish with bones
Fruits	Soft canned fruits with seeds, pits, and skin removed; ripe bananas, chilled, thick puréed fruits, soft fruits in gelatin	Raw fruits except bananas, thin puréed fruits, stringy pineapple
Vegetables	Soft canned vegetables, baked, mashed, or boiled potatoes with margarine or gravy, whipped squash with margarine, scalloped potatoes, thick puréed vegetables, minced vegetables in gelatin	Raw vegetables, chunky vegetables such as diced beets, stringy vegetables such as spinach, corn, firm peas
Soups	Thick soups (blenderized)	Thin soups or chunky style soups
Desserts	Fruit whip, gelatin,* apple or peach crisp, moist cookies without nuts or raisins, custard, pudding, sherbet, ice cream if tolerated	Dry cakes and cookies, dessert with raisins, nuts, seeds, or coconut, hard candies and chocolate

* Safety with these foods may depend on oral retention times because they melt in the mouth and become thin liquids and difficult to manage.
† Thick-It is a modified cornstarch used to thicken both hot and cold liquids. Made by Milani and available nationwide.

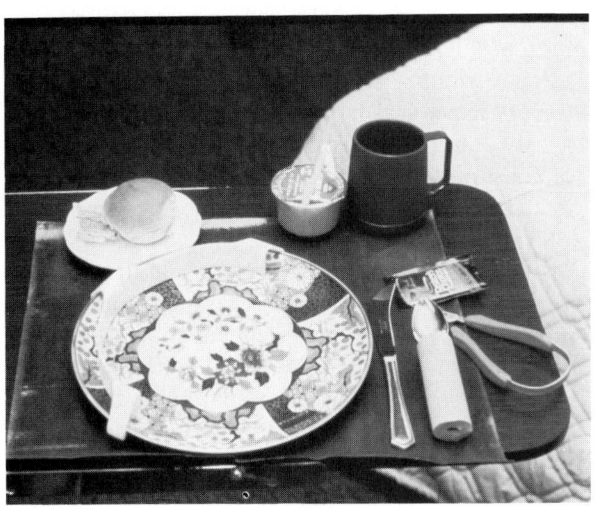
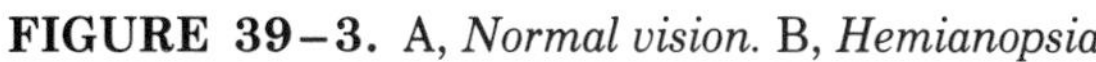
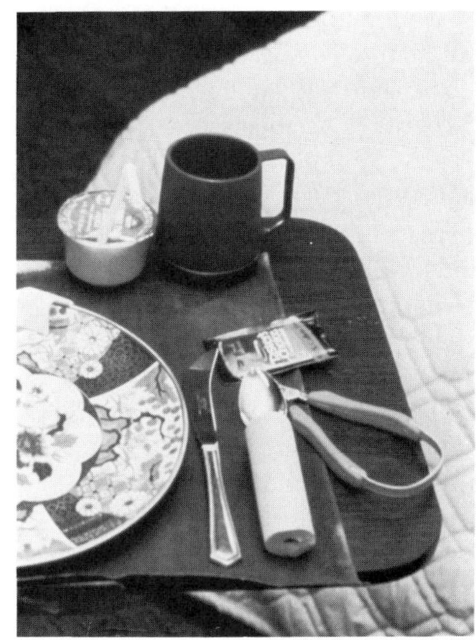

A B

FIGURE 39–3. A, *Normal vision.* B, *Hemianopsia.*

NEUROLOGIC DISEASES WITH NUTRITIONAL IMPLICATIONS

Stroke

Stroke is the result of complete ischemia, in which the brain is deprived of blood and oxygen and permanent damage occurs. It can be either *focal* (*regional*) or *global* (*generalized*). Ischemia is only partially complete in *transient ischemic attack* (*TIA*). Although blood flow is interrupted temporarily, no permanent damage occurs; however, the risk of further TIA or subsequent stroke is increased.

Strokes are the third leading cause of death in the United States, and approximately 1 million American citizens are disabled by stroke at any given time. Risk factors include hypertension, diabetes mellitus, hyperlipidemia, coronary artery disease, cardiac failure, left ventricular hypertrophy, smoking, obesity, elevated serum hematocrit, and bruits (Altman et al, 1987). The incidence of stroke has declined during the last 30 years, an improvement due in part to more effective diagnosis and treatment of hypertension.

Most strokes are caused by infarcts of the internal carotid artery and its branches. Seventy-five per cent are thromboembolic in origin, and 60% of these occur during sleep. Death occurs within 11 months of a stroke for 27% of all patients, and 80% of the survivors have a significant neurologic disability (Rivera, 1985; Wilkerson and Carter, 1984).

Medical therapy during the acute phase of stroke includes recognition and control of cerebral edema. Steroids and fluid restriction may be used. Physical rehabilitation using the team approach should begin immediately.

Nutritional Concerns

The nature and extent of feeding difficulties experienced by stroke victims is determined by the extent of the stroke and the area of the brain affected. Some or all of the factors discussed in Tables 39–1 and 39–2 apply to the assessment and care of these patients.

Warfarin is the most commonly prescribed oral anticoagulant. Because the effectiveness of the drug is reversed by vitamin K, intake of this vitamin must be kept at a constant level during warfarin therapy. If the amount of vitamin K consumed is suddenly altered, the patient may become overcoagulated or undercoagulated, either of which condition can be life-threatening. Common sources of vitamin K in addition to food (Table 6–12) include multivitamin tablets, oral supplements, and enteral feedings.

Multiple Sclerosis

Pathophysiology

Multiple sclerosis (MS) is a disease of nervous tissue caused by destruction of the myelin sheath, whose function is to speed electrical transmission of nerve impulses. MS is called "multiple" because it attacks many scattered areas of both the brain and spinal cord. The term "sclerosis" describes the replacement of myelin with sclera, or scar tissue. MS is characterized by remission and recurrence, known as a "come-and-go pattern." This characteristic makes an evaluation of treatments extremely difficult to do because it is difficult to know whether to attribute any change to treatment or to the natural course of the disease.

The precise cause of MS is unknown. One theory is that it is an immune-related disease of the CNS. The incidence of MS increases from the equator northward, suggesting an environmental factor. A familial tendency has been noted in a minority of cases. Onset occurs between the ages of 20 and 40 in two thirds of cases.

Treatment

Currently there is no proven treatment for changing the course of MS, preventing future attacks, or preventing deterioration. Once the functional level of a patient is lowered for a prolonged period, it is never regained (Fig. 39–4). The readiness of patients and families to embrace unconventional and unproven therapies is understandable; however, prudent clinicians as yet have not recognized anything that ultimately halts the inevitable downward progression of the disease (Scheinberg and Van der Noort, 1986).

Physical and occupational therapies are standard for weakness, spasticity, tremor, incoordination, and other symptoms. Steroid therapy is used in treatment of exacerbations; adrenocorticotrophic hormone (ACTH) and prednisolone are the drugs of choice. However, treatment is not consistently effective and tends to be more useful in cases of less than 5 years' duration. Side effects of short-term steroid treatment include increased appetite, weight gain, fluid retention, nervousness, and insomnia.

Nutritional Care

Many of the neurologic deficits unique to MS have nutritional implications, particularly with respect to self-feeding and personal care. Motor weakness, partial paralysis, and tremor are common and affect the patient's capacity for ambulation and self care (Fig. 39–5). Paresthesia and heightened sensitivity are common problems. Muscle tone can be either spastic, with steady and prolonged involuntary muscular contraction, or flaccid, with muscles that are limp and give little resistance to passive movement. *Ataxia*, a loss of motor coordination, is especially noticeable when patients attempt voluntary muscular movements.

Additional problems include visual impairment, dysarthria, dysphagia, and emotional lability. Visual impairments can include double vision and nystagmus, a constant involuntary movement of the eyeball that significantly interferes with vision. With *dysarthria*, speech can become difficult to understand due to cranial nerve damage affecting the tongue and other muscles of speech. *Dysphagia* can occur as the result of damaged cranial nerves, spasticity, ataxia, and muscle weakness. Alterations in emotional response can cause a patient to laugh or cry inappropriately and uncontrollably, often with subsequent embarrassment.

Neurogenic bladder is common, causing urinary incontinence, urgency, and frequency. To minimize these problems, it is helpful to distribute fluids evenly throughout the waking hours and limit them before bed. Some patients limit fluid intake severely to decrease frequency of urination. This increases the risk of urinary tract infection (UTI). UTI is common in patients with MS, and some patients increase their intake of cranberry juice as a form of self-treatment, although this is of questionable effectiveness.

Neurogenic bowel can cause either constipation or diarrhea. Incidence of fecal impaction is increased in MS. A diet that is high in fiber with adequate fluid can moderate both problems.

A major nutritional goal is maintenance of appropriate body weight (see Chapter 18). Weight gain is common in MS as a consequence of decreased activity levels and depression. Increased weight compromises

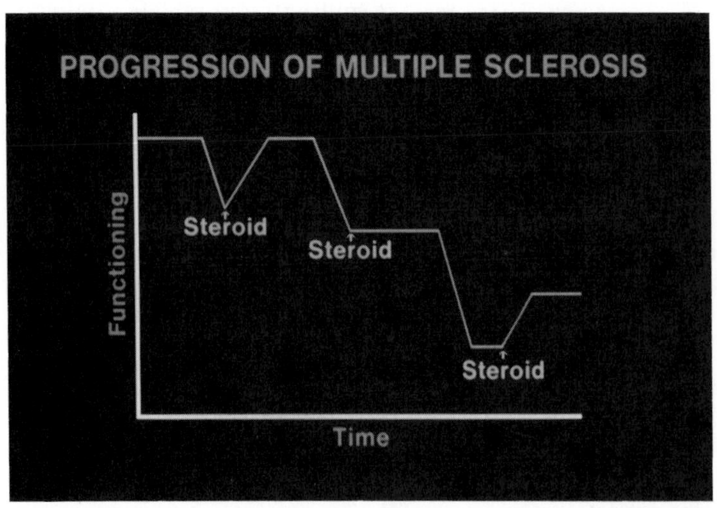

FIGURE 39–4. *The progression of multiple sclerosis.*

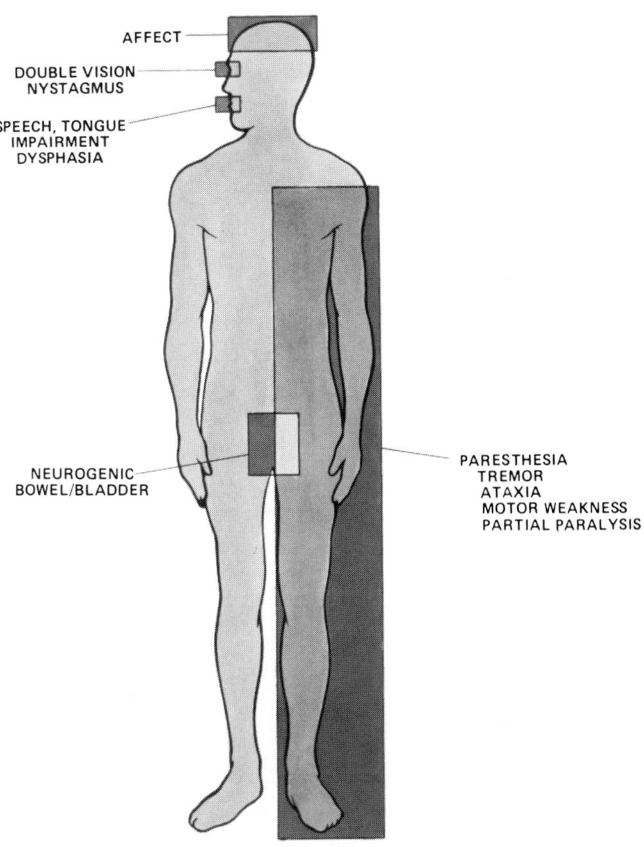

FIGURE 39–5. *The neurologic deficits in multiple sclerosis.*

ambulation even further. Another eating pattern that is typical of MS is marked by a decreased appetite and a loss of interest in food, or reliance on convenience or comfort foods. If ambulation or hand coordination is compromised, convenience foods often permit self-preparation of meals (Hewson et al, 1984).

Although many forms of diet therapy have been proposed, none have proved effective. The most popular theory is based on the report that the incidence of MS in European countries decreased during World War II when fat intake was very low. The proposed diet contains only 10 grams of saturated fat and 40 to 50 grams of polyunsaturated fat. However, a 35-year study with data supporting this theory has not been accepted because of a lack of controls (Swank, 1950, 1979, 1988).

A 3-year study that looked at the polyunsaturated fat intake, including the omega-3 fatty acids from fish, did show that those with a high polyunsaturated fatty acid (PUFA) intake remained neurologically stable, whereas those whose compliance was not as adequate experienced a decline in neurologic status (Fitzgerald et al, 1987). However, the factors of motivation and compliance could not be discounted as an element in the effectiveness of the diet.

Other dietary theories have involved gluten-free diets and high intakes of linoleic acid. However, no universal benefit from avoiding gluten has been found (Hewson, 1984), and no clear role for dietary lipid, either animal fat or linoleic acid, has been demonstrated (Bates et al, 1978; Millar et al, 1973; Paty et al, 1978; Wolfgram et al, 1975).

MS is a confusing, debilitating disease, and its sufferers often turn to unorthodox nutritional treatments in desperation. Professionals can help by providing patients and their families with consistent, sound, and nonjudgmental advice.

Amyotrophic Lateral Sclerosis

Mary Jo Adam, R.N., M.N.
Reviewed by Megan S. Veldee, M.S., R.D.

Description and Etiology

Amyotrophic lateral sclerosis (ALS) (Lou Gehrig disease) is a progressive disease involving the degeneration of motor nerves throughout the body. Peak onset occurs between 55 and 70 years of age. A familial component is apparent in 5 to 15% of cases. ALS is terminal; death occurs within 3 to 5 years of diagnosis in 50% of those afflicted (Caroscio, 1986).

The etiology of ALS is unknown. Possibilities include a latent virus, autoimmune disease, toxic metal contamination, and hormonal imbalance. Diagnosis is made from neurologic examination and electromyography (Young and Feldman, 1989).

Clinical Manifestations

Muscle weakness is the primary symptom of this disease. As the motor nerves deteriorate, almost all of the voluntary skeletal muscles are at risk for atrophy and complete loss of function. *Bulbar ALS* results from the deterioration of nerves in the motor cortex and brain stem. Because the neurons involved innervate facial muscles, the result is facial weakness. As jaw muscles weaken, chewing strength declines and mouth breathing increases. Fasciculations of the tongue are a classic symptom of bulbar involvement. Dysphagia and dysarthria result as muscles of lips, cheeks, palate, and tongue progressively weaken. Speech eventually becomes impossible, and communication becomes limited.

Spinal ALS symptoms result from deterioration of the spinal nerves. All of the voluntary muscles of the neck, trunk, and limbs may be involved. Weight loss, muscle atrophy, and loss of mobility are common.

A decline in respiratory muscle strength causes a progressive dyspnea and weak cough. The combination of an incompetent swallow and decreased ventilation frequently leads to death from respiratory failure and pneumonia (Rosen, 1986).

Eye movement and eye blink are spared, as are the sphincter muscles of the bowel and bladder. Incontinence is rare. Sensation remains intact and, except in rare cases, mental acuity is maintained. Although mechanical ventilation can extend the life of patients, the majority decline this option because the quality of life with advanced ALS is poor.

Assessment

Early assessment and intervention are critical for maintaining nutritional health in ALS. Dysphagia, psychologic upset, or a physical inability to prepare food or feed oneself can cause rapid weight loss. An unintentional weight loss of 10% or more is indicative of nutritional risk (Slowie et al, 1983).

In addition to the standard assessment data discussed in Chapter 17, the initial evaluation should include identification of any early swallowing problems. Establishing early baseline values in all areas of nutritional assessment is critical for monitoring the effectiveness of therapies in this progressive disease. There is no confirmed evidence at present to suggest increased nutrient requirements in ALS.

Atrophy of skeletal muscles follows a loss of motor innervation as ALS progresses. Reduced mobility accelerates muscle mass decline. It becomes the challenge of the nutrition professional to differentiate the unavoidable loss of muscle tissue from wasting due to malnutrition. An increased urinary excretion of creatinine, various amino acids, sulfur, phosphorus, potassium, magnesium, and zinc may occur as a result of muscular atrophy. A negative nitrogen balance can be expected and is proportional to the muscle loss (Slowie et al, 1983).

Early Nutritional Care

As bulbar symptoms progress, the tongue, cheeks, and palate become less able to control the transport of foods. Dry crumbly foods tend to break apart and cause choking. The jaw fatigues easily and the patient begins to avoid hard, dense foods, such as steak or raw vegetables. As dysphagia progresses, thin liquids become more problematic. The patient's swallowing abilities should be evaluated regularly by a speech pathologist or occupational therapist (see the discussion of dysphagia on page 672).

Instruction on proper posture for swallowing, usually sitting bolt upright with the head in a chin-down position, is helpful. Concentrating on the swallowing process can help to reduce choking. Environmental distractions and conversation during mealtime will increase risk for aspiration; however, families should be encouraged to maintain as normal mealtime behavior as possible.

Late Stage Nutritional Care

Fatigue related to dyspnea and general body weakness becomes a major obstacle to maintaining nutritional health in ALS. Meal times become excessively long, and intake is sacrificed. Changes in food consistencies to reduce the need for oral manipulation can help to conserve energy (see Table 39–3). Small, frequent meals may also increase intake (Asbeck and Burns, 1988). When the joy of eating is gone, rapid weight loss and failure to thrive soon follow.

Thin liquids frequently become difficult to swallow. Thick liquids and soft foods containing a high percentage of water need to be emphasized to maintain fluid balance. In some cases patients can be taught to intermittently pass orogastric tubes for the administration of fluids (Hillel and Miller, 1989). Gastrostomy placement may be necessary to ensure adequate hydration if other means fail.

As dysphagia progresses, the limitation of food consistencies may result in the exclusion of entire food groups. Vitamin and mineral supplementation may be necessary. If chewable supplements are not handled safely, liquid forms may be added to acceptable foods.

Enteral Feeding

Tube feeding is the most effective solution to dysphagia in ALS. Parenteral nutrition is not recommended because the patient with ALS usually has a functioning gastrointestinal tract. Placement of a feeding tube should be done before the patient becomes malnourished or exhibits weak ventilation. It may be placed to maintain adequate hydration if fluids have become difficult to take. Preventing weight loss and its associated ill effects is easier than attempting to recoup losses. A nasogastric tube can be a short-term option; however, for long-term management, a percutaneous endoscopic gastrostomy (PEG) placed under local anesthesia is the treatment of choice (see Chapter 30). Procedures requiring general anesthesia are avoided in advanced ALS due to a high incidence of perioperatic mortality (Hillel and Miller, 1989).

Many patients decline early placement of a feeding tube for fear of the emotional and physical impact of this choice. The health care team has an important role in alleviating patient concerns and in fostering informed decisions. Discussing both the advantages and disadvantages of nutritional support with the patient and family should be initiated well ahead of need. It is not unusual for the severely dysphagic and malnourished patient with ALS to refuse tube feedings, choosing not to continue life by this means.

Other Nutritional Concerns

ORAL SECRETIONS. For many, managing oral secretions is the most chronic and miserable trial during their struggle with ALS. Although the production of saliva does not increase, it tends to pool in the front of the mouth as the frequency of the automatic swallow decreases. Drooling occurs due to poor lip control and can cause fluid and electrolyte imbalances. Social dining is avoided. Removing secretions with a portable aspirator is effective, but fluids are lost in the process and must be replaced. Medical management by low doses of amitriptyline (Elavil), 25 mg/day, may be effective in drying secretions (Hillel and Miller, 1989). Giving the medication at bedtime avoids the tendency to choke on secretions during sleep.

Mouth breathing or dehydration causes phlegm to thicken and become a problem. Cleansing the oral cavity of dried secretions can be difficult. Mucous plugs may block the airway. A weak cough characteristic of ALS is not effective in dislodging thick phlegm. Management of these secretions may include swabbing the palate with dilute lemon juice. Papain, an enzyme found in meat tenderizer, helps to dissolve phlegm, and can also be applied by a cotton swab. Medications such as SSKI and Robitussin thin out secretions and may be helpful to some people (Hillel and Miller, 1989). Patients frequently avoid dairy products, believing that they increase phlegm. Supplementation with calcium, riboflavin, and vitamins A and D should be considered if adequate dietary sources are not present. A multiple vitamin/mineral supplement is usually used.

CONSTIPATION. Constipation in ALS can be both acute and chronic in nature. Poor dietary fiber intake and dehydration frequently contribute to constipation. Other factors include progressive immobility and loss of Valsalva maneuver as skeletal and abdominal muscles weaken. Inclusion of adequate dietary fiber and fluids will help avoid constipation. Under normal circumstances, 1,500 to 2,500 ml of fluids should be consumed daily. Additional fluids may be needed to compensate for salivary losses. Caffeine-containing beverages should be avoided because of their diuretic effects. Records of daily fluid intake, weight, and urine osmolality are helpful in monitoring hydration status.

Fiber intake can be increased by adding blended raw fruits to shakes or other frozen drinks. Whole-grain pastas, cereals, and legumes are also effective. If needed, additional fiber can also be incorporated by adding 1 to 2 tablespoons of bran each day to usual foods. The use of prunes or prune juice, which contain a natural laxative (dihydroxyphenylisatin), may be helpful. Use of fiber-containing commercial formulas for those on tube feeding may be indicated. While the swallow is intact, natural bulk laxatives and stool softeners may be used daily. Ducolax suppositories are commonly given if a bowel movement is delayed by a few days. Warm tap water enemas are preferred over chemical products, and disimpaction is administered by a health professional if necessary.

Alzheimer's Disease

Etiology

Some shrinkage in both the size and weight of the brain inevitably occurs with aging, but this shrinkage has little clinical significance. However, one fifth of the population over the age of 80 has moderate to severe dementia (Staehelin, 1986).

Alzheimer's disease (AD), or *primary degenerative dementia of senile onset,* is the most common form of dementia in the elderly, characterizing 20% of all patients in psychiatric hospitals. It can occur in adults at any age, but onset is typically in the late fifties or sixties. It is characterized by neuron loss and neurofibrillary tangles. These changes are seen in the hypothalamus and the cerebral cortex, the areas of the brain essential for memory and cognition. Typical deficits include dysnomia (forgetting names), poor retentive memory, spatial disorientation, paranoia and other personality changes, and gait disorder.

Animal studies have shown that diets deficient in pyridoxine, folacin, or magnesium have resulted in changes in brain tissue. However, diets deficient in these nutrients have not produced the characteristic senile plaques or neurofibrillary tangles of AD (Root and Longenecker, 1988). Brain tissue of patients with

AD has been shown to have unusually high levels of aluminum, but a causal relationship has not been clearly established. In addition, increased levels of aluminum have been found in the brains of normal elderly controls (Shore and Wyatt, 1983).

Nutritional Concerns

Weight loss is frequently mentioned as a feature common to AD. Possible causes include a higher rate of infection, increased energy output associated with constant pacing, and inadequate food intake (Sandman et al, 1987).

Infection not only increases energy needs but may also lead to a concomitant decrease in food intake. Constant pacing has been shown to require an additional 1,600 kcal/day on average when compared with sedentary patients with AD (Rheaume et al, 1988). Inadequate food intake may result from a variety of factors. Patients may refuse or forget to eat, or have difficulty eating. They may not be able to communicate their need for food. Temperament may change abruptly; patients may suddenly hide or throw their food. Other kinds of inappropriate behavior include eating spoiled food or nonfood substances, and eating favorite foods to the exclusion of almost everything else. As the dementia progresses, patients are unable to provide their own meals and may need to be fed. Patients with AD may have dysphagia and may require more time to eat.

Parkinson's Disease

Parkinson's disease (PD) affects about 1% of the population in the United States over 50 years of age (Adams and Victor, 1985). It manifests between the ages of 40 and 70 years, usually during the sixth decade. PD is characterized by involuntary tremulous action. Signs and symptoms include an expressionless face which conveys the impression that patients are cold and emotionless. Incidence of depression is increased. Other characteristics are slowness and decrease of voluntary movement, resting tremor, stooped posture and characteristic gait, along with slowness and decrease of voluntary movement. The voice is soft, and speech is hurried and monotonous. The disease is progressive and eventually disabling, usually within 5 to 10 years. PD is not fatal, however.

Etiology and Treatment

PD is characterized by neuronal degeneration from unknown causes. The resultant symptoms reflect the gradual depletion of dopamine, a neurotransmitter (Further Reading, page 685). No therapy exists to halt or slow the degeneration. However, the medication levodopa provides symptomatic relief. Symptoms of PD can occur as a side effect of some drugs.

PHARMACOLOGY. Treatment with levodopa, even for patients in very advanced stages, is more effective than any other drug. However, a common response to this drug is the "on-off" phenomenon, in which patients may go from a state of relatively good mobility to being nearly immobile in a matter of minutes or hours. This occurs frequently and unpredictably in 50 to 80% of long-term levodopa users (Riley and Lang, 1988). The development of fluctuations and the lack of response to levodopa that develops over time are the two major problems in long-term treatment of this disease.

Nutritional Considerations

As the disease progresses, rigidity of the extremities can interfere with the patient's ability to care for himself or herself, including self-feeding. Rigidity also interferes with the ability to control the position of the head and trunk, necessary for eating. Eating is slowed; it can take up to 1 hour to ingest a meal. Simultaneous movements such as those required to handle both a knife and fork become difficult. Tremor in the arms and hands may make self-feeding of liquids impossible without spilling. Perception, including spatial organization, can become impaired (Norberg and Winblad, 1987). Dysphagia is a late complication.

Side effects of medications for PD include anorexia, nausea, reduced sensitivity to smell, constipation, dry mouth, and psychiatric symptoms. If levodopa is taken with meals, the gastrointestinal side effects are diminished. Pyridoxine supplementation, even as low as 5 mg/day, reduces the effectiveness of levodopa; however, the combination of the drugs levodopa and carbidopa, the more common form of the drug, is not affected by pyridoxine intake (Roe, 1985).

MODIFIED PROTEIN DIET. Because levodopa appears to compete with large neutral amino acids (LNAA) for carriers at a level of gastrointestinal absorption and also at the site where the drug must cross the blood-brain barrier, controversy exists as to the optimal amount and distribution of dietary protein (Riley and Lang, 1988). Current therapy, which is largely experimental, is based on the results of a long-term study that claimed to achieve benefits by redistributing the protein intake so that the RDA would be met primarily in the evening meal. By restricting daytime protein to only 7 grams, daytime mobility was improved at the cost of increased rigidity overnight (Pincus and Barry, 1988; Riley and Lang, 1988). Table 39–4 presents a sample menu from this diet. Any benefit from this diet should be apparent within 1 week.

TABLE 39–4. Protein Redistribution in L-Dopa Therapy

Breakfast	Amount of Protein (g)
½ cup oatmeal	2
1 orange	0.5
1 cup Polyrich (nondairy creamer)	0.5
Egg Replacer (unlimited)	0
Low protein bread, toasted	0
Margarine or butter (unlimited)	0
Jelly or jam (unlimited)	0
Sugar or sugar substitute (unlimited)	0
Coffee or tea (unlimited)	0
Lunch	
½ cup vegetable soup	2
1 cup tossed salad	1
Salad dressing (unlimited)	0
1 banana	1
Low protein pasta (unlimited)	0
Margarine or butter (unlimited)	0
Low protein cookies (unlimited)	0
Soda pop, coffee, tea, or water	0
Afternoon Snack	
Gum drops or hard candy (unlimited)	0
Apple or cranberry juice (unlimited)	0
TOTAL	7
Dinner	
4 oz of beef, pork, veal, chicken (at least)	28 or more
1 cup stuffing	4
Gravy	0
½ cup peas	2
1 cup pudding	8
1 cup milk	8
Evening Snack	
1 oz cheese	7
4 crackers	2
Soda pop	0
DAILY TOTAL	66 or more

Epilepsy

Epilepsy is second only to stroke as the major neurologic disorder; more than 1 million Americans have recurrent seizures. *Epilepsy* is defined as an intermittent derangement of the nervous system due to sudden, excessive, disorderly electrical discharge of cerebral neurons. This electrical discharge causes convulsive movements, disturbance of sensation, loss of consciousness, or a combination of these.

Nutrient-Drug Interactions

Medications used for anticonvulsant therapy have several nutritional effects. Phenobarbital, phenytoin, and primidone interfere with intestinal absorption of calcium by increasing metabolism of vitamin D in the liver. Long-term therapy with these drugs over years may lead to osteomalacia in adults or to rickets in children. Recommended therapy is 10 to 40 μg/day of vitamin D for children and 5 μg/day for adults (Roe, 1984) (see Chapter 25).

Phenytoin metabolism requires folic acid and is accelerated by supplementation with the vitamin, possibly resulting in subtherapeutic levels of the drug. For this reason, sporadic folic acid supplementation should be avoided. Phenobarbital, however, is not affected by folate. Phenytoin and phenobarbital are bound primarily to albumin in the blood stream. Decrease of serum albumin levels (e.g., in malnutrition or reduced albumin synthesis secondary to advanced cirrhosis) limits the amount of drug that can be bound, resulting in an increase in free drug concentration and the possibility of overmedication on a standard dosage.

Continuous enteral feeding inhibits the absorption of phenytoin, necessitating a large increase in the dose to achieve a therapeutic level. Holding the tube feeding for 1 hour before and after administration of medication allows increased absorption of the phenytoin so that the dosage may not need to be increased. Toxicity can result if the enteral feeding is abruptly stopped, which might occur if a patient pulled out his or her own feeding tube. If the enteral feeding is to be reduced, it should be tapered concomitantly with the dose of phenytoin (Krueger et al, 1987).

Alcohol consumption results in the loss of the intended effect of phenytoin, possibly causing seizures. Absorption of phenobarbital is delayed by consumption of food; therefore, administration of the drug must be planned around mealtimes.

Ketogenic Diet

The ketogenic diet is used for the treatment of akinetic, myoclonic, petit mal, or psychomotor (temporal lobe) seizures in children as a last resort when they cannot be controlled by the use of medication alone. The diet is designed to create and maintain a state of ketosis; however, the mechanism of action of the diet is not clearly understood. Benefits of the diet generally last less than 2 to 3 years and are less apparent in older children.

Eighty to 90 per cent of the total energy intake in the ketogenic diet is derived from fat. The energy ratio of fat to carbohydrate plus protein should be 3 : 1 to 4 : 1. If medium-chain triglyceride (MCT) oil is used, the percentage of energy from fat can be reduced. This is because MCT oil is absorbed more rapidly than other fats, is transported directly to the liver, and thus induces ketosis more rapidly. Corn oil, which is much less expensive and more available, has been sucessfully substituted for MCT oil (Woody et al, 1988). Satisfactory weight gain for children on the diet has required 150% of the estimated energy requirements, compared with normal children of the same age and size.

Meeting the RDA for protein for the child (1 to 1.2 g/kg body weight, depending on age) leaves little room in the diet for carbohydrate (Table 39–5). Even medications must be evaluated for carbohydrate content. In addition, the carbohydrate, protein, and fat, including the MCT oil, must be divided evenly into three meals

TABLE 39–5. Typical Ketogenic Diet Menu

Food Item	Amount (g)	Carbohydrate (g)	Protein (g)	Fat (g)	Energy (kcal)
Breakfast					
White bread	5	2.8	0.4	0.2	13
Egg, scrambled	48		6.1	5.5	74
Cream, heavy whipping	10	0.3	0.3	3.8	36
Margarine	5			5	45
MCT oil	12			12	108
Fat	11			11	99
Koolaid, with non-nutritive sweetener	240				
Total		2.8	6.8	37.5	375
Lunch					
American cheese	12	2.2	2.8	3.6	52
Ham	23	0.7	3.7	3.9	53
MCT oil mayonnaise	11			11	99
Fat	19			19	171
Koolaid, with non-nutritive sweetener	240				
Total		2.9	6.5	37.5	375
Dinner					
Turkey	19		6.3	0.7	32
Tomato	10	0.5	0.1	0.0	3
Green beans	10	0.6	0.2	0.0	3
Potatoes	12	1.7	0.2	0.0	8
Margarine	15			15	135
MCT oil mayonnaise	11			11	99
Fat	10			10	90
Koolaid, with non-nutritive sweetener	240				
Total		2.8	6.8	36.7	370
Daily Total:		8.5	20.1	111.7	1120

and planned snacks. Vitamin and mineral supplementation is required.

The diet is extremely unpalatable and, because of its complex nature, is difficult to follow. If the child is ambulatory and can obtain his or her own food, compliance is usually lower. Side effects include nausea, vomiting, diarrhea, weight loss, irritability, and possibly abnormal neutrophil function leading to increased vulnerability to infection (Woody et al, 1989). Some children may simply refuse to eat the diet. For long-term compliance, parents often require substantial psychosocial support.

If no further attacks are noticed after the child has been on the diet for 3 months, carbohydrate intake can be increased gradually in steps of 5 grams as long as a state of ketosis is maintained as monitored by urinalysis. The fat is reduced to maintain an appropriate energy intake.

Polyneuropathy

Nutritional Neuropathies

Nutritional neuropathy affects the peripheral nervous system. Symptoms include progressive weakness and muscle wasting of legs (rather than arms) and distal (rather than proximal) muscles. Early signs are anorexia, constipation, abdominal discomfort, irritability, memory loss, and disturbance of sleep. Long-term consequences include paralysis, numbness, tingling, severe pain, coldness, hotness, and sensitive feet.

Two well-known forms of nutritional neuropathy are *dry beriberi* and *alcoholic neuropathy.* Although a common nutritional factor is deficient in both disorders, the exact B vitamin involved is unclear. Possibilities are pantothenic acid, thiamin, pyridoxine, niacin, and riboflavin. Standard therapy is a balanced diet with supplementation of the B-complex vitamins. In addition, 50 to 100 mg of thiamin may be added daily for alcoholic neuropathy. Treatment should cease when therapeutic response is achieved.

Prognosis for beriberi is good, but in advanced cases paralysis may be permanent. Alcoholic neuropathy is very difficult to treat; recovery is slow and may take up to 6 months. Recovery from alcoholic neuropathy requires abstinence from all alcohol (D'Orazio and D'Orazio, 1985; Shields, 1985).

Guillain-Barré Syndrome

Guillain-Barré syndrome is a rare type of polyneuropathy. The disease has been described by various terms, including Landry's paralysis, Landry-Guillain-Barré syndrome, acute infectious polyneuritis, and acute idiopathic polyneuritis. The etiology is unknown, but most research indicates that the symptoms result from a cell-mediated immunologic reaction directed at pe-

FURTHER READING: Neurotransmitters and Their Precursors

Neurotransmitters are substances that transmit signals across neuronal synapses. Four of the neurotransmitters—serotonin, dopamine, norepinephrine, and acetylcholine—are synthesized from amino acid precursors and appear to be influenced to some degree by diet (see table below).

The role of dietary manipulation is not clear because of interactions of neurotransmitters with hormones and with the precursors themselves. For example, although a high-protein meal increases plasma levels of tryptophan, the precursor of serotonin, it also increases levels of other amino acids that compete with tryptophan for absorption at the blood-brain interface. The net effect is lower levels of serotonin in the brain. Conversely, a high-carbohydrate meal stimulates production of insulin, which leads to a reduction of the competing amino acids and an increase in brain serotonin levels. Attempts to manipulate neurotransmitter levels with pharmaceutical doses of amino acids are complicated by the fact that large amounts of precursors may be toxic (Centers for Disease Control, 1990).

Neurotransmitter	Metabolic Precursor
Acetylcholine	Choline or lecithin (which contains choline)
Serotonin	Tryptophan
Catecholamines	Tyrosine and possibly phenylalanine
Dopamine	
Norepinephrine	
Epinephrine	

ripheral nerves. The major manifestation is rapidly progressive weakness.

Onset is usually preceded by a gastrointestinal or respiratory infection, surgery, or immunization, with symptoms and signs of multiple nerve involvement developing 1 to 3 weeks later. Characteristics are symmetric pain and weakness beginning in the legs. The weakness ascends to the trunk, intercostal and neck muscles, and finally to the cranial muscles. Total motor paralysis can occur within a few days. Tracheostomy and mechanical ventilation are required in severe cases. Death due to respiratory failure is no longer common, and 95% of survivors recover completely. Speed of recovery varies from a few weeks to months, but if nerves have degenerated, regeneration may require 6 to 18 months.

TREATMENT. During the acute phase, respiratory support is the primary concern. Plasma exchange should be used in early and severe cases. Physical therapy, occupational therapy, and intensive psychologic support are required for most cases. Patients who develop difficulty in chewing or dysphagia should be evaluated by a swallowing therapist who will recommend a diet of the appropriate texture or the initiation of enteral feeding. The role of the nutritionist is to ensure adequate intake of fluid, energy, protein, and other nutrients.

Ventilator-dependent patients are enterally fed. Parenteral nutrition is not indicated, as the gastrointestinal system is usually not affected by Guillain-Barré syndrome. At the time of weaning from the ventilator, the correct fat-to-carbohydrate ratio will maintain a favorable respiratory quotient, as discussed in Chapter 34. It is the responsibility of the nutritionist to recommend the appropriate enteral prescription with the addition of fat as needed.

Migraine Headache

The severe, throbbing pain of *migraine headache* is typically localized on one side of the head. The headache is periodic and lasts for a few hours to a few days. The intense pain is disabling and may require the sufferer to remain in a darkened room or in bed. Migraine attacks are often accompanied by anorexia, nausea, and vomiting. Onset of the disorder, which is familial, can be in childhood, adolescence, or adulthood, and frequency diminishes with advancing age (Adams and Victor, 1985).

A migraine attack may be triggered by psychologic, pharmacologic, environmental, or dietary factors. Documenting the link between the migraine and diet has been difficult, and the controversy continues. Among the proposed modes of action is the theory that migraine may be triggered through an allergic reaction. Elimination diets have shown improvement in both large and small studies; however, this type of study does not prove that an allergic reaction has occurred. More recent studies using RAST (see Chapter 38) have demonstrated a food allergy in some patients; however, more research is needed before definite conclusions can be drawn (Egger et al, 1989; Perkin and Hartje, 1983; Pryse-Phillips, 1987).

A second mode of action is through a chemical reaction affecting the vascular system. Chocolate and aged cheese have been shown to trigger migraine in susceptible persons, and both the tyramine and phenylethylamine have been implicated (Diamond et al, 1987) (see Chapter 25 and Clinical Insight, page 436).

Other substances that appear to have some link with migraine include alcohol, nitrites, and monosodium glutamate. Aspartame has been determined to trigger migraine in some individuals (Koehler and Glaros, 1988; Lipton et al, 1989).

One difficulty with making general recommendations about food avoidance is that the tolerance threshold varies among individuals, and the foods that have been implicated in some do not trigger attacks in most migraine sufferers. Another difficulty is that restricting intake of offending foods results in a limited food intake. Patients restricting intake of certain foods should be followed regularly by a dietitian to ensure adequate food intake and nutritional status.

Myasthenia Gravis

Myasthenia gravis (MG) is muscular weakness which, as the name implies, once carried a grave prognosis. MG is characterized by abnormal fatigue in the skeletal muscles. Muscles of the eyes, face, pharynx, larynx, and respiratory system are most commonly affected. The weakness is the result of an autoimmune defect at the neuromuscular junction that allows antibodies to destroy the receptor sites for acetylcholine at a rate faster than they can be replenished. Without adequate receptor sites, nerve impulses to the muscle are reduced, resulting in extreme fatigue. The muscle weakness is greater after periods of activity and improves after rest. A severe episode of muscular weakness, called a myasthenic crisis, may require hospitalization.

Treatment

Although there is no cure for the disease, medications, thymectomy, and plasmapheresis can maximize muscle function. Anticholinesterase drugs are most commonly given, sometimes in conjunction with immunosuppressive drugs such as steroids. Medications should be given 30 minutes to 1 hour before meals to maximize intake.

A standard treatment removes the thymus, which is a center of antibody production. Plasmapheresis removes antibodies from the blood stream.

Meals should be small, frequent, and nutritionally dense and should be made up of soft-textured foods. A half-hour rest period will defer mealtime fatigue. The first meal of the day is the most critical, because muscle strength is greatest after overnight rest. Therefore, breakfast should be the most nutritionally dense meal. Symptoms of dysphagia, difficulty in chewing, drooling, choking, and aspiration require a swallowing evaluation.

Brain Tumor

Pathophysiology of Central Nervous System Tumors

The overwhelming majority of CNS tumors occur in the brain. Most are primary brain tumors, meaning they originate in the brain as opposed to metastasizing from outside the CNS. However, 20% of patients diagnosed with cancer eventually have brain neoplasm involvement.

Tumor location and elevation of intracranial pressure (ICP) are responsible for the changes that occur in the clinical picture. Symptoms include headache, vomiting, seizures, and personality changes. Additionally, there may be changes in mental functioning, including decreased ability to perform routine tasks. Progression of the disease may lead to decreased motor function and weakness, lethargy, and cranial nerve dysfunction, including dysphagia, visual problems, decreased memory, dementia, and ataxia.

The location of the tumor determines the types of symptoms that develop (Fig. 39–6). Cerebral hemisphere tumors produce a hemiparesis in the side of the body opposite from the tumor. Focal motor seizures are commonly a result of tumors located in the motor strip. Changes in behavior are typical of temporal lobe lesions. In general, the more posterior the lesion, the milder will be the deficit. Bifrontal, subfrontal, and corpus callosum tumors often cause both dementia and behavior changes. Ataxia is typical of tumors in the posterior fossa, including the brain stem and cerebellum. Dysphagia with paralysis of the vocal cords and palate is common in medullary tumors. Symptoms of hearing loss, facial weakness, and sensory changes are typical for a neoplasm located in the pons.

ICP increases because the cranial cavity has a finite space and thus a restricted volume. Therefore, a histologically benign tumor is not medically benign. Tumor growth displaces blood and cerebrospinal fluid (CSF), causing increased pressure. Cerebral edema surrounds the tumor, causing further displacement. ICP increases directly with the rate of tumor growth, edema within the tumor, and hydrocephalus. As ICP increases, so do the frequency and severity of symptoms.

Treatment of Central Nervous System Tumors

Therapy for brain tumors includes surgery, steroids, radiation, and chemotherapy. Tissue diagnosis and debulking the tumor require surgery.

Steroids control edema both preoperatively and postoperatively. Protein needs are increased during steroid therapy due to catabolic side effects. Steroids often increase the appetite, and the patient may gain weight. This is a problem especially if the patient is

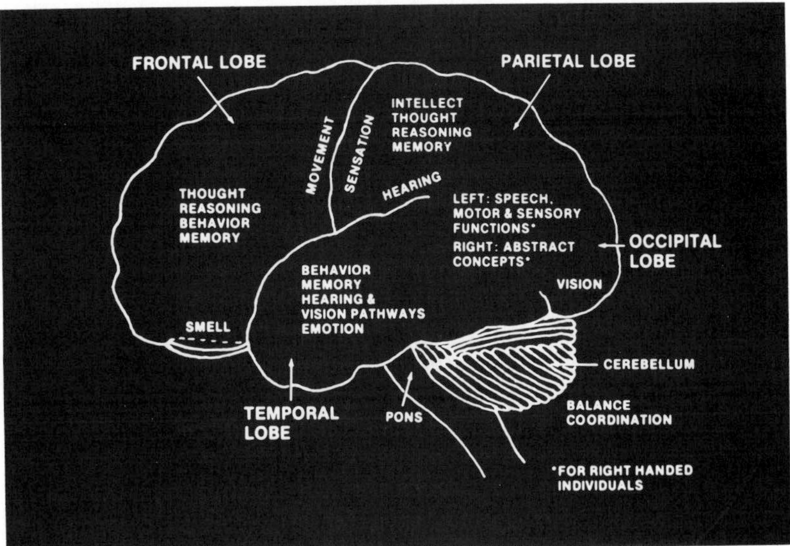

FIGURE 39–6. *Areas of the brain and neurologic function.*

hemiparetic or lethargic and is not ambulating normally.

A typical course of radiation to shrink the tumor lasts 6 weeks. Side effects often appearing 3 weeks into the treatment include nausea, anorexia, and early satiety. If other forms of therapy are ineffective, chemotherapy may be considered as an alternative. Chapter 36 discusses the nutritional implications of radiation and chemotherapy.

Closed Head Injury

Closed head injury (CHI) occurs as the result of a sudden impact to the head, with or without loss of consciousness. It can occur as the result of motor vehicle or industrial accidents, explosions, fights, falls, sports accidents, and gunshot wounds. CHI is often accompanied by multiple fractures or internal injuries.

Signs and symptoms mirror those of brain injury, including nausea, seizures, weakness or paralysis, vertigo, dyspnea, altered blood pressure, and aphasia.

Nutritional Implications

The nutritional implications of CHI are second only to those of a major burn. Both energy and protein requirements skyrocket. Resting energy expenditure (REE) increases by 140% and remains at this level for at least 1 1/2 weeks after the injury. Nitrogen metabolism increases; 22% of energy needs are consumed as protein, compared with a normal rate of 10%. This translates to an energy requirement of 50 kcal/kg body weight/day and a kcal : nitrogen ratio of less than 150 : 1, or 1.5 to 2.5 grams of protein per kilogram of body weight per day (Clifton et al, 1984).

Withholding significant energy and protein intake during the first 2 weeks after CHI increases early mortality rate (Rapp et al, 1983). Marked nitrogen losses occur when energy intake is only 100% of the REE (Butcher, 1985; Clifton et al, 1985).

Goals of nutritional care are (1) minimization of nitrogen losses, (2) full replacement of expended energy, and (3) avoidance of hyperglycemia. Aggressive nutritional assessment and early intervention are vital if visceral and somatic protein stores are to be retained. Positive nitrogen balance or even equilibrium cannot be achieved during the first 2 weeks after injury.

A thorough evaluation is required to choose the optimal route of feeding. Although early research favored total parenteral nutrition (TPN), 70 to 80% of patients can meet nutritional requirements with enteral feeding within the first week after the injury. Sepsis, barbiturates, and morphine administration can cause gastric intolerance sufficient to prevent enteral feeding. However, almost all patients can tolerate adequate levels of tube feeding by the second week. If enteral feeding is not well tolerated within 72 hours, then TPN should be started immediately. Use of TPN is complicated by the need for a severe fluid restriction to minimize brain edema (Clifton et al, 1985; Kocan and Hicklisch, 1986).

Indicators to monitor include nitrogen balance, weight, serum electrolytes, blood gases, serum glucose, serum transferrin, temperature, and fluid input and output. Common medications include steroids to reduce brain swelling, and anticonvulsants. (See Chapter 29 for further discussion.)

Patients with CHI typically are hospitalized for long periods. Adequate nutrition initially, and for sustained periods, can deter the decubitus ulcers and infection that are common to this population (Butcher, 1985). Changes in behavior and personality can interfere with oral intake and can make mealtimes difficult.

CITED REFERENCES

Adams RD and Victor M: Principles of Neurology. New York, McGraw-Hill, 1985.

Altman J, Kornhuber AW, and Kornhuber HH: Stroke: Cardiovascular risk factors and the quantitative effects of dietary treatment on them. Eur Neurol 26:90, 1987.

Asbeck C and Burns BL: Nutritional management of amyotrophic lateral sclerosis. Diet Nutr Support 10(9):11, 1988.

Bates D et al: Polyunsaturated fatty acids in the treatment of acute remitting multiple sclerosis. Br Med J 2:1390, 1978.

Butcher SK: Nutritional management in acute head injury. Diet Crit Care 7:1, 1985.

Caroscio J: Amyotrophic lateral sclerosis: The disease. *In* Caroscio J (ed): Amyotrophic Lateral Sclerosis: A Guide to Patient Care. New York, Thieme Medical Publishers, 1986.

Centers for Disease Control: Update: Eosinophilia-myalgia syndrome associated with ingestion of L-tryptophan — United States, as of January 9, 1990. JAMA 263:633, 1990.

Clifton GL et al: The metabolic response to severe head injury. J Neurosurg 60:687, 1984.

Clifton GL, Robertson CS, and Contant CF: Enteral hyperalimentation in head injury. J Neurosurg 62:186, 1985.

Diamond S et al: Migraine headache: Working for the best outcome. Postgrad Med 81(8):174, 1987.

D'Orazio L and D'Orazio P: Nutritional polyneuritis and its manifestations in the lower extremity. J Am Podiatr Med Assoc 75:28, 1985.

Egger J et al: Oligoantigenic diet treatment of children with epilepsy and migraine. J Pediatr 114:51, 1989.

Fitzgerald G et al: The effect of nutritional counseling on diet and plasma EFA status in multiple sclerosis patients over 3 years. Hum Nutr: Appl Nut 41A:297, 1987.

Hewson DC: Is there a role for gluten-free diets in multiple sclerosis? Hum Nutr: Appl Nutr 38:417, 1984.

Hewson DC et al: Food intake in multiple sclerosis. Hum Nutr: Appl Nutr 38:355, 1984.

Hillel A and Miller R: Bulbar amyotrophic lateral sclerosis: Patterns of progression and clinical management. Head Neck 11:51, 1989.

Hynak-Hankinson MT et al: Dysphagia evaluation and treatment: The team approach, Parts I and II. Nutr Supp Serv 4(5):33, 1984 and 4(6):30, 1984.

Kocan MJ and Hicklisch SM: A comparison of continuous intermittent enteral nutrition in NICU patients. J Neurosci Nurs 18:333, 1986.

Koehler SM and Glaros A: The effect of aspartame on migraine headache. Headache 28:10, 1988.

Krueger KA et al: Effect of two administration schedules of an enteral nutrient formula on phenytoin bioavailability. Epilepsia 28:706, 1987.

Lipton RB et al: Aspartame as a dietary trigger of headache. Headache 29:90, 1989.

Logemann J: Evaluation and treatment of swallowing disorders. San Diego, College-Hill Press, 1983.

Millar JHD et al: Double blind trial of linoleate supplementation of the diet in multiple sclerosis. Br Med J 1:765, 1973.

Norberg A and Winblad B: A model for the assessment of eating problems in patients with Parkinson's disease. J Adv Nurs 12:473, 1987.

Paty DW et al: Linoleic acid in multiple sclerosis: Failure to show any therapeutic benefit. Acta Neurol Scand 58:53, 1978.

Perkin JE and Hartje J: Diet and migraine: A review of the literature. J Am Diet Ass 83:459, 1983.

Pincus JH and Barry KM: Protein redistribution diet restores motor function in patients with dopa-resistant "off" periods. Neurology 38:481, 1988.

Pryse-Phillips W: Dietary precipitation of vascular headaches. *In* Chandra RK (ed): Food Allergy, St. John's, Newfoundland. Nutr Research Educ Found 1987.

Rapp RP et al: The favorable effect of early parenteral feeding on survival in head-injured patients. J Neurosurg 58:906, 1983.

Rheaume Y, Riley ME, and Volicer L: Meeting the nutritional needs of Alzheimer's patients who pace constantly. J Nutr Elderly 7:43, 1988.

Riley D and Lang AE: Practical application of a low-protein diet for Parkinson's disease. Neurology 38:1026, 1988.

Rivera VM: Stroke: A guide to differential diagnosis and prevention. Postgrad Med 77:81, 1985.

Roe DA: Nutrient and drug interactions. Nutr Rev 42:141, 1984.

Roe DA: Drug-Induced Nutritional Deficiencies, 2nd ed. Westport, CT, AVI Publ Co, 1985, p 296.

Root EJ and Longenecker JB: Nutrition, the brain, and Alzheimer's disease. Nutr Today 23(4):11, 1988.

Rosen M: Respiratory failure in amyotrophic lateral sclerosis. *In* Caroscio J (ed): Amyotrophic Lateral Sclerosis: A Guide to Patient Care. New York, Thieme Medical Publishers, 1986, p 48.

Sandman PO et al: Nutritional status and dietary intake in institutionalized patients with Alzheimer's disease and multiinfarct dementia. J Am Geriatr Soc 35:31, 1987.

Scheinberg LC and Van der Noort S: Editorial on multiple sclerosis treatments. Neurology 36:703, 1986.

Segar W: Parenteral fluid therapy. Curr Probl Pediatr 3:30, 1972.

Shields RW: Alcoholic polyneuropathy. Muscle Nerve 8:183, 1985.

Shore D and Wyatt JD: Aluminum and Alzheimer's disease. J Nerv Ment Dis 171:553, 1983.

Slowie L, Paige M, and Antel J: Nutritional considerations in the management of patients with amyotrophic lateral sclerosis (ALS). J Am Diet Assoc 83:44, 1983.

Staehelin HB: Senile dementia in relation to nutritional factors. Bibl Nutr Dieta 38:136, 1986.

Swank RL: Multiple sclerosis: A correlation of its incidence with dietary fat. Am J Med Sci 220:421, 1950.

Swank RL: Multiple sclerosis: 20 years on low fat diet. Arch Neurol 23:460, 1979.

Swank RL and Grimsgaard A: Multiple sclerosis: The lipid relationship. Am J Clin Nutr 48:1387, 1988.

Wilkerson RJ and Carter WJ: Current therapy of cerebrovascular disease. J Arkansas Med Soc 80:539, 1984.

Wolfgram F et al: Serum linoleic acid in multiple sclerosis. Neurology 25:786, 1975.

Woody RC et al: Corn oil ketogenic diet for children with intractable seizures. J Child Neurol 3:21, 1988.

Woody RC et al: Impaired neutrophil function in children with seizures treated with the ketogenic diet. J Pediatr 115:427, 1989.

Young D and Feldman R: Amyotrophic lateral sclerosis: Clinical features, pathogenesis and management. Intern Med 10:99, 1989.

ADDITIONAL REFERENCES

Asbeck C and Burns BL: What is the status of diet therapy in multiple sclerosis? Diet Nutr Supp 10:10, 1989.

Baugh S: The role of the dietitian in nutritional management of ALS. *In* Adam M (ed): Amyotrophic Lateral Sclerosis: A Teaching Manual for Health Professionals. Kirkland, WA, ALS Support Services, 1985.

Beal B: ALS and constipation. ALS Newslett (Orange County, CA) Mar/Apr 1989, p 5.

Brooks J: Swallowing difficulties in amyotrophic lateral sclerosis. *In* Caroscio J (ed): Amyotrophic Lateral Sclerosis: A Guide to Patient Care. New York, Thieme Medical Publishers, 1986.

Claggett MS: Nutritional factors relevant to Alzheimer's disease. J Am Diet Assoc 89:392, 1989.

DeGruyne LK: Nutrition and the aging brain. Nutr Clin 3(6):1, 1988.

Douglas JB and Edwards V: Nutritional practices, attitudes and knowledge of outpatients with multiple sclerosis. J Can Diet Assoc 49(Fall):246, 1988.

Erickson T et al: "On-off" phenomenon in Parkinson's disease: Relation between dopa and other large neutral amino acids in plasma. Neurology 38:1245, 1988.

Freidberg SR: Tumors of the brain. Clin Symp 38:1, 1986.

Gray GE: Nutrition and dementia. J Am Diet Assoc 89:1795, 1989.

Hillel A and Miller R: Management of bulbar symptoms in amyotrophic lateral sclerosis. Adv Exp Med Biol 209:201, 1987.

Howard PA and Hannaman KN: Warfarin resistance linked to enteral nutrition products. J Am Diet Assoc 85:713, 1985.

Juncos JL et al: Dietary influences on the antiparkinsonian response to levodopa. Arch Neurol 44:1003, 1987.

Lieberman DA: Nutritional management of the patient with Parkinson's disease. Top Clin Nutr 4(1):1, 1989.

Lione A: The reduction of aluminum intake in patients with Alzheimer's disease. J Environ Pathol Toxicol Oncol 6:21, 1985.

Loney LA et al: Nutritional concerns for patients with Alzheimer's disease. Tex Med 83:40, 1987.

Maloney FP, Burks JS, and Ringel SP (eds): Interdisciplinary Rehabilitation of Multiple Sclerosis and Neuromuscular Disorders. Philadelphia, JB Lippincott, 1985.

Miller RG: Guillain-Barré syndrome: Current methods of diagnosis and treatment. Postgrad Med 77:57, 1985.

Noroian EL: Myasthenia gravis: A nursing perspective. J Neurosci Nurs 18:74, 1986.

Nutritional status of patients with Alzheimer's dementia. Nutr MD 16(2):4, 1990.

Pincus JH and Barry KM: Influence of dietary protein on motor fluctuations in Parkinson's disease. Arch Neurol 44:270, 1987.

Pincus JH and Barry KM: Dietary method for reducing fluctuations in Parkinson's disease. Yale J Biol Med 60:133, 1987.

Scholl DE: Nutritional implications of various neurological disorders. Diet Nutr Suppl 9(9):13, 1988.

Sills MA et al: The medium-chain triglyceride diet and intractable epilepsy. Arch Dis Child 61:1168, 1986.

Slowie L: Nutritional management of dysphagia. *In* Caroscio J (ed): Amyotrophic Lateral Sclerosis: A Guide to Patient Care. New York, Thieme Medical Publishers, 1986.

Smith BR: Diet adjunct to the clinical treatment of Parkinson's disease. Nutr Today 26(1):25, 1991.

Trauner DA: Medium chain triglyceride (MCT) in intractable seizure disorders. Neurology 35:237, 1985.

Welnetz K: Maintaining adequate nutrition and hydration in the dysphagic ALS patient. Can Nurse 79:30, 1983.

CHAPTER 40

NUTRITIONAL CARE IN ARTHRITIC DISEASE

CHAPTER OUTLINE

KEY TERMS

AUTOIMMUNE—specific type of humoral or cell-mediated immune response against constituents of the body's own tissues

GOUT—a group of disorders of purine and pyrimidine metabolism characterized by hyperuricemia and deposition of urate crystals

NUCLEOPROTEIN—a substance composed of a simple basic protein combined with either deoxyribonucleic acid (DNA) or ribonucleic acid (RNA)

OSTEOARTHRITIS (DEGENERATIVE ARTHRITIS)—non-inflammatory degenerative joint disease occurring mainly in older persons, characterized by degeneration of the joint cartilage, hypertrophy of bone at the margins, and changes in the synovial membrane

PROSTAGLANDIN (PG)—any of a group of components derived from unsaturated 20-carbon fatty acids, primarily arachidonic acid, that are extremely potent mediators of a diverse group of physiologic processes; the series is designated with a subscript 1, 2, or 3, depending on the number of double bonds in the hydrocarbon skeleton and the fatty acid from which it was synthesized

PURINES—the nitrogenous bases adenine and guanine, which are constituents of nucleoproteins, whose metabolic end-product is uric acid

RHEUMATOID ARTHRITIS—chronic inflammatory systemic disease primarily of the joints marked by changes in the synovial membranes and joint structures and by atrophy and rarefaction of the bones

Arthritis is a general term describing more than 100 different manifestations of connective tissue disease marked by pain and degeneration or inflammation of the joints. The tissues most frequently affected are the interstitial tissues, blood vessels, cartilage, bone, tendons and ligaments, and the synovial membrane lining joint surfaces. The etiology is unknown.

Arthritis may be acute or chronic. An acute attack is of short duration but may recur and develop into a chronic condition. The disease may also be secondary to another condition, such as inflammatory bowel disease, celiac sprue, intestinal bypass surgery, or malabsorption. The most common forms of chronic arthritis are rheumatoid arthritis, osteoarthritis, and gout.

Because many of the pathologic processes involved in arthritic disease are temporary and spontaneous, improvement often occurs. As a result, it is common for the condition to be exploited by hucksters and by the less well-informed who are eager to offer "the latest cure" (New Directions, page 694). At present, unfortunately, arthritic diseases are only managed; they are never cured.

INFLAMMATION IN ARTHRITIC DISEASE

Inflammation is the most debilitating component of arthritis. As in other "autoimmune" diseases, antibodies are formed that react with tissue components and cause inflammation and other problems.

The inflammatory process is initiated by the production of biologically active fatty acids, prostaglandins, and leukotrienes. Most of the drugs used in the treatment of rheumatic diseases affect the synthesis of prostaglandins, usually diminishing their production. Nonsteroidal anti-inflammatory drugs (NSAIDs) inhibit an early step in the conversion of arachidonic acid to prostaglandins, and corticosteroids decrease the release of arachidonic acid from the membrane lipids.

Prostaglandins are produced from dietary omega-3 and omega-6 fatty acids. Linoleic acid, which occurs abundantly in vegetable oils, is the predominant omega-6 fatty acid. It is converted to arachidonic acid, the precursor of the prostaglandins of the 2-series (e.g., PGE_2). The most common omega-3 fatty acid, eicosapentaenoic acid (EPA), is found primarily in fish oils. Prostaglandins produced from EPA, those of the 3-series, contribute less to the inflammatory process than do those produced from arachidonic acid.

The type of prostaglandin produced is determined by the composition of cellular membrane lipids, which in turn is influenced by the nature of dietary fatty acids. Diets rich in omega-3 fatty acids can produce a dose-related change resulting in decreased severity of inflammation. In the future, alterations of the fatty acid content of the diet may be useful in the management of inflammation.

RHEUMATOID ARTHRITIS

The etiology of rheumatoid arthritis is unknown. It is a chronic, debilitating, and frequently crippling disease with overwhelming personal, social, and economic effects. Although much less common than osteoarthritis, the rheumatoid form is more severe. It is also more susceptible to amelioration by dietary intervention. Any joint may be affected by rheumatoid arthritis, but multiple involvement of the small joints of the extremities, most frequently the proximal interphalangeal joints of the hands and feet, is the rule. Pain, stiffness, and swelling are the common complaints. The swelling or puffiness shown in Figure 40–1 is caused by the accumulation of fluid in the lining membranes of the joints and inflammation of the surrounding tissues.

The incidence of rheumatoid arthritis is reported to increase twofold in the later decades of life and may reach 15% in females over 60 years of age in some populations. It occurs more frequently in women than in men, the proportion averaging three to one. Onset occurs commonly around 35 years of age and is followed generally by numerous remissions and exacerbations.

Patients with rheumatoid arthritis are frequently underweight, in contrast to those with osteoarthritis who are often overweight.

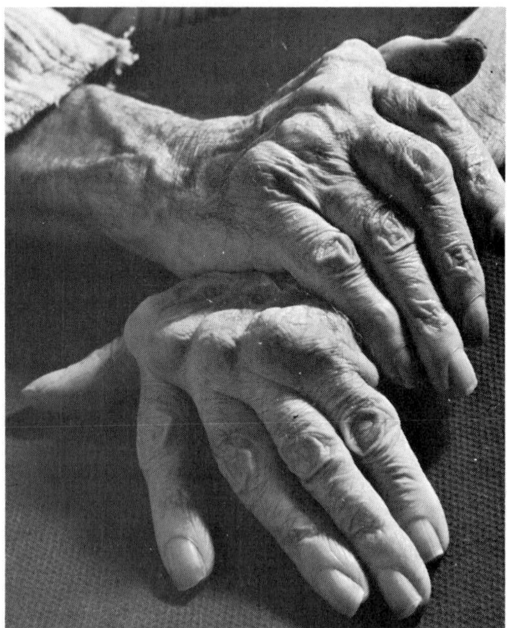

FIGURE 40–1. *A patient with advanced rheumatoid arthritis. The twisted hands and the puffiness of the metacarpal joints are typical of the disease. (Courtesy of George E. Pickow, Three Lions, Inc.)*

Nutritional Care

Rheumatoid arthritis affects the nutritional status of individuals in several ways. The inflammatory process is accompanied by an elevated metabolic rate that leads to increased nutritional requirements. Changes in the gastrointestinal mucosa lead to malabsorption. Peptic ulcer and gastritis are often present as a result of either the disease or necessary medication. *Sjögren's syndrome*, a decrease in quantity of saliva and other secretions, is a complication that interferes with swallowing and leads to severe dental decay as well as to altered taste and smell and dysphagia. Involvement of the temporomandibular joint may limit opening and closing of the mouth. All of these factors, along with the crippling nature of the disease that frequently hinders the preparation and eating of adequate meals, lead to a nutritional status that is frequently poor.

Under these circumstances, an assessment of the nutritional status of patients with rheumatoid arthritis becomes very important. A thorough nutritional assessment includes not only the usual parameters (see Chapter 17) but also the impact of the disease on food preparation and self-feeding. A physical or occupational therapy evaluation can be useful. The nutritional side effects of medications are also important, because large amounts of medication are taken daily for years. Weight change is the most reliable parameter of nutritional status. Nutritional status usually improves with control of the disease.

Diet Composition

ENERGY. Energy requirements can be determined by using the Harris-Benedict formula (see Table 2–5) or the Long equation (see Table 29–2) for resting energy expenditure (REE) with an additional factor for injury. During active disease, a factor of 1.14–1.35 × REE should be used to cover the effects of hypermetabolism. An activity factor of 1.2 × REE can be used for patients with limited mobility who are receiving physical therapy, and a factor of 1.3 × REE can be used for those receiving intensive daily physical therapy (Touger-Decker, 1988).

PROTEIN. Well-nourished individuals require protein at the level of the recommended daily allowance (RDA). Requirements of patients who are poorly nourished or who are in an inflammatory phase of the disease increase to 1.5 to 2 g/kg/day with a nonprotein calorie:nitrogen ratio of 150:1 (Touger-Decker, 1988).

LIPIDS. Omega-3 fatty acids, either in tablet form or as they occur in marine oils, are popular for use in the management of rheumatoid arthritis because of their role in inflammatory pathways. The daily use of 1.8 grams of EPA has been shown to diminish morning stiffness and the number of tender joints and to improve fatigue time in patients with rheumatoid arthritis (Kremer et al, 1985 and 1987). EPA is not recommended as the sole basis of arthritic management, however, because better symptomatic relief is available from NSAID. In addition, omega-3 fatty acids have other effects on clotting time that should be considered. However, it does appear to be worthwhile to recommend an increase in the consumption of seafoods and fish oils that are rich in omega-3 fatty acids (see Appendix Table 40).

VITAMINS. Low-serum pyridoxal (vitamin B_6) levels have been reported in patients with rheumatoid arthritis, possibly as an effect of prolonged drug therapy. Gastric mucosal lesions commonly seen in rheumatoid arthritis may also increase the need for pyridoxal-5-phosphate.

Low levels of ascorbic acid in white blood cells are also seen frequently in patients with rheumatoid arthritis. This may be related to the ingestion of large quantities of aspirin, although how this occurs is not clear. Some individuals manifest a cutaneous bruising that improves when the diet is supplemented with ascorbic acid, suggesting a vitamin C deficiency. However, massive doses of vitamin C are inappropriate in the absence of a true deficiency state.

MINERALS. Hypochromic anemia of the type associated with chronic infection or inflammation is frequently associated with arthritis. This anemia, which probably reflects a defect in the reuse of iron after destruction of the red blood cells, is not related to dietary iron deficiency. Total iron-binding capacity (TIBC) is not increased, and total iron stores in the bone marrow are normal. The anemia does not respond to iron therapy; in fact, iron supplementation may exacerbate the arthritis (Blake and Balon, 1982).

Osteoporosis and osteomalacia are frequently seen in patients with rheumatoid arthritis. Calcium and vitamin D malabsorption are characteristic of advanced stages of the disease. Other contributing factors include aging, diets deficient in calcium and vitamin D, decreased physical activity, corticosteroid therapy, and lack of sunlight (Wordsworth et al, 1984).

Elevated copper and ceruloplasmin levels in serum and joint fluid are seen in rheumatoid arthritis. Plasma copper levels correlate with the degree of joint inflammation and decrease as the inflammation is diminished. Elevated plasma ceruloplasmin levels may have a protective role through antioxidant activity against toxic oxygen radicals released during inflammation. It has been suggested that the folk remedy of wearing a

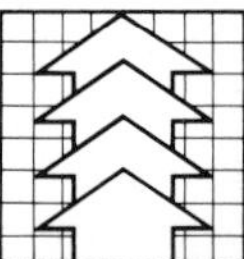

NEW DIRECTIONS: Unproven Remedies for Arthritis

Eventually almost everyone is affected to some degree by arthritis — 97% of adults over 60 years of age have arthritis that is detectable by x-ray, although not all are severely symptomatic. Because modern medicine often does not have anything to offer in the way of a cure or even relief of symptoms, many understandably turn to folk medicine and even unprincipled quackery for help. Surveys in the United States and in other countries show that from well over one half to 94% of sufferers try at least one self-help remedy and usually try more than one (Jarvis, 1990).

Favorable effects of self-help treatments are often reported, but as a rule a case cannot be established for cause-and-effect. Any amelioration can usually be attributed to the placebo effect or to the characteristic arthritis cycle of worsening followed by periods of improvement. When a home remedy coincides with a period of remission, the remedy is often continued indefinitely, even when it fails to perform through a later period of worsening.

Megavitamins and special foods or diets are among the most popular of the self-help remedies. Dietary variations are frequently bizarre, such as the honey and apple cider vinegar treatment. Few controlled trials of the effects of diet on the symptoms of arthritis are available. Among those are a few in which favorable results cannot be explained on the basis of the placebo effect. Weight loss, of course, produces a favorable response by reducing stresses on affected joints. Others are harder to explain. Theories include exposing and eliminating unrecognized allergies or modifying the immune system response to inflammation. With the exception of weight loss, there has never been a proven advantage of any particular diet program or adjunct.

Although much of the dietary experimentation is harmless except for the cost of special foods or popular diet books, some self-treatment can be harmful. This usually involves the excessive use of supplements such as fish oil, herbal remedies, or megavitamin dosages.

copper bracelet to relieve arthritis pain may be related to absorption of copper through the skin (Bollet, 1988).

In contrast to copper, serum zinc levels are lower than normal in individuals with rheumatoid arthritis. Because zinc has been shown to inhibit prostaglandin synthesis and to impair macrophage function, its low level in the manifestation of rheumatoid arthritis could be significant. However, zinc supplementation has not resulted in consistently positive results.

Low blood selenium levels in patients with rheumatoid arthritis are inversely related to the severity of the disease (Borglund et al, 1988). This finding may be related to selenium as a component of glutathione peroxidase and its activity as an antioxidant. Overproduction of peroxides may be involved in the etiology of inflammatory disorders. Supplementation of rheumatoid arthritis patients with selenium has resulted in increased blood selenium levels but without change in the disease (Tarp et al, 1987).

WATER AND ELECTROLYTES. Some arthritic patients retain salt and water because of immobility resulting from joint pain or secondary to medication. Sodium restriction is often helpful to these patients, as is the use of diuretics (see Chapter 33 for discussion of sodium-controlled diets).

Food Allergies

Joint pain can be a manifestation of food allergy. Patients with established allergic reactions can benefit from the elimination of offending foods from the diet. However, this relationship should be well documented with blinded food challenges so that foods are not eliminated unnecessarily simply because their consumption just happened to coincide with an arthritic flare-up (see Chapter 38).

Placebo-controlled studies have shown that some patients show improvement in their arthritic symptoms when placed on an elimination diet (Darlington et al, 1986; Hicklin et al, 1980). Whether this was a response to the removal of a food from an allergic reaction, the weight reduction that accompanied the elimination diet, or some other change in absorption of food or bacterial antigens is not known.

It is important to recognize that psychologic processes may produce pathophysiologic changes indistinguishable from genuine immunologic reactions. The potential for suffering such a "pseudo food allergy" can be significant in patients with rheumatoid arthritis, 40% of whom have been described as placebo responders (Pearson, 1985).

Pharmacologic Therapy

Pharmacologic therapy to control pain and inflammation is the mainstay of treatment for the arthritic. Of the seven primary drug classifications used to treat rheumatoid arthritis, salicylates and NSAID are the most widely used. The other five types are antimalarials, gold salts, D-penicillamine, steroids, and immunosuppressive agents.

The symptoms of rheumatoid arthritis are usually controlled by large daily doses of aspirin. However, side effects of chronic aspirin ingestion are gastric mucosal injury and bleeding, audiologic problems, increased bleeding time, and increased urinary excretion of vitamin C. The gastrointestinal symptoms of gastritis can frequently be alleviated by taking aspirin with milk, food, or an antacid. Vitamin C supplementation is prescribed when serum and platelet levels of ascorbic acid are below normal.

The second line of medication is made up of the NSAID, such as indomethacin. The effectiveness of aspirin and NSAID lies in the inhibition of prostaglandin synthesis. Associated with this inhibition is a change in kidney function that favors salt and water retention. Although azotemia can result in some individuals, the salt and water retention rarely causes serious problems unless congestive heart failure or hypertension are also present.

Corticosteroids are reserved for patients whose pain cannot be managed by aspirin or the NSAID. High-dose corticosteroid therapy is commonly used with systemic lupus erythematosus and other systemic connective tissue diseases, but is rarely prescribed in rheumatoid arthritis. These drugs are very effective in reducing inflammation and can be given as local injections or taken orally. However, side effects, such as cushingoid symptoms, sodium retention and potassium excretion, gastrointestinal complications, diabetes mellitus, and osteoporosis, are common. Nutritional care, in the form of sodium restriction, potassium supplementation, or a diabetic diet, may be needed for patients taking steroids.

Gold salt therapy, antimalarials, and D-penicillamine can cause a remission of rheumatoid arthritis. Toxicity from these drugs must be monitored continually.

The nutritional side effects of arthritis medications are discussed in Chapter 25.

Other Treatment

Surgery replaces irreversibly damaged joints, improves the functional capacity of damaged joints, and prevents damage to normal joints. Circulating antibodies and lymphocytes are sometimes removed by a process called aphoresis.

OSTEOARTHRITIS (DEGENERATIVE ARTHRITIS)

Osteoarthritis, also known as degenerative arthritis, is the most common form of arthritis. It occurs with over twice the frequency of rheumatoid arthritis. It probably does not have a single cause but appears to develop from the stresses and strains experienced during the normal course of life. It may follow injuries and other diseases of the joints and may be influenced by congenital and mechanical derangements of the joints. Degeneration of the articular (joint) cartilage, followed by sclerosis of the underlying bone, triggers inflammation and pain of the surrounding joint.

The joints most likely to be attacked in osteoarthritis are the distal interphalangeal joints, the thumb joint, and especially the joints of the knees, hips, ankles, and spine that bear the bulk of the body weight. The early stage of the disease is marked by stiffness, usually on arising from a chair or after standing. Later, definite soreness may be experienced. This feeling worsens at first with motion but then subsides. One or more joints may be affected, and symptoms are usually confined to the afflicted parts. In this respect, the condition differs from rheumatoid arthritis in which the general health may suffer.

Nutritional Care

Diet is important in the common circumstance in which weight reduction is necessary. The prevalence of osteoarthritis among the obese is about twice that among people of normal weight (Mascioli and Blackburn, 1985). Obesity or unknown factors associated with obesity may cause knee osteoarthritis (Felson et al, 1988). Excess weight means an added burden for the weight-bearing joints; however, the benefits of weight reduction are not specifically confined to these areas. Thus, the main dietary treatment is to achieve and maintain normal weight (see Chapter 18). Weight reduction is especially difficult for patients because the disease limits their exercise potential and energy expenditure.

Intakes of calcium and vitamin D should be at levels specified in the RDA to prevent or manage osteoporosis as much as possible. Many patients with osteoarthritis do not consume enough dairy products and calcium (White-O'Connor et al, 1989).

Pharmacologic Therapy

Osteoarthritis is treated with the same medications that are used for rheumatoid arthritis, namely aspirin and NSAID. In addition, corticosteroids may be given as local injections.

Other Treatment

Patients with osteoarthritis or rheumatoid arthritis should be encouraged to lie down at least once during the day to relieve the joints of pressure and to allow a period of rest. Regular exercise periods should be observed. Massage and heat can also relieve pain.

GOUT

Gout, one of the oldest diseases in recorded medical history, is an inherited disorder of purine metabolism in which abnormal levels of *uric acid* accumulate in the blood. As a consequence, sodium urates are formed and deposited as *tophi* in the small joints and surrounding tissues; in chronic gout, the most common site is the helix of the ear (Fig. 40–2). These deposits can cause destruction of joint tissues, leading to chronic arthritis.

The disease, which usually occurs after 35 years of age, is characterized by arthritic pain which is usually localized in a sudden attack that begins in the big toe and that continues up the leg. As the disease advances, symptoms occur more frequently and are more prolonged. Trivial injury or unaccustomed exertion may encourage the episodes, and attacks have been related to excessive eating, drinking, and exercise. Obesity is commonly associated with a gouty condition. Occasionally the disturbance is a sequel to surgery. Ketosis associated with fasting or a low-carbohydrate diet can also precipitate an attack.

Nutritional Care

Purines

Uric acid is derived from the metabolism of purines, which constitute a part of nucleoproteins. Although traditionally gout has been treated with a low-purine diet, drugs have largely replaced the need for rigid restriction of dietary purines. Endogenous formation of uric acid from simple metabolites as well as from purine breakdown accounts for 85% of the urate formed and is apparently influenced very little by dietary regulation. Even though it is thus unlikely that severe limitation of dietary purines will significantly decrease the uric acid

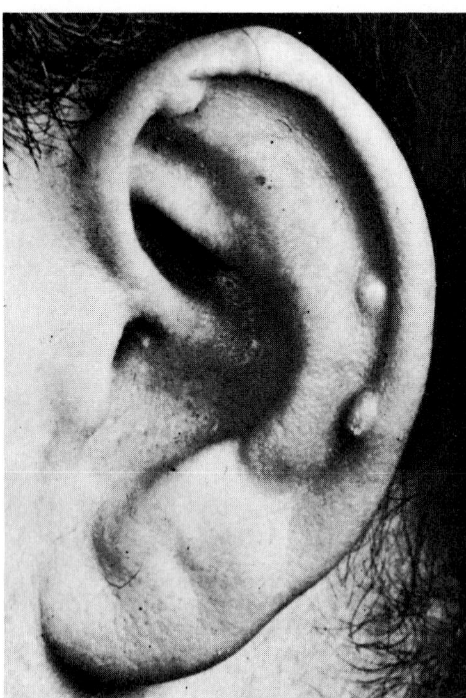

FIGURE 40–2. *Tophi on the ear of a patient who had had gout for many years. (Courtesy of John H. Talbott, M.D. From Seminar Report, Merck, Sharp and Dohme, Div. of Merck and Co, Inc, Fall 1956.)*

TABLE 40–1. Foods Grouped According to Purine Content

Group 1: High Purine Content (100 to 1,000 mg of purine nitrogen per 100 g of food)

Anchovies	Mackerel
Bouillon	Meat extracts
Brains	Mincemeat
Broth	Mussels
Consommé	Partridge
Goose	Roe
Gravy	Sardines
Heart	Scallops
Herring	Sweetbreads
Kidney	Yeast, baker's and brewer's as supplement
Liver	

Foods in this list should be omitted from the diet of patients who have gout (acute and remission stages).

Group 2: Moderate Purine Content (9 to 100 mg of purine nitrogen per 100 g of food)

Meat and Fish (except in those in group 1):	*Vegetables*
Fish	Asparagus
Poultry	Beans, dried
Meat	Lentils
Shellfish	Mushrooms
	Peas, dried
	Spinach

One serving (2 to 3 oz) of meat, fish or fowl or 1 serving (½ cup) of vegetable from this group is allowed each day or 5 days a week (depending on condition) during remissions.

Group 3: Negligible Purine Content

Bread, white and crackers	Fruit
Butter or margarine (in moderation)*	Gelatin desserts
Cake and cookies	Herbs
Carbonated beverages	Ice cream
Cereal beverage	Milk
Cereals and cereal products	Macaroni products
Cheese	Noodles
Chocolate	Nuts
Coffee	Oil
Condiments	Olives
Cornbread	Pickles
Cream (in moderation)	Popcorn
Custard	Puddings
Eggs	Relishes
Fats (in moderation)	Rennet desserts
	Rice
	Salt
	Sugar and sweets
	Tea
	Vegetables (except those in group 2)
	Vinegar
	White sauce

Foods included in this group may be used daily.

*Recommended in moderation due to fat content.

pool, it is often recommended that patients should avoid foods that are high in purines in order to reduce metabolic stress and to necessitate less medication (Table 40–1).

Rigid restriction of foods containing purines is generally recommended in the *acute stage* of gout to avoid adding exogenous purines to the existing high uric acid load. Fluids (up to 3 l/day) should be forced to assist the excretion of uric acid and to minimize the possibility of calculi formation. Because excretion of urates tends to be reduced by fats and is enhanced by carbohydrates, the diet should be relatively high in carbohydrate, moderate in protein, and low in fat. Bicarbonate or citrate can be given to alkalinize the urine and to increase the solubility of uric acid in the urine (see Chapter 35).

During the *interval stage* between attacks, dietary treatment for patients maintained on medication for gout is in the form of a normal adequate diet adjusted to achieve and maintain a body weight 10 to 15% below ideal levels. Weight loss should not be drastic but should occur gradually; a reduction in energy intake sufficient to cause ketonemia is recognized as a precipitating factor of acute attacks. Weight reduction also helps to reduce the hypertriglyceridemia that exists in 75% of patients with gout (Kelley and Fox, 1985).

The diet should be moderate in protein (0.8 g/kg/day), increased in carbohydrate, and relatively low in fat and should exclude foods of high-purine content (Table 40–1; Fig. 40–3). Most of the proteins in the therapeutic diet come from cheese, eggs, milk, and vegetables, which are low in nucleoproteins. Fluids should be adjusted to produce a normal urinary output (2,000 ml).

LOW-PURINE DIET. An ordinary diet contains from 600 to 1,000 mg of purines daily. In cases of severe or advanced gout, the purine content of the daily diet is restricted to approximately 100 to 150 mg, with fat at 30% of the energy intake. The diet may be prescribed according to the groupings in Table 40–1, allowing for considerable individualization among patients. Nutritional care for gout is summarized in Table 40–2.

Alcohol

It is now believed that mild or moderate use of alcohol by the patient with gout does not necessarily induce an

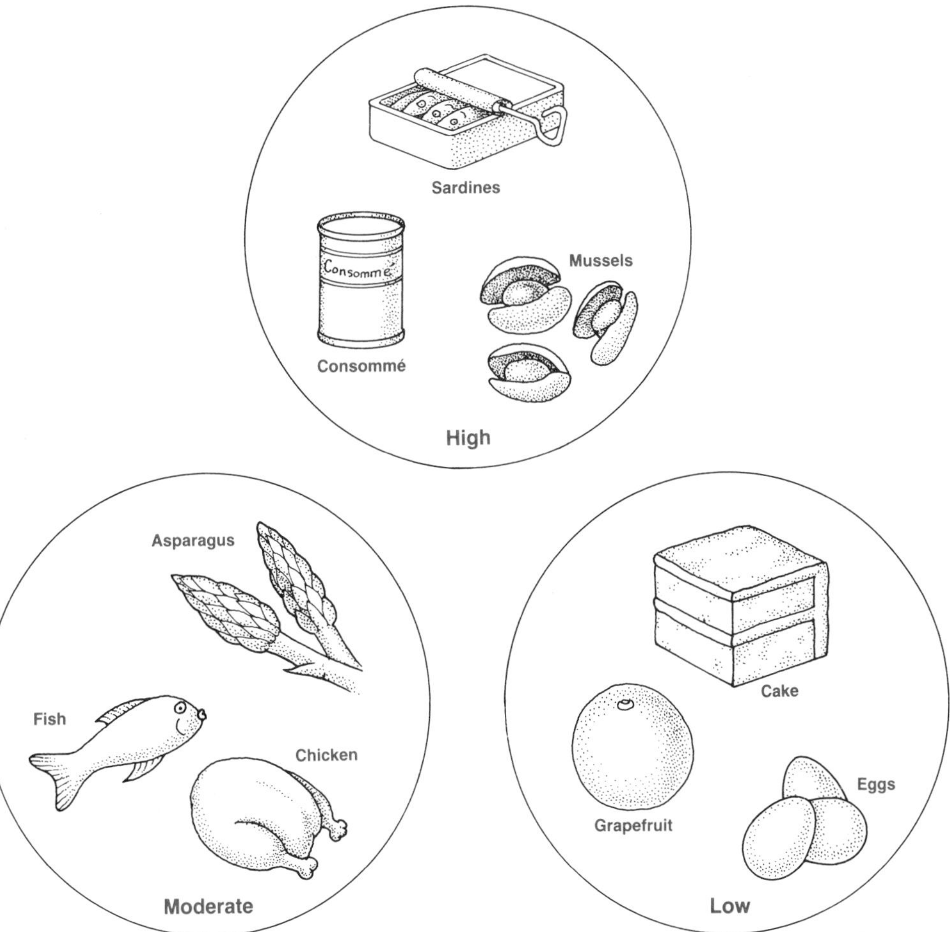

FIGURE 40–3. *Purine content of food; the foods in the "high" group should be avoided by people who have gout.*

TABLE 40–2. Summary of Nutritional Care for Gout

1. Elimination of foods high in purines as shown in Table 40–1.
2. Moderate protein intake with large proportion of protein coming from milk, cheese, vegetables, and bread.
3. Liberal carbohydrate intake (at least 100 g/day) to prevent tissue catabolism and ketosis.
4. Low to moderate fat intake.
5. Maintenance of, or gradual reduction to, ideal body weight.
6. Restriction or elimination of alcohol.
7. Liberal fluid intake to keep urine dilute.

acute attack. However, ethanol does increase uric acid production. Ideally, the patient would be wise not to consume alcohol, but moderate, infrequent consumption could be allowed depending on the patient's condition.

Pharmacologic Therapy

Gout is treated with urate eliminants or with drugs that inhibit synthesis of uric acid. Probenecid (Benemid) or sulfinpyrazone decrease the blood uric acid level by increasing elimination through the kidneys. Allopurinol inhibits uric acid production. Both probenecid and sulfinpyrazone are frequently used with colchicine, a drug that has no effect on uric acid metabolism but has been helpful in relieving the joint pains of gouty arthritis. Colchicine has most value during the acute stage, but may be needed during symptom-free periods as a preventive measure. (For nutritional effects of colchicine, see Chapter 25.) Anti-inflammatory agents such as indomethacin or phenylbutazone are sometimes used in the acute stage.

CITED REFERENCES

Blake D and Bacon PA: Iron and rheumatoid disease. Lancet 1:623, 1982.

Bollet AJ: Nutrition and diet in rheumatic disease. *In* Shils ME and Young VR (eds): Modern Nutrition in Health and Disease, 7th ed. Philadelphia, Lea & Febiger, 1988.

Borglund M, Akesson A, and Akesson B: Distribution of selenium and glutathione peroxidase in plasma compared in healthy subjects and rheumatoid arthritis patients. Scand J Clin Lab Invest 48:27, 1988.

Darlington LG, Ramsey NW, and Mansfield JR: Placebo-controlled, blind study of dietary manipulation therapy in rheumatoid arthritis. Lancet, 1:236, 1986.

Felson DT et al: Obesity and knee osteoarthritis. Ann Intern Med 109:18, 1988.

Hicklin JA, McEwen LM, and Morgan JE: The effect of diet in rheumatoid arthritis. Clin Allergy 10:463, 1980.

Jarvis WT: Arthritis: Folk remedies and quackery. Nutr Forum 7(1):1, 1990.

Kelley WN and Fox IH: Gout and related disorders of purine metabolism. *In* Kelley WN et al (eds): Textbook of Rheumatology, 2nd ed. Philadelphia, WB Saunders, 1985.

Kremer JM et al: Effects of manipulation of dietary fatty acids on clinical manifestations of rheumatoid arthritis. Lancet 1:184, 1985.

Kremer JM et al: Fish-oil fatty acid supplementation in active rheumatoid arthritis. Ann Intern Med 106:497, 1987.

Mascioli EA and Blackburn GL: Nutrition and rheumatic disease. *In* Kelley WN et al (eds): Textbook of Rheumatology, 2nd ed. Philadelphia, WB Saunders 1985.

Pearson DJ: Food allergy, hypersensitivity and food intolerance. J Roy Coll Phys Lond 19:154, 1985.

Tarp U et al: Glutathione peroxidase activity in patients with rheumatoid arthritis and in normal subjects: Effects of long-term selenium supplementation. Arthritis Rheum 30:1162, 1987.

Touger-Decker R: Nutritional considerations in rheumatoid arthritis. J Am Diet Assoc 88:327, 1988.

White-O'Connor B, Sobal J, and Muncie HL: Dietary habits, weight history, and vitamin supplement use in elderly osteoarthritis patients. J Am Diet Assoc 89:378, 1989.

Wordsworth B et al: Metabolic bone disease among patients with rheumatoid arthritis. Br J Rheum 23:251, 1984.

ADDITIONAL REFERENCES

Anderson JJ and Felson DT: Factors associated with osteoarthritis of the knee in the First National Health and Nutrition Examination Survey (HANES I). Am J Epidemiol 128:179, 1988.

Fish oils in rheumatoid arthritis. Lancet 2:720, 1987.

Hamerman D: The biology of osteoarthritis. N Engl J Med 320:1322, 1989.

Kurki P et al: Food intolerance and rheumatoid arthritis. Lancet 2:1419, 1988.

McCarty DJ (ed): Arthritis and Allied Conditions, 11th ed. Philadelphia, Lea & Febiger, 1989.

Nutrition, immune function and inflammation. Proc Nutr Soc 48:315, 1989.

Panush RS: Possible role of food sensitivity in arthritis. Ann Allergy 61(6, Part II):31, 1988.

Peyron JG: Osteoarthritis: The epidemiological viewpoint. Clin Orthop 213:13, 1986.

Rheumatoid arthritis and selenium. Nutr Rev 46:284, 1988.

Wolman PG: Management of patients using unproven regimens for arthritis. J Am Diet Assoc 87:1211, 1987.

CHAPTER 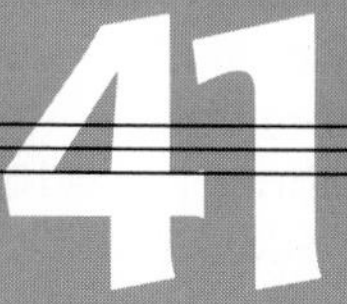

NUTRITIONAL CARE IN METABOLIC DISORDERS

Cristine M. Trahms, M.S., R.D.

CHAPTER OUTLINE

Goals of Nutritional Care

Amino Acid Disorders and Their Management

Disorders of Carbohydrate Metabolism

KEY TERMS

AUTOSOMAL RECESSIVE—incapable of expression unless the responsible allele is carried by both members of a pair of homologous chromosomes that are not sex chromosomes

ARGININOSUCCINIC ACIDURIA (ASA)—the presence of argininosuccinic acid in the blood and urine due to a deficiency or argininosuccinate lyase

CARBAMYL PHOSPHATE SYNTHETASE (CPS) DEFICIENCY—a urea cycle defect

CITRULLINEMIA—elevated citrulline in the blood and urine due to a deficiency of argininosuccinic acid synthetase in the metabolism of citrulline to argininosuccinic acid

GALACTOSEMIA—elevated plasma glucose due to a disturbance in the conversion of galactose to glucose because of the absence of the enzyme galactokinase or galactose-1-phosphate uridyl transferase

LOFENALAC—a formula composed of a 95% phenylalanine-free protein hydrolysate; used for infants with phenylketonuria

MALIGNANT PHENYLKETONURIA—hyperphenylalaninemia in which low-phenylalanine diet does not prevent neurologic deterioration

MAPLE SYRUP URINE DISEASE (MSUD) OR BRANCHED-CHAIN KETOACIDURIA—autosomal recessive metabolic defect in decarboxylation that affects the metabolism of the branched-chain amino acids

METHYLMALONIC ACIDEMIA—an excess of methylmalonic acid in the blood and urine due to a defect of methylmalonyl CoA mutase

ORNITHINE TRANSCARBAMYLASE (OTC) DEFICIENCY—a sex-linked recessive disorder in the conversion of ornithine and carbamyl phosphate to citrulline; usually lethal in males

PHENYL-FREE—a 100% phenylalanine-free formula appropriate for an older child

PHENYLKETONURIA—hyperphenylalaninemia in which phenylalanine is not metabolized to tyrosine because of a deficiency of phenylalanine hydroxylase

PROPIONIC ACIDEMIA—an excess of propionic acid in the blood due to defective propionyl CoA reductase

Metabolic disorders are inherited traits that result in the absence or reduced activity of a specific enzyme or cofactor. Most metabolic disorders are inherited as autosomal recessive traits.

It is important to remember that not all biochemical "disorders" are diseases; some, such as histidinemia, may be normal variations that are benign and do not require treatment (Snyderman et al, 1979). Significant questions related to diagnosis and treatment still need to be answered for many of the metabolic disorders.

Most inherited metabolic disorders are associated with severe clinical manifestations, often appearing soon after birth. Mental retardation and severe neurologic involvement may be the result of delayed diagnosis and treatment. Prenatal diagnosis is available for many metabolic disorders, but it usually requires the identification of a family at risk, which can be done only after the birth of an affected child. However, the efficacy of newborn screening programs as well as advanced diagnostic techniques and treatment modalities have improved the outcome for many of these infants (Further Reading, see below). Affected infants should be identified as soon as possible and should receive the advantages of care offered by centers with expertise in the treatment of these disorders. Infants who are afebrile but who for no apparent reason are lethargic, vomiting, having seizures, or are in respiratory distress should be evaluated for an undiagnosed metabolic disorder. The initial assessment should include blood gases, electrolytes, glucose and ammonia, and a urine check for ketones.

GOALS OF NUTRITIONAL CARE

The goals of nutritional therapy are maintenance of biochemical equilibrium for the affected pathway, provision of adequate nutrients to support normal growth and development, and provision of support for social and emotional development.

Nutritional treatment is designed to circumvent the missing or inactive enzyme by (1) restricting the amount of substrate available, (2) supplementing the amount of product, (3) supplementing the enzymatic cofactor, or (4) combining any or all of these approaches.

AMINO ACID DISORDERS AND THEIR MANAGEMENT

Nutritional therapy for amino acid disorders most frequently consists of substrate restriction, which involves limiting one or more essential amino acids to the minimum requirement while providing adequate energy and nutrients to promote normal growth and development. However, care must be exercised because an inadequate intake of an essential amino acid can often be as detrimental as an excess (Hanley et al, 1970). Dietary supplementation of the product is the second most common type of nutritional therapy for amino acid disorders.

Requirements for individual amino acids are difficult to determine because normal growth and develop-

FURTHER READING: PKU Time Line

HISTORICAL EVENTS IN DIAGNOSIS AND TREATMENT OF PHENYLKETONURIA

1934 A. Folling identifies phenylpyruvic acid in urine of retarded siblings in institutions. One per cent of institutionalized population excreted phenylpyruvic acid.

1953 G. Jervis demonstrates deficiency of phenylalanine oxidation in liver tissue of affected patient. H. Bickel demonstrates dietary phenylalanine restrictions will lower blood concentration of phenylalanine.

1961 R. Guthrie develops bacterial inhibition assay method to measure blood phenylalanine.

Mid–1960s Semisynthetic formulas restricted in phenylalanine become commercially available.

1965–1970 States adopt newborn screening programs to detect phenylketonuria.

1967–1980 Collaborative Study of Children Treated for Phenylketonuria. Data from this study form the basis for treatment protocols for PKU clinics in the United States.

Late 1970s Life-time restriction of phenylalanine intake becomes standard of care for PKU clinics in the United States.

Late 1970s Detrimental effects of maternal phenylketonuria are recognized as a significant public health problem.

1983 Maternal PKU Collaborative Study begins to study effects of treatment on pregnancy outcome of women with phenylketonuria.

1987 Techniques for carrier detection and prenatal diagnosis of phenylketonuria are developed.

ment can be achieved over a wide range of intake. The data of Holt and Snyderman (1967) are often used as the basis for prescribing amino acid therapy (Table 41–1). Careful and frequent monitoring are required to ensure the adequacy of the prescription. Although nitrogen studies would be the most precise, weight gain in infants is a sensitive and easily monitored index of well-being and nutritional adequacy.

Hyperphenylalaninemias

Of the amino acid disorders listed in Table 41–2, the hyperphenylalaninemias are the most frequent. They provide a reasonable model for detailed discussion because (1) they are relatively frequent and most newborns are screened for these disorders; (2) they have a predictable course, with the greatest available docu-

TABLE 41–1. Approximate Daily Requirements for Selected Nutrients and Amino Acids in Infancy and Childhood*†

		Age			
Amino Acid	Unit	*0 to 2 mo*	*2 to 5 mo*	*6 to 12 mo*	*1 to 10 yr*
Phenylalanine					
Infants	mg/kg	47–90	47–90	25–47	—
Children	mg/day	—	—	—	200 –500‡
Histidine	mg/kg	16–34	16–34	16–34	—
Tyrosine§	mg/kg	60–80	60–80	40–60	25–85
Leucine					
Infants	mg/kg	76–150	76–150	76–150	—
Children	mg/day	—	—	—	1,000
Isoleucine					
Infants	mg/kg	79–110	79–110	50–75	—
Children	mg/day	—	—	—	1,000
Valine					
Infants	mg/kg	65–105	65–105	50–80	—
Children	mg/day	—	—	—	400–600
Methionine‖					
Infants	mg/kg	20–45	20–45	20–45	—
Children	mg/day	—	—	—	400–800
Cyst(e)ine¶					
Infants	mg/kg	15–50	15–50	15–50	—
Children	mg/day	—	—	—	400–800
Lysine					
Infants	mg/kg	90–120	90–120	90–120	—
Children	mg/day	—	—	—	1,200–1,600
Threonine					
Infants	mg/kg	45–87	45–87	45–87	—
Children	mg/day	—	—	—	800–1,000
Tryptophan					
Infants	mg/kg	13–22	13–22	13–22	—
Children	mg/day	—	—	—	60–120
Energy					
Infants	kcal/kg	108	108	98	—
Children	kcal/kg	—	—	—	70–102
Water					
Infants	ml/kg	100	110	100	—
Children	ml/day	—	—	—	1,100
Carbohydrate	g/day	← Kcal × .50 →			
Protein					
Infants	g/kg	2.2	2.2	1.6	—
Children	g/day	—	—	—	16–28
Fat	g/day	← Kcal × .35 →			

* Adapted from Committee on Nutrition, American Academy of Pediatrics: Special diets for infants with inborn errors of metabolism. Pediatrics *57:783*, 1976 and Food and Nutrition Board, National Research Council, NAS: Recommended Dietary Allowances, 10th ed, Washington, DC, National Academy Press, 1989.

† Compiled from amino acid data of Holt and Snyderman. There is limited information on amino acid requirements of infants and children at different ages; the figures given here are in excess of minimum requirements. Consequently, this table should be used only as a guide and should not be regarded as an authoritative statement to which individual patients must conform.

‡ More phenylalanine (>800 mg) is required in the absence of tyrosine.

§ Total phenylalanine plus tyrosine should be considered in the prescription since most phenylalanine is converted to tyrosine.

‖ More methionine is required in the absence of cyst(e)ine.

¶ More cyst(e)ine is required in the presence of a blocked trans-sulfuration outflow pathway for methionine metabolism.

TABLE 41–2. Metabolic Disorders That Respond to Dietary Treatment

Disorder	Enzyme Defect	Incidence	Clinical/Biochemical Features	Dietary Treatment
Hyperphenylalaninemias				
"Classic" phenylketonuria	Phenylalanine hydroxylase	1:5,000	Blood Phe > 20 mg/dl ↑ Phenylketones in urine Progressive severe MR, prevented by early treatment	↓ Phe, ↑ tyrosine diet to maintain serum Phe at 2–10 mg/dl
"Atypical" phenylketonuria	Phenylalanine hydroxylase	?1:13,000	Blood Phe > 12 mg/dl ↑ Phe in urine MR less severe than in classic PKU	↓ Phe diet (less restrictive than for classic disease)
Hyperphenylalaninemia, benign	Phenylalanine hydroxylase	?1:19,000	Blood Phe < 10 mg/dl ?No effect	?Not necessary
Neonatal hyperphenylalaninemia	Phenylalanine hydroxylase Not inherited		Apparently benign	Not necessary
Offspring of maternal phenylketonuria	None	—	Fetal brain damage	None
Dihydropteridine reductase deficiency	Dihydropteridine reductase	Rare	Blood Phe < 20 mg/dl Irritability, developmental delay, seizures	None 5-hydroxytryptophan, l-3,4-dihydroxyphenylalanine carbidopa may help
Tyrosinemias				
Hereditary tyrosinemia	?	Rare	Vomiting, acidosis, diarrhea, FTT, hepatomegaly, rickets, often fatal ↑ Blood/urine tyrosine, methionine, ↑ urine parahydroxy derivatives of tyrosine	? ↓ Tyrosine, ↓ Phe diet, vitamin D for rickets
Hypertyrosinemia	Cytosol tyrosine aminotransferase	Rare	Keratosis, MR, corneal dystrophy ↑ Blood/urine tyrosine ↑ Urine parahydroxy derivatives of tyrosine	↓ Tyrosine, ↓ Phe diet
Transient neonatal tyrosinemia	?Para-hydroxyphenylpyruvic acid oxidase (appears slowly after birth) Not inherited	?	Initial lethargy ?Long-term effects ↑ Blood/urine tyrosine	Vitamin C 100 mg/day ?↓ Protein intake until tyrosine cleared
Maple Syrup Urine Diseases				
Classic MSUD	Keto acid decarboxylase <5% activity	1:225,000	Early onset, convulsions, acidosis, severe MR, often death Plasma leucine, isoleucine, valine levels 10× normal	Low leucine, isoleucine, valine diet
Intermediate MSUD	Keto acid decarboxylase 25% activity	?1:600,000	Later onset, moderate MR Plasma leucine, isoleucine, and valine levels 5–15× normal	As above
Intermittent MSUD	Keto acid decarboxylase 10–20% activity between episodes	Rare	Intermittent symptoms, can cause death, some MR Plasma leucine, isoleucine, and valine levels 10× normal during episodes	As above
Thiamin-responsive MSUD		Rare	Mild MR Plasma leucine, isoleucine and valine levels 3× normal	Thiamin 100 mg/day Diet as above
Other Amino Acid Disorders				
Homocystinuria	Cystathionine synthase	1:300,000	Arterial and venous thromboses, bony abnormalities, dislocated lens, fair hair and skin, mild to moderate MR ↑ Methionine, ↑ homocystine dislocated lens, fair hair and skin, mild to moderate MR ↑ Methionine, ↑ homocystine	Trial of 500 mg of vitamin B_6/day for 1 mo (if normal folate levels) ?Low-protein, low-methionine diet with added L-cystine
Hyperlysinuria	Lysine ketoglutarate reductase, saccharopine oxido-reductase, saccharopine dehydrogenase	Rare	Probably benign ↑ Blood/urine lysine	Does not require dietary treatment
Histidinemia	Histidinase	1:18,000	Benign ↑ Blood/urine histidine	Does not require dietary treatment

TABLE 41–2. Metabolic Disorders That Respond to Dietary Treatment *Continued*

Disorder	Enzyme Defect	Incidence	Clinical/Biochemical Features	Dietary Treatment
Urea Cycle Disorders				
Carbamyl phosphate synthetase deficiency	Carbamyl phosphate synthetase	Rare	Vomiting, seizures, coma → death Survivors usually have MR ↑ Plasma ammonia, glutamine	Long-term treatment: Low-protein diet as tolerated and sodium benzoate Acute treatment: hemodialysis or peritoneal dialysis with calories and fluids
Ornithine transcarbamylase deficiency	Ornithine transcarbamylase (X-linked)	Rare	Vomiting, seizures, coma → death as newborn usual in males ↑ Plasma ammonia, glutamine, glutamic acid, alanine	?Low-protein diet and sodium benzoate
Citrullinemia	Argininosuccinic acid synthetase	Rare	Neonatal: vomiting, seizures, coma → death Infantile: vomiting, seizures, progressive developmental delay ↑ Plasma citrulline, ammonia, alanine	Low-protein diet, arginine supplements Sodium benzoate
Argininosuccinic aciduria	Argininosuccinic acid lyase	Rare	Neonatal: hypotonia, seizures Subacute: vomiting, FTT, progressive developmental delay ↑ Plasma argininosuccinic acid, citrulline, ammonia	Neonatal: low-protein diet, although often untreatable Subacute: low-protein diet, arginine supplement, dialysis for crisis Sodium benzoate
Argininemia	Arginase	Rare	Periodic vomiting, seizures, coma Progressive spastic diplegia and developmental delay ↑ Arginine, ↑ ammonia with protein intake	?Low-protein diet
Organic Acidemias				
Methylmalonic acidemia	Methylmalonyl CoA mutase or coenzyme B_{12}	Rare	Metabolic acidosis Vomiting, seizures, coma, often death Progressive developmental delay in survivors ↑ Organic acids, ammonia	Long-term: ↑ kcal, ↓ protein diet, B_{12} supplements Acute: IV fluid, bicarbonate
Propionic acidemia	Propionyl CoA carboxylase	Rare	Metabolic acidosis, ↑ ammonia, ↑ propionic acid in blood, ↑ methylcitric acid in urine	Long-term: ↑ kcal, ↓ protein diet Acute: IV fluid, bicarbonate
Carbohydrate Disorders				
Galactosemia	Galactose-1-phosphate uridyl transferase	1:65,000	Vomiting, hepatomegaly, hypoglycemia, FTT, cataracts, MR, often early sepsis ↑ Urine/blood galactose	Galactose- and lactose-free diet
Galactokinase deficiency	Galactokinase	1:40,000	Cataracts ↑ Blood/urine galactose after lactose feeding	As above
Hereditary fructose intolerance	Fructose-1-phosphate aldolase	Rare	Vomiting, hepatomegaly, hypoglycemia, FTT, renal tubular defects after fructose introduction ↑ Blood/urine fructose after fructose feeds	Fructose-, sucrose-, and sorbitol-free diet
Fructose 1,6-diphosphate deficiency	Fructose 1,6-diphosphate	Rare	Hypoglycemia, hepatomegaly, hypotonia, metabolic acidosis → fructose introduction No ↑ fructose in blood or urine	As above
Other Disorders				
Gyrate atrophy of the choroid and retina	Ornithine keto acid transferase	Rare	Progressive gyrate atrophy of choroid and retina with cataracts May also have FTT, hepatic cirrhosis, seizures, MR ↑ Blood/urine ornithine ↓ Blood lysine	?Low-protein diet (low ornithine) with lysine supplements
Cystinuria	Defective proximal renal tubular transport of cystine and dibasic amino acids	1:13,000	Urinary tract calculi ↑ Cystine, ornithine, lysine, and arginine in urine	↑ Fluid intake Bicarbonate to alkalinize urine

Dev = developmental; FTT = failure to thrive; MR = mental retardation; Phe = phenylalanine.

mentation of "natural" and "intervention" history; (3) nutritional therapy is successful; (4) the effects of various therapies, positive or negative, have been observed over time; and (5) the effect on the next generation can be observed.

Phenylketonuria (PKU) is the most common of the hyperphenylalaninemias. In this disorder, phenylalanine (PHE) is not metabolized to tyrosine because of a deficiency or inactivity of phenylalanine hydroxylase, as shown in Figure 41-1. Nutritional treatment involves restriction of the substrate (PHE) and supplementation of the product (tyrosine). Approximately 97% of the cases exhibit the phenylalanine hydroxylase deficiency; the remainder have a defect in associated pathways, either in activity of dihydropteridine reductase (DHPR deficiency) or in the synthesis of biopterin (BH_4). These rare types have been labeled "malignant PKU" because the low-phenylalanine diet does not prevent neurologic deterioration (Early . . . , 1980; New . . . , 1979). However, therapies including administration of tetrahydrofolate for DHPR deficiency and large amounts of BH_4 or neurotransmitter precursors in BH_4 deficiency have been helpful (Irons et al, 1987; Kaufman, 1986) (see Table 41-2).

Diagnosis and Outcome

Currently, most states have newborn screening programs for PKU and other disorders. The Guthrie bacterial inhibition assay, performed on blood, is the most frequently used screening test. The American Academy of Pediatrics has recommended that newborns with a positive screening result should be tested again by both qualitative and quantitative methods (American Academy of Pediatrics, 1982)

Diagnostic criteria are blood levels of phenylalanine consistently above 16 to 20 mg/dl, tyrosine less than about 3 mg/dl, and the presence of phenylpyruvic acid and *o*-hydroxyphenylacetic acid in the urine (Koch et al, 1970). Confirmation of the diagnosis requires quantitative elevations of phenylalanine compounds in both blood and urine. A 72-hour phenylalanine challenge load may be administered at the end of the first year of life to reconfirm the diagnosis if necessary.

Outcome, measured in terms of intelligence quotient (IQ) attainment or intellectual functioning, depends on the age at diagnosis and the start of nutritional therapy, biochemical control over time, and the ability of the family to comply with the regimen. The age at diagnosis and start of nutritional therapy depend on an effective screening program and an organized follow-up program, since infants with PKU do not manifest any clinical signs of abnormality in the immediate postnatal period. Comparisons of treated and untreated children have demonstrated the advantage of rigorous nutritional therapy. Children who have not received diet therapy are severely retarded (mean IQ about 40), whereas children treated since birth have IQs in the normal range of intellectual functioning (Dobson et al, 1977; Williamson et al, 1981).

Nutritional Care for Infants and Children

FORMULA. The restricted phenylalanine diet is planned around the use of a formula with reduced phenylalanine content. The formulas described in Table 41-3 provide a major portion of the daily protein and energy needs for affected infants and children. The most commonly used are Lofenalac, a 95% phenylalanine-free protein hydrolysate used for infants, and Phenyl-free, a 100% phenylalanine-free formula for children and adolescents. Several new products have also been introduced. The Mead Johnson Metabolic Modules and the Ross Metabolic System formulas are described in Table 41-3.

The formula is supplemented with evaporated milk

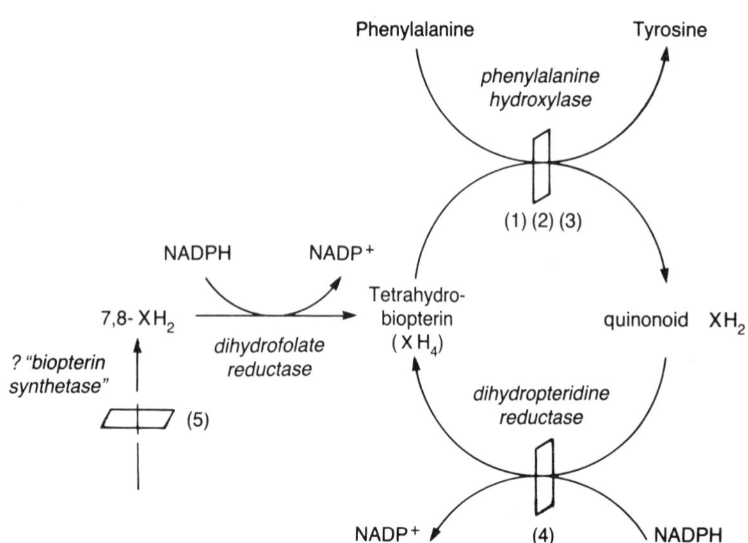

FIGURE 41-1. *Hyperphenylalaninemias: (1) "classic" phenylketonuria, (2) "atypical" phenylketonuria, (3) benign hyperphenylalaninemia, (4) dihydropteridine reductase deficiency, and (5) "biopterin synthetase" deficiency.*

TABLE 41–3. Dietary Products for the Management of Inborn Errors of Metabolism

Disorder	Product	Formulated for Infant	Formulated for Child
Phenylketonuria	Lofenalac*	X	
	Phenyl-free*		X
	PKU 1†	X	
	PKU 2†		X
	PKU 3†	Maternal PKU	
	Maxamaid XP‡		X
	Maxamum XP‡	Women	X
Tyrosinemia	3200AB*	X	X
	TYR 1†	X	
	TYR 2†		X
	Maxamaid XPHEN, TYR‡		X
MSUD and branched-chain amino acid disorders	MSUD Diet Powder*	X	X
	MSUD 1†	X	
	MSUD 2†		X
	Maxamaid MSUD‡		X
	Maxamum MSUD‡	Women and	X
Homocystinuria	3200K*	X	X
	HDM 1†	X	
	HDM 2†		X
	Maxamaid XMET‡		X
Organic acid disorders	OS 1†	X	
	OS 2†		X
	80056*	X	X
	Maxamaid XMET, THRE, VAL, ISOLEU	X	
Histidenemia (special cases only)	HIST 1†	X	
	HIST 2†		X
Hyperlysinemia	LYS 1†	X	
	LYS 2†		X
Urea cycle disorders	UCD 1†	X	
	UCD 2†		X
Carbohydrate	RCF	X	

* Formulas produced by Mead Johnson & Co, Evansville, IN 47221, are primarily a mixture of amino acids and hydrolyzed protein; corn syrup solids and modified tapioca starch to provide carbohydrate; and corn oil to provide fat, plus vitamin and mineral supplements. 80056 is similar in composition but is protein-free. There is some variation in ingredients and supplementation levels among products, thus each intake must be monitored carefully to meet individual needs according to age and metabolic requirements.

† Mead Johnson Special Metabolic Modules are produced by Milupa AG and distributed by Mead Johnson. They are amino acid, vitamin, and mineral mixes that contain no fat and small amounts of carbohydrate from sucrose. Generally, they are supplemented with vegetable oil and a carbohydrate source such as corn syrup to meet individual energy needs. It is necessary to carefully monitor the osmolarity of these formula mixtures for the young infant.

‡ The Ross Metabolic System is distributed by Ross Laboratories, Columbus, OH 43216. They are restricted amino acid, fat-free, vitamin, and mineral mixtures.

or regular infant formula during infancy and early childhood to provide high biologic value protein, nonessential amino acids, and sufficient phenylalanine to meet the individualized requirements of the growing child. The restricted phenylalanine formula and milk mixture should provide 90% of the protein and 80% of the energy needed by infants and toddlers. A method for calculating restricted phenylalanine formula intake is shown in Table 41–4. It must be stressed that formula calculations should provide adequate but not excessive energy intake for infants and should provide appropriate fluid to maintain hydration.

Blood Phenylalanine Control. The blood phenylalanine level must be checked frequently to maintain it within the range of 2 to 10 mg/dl. Phenylalanine-containing foods are offered as tolerated as long as this level remains in the range of good control. The child's rate of growth and mental development must be monitored carefully. Effective management requires a cohesive team in which the child, parents, dietitian, pediatrician, psychologist, social worker, and nurse work together to achieve and maintain biochemical control and to provide an atmosphere for normal mental and emotional development.

Elevations in blood phenylalanine level are generally caused by excessive intake or tissue catabolism. Intakes of phenylalanine in excess of the amount required for growth accumulate in the blood. Deficient energy intake or the trauma of illness or infection result

TABLE 41–4. Guidelines for Low-Protein Food Pattern Calculations

Case Study

M.S. is a 6-month-old infant with phenylketonuria. The information provided in Tables 41–1 and 41–5 can be utilized in planning a food and formula pattern for this child.

Baseline Data

Age	6 months
Sex	Male
Weight (kg)	7.7
Weight percentile	50th
Height (cm)	67.8
Height percentile	50th
Head circumference (cm)	43.3
General health	Good
Activity	Very active

Step 1. Calculate the child's requirement for phenylalanine, protein, and kilocalories (kcal) using Table 41–1.

A. Phenylalanine
7.7 kg body weight × 60* mg phenylalanine/kg/day = 462 mg phenylalanine/day

B. Protein
7.7 kg body weight × 3.3† g protein/kg/day = 25.4 g protein/day

C. Kilocalories
7.7 kg body weight × 115† kcal/kg/day = 885 kcal/day

Step 2. Determine the amount of restricted phenylalanine formula required per day. This information is determined from the infant's or child's protein requirement.

For example: 25.4 g protein/day × 90% of protein from Lofenalac = 22.9 g protein ÷ 1.5 g protein/ms‡ Lofenalac = 15 ms which is equal to 150 g of Lofenalac per day.

Step 3. Determine the amount of evaporated milk to be included in the food pattern. 2 to 2½ oz of evaporated milk is recommended for an infant 4 to 6 months of age.

Step 4. Determine the amount of water to mix with the restricted phenylalanine formula. The consistency of the formula varies according to the infant's age and fluid requirements.

For example: To prepare formula for the infant described in the case study, mix 15 ms (150 g) of Lofenalac and 2½ oz (75 ml) of evaporated milk with 4 oz of water to prevent lumps from forming. Then add water to make a total of 32 oz of formula. This provides 4 bottles of 8 oz each.

Step 5. Determine the amounts of phenylalanine, protein, and kcal in the restricted phenylalanine formula and evaporated milk.

For example:	*Phenylalanine (mg)*	*Protein (g)*	*Kcal*
Lofenalac, 15 ms	120	22.5	681
Evaporated milk, 2½ oz	265	5.5	97
Total	385	28.0	778

Step 6. Determine the amount of phenylalanine, protein, and kilocalories§ to be obtained from foods other than the formula.

Total phenylalanine = 462 mg/day
Phenylalanine in formula = 385 mg/day
Phenylalanine from other foods = 77 mg/day

Total protein	25.4 g/day
Protein in formula	28.0 g/day
Protein from other foods	1.0–2.0 g/day
Total kcal	885 kcal/day
Kcal in formula	778 kcal/day
Kcal from other foods	107 kcal/day

Step 7. Determine the amount of foods other than formula to be included in the dietary plan.§ Use exchange lists in Table 41–5.

	Phenylalanine (mg)	*Protein (g)*	*Kcal*
Baby rice cereal	18	0.4	18
Applesauce, 6 T	8	0.2	72
Green beans, strained, 2 T	18	0.4	8
Banana, mashed, 50 g	22	0.6	44
Carrots, strained, 3 T	9	0.3	12
Total	75	1.9	154

Step 8. Determine the actual amounts of phenylalanine, protein and kcal per kg of body weight by dividing the body weight (in kg) into the total available nutrients:

Phenylalanine (mg)
460 mg phenylalanine ÷ 7.7 kg body weight = 60 mg phenylalanine/kg/day

Protein
29.9 g protein ÷ 7.7 kg body weight = 3.9 g protein/kg/day

Kcal
932 kcal ÷ 7.7 kg body weight = 121 kcal/kg/day

* 60 mg of phenylalanine/kg/day is chosen as a moderate phenylalanine intake. The prescription for phenylalanine must be adapted to individual needs as judged by growth and blood levels.

† Although these intakes are higher than the RDA, they are the intakes found by the Collaborative Study to promote normal growth on protein hydrolysate-based formula. (From Acosta PB et al: Nutrient intake of treated infants with phenylketonuria (PKU). Am J Clin Nutr 30:198, 1977.)

‡ ms = measure, 1 ms of Lofenalac = 1 packed tablespoon

§ Total energy intake must be adjusted to meet individual needs, and an excess must be avoided.

in protein breakdown that releases amino acids into the blood. In general, the anorexia of illness limits phenylalanine intake, and the essential concept is to prevent tissue catabolism by maintaining the intake of formula as much as possible. Although occasionally it may be necessary to offer only clear liquids during an illness, the low-phenylalanine formula should be reintroduced as soon as it is feasible.

LOW-PHENYLALANINE FOODS. Foods of moderate or low phenylalanine content are used as a supplement to the formula mixture. These foods are offered at the appropriate ages to support developmental readiness and also to meet energy needs. Puréed foods from a spoon might be introduced at 5 to 6 months, finger foods at 7 to 8 months, and the cup at 8 to 9 months of age, using the same timing and progression of texture as recommended in Tables 10–8, 10–9, and 12–2 for children on free-choice food patterns. Table 41–5 lists phenylalanine and tyrosine values for selected food groups.

Low-protein pastas, breads, and baked goods made from wheat starch add variety to the food pattern and allow children to eat some foods "to appetite." Sources for low-protein products and cookbooks providing recipes low in phenylalanine content are given in Clinical Insight, page 711. In many cases, parents have created recipes or adapted family favorites to meet the needs of their children. These recipes enable the children to have a variety of textures and food choices and to participate in family meals. Families are also able to meet the energy and phenylalanine needs of their children without resorting to excessive intakes of sugars and concentrated sweets. The availability of aspartame (Nutrasweet), an artificial sweetener that contains phenylalanine, has made food choices more difficult as it now occurs unnoticed or unlabeled in many foods.

A restricted phenylalanine formula (Phenyl-Free) with a more appropriate amino acid, vitamin, and mineral composition for an older child is generally introduced between 3 and 8 years of age. The criteria for introduction are that the child accept the food pattern and formula well and that the child should reliably consume a wide variety of foods from the low-phenylalanine food lists. For example, Phenyl-Free provides a greater flexibility in food choices and menu planning for children and families, which is particularly important as the child enters school or other group settings. Most children and families who are not compliant on their current food pattern are unlikely to be compliant with a different formula. The appropriate use of formulas for older children generally allows a slight liberalization in low-protein food choices. The comparison of a food pattern using Phenyl-Free with a regular food pattern of a child is shown in Table 41–6.

The necessity of continuing the restricted phenylalanine diet beyond 4 to 6 years of age is a consideration in the management of children with PKU. Progressively decreasing IQs, learning difficulties, poor attention span, and behavioral difficulties have been reported in some of the children who have discontinued the dietary regimen (Cabalska et al, 1977; Koch et al, 1982; Smith et al, 1978). As the cohort of children enrolled in the National Collaborative Study matures, those who have maintained well-controlled blood phenylalanine levels are seen to also have higher intellectual achievement (Michals et al, 1988). Good dietary control of blood phenylalanine levels is the best predictor of IQ, whereas "off-diet" blood phenylalanine levels

TABLE 41–5. Serving Lists for PHE-Restricted Diets: Approximate PHE, TYR, Protein, Fat, and Energy Content per Serving*

	Nutrients				
List	*PHE (mg)*	*TYR (mg)*	*Protein (g)*	*Fat (g)*	*Energy (kcal)*
Breads/cereals	30	20	0.6	0	30
Fats	5	4	0.1	5	60
Fruits	15	10	0.5	0	60
Vegetables	15	10	0.5	0	10
Free foods A	5	4	0.1	0	65
Free foods B	0	0	0	Varies	55
Milk, whole (100 ml)	160	160	3.4	3.4	62

* From Acosta PB: Ross Metabolic Formula System Nutrition Support Protocols. © 1989 Columbus, OH, Ross Laboratories.

TABLE 41–6. Comparison of Menus for Children With and Those Without Phenylketonuria

	PKU Menu	Phenylalanine (mg)*	Regular Menu	Phenylalanine (mg)*
Breakfast	Phenyl-Free	0	Milk	450
	Rice Krispies		Rice Krispies	
	Orange juice		Orange juice	
Lunch	Jelly sandwich with low-protein bread	18	Jelly sandwich with white bread	260
	Banana		Banana	
	Carrot and celery sticks		Carrot and celery sticks	
	Low-protein chocolate chip cookies	4	Chocolate chip cookies	60
	Juice		Juice	
Snack	Phenyl-Free	0	Milk	450
	Orange		Orange	
	Potato chips (small bag)		Potato chips	
Dinner	Phenyl-Free	0	Milk	450
	Salad		Salad	
	Low-protein spaghetti with tomato sauce	8	Spaghetti with meatballs	240
				600
	Baskin-Robbins fruit ice	10	Ice cream	120
Estimated intake		400		2900

* Phenylalanine values provided only for those foods that differ between the two patterns.

are the best predictors of IQ loss (Waisbren et al, 1987). The current recommendation from most treatment centers is that the restricted phenylalanine diet should be continued for life.

Education on Diet Management. The energy needs and amino acid requirements of children with PKU do not differ appreciably from children in general. With proper diet management, normal growth can be expected. However, parents may tend to offer excessive energy as sweets because they feel that the child is being deprived of food experiences. Health care providers should stress to parents that children with PKU are well children who must make careful food choices for themselves as opposed to chronically ill children who require food indulgences. Appropriate clinical interaction with the family provides them with the information and skills to differentiate between food behaviors that are normal to the age and developmental level of the child and those related specifically to PKU (Trahms, 1986). To avoid power struggles and conflicts over food, it is advisable to involve the child in choosing appropriate foods at an early age. Two- and 3-year old children can master the concept of appropriate choices when foods are categorized as YES foods and NO foods. The concept of an appropriate quantity of a food can be introduced to a 3- or 4-year-old child as "how many" by counting crackers or raisins, and then as "how much" by weighing or measuring foods such as cereal or fruit (Heffernan and Trahms, 1981). The child then moves to more complex tasks (e.g., formula and food preparation) and planning meals (e.g., breakfast or a packed lunch). Responsibility for planning a full day's menu by calculating the quantity of phenylalanine in portions of food and compiling the daily total is the ultimate goal. These age-related tasks are shown in Table 41–7.

Psychosocial Development. The necessity for maintaining a carefully controlled food intake may encourage parents to overprotect their children and perhaps to restrict their social activities (Smith et al, 1988). The children, in turn, may react against their parents and their nutritional therapy. The ability of the family to respond to the stresses of PKU as reflected in adaptability and cohesion scores is shown by better blood phenylalanine levels and in the positive coping behaviors of the older children with PKU (Kazak et al, 1988; Nowak-Cooperman et al, 1987; Trahms et al, 1987). Thus, continuation of nutritional therapy beyond early childhood requires that children become knowledgeable about and responsible for management of their own food choices (Fig. 41–2). It also becomes the responsibility of the health care team to work with families and children to provide them with strategies that enable children and adolescents to participate in social and school activities, interact with peers, and progress through the usual developmental stages with self-confidence and self-esteem (Rees and Trahms, 1987; Trahms, 1986).

TABLE 41–7. Tasks to be Expected by Age Level

Age	School-Level	Task
2–3 years	Preschool	Distinguish yes/no foods
3–4 years	Preschool	Counting: how many?
4–5 years	Preschool	Measuring: how much?
5–6	K'garten	Prepare own formula; use of scale
	Grade 1–2	Basic notes on food diaries
	Grade 2	Some decisions on after school snack
	Grade 3	Breakfast preparation
	Grade 4	Packing lunches
	Middle school	Increasingly independent management of food choices
	High school	Independent management of PKU

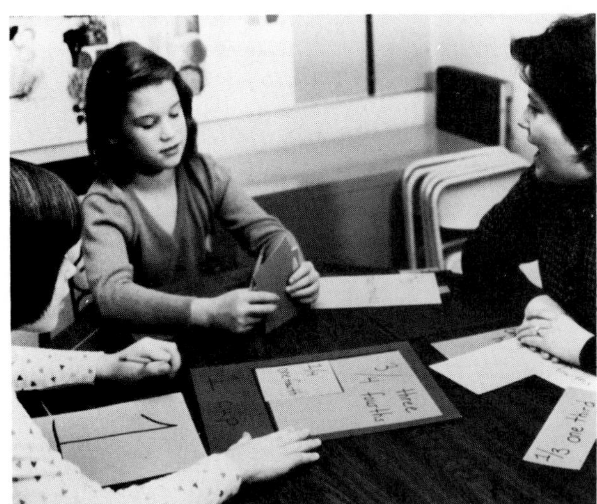

FIGURE 41–2. *Older children learning to manage their own low-phenylalanine diets by calculating their intakes and by sharing with peers.*

Children require parental and professional support as they begin to assume responsibility for their food management. Self-management of food choices avoids the risk of the child using dietary noncompliance as a wedge against parental restrictions. Normal intellectual development is a laudable goal of management of PKU, but to be entirely successful, the children with PKU need to concomitantly develop self-assurance and a strong self-image. This can be achieved in part by fostering self-management, independence, and a normal lifestyle for these children.

Nutritional Care in Maternal Phenylketonuria

A pregnant woman with elevated blood phenylalanine levels endangers her fetus because of the amplified transport of amino acids across the placenta. The fetus is exposed to about twice the phenylalanine level of normal maternal blood. Babies whose mothers have elevated blood phenylalanine levels have an increased occurrence of cardiac defects, retarded growth, microcephaly, and mental retardation, as listed in Table 41–8. It appears that the fetus is at risk of damage with only minor elevations in maternal blood phenylalanine levels and that the higher the level, the more severe will be the effect (Lenke and Levy, 1980; Rohr et al, 1987).

The management of nutritional therapy during pregnancy for a women with hyperphenylalaninemia is complex. The changing physiology of pregnancy and concomitant changing nutritional needs are difficult to monitor with the precision required to maintain appropriately low blood phenylalanine levels. Even with meticulous attention to phenylalanine intake, blood levels, and the nutritional requirements of pregnancy, a woman cannot be assured of a normal infant. Prepregnancy management of blood phenylalanine levels may decrease the risk to the fetus, but success cannot be ensured. When prepregnancy management is not possible, the restricted phenylalanine diet should be started as soon as possible after conception (Lenke and Levy, 1982; Rohr et al, 1987). The risks of abnormal development of the fetus even with dietary management are an important consideration for young women with PKU who are considering pregnancy. The only risk-free choice is to avoid pregnancy (Lowitzer, 1987).

Nutritional management during pregnancy is difficult even for women who have consistently been on a low-phenylalanine diet since infancy. Women who have been off the diet generally find that reinstitution of formula consumption and limitation of food choices constitute a difficult if not an overwhelming task. Compliance with nutritional therapy during pregnancy for even the well-motivated woman requires family and professional support as well as frequent monitoring of biochemical and nutritional aspects of both pregnancy and phenylketonuria.

Nutritional Care for Adults with Phenylketonuria

With improvements in diagnosis and treatment, adults with PKU are less likely to be affected by neurologic damage. However, among those who have had some degree of mental retardation, hyperactivity and self-abuse are often major concerns. Not all patients have

TABLE 41–8. Frequency of Abnormalities in Children Born to Mothers with Phenylketonuria (%)*

	Maternal Phenylalanine Levels (mg/dl)				
Complication	*20*	*16–19*	*11–15*	*3–10*	**Non-PKU Mother**
Mental retardation	92	73	22	21	5.0
Microcephaly	73	68	35	24	4.8
Congenital heart disease	12	15	6	0	0.8
Low birthweight	40	52	56	13	9.6

* Adapted from Lenke RR and Levy HL: Maternal phenylketonuria and hyperphenylalaninemia: An international survey of the outcome of untreated and treated pregnancies. N Engl J Med 303:1202, 1980. Adapted from information appearing in NEJM.

responded with improved behavior or intellectual functioning to the institution of a low-phenylalanine food pattern. However, it has been recommended that for the older patient who is difficult to manage, a trial of the low-phenylalanine food pattern should be tried. If successful, continued diet therapy may aid in management.

Organic Acid Disorders

In the past 10 years, organic acid disorders have been increasingly identified. This is a function of more effective diagnosis and a better understanding of the genetic basis of these disorders. Treatment modalities have been refined and involve the increased or decreased intake of specific nutrients. L-Carnitine is currently being evaluated for its efficacy in treatment (Bartholomew et al, 1988).

Propionic acidemia is a defect of propionyl CoA carboxylase in the pathway of propionyl CoA to methylmalonyl CoA, as illustrated in Figure 41–3. The clinical course can be varied but is generally marked by vomiting, lethargy, hypotonia, dehydration, seizures, and coma. Survivors often have permanent neurologic damage. Metabolic acidosis with a marked anion gap and hyperammonemia are characteristic. Long-chain ketonuria may also be present. Some patients with propionic acidemia may respond to pharmacologic doses of biotin. A dose of 10 mg/day of biotin has been suggested. Careful assessment of responsiveness is required (Wolf et al, 1981).

At least five separate enzyme deficiencies have been identified that result in *methylmalonic acidemia.* The defect of methylmalonyl CoA mutase apoenzyme is identified most frequently (see Fig. 41–3). The clinical features are similar to those of propionic acidemia. Acidosis is common, and diagnosis is documented by large amounts of methylmalonic acid in blood and urine. Other findings include hypoglycemia, ketonuria, and elevation of plasma ammonia and lactate. There is also a need to rule out frank vitamin B_{12} deficiency, since vitamin B_{12} yields two cofactors that are required to convert methylmalonate to succinate and homocysteine to methionine. The vitamin B_{12}-responsive patient may respond to pharmacologic doses of 1 to 2 mg/day (Walsher and Stewart, 1981).

The goals of management of acute episodes of propionic acidemia and methylmalonic acidemia are to achieve and maintain normal nutrient intake and biochemical balance. Maintenance of energy and fluid in-

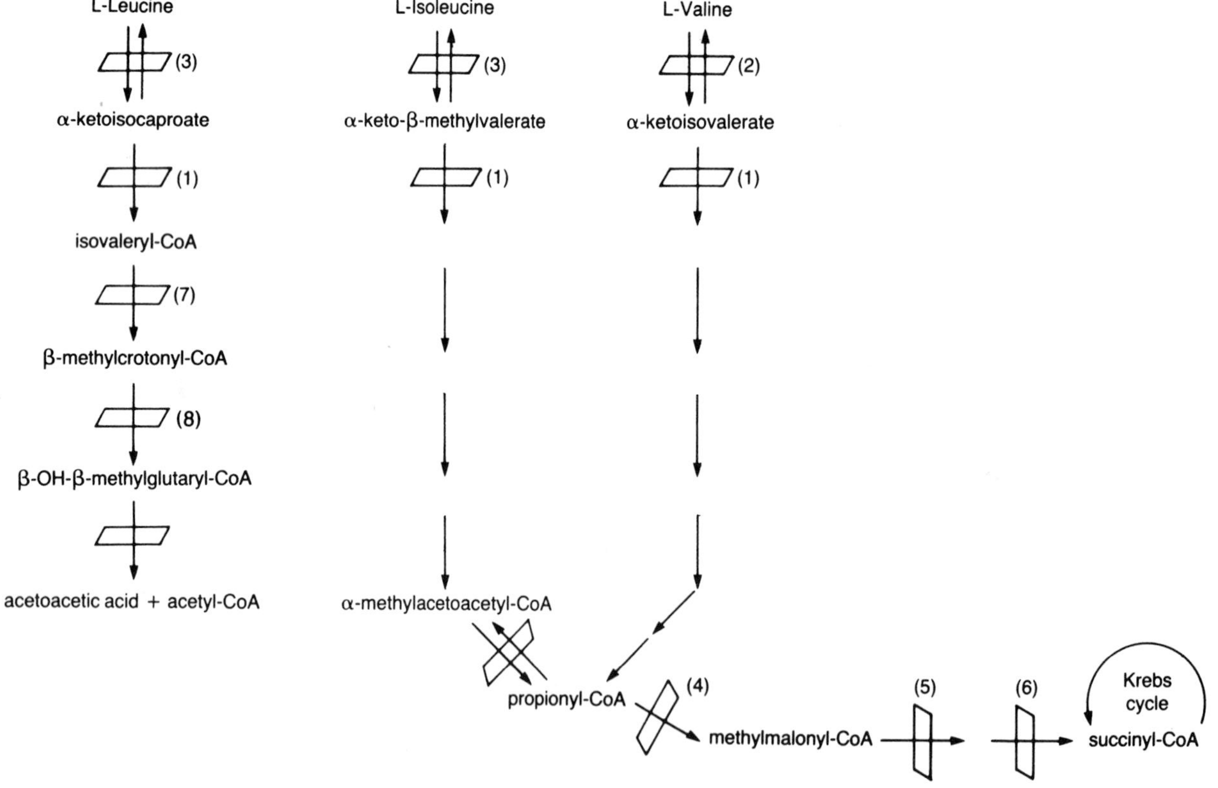

FIGURE 41–3. *Organic acidemias and MSUD: (1) branched-chain ketoacid decarboxylase (MSUD), (2) valine aminotransferase, (3) leucine-isoleucine aminotransferase, (4) propionyl CoA carboxylase (propionic acidemia), (5) methylmalonyl CoA racemase (methylmalonic aciduria), (6) methylmalonyl CoA mutase (methylmalonic aciduria), (7) isovaleryl CoA dehydrogenase (isovaleric acidemia), and (8) beta-methylcroteryl CoA carboxylase (biotin-responsive multiple carboxylase deficiency).*

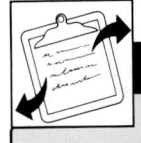

CLINICAL INSIGHT: Sources of Low-Protein Foods

Source	Products
Dietary Specialities PO Box 227 Rochester, NY 14601 (716-263-2787)	Low-protein pastas Low-protein rusks Wheat starch Prono (Gelled Dessert Mix) Porridge
Ener-G Foods, Inc 5960 1st Ave S PO Box 84487 Seattle, WA 98124-5787 (1-800-331-5222)	Ener-G low-protein bread and mix Egg replacer Low-protein pastas and cookies
Med-Diet Inc. 3050 Ranchview Ln. Plymouth, MN 55447 (1-800-633-3438)	Unimix low-protein bread and mix Low-protein pastas and cookies

take is important to prevent tissue catabolism and dehydration. Electrolyte imbalances are corrected by the usual methods, and abnormal metabolites are removed by urinary excretion promoted by a large fluid intake. Relapses of metabolic acidoses may result from excessive protein intake, infection, or unidentified reasons. Parents become skilled at identifying early signs of illness. Treatment for these episodes must be rapid because coma and death can occur quickly.

Long-term nutritional therapy includes an appropriate balance of essential nutrients and a protein intake restricted to 1 to 1.5 g/kg/day. Response to protein intake varies; some patients require little or no protein restriction and can be self-regulated, whereas others may require severe protein restrictions (Trahms, 1987). An adequate fluid intake is required to normalize blood ammonia levels. Nutritional therapy may be complicated by food refusal and by lack of appetite, which compromise medical management (Hyman et al, 1987). Information on long-term prognosis is very limited.

Urea Cycle Defects

Diagnosis and treatment of defects in the urea cycle have also advanced (Ohtani et al, 1988). All such defects result in an accumulation of ammonia in the blood. The clinical signs of elevated ammonia are vomiting and lethargy, which may progress to seizures, coma, and ultimately death. In infants, the adverse effects of elevated ammonia levels are rapid and devastating. In older children, symptoms of elevated ammonia may be preceded by hyperactivity and irritability. The severity and variation of the clinical course of all of the urea cycle defects may be related to the degree of residual enzyme activity. The common urea cycle defects are discussed in a progression that proceeds around the urea cycle as shown in Figure 41–4.

Ornithine transcarbamylase deficiency (OTC deficiency) is an X-linked recessive disorder marked by a block in the conversion of ornithine and carbamyl phosphate to citrulline. OTC deficiency is identified by hyperammonemia, increased urinary orotic acid, and normal levels of citrulline, argininosuccinic acid, and arginine (Brubakk et al, 1982). OTC deficiency is usually lethal in males, whereas heterozygous females with various degrees of enzyme activity may not demonstrate symptoms of this defect until placed under stress by infection or by a significant increase in the protein content of the diet.

Citrullinemia is the result of a deficiency of argininosuccinic acid synthetase in the metabolism of citrulline to argininosuccinic acid. Citrullinemia is identified by markedly elevated citrulline in the urine and blood. Argininosuccinic acid synthetase activity is absent or decreased in cultured skin fibroblasts. Symptoms may be present in the neonatal period or may develop gradually in early infancy. These symptoms are poor feeding and recurrent vomiting which, without immediate treatment, progress to seizures, neurologic abnormalities, and coma.

Argininosuccinic aciduria (ASA) is the result of a deficiency of argininosuccinate lyase, which is involved in the metabolism of argininosuccinic acid to arginine. ASA is identified by the presence of argininosuccinic acid in urine and blood. Citrulline may be moderately elevated in blood and urine. Argininosuccinate lyase activity is absent or decreased in cultured fibroblasts or in red blood cells.

Citrullinemia and ASA have essentially the same

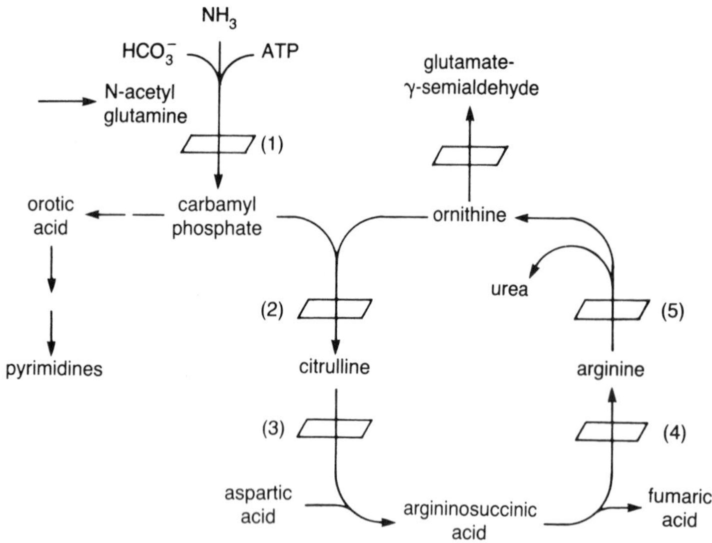

FIGURE 41–4. *Urea cycle disorders: (1) carbamyl phosphate synthetase (CPS deficiency), (2) ornithine carbamyl transferase (OTC deficiency), (3) argininosuccinic acid synthetase (citrullinemia), (4) argininosuccinic acid lyase (argininosuccinic aciduria), and (5) arginase (arginemia).*

clinical presentation. The aim of therapy for both of these defects is to prevent or decrease hyperammonemia and the detrimental neurologic consequences associated with the high amino acid levels. Acute episodes of illness are managed by the discontinuation of protein intake and by the administration of intravenous fluids and glucose to correct the dehydration and provide energy. If hyperammonemia is severe, peritoneal dialysis, hemodialysis, or exchange transfusion may be required. Intravenous arginine and sodium benzoate have also been beneficial in reducing the hyperammonemia.

Long-term therapy consists of a restricted protein diet at 1 to 2 g/kg/day, depending on individual tolerance. The food pattern should be supplemented with L-arginine (1 g/day for infants, 2 g/day for older children) to prevent arginine deficiency and to assist in waste nitrogen excretion (Brusilow and Batshaw, 1979). Sodium benzoate at 0.25 g/kg/day is frequently prescribed to aid in ammonia excretion. Keto analogues of essential amino acids have also been tried but are reported to be no more effective than a low-protein diet plus arginine (Batshaw et al, 1982). Because of the effect of infection and illness on the urea cycle, infections should be treated aggressively.

Carbamyl phosphate synthetase (CPS) deficiency is manifested in a very similar manner with hyperammonemic episodes. The onset is usually in the early neonatal period with vomiting, irritability, hypothermia, respiratory distress, altered muscle tone, lethargy, and often coma. Specific laboratory findings usually include elevated plasma glutamine and normal or low orotic acid in urine. Therapy for carbamyl phosphate synthetase deficiency is essentially the same as that described for citrullinemia and ASA, except that arginine in high doses is not indicated.

Neurologic outcome and intellectual development in those with urea cycle defects vary, with a range from normal IQ and motor function to severe mental retardation and cerebral palsy. Although information on a long-term follow-up is limited, the use of alternate pathways for waste nitrogen excretion and a protein-restricted diet to control ammonia levels may improve the outcome.

Maple Syrup Urine Disease

Classic *maple syrup urine disease (MSUD)* or *branched-chain ketoaciduria* results from a defect in decarboxylation that affects the metabolism of the branched-chain amino acids (BCAA) leucine, isoleucine, and valine (see Fig. 41–3). This rare autosomal recessive metabolic defect is estimated to occur in 1 in 225,000 newborns. Infants appear normal at birth, but by 4 or 5 days of age they demonstrate poor feeding, vomiting, lethargy, and periodic hypertonia. A characteristic sweet, malty odor from urine and perspiration appears toward the end of the first week of life. Failure to treat this condition leads to acidosis, neurologic deterioration, seizures, and coma, proceeding eventually to death. Because of the rapid onset of symptoms, results of newborn screening are often too late to initiate treatment before symptoms appear. Management of acute disease requires peritoneal dialysis and hydration. BCAA are introduced gradually into the diet when plasma leucine levels are decreased to 1 mM (Clow et al, 1981).

The precise mechanism of the complete decarboxylase reaction and the resultant neurologic damage are not known. Neither is it understood why leucine metabolism is significantly more abnormal than the other two BCAA. Clinical relapse is most often related to the degree of abnormality of the leucine level, and these relapses are frequently related to infection. Acute infections are a medical emergency; most children who have died despite being on therapy have done so during an episode of infection. If the plasma leucine level rises to over 20 mg/dl, BCAA should be removed immediately from the diet and intravenous therapy should be started.

Reports have indicated that early intervention and meticulous biochemical control can provide a more hopeful prognosis than was realized earlier. Reasonable growth and intellectual development in the normal to low-normal range have been described in a series of four patients, the oldest being 9 years of age (Clow et al, 1981). It is recommended that plasma leucine levels be maintained between 2 and 5 mg/dl. Levels above 10 mg/dl are associated with alpha-ketoacidemia and with neurologic symptoms.

Nutritional therapy requires very careful monitoring of blood levels (especially leucine), growth, and general nutritional adequacy. Several formulas specifically designed for the treatment of this disorder are now available to provide a reasonable amino acid and vitamin mixture (see Table 41-3). These generally are supplemented with a small quantity of infant formula or cow's milk to provide the BCAA needed to support growth and development. The relative leucine, isoleucine, and valine values of food groups are given in Table 41-9.

Protein-Restricted Diets

Infants and children with metabolic disorders such as urea cycle defects or organic acidemias may require diets that are restricted in protein. The most usual restrictions are for 0.5, 1, 1.5, and 2 grams of protein per kilogram of body weight. The appropriate prescription for protein level is based on the individual's tolerance. The highest level tolerated should be fed to ensure adequate growth and a margin of nutritional safety.

In general, low-protein or restricted-protein diets can be formulated from readily available infant and toddler foods. Infant formula can be diluted to meet the prescribed protein level. The resultant energy deficit is made up by supplementing carbohydrate and fat. Specialty modular formulas may also be feasible (see Table 41-3). The appropriate choice depends on the level of restriction, age, and condition of the child. Formulas should be at 20 kcal/oz and should supply at least 100 kcal/kg of energy. Osmolality of the formula must be considered; feedings of no more than 400 mOsm/l of solution have been recommended, although it must be noted that measurement of specific product osmolalities is not always possible (Martin and Acosta, 1987). Usual recommendations for vitamins and minerals are appropriate.

DISORDERS OF CARBOHYDRATE METABOLISM

Galactosemia

Galactosemia, a high level of plasma galactose combined with galactosuria, is found in two metabolic disorders that are both of autosomal recessive inheritance. The disorders are *galactokinase deficiency* and *galactose-1-phosphate uridyl transferase deficiency,* which is also called *classic galactosemia.*

Galactosemia results from a disturbance in the conversion of galactose to glucose because of the absence of one of the enzyme activities shown in Figure 41-5. The deficiencies cause an accumulation of galactose, or galactose and galactose-1-phosphate in body tissues. It is believed that galactose-1-phosphate in intercellular fluids causes the cellular disturbances in classic galactosemia.

If an infant has no galactose-1-phosphate uridyl transferase activity, illness generally occurs within the first 2 weeks of life. Symptoms are vomiting, diarrhea,

TABLE 41-9. Equivalency Lists for BCAA-Restricted Diets: Average ILE, LEU, VAL, Protein, Fat and Energy Content per Serving*

List	ILE (mg)	LEU (mg)	VAL (mg)	Protein (g)	Fat (g)	Energy (kcal)
Breads/cereals	18	35	25	0.5	0	30
Fats	7	10	7	0.1	8	70
Fruits	17	25	22	0.6	0	75
Vegetables	22	30	24	0.6	0	15
Free foods A	3	5	4	0.1	Varies	50
Free foods B	0	0	0	0	Varies	55
Milk, whole (100 ml)	203	329	224	3.4	3.4	62

* From Acosta PB: Ross Metabolic Formula System Nutrition Support Protocols. © 1989 Columbus, OH, Ross Laboratories.

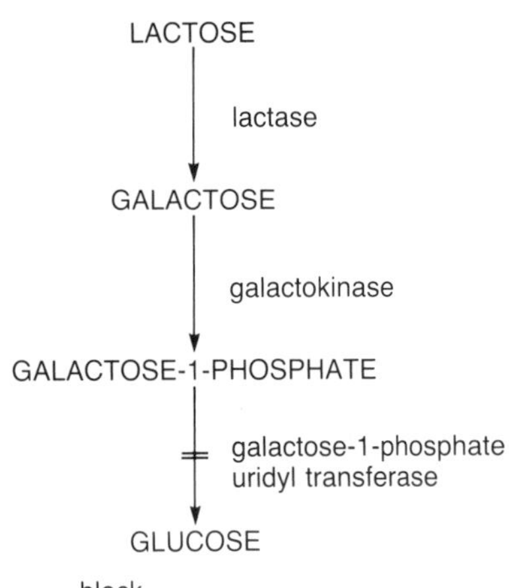

FIGURE 41–5. *Schematic metabolism of galactose in galactosemia.*

lethargy, failure to thrive, jaundice, hepatomegaly, and cataracts. Infants with galactosemia may be hypoglycemic and are susceptible to infection from gram-negative organisms. If the condition is not treated, death is frequently caused by septicemia. If diagnosis and therapy are delayed, mental retardation can result.

Diagnosis of transferase deficiency is accomplished in a stepwise fashion. Sick newborns are first screened for urinary non–glucose-reducing sugars, which are identified by a positive result on Benedict's test and a negative result on a glucose paper strip test. This is followed by the Beutler test for transferase enzyme activity and by confirmation of diagnosis by specific enzyme tests.

Galactosemia is treated by lifelong galactose restriction. Although galactose is required for the production of galactolipids and cerebrosides, it can be produced by an alternative pathway if all galactose is omitted from the food intake. Galactose restriction mandates that all milk and milk products and lactose-containing foods should be strictly avoided, because lactose is hydrolyzed into galactose and glucose. Recent data suggest the additional restriction of fruits and vegetables that contain significant amounts of galactose. Dates, papayas, bell peppers, persimmons, tomatoes and watermelon all contain more than 10 mg galactose/100 g fresh weight of product (Gross and Acosta, 1991). Effective galactose restriction makes it essential to read labels on all food products carefully. Milk is added to many products, and lactose often appears in the coating of the tablet form of medications. Table 41–10 presents a galactose-free food pattern.

With early diagnosis and treatment, physical progress should be good with resolution of physical problems, sometimes even of cataracts. Mental development is generally slightly less than expected; patients often have an IQ of 85 to 100, and visual-perceptual difficulties are common (Fischler et al, 1980).

A few treated women with galactosemia have become pregnant and have given birth to healthy babies, although ovarian failure is a recognized problem in women who are affected with galactosemia (Kaufman et al, 1988).

Galactokinase deficiency requires the same galactose-restricted regimen as galactosemia. Cataracts form, but the other sequelae of galactosemia have not been described.

TABLE 41–10. Food List for Galactose-Free Food Pattern

Foods Allowed	Foods Not Allowed
Milk and Milk Substitutes	
Isomil Neo-Mull-Soy Nutramigen Prosobee Soyalac	Breast milk All forms of animal milk Imitation or filled milk Cream, butter, some margarines Cottage cheese, cream cheese Hard cheeses Yogurt Ice cream, ice milk, sherbert
Fruits	
All fresh, frozen, canned, or dried except those processed with unsafe ingredients*	Dates, papaya, bell pepper, persimmon, tomato and watermelon contain >10 mg galactose/100 g fresh weight. Intake of fruits and vegetables that contain galactose needs to be monitored carefully.
Vegetables	
All fresh, frozen, canned, or dried except those processed with unsafe ingredients,* seasoned with butter or margarine, breaded or creamed	
Meat, Poultry, Fish, Eggs, Nuts	
Plain beef, lamb, veal, pork, ham, fish, turkey, chicken, game, fowl Kosher frankfurters Eggs Nut butters, nuts	
Breads and Cereals	
Cooked and dry cereals, bread or crackers without milk or unsafe ingredients* Macaroni, spaghetti, noodles, rice, tortillas	
Fats	
All vegetable oils All shortening, lard, margarines, salad dressings except those made with unsafe ingredients* Mayonnaise Olives	

* Unsafe ingredients are milk, buttermilk, cream, lactose, galactose, casein, caseinate, whey, dry milk solids, or curds. Labels should be regularly and carefully checked, because formulations of products change frequently.

NOTE: Lactose is often used as a pharmaceutical bulking agent, filler, or excipient, thus tablets, tinctures, and vitamin and mineral mixtures should be carefully evaluated. The PDR (Physician's Desk Reference) now lists active and inactive ingredients in medications. Manufacturers' telephone numbers are also listed.

Other Disorders

Table 41–2 outlines additional disorders with respect to the enzymatic defects involved, the outstanding clinical and biochemical features, and the current dietary treatment.

CITED REFERENCES

American Academy of Pediatrics, Committee on Genetics: New issues in newborn screening for phenylketonuria and hypothyroidism: A commentary. Pediatrics 69:104, 1982.

Bartholomew DW et al: Therapeutic approaches to cobalamin-C methylmalonic acidemia and homocystinuria. J Pediatr 112:32, 1988.

Batshaw ML et al: Treatment of inborn errors of urea synthesis: Activation of alternative pathways of waste nitrogen synthesis and excretion. N Engl J Med 306:1387, 1982.

Brubakk AM et al: Successful treatment of severe OTC deficiency. J Pediatr 100:929, 1982.

Brusilow SW and Batshaw ML: Arginine therapy of arginine-succinase deficiency. Lancet 1:124, 1979.

Cabalska B et al: Termination of dietary treatment in phenylketonuria. Eur J Pediatr 126:253, 1977.

Clow CL, Reade TM, and Scriver CR: Outcome of early and long-term management of classical maple syrup urine disease. Pediatrics 68:856, 1981.

Dobson JC et al: Intellectual assessment of 111 4-year-old children with phenylketonuria. Pediatrics 60:885, 1977.

Early diagnosis of hyperphenylalaninemia due to tetrahydrobiopterin deficiency (malignant hyperphenylalaninemia). J Pediatr 96:854, 1980.

Fischler K et al: Developmental aspects of galactosemia from infancy to childhood. Clin Pediatr 19:38, 1980.

Gross KC and Acosta PB: Fruits and vegetables are a source of galactose: Implication in planning the diets of patients with galactosaemia. J Inher Metab Dis 14:253, 1991.

Hanley WB et al: Malnutrition with early treatment of phenylketonuria. Pediatr Res 4:318, 1970.

Heffernan JF and Trahms CM: A model preschool for patients with phenylketonuria. J Am Diet Assoc 79:306, 1981.

Holt LE and Snyderman SE: The amino acid requirements of children. *In* Nyhan WL (ed): Amino Acid Metabolism and Genetic Variation. New York, McGraw-Hill, 1967, pp 381–390.

Hyman SL et al: Behavior management of feeding disturbances in urea cycle and organic acid disorders. J Pediatr 111:558, 1987.

Irons M et al: Folinic acid therapy in treatment of dihydropteridine reductase deficiency. J Pediatr 110:61, 1987.

Kaufman FR et al: Correlation of ovarian function with galactose-1-phosphate uridyl transferase levels in galactosemia. J Pediatr 112:754, 1988.

Kaufman, S: Unsolved problems in diagnosis and therapy of hyperphenylalaninemia caused by defects in tetrahydrobiopterin metabolism. J Pediatr 109:572, 1986.

Kazak AE et al: Childhood chronic disease and family functioning: A study of phenylketonuria. Pediatrics 81:224, 1988.

Koch R et al: An approach to management of phenylketonuria. J Pediatr 76:815, 1970.

Koch R et al: Preliminary report on the effects of diet discontinuation on PKU. J Pediatr 100:870, 1982.

Lenke RR and Levy HL: Maternal phenylketonuria and hyperphenylalaninemia: An international survey of the outcome of untreated and treated pregnancies. N Engl J Med 303:1202, 1980.

Lenke RR and Levy HL: Maternal phenylketonuria: Results of dietary therapy. Am J Obstet Gynecol 142:548, 1982.

Lowitzer AC: Maternal phenylketonuria: Cause for concern among women with PKU. Res Dev Dis 8:1, 1987.

Martin SB and Acosta PB: Osmolalities of selected enteral products and carbohydrate modules used to treat inherited metabolic disorders. J Am Diet Assoc 87:48, 1987.

Michals K et al: Blood phenylalanine levels and intelligence of 10-year-old children with PKU in the National Collaborative Study. J Am Diet Assoc 88:1226, 1988.

New varieties of PKU (Editorial). Lancet 1:304, 1979.

Nowak-Cooperman KM et al: The impact of assertiveness, self-concept and coping behavior on self-management abilities in adolescents with phenylketonuria (Abstract). J Adolesc Health Care 8:305, 1987.

Ohtani Y et al: Secondary carnitine deficiency in hyperammonemic attacks of ornithine transcarbamylase deficiency. J Pediatr 112:409, 1988.

Rees JM and Trahms CM: The adolescent and phenylketonuria: Promoting self-management. Top Clin Nutr 2(3):35, 1987.

Rohr FJ et al: New England Maternal PKU Project: Prospective study of untreated and treated pregnancies and their outcomes. J Pediatr 110:391, 1987.

Smith I et al: Behavior disturbance in 8-year-old children with early treated phenylketonuria. J Pediatr 112:403, 1988.

Smith I et al: Effect of stopping low-phenylalanine diet on intellectual progress of children with phenylketonuria. Br Med J 2:723, 1978.

Snyderman SE et al: The nutritional therapy of histidinemia. J Pediatr 95:712, 1979.

Trahms CM et al: Impact of patient attitudes and family function on compliance with treatment for phenylketonuria (Abstract). J Adolesc Health Care 8:305, 1987.

Trahms CM: Long-term nutrition intervention model: The treatment of phenylketonuria. Top Clin Nutr 1(1):62:1986.

Trahms CM: Low protein diets for children: Guidelines for treatment of common organic acidemias and urea cycle disorders. Top Clin Nutr 2(3):49, 1987.

Waisbren SE et al: Predictors of intelligence quotient and intelligence quotient change in persons treated for phenylketonuria early in life. Pediatrics 79:351, 1987.

Walsher M and Stewart PM: Organic acidemia and hyperammonaemia: A review. J Inher Metab Dis 4:177, 1981.

Williamson MS et al: Correlates of intelligence tests results in treated phenylketonuric children. Pediatrics 68:161, 1981.

Wolf B et al: Propionic acidemia: A clinical update. J Pediatr 99:835, 1981.

ADDITIONAL REFERENCES

Guides for Professionals

Acosta PB and Wenz E: Diet Management of PKU for infants and preschool children. DHEW Publ No (HSA) 78-5209, 1978.

Ampola MG: Metabolic Disease in Pediatric Practice. Boston, Little, Brown, 1982.

An overview of Newborn Screening Programs in the United States and Canada: 1988, Genetic Diseases Program. Springfield, IL, Division of Family Health, Dept of Public Health, 1988.

Available from Clinical Investigation Unit, Nutrition Division, The Hospital for Sick Children, 555 University Avenue, Toronto, Ontario, Canada, M5X 1G8:

Bell L: Arginine Equivalency System, 1980.

Bell L: HSC Equivalency System for Dietary Treatment of Maple Syrup Urine Disease, 1979.

Bell L: Low Protein Equivalency System, 1981.

Bell L: The Phenylalanine Content of Foods, 1980.

Burton BK: Inborn errors of metabolism: The clinical diagnosis in early infancy. Pediatrics 79:359, 1987.

Henderson RA et al: PKU and the Schools: Information for Teachers, Administrators, and Other School Personnel. DHEW Publ No (HSA) 80-5233, 1980.

Holm VA et al: Physical growth in phenylketonuria. II: Growth of treated children in the PKU Collaborative Study from birth to 4 years of age. Pediatrics 63:700, 1979.

Management of Newborn Infants with Phenylketonuria. DHEW Publ No (HSA)70-5211, 1979.

Products for Dietary Management of Inborn Errors of Metabolism and Other Special Feeding Problems. Evansville, IN, Mead Johnson, 1983.

Schuett VE: Low protein cookery for PKU. Madison, WI, University of Wisconsin Press, 1982.

State Treatment Centers for Metabolic Disorders. Washington, DC, National Center for Education in Maternal and Child Health, 1986.

Guides for Parents

Available from National Maternal and Child Health Clearinghouse, 38th and R streets, NW, Washington, DC 20057, (202)625-8410:
Barr LA and Trahms CM: Chef Lophe's Phe-nominal Cookbook.
Trahms CM and Cox C: A Babysitter's Guide to PKU.
Trahms CM, Cox C and Luce P: Games that Teach: Learning by Doing for Preschoolers with PKU.
Trahms CM et al: Finger Foods are Fun.
Trahms CM and Luce P: New Parents' Guide to PKU.

Available from Florida State University, Center for Family Studies, 103 Sandels Bldg, Tallahassee, FL 32306:
Acosta, PB et al: A Parent's Guide to the Child with Maple Syrup Urine Disease.
Acosta, PB et al: Parent's Guide to the Child with PKU.

Available from University of Wisconsin Press, 114 N Murray Street, Madison, WI 53715:
Schuett VE: Low-Protein Cookery for Phenylketonuria, 2nd ed.
Taylor M and Schuett VE: You and PKU.

APPENDICES

APPENDIX 1. Nutritive Value of the Edible Part of Food*

Item No.	Foods, Approximate Measures, Units, and Weight (Weight of Edible Portion Only)			Water	Food energy	Protein	Fat	Fatty Acids: Saturated	Fatty Acids: Monounsaturated	Fatty Acids: Polyunsaturated
	BEVERAGES		Grams	%	Calories	Grams	Grams	Grams	Grams	Grams
	Alcoholic:									
	Beer:									
1	Regular	12 fl oz	360	92	150	1	0	0.0	0.0	0.0
2	Light	12 fl oz	355	95	95	1	0	0.0	0.0	0.0
	Gin, rum, vodka, whiskey:									
3	80-proof	1½ fl oz	42	67	95	0	0	0.0	0.0	0.0
4	86-proof	1½ fl oz	42	64	105	0	0	0.0	0.0	0.0
5	90-proof	1½ fl oz	42	62	110	0	0	0.0	0.0	0.0
	Wines:									
6	Dessert	3½ fl oz	103	77	140	Tr†	0	0.0	0.0	0.0
	Table:									
7	Red	3½ fl oz	102	88	75	Tr	0	0.0	0.0	0.0
8	White	3½ fl oz	102	87	80	Tr	0	0.0	0.0	0.0
	Carbonated:[2]									
9	Club soda	12 fl oz	355	100	0	0	0	0.0	0.0	0.0
	Cola type:									
10	Regular	12 fl oz	369	89	160	0	0	0.0	0.0	0.0
11	Diet, artificially sweetened	12 fl oz	355	100	Tr	0	0	0.0	0.0	0.0
12	Ginger ale	12 fl oz	366	91	125	0	0	0.0	0.0	0.0
13	Grape	12 fl oz	372	88	180	0	0	0.0	0.0	0.0
14	Lemon-lime	12 fl oz	372	89	155	0	0	0.0	0.0	0.0
15	Orange	12 fl oz	372	88	180	0	0	0.0	0.0	0.0
16	Pepper type	12 fl oz	369	89	160	0	0	0.0	0.0	0.0
17	Root beer	12 fl oz	370	89	165	0	0	0.0	0.0	0.0
	Cocoa and chocolate-flavored beverages. See Dairy Products (items 95–98).									
	Coffee:									
18	Brewed	6 fl oz	180	100	Tr	Tr	Tr	Tr	Tr	Tr
19	Instant, prepared (22 tsp powder plus 6 fl oz water)	6 fl oz	182	99	Tr	Tr	Tr	Tr	Tr	Tr
	Fruit drinks, noncarbonated:									
	Canned:									
20	Fruit punch drink	6 fl oz	190	88	85	Tr	0	0.0	0.0	0.0
21	Grape drink	6 fl oz	187	86	100	Tr	0	0.0	0.0	0.0
22	Pineapple-grapefruit juice drink	6 fl oz	187	87	90	Tr	Tr	Tr	Tr	Tr
	Frozen:									
	Lemonade concentrate:									
23	Undiluted	6-fl-oz can	219	49	425	Tr	Tr	Tr	Tr	Tr
24	Diluted with 4⅓ parts water by volume	6 fl oz	185	89	80	Tr	Tr	Tr	Tr	Tr
	Limeade concentrate:									
25	Undiluted	6-fl-oz can	218	50	410	Tr	Tr	Tr	Tr	Tr
26	Diluted with 4⅓ parts water by volume	6 fl oz	185	89	75	Tr	Tr	Tr	Tr	Tr
	Fruit juices. See type under Fruits and Fruit Juices.									
	Milk beverages. See Dairy Products (items 92–105).									
	Tea:									
27	Brewed	8 fl oz	240	100	Tr	Tr	Tr	Tr	Tr	Tr
	Instant, powder, prepared:									
28	Unsweetened (1 tsp powder plus 8 fl oz water)	8 fl oz	241	100	Tr	Tr	Tr	Tr	Tr	Tr
29	Sweetened (3 tsp powder plus 8 fl oz water)	8 fl oz	262	91	85	Tr	Tr	Tr	Tr	Tr

* From Nutritive Value of Foods. Home and Garden Bulletin No. 72. US Department of Agriculture. Washington, DC, US Government Printing Office, 1988.

† Tr = nutrient present in trace amount.

[1] Value not determined.

[2] Mineral content varies depending on water source.

Nutrients in Indicated Quantity

Cholesterol	Carbohydrate	Calcium	Phosphorus	Iron	Potassium	Sodium	Vitamin A Value (IU)	Vitamin A Value (RE)	Thiamin	Riboflavin	Niacin	Ascorbic acid	Item No.
Milligrams	Grams	Milligrams	Milligrams	Milligrams	Milligrams	Milligrams	International units	Retinol equivalents	Milligrams	Milligrams	Milligrams	Milligrams	
0	13	14	50	0.1	115	18	0	0	0.02	0.09	1.8	0	1
0	5	14	43	0.1	64	11	0	0	0.03	0.11	1.4	0	2
0	Tr	Tr	Tr	Tr	1	Tr	0	0	Tr	Tr	Tr	0	3
0	Tr	Tr	Tr	Tr	1	Tr	0	0	Tr	Tr	Tr	0	4
0	Tr	Tr	Tr	Tr	1	Tr	0	0	Tr	Tr	Tr	0	5
0	8	8	9	0.2	95	9	([1])	([1])	0.01	0.02	0.2	0	6
0	3	8	18	0.4	113	5	([1])	([1])	0.00	0.03	0.1	0	7
0	3	9	14	0.3	83	5	([1])	([1])	0.00	0.01	0.1	0	8
0	0	18	0	Tr	0	78	0	0	0.00	0.00	0.0	0	9
0	41	11	52	0.2	7	18	0	0	0.00	0.00	0.0	0	10
0	Tr	14	39	0.2	7	32[3]	0	0	0.00	0.00	0.0	0	11
0	32	11	0	0.1	4	29	0	0	0.00	0.00	0.0	0	12
0	46	15	0	0.4	4	48	0	0	0.00	0.00	0.0	0	13
0	39	7	0	0.4	4	33	0	0	0.00	0.00	0.0	0	14
0	46	15	4	0.3	7	52	0	0	0.00	0.00	0.0	0	15
0	41	11	41	0.1	4	37	0	0	0.00	0.00	0.0	0	16
0	42	15	0	0.2	4	48	0	0	0.00	0.00	0.0	0	17
0	Tr	4	2	Tr	124	2	0	0	0.00	0.02	0.4	0	18
0	1	2	6	0.1	71	Tr	0	0	0.00	0.03	0.6	0	19
0	22	15	2	0.4	48	15	20	2	0.03	0.04	Tr	61[4]	20
0	26	2	2	0.3	9	11	Tr	Tr	0.01	0.01	Tr	64[4]	21
0	23	13	7	0.9	97	24	60	6	0.06	0.04	0.5	110[4]	22
0	112	9	13	0.4	153	4	40	4	0.04	0.07	0.7	66	23
0	21	2	2	0.1	30	1	10	1	0.01	0.02	0.2	13	24
0	108	11	13	0.2	129	Tr	Tr	Tr	0.02	0.02	0.2	26	25
0	20	2	2	Tr	24	Tr	Tr	Tr	Tr	Tr	Tr	4	26
0	Tr	0	2	Tr	36	1	0	0	0.00	0.03	Tr	0	27
0	1	1	4	Tr	61	1	0	0	0.00	0.02	0.1	0	28
0	22	1	3	Tr	49	Tr	0	0	0.00	0.04	0.1	0	29

[3] Blend of aspartame and saccharin; if only sodium saccharin is used, sodium is 75 mg; if only aspartame is used, sodium is 23 mg.
[4] With added ascorbic acid.

Table continued on following page

APPENDIX 1. Nutritive Value of the Edible Part of Food *Continued*

Item No.	Foods, Approximate Measures, Units, and Weight (Weight of Edible Portion Only)			Water	Food energy	Protein	Fat	Fatty Acids: Saturated	Fatty Acids: Monounsaturated	Fatty Acids: Polyunsaturated
	DAIRY PRODUCTS		*Grams*	*%*	*Calories*	*Grams*	*Grams*	*Grams*	*Grams*	*Grams*
	Butter. See Fats and Oils (items 128–130).									
	Cheese:									
	Natural:									
30	Blue	1 oz	28	42	100	6	8	5.3	2.2	0.2
31	Camembert (3 wedges per 4-oz container)	1 wedge	38	52	115	8	9	5.8	2.7	0.3
	Cheddar:									
32	Cut pieces	1 oz	28	37	115	7	9	6.0	2.7	0.3
33		1 in³	17	37	70	4	6	3.6	1.6	0.2
34	Shredded	1 cup	113	37	455	28	37	23.8	10.6	1.1
	Cottage (curd not pressed down):									
	Creamed (cottage cheese, 4% fat):									
35	Large curd	1 cup	225	79	235	28	10	6.4	2.9	0.3
36	Small curd	1 cup	210	79	215	26	9	6.0	2.7	0.3
37	With fruit	1 cup	226	72	280	22	8	4.9	2.2	0.2
38	Low-fat (2%)	1 cup	226	79	205	31	4	2.8	1.2	0.1
39	Uncreamed (cottage cheese dry curd, less than ½% fat)	1 cup	145	80	125	25	1	0.4	0.2	Tr
40	Cream	1 oz	28	54	100	2	10	6.2	2.8	0.4
41	Feta	1 oz	28	55	75	4	6	4.2	1.3	0.2
	Mozzarella, made with:									
42	Whole milk	1 oz	28	54	80	6	6	3.7	1.9	0.2
43	Part skim milk (low moisture)	1 oz	28	49	80	8	5	3.1	1.4	0.1
44	Muenster	1 oz	28	42	105	7	9	5.4	2.5	0.2
	Parmesan, grated:									
45	Cup, not pressed down	1 cup	100	18	455	42	30	19.1	8.7	0.7
46	Tablespoon	1 tbsp	5	18	25	2	2	1.0	0.4	Tr
47	Ounce	1 oz	28	18	130	12	9	5.4	2.5	0.2
48	Provolone	1 oz	28	41	100	7	8	4.8	2.1	0.2
	Ricotta, made with:									
49	Whole milk	1 cup	246	72	430	28	32	20.4	8.9	0.9
50	Part skim milk	1 cup	246	74	340	28	19	12.1	5.7	0.6
51	Swiss	1 oz	28	37	105	8	8	5.0	2.1	0.3
	Pasteurized process cheese:									
52	American	1 oz	28	39	105	6	9	5.6	2.5	0.3
53	Swiss	1 oz	28	42	95	7	7	4.5	2.0	0.2
54	Pasteurized process cheese food, American	1 oz	28	43	95	6	7	4.4	2.0	0.2
55	Pasteurized process cheese spread, American	1 oz	28	48	80	5	6	3.8	1.8	0.2
	Cream, sweet:									
56	Half-and-half (cream and milk)	1 cup	242	81	315	7	28	17.3	8.0	1.0
57		1 tbsp	15	81	20	Tr	2	1.1	0.5	0.1
58	Light, coffee, or table	1 cup	240	74	470	6	46	28.8	13.4	1.7
59		1 tbsp	15	74	30	Tr	3	1.8	0.8	0.1
	Whipping, unwhipped (volume about double when whipped):									
60	Light	1 cup	239	64	700	5	74	46.2	21.7	2.1
61		1 tbsp	15	64	45	Tr	5	2.9	1.4	0.1
62	Heavy	1 cup	238	58	820	5	88	54.8	25.4	3.3
63		1 tbsp	15	58	50	Tr	6	3.5	1.6	0.2
64	Whipped topping, (pressurized)	1 cup	60	61	155	2	13	8.3	3.9	0.5
65		1 tbsp	3	61	10	Tr	1	0.4	0.2	Tr
66	Cream, sour	1 cup	230	71	495	7	48	30.0	13.9	1.8
67		1 tbsp	12	71	25	Tr	3	1.6	0.7	0.1

Nutrients in Indicated Quantity

Cholesterol	Carbohydrate	Calcium	Phosphorus	Iron	Potassium	Sodium	Vitamin A Value (IU)	Vitamin A Value (RE)	Thiamin	Riboflavin	Niacin	Ascorbic acid	Item No.
Milligrams	Grams	Milligrams	Milligrams	Milligrams	Milligrams	Milligrams	International units	Retinol equivalents	Milligrams	Milligrams	Milligrams	Milligrams	
21	1	150	110	0.1	73	396	200	65	0.01	0.11	0.3	0	30
27	Tr	147	132	0.1	71	320	350	96	0.01	0.19	0.2	0	31
30	Tr	204	145	0.2	28	176	300	86	0.01	0.11	Tr	0	32
18	Tr	123	87	0.1	17	105	180	52	Tr	0.06	Tr	0	33
119	1	815	579	0.8	111	701	1,200	342	0.03	0.42	0.1	0	34
34	6	135	297	0.3	190	911	370	108	0.05	0.37	0.3	Tr	35
31	6	126	277	0.3	177	850	340	101	0.04	0.34	0.3	Tr	36
25	30	108	236	0.2	151	915	280	81	0.04	0.29	0.2	Tr	37
19	8	155	340	0.4	217	918	160	45	0.05	0.42	0.3	Tr	38
10	3	46	151	0.3	47	19	40	12	0.04	0.21	0.2	0	39
31	1	23	30	0.3	34	84	400	124	Tr	0.06	Tr	0	40
25	1	140	96	0.2	18	316	130	36	0.04	0.24	0.3	0	41
22	1	147	105	0.1	19	106	220	68	Tr	0.07	Tr	0	42
15	1	207	149	0.1	27	150	180	54	0.01	0.10	Tr	0	43
27	Tr	203	133	0.1	38	178	320	90	Tr	0.09	Tr	0	44
79	4	1,376	807	1.0	107	1,861	700	173	0.05	0.39	0.3	0	45
4	Tr	69	40	Tr	5	93	40	9	Tr	0.02	Tr	0	46
22	1	390	229	0.3	30	528	200	49	0.01	0.11	0.1	0	47
20	1	214	141	0.1	39	248	230	75	0.01	0.09	Tr	0	48
124	7	509	389	0.9	257	207	1,210	330	0.03	0.48	0.3	0	49
76	13	669	449	1.1	307	307	1,060	278	0.05	0.46	0.2	0	50
26	1	272	171	Tr	31	74	240	72	0.01	0.10	Tr	0	51
27	Tr	174	211	0.1	46	406	340	82	0.01	0.10	Tr	0	52
24	1	219	216	0.2	61	388	230	65	Tr	0.08	Tr	0	53
18	2	163	130	0.2	79	337	260	62	0.01	0.13	Tr	0	54
16	2	159	202	0.1	69	381	220	54	0.01	0.12	Tr	0	55
89	10	254	230	0.2	314	98	1,050	259	0.08	0.36	0.2	2	56
6	1	16	14	Tr	19	6	70	16	0.01	0.02	Tr	Tr	57
159	9	231	192	0.1	292	95	1,730	437	0.08	0.36	0.1	2	58
10	1	14	12	Tr	18	6	110	27	Tr	0.02	Tr	Tr	59
265	7	166	146	0.1	231	82	2,690	705	0.06	0.30	0.1	1	60
17	Tr	10	9	Tr	15	5	170	44	Tr	0.02	Tr	Tr	61
326	7	154	149	0.1	179	89	3,500	1,002	0.05	0.26	0.1	1	62
21	Tr	10	9	Tr	11	6	220	63	Tr	0.02	Tr	Tr	63
46	7	61	54	Tr	88	78	550	124	0.02	0.04	Tr	0	64
2	Tr	3	3	Tr	4	4	30	6	Tr	Tr	Tr	0	65
102	10	268	195	0.1	331	123	1,820	448	0.08	0.34	0.2	2	66
5	1	14	10	Tr	17	6	90	23	Tr	0.02	Tr	Tr	67

Table continued on following page

APPENDIX 1. Nutritive Value of the Edible Part of Food *Continued*

Item No.	Foods, Approximate Measures, Units, and Weight (Weight of Edible Portion Only)			Water	Food energy	Protein	Fat	Fatty Acids: Saturated	Fatty Acids: Monounsaturated	Fatty Acids: Polyunsaturated
	DAIRY PRODUCTS *Continued*		Grams	%	Calories	Grams	Grams	Grams	Grams	Grams
	Cream products, imitation (made with vegetable fat):									
	Sweet:									
	Creamers:									
68	Liquid (frozen)	1 tbsp	15	77	20	Tr	1	1.4	Tr	Tr
69	Powdered	1 tsp	2	2	10	Tr	1	0.7	Tr	Tr
	Whipped topping:									
70	Frozen	1 cup	75	50	240	1	19	16.3	1.2	0.4
71		1 tbsp	4	50	15	Tr	1	0.9	0.1	Tr
72	Powdered, made with whole milk	1 cup	80	67	150	3	10	8.5	0.7	0.2
73		1 tbsp	4	67	10	Tr	Tr	0.4	Tr	Tr
74	Pressurized	1 cup	70	60	185	1	16	13.2	1.3	0.2
75		1 tbsp	4	60	10	Tr	1	0.8	0.1	Tr
76	Sour dressing (filled cream type product, nonbutterfat)	1 cup	235	75	415	8	39	31.2	4.6	1.1
77		1 tbsp	12	75	20	Tr	2	1.6	0.2	0.1
	Ice cream. See Milk desserts, frozen (items 106–111).									
	Ice milk. See Milk desserts, frozen (items 112–114).									
	Milk:									
	Fluid:									
78	Whole (3.3% fat)	1 cup	244	88	150	8	8	5.1	2.4	0.3
	Low-fat (2%):									
79	No milk solids added	1 cup	244	89	120	8	5	2.9	1.4	0.2
80	Milk solids added, label claim less than 10 g of protein per cup	1 cup	245	89	125	9	5	2.9	1.4	0.2
	Low-fat (1%):									
81	No milk solids added	1 cup	244	90	100	8	3	1.6	0.7	0.1
82	Milk solids added, label claim less than 10 g of protein per cup	1 cup	245	90	105	9	2	1.5	0.7	0.1
	Nonfat (skim):									
83	No milk solids added	1 cup	245	91	85	8	Tr	0.3	0.1	Tr
84	Milk solids added, label claim less than 10 g of protein per cup	1 cup	245	90	90	9	1	0.4	0.2	Tr
85	Buttermilk	1 cup	245	90	100	8	2	1.3	0.6	0.1
	Canned:									
86	Condensed, sweetened	1 cup	306	27	980	24	27	16.8	7.4	1.0
	Evaporated:									
87	Whole milk	1 cup	252	74	340	17	19	11.6	5.9	0.6
88	Skim milk	1 cup	255	79	200	19	1	0.3	0.2	Tr
	Dried:									
89	Buttermilk	1 cup	120	3	465	41	7	4.3	2.0	0.3
	Nonfat, instantized:									
90	Envelope, 3.2 oz, net wt[6]	1 envelope	91	4	325	32	1	0.4	0.2	Tr
91	Cup	1 cup	68	4	245	24	Tr	0.3	0.1	Tr
	Milk beverages:									
	Chocolate milk (commercial):									
92	Regular	1 cup	250	82	210	8	8	5.3	2.5	0.3
93	Low-fat (2%)	1 cup	250	84	180	8	5	3.1	1.5	0.2
94	Low-fat (1%)	1 cup	250	85	160	8	3	1.5	0.8	0.1

[5] Vitamin A value is mainly from beta-carotene used for coloring.
[6] Yields 1 qt of fluid milk when reconstituted according to package directions.

Nutrients in Indicated Quantity

Cholesterol	Carbohydrate	Calcium	Phosphorus	Iron	Potassium	Sodium	Vitamin A Value (IU)	Vitamin A Value (RE)	Thiamin	Riboflavin	Niacin	Ascorbic acid	Item No.
Milligrams	Grams	Milligrams	Milligrams	Milligrams	Milligrams	Milligrams	International units	Retinol equivalents	Milligrams	Milligrams	Milligrams	Milligrams	
0	2	1	10	Tr	29	12	10[5]	1[5]	0.00	0.00	0.0	0	68
0	1	Tr	8	Tr	16	4	Tr	Tr	0.00	Tr	0.0	0	69
0	17	5	6	0.1	14	19	650[5]	65[5]	0.00	0.00	0.0	0	70
0	1	Tr	Tr	Tr	1	1	30[5]	3[5]	0.00	0.00	0.0	0	71
8	13	72	69	Tr	121	53	290[5]	39[5]	0.02	0.09	Tr	1	72
Tr	1	4	3	Tr	6	3	10[5]	2[5]	Tr	Tr	Tr	Tr	73
0	11	4	13	Tr	13	43	330[5]	33[5]	0.00	0.00	0.0	0	74
0	1	Tr	1	Tr	1	2	20[5]	2[5]	0.00	0.00	0.0	0	75
13	11	266	205	0.1	380	113	20	5	0.09	0.38	0.2	2	76
1	1	14	10	Tr	19	6	Tr	Tr	Tr	0.02	Tr	Tr	77
33	11	291	228	0.1	370	120	310	76	0.09	0.40	0.2	2	78
18	12	297	232	0.1	377	122	500	139	0.10	0.40	0.2	2	79
18	12	313	245	0.1	397	128	500	140	0.10	0.42	0.2	2	80
10	12	300	235	0.1	381	123	500	144	0.10	0.41	0.2	2	81
10	12	313	245	0.1	397	128	500	145	0.10	0.42	0.2	2	82
4	12	302	247	0.1	406	126	500	149	0.09	0.34	0.2	2	83
5	12	316	255	0.1	418	130	500	149	0.10	0.43	0.2	2	84
9	12	285	219	0.1	371	257	80	20	0.08	0.38	0.1	2	85
104	166	868	775	0.6	1,136	389	1,000	248	0.28	1.27	0.6	8	86
74	25	657	510	0.5	764	267	610	136	0.12	0.80	0.5	5	87
9	29	738	497	0.7	845	293	1,000	298	0.11	0.79	0.4	3	88
83	59	1,421	1,119	0.4	1,910	621	260	65	0.47	1.89	1.1	7	89
17	47	1,120	896	0.3	1,552	499	2,160[7]	646[7]	0.38	1.59	0.8	5	90
12	35	837	670	0.2	1,160	373	1,610[7]	483[7]	0.28	1.19	0.6	4	91
31	26	280	251	0.6	417	149	300	73	0.09	0.41	0.3	2	92
17	26	284	254	0.6	422	151	500	143	0.09	0.41	0.3	2	93
7	26	287	256	0.6	425	152	500	148	0.10	0.42	0.3	2	94

[7] With added vitamin A.

Table continued on following page

Item No.	Foods, Approximate Measures, Units, and Weight (Weight of Edible Portion Only)			Water	Food energy	Protein	Fat	Fatty Acids: Saturated	Fatty Acids: Monounsaturated	Fatty Acids: Polyunsaturated
	DAIRY PRODUCTS *Continued*		Grams	%	Calories	Grams	Grams	Grams	Grams	Grams
	Milk beverages:									
	Cocoa and chocolate-flavored beverages:									
95	Powder containing nonfat dry milk	1 oz	28	1	100	3	1	0.6	0.3	Tr
96	Prepared (6 oz water plus 1 oz powder)	1 serving	206	86	100	3	1	0.6	0.3	Tr
97	Powder without nonfat dry milk	¾ oz	21	1	75	1	1	0.3	0.2	Tr
98	Prepared (8 oz whole milk plus ¾ oz powder)	1 serving	265	81	225	9	9	5.4	2.5	0.3
99	Eggnog (commercial)	1 cup	254	74	340	10	19	11.3	5.7	0.9
	Malted milk:									
	Chocolate:									
100	Powder	¾ oz	21	2	85	1	1	0.5	0.3	0.1
101	Prepared (8 oz whole milk plus ¾ oz powder)	1 serving	265	81	235	9	9	5.5	2.7	0.4
	Natural:									
102	Powder	¾ oz	21	3	85	3	2	0.9	0.5	0.3
103	Prepared (8 oz whole milk plus ¾ oz powder)	1 serving	265	81	235	11	10	6.0	2.9	0.6
	Shakes, thick:									
104	Chocolate	10-oz container	283	72	335	9	8	4.8	2.2	0.3
105	Vanilla	10-oz container	283	74	315	11	9	5.3	2.5	0.3
	Milk desserts, frozen:									
	Ice cream, vanilla:									
	Regular (about 11% fat):									
106	Hardened	½ gal	1,064	61	2,155	38	115	71.3	33.1	4.3
107		1 cup	133	61	270	5	14	8.9	4.1	0.5
108		3 fl oz	50	61	100	2	5	3.4	1.6	0.2
109	Soft serve (frozen custard)	1 cup	173	60	375	7	23	13.5	6.7	1.0
110	Rich (about 16% fat), hardened	½ gal	1,188	59	2,805	33	190	118.3	54.9	7.1
		1 cup	148	59	350	4	24	14.7	6.8	0.9
	Ice milk, vanilla:									
112	Hardened (about 4% fat)	½ gal	1,048	69	1,470	41	45	28.1	13.0	1.7
113		1 cup	131	69	185	5	6	3.5	1.6	0.2
114	Soft serve (about 3% fat)	1 cup	175	70	225	8	5	2.9	1.3	0.2
115	Sherbert (about 2% fat)	½ gal	1,542	66	2,160	17	31	19.0	8.8	1.1
116		1 cup	193	66	270	2	4	2.4	1.1	0.1
	Yogurt:									
	With added milk solids:									
	Made with low-fat milk:									
117	Fruit-flavored[8]	8-oz container	227	74	230	10	2	1.6	0.7	0.1
118	Plain	8-oz container	227	85	145	12	4	2.3	1.0	0.1
119	Made with nonfat milk	8-oz container	227	85	125	13	Tr	0.3	0.1	Tr
	Without added milk solids:									
120	Made with whole milk	8-oz container	227	88	140	8	7	4.8	2.0	0.2
	EGGS									
	Eggs, large (24 oz per dozen):									
	Raw:									
121	Whole, without shell	1 egg	50	75	80	6	6	1.7	2.2	0.7
122	White	1 white	33	88	15	3	Tr	0.0	0.0	0.0
123	Yolk	1 yolk	17	49	65	3	6	1.7	2.2	0.7
	Cooked:									
124	Fried in butter	1 egg	46	68	95	6	7	2.7	2.7	0.8
125	Hard-cooked, shell removed	1 egg	50	75	80	6	6	1.7	2.2	0.7
126	Poached	1 egg	50	74	80	6	6	1.7	2.2	0.7
127	Scrambled (milk added) in butter. Also omelet	1 egg	64	73	110	7	8	3.2	2.9	0.8

[8] Carbohydrate content varies widely because of amount of sugar added and amount and solids content of added flavoring. Consult the label if more precise values for carbohydrate and calories are needed.

Nutrients in Indicated Quantity

Cholesterol	Carbohydrate	Calcium	Phosphorus	Iron	Potassium	Sodium	Vitamin A Value (IU)	Vitamin A Value (RE)	Thiamin	Riboflavin	Niacin	Ascorbic acid	Item No.
Milligrams	*Grams*	*Milligrams*	*Milligrams*	*Milligrams*	*Milligrams*	*Milligrams*	*International units*	*Retinol equivalents*	*Milligrams*	*Milligrams*	*Milligrams*	*Milligrams*	
1	22	90	88	0.3	223	139	Tr	Tr	0.03	0.17	0.2	Tr	95
1	22	90	88	0.3	223	139	Tr	Tr	0.03	0.17	0.2	Tr	96
0	19	7	26	0.7	136	56	Tr	Tr	Tr	0.03	0.1	Tr	97
33	30	298	254	0.9	508	176	310	76	0.10	0.43	0.3	3	98
149	34	330	278	0.5	420	138	890	203	0.09	0.48	0.3	4	99
1	18	13	37	0.4	130	49	20	5	0.04	0.04	0.4	0	100
34	29	304	265	0.5	500	168	330	80	0.14	0.43	0.7	2	101
4	15	56	79	0.2	159	96	70	17	0.11	0.14	1.1	0	102
37	27	347	307	0.3	529	215	380	93	0.20	0.54	1.3	2	103
30	60	374	357	0.9	634	314	240	59	0.13	0.63	0.4	0	104
33	50	413	326	0.3	517	270	320	79	0.08	0.55	0.4	0	105
476	254	1,406	1,075	1.0	2,052	929	4,340	1,064	0.42	2.63	1.1	6	106
59	32	176	134	0.1	257	116	540	133	0.05	0.33	0.1	1	107
22	12	66	51	Tr	96	44	200	50	0.02	0.12	0.1	Tr	108
153	38	236	199	0.4	338	153	790	199	0.08	0.45	0.2	1	109
703	256	1,213	927	0.8	1,771	868	7,200	1,758	0.36	2.27	0.9	5	110
88	32	151	115	0.1	221	108	900	219	0.04	0.28	0.1	1	111
146	232	1,409	1,035	1.5	2,117	836	1,710	419	0.61	2.78	0.9	6	112
18	29	176	129	0.2	265	105	210	52	0.08	0.35	0.1	1	113
13	38	274	202	0.3	412	163	175	44	0.12	0.54	0.2	1	114
113	469	827	594	2.5	1,585	706	1,480	308	0.26	0.71	1.0	31	115
14	59	103	74	0.3	198	88	190	39	0.03	0.09	0.1	4	116
10	43	345	271	0.2	442	133	100	25	0.08	0.40	0.2	1	117
14	16	415	326	0.2	531	159	150	36	0.10	0.49	0.3	2	118
4	17	452	355	0.2	579	174	20	5	0.11	0.53	0.3	2	119
29	11	274	215	0.1	351	105	280	68	0.07	0.32	0.2	1	120
274	1	28	90	1.0	65	69	260	78	0.04	0.15	Tr	0	121
0	Tr	4	4	Tr	45	50	0	0	Tr	0.09	Tr	0	122
272	Tr	26	86	0.9	15	8	310	94	0.04	0.07	Tr	0	123
278	1	29	91	1.1	66	162	320	94	0.04	0.14	Tr	0	124
274	1	28	90	1.0	65	69	260	78	0.04	0.14	Tr	0	125
273	1	28	90	1.0	65	146	260	78	0.03	0.13	Tr	0	126
282	2	54	109	1.0	97	176	350	102	0.04	0.18	Tr	Tr	127

Table continued on following page

Item No.	Foods, Approximate Measures, Units, and Weight (Weight of Edible Portion Only)			Water	Food energy	Protein	Fat	Fatty Acids: Saturated	Fatty Acids: Monounsaturated	Fatty Acids: Polyunsaturated
	FATS AND OILS		Grams	%	Calories	Grams	Grams	Grams	Grams	Grams
	Butter (4 sticks per lb):									
128	Stick	½ cup	113	16	810	1	92	57.1	26.4	3.4
129	Tablespoon (⅛ stick)	1 tbsp	14	16	100	Tr	11	7.1	3.3	0.4
130	Pat (1-in square, ⅓-in high; 90 per lb)	1 pat	5	16	35	Tr	4	2.5	1.2	0.2
131	Fats, cooking (vegetable shortenings)	1 cup	205	0	1,810	0	205	51.3	91.2	53.5
132		1 tbsp	13	0	115	0	13	3.3	5.8	3.4
133	Lard	1 cup	205	0	1,850	0	205	80.4	92.5	23.0
134		1 tbsp	13	0	115	0	13	5.1	5.9	1.5
	Margarine:									
135	Imitation (about 40% fat), soft	8-oz container	227	58	785	1	88	17.5	35.6	31.3
136		1 tbsp	14	58	50	Tr	5	1.1	2.2	1.9
	Regular (about 80% fat):									
	Hard (4 sticks per lb):									
137	Stick	½ cup	113	16	810	1	91	17.9	40.5	28.7
138	Tablespoon (⅛ stick)	1 tbsp	14	16	100	Tr	11	2.2	5.0	3.6
139	Pat (1-in square, ⅓-in high; 90 per lb)	1 pat	5	16	35	Tr	4	0.8	1.8	1.3
140	Soft	8-oz container	227	16	1,625	2	183	31.3	64.7	78.5
141		1 tbsp	14	16	100	Tr	11	1.9	4.0	4.8
	Spread (about 60% fat):									
	Hard (4 sticks per lb):									
142	Stick	½ cup	113	37	610	1	69	15.9	29.4	20.5
143	Tablespoon (⅛ stick)	1 tbsp	14	37	75	Tr	9	2.0	3.6	2.5
144	Pat (1-in square, ⅓-in high; 90 per lb)	1 pat	5	37	25	Tr	3	0.7	1.3	0.9
145	Soft	8-oz container	227	37	1,225	1	138	29.1	71.5	31.3
146		1 tbsp	14	37	75	Tr	9	1.8	4.4	1.9
	Oils, salad or cooking:									
147	Corn	1 cup	218	0	1,925	0	218	27.7	52.8	128.0
148		1 tbsp	14	0	125	0	14	1.8	3.4	8.2
149	Olive	1 cup	216	0	1,910	0	216	29.2	159.2	18.1
150		1 tbsp	14	0	125	0	14	1.9	10.3	1.2
151	Peanut	1 cup	216	0	1,910	0	216	36.5	99.8	69.1
152		1 tbsp	14	0	125	0	14	2.4	6.5	4.5
153	Safflower	1 cup	218	0	1,925	0	218	19.8	26.4	162.4
154		1 tbsp	14	0	125	0	14	1.3	1.7	10.4
155	Soybean oil, hydrogenated (partially hardened)	1 cup	218	0	1,925	0	218	32.5	93.7	82.0
156		1 tbsp	14	0	125	0	14	2.1	6.0	5.3
157	Soybean-cottonseed oil blend, hydrogenated	1 cup	218	0	1,925	0	218	39.2	64.3	104.9
158		1 tbsp	14	0	125	0	14	2.5	4.1	6.7
159	Sunflower	1 cup	218	0	1,925	0	218	22.5	42.5	143.2
160		1 tbsp	14	0	125	0	14	1.4	2.7	9.2
	Salad dressings:									
	Commercial:									
161	Blue cheese	1 tbsp	15	32	75	1	8	1.5	1.8	4.2
	French:									
162	Regular	1 tbsp	16	35	85	Tr	9	1.4	4.0	3.5
163	Low calorie	1 tbsp	16	75	25	Tr	2	0.2	0.3	1.0
	Italian:									
164	Regular	1 tbsp	15	34	80	Tr	9	1.3	3.7	3.2
165	Low calorie	1 tbsp	15	86	5	Tr	Tr	Tr	Tr	Tr
	Mayonnaise:									
166	Regular	1 tbsp	14	15	100	Tr	11	1.7	3.2	5.8
167	Imitation	1 tbsp	15	63	35	Tr	3	0.5	0.7	1.6
168	Mayonnaise type	1 tbsp	15	40	60	Tr	5	0.7	1.4	2.7
169	Tartar sauce	1 tbsp	14	34	75	Tr	8	1.2	2.6	3.9
	Thousand island:									
170	Regular	1 tbsp	16	46	60	Tr	6	1.0	1.3	3.2
171	Low calorie	1 tbsp	15	69	25	Tr	2	0.2	0.4	0.9

[9] For salted butter; unsalted butter contains 12 mg of sodium per stick, 2 mg per tbsp, or 1 mg per pat.

[10] Values for vitamin A are year-round average.

Nutrients in Indicated Quantity

Cholesterol	Carbohydrate	Calcium	Phosphorus	Iron	Potassium	Sodium	Vitamin A Value (IU)	Vitamin A Value (RE)	Thiamin	Riboflavin	Niacin	Ascorbic acid	Item No.
Milligrams	Grams	Milligrams	Milligrams	Milligrams	Milligrams	Milligrams	International units	Retinol equivalents	Milligrams	Milligrams	Milligrams	Milligrams	
247	Tr	27	26	0.2	29	933[9]	3,460[10]	852[10]	0.01	0.04	Tr	0	128
31	Tr	3	3	Tr	4	116[9]	430[10]	106[10]	Tr	Tr	Tr	0	129
11	Tr	1	1	Tr	1	41[9]	150[10]	38[10]	Tr	Tr	Tr	0	130
0	0	0	0	0.0	0	0	0	0	0.00	0.00	0.0	0	131
0	0	0	0	0.0	0	0	0	0	0.00	0.00	0.0	0	132
195	0	0	0	0.0	0	0	0	0	0.00	0.00	0.0	0	133
12	0	0	0	0.0	0	0	0	0	0.00	0.00	0.0	0	134
0	1	40	31	0.0	57	2,178[11]	7,510[12]	2,254[12]	0.01	0.05	Tr	Tr	135
0	Tr	2	2	0.0	4	134[11]	460[12]	139[12]	Tr	Tr	Tr	Tr	136
0	1	34	26	0.1	48	1,066[11]	3,740[12]	1,122[12]	0.01	0.04	Tr	Tr	137
0	Tr	4	3	Tr	6	132[11]	460[12]	139[12]	Tr	0.01	Tr	Tr	138
0	Tr	1	1	Tr	2	47[11]	170[12]	50[12]	Tr	Tr	Tr	Tr	139
0	1	60	46	0.0	86	2,449[11]	7,510[12]	2,254[12]	0.02	0.07	Tr	Tr	140
0	Tr	4	3	0.0	5	151[11]	460[12]	139[12]	Tr	Tr	Tr	Tr	141
0	0	24	18	0.0	34	1,123[11]	3,740[12]	1,122[12]	0.01	0.03	Tr	Tr	142
0	0	3	2	0.0	4	139[11]	460[12]	139[12]	Tr	Tr	Tr	Tr	143
0	0	1	1	0.0	1	50[11]	170[12]	50[12]	Tr	Tr	Tr	Tr	144
0	0	47	37	0.0	68	2,256[11]	7,510[12]	2,254[12]	0.02	0.06	Tr	Tr	145
0	0	3	2	0.0	4	139[11]	460[12]	139[12]	Tr	Tr	Tr	Tr	146
0	0	0	0	0.0	0	0	0	0	0.00	0.00	0.0	0	147
0	0	0	0	0.0	0	0	0	0	0.00	0.00	0.0	0	148
0	0	0	0	0.0	0	0	0	0	0.00	0.00	0.0	0	149
0	0	0	0	0.0	0	0	0	0	0.00	0.00	0.0	0	150
0	0	0	0	0.0	0	0	0	0	0.00	0.00	0.0	0	151
0	0	0	0	0.0	0	0	0	0	0.00	0.00	0.0	0	152
0	0	0	0	0.0	0	0	0	0	0.00	0.00	0.0	0	153
0	0	0	0	0.0	0	0	0	0	0.00	0.00	0.0	0	154
0	0	0	0	0.0	0	0	0	0	0.00	0.00	0.0	0	155
0	0	0	0	0.0	0	0	0	0	0.00	0.00	0.0	0	156
0	0	0	0	0.0	0	0	0	0	0.00	0.00	0.0	0	157
0	0	0	0	0.0	0	0	0	0	0.00	0.00	0.0	0	158
0	0	0	0	0.0	0	0	0	0	0.00	0.00	0.0	0	159
0	0	0	0	0.0	0	0	0	0	0.00	0.00	0.0	0	160
3	1	12	11	Tr	6	164	30	10	Tr	0.02	Tr	Tr	161
0	1	2	1	Tr	2	188	Tr	Tr	Tr	Tr	Tr	Tr	162
0	2	6	5	Tr	3	306	Tr	Tr	Tr	Tr	Tr	Tr	163
0	1	1	1	Tr	5	162	30	3	Tr	Tr	Tr	Tr	164
0	2	1	1	Tr	4	136	Tr	Tr	Tr	Tr	Tr	Tr	165
8	Tr	3	4	0.1	5	80	40	12	0.00	0.00	Tr	0	166
4	2	Tr	Tr	0.0	2	75	0	0	0.00	0.00	0.0	0	167
4	4	2	4	Tr	1	107	30	13	Tr	Tr	Tr	0	168
4	1	3	4	0.1	11	182	30	9	Tr	Tr	0.0	Tr	169
4	2	2	3	0.1	18	112	50	15	Tr	Tr	Tr	0	170
2	2	2	3	0.1	17	150	50	14	Tr	Tr	Tr	0	171

[11] For salted margarine.

[12] Based on average vitamin A content of fortified margarine. Federal specifications for fortified margarine require a minimum of 15,000 IU per pound.

Table continued on following page

Item No.	Foods, Approximate Measures, Units, and Weight (Weight of Edible Portion Only)			Water	Food energy	Protein	Fat	Fatty Acids: Saturated	Fatty Acids: Monounsaturated	Fatty Acids: Polyunsaturated
	FATS AND OILS *Continued*		*Grams*	*%*	*Calories*	*Grams*	*Grams*	*Grams*	*Grams*	*Grams*
	Salad dressings:									
	Prepared from home recipe:									
172	Cooked type[13]	1 tbsp	16	69	25	1	2	0.5	0.6	0.3
173	Vinegar and oil	1 tbsp	16	47	70	0	8	1.5	2.4	3.9
	FISH AND SHELLFISH									
	Clams:									
174	Raw, meat only	3 oz	85	82	65	11	1	0.3	0.3	0.3
175	Canned, drained solids	3 oz	85	77	85	13	2	0.5	0.5	0.4
176	Crabmeat, canned	1 cup	135	77	135	23	3	0.5	0.8	1.4
177	Fish sticks, frozen, reheated (stick, 4″ by 1″ by ½″)	1 fish stick	28	52	70	6	3	0.8	1.4	0.8
	Flounder or sole, baked, with lemon juice:									
178	With butter	3 oz	85	73	120	16	6	3.2	1.5	0.5
179	With margarine	3 oz	85	73	120	16	6	1.2	2.3	1.9
180	Without added fat	3 oz	85	78	80	17	1	0.3	0.2	0.4
181	Haddock, breaded, fried[14]	3 oz	85	61	175	17	9	2.4	3.9	2.4
182	Halibut, broiled, with butter and lemon juice	3 oz	85	67	140	20	6	3.3	1.6	0.7
183	Herring, pickled	3 oz	85	59	190	17	13	4.3	4.6	3.1
184	Ocean perch, breaded, fried[14]	1 fillet	85	59	185	16	11	2.6	4.6	2.8
	Oysters:									
185	Raw, meat only (13–19 medium selects)	1 cup	240	85	160	20	4	1.4	0.5	1.4
186	Breaded, fried[14]	1 oyster	45	65	90	5	5	1.4	2.1	1.4
	Salmon:									
187	Canned (pink), solids and liquid	3 oz	85	71	120	17	5	0.9	1.5	2.1
188	Baked (red)	3 oz	85	67	140	21	5	1.2	2.4	1.4
189	Smoked	3 oz	85	59	150	18	8	2.6	3.9	0.7
190	Sardines, Atlantic, canned in oil, drained solids	3 oz	85	62	175	20	9	2.1	3.7	2.9
191	Scallops, breaded, frozen, reheated	6 scallops	90	59	195	15	10	2.5	4.1	2.5
	Shrimp:									
192	Canned, drained solids	3 oz	85	70	100	21	1	0.2	0.2	0.4
193	French fried (7 medium)[16]	3 oz	85	55	200	16	10	2.5	4.1	2.6
194	Trout, broiled, with butter and lemon juice	3 oz	85	63	175	21	9	4.1	2.9	1.6
	Tuna, canned, drained solids:									
195	Oil pack, chunk light	3 oz	85	61	165	24	7	1.4	1.9	3.1
196	Water pack, solid white	3 oz	85	63	135	30	1	0.3	0.2	0.3
197	Tuna salad[17]	1 cup	205	63	375	33	19	3.3	4.9	9.2
	FRUITS AND FRUIT JUICES									
	Apples:									
	Raw:									
	Unpeeled, without cores:									
198	2¾-in diam. (about 3 per lb with cores)	1 apple	138	84	80	Tr	Tr	0.1	Tr	0.1
199	3¼-in diam. (about 2 per lb with cores)	1 apple	212	84	125	Tr	1	0.1	Tr	0.2
200	Peeled, sliced	1 cup	110	84	65	Tr	Tr	0.1	Tr	0.1
201	Dried, sulfured	10 rings	64	32	155	1	Tr	Tr	Tr	0.1
202	Apple juice, bottled or canned[19]	1 cup	248	88	115	Tr	Tr	Tr	Tr	0.1
	Applesauce, canned:									
203	Sweetened	1 cup	255	80	195	Tr	Tr	0.1	Tr	0.1
204	Unsweetened	1 cup	244	88	105	Tr	Tr	Tr	Tr	Tr

[13] Fatty acid values apply to product made with regular margarine.
[14] Dipped in egg, milk, and breadcrumbs; fried in vegetable shortening.
[15] If bones are discarded, value for calcium will be greatly reduced.
[16] Dipped in egg, breadcrumbs, and flour; fried in vegetable shortening.

Nutrients in Indicated Quantity

Cholesterol	Carbohydrate	Calcium	Phosphorus	Iron	Potassium	Sodium	Vitamin A Value (IU)	Vitamin A Value (RE)	Thiamin	Riboflavin	Niacin	Ascorbic acid	Item No.
Milligrams	Grams	Milligrams	Milligrams	Milligrams	Milligrams	Milligrams	International units	Retinol equivalents	Milligrams	Milligrams	Milligrams	Milligrams	
9	2	13	14	0.1	19	117	70	20	0.01	0.02	Tr	Tr	172
0	Tr	0	0	0.0	1	Tr	0	0	0.00	0.00	0.0	0	173
43	2	59	138	2.6	154	102	90	26	0.09	0.15	1.1	9	174
54	2	47	116	3.5	119	102	90	26	0.01	0.09	0.9	3	175
135	1	61	246	1.1	149	1,350	50	14	0.11	0.11	2.6	0	176
26	4	11	58	0.3	94	53	20	5	0.03	0.05	0.6	0	177
68	Tr	13	187	0.3	272	145	210	54	0.05	0.08	1.6	1	178
55	Tr	14	187	0.3	273	151	230	69	0.05	0.08	1.6	1	179
59	Tr	13	197	0.3	286	101	30	10	0.05	0.08	1.7	1	180
75	7	34	183	1.0	270	123	70	20	0.06	0.10	2.9	0	181
62	Tr	14	206	0.7	441	103	610	174	0.06	0.07	7.7	1	182
85	0	29	128	0.9	85	850	110	33	0.04	0.18	2.8	0	183
66	7	31	191	1.2	241	138	70	20	0.10	0.11	2.0	0	184
120	8	226	343	15.6	290	175	740	223	0.34	0.43	6.0	24	185
35	5	49	73	3.0	64	70	150	44	0.07	0.10	1.3	4	186
34	0	167[15]	243	0.7	307	443	60	18	0.03	0.15	6.8	0	187
60	0	26	269	0.5	305	55	290	87	0.18	0.14	5.5	0	188
51	0	12	208	0.8	327	1,700	260	77	0.17	0.17	6.8	0	189
85	0	371[15]	424	2.6	349	425	190	56	0.03	0.17	4.6	0	190
70	10	39	203	2.0	369	298	70	21	0.11	0.11	1.6	0	191
128	1	98	224	1.4	104	1,955	50	15	0.01	0.03	1.5	0	192
168	11	61	154	2.0	189	384	90	26	0.06	0.09	2.8	0	193
71	Tr	26	259	1.0	297	122	230	60	0.07	0.07	2.3	1	194
55	0	7	199	1.6	298	303	70	20	0.04	0.09	10.1	0	195
48	0	17	202	0.6	255	468	110	32	0.03	0.10	13.4	0	196
80	19	31	281	2.5	531	877	230	53	0.06	0.14	13.3	6	197
0	21	10	10	0.2	159	Tr	70	7	0.02	0.02	0.1	8	198
0	32	15	15	0.4	244	Tr	110	11	0.04	0.03	0.2	12	199
0	16	4	8	0.1	124	Tr	50	5	0.02	0.01	0.1	4	200
0	42	9	24	0.9	288	56[18]	0	0	0.00	0.10	0.6	2	201
0	29	17	17	0.9	295	7	Tr	Tr	0.05	0.04	0.2	2[20]	202
0	51	10	18	0.9	156	8	30	3	0.03	0.07	0.5	4[20]	203
0	28	7	17	0.3	183	5	70	7	0.03	0.06	0.5	3[20]	204

[17] Made with drained chunk light tuna, celery, onion, pickle relish, and mayonnaise-type salad dressing.
[18] Sodium bisulfite used to preserve color; unsulfited product would contain less sodium.
[19] Also applies to pasteurized apple cider.
[20] Without added ascorbic acid. For value with added ascorbic acid, refer to label.

Table continued on following page

APPENDIX 1. Nutritive Value of the Edible Part of Food *Continued*

Item No.	Foods, Approximate Measures, Units, and Weight (Weight of Edible Portion Only)			Water	Food energy	Pro-tein	Fat	Fatty Acids: Satu-rated	Fatty Acids: Mono-unsatu-rated	Fatty Acids: Poly-unsatu-rated
	FRUITS AND FRUIT JUICES *Continued*		*Grams*	*%*	*Calories*	*Grams*	*Grams*	*Grams*	*Grams*	*Grams*
	Apricots:									
205	Raw, without pits (about 12 per lb with pits)	3 apricots	106	86	50	1	Tr	Tr	0.2	0.1
	Canned (fruit and liquid):									
206	Heavy syrup pack	1 cup	258	78	215	1	Tr	Tr	0.1	Tr
207		3 halves	85	78	70	Tr	Tr	Tr	Tr	Tr
208	Juice pack	1 cup	248	87	120	2	Tr	Tr	Tr	Tr
209		3 halves	84	87	40	1	Tr	Tr	Tr	Tr
	Dried:									
210	Uncooked (28 large or 37 medium halves per cup)	1 cup	130	31	310	5	1	Tr	0.3	0.1
211	Cooked, unsweetened, fruit and liquid	1 cup	250	76	210	3	Tr	Tr	0.2	0.1
212	Apricot nectar, canned	1 cup	251	85	140	1	Tr	Tr	0.1	Tr
	Avocados, raw, whole, without skin and seed:									
213	California (about 2 per lb with skin and seed)	1 avocado	173	73	305	4	30	4.5	19.4	3.5
214	Florida (about 1 per lb with skin and seed)	1 avocado	304	80	340	5	27	5.3	14.8	4.5
	Bananas, raw, without peel:									
215	Whole (about 2½ per lb with peel)	1 banana	114	74	105	1	1	0.2	Tr	0.1
216	Sliced	1 cup	150	74	140	2	1	0.3	0.1	0.1
217	Blackberries, raw	1 cup	144	86	75	1	1	0.2	0.1	0.1
	Blueberries:									
218	Raw	1 cup	145	85	80	1	1	Tr	0.1	0.3
219	Frozen, sweetened	10-oz container	284	77	230	1	Tr	Tr	0.1	0.2
220		1 cup	230	77	185	1	Tr	Tr	Tr	0.1
	Cantaloupe. See Melons (item 251).									
	Cherries:									
221	Sour, red, pitted, canned, water pack	1 cup	244	90	90	2	Tr	0.1	0.1	0.1
222	Sweet, raw, without pits and stems	10 cherries	68	81	50	1	1	0.1	0.2	0.2
223	Cranberry juice cocktail, bottled, sweetened	1 cup	253	85	145	Tr	Tr	Tr	Tr	0.1
224	Cranberry sauce, sweetened, canned, strained	1 cup	277	61	420	1	Tr	Tr	0.1	0.2
	Dates:									
225	Whole, without pits	10 dates	83	23	230	2	Tr	0.1	0.1	Tr
226	Chopped	1 cup	178	23	490	4	1	0.3	0.2	Tr
227	Figs, dried	10 figs	187	28	475	6	2	0.4	0.5	1.0
	Fruit cocktail, canned, fruit and liquid:									
228	Heavy syrup pack	1 cup	255	80	185	1	Tr	Tr	Tr	0.1
229	Juice pack	1 cup	248	87	115	1	Tr	Tr	Tr	Tr
	Grapefruit:									
230	Raw, without peel, membrane and seeds (3¾-in diam., 1 lb 1 oz, whole, with refuse)	½ grapefruit	120	91	40	1	Tr	Tr	Tr	Tr
231	Canned, sections with syrup	1 cup	254	84	150	1	Tr	Tr	Tr	0.1
	Grapefruit juice:									
232	Raw	1 cup	247	90	95	1	Tr	Tr	Tr	0.1
	Canned:									
233	Unsweetened	1 cup	247	90	95	1	Tr	Tr	Tr	0.1
234	Sweetened	1 cup	250	87	115	1	Tr	Tr	Tr	0.1
	Frozen concentrate, unsweetened									
235	Undiluted	6-fl-oz can	207	62	300	4	1	0.1	0.1	0.2
236	Diluted with 3 parts water by volume	1 cup	247	89	100	1	Tr	Tr	Tr	0.1

Nutrients in Indicated Quantity

Cholesterol	Carbohydrate	Calcium	Phosphorus	Iron	Potassium	Sodium	Vitamin A Value (IU)	Vitamin A Value (RE)	Thiamin	Riboflavin	Niacin	Ascorbic acid	Item No.
Milligrams	*Grams*	*Milligrams*	*Milligrams*	*Milligrams*	*Milligrams*	*Milligrams*	*International units*	*Retinol equivalents*	*Milligrams*	*Milligrams*	*Milligrams*	*Milligrams*	
0	12	15	20	0.6	314	1	2,770	277	0.03	0.04	0.6	11	205
0	55	23	31	0.8	361	10	3,170	317	0.05	0.06	1.0	8	206
0	18	8	10	0.3	119	3	1,050	105	0.02	0.02	0.3	3	207
0	31	30	50	0.7	409	10	4,190	419	0.04	0.05	0.9	12	208
0	10	10	17	0.3	139	3	1,420	142	0.02	0.02	0.3	4	209
0	80	59	152	6.1	1,791	13	9,410	941	0.01	0.20	3.9	3	210
0	55	40	103	4.2	1,222	8	5,910	591	0.02	0.08	2.4	4	211
0	36	18	23	1.0	286	8	3,300	330	0.02	0.04	0.7	2[20]	212
0	12	19	73	2.0	1,097	21	1,060	106	0.19	0.21	3.3	14	213
0	27	33	119	1.6	1,484	15	1,860	186	0.33	0.37	5.8	24	214
0	27	7	23	0.4	451	1	90	9	0.05	0.11	0.6	10	215
0	35	9	30	0.5	594	2	120	12	0.07	0.15	0.8	14	216
0	18	46	30	0.8	282	Tr	240	24	0.04	0.06	0.6	30	217
0	20	9	15	0.2	129	9	150	15	0.07	0.07	0.5	19	218
0	62	17	20	1.1	170	3	120	12	0.06	0.15	0.7	3	219
0	50	14	16	0.9	138	2	100	10	0.05	0.12	0.6	2	220
0	22	27	24	3.3	239	17	1,840	184	0.04	0.10	0.4	5	221
0	11	10	13	0.3	152	Tr	150	15	0.03	0.04	0.3	5	222
0	38	8	3	0.4	61	10	10	1	0.01	0.04	0.1	108[21]	223
0	108	11	17	0.6	72	80	60	6	0.04	0.06	0.3	6	224
0	61	27	33	1.0	541	2	40	4	0.07	0.08	1.8	0	225
0	131	57	71	2.0	1,161	5	90	9	0.16	0.18	3.9	0	226
0	122	269	127	4.2	1,331	21	250	25	0.13	0.16	1.3	1	227
0	48	15	28	0.7	224	15	520	52	0.05	0.05	1.0	5	228
0	29	20	35	0.5	236	10	760	76	0.03	0.04	1.0	7	229
0	10	14	10	0.1	167	Tr	10[22]	1[22]	0.04	0.02	0.3	41	230
0	39	36	25	1.0	328	5	Tr	Tr	0.10	0.05	0.6	54	231
0	23	22	37	0.5	400	2	20	2	0.10	0.05	0.5	94	232
0	22	17	27	0.5	378	2	20	2	0.10	0.05	0.6	72	233
0	28	20	28	0.9	405	5	20	2	0.10	0.06	0.8	67	234
0	72	56	101	1.0	1,002	6	60	6	0.30	0.16	1.6	248	235
0	24	20	35	0.3	336	2	20	2	0.10	0.05	0.5	83	236

[21] With added ascorbic acid.

[22] For white grapefruit; pink grapefruit have about 310 IU or 31 RE.

Table continued on following page

APPENDIX 1. Nutritive Value of the Edible Part of Food *Continued*

Item No.	Foods, Approximate Measures, Units, and Weight (Weight of Edible Portion Only)			Water	Food energy	Protein	Fat	Fatty Acids: Saturated	Fatty Acids: Monounsaturated	Fatty Acids: Polyunsaturated
	FRUITS AND FRUIT JUICES *Continued*		*Grams*	*%*	*Calories*	*Grams*	*Grams*	*Grams*	*Grams*	*Grams*
	Grapes, European type (adherent skin), raw:									
237	Thompson Seedless	10 grapes	50	81	35	Tr	Tr	0.1	Tr	0.1
238	Tokay and Emperor, seeded types	10 grapes	57	81	40	Tr	Tr	0.1	Tr	0.1
	Grape juice:									
239	Canned or bottled	1 cup	253	84	155	1	Tr	0.1	Tr	0.1
	Frozen concentrate, sweetened:									
240	Undiluted	6-fl-oz can	216	54	385	1	1	0.2	Tr	0.2
241	Diluted with 3 parts water by volume	1 cup	250	87	125	Tr	Tr	0.1	Tr	0.1
242	Kiwifruit, raw, without skin (about 5 per lb with skin)	1 kiwifruit	76	83	45	1	Tr	Tr	0.1	0.1
243	Lemons, raw, without peel and seeds (about 4 per lb with peel and seeds)	1 lemon	58	89	15	1	Tr	Tr	Tr	0.1
	Lemon juice:									
244	Raw	1 cup	244	91	60	1	Tr	Tr	Tr	Tr
245	Canned or bottled, unsweetened	1 cup	244	92	50	1	1	0.1	Tr	0.2
246		1 tbsp	15	92	5	Tr	Tr	Tr	Tr	Tr
247	Frozen, single-strength, unsweetened	6-fl-oz can	244	92	55	1	1	0.1	Tr	0.2
	Lime juice:									
248	Raw	1 cup	246	90	65	1	Tr	Tr	Tr	0.1
249	Canned, unsweetened	1 cup	246	93	50	1	1	0.1	0.1	0.2
250	Mangos, raw, without skin and seed (about 1½ per lb with skin and seed)	1 mango	207	82	135	1	1	0.1	0.2	0.1
	Melons, raw, without rind and cavity contents:									
251	Cantaloupe, orange-fleshed (5-in diam., 2⅓ lb, whole, with rind and cavity contents)	½ melon	267	90	95	2	1	0.1	0.1	0.3
252	Honeydew (6½-in diam., 5¼ lb, whole, with rind and cavity contents)	⅒ melon	129	90	45	1	Tr	Tr	Tr	0.1
253	Nectarines, raw, without pits (about 3 per lb with pits)	1 nectarine	136	86	65	1	1	0.1	0.2	0.3
	Oranges, raw:									
254	Whole, without peel and seeds (2⅝-in diam., about 2½ per lb, with peel and seeds)	1 orange	131	87	60	1	Tr	Tr	Tr	Tr
255	Sections without membranes	1 cup	180	87	85	2	Tr	Tr	Tr	Tr
	Orange juice:									
256	Raw, all varieties	1 cup	248	88	110	2	Tr	0.1	0.1	0.1
257	Canned, unsweetened	1 cup	249	89	105	1	Tr	Tr	0.1	0.1
258	Chilled	1 cup	249	88	110	2	1	0.1	0.1	0.2
	Frozen concentrate:									
259	Undiluted	6-fl-oz can	213	58	340	5	Tr	0.1	0.1	0.1
260	Diluted with 3 parts water by volume	1 cup	249	88	110	2	Tr	Tr	Tr	Tr
261	Orange and grapefruit juice, canned	1 cup	247	89	105	1	Tr	Tr	Tr	Tr
262	Papayas, raw, ½-in cubes	1 cup	140	86	65	1	Tr	0.1	0.1	Tr
	Peaches:									
	Raw:									
263	Whole, 2½-in diam., peeled, pitted (about 4 per lb with peels and pits)	1 peach	87	88	35	1	Tr	Tr	Tr	Tr
264	Sliced	1 cup	170	88	75	1	Tr	Tr	0.1	0.1
	Canned, fruit and liquid:									
265	Heavy syrup pack	1 cup	256	79	190	1	Tr	Tr	0.1	0.1
266		1 half	81	79	60	Tr	Tr	Tr	Tr	Tr
267	Juice pack	1 cup	248	87	110	2	Tr	Tr	Tr	Tr
268		1 half	77	87	35	Tr	Tr	Tr	Tr	Tr

Nutrients in Indicated Quantity

Cholesterol	Carbohydrate	Calcium	Phosphorus	Iron	Potassium	Sodium	Vitamin A Value (IU)	Vitamin A Value (RE)	Thiamin	Riboflavin	Niacin	Ascorbic acid	Item No.
Milligrams	Grams	Milligrams	Milligrams	Milligrams	Milligrams	Milligrams	International units	Retinol equivalents	Milligrams	Milligrams	Milligrams	Milligrams	
0	9	6	7	0.1	93	1	40	4	0.05	0.03	0.2	5	237
0	10	6	7	0.1	105	1	40	4	0.05	0.03	0.2	6	238
0	38	23	28	0.6	334	8	20	2	0.07	0.09	0.7	Tr[20]	239
0	96	28	32	0.8	160	15	60	6	0.11	0.20	0.9	179[21]	240
0	32	10	10	0.3	53	5	20	2	0.04	0.07	0.3	60[21]	241
0	11	20	30	0.3	252	4	130	13	0.02	0.04	0.4	74	242
0	5	15	9	0.3	80	1	20	2	0.02	0.01	0.1	31	243
0	21	17	15	0.1	303	2	50	5	0.07	0.02	0.2	112	244
0	16	27	22	0.3	249	51[23]	40	4	0.10	0.02	0.5	61	245
0	1	2	1	Tr	15	3[23]	Tr	Tr	0.01	Tr	Tr	4	246
0	16	20	20	0.3	217	2	30	3	0.14	0.03	0.3	77	247
0	22	22	17	0.1	268	2	20	2	0.05	0.02	0.2	72	248
0	16	30	25	0.6	185	39[23]	40	4	0.08	0.01	0.4	16	249
0	35	21	23	0.3	323	4	8,060	806	0.12	0.12	1.2	57	250
0	22	29	45	0.6	825	24	8,610	861	0.10	0.06	1.5	113	251
0	12	8	13	0.1	350	13	50	5	0.10	0.02	0.8	32	252
0	16	7	22	0.2	288	Tr	1,000	100	0.02	0.06	1.3	7	253
0	15	52	18	0.1	237	Tr	270	27	0.11	0.05	0.4	70	254
0	21	72	25	0.2	326	Tr	370	37	0.16	0.07	0.5	96	255
0	26	27	42	0.5	496	2	500	50	0.22	0.07	1.0	124	256
0	25	20	35	1.1	436	5	440	44	0.15	0.07	0.8	86	257
0	25	25	27	0.4	473	2	190	19	0.28	0.05	0.7	82	258
0	81	68	121	0.7	1,436	6	590	59	0.60	0.14	1.5	294	259
0	27	22	40	0.2	473	2	190	19	0.20	0.04	0.5	97	260
0	25	20	35	1.1	390	7	290	29	0.14	0.07	0.8	72	261
0	17	35	12	0.3	247	9	400	40	0.04	0.04	0.5	92	262
0	10	4	10	0.1	171	Tr	470	47	0.01	0.04	0.9	6	263
0	19	9	20	0.2	335	Tr	910	91	0.03	0.07	1.7	11	264
0	51	8	28	0.7	236	15	850	85	0.03	0.06	1.6	7	265
0	16	2	9	0.2	75	5	270	27	0.01	0.02	0.5	2	266
0	29	15	42	0.7	317	10	940	94	0.02	0.04	1.4	9	267
0	9	5	13	0.2	99	3	290	29	0.01	0.01	0.4	3	268

[23] Sodium benzoate and sodium bisulfite added as preservatives.

Table continued on following page

APPENDIX 1. Nutritive Value of the Edible Part of Food *Continued*

Item No.	Foods, Approximate Measures, Units, and Weight (Weight of Edible Portion Only)			Water	Food energy	Protein	Fat	Fatty Acids: Saturated	Fatty Acids: Monounsaturated	Fatty Acids: Polyunsaturated
	FRUITS AND FRUIT JUICES *Continued*		*Grams*	*%*	*Calories*	*Grams*	*Grams*	*Grams*	*Grams*	*Grams*
	Peaches:									
	Dried:									
269	Uncooked	1 cup	160	32	380	6	1	0.1	0.4	0.6
270	Cooked, unsweetened, fruit and liquid	1 cup	258	78	200	3	1	0.1	0.2	0.3
271	Frozen, sliced, sweetened	10-oz container	284	75	265	2	Tr	Tr	0.1	0.2
272		1 cup	250	75	235	2	Tr	Tr	0.1	0.2
	Pears:									
	Raw, with skin, cored:									
273	Bartlett, 2½-in diam. (about 2½ per lb with cores and stems)	1 pear	166	84	100	1	1	Tr	0.1	0.2
274	Bosc, 2½-in diam. (about 3 per lb with cores and stems)	1 pear	141	84	85	1	1	Tr	0.1	0.1
275	D'Anjou, 3-in diam. (about 2 per lb with cores and stems)	1 pear	200	84	120	1	1	Tr	0.2	0.2
	Canned, fruit and liquid:									
276	Heavy syrup pack	1 cup	255	80	190	1	Tr	Tr	0.1	0.1
277		1 half	79	80	60	Tr	Tr	Tr	Tr	Tr
278	Juice pack	1 cup	248	86	125	1	Tr	Tr	Tr	Tr
279		1 half	77	86	40	Tr	Tr	Tr	Tr	Tr
	Pineapple:									
280	Raw, diced	1 cup	155	87	75	1	1	Tr	0.1	0.2
	Canned, fruit and liquid:									
	Heavy syrup pack:									
281	Crushed, chunks, tidbits	1 cup	255	79	200	1	Tr	Tr	Tr	0.1
282	Slices	1 slice	58	79	45	Tr	Tr	Tr	Tr	Tr
	Juice pack:									
283	Chunks or tidbits	1 cup	250	84	150	1	Tr	Tr	Tr	0.1
284	Slices	1 slice	58	84	35	Tr	Tr	Tr	Tr	Tr
285	Pineapple juice, unsweetened, canned	1 cup	250	86	140	1	Tr	Tr	Tr	0.1
	Plantains, without peel:									
286	Raw	1 plantain	179	65	220	2	1	0.3	0.1	0.1
287	Cooked, boiled, sliced	1 cup	154	67	180	1	Tr	0.1	Tr	0.1
	Plums, without pits:									
	Raw:									
288	2⅛-in diam. (about 6½ per lb with pits)	1 plum	66	85	35	1	Tr	Tr	0.3	0.1
289	1½-in diam. (about 15 per lb with pits)	1 plum	28	85	15	Tr	Tr	Tr	0.1	Tr
	Canned, purple, fruit and liquid:									
290	Heavy syrup pack	1 cup	258	76	230	1	Tr	Tr	0.2	0.1
291		3 plums	133	76	120	Tr	Tr	Tr	0.1	Tr
292	Juice pack	1 cup	252	84	145	1	Tr	Tr	Tr	Tr
293		3 plums	95	84	55	Tr	Tr	Tr	Tr	Tr
	Prunes, dried:									
294	Uncooked	4 extra large or 5 large prunes	49	32	115	1	Tr	Tr	0.2	0.1
295	Cooked, unsweetened, fruit and liquid	1 cup	212	70	225	2	Tr	Tr	0.3	0.1
296	Prune juice, canned or bottled	1 cup	256	81	180	2	Tr	Tr	0.1	Tr
	Raisins, seedless:									
297	Cup, not pressed down	1 cup	145	15	435	5	1	0.2	Tr	0.2
298	Packet, ½ oz (1½ tbsp)	1 packet	14	15	40	Tr	Tr	Tr	Tr	Tr
	Raspberries:									
299	Raw	1 cup	123	87	60	1	1	Tr	0.1	0.4
300	Frozen, sweetened	10-oz container	284	73	295	2	Tr	Tr	Tr	0.3
301		1 cup	250	73	255	2	Tr	Tr	Tr	0.2

Nutrients in Indicated Quantity														
Cholesterol	*Carbohydrate*	*Calcium*	*Phosphorus*	*Iron*	*Potassium*	*Sodium*	*Vitamin A Value* (IU)	*Vitamin A Value* (RE)	*Thiamin*	*Riboflavin*	*Niacin*	*Ascorbic acid*	**Item No.**
Milligrams	*Grams*	*Milligrams*	*Milligrams*	*Milligrams*	*Milligrams*	*Milligrams*	*International units*	*Retinol equivalents*	*Milligrams*	*Milligrams*	*Milligrams*	*Milligrams*	
0	98	45	190	6.5	1,594	11	3,460	346	Tr	0.34	7.0	8	269
0	51	23	98	3.4	826	5	510	51	0.01	0.05	3.9	10	270
0	68	9	31	1.1	369	17	810	81	0.04	0.10	1.9	268[21]	271
0	60	8	28	0.9	325	15	710	71	0.03	0.09	1.6	236[21]	272
0	25	18	18	0.4	208	Tr	30	3	0.03	0.07	0.2	7	273
0	21	16	16	0.4	176	Tr	30	3	0.03	0.06	0.1	6	274
0	30	22	22	0.5	250	Tr	40	4	0.04	0.08	0.2	8	275
0	49	13	18	0.6	166	13	10	1	0.03	0.06	0.6	3	276
0	15	4	6	0.2	51	4	Tr	Tr	0.01	0.02	0.2	1	277
0	32	22	30	0.7	238	10	10	1	0.03	0.03	0.5	4	278
0	10	7	9	0.2	74	3	Tr	Tr	0.01	0.01	0.2	1	279
0	19	11	11	0.6	175	2	40	4	0.14	0.06	0.7	24	280
0	52	36	18	1.0	265	3	40	4	0.23	0.06	0.7	19	281
0	12	8	4	0.2	60	1	10	1	0.05	0.01	0.2	4	282
0	39	35	15	0.7	305	3	100	10	0.24	0.05	0.7	24	283
0	9	8	3	0.2	71	1	20	2	0.06	0.01	0.2	6	284
0	34	43	20	0.7	335	3	10	1	0.14	0.06	0.6	27	285
0	57	5	61	1.1	893	7	2,020	202	0.09	0.10	1.2	33	286
0	48	3	43	0.9	716	8	1,400	140	0.07	0.08	1.2	17	287
0	9	3	7	0.1	114	Tr	210	21	0.03	0.06	0.3	6	288
0	4	1	3	Tr	48	Tr	90	9	0.01	0.03	0.1	3	289
0	60	23	34	2.2	235	49	670	67	0.04	0.10	0.8	1	290
0	31	12	17	1.1	121	25	340	34	0.02	0.05	0.4	1	291
0	38	25	38	0.9	388	3	2,540	254	0.06	0.15	1.2	7	292
0	14	10	14	0.3	146	1	960	96	0.02	0.06	0.4	3	293
0	31	25	39	1.2	365	2	970	97	0.04	0.08	1.0	2	294
0	60	49	74	2.4	708	4	650	65	0.05	0.21	1.5	6	295
0	45	31	64	3.0	707	10	10	1	0.04	0.18	2.0	10	296
0	115	71	141	3.0	1,089	17	10	1	0.23	0.13	1.2	5	297
0	11	7	14	0.3	105	2	Tr	Tr	0.02	0.01	0.1	Tr	298
0	14	27	15	0.7	187	Tr	160	16	0.04	0.11	1.1	31	299
0	74	43	48	1.8	324	3	170	17	0.05	0.13	0.7	47	300
0	65	38	43	1.6	285	3	150	15	0.05	0.11	0.6	41	301

Table continued on following page

APPENDIX 1. Nutritive Value of the Edible Part of Food *Continued*

Item No.	Foods, Approximate Measures, Units, and Weight (Weight of Edible Portion Only)			Water	Food energy	Protein	Fat	Fatty Acids Saturated	Fatty Acids Monounsaturated	Fatty Acids Polyunsaturated
	FRUITS AND FRUIT JUICES *Continued*		*Grams*	*%*	*Calories*	*Grams*	*Grams*	*Grams*	*Grams*	*Grams*
302	Rhubarb, cooked, added sugar	1 cup	240	68	280	1	Tr	Tr	Tr	0.1
	Strawberries:									
303	Raw, capped, whole	1 cup	149	92	45	1	1	Tr	0.1	0.3
304	Frozen, sweetened, sliced	10-oz container	284	73	275	2	Tr	Tr	0.1	0.2
305		1 cup	255	73	245	1	Tr	Tr	Tr	0.2
	Tangerines:									
306	Raw, without peel and seeds (2⅜-in diam., about 4 per lb, with peel and seeds)	1 tangerine	84	88	35	1	Tr	Tr	Tr	Tr
307	Canned, light syrup, fruit and liquid	1 cup	252	83	155	1	Tr	Tr	Tr	0.1
308	Tangerine juice, canned, sweetened	1 cup	249	87	125	1	Tr	Tr	Tr	0.1
	Watermelon, raw, without rind and seeds:									
309	Piece (4- by 8-in wedge with rind and seeds; 1/16 of 32⅔-lb melon, 10 by 16 in)	1 piece	482	92	155	3	2	0.3	0.2	1.0
310	Diced	1 cup	160	92	50	1	1	0.1	0.1	0.3
	GRAIN PRODUCTS									
311	Bagels, plain or water, enriched, 3½-in diam.[24]	1 bagel	68	29	200	7	2	0.3	0.5	0.7
312	Barley, pearled, light, uncooked	1 cup	200	11	700	16	2	0.3	0.2	0.9
	Biscuits, baking powder, 2-in diam. (enriched flour, vegetable shortening):									
313	From home recipe	1 biscuit	28	28	100	2	5	1.2	2.0	1.3
314	From mix	1 biscuit	28	29	95	2	3	0.8	1.4	0.9
315	From refrigerated dough	1 biscuit	20	30	65	1	2	0.6	0.9	0.6
	Breadcrumbs, enriched:									
316	Dry, grated	1 cup	100	7	390	13	5	1.5	1.6	1.0
	Soft. See White bread (item 351).									
	Breads:									
317	Boston brown bread, canned, slice, 3¼ in by ½ in[25]	1 slice	45	45	95	2	1	0.3	0.1	0.1
	Cracked-wheat bread (¾ enriched wheat flour, ¼ cracked wheat flour):[25]									
318	Loaf, 1 lb.	1 loaf	454	35	1,190	42	16	3.1	4.3	5.7
319	Slice (18 per loaf)	1 slice	25	35	65	2	1	0.2	0.2	0.3
320	Toasted	1 slice	21	26	65	2	1	0.2	0.2	0.3
	French or Vienna bread, enriched:[25]									
321	Loaf, 1 lb.	1 loaf	454	34	1,270	43	18	3.8	5.7	5.9
	Slice:									
322	French, 5 by 2½ by 1 in	1 slice	35	34	100	3	1	0.3	0.4	0.5
323	Vienna, 4¾ by 4 by ½ in	1 slice	25	34	70	2	1	0.2	0.3	0.3
	Italian bread, enriched:									
324	Loaf, 1 lb.	1 loaf	454	32	1,255	41	4	0.6	0.3	1.6
325	Slice, 4½ by 3¼ by ¾ in	1 slice	30	32	85	3	Tr	Tr	Tr	0.1
	Mixed grain bread, enriched:[25]									
326	Loaf, 1 lb.	1 loaf	454	37	1,165	45	17	3.2	4.1	6.5
327	Slice (18 per loaf)	1 slice	25	37	65	2	1	0.2	0.2	0.4
328	Toasted	1 slice	23	27	65	2	1	0.2	0.2	0.4

[24] Egg bagels have 44 mg cholesterol and 22 IU or 7 RE vitamin A per bagel.
[25] Made with vegetable shortening.

Nutrients in Indicated Quantity

Cholesterol	*Carbohydrate*	*Calcium*	*Phosphorus*	*Iron*	*Potassium*	*Sodium*	*Vitamin A Value* (IU)	*Vitamin A Value* (RE)	*Thiamin*	*Riboflavin*	*Niacin*	*Ascorbic acid*	Item No.
Milligrams	Grams	Milligrams	Milligrams	Milligrams	Milligrams	Milligrams	International units	Retinol equivalents	Milligrams	Milligrams	Milligrams	Milligrams	
0	75	348	19	0.5	230	2	170	17	0.04	0.06	0.5	8	302
0	10	21	28	0.6	247	1	40	4	0.03	0.10	0.3	84	303
0	74	31	37	1.7	278	9	70	7	0.05	0.14	1.1	118	304
0	66	28	33	1.5	250	8	60	6	0.04	0.13	1.0	106	305
0	9	12	8	0.1	132	1	770	77	0.09	0.02	0.1	26	306
0	41	18	25	0.9	197	15	2,120	212	0.13	0.11	1.1	50	307
0	30	45	35	0.5	443	2	1,050	105	0.15	0.05	0.2	55	308
0	35	39	43	0.8	559	10	1,760	176	0.39	0.10	1.0	46	309
0	11	13	14	0.3	186	3	590	59	0.13	0.03	0.3	15	310
0	38	29	46	1.8	50	245	0	0	0.26	0.20	2.4	0	311
0	158	32	378	4.2	320	6	0	0	0.24	0.10	6.2	0	312
Tr	13	47	36	0.7	32	195	10	3	0.08	0.08	0.8	Tr	313
Tr	14	58	128	0.7	56	262	20	4	0.12	0.11	0.8	Tr	314
1	10	4	79	0.5	18	249	0	0	0.08	0.05	0.7	0	315
5	73	122	141	4.1	152	736	0	0	0.35	0.35	4.8	0	316
3	21	41	72	0.9	131	113	0[26]	0[26]	0.06	0.04	0.7	0	317
0	227	295	581	12.1	608	1,966	Tr	Tr	1.73	1.73	15.3	Tr	318
0	12	16	32	0.7	34	106	Tr	Tr	0.10	0.09	0.8	Tr	319
0	12	16	32	0.7	34	106	Tr	Tr	0.07	0.09	0.8	Tr	320
0	230	499	386	14.0	409	2,633	Tr	Tr	2.09	1.59	18.2	Tr	321
0	18	39	30	1.1	32	203	Tr	Tr	0.16	0.12	1.4	Tr	322
0	13	28	21	0.8	23	145	Tr	Tr	0.12	0.09	1.0	Tr	323
0	256	77	350	12.7	336	2,656	0	0	1.80	1.10	15.0	0	324
0	17	5	23	0.8	22	176	0	0	0.12	0.07	1.0	0	325
0	212	472	962	14.8	990	1,870	Tr	Tr	1.77	1.73	18.9	Tr	326
0	12	27	55	0.8	56	106	Tr	Tr	0.10	0.10	1.1	Tr	327
0	12	27	55	0.8	56	106	Tr	Tr	0.08	0.10	1.1	Tr	328

[26] Made with white cornmeal. If made with yellow cornmeal, value is 32 IU or 3 RE.

Table continued on following page

APPENDIX 1. Nutritive Value of the Edible Part of Food *Continued*

Item No.	Foods, Approximate Measures, Units, and Weight (Weight of Edible Portion Only)			Water	Food energy	Protein	Fat	Fatty Acids: Saturated	Fatty Acids: Monounsaturated	Fatty Acids: Polyunsaturated
	GRAIN PRODUCTS *Continued*		Grams	%	Calories	Grams	Grams	Grams	Grams	Grams
	Breads:									
	Oatmeal bread, enriched:[25]									
329	Loaf, 1 lb.	1 loaf	454	37	1,145	38	20	3.7	7.1	8.2
330	Slice (18 per loaf)	1 slice	25	37	65	2	1	0.2	0.4	0.5
331	Toasted	1 slice	23	30	65	2	1	0.2	0.4	0.5
332	Pita bread, enriched, white, 6½-in diam.	1 pita	60	31	165	6	1	0.1	0.1	0.4
	Pumpernickel (⅔ rye flour, ⅓ enriched wheat flour):[25]									
333	Loaf, 1 lb.	1 loaf	454	37	1,160	42	16	2.6	3.6	6.4
334	Slice, 5 by 4 by ⅜ in.	1 slice	32	37	80	3	1	0.2	0.3	0.5
335	Toasted	1 slice	29	28	80	3	1	0.2	0.3	0.5
	Raisin bread, enriched:[25]									
336	Loaf, 1 lb.	1 loaf	454	33	1,260	37	18	4.1	6.5	6.7
337	Slice (18 per loaf)	1 slice	25	33	65	2	1	0.2	0.3	0.4
338	Toasted	1 slice	21	24	65	2	1	0.2	0.3	0.4
	Rye bread, light (⅔ enriched wheat flour, ⅓ rye flour):[25]									
339	Loaf, 1 lb.	1 loaf	454	37	1,190	38	17	3.3	5.2	5.5
340	Slice, 4¾ by 3¾ by 7/16 in	1 slice	25	37	65	2	1	0.2	0.3	0.3
341	Toasted	1 slice	22	28	65	2	1	0.2	0.3	0.3
	Wheat bread, enriched:[25]									
342	Loaf, 1 lb.	1 loaf	454	37	1,160	43	19	3.9	7.3	4.5
343	Slice (18 per loaf)	1 slice	25	37	65	2	1	0.2	0.4	0.3
344	Toasted	1 slice	23	28	65	3	1	0.2	0.4	0.3
	White bread, enriched:[25]									
345	Loaf, 1 lb.	1 loaf	454	37	1,210	38	18	5.6	6.5	4.2
346	Slice (18 per loaf)	1 slice	25	37	65	2	1	0.3	0.4	0.2
347	Toasted	1 slice	22	28	65	2	1	0.3	0.4	0.2
348	Slice (22 per loaf)	1 slice	20	37	55	2	1	0.2	0.3	0.2
349	Toasted	1 slice	17	28	55	2	1	0.2	0.3	0.2
350	Cubes	1 cup	30	37	80	2	1	0.4	0.4	0.3
351	Crumbs, soft	1 cup	45	37	120	4	2	0.6	0.6	0.4
	Whole-wheat bread:[25]									
352	Loaf, 1 lb.	1 loaf	454	38	1,110	44	20	5.8	6.8	5.2
353	Slice (16 per loaf)	1 slice	28	38	70	3	1	0.4	0.4	0.3
354	Toasted	1 slice	25	29	70	3	1	0.4	0.4	0.3
	Bread stuffing (from enriched bread), prepared from mix:									
355	Dry type	1 cup	140	33	500	9	31	6.1	13.3	9.6
356	Moist type	1 cup	203	61	420	9	26	5.3	11.3	8.0
	Breakfast cereals:									
	Hot type, cooked:									
	Corn (hominy) grits:									
357	Regular and quick, enriched	1 cup	242	85	145	3	Tr	Tr	0.1	0.2
358	Instant, plain	1 pkt	137	85	80	2	Tr	Tr	Tr	0.1
	Cream of Wheat:									
359	Regular, quick, instant	1 cup	244	86	140	4	Tr	0.1	Tr	0.2
360	Mix'n Eat, plain	1 pkt	142	82	100	3	Tr	Tr	Tr	0.1
361	Malt-O-Meal	1 cup	240	88	120	4	Tr	Tr	Tr	0.1
	Oatmeal or rolled oats:									
362	Regular, quick, instant, nonfortified	1 cup	234	85	145	6	2	0.4	0.8	1.0
	Instant, fortified:									
363	Plain	1 pkt	177	86	105	4	2	0.3	0.6	0.7
364	Flavored	1 pkt	164	76	160	5	2	0.3	0.7	0.8

[27] Nutrient added.
[28] Cooked without salt. If salt is added according to label recommendations, sodium content is 540 mg.
[29] For white corn grits. Cooked yellow grits contain 145 IU or 14 RE.
[30] Value based on label declaration for added nutrients.

Nutrients in Indicated Quantity

Cholesterol	Carbohydrate	Calcium	Phosphorus	Iron	Potassium	Sodium	Vitamin A Value (IU)	Vitamin A Value (RE)	Thiamin	Riboflavin	Niacin	Ascorbic acid	Item No.
Milligrams	*Grams*	*Milligrams*	*Milligrams*	*Milligrams*	*Milligrams*	*Milligrams*	*International units*	*Retinol equivalents*	*Milligrams*	*Milligrams*	*Milligrams*	*Milligrams*	
0	212	267	563	12.0	707	2,231	0	0	2.09	1.20	15.4	0	329
0	12	15	31	0.7	39	124	0	0	0.12	0.07	0.9	0	330
0	12	15	31	0.7	39	124	0	0	0.09	0.07	0.9	0	331
0	33	49	60	1.4	71	339	0	0	0.27	0.12	2.2	0	332
0	218	322	990	12.4	1,966	2,461	0	0	1.54	2.36	15.0	0	333
0	16	23	71	0.9	141	177	0	0	0.11	0.17	1.1	0	334
0	16	23	71	0.9	141	177	0	0	0.09	0.17	1.1	0	335
0	239	463	395	14.1	1,058	1,657	Tr	Tr	1.50	2.81	18.6	Tr	336
0	13	25	22	0.8	59	92	Tr	Tr	0.08	0.15	1.0	Tr	337
0	13	25	22	0.8	59	92	Tr	Tr	0.06	0.15	1.0	Tr	338
0	218	363	658	12.3	926	3,164	0	0	1.86	1.45	15.0	0	339
0	12	20	36	0.7	51	175	0	0	0.10	0.08	0.8	0	340
0	12	20	36	0.7	51	175	0	0	0.08	0.08	0.8	0	341
0	213	572	835	15.8	627	2,447	Tr	Tr	2.09	1.45	20.5	Tr	342
0	12	32	47	0.9	35	138	Tr	Tr	0.12	0.08	1.2	Tr	343
0	12	32	47	0.9	35	138	Tr	Tr	0.10	0.08	1.2	Tr	344
0	222	572	490	12.9	508	2,334	Tr	Tr	2.13	1.41	17.0	Tr	345
0	12	32	27	0.7	28	129	Tr	Tr	0.12	0.08	0.9	Tr	346
0	12	32	27	0.7	28	129	Tr	Tr	0.09	0.08	0.9	Tr	347
0	10	25	21	0.6	22	101	Tr	Tr	0.09	0.06	0.7	Tr	348
0	10	25	21	0.6	22	101	Tr	Tr	0.07	0.06	0.7	Tr	349
0	15	38	32	0.9	34	154	Tr	Tr	0.14	0.09	1.1	Tr	350
0	22	57	49	1.3	50	231	Tr	Tr	0.21	0.14	1.7	Tr	351
0	206	327	1,180	15.5	799	2,887	Tr	Tr	1.59	0.95	17.4	Tr	352
0	13	20	74	1.0	50	180	Tr	Tr	0.10	0.06	1.1	Tr	353
0	13	20	74	1.0	50	180	Tr	Tr	0.08	0.06	1.1	Tr	354
0	50	92	136	2.2	126	1,254	910	273	0.17	0.20	2.5	0	355
67	40	81	134	2.0	118	1,023	850	256	0.10	0.18	1.6	0	356
0	31	0	29	1.5[27]	53	0[28]	0[29]	0[29]	0.24[27]	0.15[27]	2.0[27]	0	357
0	18	7	16	1.0[27]	29	343	0	0	0.18[27]	0.08[27]	1.3[27]	0	358
0	29	54[30]	43[31]	10.9[30]	46	5[31,32]	0	0	0.24[30]	0.07[30]	1.5[30]	0	359
0	21	20[30]	20[30]	8.1[30]	38	241	1,250[30]	376[30]	0.43[30]	0.28[30]	5.0[30]	0	360
0	26	5	24[30]	9.6[30]	31	2[33]	0	0	0.48[30]	0.24[30]	5.8[30]	0	361
0	25	19	178	1.6	131	2[34]	40	4	0.26	0.05	0.3	0	362
0	18	163[27]	133	6.3[27]	99	285[27]	1,510[27]	453[27]	0.53[27]	0.28[27]	5.5[27]	0	363
0	31	168[27]	148	6.7[27]	137	254[27]	1,530[27]	460[27]	0.53[27]	0.38[27]	5.9[27]	Tr	364

[31] For regular and instant cereal. For quick cereal, phosphorus is 102 mg and sodium is 142 mg.
[32] Cooked without salt. If salt is added according to label recommendations, sodium content is 390 mg.
[33] Cooked without salt. If salt is added according to label recommendations, sodium content is 324 mg.
[34] Cooked without salt. If salt is added according to label recommendations, sodium content is 374 mg.

Table continued on following page

APPENDIX 1. Nutritive Value of the Edible Part of Food *Continued*

Item No.	Foods, Approximate Measures, Units, and Weight (Weight of Edible Portion Only)			Water	Food energy	Protein	Fat	Fatty Acids: Saturated	Fatty Acids: Monounsaturated	Fatty Acids: Polyunsaturated
	GRAIN PRODUCTS *Continued*		*Grams*	*%*	*Calories*	*Grams*	*Grams*	*Grams*	*Grams*	*Grams*
	Breakfast cereals:									
	Ready to eat:									
365	All-Bran (about ⅓ cup)	1 oz	28	3	70	4	1	0.1	0.1	0.3
366	Cap'n Crunch (about ¾ cup)	1 oz	28	3	120	1	3	1.7	0.3	0.4
367	Cheerios (about 1¼ cups)	1 oz	28	5	110	4	2	0.3	0.6	0.7
	Corn Flakes (about 1¼ cups):									
368	Kellogg's	1 oz	28	3	110	2	Tr	Tr	Tr	Tr
369	Toasties	1 oz	28	3	110	2	Tr	Tr	Tr	Tr
	40% Bran Flakes:									
370	Kellogg's (about ¾ cup)	1 oz	28	3	90	4	1	0.1	0.1	0.3
371	Post (about ⅔ cup)	1 oz	28	3	90	3	Tr	0.1	0.1	0.2
372	Froot Loops (about 1 cup)	1 oz	28	3	110	2	1	0.2	0.1	0.1
373	Golden Grahams (about ¾ cup)	1 oz	28	2	110	2	1	0.7	0.1	0.2
374	Grape-Nuts (about ¼ cup)	1 oz	28	3	100	3	Tr	Tr	Tr	0.1
375	Honey Nut Cheerios (about ¾ cup)	1 oz	28	3	105	3	1	0.1	0.3	0.3
376	Lucky Charms (about 1 cup)	1 oz	28	3	110	3	1	0.2	0.4	0.4
377	Nature Valley Granola (about ⅓ cup)	1 oz	28	4	125	3	5	3.3	0.7	0.7
378	100% Natural Cereal (about ¼ cup)	1 oz	28	2	135	3	6	4.1	1.2	0.5
379	Product 19 (about ¾ cup)	1 oz	28	3	110	3	Tr	Tr	Tr	0.1
	Raisin Bran:									
380	Kellogg's (about ¾ cup)	1 oz	28	8	90	3	1	0.1	0.1	0.3
381	Post (about ½ cup)	1 oz	28	9	85	3	1	0.1	0.1	0.3
382	Rice Krispies (about 1 cup)	1 oz	28	2	110	2	Tr	Tr	Tr	0.1
383	Shredded Wheat (about ⅔ cup)	1 oz	28	5	100	3	1	0.1	0.1	0.3
384	Special K (about 1⅓ cups)	1 oz	28	2	110	6	Tr	Tr	Tr	Tr
385	Super Sugar Crisp (about ⅞ cup)	1 oz	28	2	105	2	Tr	Tr	Tr	0.1
386	Sugar Frosted Flakes, Kellogg's (about ¾ cup)	1 oz	28	3	110	1	Tr	Tr	Tr	Tr
387	Sugar Smacks (about ¾ cup)	1 oz	28	3	105	2	1	0.1	0.1	0.2
388	Total (about 1 cup)	1 oz	28	4	100	3	1	0.1	0.1	0.3
389	Trix (about 1 cup)	1 oz	28	3	110	2	Tr	0.2	0.1	0.1
390	Wheaties (about 1 cup)	1 oz	28	5	100	3	Tr	0.1	Tr	0.2
391	Buckwheat flour, light, sifted	1 cup	98	12	340	6	1	0.2	0.4	0.4
392	Bulgur, uncooked	1 cup	170	10	600	19	3	1.2	0.3	1.2
	Cakes prepared from cake mixes with enriched flour:[35]									
	Angel food:									
393	Whole cake, 9¾-in diam. tube cake	1 cake	635	38	1,510	38	2	0.4	0.2	1.0
394	Piece, 1/12 of cake	1 piece	53	38	125	3	Tr	Tr	Tr	0.1
	Coffeecake, crumb:									
395	Whole cake, 7¾ by 5⅝ by 1¼ in	1 cake	430	30	1,385	27	41	11.8	16.7	9.6
396	Piece, ⅙ of cake	1 piece	72	30	230	5	7	2.0	2.8	1.6
	Devil's food with chocolate frosting:									
397	Whole, 2-layer cake, 8- or 9-in diam	1 cake	1,107	24	3,755	49	136	55.6	51.4	19.7
398	Piece, 1/16 of cake	1 piece	69	24	235	3	8	3.5	3.2	1.2
399	Cupcake, 2½-in diam.	1 cupcake	35	24	120	2	4	1.8	1.6	0.6
	Gingerbread:									
400	Whole cake, 8 in square	1 cake	570	37	1,575	18	39	9.6	16.4	10.5
401	Piece, ⅑ of cake	1 piece	63	37	175	2	4	1.1	1.8	1.2

[27] Nutrient added.
[30] Value based on label declaration for added nutrients.

Nutrients in Indicated Quantity

Cholesterol	Carbohydrate	Calcium	Phosphorus	Iron	Potassium	Sodium	Vitamin A Value (IU)	Vitamin A Value (RE)	Thiamin	Riboflavin	Niacin	Ascorbic acid	Item No.
Milligrams	*Grams*	*Milligrams*	*Milligrams*	*Milligrams*	*Milligrams*	*Milligrams*	*International units*	*Retinol equivalents*	*Milligrams*	*Milligrams*	*Milligrams*	*Milligrams*	
0	21	23	264	4.5[30]	350	320	1,250[30]	375[30]	0.37[30]	0.43[30]	5.0[30]	15[30]	365
0	23	5	36	7.5[27]	37	213	40	4	0.50[27]	0.55[27]	6.6[27]	0	366
0	20	48	134	4.5[30]	101	307	1,250[30]	375[30]	0.37[30]	0.43[30]	5.0[30]	15[30]	367
0	24	1	18	1.8[30]	26	351	1,250[30]	375[30]	0.37[30]	0.43[30]	5.0[30]	15[30]	368
0	24	1	12	0.7[27]	33	297	1,250[30]	375[30]	0.37[30]	0.43[30]	5.0[30]	0	369
0	22	14	139	8.1[30]	180	264	1,250[30]	375[30]	0.37[30]	0.43[30]	5.0[30]	0	370
0	22	12	179	4.5[30]	151	260	1,250[30]	375[30]	0.37[30]	0.43[30]	5.0[30]	0	371
0	25	3	24	4.5[30]	26	145	1,250[30]	375[30]	0.37[30]	0.43[30]	5.0[30]	15[30]	372
Tr	24	17	41	4.5[30]	63	346	1,250[30]	375[30]	0.37[30]	0.43[30]	5.0[30]	15[30]	373
0	23	11	71	1.2	95	197	1,250[30]	375[30]	0.37[30]	0.43[30]	5.0[30]	0	374
0	23	20	105	4.5[30]	99	257	1,250[30]	375[30]	0.37[30]	0.43[30]	5.0[30]	15[30]	375
0	23	32	79	4.5[30]	59	201	1,250[30]	375[30]	0.37[30]	0.43[30]	5.0[30]	15[30]	376
0	19	18	89	0.9	98	58	20	2	0.10	0.05	0.2	0	377
Tr	18	49	104	0.8	140	12	20	2	0.09	0.15	0.6	0	378
0	24	3	40	18.0[30]	44	325	5,000[30]	1,501[30]	1.50[30]	1.70[30]	20.0[30]	60[30]	379
0	21	10	105	3.5[30]	147	207	960[30]	288[30]	0.28[30]	0.34[30]	3.9[30]	0	380
0	21	13	119	4.5[30]	175	185	1,250[30]	375[30]	0.37[30]	0.43[30]	5.0[30]	0	381
0	25	4	34	1.8[30]	29	340	1,250[30]	375[30]	0.37[30]	0.43[30]	5.0[30]	15[30]	382
0	23	11	100	1.2	102	3	0	0	0.07	0.08	1.5	0	383
Tr	21	8	55	4.5[30]	49	265	1,250[30]	375[30]	0.37[30]	0.43[30]	5.0[30]	15[30]	384
0	26	6	52	1.8[30]	105	25	1,250[30]	375[30]	0.37[30]	0.43[30]	5.0[30]	0	385
0	26	1	21	1.8[30]	18	230	1,250[30]	375[30]	0.37[30]	0.43[30]	5.0[30]	15[30]	386
0	25	3	31	1.8[30]	42	75	1,250[30]	375[30]	0.37[30]	0.43[30]	5.0[30]	15[30]	387
0	22	48	118	18.0[30]	106	352	5,000[30]	1,501[30]	1.50[30]	1.70[30]	20.0[30]	60[30]	388
0	25	6	19	4.5[30]	27	181	1,250[30]	375[30]	0.37[30]	0.43[30]	5.0[30]	15[30]	389
0	23	43	98	4.5[30]	106	354	1,250[30]	375[30]	0.37[30]	0.43[30]	5.0[30]	15[30]	390
0	78	11	86	1.0	314	2	0	0	0.08	0.04	0.4	0	391
0	129	49	575	9.5	389	7	0	0	0.48	0.24	7.7	0	392
0	342	527	1,086	2.7	845	3,226	0	0	0.32	1.27	1.6	0	393
0	29	44	91	0.2	71	269	0	0	0.03	0.11	0.1	0	394
279	225	262	748	7.3	469	1,853	690	194	0.82	0.90	7.7	1	395
47	38	44	125	1.2	78	310	120	32	0.14	0.15	1.3	Tr	396
598	645	653	1,162	22.1	1,439	2,900	1,660	498	1.11	1.66	10.0	1	397
37	40	41	72	1.4	90	181	100	31	0.07	0.10	0.6	Tr	398
19	20	21	37	0.7	46	92	50	16	0.04	0.05	0.3	Tr	399
6	291	513	570	10.8	1,562	1,733	0	0	0.86	1.03	7.4	1	400
1	32	57	63	1.2	173	192	0	0	0.09	0.11	0.8	Tr	401

[35] With the exception of angel food cake, cakes were made from mixes containing vegetable shortening and frostings were made with margarine.

Table continued on following page

APPENDIX 1. Nutritive Value of the Edible Part of Food *Continued*

Item No.	Foods, Approximate Measures, Units, and Weight (Weight of Edible Portion Only)			Water	Food energy	Protein	Fat	Fatty Acids: Saturated	Fatty Acids: Monounsaturated	Fatty Acids: Polyunsaturated
	GRAIN PRODUCTS *Continued*		Grams	%	Calories	Grams	Grams	Grams	Grams	Grams
	Cakes prepared from cake mixes with enriched flour:[35]									
	Yellow with chocolate frosting:									
402	Whole, 2-layer cake, 8- or 9-in diam.	1 cake	1,108	26	3,735	45	125	47.8	48.8	21.8
403	Piece, 1/16 of cake	1 piece	69	26	235	3	8	3.0	3.0	1.4
	Cakes prepared from home recipes using enriched flour:									
	Carrot, with cream cheese frosting:[36]									
404	Whole cake, 10-in diam. tube cake	1 cake	1,536	23	6,175	63	328	66.0	135.2	107.5
405	Piece, 1/16 of cake	1 piece	96	23	385	4	21	4.1	8.4	6.7
	Fruitcake, dark:[36]									
406	Whole cake, 7½-in diam., 2¼-in-high tube cake	1 cake	1,361	18	5,185	74	228	47.6	113.0	51.7
407	Piece, 1/32 of cake, ⅔-in arc	1 piece	43	18	165	2	7	1.5	3.6	1.6
	Plain sheet cake:[37]									
	Without frosting:									
408	Whole cake, 9-in square	1 cake	777	25	2,830	35	108	29.5	45.1	25.6
409	Piece, 1/9 of cake	1 piece	86	25	315	4	12	3.3	5.0	2.8
	With uncooked white frosting:									
410	Whole cake, 9-in square	1 cake	1,096	21	4,020	37	129	41.6	50.4	26.3
411	Piece, 1/9 of cake	1 piece	121	21	445	4	14	4.6	5.6	2.9
	Pound:[38]									
412	Loaf, 8½ by 3½ by 3¼ in	1 loaf	514	22	2,025	33	94	21.1	40.9	26.7
413	Slice, 1/17 of loaf	1 slice	30	22	120	2	5	1.2	2.4	1.6
	Cakes, commercial, made with enriched flour:									
	Pound:									
414	Loaf, 8½ by 3½ by 3 in	1 loaf	500	24	1,935	26	94	52.0	30.0	4.0
415	Slice, 1/17 of loaf	1 slice	29	24	110	2	5	3.0	1.7	0.2
	Snack cakes:									
416	Devil's food with creme filling (2 small cakes per pkg)	1 small cake	28	20	105	1	4	1.7	1.5	0.6
417	Sponge with creme filling (2 small cakes per pkg)	1 small cake	42	19	155	1	5	2.3	2.1	0.5
	White with white frosting:									
418	Whole, 2-layer cake, 8- or 9-in diam	1 cake	1,140	24	4,170	43	148	33.1	61.6	42.2
419	Piece, 1/16 of cake	1 piece	71	24	260	3	9	2.1	3.8	2.6
	Yellow with chocolate frosting:									
420	Whole, 2-layer cake, 8- or 9-in diam.	1 cake	1,108	23	3,895	40	175	92.0	58.7	10.0
421	Piece, 1/16 of cake	1 piece	69	23	245	2	11	5.7	3.7	0.6
	Cheesecake:									
422	Whole cake, 9-in diam.	1 cake	1,110	46	3,350	60	213	119.9	65.5	14.4
423	Piece, 1/12 of cake	1 piece	92	46	280	5	18	9.9	5.4	1.2
	Cookies made with enriched flour:									
	Brownies with nuts:									
424	Commercial, with frosting, 1½ by 1¾ by ⅞ in	1 brownie	25	13	100	1	4	1.6	2.0	0.6
425	From home recipe, 1¾ by 1¾ by ⅞ in[36]	1 brownie	20	10	95	1	6	1.4	2.8	1.2
	Chocolate chip:									
426	Commercial, 2¼-in diam., ⅜ in thick	4 cookies	42	4	180	2	9	2.9	3.1	2.6

[35] With the exception of angel food cake, cakes were made from mixes containing vegetable shortening and frostings were made with margarine.
[36] Made with vegetable oil.

Nutrients in Indicated Quantity

Cholesterol	Carbohydrate	Calcium	Phosphorus	Iron	Potassium	Sodium	Vitamin A Value (IU)	Vitamin A Value (RE)	Thiamin	Riboflavin	Niacin	Ascorbic acid	Item No.
Milligrams	*Grams*	*Milligrams*	*Milligrams*	*Milligrams*	*Milligrams*	*Milligrams*	*International units*	*Retinol equivalents*	*Milligrams*	*Milligrams*	*Milligrams*	*Milligrams*	
576	638	1,008	2,017	15.5	1,208	2,515	1,550	465	1.22	1.66	11.1	1	402
36	40	63	126	1.0	75	157	100	29	0.08	0.10	0.7	Tr	403
1183	775	707	998	21.0	1,720	4,470	2,240	246	1.83	1.97	14.7	23	404
74	48	44	62	1.3	108	279	140	15	0.11	0.12	0.9	1	405
640	783	1,293	1,592	37.6	6,138	2,123	1,720	422	2.41	2.55	17.0	504	406
20	25	41	50	1.2	194	67	50	13	0.08	0.08	0.5	16	407
552	434	497	793	11.7	614	2,331	1,320	373	1.24	1.40	10.1	2	408
61	48	55	88	1.3	68	258	150	41	0.14	0.15	1.1	Tr	409
636	694	548	822	11.0	669	2,488	2,190	647	1.21	1.42	9.9	2	410
70	77	61	91	1.2	74	275	240	71	0.13	0.16	1.1	Tr	411
555	265	339	473	9.3	483	1,645	3,470	1,033	0.93	1.08	7.8	1	412
32	15	20	28	0.5	28	96	200	60	0.05	0.06	0.5	Tr	413
1100	257	146	517	8.0	443	1,857	2,820	715	0.96	1.12	8.1	0	414
64	15	8	30	0.5	26	108	160	41	0.06	0.06	0.5	0	415
15	17	21	26	1.0	34	105	20	4	0.06	0.09	0.7	0	416
7	27	14	44	0.6	37	155	30	9	0.07	0.06	0.6	0	417
46	670	536	1,585	15.5	832	2,827	640	194	3.19	2.05	27.6	0	418
3	42	33	99	1.0	52	176	40	12	0.20	0.13	1.7	0	419
609	620	366	1,884	19.9	1,972	3,080	1,850	488	0.78	2.22	10.0	0	420
38	39	23	117	1.2	123	192	120	30	0.05	0.14	0.6	0	421
2053	317	622	977	5.3	1,088	2,464	2,820	833	0.33	1.44	5.1	56	422
170	26	52	81	0.4	90	204	230	69	0.03	0.12	0.4	5	423
14	16	13	26	0.6	50	59	70	18	0.08	0.07	0.3	Tr	424
18	11	9	26	0.4	35	51	20	6	0.05	0.05	0.3	Tr	425
5	28	13	41	0.8	68	140	50	15	0.10	0.23	1.0	Tr	426

Table continued on following page

APPENDIX 1. Nutritive Value of the Edible Part of Food *Continued*

Item No.	Foods, Approximate Measures, Units, and Weight (Weight of Edible Portion Only)			Water	Food energy	Protein	Fat	Fatty Acids: Saturated	Fatty Acids: Monounsaturated	Fatty Acids: Polyunsaturated
	GRAIN PRODUCTS *Continued*		Grams	%	Calories	Grams	Grams	Grams	Grams	Grams
	Cookies made with enriched flour:									
	Chocolate chip:									
427	From home recipe, 2¼-in diam.[25]	4 cookies	40	3	185	2	11	3.9	4.3	2.0
428	From refrigerated dough, 2¼-in diam., ⅜ in thick	4 cookies	48	5	225	2	11	4.0	4.4	2.0
429	Fig bars, square, 1⅝ by 1⅝ by ⅜ in or rectangular, 1½ by 1¾ by ½ in	4 cookies	56	12	210	2	4	1.0	1.5	1.0
430	Oatmeal with raisins, 2⅝-in diam., ¼ in thick	4 cookies	52	4	245	3	10	2.5	4.5	2.8
431	Peanut butter cookie, from home recipe, 2⅝-in diam.[25]	4 cookies	48	3	245	4	14	4.0	5.8	2.8
432	Sandwich type (chocolate or vanilla), 1¾-in diam., ⅜ in thick	4 cookies	40	2	195	2	8	2.0	3.6	2.2
	Shortbread:									
433	Commercial	4 small cookies	32	6	155	2	8	2.9	3.0	1.1
434	From home recipe[38]	2 large cookies	28	3	145	2	8	1.3	2.7	3.4
435	Sugar cookie, from refrigerated dough, 2½-in diam., ¼ in thick	4 cookies	48	4	235	2	12	2.3	5.0	3.6
436	Vanilla wafers, 1¾-in diam., ¼ in thick	10 cookies	40	4	185	2	7	1.8	3.0	1.8
437	Corn chips	1-oz package	28	1	155	2	9	1.4	2.4	3.7
	Cornmeal:									
438	Whole-ground, unbolted, dry form	1 cup	122	12	435	11	5	0.5	1.1	2.5
439	Bolted (nearly whole-grain), dry form	1 cup	122	12	440	11	4	0.5	0.9	2.2
	Degermed, enriched:									
440	Dry form	1 cup	138	12	500	11	2	0.2	0.4	0.9
441	Cooked	1 cup	240	88	120	3	Tr	Tr	0.1	0.2
	Crackers:[39]									
	Cheese:									
442	Plain, 1 in square	10 crackers	10	4	50	1	3	0.9	1.2	0.3
443	Sandwich type (peanut butter)	1 sandwich	8	3	40	1	2	0.4	0.8	0.3
444	Graham, plain, 2½ in square	2 crackers	14	5	60	1	1	0.4	0.6	0.4
445	Melba toast, plain	1 piece	5	4	20	1	Tr	0.1	0.1	0.1
446	Rye wafers, whole-grain, 1⅞ by 3½ in	2 wafers	14	5	55	1	1	0.3	0.4	0.3
447	Saltines[40]	4 crackers	12	4	50	1	1	0.5	0.4	0.2
448	Snack-type, standard	1 round cracker	3	3	15	Tr	1	0.2	0.4	0.1
449	Wheat, thin	4 crackers	8	3	35	1	1	0.5	0.5	0.4
450	Whole-wheat wafers	2 crackers	8	4	35	1	2	0.5	0.6	0.4
451	Croissants, made with enriched flour, 4½ by 4 by 1¾ in	1 croissant	57	22	235	5	12	3.5	6.7	1.4
	Danish pastry, made with enriched flour:									
	Plain without fruit or nuts:									
452	Packaged ring, 12 oz	1 ring	340	27	1,305	21	71	21.8	28.6	15.6
453	Round piece, about 4¼-in diam., 1 in high	1 pastry	57	27	220	4	12	3.6	4.8	2.6
454	Ounce	1 oz	28	27	110	2	6	1.8	2.4	1.3
455	Fruit, round piece	1 pastry	65	30	235	4	13	3.9	5.2	2.9
	Doughnuts, made with enriched flour:									
456	Cake type, plain, 3¼-in diam., 1 in high	1 doughnut	50	21	210	3	12	2.8	5.0	3.0
457	Yeast-leavened, glazed, 3¾-in diam., 1¼ in high	1 doughnut	60	27	235	4	13	5.2	5.5	0.9
458	English muffins, plain, enriched	1 muffin	57	42	140	5	1	0.3	0.2	0.3
459	Toasted	1 muffin	50	29	140	5	1	0.3	0.2	0.3

[37] Cake made with vegetable shortening; frosting with margarine.
[38] Made with margarine.

Nutrients in Indicated Quantity													
							Vitamin A Value						
Cholesterol	Carbohydrate	Calcium	Phosphorus	Iron	Potassium	Sodium	(IU)	(RE)	Thiamin	Riboflavin	Niacin	Ascorbic acid	Item No.
Milligrams	Grams	Milligrams	Milligrams	Milligrams	Milligrams	Milligrams	International units	Retinol equivalents	Milligrams	Milligrams	Milligrams	Milligrams	
18	26	13	34	1.0	82	82	20	5	0.06	0.06	0.6	0	427
22	32	13	34	1.0	62	173	30	8	0.06	0.10	0.9	0	428
27	42	40	34	1.4	162	180	60	6	0.08	0.07	0.7	Tr	429
2	36	18	58	1.1	90	148	40	12	0.09	0.08	1.0	0	430
22	28	21	60	1.1	110	142	20	5	0.07	0.07	1.9	0	431
0	29	12	40	1.4	66	189	0	0	0.09	0.07	0.8	0	432
27	20	13	39	0.8	38	123	30	8	0.10	0.09	0.9	0	433
0	17	6	31	0.6	18	125	300	89	0.08	0.06	0.7	Tr	434
29	31	50	91	0.9	33	261	40	11	0.09	0.06	1.1	0	435
25	29	16	36	0.8	50	150	50	14	0.07	0.10	1.0	0	436
0	16	35	52	0.5	52	233	110	11	0.04	0.05	0.4	1	437
0	90	24	312	2.2	346	1	620	62	0.46	0.13	2.4	0	438
0	91	21	272	2.2	303	1	590	59	0.37	0.10	2.3	0	439
0	108	8	137	5.9	166	1	610	61	0.61	0.36	4.8	0	440
0	26	2	34	1.4	38	0	140	14	0.14	0.10	1.2	0	441
6	6	11	17	0.3	17	112	20	5	0.05	0.04	0.4	0	442
1	5	7	25	0.3	17	90	Tr	Tr	0.04	0.03	0.6	0	443
0	11	6	20	0.4	36	86	0	0	0.02	0.03	0.6	0	444
0	4	6	10	0.1	11	44	0	0	0.01	0.01	0.1	0	445
0	10	7	44	0.5	65	115	0	0	0.06	0.03	0.5	0	446
4	9	3	12	0.5	17	165	0	0	0.06	0.05	0.6	0	447
0	2	3	6	0.1	4	30	Tr	Tr	0.01	0.01	0.1	0	448
0	5	3	15	0.3	17	69	Tr	Tr	0.04	0.03	0.4	0	449
0	5	3	22	0.2	31	59	0	0	0.02	0.03	0.4	0	450
13	27	20	64	2.1	68	452	50	13	0.17	0.13	1.3	0	451
292	152	360	347	6.5	316	1,302	360	99	0.95	1.02	8.5	Tr	452
49	26	60	58	1.1	53	218	60	17	0.16	0.17	1.4	Tr	453
24	13	30	29	0.5	26	109	30	8	0.08	0.09	0.7	Tr	454
56	28	17	80	1.3	57	233	40	11	0.16	0.14	1.4	Tr	455
20	24	22	111	1.0	58	192	20	5	0.12	0.12	1.1	Tr	456
21	26	17	55	1.4	64	222	Tr	Tr	0.28	0.12	1.8	0	457
0	27	96	67	1.7	331	378	0	0	0.26	0.19	2.2	0	458
0	27	96	67	1.7	331	378	0	0	0.23	0.19	2.2	0	459

[39] Crackers made with enriched flour except for rye wafers and whole-wheat wafers.
[40] Made with lard.

Table continued on following page

APPENDIX 1. Nutritive Value of the Edible Part of Food *Continued*

Item No.	Foods, Approximate Measures, Units, and Weight (Weight of Edible Portion Only)			Water	Food energy	Protein	Fat	Fatty Acids Saturated	Fatty Acids Monounsaturated	Fatty Acids Polyunsaturated
	GRAIN PRODUCTS *Continued*		*Grams*	*%*	*Calories*	*Grams*	*Grams*	*Grams*	*Grams*	*Grams*
460	French toast, from home recipe	1 slice	65	53	155	6	7	1.6	2.0	1.6
	Macaroni, enriched, cooked (cut lengths, elbows, shells):									
461	Firm stage (hot)	1 cup	130	64	190	7	1	0.1	0.1	0.3
	Tender stage:									
462	Cold	1 cup	105	72	115	4	Tr	0.1	0.1	0.2
463	Hot	1 cup	140	72	155	5	1	0.1	0.1	0.2
	Muffins made with enriched flour, 2½-in diam., 1½ in high:									
	From home recipe:									
464	Blueberry[25]	1 muffin	45	37	135	3	5	1.5	2.1	1.2
465	Bran[36]	1 muffin	45	35	125	3	6	1.4	1.6	2.3
466	Corn (enriched, degermed cornmeal and flour)[25]	1 muffin	45	33	145	3	5	1.5	2.2	1.4
	From commercial mix (egg and water added):									
467	Blueberry	1 muffin	45	33	140	3	5	1.4	2.0	1.2
468	Bran	1 muffin	45	28	140	3	4	1.3	1.6	1.0
469	Corn	1 muffin	45	30	145	3	6	1.7	2.3	1.4
470	Noodles (egg noodles), enriched, cooked	1 cup	160	70	200	7	2	0.5	0.6	0.6
471	Noodles, chow mein, canned	1 cup	45	11	220	6	11	2.1	7.3	0.4
	Pancakes, 4-in diam.:									
472	Buckwheat, from mix (with buckwheat and enriched flours), egg and milk added	1 pancake	27	58	55	2	2	0.9	0.9	0.5
	Plain:									
473	From home recipe using enriched flour	1 pancake	27	50	60	2	2	0.5	0.8	0.5
474	From mix (with enriched flour), egg, milk, and oil added	1 pancake	27	54	60	2	2	0.5	0.9	0.5
	Piecrust, made with enriched flour and vegetable shortening, baked:									
475	From home recipe, 9-in diam.	1 pie shell	180	15	900	11	60	14.8	25.9	15.7
476	From mix, 9-in diam	Piecrust for 2-crust pie	320	19	1,485	20	93	22.7	41.0	25.0
	Pies, piecrust made with enriched flour, vegetable shortening, 9-in diam.:									
	Apple:									
477	Whole	1 pie	945	48	2,420	21	105	27.4	44.4	26.5
478	Piece, ⅙ of pie	1 piece	158	48	405	3	18	4.6	7.4	4.4
	Blueberry:									
479	Whole	1 pie	945	51	2,285	23	102	25.5	44.4	27.4
480	Piece, ⅙ of pie	1 piece	158	51	380	4	17	4.3	7.4	4.6
	Cherry:									
481	Whole	1 pie	945	47	2,465	25	107	28.4	46.3	27.4
482	Piece, ⅙ of pie	1 piece	158	47	410	4	18	4.7	7.7	4.6
	Creme:									
483	Whole	1 pie	910	43	2,710	20	139	90.1	23.7	6.4
484	Piece, ⅙ of pie	1 piece	152	43	455	3	23	15.0	4.0	1.1
	Custard:									
485	Whole	1 pie	910	58	1,985	56	101	33.7	40.0	19.1
486	Piece, ⅙ of pie	1 piece	152	58	330	9	17	5.6	6.7	3.2
	Lemon meringue:									
487	Whole	1 pie	840	47	2,140	31	86	26.0	34.4	17.6
488	Piece, ⅙ of pie	1 piece	140	47	355	5	14	4.3	5.7	2.9
	Peach:									
489	Whole	1 pie	945	48	2,410	24	101	24.6	43.5	26.5
490	Piece, ⅙ of pie	1 piece	158	48	405	4	17	4.1	7.3	4.4

[25] Made with vegetable shortening.

Nutrients in Indicated Quantity

Cholesterol	Carbohydrate	Calcium	Phosphorus	Iron	Potassium	Sodium	Vitamin A Value (IU)	Vitamin A Value (RE)	Thiamin	Riboflavin	Niacin	Ascorbic acid	Item No.
Milligrams	Grams	Milligrams	Milligrams	Milligrams	Milligrams	Milligrams	International units	Retinol equivalents	Milligrams	Milligrams	Milligrams	Milligrams	
112	17	72	85	1.3	86	257	110	32	0.12	0.16	1.0	Tr	460
0	39	14	85	2.1	103	1	0	0	0.23	0.13	1.8	0	461
0	24	8	53	1.3	64	1	0	0	0.15	0.08	1.2	0	462
0	32	11	70	1.7	85	1	0	0	0.20	0.11	1.5	0	463
19	20	54	46	0.9	47	198	40	9	0.10	0.11	0.9	1	464
24	19	60	125	1.4	99	189	230	30	0.11	0.13	1.3	3	465
23	21	66	59	0.9	57	169	80	15	0.11	0.11	0.9	Tr	466
45	22	15	90	0.9	54	225	50	11	0.10	0.17	1.1	Tr	467
28	24	27	182	1.7	50	385	100	14	0.08	0.12	1.9	0	468
42	22	30	128	1.3	31	291	90	16	0.09	0.09	0.8	Tr	469
50	37	16	94	2.6	70	3	110	34	0.22	0.13	1.9	0	470
5	26	14	41	0.4	33	450	0	0	0.05	0.03	0.6	0	471
20	6	59	91	0.4	66	125	60	17	0.04	0.05	0.2	Tr	472
16	9	27	38	0.5	33	115	30	10	0.06	0.07	0.5	Tr	473
16	8	36	71	0.7	43	160	30	7	0.09	0.12	0.8	Tr	474
0	79	25	90	4.5	90	1,100	0	0	0.54	0.40	5.0	0	475
0	141	131	272	9.3	179	2,602	0	0	1.06	0.80	9.9	0	476
0	360	76	208	9.5	756	2,844	280	28	1.04	0.76	9.5	9	477
0	60	13	35	1.6	126	476	50	5	0.17	0.13	1.6	2	478
0	330	104	217	12.3	945	2,533	850	85	1.04	0.85	10.4	38	479
0	55	17	36	2.1	158	423	140	14	0.17	0.14	1.7	6	480
0	363	132	236	9.5	992	2,873	4,160	416	1.13	0.85	9.5	0	481
0	61	22	40	1.6	166	480	700	70	0.19	0.14	1.6	0	482
46	351	273	919	6.8	796	2,207	1,250	391	0.36	0.89	6.4	0	483
8	59	46	154	1.1	133	369	210	65	0.06	0.15	1.1	0	484
1010	213	874	1,028	9.1	1,247	2,612	2,090	573	0.82	1.91	5.5	0	485
169	36	146	172	1.5	208	436	350	96	0.14	0.32	0.9	0	486
857	317	118	412	8.4	420	2,369	1,430	395	0.59	0.84	5.0	25	487
143	53	20	69	1.4	70	395	240	66	0.10	0.14	0.8	4	488
0	361	95	274	11.3	1,408	2,533	6,900	690	1.04	0.95	14.2	28	489
0	60	16	46	1.9	235	423	1,150	115	0.17	0.16	2.4	5	490

[36] Made with vegetable oil.

Table continued on following page

APPENDIX 1. Nutritive Value of the Edible Part of Food *Continued*

Item No.	Foods, Approximate Measures, Units, and Weight (Weight of Edible Portion Only)			Water	Food energy	Protein	Fat	Fatty Acids: Saturated	Fatty Acids: Monounsaturated	Fatty Acids: Polyunsaturated
	GRAIN PRODUCTS *Continued*		Grams	%	Calories	Grams	Grams	Grams	Grams	Grams
	Pies, piecrust made with enriched flour, vegetable shortening, 9-inch diam.:									
	Pecan:									
491	Whole	1 pie	825	20	3,450	42	189	28.1	101.5	47.0
492	Piece, ⅙ of pie	1 piece	138	20	575	7	32	4.7	17.0	7.9
	Pumpkin:									
493	Whole	1 pie	910	59	1,920	36	102	38.2	40.0	18.2
494	Piece, ⅙ of pie	1 piece	152	59	320	6	17	6.4	6.7	3.0
	Pies, fried:									
495	Apple	1 pie	85	43	255	2	14	5.8	6.6	0.6
496	Cherry	1 pie	85	42	250	2	14	5.8	6.7	0.6
	Popcorn, popped:									
497	Air-popped, unsalted	1 cup	8	4	30	1	Tr	Tr	0.1	0.2
498	Popped in vegetable oil, salted	1 cup	11	3	55	1	3	0.5	1.4	1.2
499	Sugar syrup coated	1 cup	35	4	135	2	1	0.1	0.3	0.6
	Pretzels, made with enriched flour:									
500	Stick, 2¼ in long	10 pretzels	3	3	10	Tr	Tr	Tr	Tr	Tr
501	Twisted, Dutch, 2¾ by 2⅝ in	1 pretzel	16	3	65	2	1	0.1	0.2	0.2
502	Twisted, thin, 3¼ by 2¼ by ¼ in	10 pretzels	60	3	240	6	2	0.4	0.8	0.6
	Rice:									
503	Brown, cooked, served hot	1 cup	195	70	230	5	1	0.3	0.3	0.4
	White, enriched:									
	Commercial varieties, all types:									
504	Raw	1 cup	185	12	670	12	1	0.2	0.2	0.3
505	Cooked, served hot	1 cup	205	73	225	4	Tr	0.1	0.1	0.1
506	Instant, ready-to-serve, hot	1 cup	165	73	180	4	0	0.1	0.1	0.1
	Parboiled:									
507	Raw	1 cup	185	10	685	14	1	0.1	0.1	0.2
508	Cooked, served hot	1 cup	175	73	185	4	Tr	Tr	Tr	0.1
	Rolls, enriched:									
	Commercial:									
509	Dinner, 2½-in diam., 2 in high	1 roll	28	32	85	2	2	0.5	0.8	0.6
510	Frankfurter and hamburger (8 per 11½-oz pkg.)	1 roll	40	34	115	3	2	0.5	0.8	0.6
511	Hard, 3¾-in diam., 2 in high	1 roll	50	25	155	5	2	0.4	0.5	0.6
512	Hoagie or submarine, 11½ by 3 by 2½ in	1 roll	135	31	400	11	8	1.8	3.0	2.2
	From home recipe:									
513	Dinner, 2½-in diam., 2 in high	1 roll	35	26	120	3	3	0.8	1.2	0.9
	Spaghetti, enriched, cooked:									
514	Firm stage, "al dente," served hot	1 cup	130	64	190	7	1	0.1	0.1	0.3
515	Tender stage, served hot	1 cup	140	73	155	5	1	0.1	0.1	0.2
516	Toaster pastries	1 pastry	54	13	210	2	6	1.7	3.6	0.4
517	Tortillas, corn	1 tortilla	30	45	65	2	1	0.1	0.3	0.6
	Waffles, made with enriched flour, 7-in diam.:									
518	From home recipe	1 waffle	75	37	245	7	13	4.0	4.9	2.6
519	From mix, egg and milk added	1 waffle	75	42	205	7	8	2.7	2.9	1.5
	Wheat flours:									
	All-purpose or family flour, enriched:									
520	Sifted, spooned	1 cup	115	12	420	12	1	0.2	0.1	0.5
521	Unsifted, spooned	1 cup	125	12	455	13	1	0.2	0.1	0.5
522	Cake or pastry flour, enriched, sifted, spooned	1 cup	96	12	350	7	1	0.1	0.1	0.3
523	Self-rising, enriched, unsifted, spooned	1 cup	125	12	440	12	1	0.2	0.1	0.5
524	Whole-wheat, from hard wheats, stirred	1 cup	120	12	400	16	2	0.3	0.3	1.1

Nutrients in Indicated Quantity

Cholesterol	Carbohydrate	Calcium	Phosphorus	Iron	Potassium	Sodium	Vitamin A Value (IU)	Vitamin A Value (RE)	Thiamin	Riboflavin	Niacin	Ascorbic acid	Item No.
Milligrams	*Grams*	*Milligrams*	*Milligrams*	*Milligrams*	*Milligrams*	*Milligrams*	*International units*	*Retinol equivalents*	*Milligrams*	*Milligrams*	*Milligrams*	*Milligrams*	
569	423	388	850	27.2	1,015	1,823	1,320	322	1.82	0.99	6.6	0	491
95	71	65	142	4.6	170	305	220	54	0.30	0.17	1.1	0	492
655	223	464	628	8.2	1,456	1,947	22,480	2,493	0.82	1.27	7.3	0	493
109	37	78	105	1.4	243	325	3,750	416	0.14	0.21	1.2	0	494
14	31	12	34	0.9	42	326	30	3	0.09	0.06	1.0	1	495
13	32	11	41	0.7	61	371	190	19	0.06	0.06	0.6	1	496
0	6	1	22	0.2	20	Tr	10	1	0.03	0.01	0.2	0	497
0	6	3	31	0.3	19	86	20	2	0.01	0.02	0.1	0	498
0	30	2	47	0.5	90	Tr	30	3	0.13	0.02	0.4	0	499
0	2	1	3	0.1	3	48	0	0	0.01	0.01	0.1	0	500
0	13	4	15	0.3	16	258	0	0	0.05	0.04	0.7	0	501
0	48	16	55	1.2	61	966	0	0	0.19	0.15	2.6	0	502
0	50	23	142	1.0	137	0	0	0	0.18	0.04	2.7	0	503
0	149	44	174	5.4	170	9	0	0	0.81	0.06	6.5	0	504
0	50	21	57	1.8	57	0	0	0	0.23	0.02	2.1	0	505
0	40	5	31	1.3	0	0	0	0	0.21	0.02	1.7	0	506
0	150	111	370	5.4	278	17	0	0	0.81	0.07	6.5	0	507
0	41	33	100	1.4	75	0	0	0	0.19	0.02	2.1	0	508
Tr	14	33	44	0.8	36	155	Tr	Tr	0.14	0.09	1.1	Tr	509
Tr	20	54	44	1.2	56	241	Tr	Tr	0.20	0.13	1.6	Tr	510
Tr	30	24	46	1.4	49	313	0	0	0.20	0.12	1.7	0	511
Tr	72	100	115	3.8	128	683	0	0	0.54	0.33	4.5	0	512
12	20	16	36	1.1	41	98	30	8	0.12	0.12	1.2	0	513
0	39	14	85	2.0	103	1	0	0	0.23	0.13	1.8	0	514
0	32	11	70	1.7	85	1	0	0	0.20	0.11	1.5	0	515
0	38	104	104	2.2	91	248	520	52	0.17	0.18	2.3	4	516
0	13	42	55	0.6	43	1	80	8	0.05	0.03	0.4	0	517
102	26	154	135	1.5	129	445	140	39	0.18	0.24	1.5	Tr	518
59	27	179	257	1.2	146	515	170	49	0.14	0.23	0.9	Tr	519
0	88	18	100	5.1	109	2	0	0	0.73	0.46	6.1	0	520
0	95	20	109	5.5	119	3	0	0	0.80	0.50	6.6	0	521
0	76	16	70	4.2	91	2	0	0	0.58	0.38	5.1	0	522
0	93	331	583	5.5	113	1,349	0	0	0.80	0.50	6.6	0	523
0	85	49	446	5.2	444	4	0	0	0.66	0.14	5.2	0	524

Table continued on following page

Item No.	Foods, Approximate Measures, Units, and Weight (Weight of Edible Portion Only)			Water	Food energy	Protein	Fat	Fatty Acids: Saturated	Fatty Acids: Monounsaturated	Fatty Acids: Polyunsaturated
	LEGUMES, NUTS, AND SEEDS		Grams	%	Calories	Grams	Grams	Grams	Grams	Grams
	Almonds, shelled:									
525	Slivered, packed	1 cup	135	4	795	27	70	6.7	45.8	14.8
526	Whole	1 oz	28	4	165	6	15	1.4	9.6	3.1
	Beans, dry:									
	Cooked, drained:									
527	Black	1 cup	171	66	225	15	1	0.1	0.1	0.5
528	Great Northern	1 cup	180	69	210	14	1	0.1	0.1	0.6
529	Lima	1 cup	190	64	260	16	1	0.2	0.1	0.5
530	Pea (navy)	1 cup	190	69	225	15	1	0.1	0.1	0.7
531	Pinto	1 cup	180	65	265	15	1	0.1	0.1	0.5
	Canned, solids and liquid:									
	White with:									
532	Frankfurters (sliced)	1 cup	255	71	365	19	18	7.4	8.8	0.7
533	Pork and tomato sauce	1 cup	255	71	310	16	7	2.4	2.7	0.7
534	Pork and sweet sauce	1 cup	255	66	385	16	12	4.3	4.9	1.2
535	Red kidney	1 cup	255	76	230	15	1	0.1	0.1	0.6
536	Black-eyed peas, dry, cooked (with residual cooking liquid)	1 cup	250	80	190	13	1	0.2	Tr	0.3
537	Brazil nuts, shelled	1 oz	28	3	185	4	19	4.6	6.5	6.8
538	Carob flour	1 cup	140	3	255	6	Tr	Tr	0.1	0.1
	Cashew-nuts, salted:									
539	Dry roasted	1 cup	137	2	785	21	63	12.5	37.4	10.7
540		1 oz	28	2	165	4	13	2.6	7.7	2.2
541	Roasted in oil	1 cup	130	4	750	21	63	12.4	36.9	10.6
542		1 oz	28	4	165	5	14	2.7	8.1	2.3
543	Chestnuts, European (Italian), roasted, shelled	1 cup	143	40	350	5	3	0.6	1.1	1.2
544	Chickpeas, cooked, drained	1 cup	163	60	270	15	4	0.4	0.9	1.9
	Coconut:									
	Raw:									
545	Piece, about 2 by 2 by ½ in	1 piece	45	47	160	1	15	13.4	0.6	0.2
546	Shredded or grated	1 cup	80	47	285	3	27	23.8	1.1	0.3
547	Dried, sweetened, shredded	1 cup	93	13	470	3	33	29.3	1.4	0.4
548	Filberts (hazelnuts), chopped	1 cup	115	5	725	15	72	5.3	56.5	6.9
549		1 oz	28	5	180	4	18	1.3	13.9	1.7
550	Lentils, dry, cooked	1 cup	200	72	215	16	1	0.1	0.2	0.5
551	Macadamia nuts, roasted in oil, salted	1 cup	134	2	960	10	103	15.4	80.9	1.8
552		1 oz	28	2	205	2	22	3.2	17.1	0.4
	Mixed nuts, with peanuts, salted:									
553	Dry roasted	1 oz	28	2	170	5	15	2.0	8.9	3.1
554	Roasted in oil	1 oz	28	2	175	5	16	2.5	9.0	3.8
555	Peanuts, roasted in oil, salted	1 cup	145	2	840	39	71	9.9	35.5	22.6
556		1 oz	28	2	165	8	14	1.9	6.9	4.4
557	Peanut butter	1 tbsp	16	1	95	5	8	1.4	4.0	2.5
558	Peas, split, dry, cooked	1 cup	200	70	230	16	1	0.1	0.1	0.3
559	Pecans, halves	1 cup	108	5	720	8	73	5.9	45.5	18.1
560		1 oz	28	5	190	2	19	1.5	12.0	4.7
561	Pine nuts (pinyons), shelled	1 oz	28	6	160	3	17	2.7	6.5	7.3
562	Pistachio nuts, dried, shelled	1 oz	28	4	165	6	14	1.7	9.3	2.1
563	Pumpkin and squash kernels, dry, hulled	1 oz	28	7	155	7	13	2.5	4.0	5.9
564	Refried beans, canned	1 cup	290	72	295	18	3	0.4	0.6	1.4
565	Sesame seeds, dry, hulled	1 tbsp	8	5	45	2	4	0.6	1.7	1.9
566	Soybeans, dry, cooked, drained	1 cup	180	71	235	20	10	1.3	1.9	5.3
	Soy products:									
567	Miso	1 cup	276	53	470	29	13	1.8	2.6	7.3
568	Tofu, piece 2½ by 2¾ by 1 in	1 piece	120	85	85	9	5	0.7	1.0	2.9
569	Sunflower seeds, dry, hulled	1 oz	28	5	160	6	14	1.5	2.7	9.3
570	Tahini	1 tbsp	15	3	90	3	8	1.1	3.0	3.5

Nutrients in Indicated Quantity

Cholesterol	*Carbohydrate*	*Calcium*	*Phosphorus*	*Iron*	*Potassium*	*Sodium*	*Vitamin A Value (IU)*	*Vitamin A Value (RE)*	*Thiamin*	*Riboflavin*	*Niacin*	*Ascorbic acid*	**Item No.**
Milligrams	*Grams*	*Milligrams*	*Milligrams*	*Milligrams*	*Milligrams*	*Milligrams*	*International units*	*Retinol equivalents*	*Milligrams*	*Milligrams*	*Milligrams*	*Milligrams*	
0	28	359	702	4.9	988	15	0	0	0.28	1.05	4.5	1	525
0	6	75	147	1.0	208	3	0	0	0.06	0.22	1.0	Tr	526
0	41	47	239	2.9	608	1	Tr	Tr	0.43	0.05	0.9	0	527
0	38	90	266	4.9	749	13	0	0	0.25	0.13	1.3	0	528
0	49	55	293	5.9	1,163	4	0	0	0.25	0.11	1.3	0	529
0	40	95	281	5.1	790	13	0	0	0.27	0.13	1.3	0	530
0	49	86	296	5.4	882	3	Tr	Tr	0.33	0.16	0.7	0	531
30	32	94	303	4.8	668	1,374	330	33	0.18	0.15	3.3	Tr	532
10	48	138	235	4.6	536	1,181	330	33	0.20	0.08	1.5	5	533
10	54	161	291	5.9	536	969	330	33	0.15	0.10	1.3	5	534
0	42	74	278	4.6	673	968	10	1	0.13	0.10	1.5	0	535
0	35	43	238	3.3	573	20	30	3	0.40	0.10	1.0	0	536
0	4	50	170	1.0	170	1	Tr	Tr	0.28	0.03	0.5	Tr	537
0	126	390	102	5.7	1,275	24	Tr	Tr	0.07	0.07	2.2	Tr	538
0	45	62	671	8.2	774	877[41]	0	0	0.27	0.27	1.9	0	539
0	9	13	139	1.7	160	181[41]	0	0	0.06	0.06	0.4	0	540
0	37	53	554	5.3	689	814[42]	0	0	0.55	0.23	2.3	0	541
0	8	12	121	1.2	150	177[42]	0	0	0.12	0.05	0.5	0	542
0	76	41	153	1.3	847	3	30	3	0.35	0.25	1.9	37	543
0	45	80	273	4.9	475	11	Tr	Tr	0.18	0.09	0.9	0	544
0	7	6	51	1.1	160	9	0	0	0.03	0.01	0.2	1	545
0	12	11	90	1.9	285	16	0	0	0.05	0.02	0.4	3	546
0	44	14	99	1.8	313	244	0	0	0.03	0.02	0.4	1	547
0	18	216	359	3.8	512	3	80	8	0.58	0.13	1.3	1	548
0	4	53	88	0.9	126	1	20	2	0.14	0.03	0.3	Tr	549
0	38	50	238	4.2	498	26	40	4	0.14	0.12	1.2	0	550
0	17	60	268	2.4	441	348[43]	10	1	0.29	0.15	2.7	0	551
0	4	13	57	0.5	93	74[43]	Tr	Tr	0.06	0.03	0.6	0	552
0	7	20	123	1.0	169	190[44]	Tr	Tr	0.06	0.06	1.3	0	553
0	6	31	131	0.9	165	185[44]	10	1	0.14	0.06	1.4	Tr	554
0	27	125	734	2.8	1,019	626[45]	0	0	0.42	0.15	21.5	0	555
0	5	24	143	0.5	199	122[45]	0	0	0.08	0.03	4.2	0	556
0	3	5	60	0.3	110	75	0	0	0.02	0.02	2.2	0	557
0	42	22	178	3.4	592	26	80	8	0.30	0.18	1.8	0	558
0	20	39	314	2.3	423	1	140	14	0.92	0.14	1.0	2	559
0	5	10	83	0.6	111	Tr	40	4	0.24	0.04	0.3	1	560
0	5	2	10	0.9	178	20	10	1	0.35	0.06	1.2	1	561
0	7	38	143	1.9	310	2	70	7	0.23	0.05	0.3	Tr	562
0	5	12	333	4.2	229	5	110	11	0.06	0.09	0.5	Tr	563
0	51	141	245	5.1	1,141	1,228	0	0	0.14	0.16	1.4	17	564
0	1	11	62	0.6	33	3	10	1	0.06	0.01	0.4	0	565
0	19	131	322	4.9	972	4	50	5	0.38	0.16	1.1	0	566
0	65	188	853	4.7	922	8,142	110	11	0.17	0.28	0.8	0	567
0	3	108	151	2.3	50	8	0	0	0.07	0.04	0.1	0	568
0	5	33	200	1.9	195	1	10	1	0.65	0.07	1.3	Tr	569
0	3	21	119	0.7	69	5	10	1	0.24	0.02	0.8	1	570

[41] Cashews without salt contain 21 mg of sodium per cup or 4 mg per oz.
[42] Cashews without salt contain 22 mg of sodium per cup or 5 mg per oz.
[43] Macadamia nuts with salt contain 9 mg of sodium per cup or 2 mg per oz.
[44] Mixed nuts without salt contain 3 mg of sodium per oz.
[45] Peanuts without salt contain 22 mg of sodium per cup or 4 mg per oz.

Table continued on following page

APPENDIX 1. Nutritive Value of the Edible Part of Food *Continued*

Item No.	Foods, Approximate Measures, Units, and Weight (Weight of Edible Portion Only)			Water	Food energy	Protein	Fat	Fatty Acids: Saturated	Fatty Acids: Monounsaturated	Fatty Acids: Polyunsaturated
	LEGUMES, NUTS, AND SEEDS *Continued*		Grams	%	Calories	Grams	Grams	Grams	Grams	Grams
	Walnuts:									
571	Black, chopped	1 cup	125	4	760	30	71	4.5	15.9	46.9
572		1 oz	28	4	170	7	16	1.0	3.6	10.6
573	English or Persian, pieces or chips	1 cup	120	4	770	17	74	6.7	17.0	47.0
574		1 oz	28	4	180	4	18	1.6	4.0	11.1
	MEAT AND MEAT PRODUCTS									
	Beef, cooked:[46]									
	Cuts braised, simmered, or pot roasted:									
	Relatively fat such as chuck blade:									
575	Lean and fat, piece, 2½ by 2½ by ¾ in	3 oz	85	43	325	22	26	10.8	11.7	0.9
576	Lean only from item 575	2.2 oz	62	53	170	19	9	3.9	4.2	0.3
	Relatively lean, such as bottom round:									
577	Lean and fat, piece, 4⅛ by 2¼ by ½ in	3 oz	85	54	220	25	13	4.8	5.7	0.5
578	Lean only from item 577	2.8 oz	78	57	175	25	8	2.7	3.4	0.3
	Ground beef, broiled, patty, 3 by ⅝ in:									
579	Lean	3 oz	85	56	230	21	16	6.2	6.9	0.6
580	Regular	3 oz	85	54	245	20	18	6.9	7.7	0.7
581	Heart, lean, braised	3 oz	85	65	150	24	5	1.2	0.8	1.6
582	Liver, fried, slice, 6½ by 2⅜ by ⅜ in[47]	3 oz	85	56	185	23	7	2.5	3.6	1.3
	Roast, oven cooked, no liquid added:									
	Relatively fat, such as rib:									
583	Lean and fat, 2 pieces, 4⅛ by 2¼ by ¼ in	3 oz	85	46	315	19	26	10.8	11.4	0.9
584	Lean only from item 583	2.2 oz	61	57	150	17	9	3.6	3.7	0.3
	Relatively lean, such as eye of round:									
585	Lean and fat, 2 pieces, 2½ by 2½ by ⅜ in	3 oz	85	57	205	23	12	4.9	5.4	0.5
586	Lean only from item 585	2.6 oz	75	63	135	22	5	1.9	2.1	0.2
	Steak:									
	Sirloin, broiled:									
587	Lean and fat, piece, 2½ by 2½ by ¾ in	3 oz	85	53	240	23	15	6.4	6.9	0.6
588	Lean only from item 587	2.5 oz	72	59	150	22	6	2.6	2.8	0.3
589	Beef, canned, corned	3 oz	85	59	185	22	10	4.2	4.9	0.4
590	Beef, dried, chipped	2.5 oz	72	48	145	24	4	1.8	2.0	0.2
	Lamb, cooked:									
	Chops, (3 per lb with bone):									
	Arm, braised:									
591	Lean and fat	2.2 oz	63	44	220	20	15	6.9	6.0	0.9
592	Lean only from item 591	1.7 oz	48	49	135	17	7	2.9	2.6	0.4
	Loin, broiled:									
593	Lean and fat	2.8 oz	80	54	235	22	16	7.3	6.4	1.0
594	Lean only from item 593	2.3 oz	64	61	140	19	6	2.6	2.4	0.4
	Leg, roasted:									
595	Lean and fat, 2 pieces, 4⅛ by 2¼ by ¼ in	3 oz	85	59	205	22	13	5.6	4.9	0.8
596	Lean only from item 595	2.6 oz	73	64	140	20	6	2.4	2.2	0.4
	Rib, roasted:									
597	Lean and fat, 3 pieces, 2½ by 2½ by ¼ in	3 oz	85	47	315	18	26	12.1	10.6	1.5
598	Lean only from item 597	2 oz	57	60	130	15	7	3.2	3.0	0.5

[46] Outer layer of fat was removed to within approximately ½ in. of the lean. Deposits of fat within the cut were not removed.
[47] Fried in vegetable shortening.

Nutrients in Indicated Quantity

Cholesterol	Carbohydrate	Calcium	Phosphorus	Iron	Potassium	Sodium	Vitamin A Value (IU)	Vitamin A Value (RE)	Thiamin	Riboflavin	Niacin	Ascorbic acid	Item No.
Milligrams	Grams	Milligrams	Milligrams	Milligrams	Milligrams	Milligrams	International units	Retinol equivalents	Milligrams	Milligrams	Milligrams	Milligrams	
0	15	73	580	3.8	655	1	370	37	0.27	0.14	0.9	Tr	571
0	3	16	132	0.9	149	Tr	80	8	0.06	0.03	0.2	Tr	572
0	22	113	380	2.9	602	12	150	15	0.46	0.18	1.3	4	573
0	5	27	90	0.7	142	3	40	4	0.11	0.04	0.3	1	574
87	0	11	163	2.5	163	53	Tr	Tr	0.06	0.19	2.0	0	575
66	0	8	146	2.3	163	44	Tr	Tr	0.05	0.17	1.7	0	576
81	0	5	217	2.8	248	43	Tr	Tr	0.06	0.21	3.3	0	577
75	0	4	212	2.7	240	40	Tr	Tr	0.06	0.20	3.0	0	578
74	0	9	134	1.8	256	65	Tr	Tr	0.04	0.18	4.4	0	579
76	0	9	144	2.1	248	70	Tr	Tr	0.03	0.16	4.9	0	580
164	0	5	213	6.4	198	54	Tr	Tr	0.12	1.31	3.4	5	581
410	7	9	392	5.3	309	90	30,690[48]	9,120[48]	0.18	3.52	12.3	23	582
72	0	8	145	2.0	246	54	Tr	Tr	0.06	0.16	3.1	0	583
49	0	5	127	1.7	218	45	Tr	Tr	0.05	0.13	2.7	0	584
62	0	5	177	1.6	308	50	Tr	Tr	0.07	0.14	3.0	0	585
52	0	3	170	1.5	297	46	Tr	Tr	0.07	0.13	2.8	0	586
77	0	9	186	2.6	306	53	Tr	Tr	0.10	0.23	3.3	0	587
64	0	8	176	2.4	290	48	Tr	Tr	0.09	0.22	3.1	0	588
80	0	17	90	3.7	51	802	Tr	Tr	0.02	0.20	2.9	0	589
46	0	14	287	2.3	142	3,053	Tr	Tr	0.05	0.23	2.7	0	590
77	0	16	132	1.5	195	46	Tr	Tr	0.04	0.16	4.4	0	591
59	0	12	111	1.3	162	36	Tr	Tr	0.03	0.13	3.0	0	592
78	0	16	162	1.4	272	62	Tr	Tr	0.09	0.21	5.5	0	593
60	0	12	145	1.3	241	54	Tr	Tr	0.08	0.18	4.4	0	594
78	0	8	162	1.7	273	57	Tr	Tr	0.09	0.24	5.5	0	595
65	0	6	150	1.5	247	50	Tr	Tr	0.08	0.20	4.6	0	596
77	0	19	139	1.4	224	60	Tr	Tr	0.08	0.18	5.5	0	597
50	0	12	111	1.0	179	46	Tr	Tr	0.05	0.13	3.5	0	598

[48] Value varies widely.

Table continued on following page

APPENDIX 1. Nutritive Value of the Edible Part of Food *Continued*

Item No.	Foods, Approximate Measures, Units, and Weight (Weight of Edible Portion Only)			Water	Food energy	Protein	Fat	Fatty Acids: Saturated	Fatty Acids: Monounsaturated	Fatty Acids: Polyunsaturated
	MEAT AND MEAT PRODUCTS *Continued*		Grams	%	Calories	Grams	Grams	Grams	Grams	Grams
	Pork, cured, cooked:									
	Bacon:									
599	Regular	3 medium slices	19	13	110	6	9	3.3	4.5	1.1
600	Canadian-style	2 slices	46	62	85	11	4	1.3	1.9	0.4
	Ham, light cure, roasted:									
601	Lean and fat, 2 pieces, 4⅛ by 2¼ by ¼ in	3 oz	85	58	205	18	14	5.1	6.7	1.5
602	Lean only from item 601	2.4 oz	68	66	105	17	4	1.3	1.7	0.4
603	Ham, canned, roasted, 2 pieces, 4⅛ by 2¼ by ¼ in	3 oz	85	67	140	18	7	2.4	3.5	0.8
	Luncheon meat:									
604	Canned, spiced or unspiced, slice, 3 by 2 by ½ in	2 slices	42	52	140	5	13	4.5	6.0	1.5
605	Chopped ham (8 slices per 6 oz pkg)	2 slices	42	64	95	7	7	2.4	3.4	0.9
	Cooked ham (8 slices per 8-oz pkg.):									
606	Regular	2 slices	57	65	105	10	6	1.9	2.8	0.7
607	Extra lean	2 slices	57	71	75	11	3	0.9	1.3	0.3
	Pork, fresh, cooked:									
	Chop, loin (cut 3 per lb with bone):									
	Broiled:									
608	Lean and fat	3.1 oz	87	50	275	24	19	7.0	8.8	2.2
609	Lean only from item 608	2.5 oz	72	57	165	23	8	2.6	3.4	0.9
	Pan fried:									
610	Lean and fat	3.1 oz	89	45	335	21	27	9.8	12.5	3.1
611	Lean only from item 610	2.4 oz	67	54	180	19	11	3.7	4.8	1.3
	Ham (leg), roasted:									
612	Lean and fat, piece, 2½ by 2½ by ¾ in	3 oz	85	53	250	21	18	6.4	8.1	2.0
613	Lean only from item 612	2.5 oz	72	60	160	20	8	2.7	3.6	1.0
	Rib, roasted:									
614	Lean and fat, piece, 2½ by ¾ in	3 oz	85	51	270	21	20	7.2	9.2	2.3
615	Lean only from item 614	2.5 oz	71	57	175	20	10	3.4	4.4	1.2
	Shoulder cut, braised:									
616	Lean, and fat, 3 pieces, 2½ by 2½ by ¼ in	3 oz	85	47	295	23	22	7.9	10.0	2.4
617	Lean only from item 616	2.4 oz	67	54	165	22	8	2.8	3.7	1.0
	Sausages (See also Luncheon meats, items 604–607):									
618	Bologna, slice (8 per 8-oz pkg)	2 slices	57	54	180	7	16	6.1	7.6	1.4
619	Braunschweiger, slice (6 per 6-oz pkg)	2 slices	57	48	205	8	18	6.2	8.5	2.1
620	Brown and serve (10–11 per 8-oz pkg), browned	1 link	13	45	50	2	5	1.7	2.2	0.5
621	Frankfurter (10 per 1-lb pkg), cooked (reheated)	1 frankfurter	45	54	145	5	13	4.8	6.2	1.2
622	Pork link (16 per 1-lb pkg), cooked[50]	1 link	13	45	50	3	4	1.4	1.8	0.5
	Salami:									
623	Cooked type, slice (8 per 8-oz pkg)	2 slices	57	60	145	8	11	4.6	5.2	1.2
624	Dry type, slice (12 per 4-oz pkg)	2 slices	20	35	85	5	7	2.4	3.4	0.6
625	Sandwich spread (pork, beef)	1 tbsp	15	60	35	1	3	0.9	1.1	0.4
626	Vienna sausage (7 per 4-oz can)	1 sausage	16	60	45	2	4	1.5	2.0	0.3
	Veal, medium fat, cooked, bone removed:									
627	Cutlet, 4⅛ by 2¼ by ½ in, braised or broiled	3 oz	85	60	185	23	9	4.1	4.1	0.6
628	Rib, 2 pieces, 4⅛ by 2¼ by ¼ in, roasted	3 oz	85	55	230	23	14	6.0	6.0	1.0

[49] Contains added sodium ascorbate. If sodium ascorbate is not added, abscorbic acid content is negligible.
[50] One patty (8 per lb) of bulk sausage is equivalent to 2 links.

Nutrients in Indicated Quantity

Cholesterol	Carbohydrate	Calcium	Phosphorus	Iron	Potassium	Sodium	Vitamin A Value (IU)	Vitamin A Value (RE)	Thiamin	Riboflavin	Niacin	Ascorbic acid	Item No.
Milligrams	*Grams*	*Milligrams*	*Milligrams*	*Milligrams*	*Milligrams*	*Milligrams*	*International units*	*Retinol equivalents*	*Milligrams*	*Milligrams*	*Milligrams*	*Milligrams*	
16	Tr	2	64	0.3	92	303	0	0	0.13	0.05	1.4	6	599
27	1	5	136	0.4	179	711	0	0	0.38	0.09	3.2	10	600
53	0	6	182	0.7	243	1,009	0	0	0.51	0.19	3.8	0	601
37	0	5	154	0.6	215	902	0	0	0.46	0.17	3.4	0	602
35	Tr	6	188	0.9	298	908	0	0	0.82	0.21	4.3	19[49]	603
26	1	3	34	0.3	90	541	0	0	0.15	0.08	1.3	Tr	604
21	0	3	65	0.3	134	576	0	0	0.27	0.09	1.6	8[49]	605
32	2	4	141	0.6	189	751	0	0	0.49	0.14	3.0	16[49]	606
27	1	4	124	0.4	200	815	0	0	0.53	0.13	2.8	15[49]	607
84	0	3	184	0.7	312	61	10	3	0.87	0.24	4.3	Tr	608
71	0	4	176	0.7	302	56	10	1	0.83	0.22	4.0	Tr	609
92	0	4	190	0.7	323	64	10	3	0.91	0.24	4.6	Tr	610
72	0	3	178	0.7	305	57	10	1	0.84	0.22	4.0	Tr	611
79	0	5	210	0.9	280	50	10	2	0.54	0.27	3.9	Tr	612
68	0	5	202	0.8	269	46	10	1	0.50	0.25	3.6	Tr	613
69	0	9	190	0.8	313	37	10	3	0.50	0.24	4.2	Tr	614
56	0	8	182	0.7	300	33	10	2	0.45	0.22	3.8	Tr	615
93	0	6	162	1.4	286	75	10	3	0.46	0.26	4.4	Tr	616
76	0	5	151	1.3	271	68	10	1	0.40	0.24	4.0	Tr	617
31	2	7	52	0.9	103	581	0	0	0.10	0.08	1.5	12[49]	618
89	2	5	96	5.3	113	652	8,010	2,405	0.14	0.87	4.8	6[49]	619
9	Tr	1	14	0.1	25	105	0	0	0.05	0.02	0.4	0	620
23	1	5	39	0.5	75	504	0	0	0.09	0.05	1.2	12[49]	621
11	Tr	4	24	0.2	47	168	0	0	0.10	0.03	0.6	Tr	622
37	1	7	66	1.5	113	607	0	0	0.14	0.21	2.0	7[49]	623
16	1	2	28	0.3	76	372	0	0	0.12	0.06	1.0	5[49]	624
6	2	2	9	0.1	17	152	10	1	0.03	0.02	0.3	0	625
8	Tr	2	8	0.1	16	152	0	0	0.01	0.02	0.3	0	626
109	0	9	196	0.8	258	56	Tr	Tr	0.06	0.21	4.6	0	627
109	0	10	211	0.7	259	57	Tr	Tr	0.11	0.26	6.6	0	628

Table continued on following page

APPENDIX 1. Nutritive Value of the Edible Part of Food *Continued*

Item No.	Foods, Approximate Measures, Units, and Weight (Weight of Edible Portion Only)			Water	Food energy	Protein	Fat	Fatty Acids Saturated	Fatty Acids Monounsaturated	Fatty Acids Polyunsaturated
	MIXED DISHES AND FAST FOODS		Grams	%	Calories	Grams	Grams	Grams	Grams	Grams
	Mixed dishes:									
629	Beef and vegetable stew, from home recipe	1 cup	245	82	220	16	11	4.4	4.5	0.5
630	Beef potpie, from home recipe, baked, piece, ⅓ of 9-in diam. pie[51]	1 piece	210	55	515	21	30	7.9	12.9	7.4
631	Chicken a la king, cooked, from home recipe	1 cup	245	68	470	27	34	12.9	13.4	6.2
632	Chicken and noodles, cooked, from home recipe	1 cup	240	71	365	22	18	5.1	7.1	3.9
	Chicken chow mein:									
633	Canned	1 cup	250	89	95	7	Tr	0.1	0.1	0.8
634	From home recipe	1 cup	250	78	255	31	10	4.1	4.9	3.5
635	Chicken potpie, from home recipe, baked, piece, ⅓ of 9-in diam. pie[51]	1 piece	232	57	545	23	31	10.3	15.5	6.6
636	Chili con carne with beans, canned	1 cup	255	72	340	19	16	5.8	7.2	1.0
637	Chop suey with beef and pork, from home recipe	1 cup	250	75	300	26	17	4.3	7.4	4.2
	Macaroni (enriched) and cheese:									
638	Canned[52]	1 cup	240	80	230	9	10	4.7	2.9	1.3
639	From home recipe[38]	1 cup	200	58	430	17	22	9.8	7.4	3.6
640	Quiche Lorraine, ⅛ of 8-in diam. quiche[51]	1 slice	176	47	600	13	48	23.2	17.8	4.1
	Spaghetti (enriched) in tomato sauce with cheese:									
641	Canned	1 cup	250	80	190	6	2	0.4	0.4	0.5
642	From home recipe	1 cup	250	77	260	9	9	3.0	3.6	1.2
	Spaghetti (enriched) with meatballs and tomato sauce:									
643	Canned	1 cup	250	78	260	12	10	2.4	3.9	3.1
644	From home recipe	1 cup	248	70	330	19	12	3.9	4.4	2.2
	Fast food entrees:									
	Cheeseburger:									
645	Regular	1 sandwich	112	46	300	15	15	7.3	5.6	1.0
646	4 oz patty	1 sandwich	194	46	525	30	31	15.1	12.2	1.4
	Chicken, fried. See Poultry and Poultry Products (items 656–659).									
647	Enchilada	1 enchilada	230	72	235	20	16	7.7	6.7	0.6
648	English muffin, egg, cheese, and bacon	1 sandwich	138	49	360	18	18	8.0	8.0	0.7
	Fish sandwich:									
649	Regular, with cheese	1 sandwich	140	43	420	16	23	6.3	6.9	7.7
650	Large, without cheese	1 sandwich	170	48	470	18	27	6.3	8.7	9.5
	Hamburger:									
651	Regular	1 sandwich	98	46	245	12	11	4.4	5.3	0.5
652	4-oz patty	1 sandwich	174	50	445	25	21	7.1	11.7	0.6
653	Pizza, cheese, ⅛ of 15-in diam., pizza[51]	1 slice	120	46	290	15	9	4.1	2.6	1.3
654	Roast beef sandwich	1 sandwich	150	52	345	22	13	3.5	6.9	1.8
655	Taco	1 taco	81	55	195	9	11	4.1	5.5	0.8

[51] Crust made with vegetable shortening and enriched flour.
[52] Made with corn oil.

Nutrients in Indicated Quantity

Cholesterol	Carbohydrate	Calcium	Phosphorus	Iron	Potassium	Sodium	Vitamin A Value (IU)	Vitamin A Value (RE)	Thiamin	Riboflavin	Niacin	Ascorbic acid	Item No.
Milligrams	Grams	Milligrams	Milligrams	Milligrams	Milligrams	Milligrams	International units	Retinol equivalents	Milligrams	Milligrams	Milligrams	Milligrams	
71	15	29	184	2.9	613	292	5,690	568	0.15	0.17	4.7	17	629
42	39	29	149	3.8	334	596	4,220	517	0.29	0.29	4.8	6	630
221	12	127	358	2.5	404	760	1,130	272	0.10	0.42	5.4	12	631
103	26	26	247	2.2	149	600	430	130	0.05	0.17	4.3	Tr	632
8	18	45	85	1.3	418	725	150	28	0.05	0.10	1.0	13	633
75	10	58	293	2.5	473	718	280	50	0.08	0.23	4.3	10	634
56	42	70	232	3.0	343	594	7,220	735	0.32	0.32	4.9	5	635
28	31	82	321	4.3	594	1,354	150	15	0.08	0.18	3.3	8	636
68	13	60	248	4.8	425	1,053	600	60	0.28	0.38	5.0	33	637
24	26	199	182	1.0	139	730	260	72	0.12	0.24	1.0	Tr	638
44	40	362	322	1.8	240	1,086	860	232	0.20	0.40	1.8	1	639
285	29	211	276	1.0	283	653	1,640	454	0.11	0.32	Tr	Tr	640
3	39	40	88	2.8	303	955	930	120	0.35	0.28	4.5	10	641
8	37	80	135	2.3	408	955	1,080	140	0.25	0.18	2.3	13	642
23	29	53	113	3.3	245	1,220	1,000	100	0.15	0.18	2.3	5	643
89	39	124	236	3.7	665	1,009	1,590	159	0.25	0.30	4.0	22	644
44	28	135	174	2.3	219	672	340	65	0.26	0.24	3.7	1	645
104	40	236	320	4.5	407	1,224	670	128	0.33	0.48	7.4	3	646
19	24	97	198	3.3	653	1,332	2,720	352	0.18	0.26	Tr	Tr	647
213	31	197	290	3.1	201	832	650	160	0.46	0.50	3.7	1	648
56	39	132	223	1.8	274	667	160	25	0.32	0.26	3.3	2	649
91	41	61	246	2.2	375	621	110	15	0.35	0.23	3.5	1	650
32	28	56	107	2.2	202	463	80	14	0.23	0.24	3.8	1	651
71	38	75	225	4.8	404	763	160	28	0.38	0.38	7.8	1	652
56	39	220	216	1.6	230	699	750	106	0.34	0.29	4.2	2	653
55	34	60	222	4.0	338	757	240	32	0.40	0.33	6.0	2	654
21	15	109	134	1.2	263	456	420	57	0.09	0.07	1.4	1	655

Table continued on following page

APPENDIX 1. Nutritive Value of the Edible Part of Food *Continued*

Item No.	Foods, Approximate Measures, Units, and Weight (Weight of Edible Portion Only)			Water	Food energy	Protein	Fat	Fatty Acids Saturated	Fatty Acids Monounsaturated	Fatty Acids Polyunsaturated
	POULTRY AND POULTRY PRODUCTS		Grams	%	Calories	Grams	Grams	Grams	Grams	Grams
	Chicken:									
	Fried, flesh, with skin:[53]									
	Batter dipped:									
656	Breast, ½ breast (5.6 oz with bones)	4.9 oz	140	52	365	35	18	4.9	7.6	4.3
657	Drumstick (3.4 oz with bones)	2.5 oz	72	53	195	16	11	3.0	4.6	2.7
	Flour coated:									
658	Breast, ½ breast (4.2 oz with bones)	3.5 oz	98	57	220	31	9	2.4	3.4	1.9
659	Drumstick (2.6 oz with bones)	1.7 oz	49	57	120	13	7	1.8	2.7	1.6
	Roasted, flesh only:									
660	Breast, ½ breast (4.2 oz with bones and skin)	3.0 oz	86	65	140	27	3	0.9	1.1	0.7
661	Drumstick, (2.9 oz with bones and skin	1.6 oz	44	67	75	12	2	0.7	0.8	0.6
662	Stewed, flesh only, light and dark meat, chopped or diced	1 cup	140	67	250	38	9	2.6	3.3	2.2
663	Chicken liver, cooked	1 liver	20	68	30	5	1	0.4	0.3	0.2
664	Duck, roasted, flesh only	½ duck	221	64	445	52	25	9.2	8.2	3.2
	Turkey, roasted, flesh only:									
665	Dark meat, piece, 2½ by 1⅝ by ¼ in	4 pieces	85	63	160	24	6	2.1	1.4	1.8
666	Light meat, piece, 4 by 2 by ¼ in	2 pieces	85	66	135	25	3	0.9	0.5	0.7
	Light and dark meat:									
667	Chopped or diced	1 cup	140	65	240	41	7	2.3	1.4	2.0
668	Pieces (1 slice white meat, 4 by 2 by ¼ in and 2 slices dark meat, 2½ by 1⅝ by ¼ in)	3 pieces	85	65	145	25	4	1.4	0.9	1.2
	Poultry food products:									
	Chicken:									
669	Canned, boneless	5 oz	142	69	235	31	11	3.1	4.5	2.5
670	Frankfurter (10 per 1-lb pkg)	1 frankfurter	45	58	115	6	9	2.5	3.8	1.8
671	Roll, light (6 slices per 6-oz pkg)	2 slices	57	69	90	11	4	1.1	1.7	0.9
	Turkey:									
672	Gravy and turkey, frozen	5-oz package	142	85	95	8	4	1.2	1.4	0.7
673	Ham, cured turkey thigh meat (8 slices per 8-oz pkg)	2 slices	57	71	75	11	3	1.0	0.7	0.9
674	Loaf, breast meat (8 slices per 6-oz pkg)	2 slices	42	72	45	10	1	0.2	0.2	0.1
675	Patties, breaded, battered, fried (2.25 oz)	1 patty	64	50	180	9	12	3.0	4.8	3.0
676	Roast, boneless, frozen, seasoned, light and dark meat, cooked	3 oz	85	68	130	18	5	1.6	1.0	1.4
	SOUPS, SAUCES, AND GRAVIES									
	Soups:									
	Canned, condensed:									
	Prepared with equal volume of milk:									
677	Clam chowder, New England	1 cup	248	85	165	9	7	3.0	2.3	1.1
678	Cream of chicken	1 cup	248	85	190	7	11	4.6	4.5	1.6
679	Cream of mushroom	1 cup	248	85	205	6	14	5.1	3.0	4.6
680	Tomato	1 cup	248	85	160	6	6	2.9	1.6	1.1

[53] Fried in vegetable shortening.

Nutrients in Indicated Quantity

Cholesterol	Carbohydrate	Calcium	Phosphorus	Iron	Potassium	Sodium	Vitamin A Value (IU)	Vitamin A Value (RE)	Thiamin	Riboflavin	Niacin	Ascorbic acid	Item No.
Milligrams	Grams	Milligrams	Milligrams	Milligrams	Milligrams	Milligrams	International units	Retinol equivalents	Milligrams	Milligrams	Milligrams	Milligrams	
119	13	28	259	1.8	281	385	90	28	0.16	0.20	14.7	0	656
62	6	12	106	1.0	134	194	60	19	0.08	0.15	3.7	0	657
87	2	16	228	1.2	254	74	50	15	0.08	0.13	13.5	0	658
44	1	6	86	0.7	112	44	40	12	0.04	0.11	3.0	0	659
73	0	13	196	0.9	220	64	20	5	0.06	0.10	11.8	0	660
41	0	5	81	0.6	108	42	30	8	0.03	0.10	2.7	0	661
116	0	20	210	1.6	252	98	70	21	0.07	0.23	8.6	0	662
126	Tr	3	62	1.7	28	10	3,270	983	0.03	0.35	0.9	3	663
197	0	27	449	6.0	557	144	170	51	0.57	1.04	11.3	0	664
72	0	27	173	2.0	246	67	0	0	0.05	0.21	3.1	0	665
59	0	16	186	1.1	259	54	0	0	0.05	0.11	5.8	0	666
106	0	35	298	2.5	417	98	0	0	0.09	0.25	7.6	0	667
65	0	21	181	1.5	253	60	0	0	0.05	0.15	4.6	0	668
88	0	20	158	2.2	196	714	170	48	0.02	0.18	9.0	3	669
45	3	43	48	0.9	38	616	60	17	0.03	0.05	1.4	0	670
28	1	24	89	0.6	129	331	50	14	0.04	0.07	3.0	0	671
26	7	20	115	1.3	87	787	60	18	0.03	0.18	2.6	0	672
32	Tr	6	108	1.6	184	565	0	0	0.03	0.14	2.0	0	673
17	0	3	97	0.2	118	608	0	0	0.02	0.05	3.5	0[54]	674
40	10	9	173	1.4	176	512	20	7	0.06	0.12	1.5	0	675
45	3	4	207	1.4	253	578	0	0	0.04	0.14	5.3	0	676
22	17	186	156	1.5	300	992	160	40	0.07	0.24	1.0	3	677
27	15	181	151	0.7	273	1,047	710	94	0.07	0.26	0.9	1	678
20	15	179	156	0.6	270	1,076	150	37	0.08	0.28	0.9	2	679
17	22	159	149	1.8	449	932	850	109	0.13	0.25	1.5	68	680

[54] If sodium ascorbate is added, product contains 11 mg of ascorbic acid.

Table continued on following page

APPENDIX 1. Nutritive Value of the Edible Part of Food *Continued*

Item No.	Foods, Approximate Measures, Units, and Weight (Weight of Edible Portion Only)			Water	Food energy	Protein	Fat	Fatty Acids Saturated	Fatty Acids Monounsaturated	Fatty Acids Polyunsaturated
	SOUPS, SAUCES, AND GRAVIES *Continued*		Grams	%	Calories	Grams	Grams	Grams	Grams	Grams
	Soups:									
	Canned, condensed:									
	Prepared with equal volume of water:									
681	Bean with bacon	1 cup	253	84	170	8	6	1.5	2.2	1.8
682	Beef broth, bouillon, consomme	1 cup	240	98	15	3	1	0.3	0.2	Tr
683	Beef noodle	1 cup	244	92	85	5	3	1.1	1.2	0.5
684	Chicken noodle	1 cup	241	92	75	4	2	0.7	1.1	0.6
685	Chicken rice	1 cup	241	94	60	4	2	0.5	0.9	0.4
686	Clam chowder, Manhattan	1 cup	244	90	80	4	2	0.4	0.4	1.3
687	Cream of chicken	1 cup	244	91	115	3	7	2.1	3.3	1.5
688	Cream of mushroom	1 cup	244	90	130	2	9	2.4	1.7	4.2
689	Minestrone	1 cup	241	91	80	4	3	0.6	0.7	1.1
690	Pea, green	1 cup	250	83	165	9	3	1.4	1.0	0.4
691	Tomato	1 cup	244	90	85	2	2	0.4	0.4	1.0
692	Vegetable beef	1 cup	244	92	80	6	2	0.9	0.8	0.1
693	Vegetarian	1 cup	241	92	70	2	2	0.3	0.8	0.7
	Dehydrated:									
	Unprepared:									
694	Bouillon	1 packet	6	3	15	1	1	0.3	0.2	Tr
695	Onion	1 packet	7	4	20	1	Tr	0.1	0.2	Tr
	Prepared with water:									
696	Chicken noodle	1 packet (6 fl oz)	188	94	40	2	1	0.2	0.4	0.3
697	Onion	1 packet (6 fl oz)	184	96	20	1	Tr	0.1	0.2	0.1
698	Tomato vegetable	1 packet (6 fl oz)	189	94	40	1	1	0.3	0.2	0.1
	Sauces:									
	From dry mix:									
699	Cheese, prepared with milk	1 cup	279	77	305	16	17	9.3	5.3	1.6
700	Hollandaise, prepared with water	1 cup	259	84	240	5	20	11.6	5.9	0.9
701	White sauce, prepared with milk	1 cup	264	81	240	10	13	6.4	4.7	1.7
	From home recipe:									
702	White sauce, medium[55]	1 cup	250	73	395	10	30	9.1	11.9	7.2
	Ready to serve:									
703	Barbecue	1 tbsp	16	81	10	Tr	Tr	Tr	0.1	0.1
704	Soy	1 tbsp	18	68	10	2	0	0.0	0.0	0.0
	Gravies:									
	Canned:									
705	Beef	1 cup	233	87	125	9	5	2.7	2.3	0.2
706	Chicken	1 cup	238	85	190	5	14	3.4	6.1	3.6
707	Mushroom	1 cup	238	89	120	3	6	1.0	2.8	2.4
	From dry mix:									
708	Brown	1 cup	261	91	80	3	2	0.9	0.8	0.1
709	Chicken	1 cup	260	91	85	3	2	0.5	0.9	0.4
	SUGARS AND SWEETS									
	Candy:									
710	Caramels, plain or chocolate	1 oz	28	8	115	1	3	2.2	0.3	0.1
	Chocolate:									
711	Milk, plain	1 oz	28	1	145	2	9	5.4	3.0	0.3
712	Milk, with almonds	1 oz	28	2	150	3	10	4.8	4.1	0.7
713	Milk, with peanuts	1 oz	28	1	155	4	11	4.2	3.5	1.5
714	Milk, with rice cereal	1 oz	28	2	140	2	7	4.4	2.5	0.2
715	Semisweet, small pieces (60 per oz)	1 cup or 6 oz	170	1	860	7	61	36.2	19.9	1.9
716	Sweet (dark)	1 oz	28	1	150	1	10	5.9	3.3	0.3
717	Fondant, uncoated (mints, candy corn, other)	1 oz	28	3	105	Tr	0	0.0	0.0	0.0
718	Fudge, chocolate, plain	1 oz	28	8	115	1	3	2.1	1.0	0.1
719	Gum drops	1 oz	28	12	100	Tr	Tr	Tr	Tr	0.1

[55] Made with enriched flour, margarine, and whole milk.

Nutrients in Indicated Quantity

Cholesterol	Carbohydrate	Calcium	Phosphorus	Iron	Potassium	Sodium	Vitamin A Value (IU)	Vitamin A Value (RE)	Thiamin	Riboflavin	Niacin	Ascorbic acid	Item No.
Milligrams	Grams	Milligrams	Milligrams	Milligrams	Milligrams	Milligrams	International units	Retinol equivalents	Milligrams	Milligrams	Milligrams	Milligrams	
3	23	81	132	2.0	402	951	890	89	0.09	0.03	0.6	2	681
Tr	Tr	14	31	0.4	130	782	0	0	Tr	0.05	1.9	0	682
5	9	15	46	1.1	100	952	630	63	0.07	0.06	1.1	Tr	683
7	9	17	36	0.8	55	1,106	710	71	0.05	0.06	1.4	Tr	684
7	7	17	22	0.7	101	815	660	66	0.02	0.02	1.1	Tr	685
2	12	34	59	1.9	261	1,808	920	92	0.06	0.05	1.3	3	686
10	9	34	37	0.6	88	986	560	56	0.03	0.06	0.8	Tr	687
2	9	46	49	0.5	100	1,032	0	0	0.05	0.09	0.7	1	688
2	11	34	55	0.9	313	911	2,340	234	0.05	0.04	0.9	1	689
0	27	28	125	2.0	190	988	200	20	0.11	0.07	1.2	2	690
0	17	12	34	1.8	264	871	690	69	0.09	0.05	1.4	66	691
5	10	17	41	1.1	173	956	1,890	189	0.04	0.05	1.0	2	692
0	12	22	34	1.1	210	822	3,010	301	0.05	0.05	0.9	1	693
1	1	4	19	0.1	27	1,019	Tr	Tr	Tr	0.01	0.3	0	694
Tr	4	10	23	0.1	47	627	Tr	Tr	0.02	0.04	0.4	Tr	695
2	6	24	24	0.4	23	957	50	5	0.05	0.04	0.7	Tr	696
0	4	9	22	0.1	48	635	Tr	Tr	0.02	0.04	0.4	Tr	697
0	8	6	23	0.5	78	856	140	14	0.04	0.03	0.6	5	698
53	23	569	438	0.3	552	1,565	390	117	0.15	0.56	0.3	2	699
52	14	124	127	0.9	124	1,564	730	220	0.05	0.18	0.1	Tr	700
34	21	425	256	0.3	444	797	310	92	0.08	0.45	0.5	3	701
32	24	292	238	0.9	381	888	1,190	340	0.15	0.43	0.8	2	702
0	2	3	3	0.1	28	130	140	14	Tr	Tr	0.1	1	703
0	2	3	38	0.5	64	1,029	0	0	0.01	0.02	0.6	0	704
7	11	14	70	1.6	189	117	0	0	0.07	0.08	1.5	0	705
5	13	48	69	1.1	259	1,373	880	264	0.04	0.10	1.1	0	706
0	13	17	36	1.6	252	1,357	0	0	0.08	0.15	1.6	0	707
2	14	66	47	0.2	61	1,147	0	0	0.04	0.09	0.9	0	708
3	14	39	47	0.3	62	1,134	0	0	0.05	0.15	0.8	3	709
1	22	42	35	0.4	54	64	Tr	Tr	0.01	0.05	0.1	Tr	710
6	16	50	61	0.4	96	23	30	10	0.02	0.10	0.1	Tr	711
5	15	65	77	0.5	125	23	30	8	0.02	0.12	0.2	Tr	712
5	13	49	83	0.4	138	19	30	8	0.07	0.07	1.4	Tr	713
6	18	48	57	0.2	100	46	30	8	0.01	0.08	0.1	Tr	714
0	97	51	178	5.8	593	24	30	3	0.10	0.14	0.9	Tr	715
0	16	7	41	0.6	86	5	10	1	0.01	0.04	0.1	Tr	716
0	27	2	Tr	0.1	1	57	0	0	Tr	Tr	Tr	0	717
1	21	22	24	0.3	42	54	Tr	Tr	0.01	0.03	0.1	Tr	718
0	25	2	Tr	0.1	1	10	0	0	0.00	Tr	Tr	0	719

Table continued on following page

APPENDIX 1. Nutritive Value of the Edible Part of Food *Continued*

Item No.	Foods, Approximate Measures, Units, and Weight (Weight of Edible Portion Only)			Water	Food energy	Protein	Fat	Fatty Acids Saturated	Fatty Acids Monounsaturated	Fatty Acids Polyunsaturated
	SUGARS AND SWEETS *Continued*		Grams	%	Calories	Grams	Grams	Grams	Grams	Grams
	Candy:									
720	Hard	1 oz	28	1	110	0	0	0.0	0.0	0.0
721	Jelly beans	1 oz	28	6	105	Tr	Tr	Tr	Tr	0.1
722	Marshmallows	1 oz	28	17	90	1	0	0.0	0.0	0.0
723	Custard, baked	1 cup	265	77	305	14	15	6.8	5.4	0.7
724	Gelatin dessert prepared with gelatin dessert powder and water	½ cup	120	84	70	2	0	0.0	0.0	0.0
725	Honey, strained or extracted	1 cup	339	17	1,030	1	0	0.0	0.0	0.0
726		1 tbsp	21	17	65	Tr	0	0.0	0.0	0.0
727	Jams and preserves	1 tbsp	20	29	55	Tr	Tr	0.0	Tr	Tr
728		1 packet	14	29	40	Tr	Tr	0.0	Tr	Tr
729	Jellies	1 tbsp	18	28	50	Tr	Tr	Tr	Tr	Tr
730		1 packet	14	28	40	Tr	Tr	Tr	Tr	Tr
731	Popsicle, 3-fl-oz size	1 popsicle	95	80	70	0	0	0.0	0.0	0.0
	Puddings:									
	Canned:									
732	Chocolate	5-oz can	142	68	205	3	11	9.5	0.5	0.1
733	Tapioca	5-oz can	142	74	160	3	5	4.8	Tr	Tr
734	Vanilla	5-oz can	142	69	220	2	10	9.5	0.2	0.1
	Dry mix, prepared with whole milk:									
	Chocolate:									
735	Instant	½ cup	130	71	155	4	4	2.3	1.1	0.2
736	Regular (cooked)	½ cup	130	73	150	4	4	2.4	1.1	0.1
737	Rice	½ cup	132	73	155	4	4	2.3	1.1	0.1
738	Tapioca	½ cup	130	75	145	4	4	2.3	1.1	0.1
	Vanilla:									
739	Instant	½ cup	130	73	150	4	4	2.2	1.1	0.2
740	Regular (cooked)	½ cup	130	74	145	4	4	2.3	1.0	0.1
	Sugars:									
741	Brown, pressed down	1 cup	220	2	820	0	0	0.0	0.0	0.0
	White:									
742	Granulated	1 cup	200	1	770	0	0	0.0	0.0	0.0
743		1 tbsp	12	1	45	0	0	0.0	0.0	0.0
744		1 packet	6	1	25	0	0	0.0	0.0	0.0
745	Powered, sifted, spooned into cup	1 cup	100	1	385	0	0	0.0	0.0	0.0
	Syrups:									
	Chocolate-flavored syrup or topping:									
746	Thin type	2 tbsp	38	37	85	1	Tr	0.2	0.1	0.1
747	Fudge type	2 tbsp	38	25	125	2	5	3.1	1.7	0.2
748	Molasses, cane, blackstrap	2 tbsp	40	24	85	0	0	0.0	0.0	0.0
749	Table syrup (corn and maple)	2 tbsp	42	25	122	0	0	0.0	0.0	0.0
	VEGETABLES AND VEGETABLE PRODUCTS									
750	Alfalfa seeds, sprouted, raw	1 cup	33	91	10	1	Tr	Tr	Tr	0.1
751	Artichokes, globe or French, cooked, drained	1 artichoke	120	87	55	3	Tr	Tr	Tr	0.1
	Asparagus, green:									
	Cooked, drained:									
	From raw:									
752	Cuts and tips	1 cup	180	92	45	5	1	0.1	Tr	0.2
753	Spears, ½-in diam. at base	4 spears	60	92	15	2	Tr	Tr	Tr	0.1
	From frozen:									
754	Cuts and tips	1 cup	180	91	50	5	1	0.2	Tr	0.3
755	Spears, ½-in diam. at base	4 spears	60	91	15	2	Tr	0.1	Tr	0.1
756	Canned, spears, ½-in diam. at base	4 spears	80	95	10	1	Tr	Tr	Tr	0.1
757	Bamboo shoots, canned, drained	1 cup	131	94	25	2	1	0.1	Tr	0.2

Nutrients in Indicated Quantity

Cholesterol	Carbohydrate	Calcium	Phosphorus	Iron	Potassium	Sodium	Vitamin A Value (IU)	Vitamin A Value (RE)	Thiamin	Riboflavin	Niacin	Ascorbic acid	Item No.
Milligrams	Grams	Milligrams	Milligrams	Milligrams	Milligrams	Milligrams	International units	Retinol equivalents	Milligrams	Milligrams	Milligrams	Milligrams	
0	28	Tr	2	0.1	1	7	0	0	0.10	0.00	0.0	0	720
0	26	1	1	0.3	11	7	0	0	0.00	Tr	Tr	0	721
0	23	1	2	0.5	2	25	0	0	0.00	Tr	Tr	0	722
278	29	297	310	1.1	387	209	530	146	0.11	0.50	0.3	1	723
0	17	2	23	Tr	Tr	55	0	0	0.00	0.00	0.0	0	724
0	279	17	20	1.7	173	17	0	0	0.02	0.14	1.0	3	725
0	17	1	1	0.1	11	1	0	0	Tr	0.01	0.1	Tr	726
0	14	4	2	0.2	18	2	Tr	Tr	Tr	0.01	Tr	Tr	727
0	10	3	1	0.1	12	2	Tr	Tr	Tr	Tr	Tr	Tr	728
0	13	2	Tr	0.1	16	5	Tr	Tr	Tr	0.01	Tr	1	729
0	10	1	Tr	Tr	13	4	Tr	Tr	Tr	Tr	Tr	1	730
0	18	0	0	Tr	4	11	0	0	0.00	0.00	0.0	0	731
1	30	74	117	1.2	254	285	100	31	0.04	0.17	0.6	Tr	732
Tr	28	119	113	0.3	212	252	Tr	Tr	0.03	0.14	0.4	Tr	733
1	33	79	94	0.2	155	305	Tr	Tr	0.03	0.12	0.6	Tr	734
14	27	130	329	0.3	176	440	130	33	0.04	0.18	0.1	1	735
15	25	146	120	0.2	190	167	140	34	0.05	0.20	0.1	1	736
15	27	133	110	0.5	165	140	140	33	0.10	0.18	0.6	1	737
15	25	131	103	0.1	167	152	140	34	0.04	0.18	0.1	1	738
15	27	129	273	0.1	164	375	140	33	0.04	0.17	0.1	1	739
15	25	132	102	0.1	166	178	140	34	0.04	0.18	0.1	1	740
0	212	187	56	4.8	757	97	0	0	0.02	0.07	0.2	0	741
0	199	3	Tr	0.1	7	5	0	0	0.00	0.00	0.0	0	742
0	12	Tr	Tr	Tr	Tr	Tr	0	0	0.00	0.00	0.0	0	743
0	6	Tr	Tr	Tr	Tr	Tr	0	0	0.00	0.00	0.0	0	744
0	100	1	Tr	Tr	4	2	0	0	0.00	0.00	0.0	0	745
0	22	6	49	0.8	85	36	Tr	Tr	Tr	0.02	0.1	0	746
0	21	38	60	0.5	82	42	40	13	0.02	0.08	0.1	0	747
0	22	274	34	10.1	1,171	38	0	0	0.04	0.08	0.8	0	748
0	32	1	4	Tr	7	19	0	0	0.00	0.00	0.0	0	749
0	1	11	23	0.3	26	2	50	5	0.03	0.04	0.2	3	750
0	12	47	72	1.6	316	79	170	17	0.07	0.06	0.7	9	751
0	8	43	110	1.2	558	7	1,490	149	0.18	0.22	1.9	49	752
0	3	14	37	0.4	186	2	500	50	0.06	0.07	0.6	16	753
0	9	41	99	1.2	392	7	1,470	147	0.12	0.19	1.9	44	754
0	3	14	33	0.4	131	2	490	49	0.04	0.06	0.6	15	755
0	2	11	30	0.5	122	278[56]	380	38	0.04	0.07	0.7	13	756
0	4	10	33	0.4	105	9	10	1	0.03	0.03	0.2	1	757

[56] For regular pack; special dietary pack contains 3 mg sodium.

Table continued on following page

APPENDIX 1. Nutritive Value of the Edible Part of Food *Continued*

Item No.	Foods, Approximate Measures, Units, and Weight (Weight of Edible Portion Only)			Water	Food energy	Pro-tein	Fat	Fatty Acids: Satu-rated	Fatty Acids: Mono-unsatu-rated	Fatty Acids: Poly-unsatu-rated
	VEGETABLES AND VEGETABLE PRODUCTS *Continued*		*Grams*	*%*	*Calories*	*Grams*	*Grams*	*Grams*	*Grams*	*Grams*
	Beans:									
	Lima, immature seeds, frozen, cooked, drained:									
758	Thick-seeded types (Fordhooks)	1 cup	170	74	170	10	1	0.1	Tr	0.3
759	Thin-seeded types (baby limas)	1 cup	180	72	190	12	1	0.1	Tr	0.3
	Snap:									
	Cooked, drained:									
760	From raw (cut and French style)	1 cup	125	89	45	2	Tr	0.1	Tr	0.2
761	From frozen (cut)	1 cup	135	92	35	2	Tr	Tr	Tr	0.1
762	Canned, drained solids (cut)	1 cup	135	93	25	2	Tr	Tr	Tr	0.1
	Beans, mature. See Beans, dry (items 527–535) and Black-eyed peas, dry (item 536).									
	Bean sprouts (mung):									
763	Raw	1 cup	104	90	30	3	Tr	Tr	Tr	0.1
764	Cooked, drained	1 cup	124	93	25	3	Tr	Tr	Tr	Tr
	Beets:									
	Cooked, drained:									
765	Diced or sliced	1 cup	170	91	55	2	Tr	Tr	Tr	Tr
766	Whole beets, 2-in diam.	2 beets	100	91	30	1	Tr	Tr	Tr	Tr
767	Canned, drained solids, diced or sliced	1 cup	170	91	55	2	Tr	Tr	Tr	0.1
768	Beet greens, leaves and stems, cooked, drained	1 cup	144	89	40	4	Tr	Tr	0.1	0.1
	Black-eyed peas, immature seeds, cooked and drained:									
769	From raw	1 cup	165	72	180	13	1	0.3	0.1	0.6
770	From frozen	1 cup	170	66	225	14	1	0.3	0.1	0.5
	Broccoli:									
771	Raw	1 spear	151	91	40	4	1	0.1	Tr	0.3
	Cooked, drained:									
	From raw:									
772	Spear, medium	1 spear	180	90	50	5	1	0.1	Tr	0.2
773	Spears, cut into ½-in pieces	1 cup	155	90	45	5	Tr	0.1	Tr	0.2
	From frozen:									
774	Piece, 4½ to 5 in long	1 piece	30	91	10	1	Tr	Tr	Tr	Tr
775	Chopped	1 cup	185	91	50	6	Tr	Tr	Tr	0.1
	Brussels sprouts, cooked, drained:									
776	From raw, 7–8 sprouts, 1¼ to 1½ in diam.	1 cup	155	87	60	4	1	0.2	0.1	0.4
777	From frozen	1 cup	155	87	65	6	1	0.1	Tr	0.3
	Cabbage, common varieties:									
778	Raw, coarsely shredded or sliced	1 cup	70	93	15	1	Tr	Tr	Tr	0.1
779	Cooked, drained	1 cup	150	94	30	1	Tr	Tr	Tr	0.2
	Cabbage, Chinese:									
780	Bok-choi, cooked, drained	1 cup	170	96	20	3	Tr	Tr	Tr	0.1
781	Pe-tsai, raw, 1-in pieces	1 cup	76	94	10	1	Tr	Tr	Tr	0.1
782	Cabbage, red, raw, coarsely shredded or sliced	1 cup	70	92	20	1	Tr	Tr	Tr	0.1
783	Cabbage, savoy, raw, coarsely shredded or sliced	1 cup	70	91	20	1	Tr	Tr	Tr	Tr

[57] For green varieties; yellow varieties contain 101 IU or 10 RE.
[58] For green varieties; yellow varieties contain 151 IU or 15 RE.
[59] For regular pack; special dietary pack contains 3 mg of sodium.

Nutrients in Indicated Quantity

Cholesterol	Carbohydrate	Calcium	Phosphorus	Iron	Potassium	Sodium	Vitamin A Value (IU)	Vitamin A Value (RE)	Thiamin	Riboflavin	Niacin	Ascorbic acid	Item No.
Milligrams	*Grams*	*Milligrams*	*Milligrams*	*Milligrams*	*Milligrams*	*Milligrams*	*International units*	*Retinol equivalents*	*Milligrams*	*Milligrams*	*Milligrams*	*Milligrams*	
0	32	37	107	2.3	694	90	320	32	0.13	0.10	1.8	22	758
0	35	50	202	3.5	740	52	300	30	0.13	0.10	1.4	10	759
0	10	58	49	1.6	374	4	830[57]	83[57]	0.09	0.12	0.8	12	760
0	8	61	32	1.1	151	18	710[58]	71[58]	0.06	0.10	0.6	11	761
0	6	35	26	1.2	147	339[59]	470[60]	47[60]	0.02	0.08	0.3	6	762
0	6	14	56	0.9	155	6	20	2	0.09	0.13	0.8	14	763
0	5	15	35	0.8	125	12	20	2	0.06	0.13	1.0	14	764
0	11	19	53	1.1	530	83	20	2	0.05	0.02	0.5	9	765
0	7	11	31	0.6	312	49	10	1	0.03	0.01	0.3	6	766
0	12	26	29	3.1	252	466[61]	20	2	0.02	0.07	0.3	7	767
0	8	164	59	2.7	1,309	347	7,340	734	0.17	0.42	0.7	36	768
0	30	46	196	2.4	693	7	1,050	105	0.11	0.18	1.8	3	769
0	40	39	207	3.6	638	9	130	13	0.44	0.11	1.2	4	770
0	8	72	100	1.3	491	41	2,330	233	0.10	0.18	1.0	141	771
0	10	205	86	2.1	293	20	2,540	254	0.15	0.37	1.4	113	772
0	9	177	74	1.8	253	17	2,180	218	0.13	0.32	1.2	97	773
0	2	15	17	0.2	54	7	570	57	0.02	0.02	0.1	12	774
0	10	94	102	1.1	333	44	3,500	350	0.10	0.15	0.8	74	775
0	13	56	87	1.9	491	33	1,110	111	0.17	0.12	0.9	96	776
0	13	37	84	1.1	504	36	910	91	0.16	0.18	0.8	71	777
0	4	33	16	0.4	172	13	90	9	0.04	0.02	0.2	33	778
0	7	50	38	0.6	308	29	130	13	0.09	0.08	0.3	36	779
0	3	158	49	1.8	631	58	4,370	437	0.05	0.11	0.7	44	780
0	2	59	22	0.2	181	7	910	91	0.03	0.04	0.3	21	781
0	4	36	29	0.3	144	8	30	3	0.04	0.02	0.2	40	782
0	4	25	29	0.3	161	20	700	70	0.05	0.02	0.2	22	783

[60] For green varieties; yellow varieties contain 142 IU or 14 RE.
[61] For regular pack; special dietary pack contains 78 mg of sodium.

Table continued on following page

APPENDIX 1. Nutritive Value of the Edible Part of Food *Continued*

Item No.	Foods, Approximate Measures, Units, and Weight (Weight of Edible Portion Only)			Water	Food energy	Protein	Fat	Fatty Acids Saturated	Fatty Acids Monounsaturated	Fatty Acids Polyunsaturated
	VEGETABLES AND VEGETABLE PRODUCTS *Continued*		Grams	%	Calories	Grams	Grams	Grams	Grams	Grams
	Carrots:									
	Raw, without crowns and tips, scraped:									
784	Whole, 7½ by 1⅛ in, or strips, 2½ to 3 in long	1 carrot or 18 strips	72	88	30	1	Tr	Tr	Tr	0.1
785	Grated	1 cup	110	88	45	1	Tr	Tr	Tr	0.1
	Cooked, sliced, drained:									
786	From raw	1 cup	156	87	70	2	Tr	0.1	Tr	0.1
787	From frozen	1 cup	146	90	55	2	Tr	Tr	Tr	0.1
788	Canned, sliced, drained solids	1 cup	146	93	35	1	Tr	0.1	Tr	0.1
	Cauliflower:									
789	Raw (flowerets)	1 cup	100	92	25	2	Tr	Tr	Tr	0.1
	Cooked, drained:									
790	From raw (flowerets)	1 cup	125	93	30	2	Tr	Tr	Tr	0.1
791	From frozen (flowerets)	1 cup	180	94	35	3	Tr	0.1	Tr	0.2
	Celery, pascal type, raw:									
792	Stalk, large outer, 8 by 1½ in (at root end)	1 stalk	40	95	5	Tr	Tr	Tr	Tr	Tr
793	Pieces, diced	1 cup	120	95	20	1	Tr	Tr	Tr	0.1
	Collards, cooked, drained:									
794	From raw (leaves without stems)	1 cup	190	96	25	2	Tr	0.1	Tr	0.2
795	From frozen (chopped)	1 cup	170	88	60	5	1	0.1	0.1	0.4
	Corn, sweet:									
	Cooked, drained:									
796	From raw, ear 5 by 1¾ in	1 ear	77	70	85	3	1	0.2	0.3	0.5
	From frozen:									
797	Ear, trimmed to about 3½ in long	1 ear	63	73	60	2	Tr	0.1	0.1	0.2
798	Kernels	1 cup	165	76	135	5	Tr	Tr	Tr	0.1
	Canned:									
799	Cream style	1 cup	256	79	185	4	1	0.2	0.3	0.5
800	Whole kernel, vacuum pack	1 cup	210	77	165	5	1	0.2	0.3	0.5
	Cowpeas. See Black-eyed peas, immature (items 769, 770), mature (item 536).									
801	Cucumber, with peel, slices, ⅛ in thick (large, 2⅛-in diam.; small, 1¾-in diam.)	6 large or 8 small slices	28	96	5	Tr	Tr	Tr	Tr	Tr
802	Dandelion greens, cooked, drained	1 cup	105	90	35	2	1	0.1	Tr	0.3
803	Eggplant, cooked, steamed	1 cup	96	92	25	1	Tr	Tr	Tr	0.1
804	Endive, curly (including escarole), raw, small pieces	1 cup	50	94	10	1	Tr	Tr	Tr	Tr
805	Jerusalem-artichoke, raw, sliced	1 cup	150	78	115	3	Tr	0.0	Tr	Tr
	Kale, cooked, drained:									
806	From raw, chopped	1 cup	130	91	40	2	1	0.1	Tr	0.3
807	From frozen, chopped	1 cup	130	91	40	4	1	0.1	Tr	0.3
808	Kohlrabi, thickened bulb-like stems, cooked, drained, diced	1 cup	165	90	50	3	Tr	Tr	Tr	0.1
	Lettuce, raw:									
	Butterhead, as Boston types:									
809	Head, 5-in diam	1 head	163	96	20	2	Tr	Tr	Tr	0.2
810	Leaves	1 outer or 2 inner leaves	15	96	Tr	Tr	Tr	Tr	Tr	Tr
	Crisphead, as iceberg:									
811	Head, 6-in diam	1 head	539	96	70	5	1	0.1	Tr	0.5
812	Wedge, ¼ of head	1 wedge	135	96	20	1	Tr	Tr	Tr	0.1
813	Pieces, chopped or shredded	1 cup	55	96	5	1	Tr	Tr	Tr	0.1
814	Looseleaf (bunching varieties including romaine or cos), chopped or shredded pieces	1 cup	56	94	10	1	Tr	Tr	Tr	0.1

[62] For regular pack; special dietary pack contains 61 mg of sodium.
[63] For yellow varieties; white varieties contain only a trace of vitamin A.

Nutrients in Indicated Quantity

Cholesterol	Carbohydrate	Calcium	Phosphorus	Iron	Potassium	Sodium	Vitamin A Value (IU)	Vitamin A Value (RE)	Thiamin	Riboflavin	Niacin	Ascorbic acid	Item No.
Milligrams	*Grams*	*Milligrams*	*Milligrams*	*Milligrams*	*Milligrams*	*Milligrams*	*International units*	*Retinol equivalents*	*Milligrams*	*Milligrams*	*Milligrams*	*Milligrams*	
0	7	19	32	0.4	233	25	20,250	2,025	0.07	0.04	0.7	7	784
0	11	30	48	0.6	355	39	30,940	3,094	0.11	0.06	1.0	10	785
0	16	48	47	1.0	354	103	38,300	3,830	0.05	0.09	0.8	4	786
0	12	41	38	0.7	231	86	25,850	2,585	0.04	0.05	0.6	4	787
0	8	37	35	0.9	261	352[62]	20,110	2,011	0.03	0.04	0.8	4	788
0	5	29	46	0.6	355	15	20	2	0.08	0.06	0.6	72	789
0	6	34	44	0.5	404	8	20	2	0.08	0.07	0.7	69	790
0	7	31	43	0.7	250	32	40	4	0.07	0.10	0.6	56	791
0	1	14	10	0.2	114	35	50	5	0.01	0.01	0.1	3	792
0	4	43	31	0.6	341	106	150	15	0.04	0.04	0.4	8	793
0	5	148	19	0.8	177	36	4,220	422	0.03	0.08	0.4	19	794
0	12	357	46	1.9	427	85	10,170	1,017	0.08	0.20	1.1	45	795
0	19	2	79	0.5	192	13	170[63]	17[63]	0.17	0.06	1.2	5	796
0	14	2	47	0.4	158	3	130[63]	13[63]	0.11	0.04	1.0	3	797
0	34	3	78	0.5	229	8	410[63]	41[63]	0.11	0.12	2.1	4	798
0	46	8	131	1.0	343	730[64]	250[63]	25[63]	0.06	0.14	2.5	12	799
0	41	11	134	0.9	391	571[65]	510[63]	51[63]	0.09	0.15	2.5	17	800
0	1	4	5	0.1	42	1	10	1	0.01	0.01	0.1	1	801
0	7	147	44	1.9	244	46	12,290	1,229	0.14	0.18	0.5	19	802
0	6	6	21	0.3	238	3	60	6	0.07	0.02	0.6	1	803
0	2	26	14	0.4	157	11	1,030	103	0.04	0.04	0.2	3	804
0	26	21	117	5.1	644	6	30	3	0.30	0.09	2.0	6	805
0	7	94	36	1.2	296	30	9,620	962	0.07	0.09	0.7	53	806
0	7	179	36	1.2	417	20	8,260	826	0.06	0.15	0.9	33	807
0	11	41	74	0.7	561	35	60	6	0.07	0.03	0.6	89	808
0	4	52	38	0.5	419	8	1,580	158	0.10	0.10	0.5	13	809
0	Tr	5	3	Tr	39	1	150	15	0.01	0.01	Tr	1	810
0	11	102	108	2.7	852	49	1,780	178	0.25	0.16	1.0	21	811
0	3	26	27	0.7	213	12	450	45	0.06	0.04	0.3	5	812
0	1	10	11	0.3	87	5	180	18	0.03	0.02	0.1	2	813
0	2	38	14	0.8	148	5	1,060	106	0.03	0.04	0.2	10	814

[64] For regular pack; special dietary pack contains 8 mg of sodium.
[65] For regular pack; special dietary pack contains 6 mg of sodium.

Table continued on following page

Item No.	Foods, Approximate Measures, Units, and Weight (Weight of Edible Portion Only)			Water	Food energy	Protein	Fat	Fatty Acids: Saturated	Fatty Acids: Monounsaturated	Fatty Acids: Polyunsaturated
	VEGETABLES AND VEGETABLE PRODUCTS *Continued*		*Grams*	*%*	*Calories*	*Grams*	*Grams*	*Grams*	*Grams*	*Grams*
	Mushrooms:									
815	Raw, sliced or chopped	1 cup	70	92	20	1	Tr	Tr	Tr	0.1
816	Cooked, drained	1 cup	156	91	40	3	1	0.1	Tr	0.3
817	Canned, drained solids	1 cup	156	91	35	3	Tr	0.1	Tr	0.2
818	Mustard greens, without stems and midribs, cooked, drained	1 cup	140	94	20	3	Tr	Tr	0.2	0.1
819	Okra pods, 3 by 5/8 in, cooked	8 pods	85	90	25	2	Tr	Tr	Tr	Tr
	Onions:									
	Raw:									
820	Chopped	1 cup	160	91	55	2	Tr	0.1	0.1	0.2
821	Sliced	1 cup	115	91	40	1	Tr	0.1	Tr	0.1
822	Cooked (whole or sliced), drained	1 cup	210	92	60	2	Tr	0.1	Tr	0.1
823	Onions, spring, raw, bulb (3/8-in diam.) and white portion of top	6 onions	30	92	10	1	Tr	Tr	Tr	Tr
824	Onion rings, breaded, pan-fried, frozen, prepared	2 rings	20	29	80	1	5	1.7	2.2	1.0
	Parsley:									
825	Raw	10 sprigs	10	88	5	Tr	Tr	Tr	Tr	Tr
826	Freeze-dried	1 tbsp	0.4	2	Tr	Tr	Tr	Tr	Tr	Tr
827	Parsnips, cooked (diced or 2-in lengths), drained	1 cup	156	78	125	2	Tr	0.1	0.2	0.1
828	Peas, edible pod, cooked, drained	1 cup	160	89	65	5	Tr	0.1	Tr	0.2
	Peas, green:									
829	Canned, drained solids	1 cup	170	82	115	8	1	0.1	0.1	0.3
830	Frozen, cooked, drained	1 cup	160	80	125	8	Tr	0.1	Tr	0.2
	Peppers:									
831	Hot chili, raw	1 pepper	45	88	20	1	Tr	Tr	Tr	Tr
	Sweet (about 5 per lb, whole), stem and seeds removed:									
832	Raw	1 pepper	74	93	20	1	Tr	Tr	Tr	0.2
833	Cooked, drained	1 pepper	73	95	15	Tr	Tr	Tr	Tr	0.1
	Potatoes, cooked:									
	Baked (about 2 per lb, raw):									
834	With skin	1 potato	202	71	220	5	Tr	0.1	Tr	0.1
835	Flesh only	1 potato	156	75	145	3	Tr	Tr	Tr	0.1
	Boiled (about 3 per lb, raw):									
836	Peeled after boiling	1 potato	136	77	120	3	Tr	Tr	Tr	0.1
837	Peeled before boiling	1 potato	135	77	115	2	Tr	Tr	Tr	0.1
	French fried, strip, 2 to 3½ in long, frozen:									
838	Oven heated	10 strips	50	53	110	2	4	2.1	1.8	0.3
839	Fried in vegetable oil	10 strips	50	38	160	2	8	2.5	1.6	3.8
	Potato products, prepared:									
	Au gratin:									
840	From dry mix	1 cup	245	79	230	6	10	6.3	2.9	0.3
841	From home recipe	1 cup	245	74	325	12	19	11.6	5.3	0.7
842	Hashed brown, from frozen	1 cup	156	56	340	5	18	7.0	8.0	2.1
	Mashed:									
	From home recipe:									
843	Milk added	1 cup	210	78	160	4	1	0.7	0.3	0.1
844	Milk and margarine added	1 cup	210	76	225	4	9	2.2	3.7	2.5
845	From dehydrated flakes (without milk), water, milk, butter, and salt added	1 cup	210	76	235	4	12	7.2	3.3	0.5
846	Potato salad, made with mayonnaise	1 cup	250	76	360	7	21	3.6	6.2	9.3
	Scalloped:									
847	From dry mix	1 cup	245	79	230	5	11	6.5	3.0	0.5
848	From home recipe	1 cup	245	81	210	7	9	5.5	2.5	0.4

[66] For regular pack; special dietary pack contains 3 mg of sodium.
[67] For red peppers; green peppers contain 350 IU or 35 RE.
[68] For green peppers; red peppers contain 4,220 IU or 422 RE.

Nutrients in Indicated Quantity

Cho-les-terol	Carbo-hydrate	Calcium	Phos-phorus	Iron	Potas-sium	Sodium	Vitamin A Value (IU)	Vitamin A Value (RE)	Thiamin	Ribo-flavin	Niacin	Ascorbic acid	Item No.
Milli-grams	Grams	Milli-grams	Milli-grams	Milli-grams	Milli-grams	Milli-grams	Inter-national units	Retinol equiva-lents	Milli-grams	Milli-grams	Milli-grams	Milli-grams	
0	3	4	73	0.9	259	3	0	0	0.07	0.31	2.9	2	815
0	8	9	136	2.7	555	3	0	0	0.11	0.47	7.0	6	816
0	8	17	103	1.2	201	663	0	0	0.13	0.03	2.5	0	817
0	3	104	57	1.0	283	22	4,240	424	0.06	0.09	0.6	35	818
0	6	54	48	0.4	274	4	490	49	0.11	0.05	0.7	14	819
0	12	40	46	0.6	248	3	0	0	0.10	0.02	0.2	13	820
0	8	29	33	0.4	178	2	0	0	0.07	0.01	0.1	10	821
0	13	57	48	0.4	319	17	0	0	0.09	0.02	0.2	12	822
0	2	18	10	0.6	77	1	1,500	150	0.02	0.04	0.1	14	823
0	8	6	16	0.3	26	75	50	5	0.06	0.03	0.7	Tr	824
0	1	13	4	0.6	54	4	520	52	0.01	0.01	0.1	9	825
0	Tr	1	2	0.2	25	2	250	25	Tr	0.01	Tr	1	826
0	30	58	108	0.9	573	16	0	0	0.13	0.08	1.1	20	827
0	11	67	88	3.2	384	6	210	21	0.20	0.12	0.9	77	828
0	21	34	114	1.6	294	372[66]	1,310	131	0.21	0.13	1.2	16	829
0	23	38	144	2.5	269	139	1,070	107	0.45	0.16	2.4	16	830
0	4	8	21	0.5	153	3	4,840[67]	484[67]	0.04	0.04	0.4	109	831
0	4	4	16	0.9	144	2	390[68]	39[68]	0.06	0.04	0.4	95[69]	832
0	3	3	11	0.6	94	1	280[70]	28[70]	0.04	0.03	0.3	81[71]	833
0	51	20	115	2.7	844	16	0	0	0.22	0.07	3.3	26	834
0	34	8	78	0.5	610	8	0	0	0.16	0.03	2.2	20	835
0	27	7	60	0.4	515	5	0	0	0.14	0.03	2.0	18	836
0	27	11	54	0.4	443	7	0	0	0.13	0.03	1.8	10	837
0	17	5	43	0.7	229	16	0	0	0.06	0.02	1.2	5	838
0	20	10	47	0.4	366	108	0	0	0.09	0.01	1.6	5	839
12	31	203	233	0.8	537	1,076	520	76	0.05	0.20	2.3	8	840
56	28	292	277	1.6	970	1,061	650	93	0.16	0.28	2.4	24	841
0	44	23	112	2.4	680	53	0	0	0.17	0.03	3.8	10	842
4	37	55	101	0.6	628	636	40	12	0.18	0.08	2.3	14	843
4	35	55	97	0.5	607	620	360	42	0.18	0.08	2.3	13	844
29	32	103	118	0.5	489	697	380	44	0.23	0.11	1.4	20	845
170	28	48	130	1.6	635	1,323	520	83	0.19	0.15	2.2	25	846
27	31	88	137	0.9	497	835	360	51	0.05	0.14	2.5	8	847
29	26	140	154	1.4	926	821	330	47	0.17	0.23	2.6	26	848

[69] For green peppers; red peppers contain 141 mg of ascorbic acid.
[70] For green peppers; red peppers contain 2,740 IU or 274 RE.
[71] For green peppers; red peppers contain 121 mg of ascorbic acid.

Table continued on following page

APPENDIX 1. Nutritive Value of the Edible Part of Food *Continued*

Item No.	Foods, Approximate Measures, Units, and Weight (Weight of Edible Portion Only)			Water	Food energy	Protein	Fat	Fatty Acids: Saturated	Fatty Acids: Monounsaturated	Fatty Acids: Polyunsaturated
	VEGETABLES AND VEGETABLE PRODUCTS *Continued*		*Grams*	*%*	*Calories*	*Grams*	*Grams*	*Grams*	*Grams*	*Grams*
849	Potato chips	10 chips	20	3	105	1	7	1.8	1.2	3.6
	Pumpkin:									
850	Cooked from raw, mashed	1 cup	245	94	50	2	Tr	0.1	Tr	Tr
851	Canned	1 cup	245	90	85	3	1	0.4	0.1	Tr
852	Radishes, raw, stem ends, rootlets cut off	4 radishes	18	95	5	Tr	Tr	Tr	Tr	Tr
853	Sauerkraut, canned, solids and liquid	1 cup	236	93	45	2	Tr	0.1	Tr	0.1
	Seaweed:									
854	Kelp, raw	1 oz	28	82	10	Tr	Tr	0.1	Tr	Tr
855	Spirulina, dried	1 oz	28	5	80	16	2	0.8	0.2	0.6
	Southern peas. See Black-eyed peas, immature (items 769, 770), mature (item 536).									
	Spinach:									
856	Raw, chopped	1 cup	55	92	10	2	Tr	Tr	Tr	0.1
	Cooked, drained:									
857	From raw	1 cup	180	91	40	5	Tr	0.1	Tr	0.2
858	From frozen (leaf)	1 cup	190	90	55	6	Tr	0.1	Tr	0.2
859	Canned, drained solids	1 cup	214	92	50	6	1	0.2	Tr	0.4
860	Spinach souffle	1 cup	136	74	220	11	18	7.1	6.8	3.1
	Squash, cooked:									
861	Summer (all varieties), sliced, drained	1 cup	180	94	35	2	1	0.1	Tr	0.2
862	Winter (all varieties), baked, cubes	1 cup	205	89	80	2	1	0.3	0.1	0.5
	Sunchoke. See Jerusalem artichoke (item 805).									
	Sweet potatoes:									
	Cooked (raw, 5 by 2 in; about 2½ per lb):									
863	Baked in skin, peeled	1 potato	114	73	115	2	Tr	Tr	Tr	0.1
864	Boiled, without skin	1 potato	151	73	160	2	Tr	0.1	Tr	0.2
865	Candied, 2½ by 2-in piece	1 piece	105	67	145	1	3	1.4	0.7	0.2
	Canned:									
866	Solid pack (mashed)	1 cup	255	74	260	5	1	0.1	Tr	0.2
867	Vacuum pack, piece 2¾ by 1 in	1 piece	40	76	35	1	Tr	Tr	Tr	Tr
	Tomatoes:									
868	Raw, 2⅗-in diam. (3 per 12-oz pkg.)	1 tomato	123	94	25	1	Tr	Tr	Tr	0.1
869	Canned, solids and liquid	1 cup	240	94	50	2	1	0.1	0.1	0.2
870	Tomato juice, canned	1 cup	244	94	40	2	Tr	Tr	Tr	0.1
	Tomato products, canned:									
871	Paste	1 cup	262	74	220	10	2	0.3	0.4	0.9
872	Puree	1 cup	250	87	105	4	Tr	Tr	Tr	0.1
873	Sauce	1 cup	245	89	75	3	Tr	0.1	0.1	0.2
874	Turnips, cooked, diced	1 cup	156	94	30	1	Tr	Tr	Tr	0.1
	Turnip greens, cooked, drained:									
875	From raw (leaves and stems)	1 cup	144	93	30	2	Tr	0.1	Tr	0.1
876	From frozen (chopped)	1 cup	164	90	50	5	1	0.2	Tr	0.3
877	Vegetable juice cocktail, canned	1 cup	242	94	45	2	Tr	Tr	Tr	0.1
	Vegetables, mixed:									
878	Canned, drained solids	1 cup	163	87	75	4	Tr	0.1	Tr	0.2
879	Frozen, cooked, drained	1 cup	182	83	105	5	Tr	0.1	Tr	0.1
880	Water chestnuts, canned	1 cup	140	86	70	1	Tr	Tr	Tr	Tr

[72] With added salt; if none is added, sodium content is 58 mg.
[73] For regular pack; special dietary pack contains 31 mg of sodium.
[74] With added salt; if none is added, sodium content is 24 mg.

Nutrients in Indicated Quantity

Cholesterol	Carbohydrate	Calcium	Phosphorus	Iron	Potassium	Sodium	Vitamin A Value (IU)	Vitamin A Value (RE)	Thiamin	Riboflavin	Niacin	Ascorbic acid	Item No.
Milligrams	*Grams*	*Milligrams*	*Milligrams*	*Milligrams*	*Milligrams*	*Milligrams*	*International units*	*Retinol equivalents*	*Milligrams*	*Milligrams*	*Milligrams*	*Milligrams*	
0	10	5	31	0.2	260	94	0	0	0.03	Tr	0.8	8	849
0	12	37	74	1.4	564	2	2,650	265	0.08	0.19	1.0	12	850
0	20	64	86	3.4	505	12	54,040	5,404	0.06	0.13	0.9	10	851
0	1	4	3	0.1	42	4	Tr	Tr	Tr	0.01	0.1	4	852
0	10	71	47	3.5	401	1,560	40	4	0.05	0.05	0.3	35	853
0	3	48	12	0.8	25	66	30	3	0.01	0.04	0.1	([1])	854
0	7	34	33	8.1	386	297	160	16	0.67	1.04	3.6	3	855
0	2	54	27	1.5	307	43	3,690	369	0.04	0.10	0.4	15	856
0	7	245	101	6.4	839	126	14,740	1,474	0.17	0.42	0.9	18	857
0	10	277	91	2.9	566	163	14,790	1,479	0.11	0.32	0.8	23	858
0	7	272	94	4.9	740	683[72]	18,780	1,878	0.03	0.30	0.8	31	859
184	3	230	231	1.3	201	763	3,460	675	0.09	0.30	0.5	3	860
0	8	49	70	0.6	346	2	520	52	0.08	0.07	0.9	10	861
0	18	29	41	0.7	896	2	7,290	729	0.17	0.05	1.4	20	862
0	28	32	63	0.5	397	11	24,880	2,488	0.08	0.14	0.7	28	863
0	37	32	41	0.8	278	20	25,750	2,575	0.08	0.21	1.0	26	864
8	29	27	27	1.2	198	74	4,400	440	0.02	0.04	0.4	7	865
0	59	77	133	3.4	536	191	38,570	3,857	0.07	0.23	2.4	13	866
0	8	9	20	0.4	125	21	3,190	319	0.01	0.02	0.3	11	867
0	5	9	28	0.6	255	10	1,390	139	0.07	0.06	0.7	22	868
0	10	62	46	1.5	530	391[73]	1,450	145	0.11	0.07	1.8	36	869
0	10	22	46	1.4	537	881[74]	1,360	136	0.11	0.08	1.6	45	870
0	49	92	207	7.8	2,442	170[75]	6,470	647	0.41	0.50	8.4	111	871
0	25	38	100	2.3	1,050	50[76]	3,400	340	0.18	0.14	4.3	88	872
0	18	34	78	1.9	909	1,482[77]	2,400	240	0.16	0.14	2.8	32	873
0	8	34	30	0.3	211	78	0	0	0.04	0.04	0.5	18	874
0	6	197	42	1.2	292	42	7,920	792	0.06	0.10	0.6	39	875
0	8	249	56	3.2	367	25	13,080	1,308	0.09	0.12	0.8	36	876
0	11	27	41	1.0	467	883	2,830	283	0.10	0.07	1.8	67	877
0	15	44	68	1.7	474	243	18,990	1,899	0.08	0.08	0.9	8	878
0	24	46	93	1.5	308	64	7,780	778	0.13	0.22	1.5	6	879
0	17	6	27	1.2	165	11	10	1	0.02	0.03	0.5	2	880

[75] With no added salt; if salt is added, sodium content is 2,070 mg.
[76] With no added salt; if salt is added, sodium content is 998 mg.
[77] With salt added.

Table continued on following page

APPENDIX 1. Nutritive Value of the Edible Part of Food *Continued*

Item No.	Foods, Approximate Measures, Units, and Weight (Weight of Edible Portion Only)			Water	Food energy	Protein	Fat	Fatty Acids: Saturated	Fatty Acids: Monounsaturated	Fatty Acids: Polyunsaturated
	MISCELLANEOUS ITEMS		*Grams*	*%*	*Calories*	*Grams*	*Grams*	*Grams*	*Grams*	*Grams*
	Baking powders for home use:									
	Sodium aluminum sulfate:									
881	With monocalcium phosphate monohydrate	1 tsp	3	2	5	Tr	0	0.0	0.0	0.0
882	With monocalcium phosphate monohydrate, calcium sulfate	1 tsp	2.9	1	5	Tr	0	0.0	0.0	0.0
883	Straight phosphate	1 tsp	3.8	2	5	Tr	0	0.0	0.0	0.0
884	Low sodium	1 tsp	4.3	1	5	Tr	0	0.0	0.0	0.0
885	Catsup	1 cup	273	69	290	5	1	0.2	0.2	0.4
886		1 tbsp	15	69	15	Tr	Tr	Tr	Tr	Tr
887	Celery seed	1 tsp	2	6	10	Tr	1	Tr	0.3	0.1
888	Chili powder	1 tsp	2.6	8	10	Tr	Tr	0.1	0.1	0.2
	Chocolate:									
889	Bitter or baking	1 oz	28	2	145	3	15	9.0	4.9	0.5
	Semisweet, see Candy (item 715).									
890	Cinnamon	1 tsp	2.3	10	5	Tr	Tr	Tr	Tr	Tr
891	Curry powder	1 tsp	2	10	5	Tr	Tr	[1]	[1]	[1]
892	Garlic powder	1 tsp	2.8	6	10	Tr	Tr	Tr	Tr	Tr
893	Gelatin, dry	1 envelope	7	13	25	6	Tr	Tr	Tr	Tr
894	Mustard, prepared, yellow	1 tsp or individual packet	5	80	5	Tr	Tr	Tr	0.2	Tr
	Olives, canned:									
895	Green	4 medium or 3 extra large	13	78	15	Tr	2	0.2	1.2	0.1
896	Ripe, Mission, pitted	3 small or 2 large	9	73	15	Tr	2	0.3	1.3	0.2
897	Onion powder	1 tsp	2.1	5	5	Tr	Tr	Tr	Tr	Tr
898	Oregano	1 tsp	1.5	7	5	Tr	Tr	Tr	Tr	0.1
899	Paprika	1 tsp	2.1	10	5	Tr	Tr	Tr	Tr	0.2
900	Pepper, black	1 tsp	2.1	11	5	Tr	Tr	Tr	Tr	Tr
	Pickles, cucumber:									
901	Dill, medium, whole, 3¾-in long, 1¼-in diam.	1 pickle	65	93	5	Tr	Tr	Tr	Tr	0.1
902	Fresh-pack, slices 1½-in diam., ¼-in thick	2 slices	15	79	10	Tr	Tr	Tr	Tr	Tr
903	Sweet, gherkin, small, whole, about 2½-in long, ¾-in diam.	1 pickle	15	61	20	Tr	Tr	Tr	Tr	Tr
	Popcorn. See Grain Products (items 497-499).									
904	Relish, finely chopped, sweet	1 tbsp	15	63	20	Tr	Tr	Tr	Tr	Tr
905	Salt	1 tsp	5.5	0	0	0	0	0.0	0.0	0.0
906	Vinegar, cider	1 tbsp	15	94	Tr	Tr	0	0.0	0.0	0.0
	Yeast:									
907	Baker's, dry, active	1 pkg	7	5	20	3	Tr	Tr	0.1	Tr
908	Brewer's, dry	1 tbsp	8	5	25	3	Tr	Tr	Tr	0.0

Nutrients in Indicated Quantity

Cholesterol	Carbohydrate	Calcium	Phosphorus	Iron	Potassium	Sodium	Vitamin A Value (IU)	Vitamin A Value (RE)	Thiamin	Riboflavin	Niacin	Ascorbic acid	Item No.
Milligrams	*Grams*	*Milligrams*	*Milligrams*	*Milligrams*	*Milligrams*	*Milligrams*	*International units*	*Retinol equivalents*	*Milligrams*	*Milligrams*	*Milligrams*	*Milligrams*	
0	1	58	87	0.0	5	329	0	0	0.00	0.00	0.0	0	881
0	1	183	45	0.0	4	290	0	0	0.00	0.00	0.0	0	882
0	1	239	359	0.0	6	312	0	0	0.00	0.00	0.0	0	883
0	1	207	314	0.0	891	Tr	0	0	0.00	0.00	0.0	0	884
0	69	60	137	2.2	991	2,845	3,820	382	0.25	0.19	4.4	41	885
0	4	3	8	0.1	54	156	210	21	0.01	0.01	0.2	2	886
0	1	35	11	0.9	28	3	Tr	Tr	0.01	0.01	0.1	Tr	887
0	1	7	8	0.4	50	26	910	91	0.01	0.02	0.2	2	888
0	8	22	109	1.9	235	1	10	1	0.01	0.07	0.4	0	889
0	2	28	1	0.9	12	1	10	1	Tr	Tr	Tr	1	890
0	1	10	7	0.6	31	1	20	2	0.01	0.01	0.1	Tr	891
0	2	2	12	0.1	31	1	0	0	0.01	Tr	Tr	Tr	892
0	0	1	0	0.0	2	6	0	0	0.00	0.00	0.0	0	893
0	Tr	4	4	0.1	7	63	0	0	Tr	0.01	Tr	Tr	894
0	Tr	8	2	0.2	7	312	40	4	Tr	Tr	Tr	0	895
0	Tr	10	2	0.2	2	68	10	1	Tr	Tr	Tr	0	896
0	2	8	7	0.1	20	1	Tr	Tr	0.01	Tr	Tr	Tr	897
0	1	24	3	0.7	25	Tr	100	10	0.01	Tr	0.1	1	898
0	1	4	7	0.5	49	1	1,270	127	0.01	0.04	0.3	1	899
0	1	9	4	0.6	26	1	Tr	Tr	Tr	0.01	Tr	0	900
0	1	17	14	0.7	130	928	70	7	Tr	0.01	Tr	4	901
0	3	5	4	0.3	30	101	20	2	Tr	Tr	Tr	1	902
0	5	2	2	0.2	30	107	10	1	Tr	Tr	Tr	1	903
0	5	3	2	0.1	30	107	20	2	Tr	Tr	0.0	1	904
0	0	14	3	Tr	Tr	2,132	0	0	0.00	0.00	0.0	0	905
0	1	1	1	0.1	15	Tr	0	0	0.00	0.00	0.0	0	906
0	3	3	90	1.1	140	4	Tr	Tr	0.16	0.38	2.6	Tr	907
0	3	17[78]	140	1.4	152	10	Tr	Tr	1.25	0.34	3.0	Tr	908

[78] Value may vary from 6 to 60 mg.

APPENDIX 2. Provisional Table on the Dietary Fiber Content of Selected Foods (100 g of Edible Portion)*

Food Item	Moisture	Total Dietary Fiber (AOAC)†
	g per 100 g edible portion	
Baked Products		
Bagels, plain	31.6	2.1
Biscuit mix:		
Dry	8.7	1.3
Baked	29.4	1.8
Biscuits, made from refrigerated dough, baked	28.7	1.5
Breads:		
Boston brown	47.2	4.7
Bran	37.7	8.5
Cornbread mix:		
Dry	6.0	6.5
Baked	34.4	2.6
Cracked-wheat	35.9	5.3
French	33.9	2.3
Hollywood-type, light	37.8	4.8
Italian	34.1	2.7
Mixed-grain	38.2	6.3
Oatmeal	36.7	3.9
Pita:		
White	32.1	1.6
Whole-wheat	30.6	7.4
Pumpernickel	38.3	5.9
Reduced-calorie, high-fiber:		
Wheat	43.7	11.3
White	41.8	7.9
Rye	37.0	6.2
Vienna		3.2
Wheat	37.0	3.5
Toasted		5.2
White	37.1	1.9
Toasted		2.5
Whole-wheat	38.3	7.4
Toasted		8.9
Bread crumbs, plain or seasoned	5.7	4.2
Bread stuffing, flavored, from dry mix	65.1	2.9
Cake mix:		
Chocolate:		
Dry	3.8	2.4
Prepared	33.3	2.2
Yellow:		
Dry	4.1	1.1
Prepared	40.0	0.8
Cakes:		
Boston cream pie	47.6	1.4
Coffeecake:		
Crumb topping	22.3	3.3
Fruit	31.7	2.5
Fruitcake, commercial	22.0	3.7
Gingerbread, from dry mix	38.5	2.9
Cheesecake:		
Commercial	44.6	2.1
From no-bake mix	44.4	1.9
Baked Products *Continued*		
Cookies:		
Brownies	12.6	2.2
With nuts	12.6	2.6
Butter	4.7	2.4
Chocolate chip	4.0	2.7
Chocolate sandwich	2.2	2.9
Fig bars	16.7	4.6
Fortune	8.0	1.6
Oatmeal	5.7	2.9
Oatmeal, soft-type		2.7
Peanut butter	6.7	1.8
Shortbread with pecans	3.3	1.8
Vanilla sandwich	2.1	1.5
Crackers:		
Cheese, sandwich with peanut butter filling	4.0	1.1
Crisp bread, rye	6.1	16.2
Graham	4.1	3.2
Honey	4.1	1.7
Matzo:		
Plain	6.1	2.9
Egg/onion	8.0	5.0
Whole-wheat	3.0	11.8
Melba toast:		
Plain	5.6	6.3
Rye	6.7	7.9
Wheat	6.1	7.4
Rye	7.2	15.8
Saltines		2.6
Snack-type	4.2	1.2
Wheat	3.2	5.5
Whole-wheat	2.7	10.4
Croutons, plain or seasoned	5.6	4.7
Doughnuts:		
Cake	19.7	1.3
Yeast-leavened, glazed	26.7	2.2
English muffin, whole-wheat	45.7	6.7
French toast, commercial, ready-to-eat	48.1	3.1
Ice cream cones:		
Sugar, rolled type	3.0	4.6
Wafer-type	5.3	4.1
Muffins, commercial:		
Blueberry	37.3	3.6
Oat bran	35.0	7.5
Pancake/waffle mix:		
Regular:		
Dry	8.7	2.7
Prepared	50.4	1.4
Buckwheat, dry	9.1	2.3
Pastry, danish:		
Plain	19.3	1.3
Fruit	27.6	1.9
Baked Products *Continued*		
Pies, commercial:		
Apple	51.7	1.6
Cherry	46.2	0.8
Chocolate cream	43.5	2.0
Egg custard	46.5	1.6
Fruit and coconut		0.9
Lemon meringue	41.7	1.2
Pecan	19.8	3.5
Pumpkin	58.1	2.7
Rolls, dinner, egg	30.4	3.8
Taco shells	6.0	8.0
Toaster pastries	8.9	1.0
Tortillas:		
Corn	43.6	5.2
Flour, wheat	26.2	2.9
Waffles, commercial, frozen, ready-to-eat	45.0	2.4
Breakfast Cereals, Ready-to-Eat		
Bran, high fiber	2.9	35.3
Extra fiber		45.9
Bran flakes	2.9	18.8
Bran flakes with raisins	8.3	13.4
Corn flakes:		
Plain	2.8	2.0
Frosted or sugar-sparkled	1.9	2.2
Fiber cereal with fruit		14.8
Granola	3.3	10.5
Oat cereal	5.0	10.6
Oat flakes, fortified	3.1	3.0
Puffed wheat, sugar-coated	1.5	1.5
Rice, crispy	2.4	1.2
Wheat and malted barley:		
Flakes	3.4	6.8
Nuggets	3.2	6.5
With raisins		5.0
Wheat flakes	4.3	9.0
Cereal Grains		
Amaranth	9.8	15.2
Amaranth flour, whole-grain	10.4	10.2
Arrowroot flour	11.4	3.4
Barley	9.4	17.3
Barley, pearled, raw	10.1	15.6
Bulgur, dry	8.0	18.3
Corn bran, crude	4.7	84.6
Corn flour, whole-grain	10.9	13.4
Cornmeal:		
Whole-grain	10.3	11.0
Degermed	11.6	5.2

Table continued on following page

APPENDIX 2. Provisional Table on the Dietary Fiber Content of Selected Foods (100 Grams Edible Portion)* *Continued*

Food Item	Moisture	Total Dietary Fiber (AOAC)†
	g per 100 g edible portion	
Breakfast Cereals, Ready-to-Eat *Continued*		
Cornstarch	8.3	0.9
Farina, regular or instant:		
Dry	10.6	2.7
Cooked	85.8	1.4
Hominy, canned	79.8	2.5
Millet, hulled, raw		8.5
Oat bran, raw	6.6	15.9
Oat flour	7.8	9.6
Oats, rolled or oatmeal, dry	8.8	10.3
Rice, brown, long-grain:		
Raw	11.1	3.5
Cooked	73.1	1.7
Rice, white:		
Glutinous, raw	10.0	2.8
Long-grain:		
Raw	11.6	1.0
Parboiled:		
Dry	10.5	1.8
Cooked		0.5
Precooked or instant:		
Dry	8.1	1.6
Cooked	76.4	0.8
Medium-grain, raw	12.9	1.4
Rice bran, crude	6.1	21.7
Rice flour:		
Brown	12.0	4.6
White	11.9	2.4
Rye flour, medium or light	9.4	14.6
Semolina	12.7	3.9
Tapioca, pearl, dry	12.0	1.1
Triticale	10.5	18.1
Triticale flour, whole-grain	10.0	14.6
Wheat bran, crude	9.9	42.4
Wheat flour:		
White, all-purpose	11.8	2.7
Whole-grain	10.9	12.6
Wheat germ:		
Crude	11.1	15.0
Toasted	2.9	12.9
Wild rice, raw	7.8	5.2
Fruits and Fruit Products		
Apples, raw:		
With skin	83.9	2.2
Without skin	84.5	1.9
Apple juice, unsweetened	87.9	0.1
Applesauce:		
Sweetened	79.6	1.2
Unsweetened	88.4	1.5
Apricots, dried	31.1	7.8

Food Item	Moisture	Total Dietary Fiber (AOAC)†
	g per 100 g edible portion	
Legumes, Nuts, and Seeds *Continued*		
Cashews, oil-roasted	5.4	6.0
Chickpeas, canned, drained	68.2	5.8
Coconut, raw	47.0	9.0
Cowpeas (black-eyed peas):		
Raw	12.0	27.0
Cooked, drained	70.0	9.6
Hazelnuts, oil-roasted	1.2	6.4
Lima beans:		
Raw	10.2	19.0
Cooked, drained	69.8	7.2
Miso	47.4	5.4
Mixed nuts, oil-roasted, with peanuts		9.0
Peanuts:		
Dry-roasted	1.6	8.0
Oil-roasted	2.0	8.8
Peanut butter:		
Chunky	1.1	6.6
Smooth	1.4	6.0
Pecans, dried	4.8	6.5
Pistachio nuts	3.9	10.8
Sunflower seeds, oil-roasted	2.6	6.8
Tahini	3.0	9.3
Tofu	84.6	1.2
Walnuts, dried:		
Black	4.4	5.0
English	3.6	4.8
Miscellaneous		
Beer, regular	92.3	0.5
Candy:		
Caramels, vanilla	7.6	1.2
Chocolate, milk	0.8	2.8
Sugar-coated discs		3.1
Carob powder, unsweetened	1.2	32.8
Chili powder	9.1	34.2
Chocolate, baking	0.7	15.4
Cocoa, baking	1.3	29.8
Cocoa mix, prepared	79.8	1.2
Curry powder	8.7	33.2
Gravy, beef, canned	89.1	0.4
Jelly, apple	32.3	0.6
Milk, chocolate	82.3	1.5
Pepper, black	9.4	25.0
Pie filling:		
Apple	74.9	1.0
Cherry	69.7	0.6
Preserves:		
Peach	32.4	0.7
Strawberry	31.7	1.2
Soup, canned, condensed:		
Chicken with noodles or rice	86.5	0.6

Food Item	Moisture	Total Dietary Fiber (AOAC)†
	g per 100 g edible portion	
Vegetables and Vegetable Products *Continued*		
Beans, snap *Continued*		
Canned:		
Drained solids	93.3	1.3
Solids and liquid	94.5	0.8
Beets, canned:		
Drained solids, sliced	91.0	1.7
Solids and liquid	91.3	1.1
Broccoli:		
Raw	90.7	2.8
Cooked	90.2	2.6
Brussels sprouts, boiled	87.3	4.3
Cabbage, Chinese:		
Raw	94.9	1.0
Cooked	95.4	1.6
Cabbage, red:		
Raw	91.6	2.0
Cooked	93.6	2.0
Cabbage, white, raw	91.5	2.4
Carrots:		
Raw	87.8	3.2
Canned, drained solids	93.0	1.5
Cauliflower:		
Raw	92.3	2.4
Cooked	92.5	2.2
Celery, raw	94.7	1.6
Chives	92.0	3.2
Corn, sweet:		
Raw	76.0	3.2
Cooked	69.6	3.7
Canned:		
Brine pack:		
Drained solids	76.9	1.4
Solids and liquid	81.9	0.8
Cream-style	78.7	1.2
Cucumbers, raw	96.0	1.0
Pared		0.5
Lettuce:		
Butterhead or iceberg	95.7	1.0
Romaine	94.9	1.7
Mushrooms:		
Raw	91.8	1.3
Boiled	91.1	2.2
Onions, raw	90.1	1.6
Onions, spring, raw	91.9	2.4
Parsley, raw	88.3	4.4
Peas, edible-podded:		
Raw	88.9	2.6
Cooked	88.9	2.8
Peas, sweet, canned:		
Drained solids	81.7	3.4
Solids and liquid	86.5	2.0

Food		
Apricot nectar	84.9	0.6
Bananas, raw	74.3	1.6
Blueberries, raw	84.6	2.3
Cantaloupe, raw	89.8	0.8
Figs, dried	28.4	9.3
Fruit cocktail, canned in heavy syrup, drained		1.5
Grapefruit, raw	90.9	0.6
Grapes, Thompson, seedless, raw	81.3	0.7
Kiwifruit, raw	83.0	3.4
Netarines, raw	86.3	1.6
Olives:		
Green		2.6
Ripe		3.0
Oranges, raw	86.8	2.4
Orange juice, frozen concentrate:		
Undiluted	57.8	0.8
Prepared	88.1	0.2
Peaches:		
Raw	87.7	1.6
Canned in juice, drained		1.0
Dried	31.8	8.2
Pears, raw	83.8	2.6
Pineapple:		
Raw	86.5	1.2
Canned in heavy syrup, chunks, drained	79.0	1.1
Prunes:		
Dried	32.4	7.2
Stewed		6.6
Prune juice	81.2	1.0
Raisins	15.4	5.3
Strawberries	91.6	2.6
Watermelon	91.5	0.4
Legumes, Nuts, and Seeds		
Almonds, oil-roasted	3.3	11.2
Baked beans, canned:		
Barbecue-style		5.8
Sweet or tomato sauce:		
Plain	72.6	7.7
With franks	69.3	6.9
With pork	71.7	5.5
Beans, Great Northern:		
Raw	10.7	40.0
Canned, drained	69.9	5.4
Vegetable	84.9	1.3
Yeast, active, dry	6.8	31.6
Pasta		
Macaroni (see spaghetti)		
Macraroni, protein-fortified, dry	10.2	4.3
Macraroni, tricolor, dry	9.8	4.3
Noodles, Chinese, chow mein	0.7	3.9
Noodles, egg, regular:		
Dry	9.7	2.7
Cooked	68.7	2.2
Noodles, Japanese, dry:		
Somen	9.2	4.3
Udon	8.7	5.4
Noodles, spinach, dry	8.5	6.8
Spaghetti and macaroni:		
Dry	10.5	2.4
Cooked	64.7	1.6
Spaghetti, dry:		
Spinach	8.7	10.6
Whole-wheat	7.1	11.8
Snacks		
Cheese-flavored, corn-based puffs or twists		1.0
Corn, toasted		6.9
Corn chips		4.4
Barbecue-flavored		5.2
Granola bars, crunchy:		
Chocolate chip		4.4
Cinnamon		5.0
Popcorn:		
Air-popped		15.1
Oil-popped		10.0
Potato chips	2.5	4.8
Flavored		4.5
Potato chips, formulated	1.6	3.6
Pretzels		2.8
Tortilla chips		6.5
Flavored		6.2
Vegetables and Vegetable Products		
Artichokes, raw	84.4	5.2
Beans, snap:		
Raw	90.3	1.8
Peppers, sweet, raw	92.8	1.6
Pickles:		
Dill	93.8	1.2
Sweet	68.9	1.1
Potatoes:		
Raw:		
Flesh and skin	80.0	1.8
Flesh	79.0	1.6
Baked:		
Flesh	75.4	1.5
Skin	47.3	4.0
Boiled	77.0	1.5
French-fried, home-prepared from frozen	52.9	4.2
Hashed brown	56.1	2.0
Spinach:		
Raw	91.6	2.6
Boiled	91.2	2.2
Squash:		
Summer:		
Raw	93.7	1.2
Cooked	93.7	1.4
Winter:		
Raw	88.7	1.8
Cooked	89.0	2.8
Sweet potatoes:		
Raw	72.8	3.0
Cooked	72.8	3.0
Canned, drained solids	72.5	1.8
Tomatoes, raw	94.0	1.3
Tomato products:		
Catsup		1.6
Paste	74.1	4.3
Puree	87.3	2.3
Sauce	89.1	1.5
Turnip greens:		
Raw	91.1	2.4
Boiled	93.2	3.1
Turnips:		
Raw	91.9	1.8
Boiled	93.6	2.0
Vegetables, mixed, frozen, cooked	83.2	3.8
Water chestnuts, canned, drained solids	87.9	2.2
Watercress	95.1	2.3

* From United States Department of Agriculture, Human Nutrition Information Service, HNIS/PT-106, Nutrient Data Research Branch, Nutrition Monitoring Division, September 1988.
† AOAC = accepted method of dietary fiber analysis of the Association of Official Analytical Chemists.

APPENDIX 3. Folic Acid Content of Foods (μg per 100 kcal and per Serving)

	Wt (g)	Svg	Cal	Folic Acid (μg) 100 Kcal	Folic Acid (μg) Svg
Baked Goods					
Apple crisp, 3″ × 3″	78	1 ea	146	2	3
Bagel, egg/plain, 3.5″ diam	68	1 ea	180	9	16
Biscuits, average	28	1 ea	93	1.5	1+
Breads:					
Banana nut, ½″	50	1 pce	161	7	11
Boston brown, ½″ slc	45	1 pce	95	8.4	8
Cornbread muffin	45	1 ea	145	3	5
Cracked wheat	25	1 pce	65	19	12
French, 5″ × 2.5″ × 1″	35	1 pce	100	13	13
Mixed grain	25	1 pce	65	25	16
Oatmeal	25	1 pce	65	12	8
Pita pocket, 6.5″ diam.	60	1 ea	165	7	12
Pumpernickel, 4″ × 5″ × ⅜″	32	1 pce	80	20	16
Raisin	25	1 pce	68	13	9
Rye, 5″ × 3.5″	25	1 pce	65	15	10
Wheat (white and whole wheat flour)	28	1 pce	72	18	13
White	28	1 pce	75	13	10
Whole wheat	28	1 pce	70	22	16
Cakes, pce = 1/16 cake unless otherwise noted:					
Angel food, 1/12	53	1 pce	125	3	4
Boston cream pie, ⅛	120	1 pce	260	3	7
Carrot w/cream cheese frosting, 2.5″ × 3″ pce	112	1 pce	406	3	11
Cheesecake f/recipe, 1/12	92	1 pce	278	6	17
Chocolate, choc. frosting	69	1 pce	235	2	4
Coffee cake f/mix, 2.4″ × 2.8″	72	1 pce	230	2	5
Gingerbread, 3″ × 3″	63	1 pce	174	2	4
Pound cake, ½″	30	1 pce	115	3	3
Sheet cake, 3″ × 3″:					
Plain	86	1 pce	315	5	15
White frosting	121	1 pce	445	3	12
Spongecake, 1/12 tube	66	1 pce	194	6	11
Snack cake, like Twinkies	42	1 ea	155	3	4
White cake:					
Chocolate frosting	77	1 pce	291	3	8
Coconut frosting	70	1 pce	270	1.5	4
Yellow cake, choc. frosting	69	1 pce	240	2	5
Cherry crisp, 3″ × 3″	138	1 pce	157	6	10
Chips: see corn and tortillas this section, potato chips under Vegetables and Legumes.					
Cookies, average	45	4 ea	180–245	2	4
Crackers:					
Armenian cracker bread	28	4 pce	117	10	12
Graham crackers	14	2 ea	60	3	2
***Baked Goods** Continued*					
Tortillas:					
Corn, enr., fried, 6″ diam.	30	1 ea	87	6	5
Flour, 10.5″ diam.	57	1 ea	168	15	25
Flour, 8″ diam.	35	1 ea	105	15	16
Waffles, 7″ diam.:					
From recipe	75	1 ea	245	5	13
From mix	75	1 ea	205	2	4
Dairy and Dairy Products					
Cheese (1.5″ cube ≈ 1 oz):					
American	28	1 oz	106	2	2
Blue	28	1 oz	100	10	10
Brick	28	1 oz	105	6	6
Brie	28	1 oz	95	19	18
Camembert	28	1 oz	85	21	18
Cheddar	28	1 oz	114	4	5
Cheshire	28	1 oz	110	4	4
Colby	28	1 oz	112	5	5
Cottage:					
Lowfat 1%	226	1 c	164	17	28
Lowfat 2%	226	1 c	205	15	30
Creamed, large curd	225	1 c	235	12	27
Creamed, small curd	210	1 c	215	12	26
Creamed, with fruit	226	1 c	279	8	22
Dry curd	145	1 c	123	17	21
Cream (1 T = 15 g)	28	1 oz	99	4	4
Edam	28	1 oz	101	5	5
Gorgonzola	28	1 oz	111	8	9
Gouda	28	1 oz	101	6	6
Liederkranz	28	1 oz	87	39	34
Limburger	28	1 oz	93	17	16
Parmesan, grated (1 T ≈ 5 g)	100	1 c	455	2	8
Ricotta, part skim	246	1 c	340	4	14
Roquefort	28	1 oz	105	13	14
Swiss	28	1 oz	92	2	2
Cream, Sweet, fluid:					
Coffee or table	240	1 c	469	1	6
Half and half	15	1 T	20	10	2
Light whipping cream	239	1 c	699	1	9
Cream, Sweet, whipped:					
Heavy cream, whipped	119	1 c	410	1	5
Pressurized	60	1 c	154	.6	1

Food	Weight (g)	Amount	Calories	Protein	Fat
Rye wafers, whole grain	14	2 ea	55	18	10
Sesame crackers	12	4 ea	60	8	5
Wheat cracker, thin	8	4 ea	35	9	3
Crepe (no filling)	27	1 ea	47	11	5
Croissant, 4.5″ × 4″ × 2″	57	1 ea	235	8	18
Danish pastry, average	61	1 ea	228	7	15
Doughnut, yeast raised	60	1 ea	235	5	13
English muffin:					
Plain, enriched	57	1 ea	140	13	18
Sourdough	56	1 ea	129	12	15
Muffins, from mix:					
Blueberry	45	1 ea	140	10	14
Bran	45	1 ea	140	14	19
Cornmeal	45	1 ea	145	3	5
Pancakes:					
Buckwheat, f/mix, 4″ diam.	27	1 ea	55	10	6
Plain, recipe, 4″ diam.	27	1 ea	60	6	4
Whole wheat, 5″ diam.	52	1 ea	94	10	9
Pies, pce = ⅙ of 9″ pie:					
Apple	158	1 pce	405	2	8
Banana cream	198	1 pce	319	7	22
Blueberry	158	1 pce	380	4	14
Cherry	158	1 pce	410	4	16
Chocolate cream	175	1 pce	311	4	11
Coconut cream	172	1 pce	343	3	11
Coconut custard	165	1 pce	384	7	25
Cream, commercial	152	1 pce	455	4	18
Custard	152	1 pce	293	5	15
Pecan	138	1 pce	583	3	18
Lemon meringue	140	1 pce	355	4	13
Mincemeat	160	1 pce	395	2	9
Peach	158	1 pce	405	3	12
Pumpkin	200	1 pce	367	5	20
Strawberry chiffon, recipe	162	1 pce	372	6	21
Pop Tart-type pastry, fortified	54	1 ea	210	21	43
Pretzels, thin twists	60	10 ea	240	4	10
Rolls:					
Cinnamon, small	50	1 ea	158	11	18
Dinner, 2.5″ × 2″	28	1 ea	85	12	10
Hamburger bun	45	1 ea	129	13	17
Hard roll, white	50	1 ea	155	11	17
Hotdog bun	40	1 ea	115	13	15
Rye roll, dark	28	1 ea	79	15	12
Rye roll, light	28	1 ea	76	15	11
Submarine roll (hoagie)	135	1 ea	400	12	49
Whole wheat roll	35	1 ea	88	22	20
Stuffing, w/enr. bread:					
Bread stuffing fr/dry	140	1 c	500	3	14
Stove Top stuffing	108	½ c	176	13	22

Food	Weight (g)	Amount	Calories	Protein	Fat
Cream, Sour, dairy:					
Cultured, dairy	230	1 c	493	5	25
Sour dressing, dairy	235	1 c	416	7	28
Cream, sour, imitation, nondairy	230	1 c	479	0	0
Cream substitutes, nondairy:					
Coffee whitener, liq/frzn	120	½ c	163	0	0
Coffee whitener, powder	94	1 c	541	0	0
Dessert toppings, nondairy:					
Frozen, like Coolwhip	75	1 c	239	0	0
Dessert powder, dry	43	1.5 oz	245	0	0
Pressurized, nondairy	70	1 c	185	0	0
Kefir beverage	233	1 c	160	13	20
Milk (cow):					
Skim	245	1 c	86	16	14
Low-fat 1%	244	1 c	102	12	12
Low-fat 2%	244	1 c	121	10	12
Whole (3.3% fat)	244	1 c	150	8	12
Buttermilk (<1% fat)	245	1 c	99	12	12
Canned:					
Skim, evaporated	255	1 c	200	11	22
Whole, evaporated	252	1 c	340	5	18
Sweetened, condensed	306	1 c	982	4	34
Dry, instant, nonfat	68	1 c	244	14	34
Dry, instant, buttermilk	120	1 c	464	12	57
Milk (other):					
Human breast milk	246	1 c	171	14	24
Soy milk	240	1 c	79	5	3.6
Milk Beverages and mixes:					
Chocolate flavor to be mixed w/milk:					
Powder	21.6	¾ oz	75	5	4
Drink w/whole milk	266	1 c	226	5	12
Chocolate flavor to be mixed w/water:					
Powder (includes dry milk)	28	1 oz	100	3	3
Drink	206	¾ c	100	3	3
Cocoa, hot, w/whole milk	250	1 c	218	6	12
Instant Breakfast, fortified, dry	37	1 env	130	77	100
Malted milk, w/whole milk:					
Chocolate flavor	265	1 c	229	7	16
Natural flavor	265	1 c	237	9	22
Milkshakes, 10 fl oz = 1.25 c:					
Chocolate	283	1.25 c	360	3	10
Strawberry	283	1.25 c	319	3	9
Vanilla	283	1.25 c	314	3	9
Milk Desserts:					
Custard, baked	265	1 c	305	8	24
Ice cream, vanilla					
Regular	133	1 c	269	1	3
Soft serve	173	1 c	377	2	9
Ice milk, soft serve, vanilla	175	1 c	223	2	5

Table continued on following page

APPENDIX 3. Folic Acid Content of Foods (μg per 100 kcal and per Serving) *Continued*

	Wt (g)	Svg	Cal	Folic Acid (μg) 100 Kcal	Folic Acid (μg) Svg
***Dairy and Dairy Products** Continued*					
Milk Desserts *Continued*					
Puddings (5 oz can ≈ ½ c):					
Assorted flavors:					
Low calorie	130	¾ c	69	10	7
Regular	135	½ c	150–175	3-4	6
Chocolate:					
Cooked from mix	260	1 c	300	3	8
From instant	260	1 c	310	3	10
Canned	142	1 can	205	1.5	3
Lemon or coconut f/inst	149	¾ c	181	3	6
Vanilla, canned	142	1 can	220	1.4	3
Sherbet (2% fat)	193	1 c	270	6	14
Yogurt, frozen, average	174	1 c	220	6	14
Yogurt:					
Low-fat, plain	227	1 c	144	17	25
Low-fat, fruit	227	1 c	231	9	21
Low-fat, coffee or vanilla	227	1 c	193	12	23
Nonfat yogurt	227	1 c	127	22	28
Whole	227	1 c	138	12	16
Eggs					
Whole egg (chicken):					
Cooked	50	1 ea	77.5	30	23
Raw	50	1 ea	75	31	23
White, raw	33.4	1 ea	17	6	1
Yolk, raw	16.6	1 ea	59	41	24
Fruits and Fruit Juices					
Apple, 2.75″ diam:					
With peel	138	1 ea	80	5.0	4.0
Without peel	128	1 ea	72	0.7	0.5
Apricots:					
Fresh, pitted	106	3 ea	51	18	9
Canned, juice pack	248	1 c	119	4	5
Canned, heavy syrup	258	1 c	214	2	4
Dried, halves	35	10 ea	83	4	4
Avocado, whole:					
California	173	1 ea	305	37	113
Florida	304	1 ea	340	48	162
Banana, 8.75″, 176 g w/peel	114	1 ea	105	23	24
Blackberries:					
Fresh berries	144	1 c	74	66	49
Frozen, unthawed	151	1 c	97	53	51
Canned	256	1 c	236	29	68

	Wt (g)	Svg	Cal	Folic Acid (μg) 100 Kcal	Folic Acid (μg) Svg
***Fruits and Fruit Juices** Continued*					
Lime juice:					
Fresh juice	246	1 c	65	32	21
Bottled	246	1 c	50	39	20
Loganberries, fresh	100	⅔ c	70	37	26
Mandarin oranges, canned	252	1 c	155	13	20
Mango, fresh slices	165	1 c	108	29	31
Melon, cubes, see also Watermelon:					
Cantaloupe	160	1 c	57	84	48
Casaba	170	1 c	45	89	40
Honeydew	170	1 c	60	85	51
Frozen, melon balls, mixed	173	1 c	55	81	45
Nectarine (med = 1 c slc)	136	1 med	67	8	5
Orange 2-⅝″, 180 g w/peel	131	1 ea	60	66	40
Orange juice:					
Fresh juice	248	1 c	111	98	109
Chilled	249	1 c	110	41	45
Prep. frzn concentrate	249	1 c	110	99	109
Canned, unsweetened	249	1 c	105	14	15
Orange grapefruit jce, canned	247	1 c	105	19	20
Papaya, 454g w/refuse	304	1 ea	117	41	48
Papaya nectar, canned	250	1 c	142	4	5
Peaches:					
Fresh, peeled slices	170	1 c	73	8	6
Frozen, thawed slices	250	1 c	235	3	8
Canned, juice pack	77	1 half	34	8	2.6
Canned, heavy syrup	81	1 half	60	4	2.6
Pears:					
Bartlett, 180 g w/refuse	166	1 ea	98	12	12
Canned, heavy syrup	79	1 half	59	1.5	.9
Canned, juice pack	77	1 half	38	4	1.6
Persimmon, Japanese, large	168	1 ea	118	11	13
Pineapple:					
Fresh, chunks	155	1 c	76	22	16
Canned pieces, juice pack	250	1 c	150	8	12
Canned pieces, heavy syrup	255	1 c	199	6	12
Pineapple juice:					
From frozen	250	1 c	129	50	64
Canned, unsweetened	250	1 c	140	41	58
Plantain slices, fresh	148	1 c	181	18	33

Blueberries:					
Fresh berries	145	1 c	82	11	9
Frozen, unsweetened	155	1 c	78	13	10
Canned	256	1 c	225	3	7
Boysenberries:					
Frozen, unthawed	132	1 c	66	127	84
Canned	256	1 c	225	39	88
Cherries, sour:					
Frozen, unthawed	155	1 c	72	10	7
Canned	244	1 c	90	22	20
Cherries, Sweet:					
Fresh, pitted, 10 = 68 g	145	1 c	104	8	8
Canned	257	1 c	213	4	7
Cantaloupe: see Melons.					
Currants:					
Fresh, Black	112	1 c	71	6	4
Fresh, Red or white	112	1 c	63	6	4
Dried, (Zante)	144	1 c	407	4	15
Dates, fresh, pitted	83	10 ea	228	6	14
Figs, fresh, medium	50	1 med	37	4	1.5
Figs, dried	187	10 ea	477	3	16
Fruit cocktail, canned:					
Juice pack	248	1 c	115	2	1.5
Heavy syrup	255	1 c	185	.6	1.2
Gooseberries, canned w/liq.	252	1 c	185	4	8
Grapefruit, half = 241 g w/rind:					
Half, pink or red	123	1 ea	37	41	15
Half, white	118	1 ea	39	30	12
Canned, sections	254	1 c	152	14	22
Grapefruit juice:					
Fresh juice	247	1 c	96	54	52
Prep f/frzn conc.	247	1 c	102	51	52
Canned, unsweetened	247	1 c	93	28	26
Grapes:					
Thompson, seedless	50	10 ea	35	10	4
Tokay or Emperor	57	10 ea	40	10	4
Canned, heavy syrup	256	1 c	187	4	8
Grape juice:					
From frozen	250	1 c	128	3	4
Bottled or canned	253	1 c	155	4	7
Guava, raw	90	1 ea	45	28	13
Kiwi fruit	76	1 ea	46	37	17
Lemon juice:					
Fresh juice	244	1 c	60	53	32
Frozen, standard strength	244	1 c	54	43	23
Bottled	244	1 c	52	47	25
Plantain slices, cooked	154	1 c	179	22	40
Plums:					
Medium, 2⅛″ diam.	66	1 ea	36	9	3
Canned, juice pack	95	3 ea	55	5	2.8
Canned, heavy syrup	110	3 ea	98	3	2.8
Prunes, dried	84	10 ea	201	2	3.4
Raisins, dark, unpacked meas	145	1 c	435	1	5
Raspberries:					
Fresh berries	123	1 c	60	54	33
Frozen, thawed measure	250	1 c	255	26	65
Canned	256	1 c	234	12	27
Rhubarb:					
Fresh, diced	122	1 c	26	34	9
Cooked with sugar	240	1 c	279	5	13
Strawberries:					
Fresh berries	149	1 c	45	62	28
Frozen, thawed, sweetened	255	1 c	245	17	42
Frozen, unsweetened	149	1 c	52	54	28
Tangerines, medium	84	1 ea	37	46	17
Tangerine juice:					
From frozen	241	1 c	110	10	11
Canned, sweetened	249	1 c	125	6	8
Watermelon, diced pieces	160	1 cup	50	7	3.4
Grains and Grain Products					
Amaranth grain, dry	195	1 c	729	13	95
Barley, pearled, cooked	157	1 c	193	13	25
Bran: see Oat, Rice, Wheat.					
Buckwheat flour:					
Dark	98	1 c	338	37	125
Light	98	1 c	340	29	100
Bulgar wheat, cooked	182	1 c	151	22	33
Cereals, Cold (Ready To Eat): Cereals can be fortified with folacin. Amounts vary. Check the label.					
Cereals, Hot (cooked):					
Corn grits	242	1 c	145	1.4	2
Cream of Rice	244	1 c	126	6	8
Cream of Wheat	244	1 c	140	7	9
Farina, cooked	233	1 c	116	4	5
Malt-O-Meal	240	1 c	122	4	5
Maypo, cooked	180	¾ c	128	6	7
Oatmeal, regular, quick/inst.	234	1 c	145	7	9.4
Oatmeal, fortified instant:					
Plain, from packet	177	¾ c	104	144	150
Other flavors averaged	164	¾ c	160	94	150
Ralston	253	1 c	134	13	18
Roman Meal	181	¾ c	111	16	18

Table continued on following page

APPENDIX 3. Folic Acid Content of Foods (μg per 100 kcal and per Serving) *Continued*

	Wt (g)	Svg	Cal	Folic Acid (μg) 100 Kcal	Folic Acid (μg) Svg
***Grains and Grain Products** Continued*					
Cereals, Hot *Continued*					
Wheatena	243	1 c	135	13	17
Whole wheat cereal	242	1 c	150	17	25
Corn flour:					
Regular	117	1 c	422	7	29
Masa Harina, enriched	114	1 c	416	6	27
Cornmeal, dry, degermed	138	1 c	505	13	66
Flour: see specific grain, nut, or vegetable.					
Macaroni, cooked, enriched	140	1 c	197	5	10
Millet, cooked	120	½ c	143	16	23
Noodles:					
Chow mein, dry	45	1 c	237	4	10
Egg, cooked	160	1 c	213	5	11
Spinach, cooked	140	1 c	182	9	17
Oat bran (1T = 6 g)	94	1 c	132	37	49
Oats, rolled, dry	81	1 c	311	8	26
Pasta: see Macaroni, Noodles, Spaghetti.					
Popcorn, popped in oil	11	1 c	55	5	3
Rice, cooked:					
Brown rice	195	1 c	217	4	8
White, regular, enriched	205	1 c	264	2	6
White, converted, enriched	175	1 c	200	4	7
White, instant	165	1 c	162	4	7
Wild rice	164	1 c	166	26	43
Rice bran	83	1 c	262	20	52
Rice flour	158	1 c	578	1	6
Rye flour:					
Dark	128	1 c	415	19	77
Light	102	1 c	361	6	22
Soy flour, stirred:					
Full fat, raw	85	1 c	368	80	293
Full fat, roasted	85	1 c	373	52	193
Lowfat	85	1 c	326	111	361
Defatted	100	1 c	327	93	305
Spaghetti, cooked:					
Enriched	140	1 c	197	5	10
Whole-wheat spaghetti	140	1 c	174	4	7
Tapioca, dry	152	1 c	518	1	6
Wheat:					
Wheat bran	30	½ c	65	36	23.7

	Wt (g)	Svg	Cal	Folic Acid (μg) 100 Kcal	Folic Acid (μg) Svg
***Meats: Fish and Shellfish** Continued*					
Mullet, baked/broiled	85	3 oz	127	7	8
Oysters:					
Raw, Eastern	248	1 c	170	14	25
Raw, Pacific	248	1 c	200	12	24
Fried, Eastern, medium	88	6 ea	173	7	12
Simmered, Eastern	100	3.5 oz	137	13	18
Perch, Ocean:					
Baked or broiled	100	3.5 oz	121	7	9
Breaded, fried	85	3 oz	185	3	6
Pike, Northern, baked/broiled	100	3.5 oz	113	27	30
Pollock, baked or broiled	100	3.5 oz	99	13	13
Salmon, cooked:					
Broiled or baked, avg	85	3 oz	183	8	14
Smoked salmon, Chinook	85	3 oz	99	2	1.6
Canned, Atlantic, small can	220	1 can	281	12	35
Pink, No. 1 can, drained	454	1 can	631	11	70
Sockeye, No. 1 can, drained	369	1 can	566	6	36
Sardines, canned, drained:					
Atlantic, 2 ea = 24 g	92	1 can	192	6	11
Pacific, 1 ea = 38 g	100	3.5 oz	178	14	24
Scallops:					
Breaded, fried	93	6 ea	200	5	11
Steamed	100	3.5 oz	113	16	18
Seatrout or Steelhead, cooked	100	3.5 oz	131	7	10
Shrimp:					
Boiled, 2 large ≈ 11 g	100	3.5 oz	99	4	4
Breaded, fried, 2 large ≈ 15 g	90	12 ea	218	3	7
Smelt, Rainbow, cooked	85	3 oz	106	15	16
Snapper, baked or broiled	100	3.5 oz	128	7	9
Sole (Flounder):					
Baked or broiled	85	3 oz	99	10	10
Fried in batter	85	3 oz	250	3	7
Breaded, fried	100	3.5 oz	188	5	9
Steamed	100	3.5 oz	92	11	10
Swordfish, baked/broiled	100	3.5 oz	155	10	16
Tuna, canned, drained-No. ½ can:					
Light, oil pack	171	1 can	339	3	9
Light, water pack	165	1 can	216	4	8

Flour, unbleached:					
All purpose, white, unsifted	125	1 c	455	7	32.5
Cake, sifted	96	1 c	348	5.5	19
Semolina	167	1 c	601	20	120
Whole wheat	120	1 c	407	13	53
Wheat germ, raw	100	1 c	360	78	281
Wheat germ, toasted	113	1 c	432	92	398
Wheat, rolled:					
Cooked	240	1 c	142	19	27
Dry	85	1 c	289	19	54
Whole-grain wheat (wheat berries) cooked	50	⅓ c	86	7	6
Whole wheat, sprouted	108	1 c	214	21	44
Meats: Fish and Shellfish					
Bass, baked/broiled	100	3.5 oz	125	7	9
Carp, baked/broiled	100	3.5 oz	162	6	9
Catfish, fried w/cornmeal	100	3.5 oz	229	3	7
Clams:					
Breaded, fried, small	188	20 ea	379	1	5
Steamed clams, meat only	90	20 ea	133	3	4
Canned, drained	160	1 c	236	3	7
Cod:					
Baked or broiled	100	3.5 oz	105	10	10
Fried with batter	100	3.5 oz	199	4	9
Canned with liquid, 11 oz	312	1 can	327	9	28
Crayfish, cooked, moist heat	85	3 oz	97	6	6
Crab:					
Blue, canned, unpacked	135	1 c	133	17	22
Dungeness, cooked	101	¾ c	85	24	20
Eel, smoked	100	3.5 oz	330	2	8
Fish cakes, recipe	100	3.5 oz	172	5	8
Fish sticks, heated fr/frozen	57	2 ea	155	7	10
Haddock:					
Baked, broiled or poached	85	3 oz	95	14	13
Breaded, fried	85	3 oz	175	8	14
Halibut:					
Baked or broiled	85	35 oz	119	7	8
Smoked	100	3.5 oz	224	2	5
Steamed, pacific	100	3.5 oz	131	8	11
Herring:					
Baked or broiled	100	3.5 oz	203	3	5
Canned with liquid	100	3.5 oz	208	2	5
Smoked or kippered	100	3.5 oz	217	2	4
Lobster, meat only, cooked	145	1 c	142	11	16
Mackerel:					
Baked/broiled, Atlantic	100	3.5 oz	262	3	7
Baked/broiled, Spanish	100	3.5 oz	158	4	7
Canned, Jack, No. 300 can-tall	361	1 can	563	3	18

Meats: Beef, Pork, Ham, etc.					
Beef:					
Chuck blade, pot roasted:					
Lean and fat	85	3 oz	325	1.5	5
Lean only	85	3 oz	230	2.2	5
Ground beef, baked, broiled, pan-fried average:					
Extra lean, 17% fat raw	85	3 oz	215	3.6	7.7
Lean, 20.7% fat raw	85	3 oz	231	3.3	7.7
Regular, 26.6% fat, raw	85	3 oz	250	3.1	7.7
Frozen patty, broiled, 23% fat	85	3 oz	240	3.2	7.7
Rib, oven roasted:					
Lean and fat	85	3 oz	324	2	6
Lean only	85	3 oz	204	3	7
Round steak, broiled:					
Lean and fat	85	3 oz	233	3	8
Lean only	85	3 oz	165	5	9
Round tip, oven roasted:					
Lean and fat	85	3 oz	213	3	6
Lean only	85	3 oz	162	4	7
Sirloin steak, broiled:					
Lean and fat	85	3 oz	238	3	6
Lean only	85	3 oz	172	4	7
T-bone steak, broiled:					
Lean and fat	85	3 oz	276	2	6
Lean only	85	3 oz	182	4	7
Beef kidney, cooked	140	1 ea	201	68	137
Beef liver, fried	85	3 oz	184	102	187
Dried beef, cured (6–7 pieces)	28	1 oz	47	8	4
Corned beef, canned	85	3 oz	213	2	5
Ham: see Pork, cured; Lunchmeat group and Turkey ham.					
Lamb:					
Arm chop, braised:					
Lean and fat	70	1 ea	244	5	13
Lean only	55	1 ea	152	8	12
Loin chop, broiled:					
Lean and fat	64	1 ea	201	6	12
Lean only	46	1 ea	100	11	11
Cutlet, lean, cooked average	85	3 oz	175	11	19
Leg of lamb, roasted:					
Lean and fat	85	3 oz	219	8	17
Lean only	85	3 oz	162	12	20
Shoulder roast:					
Lean and fat	85	3 oz	235	8	18
Lean only	85	3 oz	173	12	21
Liver	85	3 oz	202	168	340
Pork:					
Bacon, regular, cooked	19	3 pces	109	1	1
Center loin chop:					
Braised, lean and fat	75	1 ea	266	1	3
Braised, lean only	61	1 ea	166	2	3

Table continued on following page

APPENDIX 3. Folic Acid Content of Foods (μg per 100 kcal and per Serving) *Continued*

	Wt (g)	Svg	Cal	Folic Acid (μg) 100 Kcal	Folic Acid (μg) Svg
Meats: Beef, Pork, Ham, etc. *Continued*					
Pork *Continued*					
Broiled, lean and fat	82	1 ea	284	2	4
Broiled, lean only	72	1 ea	166	3	4
Fried, lean and fat	89	1 ea	333	1	4
Fried, lean only	67	1 ea	178	2	4
Roasted, lean and fat	88	1 ea	268	<1	1
Roasted, lean only	72	1 ea	180	<1	1
Center rib chop:					
Braised, lean and fat	67	1 ea	246	2	4
Braised, lean only	53	1 ea	147	3	4
Broiled, lean and fat	77	1 ea	264	2	6
Broiled, lean only	63	1 ea	162	3	5
Fried, lean and fat	88	1 ea	343	1	5
Fried, lean only	62	1 ea	160	3	5
Roasted, lean and fat	79	1 ea	252	2	6
Roasted, lean	66	1 ea	162	4	6
Pork roast, average loin/rib:					
Lean and fat	85	3 oz	265	3	7
Lean only	85	3 oz	200	4	8
Spareribs, cooked fr/1 lb raw	177	6.25 oz	703	1	7
Pork Cured-Ham: see also Lunchmeat group and Turkey ham.					
Roasted, lean and fat	140	1 c	341	1	4
Roasted, lean only	140	1 c	219	3	6
Canned, roasted, average	85	3 oz	142	3	4
Rabbit, roasted meat	85	3 oz	175	4	7
Veal (calf):					
Cutlet, lean, cooked avg	85	3 oz	166	8	13
Liver, pan-fried	85	3 oz	208	131	272
Rib roast	85	3 oz	151	8	12
Meats: Poultry					
Chicken:					
All types of meat:					
Fried	140	1 c	307	3	10
Roasted	140	1 c	266	3	8
Stewed	140	1 c	248	3	8
Canned, boned w/broth	142	5 oz	235	1.6	4
Dark meat:					
Fried	85	3 oz	203	4	7.0
Roasted	85	3 oz	174	4	6.7
Stewed	85	3 oz	163	4	6.0
Light meat:					
Fried	85	3 oz	163	2	3.6
Roasted	85	3 oz	147	2	3.0
Stewed	85	3 oz	135	2	3.0

	Wt (g)	Svg	Cal	Folic Acid (μg) 100 Kcal	Folic Acid (μg) Svg
Mixed Dishes and Fast Foods					
Beef and vegetable stew:					
Recipe	245	1 c	220	17	37
Canned	245	1 c	194	16	31
Beef, macaroni and tomato sauce, recipe	226	1 c	189	12	23
Beef pot pie, from frozen	234	1 ea	426	4	17
Burrito:					
Bean	174	1 ea	322	17	55
Beef	177	1 ea	463	8	35
Beef and bean	175	1 ea	390	12	48
Deluxe combination	198	1 ea	424	12	51
Cheese souffle, recipe	112	1 c	221	13	29
Chicken a la king, recipe	245	1 c	470	2	11
Chicken and noodles, recipe	240	1 c	365	3	9
Chicken chow mein:					
Recipe	250	1 c	255	7	19
Canned	250	1 c	95	13	12
Chicken egg roll	100	1 ea	242	18	44
Chicken pot pie, from frozen	230	1 ea	430	7	29
Chicken salad w/celery	78	½ c	266	2	4
Chili w/beans, canned	255	1 c	286	14	41
Cole slaw	120	1 c	84	38	32
Chop suey w/beef and pork	250	1 c	300	7	22
Corn fritter, recipe	45	1 ea	116	15	17
Corn pudding	250	1 c	271	23	63
Corned beef hash, canned	220	1 c	382	4	15
Egg salad	183	1 c	438	17	74
Enchilada:					
Beef	120	1 ea	292	4	11
Cheese	120	1 ea	330	5	15
Chicken	120	1 ea	269	4	12
French toast, recipe	65	1 pce	123	15	18
Lasagna, recipe:					
With meat	245	1 pce	398	4	16
Without meat	218	1 pce	316	5	14
Macaroni and cheese:					
Recipe	200	1 c	430	2	10
Canned	240	1 c	230	3	8
Manicotti, frozen entrée	225	1 ea	271	10	28

Breast*, meat and skin:					
Batter-fried	140	1 ea	364	2	8
Flour-fried	98	1 ea	218	2	4
Roasted	98	1 ea	193	2	3
Breast*, meat only:					
Fried	86	1 ea	161	2	4
Roasted	86	1 ea	142	2	3
*Two pieces per bird					
Drumstick, meat and skin:					
Batter-fried	72	1 ea	193	3	6
Flour-fried	49	1 ea	120	3	4
Roasted	52	1 ea	112	4	4
Stewed	57	1 ea	116	3	4
Drumstick, meat:					
Fried	42	1 ea	82	5	4
Roasted	44	1 ea	76	5	4
Stewed	46	1 ea	78	5	4
Thigh, meat and skin:					
Batter-fried	86	1 ea	238	3	8
Flour-fried	62	1 ea	162	3	5
Roasted	62	1 ea	153	3	4
Stewed	68	1 ea	158	2.5	4
Thigh, meat:					
Fried	52	1 ea	113	3.5	4
Roasted	52	1 ea	109	4	4
Stewed	55	1 ea	107	4	4
Chicken gizzard	22	1 ea	34	34	12
Chicken liver	20	1 ea	30	513	154
Duck, domestic, roasted:					
Meat and skin	85	3 oz	286	2	6
Meat only	85	3 oz	171	5	8.5
Goose, domestic, roasted:					
Meat and skin	85	3 oz	259	.7	2
Meat only	85	3 oz	202	.9	2
Liver pate, canned	13	1 T	41	19	8
Turkey, roasted:					
All types	85	3 oz	145	4	6
Dark meat	85	3 oz	159	5	8
Light meat	85	3 oz	133	4	5
Turkey gizzard	67	1 ea	109	33	36
Turkey heart	16	1 ea	28	45	13
Turkey liver	75	1 ea	127	393	499
Ground turkey, cooked	100	3.5 oz	229	3	7
Meats: Sausages and Lunchmeats					
Braunschweiger	57	2 oz	205	28	57
Italian sausage link, cooked	67	1 ea	216	2	4
Liverwurst, pork	18	1 pce	59	9	5
Salami, turkey	57	2 oz	111	5	5
Turkey ham	57	2 oz	73	6	4
Turkey pastrami	57	2 oz	74	5	4

Meat loaf, average	87	1 pce	203	4	8
Moussaka, lamb and eggplant	250	1 c	250	18	44
Pizza, cheese:					
Regular crust, 1/8 of 15″ diam.	120	1 pce	290	14	40
Thick crust, ½ of 10″ diam.	208	1 pce	519	14	70
Potato salad w/mayo and eggs	250	1 c	358	5	17
Quiche Lorraine, ⅛ pie	176	1 pce	600	3	17
Ravioli, beef, canned	226	1 c	220	10	21
Sandwiches, fast food items:					
Cheeseburger, 3 oz beef	112	1 ea	300	7	20
Cheeseburger, 4 oz beef	194	1 ea	524	4	23
Chicken patty sandwich	157	1 ea	436	4	18
English muffin with egg, cheese and bacon	38	1 ea	360	10	35
Fish sandwich:					
Large without cheese	170	1 ea	470	9	43
Regular with cheese	140	1 ea	420	6	24
Hamburger, 3 oz beef	98	1 ea	245	7	16
Hamburger, 4 oz beef	174	1 ea	445	5	24
Hotdog (frankfurter) and bun	85	1 ea	260	7	17
Sandwiches (on part whole wheat bread, except when stated as rye):					
Avocado, cheese, sprouts and tomato	195	1 ea	432	18	76
Bacon, lettuce and tomato	135	1 ea	327	12	41
Chicken salad sandwich	100	1 ea	294	10	28
Egg salad sandwich	111	1 ea	319	14	44
Grilled cheese	117	1 ea	393	8	30
Ham and cheese	151	1 ea	363	9	31
Ham and swiss on rye	145	1 ea	350	7	25
Ham on rye	116	1 ea	242	10	23
Ham sandwich	122	1 ea	256	11	29
Peanut butter and jam	100	1 ea	341	14	47
Roast beef sandwich	122	1 ea	280	10	29
Tuna salad sandwich	116	1 ea	303	12	36
Turkey sandwich	122	1 ea	271	11	28
Spaghetti (pasta and tomato sauce w/cheese):					
Recipe	250	1 c	260	3	8
Canned	250	1 c	190	3	6
Spinach souffle	136	1 c	218	28	62
Taco, beef	78	1 ea	207	6	13
Taco, chicken	78	1 ea	172	8	14
Tostadas, with:					
Beans and beef	192	1 ea	332	11	37
Beans and chicken	157	1 ea	249	14	34
Refried beans only	157	1 ea	212	22	47
Tuna noodle casserole, recipe	202	1 c	251	5	13
Tuna salad, without egg	205	1 c	383	4	15
Turkey pot pie, frozen	233	1 ea	416	6	24

Table continued on following page

APPENDIX 3. Folic Acid Content of Foods (μg per 100 kcal and per Serving) *Continued*

	Wt (g)	Svg	Cal	Folic Acid (μg) 100 Kcal	Folic Acid (μg) Svg
Nuts and Seeds					
Almonds, dried, whole	142	1 c	837	10	83
Brazil nuts, dry, unsalted	140	1 c	919	.6	6
Cashew butter	16	1 T	94	12	11
Cashews:					
Dry roasted	137	1 c	787	12	95
Oil roasted	130	1 c	748	12	88
Chestnuts, roasted	143	1 c	350	29	100
Coconut:					
Raw, grated	80	1 c	283	7	21
Shredded, sweetened, pkg	93	1 c	466	2	9
Dried unsweetened	78	1 c	515	1	7
Coconut milk, raw	240	1 c	552	1	6
Filberts (hazelnuts), whole	135	1 c	853	11	97
Macadamias, dried	134	1 c	940	10	91
Mixed Nuts w/peanuts					
(cashews, peanuts, brazil nuts, filberts, almonds, pecans):					
Dry roasted	137	1 c	814	8	69
Oil roasted	142	1 c	876	13	118
Mixed Nuts w/o peanuts					
(cashews, almonds, brazil nuts, pecans and filberts) oil roasted	144	1 c	886	9	81
Peanuts:					
Dry roasted	146	1 c	855	25	212
Oil roasted	144	1 c	837	22	181
Peanut butter:					
Chunky	258	1 c	1520	16	237
Smooth	258	1 c	1517	13	202
Pecans, dried, chopped	119	1 c	794	6	47
Pine nuts, dried:					
Pignola	28	1 oz	146	13	19
Pinyon	28	1 oz	161	12	19
Pistachios, dried, shelled	128	1 c	739	10	74
Pumpkin/squash seeds:					
Kernels, roasted	227	1 c	1185	10	115
Whole, roasted	64	1 c	285	9	27
Sesame seeds:					
Kernels, dried	150	1 c	882	17	150
Whole, dried	144	1 c	825	17	139

	Wt (g)	Svg	Cal	Folic Acid (μg) 100 Kcal	Folic Acid (μg) Svg
Soups, Sauces, and Gravies *Continued*					
Soups *Continued*					
Split pea soup:					
With ham, chunky, RTS	240	1 c	184	3	5
From dry mix	255	1 c	133	11	15
Tomato soup:					
Prepared w/milk	248	1 c	160	13	21
Prepared w/water	244	1 c	86	17	15
Prepared fr/dry	265	1 c	102	7	7
Turkey soup, chunky, RTS	236	1 c	136	18	25
Vegetable beef	244	1 c	79	13	11
Vegetable, chunky, RTS	240	1 c	122	14	17
Vegetarian vegetable	241	1 c	70	15	11
Vegetables and Legumes					
Alfalfa sprouts	33	1 c	10	122	12
Amaranth leaves:					
Chopped, fresh	28	1 c	7	327	24
Cooked	132	1 c	28	328	92
Artichoke, globe, cooked	120	1 ea	60	102	61
Artichoke, hearts:					
Cooked from frozen-pkg	240	9 oz	108	264	285
Marinated-jar	170	6 oz	168	89	149
Asparagus, pieces:					
Fresh, pieces	67	½ c	15	467	70
Ckd from fresh	90	½ c	23	392	88
Ckd from frozen	180	1 c	50	349	176
Canned, drained	121	½ c	16	613	98
Canned with liquid	122	½ c	17	612	104
Bamboo shoots, sliced, canned	131	1 c	25	160	40
Beans (see also Garbanzo, Lentils, Soybeans):					
Baked beans (dry white beans w/spices and sauce):					
Home prepared	253	1 c	382	32	122
Canned, plain/vegetarian	254	1 c	235	26	61
Canned w/frankfurters	257	1 c	366	21	77
Canned w/pork	253	1 c	268	34	92
Canned w/sweet sauce	253	1 c	282	34	95
Canned w/tomato sauce	253	1 c	247	23	57
Black beans, cooked fr/dry	172	1 c	227	113	256
Broadbeans:					
Ckd from dry	170	1 c	186	95	177
Canned	256	1 c	183	46	84
Great northern:					
Ckd from dry	177	1 c	210	86	181
Canned	262	1 c	300	71	213

Sesame flour:					
High fat	28	1 oz	149	6	9
Low fat	28	1 oz	95	9	8
Soybeans, dry roasted	172	1 c	810	45	364
Sunflower seed kernels:					
Dry roasted	128	1 c	745	37	272
Oil roasted	135	1 c	830	38	316
Sunflower seed butter	16	1 T	93	37	34
Walnuts, chopped:					
Black	125	1 c	759	11	83
English	120	1 c	770	10	79
Soups, Sauces, and Gravies					
Beef gravy:					
Recipe	135	½ c	151	5	7
Canned	233	1 c	124	6	7
Sauces (also see Other):					
Cheese sauce:					
Regular	101	½ c	216	4	9
From mix w/milk	279	1 c	305	4	12
Hollandaise sauce, recipe	160	1 c	867	7	60
Spaghetti sauce, plain:					
Recipe	220	1 c	179	13	23
Canned	249	1c	272	14	39
White sauce, recipe, med	250	1 c	395	3	12
Soups: All soups are canned unless otherwise stated.					
For soups prep. w/milk, assume whole milk.					
RTS = Ready To Serve.					
Bean w/bacon	253	1 c	173	18	32
Beef broth/bouillon	240	1 c	16	10	2
Beef noodle	244	1 c	84	5	4
Beef, chunky, RTS	240	1 c	171	8	13
Black bean soup, prepared	247	1 c	116	21	25
Celery, cream of, prepared with milk	248	1 c	165	5	9
Chicken noodle	241	1 c	75	3	2.2
Chicken rice, chunky, RTS	240	1 c	127	3	4
Chicken, chunky, RTS	251	1 c	178	3	5
Chicken, cream of, w/milk	248	1 c	191	4	8
Chili beef	250	1 c	169	6	10
Clam chowder:					
New England	248	1 c	163	7	12
Manhattan style, RTS	240	1 c	133	7	9
Lentil and ham, RTS	248	1 c	140	35	50
Minestrone	241	1 c	80	20	16
Mushroom, cream of:					
Condensed	251	1 c	257	3	7
Prepared w/milk	248	1 c	205	7	15
Onion soup, canned	241	1 c	57	27	15
Oyster stew, w/milk	245	1 c	134	5	7
Potato, cream of	248	1 c	148	6	9

Green beans, snap beans:					
Fresh, uncooked	110	1 c	34	118	40
Ckd from fresh	125	1 c	44	95	42
Ckd from frozen	135	1 c	36	117	42
Canned, drained	135	1 c	26	165	43
Canned with liquid	240	1 c	36	121	44
Kidney beans:					
Ckd fr/dry	177	1 c	225	102	229
Canned with liquid	256	1 c	208	61	126
Lima beans:					
Ckd fr/fresh	170	1 c	208	41	86
Ckd fr/frozen, average	88	½ c	90	63	57
Ckd fr/dry, large	188	1 c	217	72	156
Ckd fr/dry, small	182	1 c	229	119	273
Canned, drained	170	1 c	164	24	40
Canned with liquid	241	1 c	191	63	121
Navy, ckd fr/dry	182	1 c	259	99	255
Pinto beans:					
Canned	240	1 c	186	78	145
Ckd fr/dry	171	1 c	235	125	294
Refried, canned	253	1 c	270	56	150
White, ckd from dry	179	1 c	253	97	245
Winged, ckd from dry	172	1 c	252	7	18
Yardlong, ckd from dry	171	1 c	202	123	249
Yellow wax: see green beans.					
Bean sprouts (Mung beans):					
Fresh sprouts	104	1 c	31	203	63
Boiled, drained	124	1 c	26	135	35
Stir-fried	124	1 c	62	116	72
Canned, drained	125	1 c	16	76	12
Beet greens, cooked, drained	144	1 c	40	118	47
Beets:					
Ckd from fresh, whole	100	2 ea	31	277	86
Canned, drained, diced	85	½ c	27	82	22
Pickled, slices	114	½ c	74	47	35
Broccoli, chopped:					
Fresh, chopped	88	1 c	24	260	62
Ckd from fresh	156	1 c	44	177	78
Ckd from frozen	184	1 c	51	108	55
W/cheese sauce	142	½ c	166	66	110
W/hollandaise sauce	95	½ c	105	101	106
Brussels sprouts:					
Ckd fr/fresh	156	1 c	60	156	94
Ckd fr/frozen	155	1 c	65	242	157
Cabbage:					
Common, fresh, shredded	70	1 c	16	248	40
Common, cooked	150	1 c	32	97	31
Bok choy, fresh, shredded	70	1 c	9	633	57
Bok choy, cooked	170	1 c	20	160	32
Pe-Tsai, fresh, shredded	76	1 c	12	498	60
Pe-Tsai, cooked	119	1 c	16	397	64
Red, fresh, shredded	70	1 c	19	100	19

Table continued on following page

APPENDIX 3. Folic Acid Content of Foods (μg per 100 kcal and per Serving) *Continued*

	Wt (g)	Svg	Cal	Folic Acid (μg) 100 Kcal	Folic Acid (μg) Svg
Vegetables and Legumes *Continued*					
Cabbage *Continued*					
Red, cooked	75	½ c	16	59	9
Savoy, fresh, shredded	70	1 c	20	160	32
Savoy cooked	145	1 c	35	106	37
Carrots:					
Fresh, whole, 7.5″ × 1-⅛″	72	1 ea	31	33	10
Fresh, grated	55	½ c	24	32	8
Ckd from fresh, sliced	78	½ c	35	31	11
Ckd from frozen	73	½ c	26	30	8
Canned, drained	73	½ c	17	39	7
Canned with liquid	123	½ c	28	36	10
Carrot juice	123	½ c	49	10	5
Cauliflower:					
Fresh pieces	50	½ c	12	276	33
Ckd fr/fresh	62	½ c	15	211	32
Ckd fr/frozen	180	1 c	34	217	74
Celery:					
Fresh, large outer stalk	40	1 ea	6	183	11
Ckd, diced	150	1 c	27	122	33
Chard, Swiss, fresh, chopped	36	1 c	7	285	20
Chard, Swiss, cooked	175	1 c	35	163	57
Collards:					
Fresh, chopped	36	1 c	11	36	4
Cooked fr/fresh	128	1 c	35	23	8
Cooked fr/frozen	170	1 c	63	212	129
Corn:					
Fresh kernels, uncooked	77	½ c	66	54	35
Ckd from fresh	82	½ c	89	43	38
Ckd from frozen	82	½ c	67	28	19
Canned, drained	82	½ c	66	46	30
Canned, with liquid	128	½ c	79	62	49
Canned, vacuum pack	210	1 c	166	63	104
Canned, cream style	128	½ c	93	62	57
Cucumber w/peel, ⅛″ slices	28	7 pce	4	107	4
Dandelion greens:					
Fresh	55	1 c	25	256	64
Cooked	105	1 c	35	234	82
Eggplant, cooked	160	1 c	45	51	23
Endive, fresh, chopped	25	½ c	4	888	36
Escarole/curly endive	50	1 c	9	835	71

	Wt (g)	Svg	Cal	Folic Acid (μg) 100 Kcal	Folic Acid (μg) Svg
Vegetables and Legumes *Continued*					
Peas:					
Black-eyed peas:					
Ckd from fresh	165	1 c	160	131	210
Ckd from frozen	170	1 c	224	107	240
Ckd from dry	171	1 c	198	180	356
Canned	240	1 c	184	67	123
Grean peas:					
Fresh, uncooked	145	1 c	118	80	94
Ckd from fresh	160	1 c	134	75	101
Ckd from frozen	80	½ c	63	74	47
Canned, drained	85	½ c	59	64	38
Green peas, edible-pods:					
Fresh, uncooked	145	1 c	61	71	44
Ckd from fresh	160	1 c	67	72	48
Ckd from frozen	80	½ c	42	57	24
Split, ckd fr/dry	196	1 c	231	55	127
Peas and carrots:					
Canned	128	½ c	48	49	24
Ckd from frozen	80	½ c	38	55	21
Peas, sprouted, mature:					
Fresh sprouts	120	1 c	154	112	173
Ckd from fresh	100	3.5 oz	118	31	36
Peppers, Hot, green/red:					
Fresh, chopped, 1 pod ~ 45 g	75	½ c	30	58	18
Canned, hot chili, or Jalapeno	68	½ c	17	206	35
Peppers, Sweet, green/red:					
Fresh, chopped, 1 pod ~ 74 g	50	½ c	14	79	11
Cooked fr/fresh	68	½ c	19	53	10
Potatoes:					
Baked in oven:					
Flesh and skin	202	1 ea	220	10	22
Flesh only	156	1 ea	145	10	14
Potato skin	58	1 ea	115	11	13
Baked in microwave oven:					
Flesh and skin	202	1 ea	212	11	24
Flesh only	156	1 ea	156	12	19
Potato skin	58	1 ea	77	13	10
Boiled, 2.5″ diam, flesh only:					
Cooked without skin	135	1 ea	116	10	12
Boiled in skin, then peeled	136	1 ea	119	11	14
Ckd fr/frozen, small	70	1 ea	46	13	6
French fries, fr/frozen:					
Fried in oil	50	10 pces	158	9	15

Food	Wt (g)	Measure			
Garbanzo beans (chickpeas):					
Ckd from dry	164	1 c	269	105	282
Canned	240	1 c	285	56	160
Jerusalem artichoke, slices	150	1 c	114	13	15
Jicama	100	3.5 oz	20	75	15
Kale:					
Fresh, chopped	67	1 c	33	59	20
Ckd fr/raw or frozen	130	1 c	40	75	30
Kohlrabi:					
Fresh, sliced	140	1 c	38	37	14
Ckd from fresh	165	1 c	48	28	13
Leeks, chopped:					
Fresh	104	1 c	63	105	67
Cooked	52	½ c	24	67	16
Lentils, cooked from dry	198	1 c	231	155	358
Lentils, sprouted:					
Fresh sprouts	77	1 c	81	95	77
Stir-fried	100	3.5 oz	101	83	84
Lettuce:					
Butterhead	56	1 c	7.3	563	41
Iceberg	56	1 c	7.3	431	31
Loose leaf	56	1 c	10	594	60
Romaine	56	1 c	9	848	76
Mushrooms:					
Fresh slices	35	½ c	9	82	7.4
Cooked from fresh	78	½ c	21	68	14
Canned, drained	78	½ c	18	51	10
Mustard greens:					
Fresh, chopped	56	1 c	145	226	33
Cooked from fresh	140	1 c	21	95	20
Cooked from frozen	150	1 c	29	70	20
Okra:					
Pods, ckd fr/fresh	85	8 ea	27	143	39
Slices, ckd fr/frozen	92	½ c	34	394	134
Onions:					
Fresh, chopped	160	1 c	61	49	30
Cooked fr/fresh, chopped	105	½ c	46	35	16
Dehydrated flakes	14	¼ c	45	52	23
Parsley:					
Fresh, chopped	30	½ c	10	549	55
Freeze-dried	1.4	¼ c	4	538	22
Parsnips:					
Fresh slices	133	1 c	100	89	89
Cooked	156	1 c	125	73	91
Oven heated	50	10 pces	111	8	8
Hash browned, fr/frozen	156	1 c	340	8	26
Mashed potatoes:					
Prep. w/milk	210	1 c	162	11	17
Prep. fr/instant	215	1 c	239	6	15
Potato puffs (tater tots)	62	½ c	138	7	10
Canned, 1″ diam.	70	2 ea	42	11	4
Potato chips	28	14 ea	148	9	13
Potatoes au gratin, recipe	245	1 c	322	6	20
Potatoes scalloped, recipe	245	1 c	210	10	21
Potato pancakes	76	1 ea	237	9	22
Pumpkin:					
Ckd fr/fresh, mashed	245	1 c	50	66	33
Canned	123	½ c	42	36	15
Radishes, daikon	44	½ c	8	120	10
Radishes, red	45	10 ea	7	174	12
Radish seeds, sprouted	38	1 c	16	231	36
Rutabaga, cubes:					
Fresh	140	1 c	51	56	29
Cooked	85	½ c	29	46	13
Sauerkraut, canned w/liquid	236	1 c	44	9	4
Seaweed (kelp), fresh	28	1 oz	12	418	51
Shallots, freeze-dried, chopped	3.6	¼ c	13	32	4
Spinach:					
Fresh, chopped	56	1 c	12	886	109
Ckd fr/fresh	180	1 c	41	639	262
Ckd fr/frozen	190	1 c	53	384	204
Canned, drained	214	1 c	50	418	209
Soybeans, ckd from dry	172	1 c	298	31	93
Soybeans, mature, sprouted:					
Fresh sprouts	35	½ c	45	134	60
Steamed	94	½ c	76	101	77
Soybean Products: see tofu this section; miso, and tempeh in Other; roasted soybeans in Nuts and Seeds; soy milk in Dairy; soy flour in Grains.					
Squash, Summer varieties:					
Crookneck, fresh slices	130	1 c	24	124	30
Crookneck, cooked	180	1 c	36	101	36
Scallop, fresh slices	130	1 c	24	163	39
Scallop, cooked	90	½ c	14	133	19
Zucchini, fresh slices	130	1 c	19	152	29
Zucchini, cooked	180	1 c	29	104	30
Squash, Winter, mashed:					
Acorn/Danish, baked	245	1 c	137	33	46
Acorn/Danish, boiled	245	1 c	83	33	28
Butternut, baked	245	1 c	99	48	47
Butternut, cooked fr/frozen	240	1 c	94	31	29

Table continued on following page

APPENDIX 3. Folic Acid Content of Foods (μg per 100 kcal and per Serving) *Continued*

	Wt (g)	Svg	Cal	Folic Acid (μg) 100 Kcal	Folic Acid (μg) Svg
***Vegetables and Legumes** Continued*					
Squash Winter *Continued*					
Hubbard, baked	240	1 c	120	32	39
Hubbard, boiled	236	1 c	70	33	23
Spaghetti, baked or boiled	155	1 c	45	28	12
Succotash:					
Ckd from fresh	192	1 c	222	34	75
Ckd from frozen	170	1 c	158	36	57
Sweet potatoes:					
Baked in skin	114	1 ea	118	22	26
Boiled, peeled	151	1 ea	160	14	22
Candied, recipe	105	1 pce	144	8	12
Canned, mashed	128	½ c	129	16	21
Tofu, raw (soybean product):					
Firm	126	½ c	183	20	37
Regular	124	½ c	94	20	19
Tomatoes:					
Fresh, whole	123	1 ea	26	73	19
Fresh, chopped	180	1 c	38	71	27
Cooked from fresh	240	1 c	65	48	31
Canned, whole	240	1 c	47	75	35
Tomato juice, canned	244	1 c	41.5	117	49
Tomato paste, canned	262	1 c	220	18	40
Tomato purée, canned	250	1 c	102	38	39
Tomato sauce, canned	245	1 c	74	52	39
Turnip, cubes:					
Fresh cubes	130	1 c	35	54	19
Ckd from fresh	78	½ c	14	51	7

	Wt (g)	Svg	Cal	Folic Acid (μg) 100 Kcal	Folic Acid (μg) Svg
***Other** Continued*					
Blue cheese salad dressing	15	1 T	75	11	8
Beverages (see also Dairy and Dairy Products, Fruits and Fruit Juices, and Vegetables and Legumes)					
Beer (1.5 cup = 12 fl oz)	356	1.5 c	146	15	21
Beer, light	354	1.5 c	100	15	15
Bloody mary, 5 fl oz drink	148	1 ea	116	17	20
Lemonade/Limeade fr/frzn	248	1 c	101	6	6
Pineapple grapefruit drink	250	1 c	117	22	26
Pineapple orange drink	250	1 c	125	22	27
Screwdriver, 7 fl oz drink	213	1 ea	174	43	75
Tequila sunrise, 5.5 oz drink	172	1 ea	189	31	58
Tea, brewed	240	1 c	2	500–620	10–12
Butter	227	1 c	1,626	0.4	7
Candy:					
Chocolate covered:					
Almonds	165	1 c	935	14	128
Coconut	28	1 oz	133	4	5
Peanuts	170	1 c	954	18	171
Raisins	187	1 c	733	2	17
Fudge, average, w/nuts	28	1 oz	118	3	4
M & M's plain candies	48	1 pkg	237	2	5
M & M's peanut candies	47	1 pkg	240	2	5
Milk chocolate, w/almonds	28	1 oz	150	3	4
Milk chocolate, w/peanuts	28	1 oz	155	10	16
Reese's peanut butter cup	45	2 ea	240	7	17
Snickers, 2.2 oz	61	1 bar	290	2	6
Catsup	245	1 c	255	15	37
Chili sauce, tomato based	273	1 c	284	7	20
Chocolate:					
Baking unsweetened	28	1 oz	145	12	18

Turnip greens, cooked:					
From fresh	144	1 c	29	590	171
From frozen	82	½ c	24	135	32
Vegetable juice cocktail	242	1 c	46	83	38
Vegetables, Mixed, cooked from frozen:					
Broccoli, carrots, and pasta	95	⅔ c	88	68	60
Broccoli, carrots, and water chestnuts	91	⅔ c	32	266	85
Broccoli, cauliflower, and red pepper	95	⅔ c	25	196	49
Broccoli and water chestnuts	95	½ c	33	346	114
Cantonese stir fry vegetables	95	½ c	53	87	46
Chinese stir fry vegetables	95	½ c	31	32	10
Green beans and spaetzle, Bavarian style	95	½ c	108	26	28
Japanese style vegetables	95	½ c	29	117	34
Mixed vegetables (corn, peas, carrots, greens beans, and limas):					
Canned, drained	163	1 c	77	50	39
Cooked from frozen	182	1 c	107	32	35
Peas, carrots and onions	91	½ c	54	104	56
Peas, cauliflower, and cream sce	95	½ c	118	41	48
Peas and mushrooms	95	½ c	73	111	81
Peas and onions	95	½ c	71	103	73
Peas, onions, and pasta	95	½ c	122	31	38
Peas, onions, and cheese sce	142	½ c	165	41	67
Peas, pasta, corn, and cream sce	95	½ c	132	40	5
Peas, pasta, mushrooms, and cream sauce	95	½ c	129	53	68
Peas, potatoes, and cream sce	76	½ c	140	29	41
Peas, rice, and mushrooms	66	⅔ c	108	27	29
Water chestnuts, cnd, slices	70	½ c	35	21	8
Watercress, fresh	17	½ c	2	1,700	34
Yam, orange: see Sweet potato.					
Yam, white, cooked, cubes	136	1 c	158	14	22
Zucchini: see Squash.					
	Other				
1,000 Island salad dressing	16	1 T	60	10	6
Barbecue sauce	103	1 c	185	16	30

Bittersweet	28	1 oz	141	10	14
Chocolate chips, semisweet	170	1 c	860	3	22
Hot fudge topping	300	1 c	1,020	2	23
Syrup, thin	300	1 c	680	4	24
Cocoa powder	86	1 c	224	15	33
Granola bar	28	1 ea	127	18	23
Honey	339	1 c	1,030	3	32
Hummous or Humous	246	1 c	420	35	146
Margarine, 80% fat	227	1 c	1,626	.2	2.4–3
Mayonnaise	220	1 c	1,577	.4	6
Miso (soybean product)	275	1 c	565	16	91
Molasses, blackstrap	40	2 T	85	7	6
Salsa:					
Picante by Tostitos	85	6 T	40	35	14
Recipe	108	½ c	46	36	28
Soy sauce:					
Regular (wheat and soy)	18	1 T	9	31	2.8
Tamari (soy)	18	1 T	11	30	3.3
From hydrolyzed protein	18	1 T	7	33	2.3
Spices:					
Chili powder	7.5	1 T	24	16	4
Fenugreek seed	11.1	1 T	36	18	6
Garlic cloves	9	3 cloves	13	2	0.3
Garlic powder	8.4	1 T	28	18	5
Onion powder	6.5	1 T	15	60	9
Tempeh (soybean product)	166	1 c	331	26	86
Teriyaki sauce	18	1 T	15	24	4
Tobasco sauce	15	1 T	1.6	12	.2
Yeast:					
Brewer's	8	1 T	25	1252	313
Dry active, regular	30	4 T	80	1425	1,140

APPENDIX 4. Vitamin E as Alpha-Tocopherol (mg)*

Food	Vitamin E (mg)
Chips and Snacks	
Potato chips—*1 oz (28 g)*	1.20
Potato sticks—*1 oz (28 g)*	2.23
Eggs, Chicken	
Whole, fresh/frzn—*1 large (50 g)*	0.88
Yolk, fresh—*yolk of 1 large egg (17 g)*	0.87
Entrees, Box Mix	
Pizza, cheese, from Contadina Pizzeria Kit	
Thick crust—*¼ pizza (128 g)*	0.14
Thin crust—*¼ pizza (104 g)*	0.14
Fats, Oils, and Shortenings	
Animal Fats	
Beef tallow, raw—*1 T (13 g)*	0.30
Pork fat (lard), raw—*1 T (13 g)*	0.20
Vegetable Oils	
Almond oil—*1 T (14 g)*	5.30
Coconut oil—*1 T (14 g)*	0.10
Corn oil—*1 T (14 g)*	1.90
Corn oil, Mazola—*1 T (14 g)*	3.00
Cottonseed oil—*1 T (14 g)*	4.80
Olive oil—*1 T (14 g)*	1.60
Palm oil—*1 T (14 g)*	2.60
Peanut oil—*1 T (14 g)*	1.60
Safflower oil—*1 T (14 g)*	4.60
Sesame oil—*1 T (14 g)*	0.20
Soybean oil—*1 T (14 g)*	1.50
Soybean oil, hydrogenated—*1 T (14 g)*	1.10
Sunflower oil—*1 T (14 g)*	6.10
Veg-oil spray, Mazola No Stick—*2.5 sec spray (0.7 g)*	0.51†
Wheat-germ oil—*1 T (14 g)*	20.30
Fruit and Vegetable Juices	
Apple jce, cnd/bottled—*8 fl oz (248 g)*	0.03
Grapefruit jce, cnd—*8 fl oz (247 g)*	0.10
Orange jce, fresh—*8 fl oz (248 g)*	0.10
Tomato jce—*6 fl oz (182 g)*	0.40
Fruits	
Apple	
Raw, w/skin—*1 med (138 g)*	0.81
Raw, w/o skin—*1 med (128 g)*	0.35
Apricots, cnd, in heavy syrup—*4 halves (90 g)*	0.80
Banana, raw—*1 med (114 g)*	0.31
Blackberries, raw—*½ cup (72 g)*	0.35
Cantaloupe, raw—*1 cup pieces (160 g)*	0.22
Cherries, sour, raw—*½ cup (78 g)*	0.10
Currants, European black, raw—*½ cup (56 g)*	0.56
Currants, red and white, raw—*½ cup (56 g)*	0.06
Gooseberries, raw—*1 cup (150 g)*	0.56
Grapefruit, raw, red and white—*½ med (123 g)*	0.30
Mango, raw—*1 med (207 g)*	2.32
Mixed fruit, frzn, in syrup, Birds Eye—*½ cup (142 g)*	0.06
Orange, navel or valencia, raw—*1 fruit (131 g)*	0.30
Pear, raw—*1 med (166 g)*	0.83
Pineapple, raw—*1 cup pieces (155 g)*	0.16
Raspberries	
Raw—*1 cup (123 g)*	0.37
Frzn, in lite syrup, Birds Eye—*½ cup (142 g)*	0.27
Strawberries	
Raw—*1 cup (149 g)*	0.18
Frzn, in lite syrup, Birds Eye—*½ cup (142 g)*	0.13
Frzn, sweetened or unsweetened—*1 cup (149 g)*	0.31
Grain Products	
Pasta	
Macaroni, enr, ckd—*1 cup (140 g)*	1.03
Spaghetti, enr, ckd—*1 cup (140 g)*	1.03
Nuts, Nut Products, and Seeds	
Almonds	
Dried—*1 oz (24 nuts) (28 g)*	6.72
Oil roasted—*1 oz (22 nuts) (28 g)*	1.55
Toasted—*1 oz (28 g)*	1.41
Whole, Blue Diamond—*1 oz (28 g)*	1.66
Brazilnuts, dried—*1 oz (8 med nuts) (28 g)*	2.13
Cashews, dry roasted—*1 oz (28 g)*	0.16
Coconut, raw—*1 piece (2″ × 2″ × ½″) (45 g)*	0.33
Filberts (hazelnuts), dried—*1 oz (28 g)*	6.70
Peanut butter, creamy/smooth, Skippy—*1 T (16 g)*	3.00
Peanut butter, chunk style/crunchy, Skippy—*1 T (16 g)*	3.00
Peanuts	
Dried—*1 oz (28 g)*	2.56
Dry roasted—1 oz (28 g)	2.18
Oil roasted—*1 oz (28 g)*	2.07
Pecans, dried—*1 oz (31 large nuts) (28 g)*	0.87
Pistachio nuts, dried—*1 oz (47 nuts) (28 g)*	1.46
Sesame seeds, whole, dried—*1 T (9 oz)*	0.20
Walnuts, English/Persian, dried—*1 oz (14 halves) (28 g)*	0.73
Spreads	
Butter—*1 T (15 g)*	0.20
Margarine by brand	
Mazola—*1 T (14 g)*	8.00
Mazola unsalted—*1 T (14 g)*	8.00
Margarine by form and type of oil	
Liquid, soybean and cottonseed—*1 t (5 g)*	0.20
Stick, safflower and soybean—*1 t (5 g)*	0.80
Stick soybean—*1 t (5 g)*	0.10
Stick, soybean and cottonseed—*1 t (5 g)*	0.30
Tub, corn—*1 t (5 g)*	0.50
Tub, safflower—*1 t (5 g)*	0.60
Tub, soybean—*1 t (5 g)*	0.10
Tub, soybean and cottonseed—*1 t (5 g)*	0.30
Margarine, imitation (diet) by brand	
Mazola diet—*1 T (14 g)*	3.00
Parkay, diet soft—*1 T (14 g)*	0.40
Margarine, imitation (diet) by form and type of oil	
Tub, soybean and cottonseed—*1 t (5 g)*	0.40
Mayonnaise	
Best Foods/Hellmann's—*1 T (14 g)*	11.00
Soybean—*1 T (14 g)*	2.90
Miracle whip, Kraft—*1 T (14 g)*	0.50
Miracle whip, light, Kraft—*1 T (14 g)*	0.40
Sandwich spread, Best Foods/Hellmann's—*1 T (15 g)*	5.00
Vegetables	
Asparagus	
Cnd—*½ cup (121 g)*	0.46
Frzn, boiled—*4 spears (60 g)*	0.81
Raw—*4 spears (58 g)*	1.15
Avocado, raw, Calif—*1 med (173 g)*	2.32
Beet greens, raw—*1 cup (38 g)*	0.57
Beets, cnd, harvard—*½ cup slices (123 g)*	0.04
Broccoli, raw—*½ cup chopped (44 g)*	0.20
Brussels sprouts	
Raw—*½ cup chopped (44 g)*	0.39
Boiled—*½ cup (4 sprouts) (78 g)*	0.66
Cabbage, Chinese (bok-choi), raw—*½ cup shredded (35 g)*	0.05
Cabbage, green, raw—*½ cup shredded (35 g)*	0.58
Carrots	
Raw—*1 med (72 g)*	0.32
Boiled—*½ cup slices (78 g)*	0.33
Cauliflower, raw—*½ cup pieces (50 g)*	0.02
Celery, raw—*1 stalk (7.5″ long) (40 g)*	0.14
Corn, sweet, yellow/white, cnd—*½ cup (128 g)*	0.05
Corn, sweet, yellow/white, frzn—*½ cup (82 g)*	0.02

APPENDIX 4. Vitamin E as Alpha-Tocopherol (mg)* *Continued*

Food	mg
Vegetables *Continued*	
Cucumber, raw—*½ cup slices (⅙ cucumber) (52 g)*	0.08
Dandelion greens, raw—*½ cup chopped (28 g)*	0.70
Eggplant, raw—*½ cup pieces (41 g)*	0.01
Garden cress, raw—*½ cup (25 g)*	0.18
Garlic, raw—*3 cloves (9 g)*	0.001
Green beans (snap beans)	
Raw—*½ cup (55 g)*	0.01
Cnd—*½ cup (68 g)*	0.03
Frzn—*½ cup (62 g)*	0.06
Frzn, boiled—*½ cup (68 g)*	0.09
Leeks, raw—*¼ cup chopped (26 g)*	0.24
Lettuce, iceberg, raw—*¼ head (135 g)*	0.54
Mushrooms, raw—*½ cup pieces (35 g)*	0.03
Mustard greens, raw—*½ cup chopped (28 g)*	0.56
Onion rings, frzn, heated—*7 rings (70 g)*	0.48
Onions, raw—*½ cup chopped (80 g)*	0.25
Parsley, raw—*½ cup chopped (30 g)*	0.52
Parsnips, raw—*½ cup (67 g)*	0.67
Peas, green	
Raw—*½ cup (78 g)*	0.10
Frzn—*½ cup (72 g)*	0.09
Frzn, boiled—*½ cup (80 g)*	0.10
Vegetables *Continued*	
Peppers, sweet, raw—*½ cup chopped (50 g)*	0.34
Potato	
Raw w/o skin—*1 potato (112 g)*	0.07
Baked w/o skin—*1 potato (156 g)*	0.05
Boiled w/o skin—*1 potato (135 g)*	0.05
French fried, frzn, heated—*10 pieces (50 g)*	0.10
Pumpkin, raw—*½ cup (58 g)*	0.58
Rutabaga, boiled—*½ cup cubes (85 g)*	0.13
Seaweed, kelp (kombu/tangle), raw—*3.5 oz (100 g)*	0.87
Spinach	
Raw—*½ cup chopped (28 g)*	0.53
Cnd—*½ cup (107 g)*	0.02
Squash, winter, all varieties, baked—*½ cup cubes (102 g)*	0.12
Sweet potato, raw—*1 med (130 g)*	5.93
Tomato, red, raw—*1 tomato (123 g)*	0.42
Turnip greens, raw—*½ cup chopped (28 g)*	0.63
Watercress, raw—*½ cup chopped (17 g)*	0.17

* From Pennington JAT: Bowes and Church's Food Values of Portions Commonly Used, 15th ed. Philadelphia, JB Lippincott, 1989, pp 284–285.
† Specified as tocopherols.

APPENDIX 5. Zinc Content of Foods—mg per 100 kcal and Per Serving*

	Wt (g)	Svg	Cal	Zinc (mg) 100 Cal	Zinc (mg) Svg
Baked Goods					
Breads, Cakes, Cookies, Crackers, Muffins, Pancakes, Pastries, Pies, Rolls					
Apple crisp	78	1 pce	146	.1	.088
Bagel, 3.5″ dm, plain/egg	68	1 ea	180	.3	.612
Biscuits:					
Homemade	28	1 ea	100	.2	.153
From mix	28	1 ea	94	.2	.179
From refrig dough	20	1 ea	65	.1	.094
Breads:					
Boston brown, canned	45	1 pce	95	.4	.350
Cornbread muffin, avg	45	1 ea	145	.2	.325
Cracked wheat	25	1 pce	65	.5	.350
French, 5″ × 2.5″ × 1″	35	1 pce	100	.2	.221
Mixed grain bread	25	1 pce	65	.5	.300
Oatmeal bread	25	1 pce	65	.4	.245
Pita pocket, 6.5″ dm.	60	1 ea	165	.3	.501
Pumpernickel, 5″ × 4″ × 3/8″	32	1 pce	80	.5	.400
Raisin bread	25	1 pce	68	.2	.155
Rye, light 5″ × 3.5″ × 7/16″	25	1 pce	65	.6	.380
Wheat (white and whole wheat flour)	28	1 pce	72	.4	.294
White bread	28	1 pce	75	.2	.173
Whole wheat bread	28	1 pce	70	.7	.500
Bread pudding w/raisins	165	1 c	349	.2	.863
Breadsticks, 4″ × 1/2″ dm.	100	10 ea	384	.1	.570
Brownies w/frosting and nuts	25	1 ea	100	.4	.36
Cakes: pce = 1/16th cake (3″ × 3″) unless otherwise stated. Cupcakes ≈ 42 grams.					
Angel food, 1/12 tube cake	53	1 pce	125	.1	.070
Boston cream pie, 1/8	120	1 pce	260	.1	.230
Carrot, cream cheese frosting	112	1 pce	406	.1	.45
Cheesecake:					
From recipe, 1/12 cake	92	1 pce	278	.1	.386
From mix, 1/8	103	1 pce	300	.1	.427
Chocolate, chocolate frosting	69	1 pce	235	.2	.530
Coffeecake, f/mix, 2.4″ × 2.8″	72	1 pce	230	.3	.619
Fruitcake, dark, 2/3″ arc	43	1 pce	165	.1	.215
Gingerbread, 1/9 of 8″ sq.	63	1 pce	174	.35	.610
Pound cake, commercial	29	1 pce	110	.1	.11
Sheet cake, 3″ × 3″:					
Plain cake	86	1 pce	315	.1	.306
White frosting	121	1 pce	445	.1	.322
Snack cake, cream filled:					
Chocolate, like Ding-dongs	28	1 ea	105	.2	.172
Sponge cake, like Twinkies	42	1 ea	155	.1	.210
Sponge cake, 1/12	66	1 pce	194	.2	.475
White, chocolate frosting	77	1 pce	291	.1	.323
White, coconut/white frosting	70	1 pce	270	.1	.212
Yellow, chocolate frosting, avg	69	1 pce	240	.1	.206
Cherry crisp, 3″ × 3″	138	1 pce	157	.1	.145
Chips: see Corn and Tortilla in this section; see vegetable section for Potato chips.					
Baked Goods Continued					
Cookies:					
Chocolate chip:					
Recipe	40	4 ea	185	.1	.220
Refrig dough	48	4 ea	225	.1	.240
Commercial	42	4 ea	180	.2	.304
Fig bars	56	4 ea	210	.2	.358
Lady fingers	44	4 ea	158	.4	.576
Oatmeal raisin	52	4 ea	245	.2	.530
Peanut butter, homemade	48	4 ea	245	.1	.360
Sandwich type, all	40	4 ea	195	.1	.214
Sugar, from refrigerator dough	48	4 ea	235	.1	.240
Corn chips (Fritos)	28	1 oz	155	.3	.440
Crackers:					
Armenian cracker bread	28	4 pce	117	.8	.900
Rye wafers, whole grain	14	2 ea	55	2.9	1.60
Sesame	12	4 ea	60	.2	.125
Wheat crackers, thin	8	4 ea	35	.7	.240
Whole wheat	8	2 ea	35	.7	.233
Cream puff, custard filled	110	1 ea	280	.2	.624
Croissant, 4.5″ × 4″ × 2″	57	1 ea	235	.1	.322
Danish pastry:					
Plain pastry	57	1 ea	220	.2	.479
With fruit	65	1 ea	235	.2	.546
Eclair, custard filled, choc icing	94	1 ea	262	.2	.546
English muffin, plain/sourdough	57	1 ea	135	.3	.410
Muffins:					
Blueberry:					
Recipe	45	1 ea	135	.2	.290
From mix	45	1 ea	140	.2	.210
Bran, wheat:					
Recipe	45	1 ea	125	.3	.370
From mix	45	1 ea	140	.7	.950
Cornmeal:					
Recipe	45	1 ea	145	.2	.310
From mix	45	1 ea	145	.2	.340
Pancakes:					
Plain, 4″ recipe/mix	27	1 ea	60	.4	.226
Buckwheat, 4″ dm, mix	27	1 ea	55	.9	.500
Whole-wheat, 5″ dm.	52	1 ea	94	.6	.519
Pies: piece is 1/6 of 9″ pie unless otherwise stated.					
Apple pie	158	1 pce	405	.1	.267
Banana cream, commercial	152	1 pce	333	.3	.873
Chocolate cream	175	1 pce	311	.2	.743
Coconut cream	172	1 pce	343	.2	.823
Coconut custard	165	1 pce	384	.3	1.21
Cream, commercial	152	1 pce	455	.2	.785
Custard pie	152	1 pce	293	.3	.792
Lemon meringue	140	1 pce	355	.1	.510
Peach pie	158	1 pce	405	.1	.352
Pecan pie	138	1 pce	583	.3	1.47
Pumpkin pie	200	1 pce	367	.3	.993
Poptart-type toaster pastry	54	1 ea	210	.1	.313
Pretzel, dutch twist	16	1 ea	65	.3	.173
Pretzel, thin twists	60	10 ea	240	.2	.419
Rolls:					
Cinnamon bun, small	50	1 ea	158	.3	.452
Dinner roll, 2.5″ × 2″	28	1 ea	85	.3	.223

APPENDIX 5. Zinc Content of Foods—mg per 100 kcal and Per Serving* *Continued*

	Wt (g)	Svg	Cal	Zinc (mg) 100 Cal	Zinc (mg) Svg
Baked Goods *Continued*					
Rolls *Continued:*					
Hamburger bun	45	1 ea	129	.3	.408
Hard roll, white	50	1 ea	155	.3	.438
Hotdog bun	40	1 ea	115	.3	.363
Rye roll, light	28	1 ea	76	.6	.426
Rye roll, dark	28	1 ea	79	.3	.274
Submarine roll (hoagie)	135	1 ea	400	.3	1.17
Whole wheat roll	35	1 ea	88	.7	.580
Tortillas:					
Corn, 6″ diam, fried	30	1 ea	87	.3	.300
Flour, 10.5″ diam.	57	1 ea	168	.3	.432
Flour, 8″ diam.	35	1 ea	105	.3	.269
Tortilla chips, all kinds	28	1 oz	139	.3	.420
Waffles:					
Homemade, 7″ dm.	75	1 ea	245	.3	.652
Prep f/mix, 7″ dm.	75	1 ea	205	.3	.515
Frozen, 4″ dm.	35	1 ea	98	.3	.288
Dairy and Dairy Products					
Cheese [1.5″ cube ≈ 1 oz]:					
American processed cheese	28	1 oz	106	.9	.933
American cheese food	28	1 oz	94	.9	.850
American cheese spread	28	1 oz	82	1.0	.780
Blue cheese	28	1 oz	100	.8	.750
Brick cheese	28	1 oz	105	.7	.734
Brie cheese	28	1 oz	95	.7	.700
Camembert	28	1 oz	85	.8	.675
Caraway	28	1 oz	107	.8	.882
Cheddar cheese	28	1 oz	114	.8	.924
Cheshire	28	1 oz	110	.7	.800
Colby	28	1 oz	112	.8	.870
Cottage cheese:					
Low-fat 1%	226	1 c	164	.5	.860
Low-fat 2%	226	1 c	205	.5	.950
Creamed, lrg curd	225	1 c	235	.3	.800
Creamed, sm curd	210	1 c	215	.4	.802
Cream cheese	28	1 oz	99	.3	.325
Edam cheese	28	1 oz	101	1.0	1.06
Feta cheese	28	1 oz	75	1.1	.813
Fontina	28	1 oz	110	.9	.990
Gjetost	28	1 oz	132	.7	.946
Gouda	28	1 oz	101	1.1	1.10
Gruyere	28	1 oz	117	.9	1.00
Liederkranz	28	1 oz	87	.8	.700
Limburger	28	1 oz	93	.6	.600
Monterey jack	28	1 oz	106	.8	.846
Mozzarella, low moisture:					
Part skim	28	1 oz	80	1.0	.825
Whole milk	28	1 oz	90	1.0	.895
Muenster	28	1 oz	104	.8	.843
Parmesan, grated (1 T = 5g)	28	1 oz	129	.8	1.00
Pimento, processed	28	1 oz	106	.8	.840
Port du salut	28	1 oz	100	.8	.800
Provolone	28	1 oz	100	.9	.889
Ricotta, part skim	246	1 c	340	1.0	3.29
Ricotta, whole milk	246	1 c	428	.7	2.85
Romano, grated (1 T = 5g)	28	1 oz	128	.9	1.20
Roquefort	28	1 oz	105	.5	.570
Swiss cheese	28	1 oz	107	1.0	1.10
Cream, Sweet, Fluid:					
Coffee or table	240	1 c	469	.1	.649
Dairy and Dairy Products *Continued*					
Cream, Sweet, Fluid *Continued:*					
Half and half	242	1 c	315	.4	1.23
Light whipping cream	239	1 c	699	.1	.600
Heavy whipping cream	238	1 c	821	.1	.550
Cream, Sweet, Whipped:					
Heavy cream, unsweetened	119	1 c	410	.1	.275
Pressurized	60	1 c	154	.1	.220
Cream, Sour, cultured, dairy	230	1 c	493	.1	.690
Cream, sour, imitation (nondairy)	230	1 c	479	0	0
Cream Substitutes, nondairy:					
Coffee whitener, powder	94	1 c	514	.1	.480
Coffee whitener, liquid	120	½ c	163	<.1	.020
Dessert Toppings, nondairy, Frozen (like Coolwhip)	75	1 c	239	<.1	.029
Kefir beverage	233	1 c	160	.6	.900
Milk (cow):					
Skim milk	245	1 c	86	1.1	.915
Low-fat 1%	244	1 c	102	.9	.963
Low-fat 2%	244	1 c	121	.8	.963
Whole (3.3% fat)	244	1 c	150	.6	.930
Buttermilk	245	1 c	99	1.0	1.03
Canned, evap, skim	255	1 c	200	1.1	2.18
Canned, evap, whole	252	1 c	340	.6	1.94
Dry, nonfat instant	68	1 c	244	1.3	3.06
Milk (other):					
Goat milk	244	1 c	168	.4	.730
Human breast milk	246	1 c	171	.2	.420
Soy milk	240	1 c	79	.7	.540
Milk Beverages and Mixes:					
Chocolate milk, commercial:					
Low-fat 1%	250	1 c	160	.6	1.02
Low-fat 2%	250	1 c	180	.5	.910
Whole (3.3%)	250	1 c	210	.5	1.02
Chocolate-flavored mix, to be mixed with water:					
Powder (includes dry milk)	28	1 oz	100	1.3	1.26
Drink, prepared	206	¾ c	100	1.3	1.26
Chocolate-flavored mix, to be mixed with milk:					
Powder	21.6	¾ oz	75	.4	.330
Drink, prep w/wh milk	266	1 c	226	.6	1.26
Eggnog, commercial	254	1 c	342	.3	1.17
Instant Breakfast, dry	37	1 env	130	2.3	3.00
Malted milk, prep w/ whole milk:					
Chocolate flavor	265	1 c	229	.5	1.09
Natural flavor	265	1 c	237	.5	1.14
Milkshake (10 fl oz = 1.25 c):					
Chocolate	283	1.25 c	360	.3	1.15
Strawberry	283	1.25 c	319	.3	1.00
Vanilla	283	1.25 c	314	.3	1.01

Table continued on following page

APPENDIX 5. Zinc Content of Foods—mg per 100 kcal and Per Serving* *Continued*

	Wt (g)	Svg	Cal	Zinc (mg) 100 Cal	Zinc (mg) Svg
***Dairy and Dairy Products** Continued*					
Milk Desserts:					
Custard, baked:					
Recipe	265	1 c	305	.5	1.53
Prep from mix	143	½ c	161	.4	.645
Ice cream, vanilla:					
Regular	133	1 c	269	.5	1.41
Soft serve	173	1 c	377	.5	1.99
Rich	148	1 c	349	.3	1.21
Ice milk, vanilla:					
Regular	131	1 c	184	.3	.550
Soft serve, 3% fat	175	1 c	223	.4	.860
Puddings, prepared (5-oz can ≈ 55 c)					
Chocolate:					
From mix-ckd or instant	260	1 c	305	.4	1.18
Canned	142	1 can	205	.3	.700
Coconut, f/instant	149	½ c	184	.3	.474
Lemon, f/instant	149	½ c	178	.3	.480
Rice, ckd/instant mix	141	½ c	165	.4	.577
Tapioca pudding, ckd f/mix	130	½ c	145	.3	.500
Tapioca, canned	142	1 can	160	.4	.700
Vanilla, ckd/instant mix	130	½ c	148	.3	.500
Vanilla, canned	142	1 can	220	.3	.700
Pudding Pops:					
Banana/butterscotch/van	57	1 ea	94	.3	.245
Chocolate/choc fudge	57	1 ea	99	.4	.355
Sherbet	193	1 c	270	.5	1.33
Yogurt, frozen, avg	174	1 c	220	.5	1.12
Yogurt:					
Low-fat, plain	227	1 c	144	1.4	2.02
Low-fat, with fruit	227	1 c	231	.7	1.68
Low-fat, coffee or vanilla	227	1 c	193	1.0	1.88
Nonfat	227	1 c	127	1.7	2.20
Whole	227	1 c	138	1.0	1.34
Yogurt cheese, recipe	208	1 c	222	1.7	3.72
Eggs					
Egg, chicken, raw/cooked:					
Whole egg	50	1 ea	77.5	.7	.55
White only	33.4	1 ea	17	0	0
Yolk only	16.6	1 ea	59	.9	.54
Egg substitutes (check label, products vary):					
Frozen	60	¼ c	96	.6	.590
Liquid	251	1 c	211	1.5	3.26
Fruit and Fruit Juices					
Apple, w/peel, 2.75″ dm.	138	1 ea	80	.1	.050
Apricots:					
Fresh, pitted	106	3 ea	51	.5	.280
Canned, juice pack	248	1 c	119	.2	.270
Canned, heavy syrup	258	1 c	214	.1	.270
Dried apricots	35	10 ea	83	.3	.260
Apricot nectar, canned	251	1 c	141	.2	.230
Avocado, whole:					
California	173	1 ea	305	.2	.730
Florida	304	1 ea	340	.4	1.28
Banana, 8.75″, 176 g w/peel	114	1 ea	105	.2	.190
Blackberries:					
Fresh berries	144	1 c	74	.5	.390
Frozen, unthawed	151	1 c	97	.4	.370
Canned	256	1 c	236	.2	.470
***Fruit and Fruit Juices** Continued*					
Blueberries:					
Fresh	145	1 c	82	.2	.160
Canned	256	1 c	225	.1	.170
Boysenberries:					
Frozen	132	1 c	66	.4	.290
Canned	256	1 c	225	.2	.480
Cantaloupe: see Melon.					
Cassava, fresh	100	3.5 oz	120	.8	.980
Cherries, sour:					
Frozen	155	1 c	72	.2	.160
Canned	244	1 c	90	.2	170
Cherries, Sweet:					
Fresh, pitted	68	10 ea	49	.1	.040
Canned w/liquid	257	1 c	213	.1	.260
Cranberries, fresh, whole	95	1 c	46	.3	.120
Cranberry juice cocktail	253	1 c	145	.1	.177
Currants:					
Black, fresh	112	1 c	71	.4	.300
Red or white, fresh	112	1 c	63	.4	.260
Zante, dried	144	1 c	407	.2	.940
Dates, whole, pitted	83	10 ea	228	.1	.242
Figs, fresh, medium	50	1 ea	37	.2	.070
Figs, dried	187	10 ea	477	.2	.940
Fruit cocktail, canned:					
Juice pack	248	1 c	115	.2	.210
Heavy syrup	255	1 c	185	.1	.210
Gooseberries:					
Fresh berries	150	1 c	67	.3	.180
Canned with liquid	252	1 c	185	.2	.280
Grapefruit (half = 241g w/refuse):					
Pink or red half	123	1 ea	37	.2	.090
White half	118	1 ea	39	.2	.080
Canned sections	254	1 c	152	.1	.21
Grapefruit juice, canned	247	1 c	93	.2	.220
Guava, fresh	90	1 ea	45	.5	.210
Lemon juice, bottled	244	1 c	52	.3	.150
Lime juice, bottled	246	1 c	50	.3	.150
Loganberries, frozen	147	1 c	80	.6	.500
Lychees, canned	100	3.5 oz	68	.3	.200
Mandarin oranges, canned	252	1 c	155	<.1	.075
Mango, fresh slices	165	1 c	108	.2	.260
Melon, also see Watermelon:					
Cantaloupe cubes	160	1 c	57	.4	.256
Frozen melon balls, mixed	173	1 c	55	.5	.290
Mixed fruit, dried	293	11 oz	712	.2	1.47
Orange, avg (180 g w/refuse)	131	1 ea	60	.1	.090
Orange juice:					
Fresh juice	248	1 c	111	.1	.124
Prep from frozen	249	1 c	110	.1	.128
Frozen conc, 6 oz can	213	¾ c	339	.1	.383
Canned, unsweetened	249	1 c	105	.2	.174
Orange grapefruit juice, cnd	247	1 c	105	.2	.180
Papaya (454 g w/refuse)	304	1 ea	117	.2	.220
Papaya nectar, canned	250	1 c	142	.3	.380
Peaches:					
Fresh, 2.5″ diam	87	1 ea	37	.3	.120
Canned, juice pack	77	1 half	34	.3	.085
Canned, heavy syrup	81	1 half	60	.1	.070
Peach nectar, canned	249	1 c	134	.1	.200

APPENDIX 5. Zinc Content of Foods—mg per 100 kcal and Per Serving* *Continued*

	Wt (g)	Svg	Cal	Zinc (mg) 100 Cal	Zinc (mg) Svg
Fruit and Fruit Juices *Continued*					
Pears:					
Fresh, Bartlett (180 g w/refuse)	166	1 ea	98	.2	.200
Canned, juice pack	77	1 half	38	.2	.069
Canned, heavy syrup	79	1 half	59	.1	.063
Pear nectar, canned	250	1 c	149	.1	.160
Persimmon, (Japanese)	168	1 ea	118	.2	.180
Pineapple:					
Fresh, chunks	155	1 c	76	.2	.120
Canned pieces (1 ring = 58 g):					
Juice pack	250	1 c	150	.2	.250
Heavy syrup	255	1 c	199	.2	.306
Pineapple juice	250	1 c	135	.2	.283
Plantain, fresh slices	148	1 c	181	.1	.270
Plantain, cooked slices	154	1 c	179	.1	.210
Plums:					
Fresh, med, 2-⅛″ dm.	66	1 ea	36	.2	.06
Canned, juice pack	95	3 ea	55	.2	.11
Canned, heavy syrup	110	3 ea	98	.1	.08
Prunes, dried, pitted	84	10 ea	201	.2	.445
Prune juice, bottled	256	1 c	181	.3	.538
Raisins, dark, unpacked	145	1 c	435	.1	.464
Raspberries:					
Fresh berries	123	1 c	60	.9	.566
Frozen, thawed	250	1 c	255	.2	.450
Rhubarb:					
Fresh, diced	122	1 c	26	.5	.130
Cooked with sugar	240	1 c	279	.1	.192
Strawberries:					
Fresh berries	149	1 c	45	.4	.194
Frozen, unsweetened	149	1 c	52	.4	.190
Frozen, thawed, swtnd	255	1 c	245	.1	.153
Tangerine	84	1 ea	37	1.0	.380
Watermelon cubes	160	1 c	50	.2	.112
Grains and Grain Products					
Cereals, Flour, Grains, Noodles, Pasta, and Popcorn					
Amaranth grain, dry	195	1 c	729	.85	6.20
Barley, cooked:					
Whole	200	1 c	200	.6	1.16
Pearled	157	1 c	193	.7	1.29
Bran: see Oat, Rice, Wheat.					
Buckwheat flour, light	98	1 c	340	.8	2.56
Buckwheat flour, dark	98	1 c	338	.8	2.65
Bulgar wheat, cooked	182	1 c	151	.7	1.04
Cereals, Cold (Ready to eat) Cereals are often fortified with zinc. Check the label.					
Cereals, Hot (cooked):					
Corn grits, cooked, enriched	242	1 c	145	.1	.169
Cream of Rice	244	1 c	126	.3	.390
Cream of Wheat, cooked	244	1 c	140	.2	.347
Farina	233	1 c	116	.1	.163
Malt-O-Meal	240	1 c	122	.1	.168
Maypo cereal	180	¾ c	128	.9	1.12
Oatmeal, from rolled oats (regular, quick, instant)	234	1 c	145	.8	1.15
Grains and Grain Products *Continued*					
Cereals, Hot *Continued:*					
Oatmeal, fortified, instant, prepared from packet:					
Plain	177	¾ c	104	1.0	1.00
With bran and raisin	195	¾ c	158	.9	1.35
Other flavors, avg	164	¾ c	160	.6	1.00
Ralston cereal	253	1 c	134	1.1	1.42
Roman Meal	181	¾ c	111	1.2	1.34
Wheatena	243	1 c	135	1.2	1.68
Whole wheat	242	1 c	150	.8	1.16
Corn flour	117	1 c	422	.5	2.02
Corn flour, Masa Harina, enr	114	1 c	416	.5	2.03
Cornmeal:					
Degermed, dry	138	1 c	505	.2	.994
Bolted, nearly whole	122	1 c	441	.5	2.22
Flour: see specific grain, nut, or vegetable.					
Macaroni, cooked:					
Enriched	140	1 c	197	.4	.742
Vegetable, enriched	134	1 c	172	.3	.59
Whole wheat	140	1 c	174	.6	1.13
Millet, cooked	120	½ c	143	.8	1.10
Noodles, cooked:					
Egg noodles, enriched	160	1 c	213	.5	.992
Spinach noodles	140	1 c	182	.8	1.51
Oat bran, 1 T ≈ 6 g	94	1 c	132	2.2	2.92
Oats, rolled, dry, uncooked	81	1 c	311	.8	2.49
Pasta: see Macaroni, Noodles, Spaghetti.					
Popcorn, ckd in oil, salted	11	1 c	55	.5	.285
Rice, cooked:					
Brown rice	195	1 c	217	.6	1.23
White, regular	205	1 c	264	.4	.943
White, converted	175	1 c	200	.3	.542
White, instant	165	1 c	162	.2	.396
Wild rice	164	1 c	166	1.3	2.20
Rye flour:					
Dark	128	1 c	415	1.7	7.19
Light	102	1 c	361	.5	1.79
Soy flour, stirred					
Low fat	44	½ c	163	.32	.52
Defatted	50	½ c	164	.75	1.23
Full fat, raw	42	½ c	182	.92	1.67
Spaghetti noodles, ckd:					
Enriched	140	1 c	197	.4	.742
Whole-wheat spaghetti	140	1 c	174	.7	1.14
Wheat:					
Wheat bran	30	½ c	65	3.4	2.18
Wheat flours:					
All purpose, white, unsifted	125	1 c	455	.2	.875
Cake flour, sifted	96	1 c	348	.2	.595
Self-rising	125	1 c	442	.2	.775
Semolina	167	1 c	601	.3	.175
Whole wheat	120	1 c	407	.9	3.52
Wheat germ:					
Raw	100	1 c	360	3.4	12.3
Toasted	113	1 c	432	4.4	18.9
Wheat, rolled, cooked	240	1 c	142	.9	1.22
Wheat, rolled, dry	85	1 c	289	.9	2.5

Table continued on following page

APPENDIX 5. Zinc Content of Foods—mg per 100 kcal and Per Serving* *Continued*

	Wt (g)	Svg	Cal	Zinc (mg) 100 Cal	Zinc (mg) Svg
***Grains and Grain Products** Continued*					
Wheat *Continued:*					
Whole-grain (wheat-berries) cooked	50	⅓ c	28	.9	.244
Whole-wheat, sprouted	108	1 c	214	.8	1.78
Meats: Fish and Shellfish					
Abalone, fried	85	3 oz	161	.5	.800
Anchovies cnd in oil, drained	45	11 ea	95	1.2	1.10
Bass, freshwater, baked/broiled	100	3.5 oz	125	.6	.700
Bluefish:					
Baked/broiled	100	3.5 oz	159	.7	1.04
Fried in crumbs	100	3.5 oz	205	.4	.900
Carp, baked/broiled	100	3.5 oz	162	1.2	1.90
Catfish, cornmeal fried	100	3.5 oz	229	.5	1.20
Clams, meat only:					
Canned, drained	160	1 c	236	1.9	4.37
Minced w/liquid, small can	183	1 can	145	.4	.561
Breaded, fried, small	188	20 ea	379	.7	2.74
Steamed meat	90	20 ea	133	1.8	2.46
Clam nectar, canned	240	1 c	6	4.0	.240
Cod, Atlantic:					
Broiled/baked/poached	100	3.5 oz	105	.6	.580
Batter fried	100	3.5 oz	199	.3	.500
Smoked	100	3.5 oz	79	.5	.380
Crab meat, cooked:					
Alaska King crab leg	134	1 ea	129	7.9	10.2
Blue crab, unpacked measure					
Cooked	135	1 c	138	4.1	5.70
Canned	135	1 c	133	4.1	5.42
Dungeness meat, ckd	101	¾ c	85	5.1	4.33
Crab, imitation fr/surimi	85	3 oz	87	.3	.250
Crab cakes fr/recipe	60	1 ea	93	2.6	2.46
Crayfish, ckd, moist heat	85	3 oz	97	1.5	1.42
Eel, baked/broiled	100	3.5 oz	236	.9	2.08
Eel, smoked	100	3.5 oz	330	.2	.70
Fish cakes, fried:					
Homemade	100	3.5 oz	172	.3	.480
From frozen	100	3.5 oz	213	.2	.400
Fish sticks, frzn, heated	57	2 ea	155	.2	.380
Haddock:					
Baked/broiled/poached	85	3 oz	95	.4	.410
Breaded, fried	85	3 oz	175	.5	.850
Smoked	100	3.5 oz	116	.4	.500
Halibut, baked/broiled	85	3.5 oz	119	.4	.450
Herring:					
Baked/broiled	100	3.5 oz	203	.6	1.27
Canned w/liquid	100	3.5 oz	208	.8	1.72
Canned w/tomato sce	100	3.5 oz	173	.9	1.60
Smoked, kippered	100	3.5 oz	217	.6	1.36
Pickled, 1 pce = 15 g	100	3.5 oz	262	.2	.53
Lobster meat, cooked	145	1 c	142	3.0	4.23
Mackerel:					
Baked/broiled, Atlantic	100	3.5 oz	262	.4	.94
Canned, Jack, 1 tall can	361	1 can	563	.7	3.68
Mullet, baked/broiled	85	3 oz	127	.6	.750
Ocean perch:					
Baked/broiled	100	3.5 oz	121	.5	.610
Breaded, fried	85	3 oz	185	.2	.410
***Meats: Fish and Shellfish** Continued*					
Octopus, raw	100	3.5 oz	82	2.0	1.68
Oyster:					
Raw, Eastern	248	1 c	170	133	226
Raw, Pacific	248	1 c	200	21	41.2
Simmered, Eastern	100	3.5 oz	137	133	182
Breaded, fried, med, Eastern	88	6 ea	173	44	76.7
Perch, baked/broiled	92	2 ea	108	1.2	1.32
Pike, baked/broiled, Northern	100	3.5 oz	113	.8	.860
Pollock:					
Baked/broiled, mixed	100	3.5 oz	99	.5	.536
Baked/broiled, Walleye	100	3.5 oz	113	.5	.600
Rockrish, baked/broiled	100	3.5 oz	121	.4	.530
Salmon:					
Average, baked/brld	85	3 oz	183	.2	.430
Chinook, smoked	85	3 oz	99	.3	.260
Coho, steamed/poached	100	3.5 oz	185	.3	.520
Sockeye, baked/brld	100	3.5 oz	216	.2	.510
Canned, Atlantic, small can	220	1 can	281	.6	1.58
Canned, Pink, No. 1 can	454	1 can	631	.7	4.19
Canned, Sockeye, No. 1 can	369	1 can	566	.7	3.75
Sardines, cnd, drained:					
Atlantic, 2 ≈ 24 g	92	1 can	192	.6	1.21
Pacific, 1 ≈ 38 g	100	3.5 oz	178	.8	1.40
Scallops:					
Breaded, fried	93	6 ea	200	.5	.986
Steamed	100	3.5 oz	113	1.0	1.16
Sea Bass, baked/brld	100	3.5 oz	124	.4	.520
Seatrout/Steelhead, ckd	100	3.5 oz	131	.4	.520
Shad:					
Baked w/bacon	100	3.5 oz	201	.1	.295
Batter-fried	85	3 oz	194	.2	.410
Shrimp:					
Boiled, 2 large ≈ 11 g	100	3.5 oz	99	1.6	1.56
Breaded, fried (2 large ≈ 15 g)	90	12 ea	218	.6	1.24
Canned, drained	128	1 c	154	1.0	1.61
Canned w/liquid	100	3.5 oz	102	2.3	2.30
Smelt, Rainbow, ckd	85	3 oz	106	1.7	1.80
Snapper, baked/brld	100	3.5 oz	128	.3	.440
Sole (Flounder):					
Baked/broiled	85	3 oz	99	.5	.530
Breaded, fried	100	3.5 oz	188	.2	.453
Batter-fried	85	3 oz	250	.2	.450
Squid, flour-fried	85	3 oz	149	1.0	1.50
Sturgeon:					
Cooked	85	3 oz	115	.4	.460
Smoked	85	3 oz	147	.4	.658
Surimi, processed walleye (Alaska) pollock; see imitation crab.					
Swordfish, baked/brld	100	3.5 oz	155	.9	1.47
Trout, baked/brld	85	3 oz	129	.9	1.18
Tuna:					
Light, canned, drained (No. ½ can):					
Canned in oil	171	1 can	339	.5	1.54
Water pack	165	1 can	216	.6	1.30
Bluefin, ckd f/fresh	85	3 oz	157	.4	.650

APPENDIX 5. Zinc Content of Foods—mg per 100 kcal and Per Serving* *Continued*

	Wt (g)	Svg	Cal	Zinc (mg) 100 Cal	Zinc (mg) Svg
Meats					
Beef, Ham, Pork, Frog legs, Rabbit, Venison, and Veal					
Beef:					
Breakfast strips (cured beef), cooked	34	3 pce	153	1.4	2.17
Chuck blade, pot roasted, all grades:					
Lean and fat (5.4 oz raw)	85	3 oz	325	2.0	6.66
Lean only	85	3 oz	230	3.8	8.73
Ground beef, average baked, broiled, fried:					
Extra lean (17% fat, raw)	85	3 oz	215	2.1	4.59
Lean (20.7% fat, raw)	85	3 oz	231	1.9	4.44
Regular (26.6% fat, raw)	85	3 oz	250	1.7	4.29
Frzn patty, brld (23% fat raw)	85	3 oz	240	1.9	4.59
Rib, choice, roasted:					
Lean and fat (5 oz raw)	85	3 oz	324	1.4	4.40
Lean only	85	3 oz	204	2.9	5.90
Round steak, choice, brld:					
Lean and fat (4.5 oz raw)	85	3 oz	233	1.5	3.51
Lean only	85	3 oz	165	2.4	3.97
Round tip, all grades, rstd:					
Lean and fat	85	3 oz	213	2.5	5.41
Lean only	85	3 oz	162	3.7	6.01
Sirloin steak, all grades, broiled (11.3 oz raw = 8.2 oz ckd, lean and fat; 6.9 oz lean. Cooked values follow):					
Lean and fat	85	3 oz	238	1.6	3.91
Lean only	85	3 oz	172	2.6	4.44
T-bone steak, choice, broiled (16 oz raw = 9.7 oz ckd, lean and fat; 7.4 oz lean. Cooked values follow):					
Lean and fat	85	3 oz	276	1.4	3.79
Lean only	85	3 oz	182	2.5	4.59
Variety meats:					
Corned beef, canned	85	3 oz	213	1.4	3.03
Dried beef, cured (6–7 pces)	28	1 oz	47	3.2	1.49
Heart, simmered	85	3 oz	140	1.9	2.66
Liver, fried	85	3 oz	184	2.5	4.63
Tongue, cooked	85	3 oz	241	1.7	4.08
Ham: see Pork, cured; Turkey ham; and Lunchmeat section.					
Lamb:					
Arm chop, braised (5.6 oz w/bone, raw):					
Lean and fat	70	1 chop	244	1.8	4.28
Lean only	55	1 chop	152	2.6	3.98
Loin chop, broiled (4.2 oz w/bone, raw):					
Lean and fat	64	1 chop	201	1.1	2.22
Lean only	46	1 chop	100	1.9	1.91
Cutlet lean, ckd average	85	3 oz	175	2.6	4.48
Leg of lamb, roasted:					
Lean and fat	85	3 oz	219	1.7	3.74
Lean only	85	3 oz	162	2.6	4.20
Rib roast:					
Lean and fat	85	3 oz	305	1.0	2.96
Lean only	85	3 oz	197	1.9	3.80
Shoulder roast:					
Lean and fat	85	3 oz	235	1.9	4.44
Lean only	85	3 oz	173	3.0	5.14
Lamb liver, pan-fried	85	3 oz	202	2.4	4.79
Meats *Continued*					
Pork:					
Bacon, cooked:					
Regular	19	3 pce	109	.6	.620
Canadian style	47	2 pce	86	.9	.790
Breakfast strips	34	3 pce	156	.8	1.25
Blade chop:					
Braised, lean and fat	67	1 ea	275	.9	2.58
Braised, lean only	50	1 ea	156	1.6	2.47
Broiled, lean and fat	77	1 ea	303	.8	2.35
Broiled, lean only	59	1 ea	117	1.9	2.24
Pan-fried, lean and fat	89	1 ea	368	.7	2.41
Pan-fried, lean only	62	1 ea	175	1.3	2.28
Roasted, lean and fat	88	1 ea	321	.8	2.63
Roasted, lean only	71	1 ea	198	1.3	2.55
Center loin chop:					
Braised, lean and fat	75	1 ea	266	.7	1.85
Braised, lean only	61	1 ea	166	1.1	1.78
Broiled, lean and fat	87	1 ea	275	.6	1.68
Broiled, lean only	72	1 ea	166	1.0	1.61
Pan-fried, lean and fat	89	1 ea	333	.5	1.74
Pan-fried, lean only	67	1 ea	178	.9	1.61
Roasted, lean and fat	88	1 ea	268	.7	1.80
Roasted, lean only	72	1 ea	180	1.0	1.71
Center rib chop:					
Braised, lean and fat	67	1 ea	246	.6	1.57
Braised, lean only	53	1 ea	147	1.0	1.49
Broiled, lean and fat	77	1 ea	264	.6	1.56
Broiled, lean only	63	1 ea	162	.9	1.50
Pan-fried, lean and fat	88	1 ea	343	.4	1.43
Pan-fried, lean only	62	1 ea	160	.8	1.28
Roasted, lean and fat	79	1 ea	252	.6	1.55
Roasted, lean only	66	1 ea	162	.9	1.47
Leg of pork, roasted:					
Lean and fat	85	3 oz	250	1.0	2.43
Lean only	85	3 oz	187	1.5	2.77
Pork roast, average loin and rib:					
Lean and fat	85	3 oz	265	.6	1.70
Lean only	85	3 oz	206	.9	1.92
Shoulder, braised (yield from 6.8 oz raw w/bone and skin):					
Lean and fat	85	3 oz	293	1.2	3.43
Lean only	67	2.4 oz	166	2.0	3.33
Spareribs, from 1 lb raw	177	6.25 oz	703	1.2	8.14
Pork heart	145	1 c	214	2.1	4.48
Pork liver	85	3 oz	141	4.0	5.71
Pork, Cured—Ham, also see bacon under Pork:					
Roasted, lean and fat	85	3 oz	207	1.0	1.97
Roasted, lean only	85	3 oz	133	1.6	2.19
Canned, roasted	85	3 oz	140	1.4	1.97
Rabbit, roasted	85	3 oz	131	1.2	1.51
Veal (calf):					
Cutlet, lean, ckd avg	85	3 oz	166	2.6	4.33
Rib, roasted	85	3 oz	151	2.5	3.81
Heart, braised	85	3 oz	134	1.7	2.34
Liver, pan-fried	85	3 oz	208	3.2	6.69
Venison (deer) roasted	85	3 oz	134	1.7	2.34
Meats: Poultry					
Chicken: A 3-lb chicken ≈ 1.45 lb raw; 1.1 lb cooked.					
All types:					
Fried	140	1 c	307	1.0	3.13
Roasted	140	1 c	266	1.1	2.94
Stewed	140	1 c	248	1.1	2.79

Table continued on following page

APPENDIX 5. Zinc Content of Foods—mg per 100 kcal and Per Serving* *Continued*

	Wt (g)	Svg	Cal	Zinc (mg) 100 Cal	Zinc (mg) Svg
Meats: Poultry *Continued*					
Chicken, all types *Continued:*					
Canned, boned w/ broth	142	5 oz	235	.9	2.13
Dark meat:					
Fried	85	3 oz	203	1.2	2.47
Roasted	85	3 oz	174	1.4	2.38
Stewed	85	3 oz	163	1.4	2.26
Light meat:					
Fried	85	3 oz	163	.7	1.08
Roasted	85	3 oz	147	.7	1.05
Stewed	85	3 oz	135	.7	1.01
Breast,* meat and skin (145 g raw; 181 g raw w/bone):					
Batter-fried	140	1 ea	364	.4	1.33
Flour-fried	98	1 ea	218	.5	1.07
Roasted	98	1 ea	193	.5	1.00
Stewed	110	1 ea	202	.5	1.06
Breast,* meat only (118 g raw):					
Fried	86	1 ea	161	.6	.930
Roasted	86	1 ea	142	.6	.860
Stewed	95	1 ea	144	.6	.920
***2 pieces per bird**					
Drumstick, meat and skin (73 g raw; 110 g raw w/bone):					
Batter-fried	72	1 ea	193	.9	1.67
Flour-fried	49	1 ea	120	1.2	1.42
Roasted	52	1 ea	112	1.3	1.49
Stewed	57	1 ea	116	1.3	1.51
Drumstick, meat (62 g raw):					
Fried	42	1 ea	82	1.6	1.35
Roasted	44	1 ea	76	1.8	1.40
Stewed	46	1 ea	78	1.8	1.39
Thigh, meat and skin (94 g raw; 120 g raw w/bone):					
Batter-fried	86	1 ea	238	.7	1.75
Flour-fried	62	1 ea	162	1.0	1.56
Roasted	62	1 ea	153	1.0	1.46
Stewed	68	1 ea	158	1.0	1.53
Thigh, meat (69 g raw):					
Fried	52	1 ea	113	1.3	1.45
Roasted	52	1 ea	109	1.2	1.34
Stewed	55	1 ea	107	1.3	1.42
Wing, meat and skin (49 g raw; 90 g raw w/bone):					
Batter-fried	49	1 ea	159	.4	.670
Flour-fried	32	1 ea	103	.5	.560
Roasted	34	1 ea	99	.6	.62
Stewed	40	1 ea	100	.7	.650
Wing, meat only (29 g raw):					
Fried	20	1 ea	42	1.0	.420
Roasted	21	1 ea	43	1.0	.450
Stewed	24	1 ea	43	1.1	.490
Chicken gizzard	22	1 ea	34	2.8	.963
Chicken heart	3.3	1 ea	6	4.0	.240
Chicken liver	20	1 ea	30	2.9	.867
Chicken roll, light meat	57	2 pce	90	.5	.410
Duck, domestic, roasted:					
Meat and skin	85	3 oz	286	.6	1.58
Meat only	85	3 oz	171	1.3	2.21
Goose, domestic, roasted:					
Meat and skin	85	3 oz	259	.7	1.76
Meat only	85	3 oz	202	1.1	2.30
Turkey:					
Breast meat, seasoned:					
Barbecued	28	1 oz	40	.9	.350
Hickory smoked	28	1 oz	35	.9	.300
Ground, cooked	100	3.5 oz	229	1.2	2.86

	Wt (g)	Svg	Cal	Zinc (mg) 100 Cal	Zinc (mg) Svg
Meats: Poultry *Continued*					
Turkey *Continued:*					
Roasted:					
All types	140	1 c	238	1.8	4.34
Dark meat only	85	3 oz	159	2.4	3.80
Light meat only	85	3 oz	133	1.3	1.73
Frozen slices w/gravy	142	5 oz	95	1.0	.994
Frozen slices	85	3 oz	130	1.8	2.37
Breaded, fried patty	64	1 ea	181	.8	1.50
Turkey gizzard	67	1 ea	109	2.6	2.79
Turkey heart	16	1 ea	28	3.0	.843
Turkey liver	75	1 ea	127	1.8	2.32
Meats: Sausages and Lunchmeats					
Barbeque loaf, pork and beef	23	1 pce	40	1.4	.570
Beef lunchmeat:					
Loaf or roll	28	1 oz	87	.8	.720
Thin sliced	28	1 oz	50	2.3	1.13
Beerwurst (beer salami):					
Beef salami	23	1 pce	75	.8	.610
Pork salami	23	1 pce	55	.7	.400
Berliner sausage	23	1 pce	53	1.1	.570
Bologna:					
Beef bologna	23	1 pce	72	.6	.460
Beef and pork	28	1 oz	89	.6	.550
Cured pork	23	1 pce	57	.8	.470
Turkey	28	1 oz	56	.9	.492
Braunschweiger	18	1 pce	65	.8	.510
Brotwurst, link	70	1 ea	226	.7	1.47
Cheesefurter (cheese smoki)	43	1 ea	141	.7	.970
Chicken roll, light meat	57	2 oz	90	.5	.410
Corned beef loaf, jellied	28	1 oz	46	2.3	1.08
Dutch brand loaf	28	1 oz	68	.7	.490
Frankfurter (hotdog):					
Beef, 8/pkg	57	1 ea	184	.7	1.21
Beef and pork, 8/pkg	57	1 ea	183	.6	1.05
Chicken, 10/pkg	45	1 ea	115	.9	1.00
Turkey, 10/pkg	45	1 ea	102	1.0	1.00
Ham, lunchmeat:					
Extra lean	57	2 oz	75	1.5	1.09
Regular	57	2 oz	103	1.2	1.21
Thin slices, (3 ≈ 1 oz)	28	3 pce	37	1.5	.550
Ham, chopped, packaged	42	2 pce	98	.8	.769
Ham, minced	21	1 pce	55	.7	.400
Ham patty, cooked	60	1 ea	203	.6	1.13
Ham and cheese roll/loaf	57	2 oz	147	.8	1.13
Ham salad spread	240	1 c	518	.5	2.64
Italian sausage link, cooked	67	1 ea	216	.7	1.59
Keilbasa	26	1 pce	81	.6	.520
Knockwurst, link	68	1 ea	209	.5	1.13
Liverwurst, pork	18	1 pce	59	.8	.468
Luncheon meat, canned	21	1 pce	70	.4	.310
Luncheon sausage, beef and pork	23	1 pce	60	.9	.560
Luxury loaf	57	2 oz	80	2.2	1.73
Mortadella	15	1 pce	47	.7	.320
Olive loaf	57	2 oz	133	.6	.780
Pastrami:					
Beef, cured	57	2 oz	198	.6	1.21
Turkey, cured	57	2 oz	74	2.0	1.46
Peppered loaf	28	1 pce	42	2.2	.920
Pepperoni sausage, small slice	22	4 pce	109	.5	.550

APPENDIX 5. Zinc Content of Foods—mg per 100 kcal and Per Serving* *Continued*

	Wt (g)	Svg	Cal	Zinc (mg) 100 Cal	Zinc (mg) Svg
Meats: Sausages and Lunchmeats *Continued*					
Pickle and pimento loaf	57	2 oz	149	.5	.790
Polish sausage	28	1 oz	92	.6	.550
Pork sausage:					
Link, cooked	13	1 ea	48	.7	.330
Patty, cooked	27	1 pce	100	.7	.680
Brown and serve, links	13	1 ea	50	.3	.150
Poultry sandwich spread	13	1 T	25	1.0	.250
Salami:					
Beef	23	1 pce	58	.8	.490
Pork and beef	57	2 oz	143	.8	1.21
Turkey	57	2 oz	111	1.1	1.25
Salami, dry, beef and pork	20	2 pce	85	.8	.640
Smoked link sausage:					
Beef and pork	68	1 ea	229	.6	1.44
Pork link	68	1 ea	265	.7	1.92
Turkey lunchmeats (other):					
Smoked turkey sausage	28	1 oz	55	1.3	.710
Summer sausage	23	1 pce	80	.6	.470
Breakfast sausage	28	1 oz	65	1.5	.970
Turkey ham	57	2 oz	73	2.2	1.58
Turkey roll, light and dark	57	2 oz	84	1.3	1.13
Turkey roll, light meat	57	2 oz	83	1.1	.880
Turkey summer sausage	28	1 oz	50	1.4	.720
Vienna sausage, canned	16	1 can	45	.6	.260
Mixed Dishes and Fast Foods					
Beef and vegetable stew:					
Recipe	245	1 c	220	2.4	5.29
Canned	245	1 c	194	2.2	4.23
Beef, macaroni, tomato sauce, recipe	226	1 c	189	1.1	2.07
Beef pot pie, f/frzn	234	1 ea	426	.6	2.64
Burrito:					
Bean burrito	174	1 ea	322	.7	2.37
Beef burrito	177	1 ea	463	1.3	5.80
Beef and bean	175	1 ea	390	.8	3.30
Deluxe combination	198	1 ea	424	.9	3.91
Cheese soufflé, recipe	112	1 c	221	.6	1.35
Chicken à la king, recipe	245	1 c	470	.4	1.80
Chicken chow mein:					
Recipe	250	1 c	255	.8	2.12
Canned	250	1 c	95	1.4	1.30
Chicken egg roll	100	1 ea	242	.2	.400
Chicken and noodles, recipe	240	1 c	365	.6	2.14
Chicken pot pie, f/frozen	230	1 ea	430	.3	1.22
Chili w/beans, canned	255	1 c	286	1.8	5.10
Cole slaw	120	1 c	84	.3	.240
Chicken salad w/celery	78	½ c	266	.3	.804
Chop suey w/beef and pork	250	1 c	300	1.2	3.58
Corn dog	111	1 ea	330	.4	1.44
Corn fritter, recipe	45	1 ea	116	.3	.295
Corn pudding	250	1 c	271	.5	1.26
Corned beef hash, canned	220	1 c	382	1.1	4.38
Egg salad	183	1 c	438	.5	2.24
Enchilada:					
Beef enchilada	120	1 ea	292	.8	2.25
Cheese enchilada	120	1 ea	330	.5	1.50
Chicken enchilada	120	1 ea	269	.4	1.21
French toast, recipe	65	1 pce	123	.4	.474
Lasagna:					
Recipe, w/meat	245	1 pce	398	.8	3.23
Recipe, w/o meat	218	1 pce	316	.6	1.93
Mixed Dishes and Fast Foods *Continued*					
Lasagna *Continued:*					
Frozen entrée	205	1 pce	275	.5	1.25
Macaroni and cheese:					
Recipe	200	1 c	430	.3	1.20
Canned	240	1 c	230	.5	1.20
Macaroni salad, no cheese	141	1 c	371	.1	.335
Manicotti:					
Meat and tomato sce	233	1 ea	320	.6	1.78
Frozen entree	225	1 ea	271	.7	2.00
Meat loaf:					
Beef only	87	1 pce	193	1.8	3.50
Beef and ⅓ pork	87	1 pce	212	1.3	2.86
Moussaka, (lamb and eggplant)	250	1 c	250	1.3	3.29
Pies, fried, commercial:					
Apple pie	85	1 ea	255	.1	.144
Cherry pie	85	1 ea	250	.1	.150
Pizza, cheese:					
Thick crust ½ of 10″	208	1 pce	519	.5	2.66
Regular crust ⅛ of 15″	120	1 pce	290	.6	1.81
Potato salad w/mayo and eggs	250	1 c	358	.2	.780
Quiche Lorraine, ⅛ pie	176	1 pce	600	.3	1.95
Ravioli, beef, frzn w/sce	28	2 ea	33	.5	.170
Ravioli, canned	226	1 c	220	.6	1.37
Sandwiches, Fast food:					
Cheeseburger, 3-oz patty	112	1 ea	300	.8	2.53
Cheeseburger, 4-oz patty	194	1 ea	524	1.0	5.27
Chicken patty sandwich	157	1 ea	436	.2	1.00
English muffin, egg, cheese, bacon	138	1 ea	360	.5	1.86
Fish sandwich:					
Regular w/cheese	140	1 ea	420	.2	.952
Large, w/o cheese	170	1 ea	470	.2	.884
Hamburger, 3-oz patty	98	1 ea	245	.8	2.00
Hamburger, 4-oz patty	174	1 ea	445	1.1	5.01
Hotdog (frankfurter) w/ bun	85	1 ea	260	.5	1.19
Roast beef w/bun	150	1 ea	345	1.1	3.66
Sandwiches on part whole-wheat bread unless stated as rye.					
Avocado, cheese, sprouts, tomato	195	1 ea	432	.4	1.87
Bacon, lettuce, tomato	135	1 ea	327	.4	1.30
Chicken salad sandwich	100	1 ea	294	.3	.998
Corned beef and swiss on rye	147	1 ea	429	1.0	4.37
Egg salad sandwich	111	1 ea	319	.4	1.16
Grilled cheese	117	1 ea	393	.6	2.49
Ham sandwich	122	1 ea	256	.7	1.74
Ham on rye	116	1 ea	242	.1	1.91
Ham and cheese	151	1 ea	363	.7	2.69
Ham and swiss on rye	145	1 ea	350	.9	3.03
Ham salad sandwich	125	1 ea	339	.4	1.26
Patty melt on rye	177	1 ea	567	1.2	6.63
Peanut butter and jam	100	1 ea	341	.4	1.30
Reuben sandwich, grilled	233	1 ea	480	.9	4.55
Roast beef sandwich	122	1 ea	280	1.0	2.87
Tuna salad sandwich	116	1 ea	303	.3	.893
Turkey sandwich	122	1 ea	271	.5	1.24
Turkey ham sandwich	122	1 ea	253	.9	2.20

Table continued on following page

APPENDIX 5. Zinc Content of Foods—mg per 100 kcal and Per Serving* *Continued*

	Wt (g)	Svg	Cal	Zinc (mg) 100 Cal	Zinc (mg) Svg
***Mixed Dishes and Fast Foods** Continued*					
Spaghetti (pasta, tomato sauce and cheese):					
Homemade	250	1 c	260	.5	1.30
Canned	250	1 c	190	.6	1.12
Spaghetti (pasta, tomato sauce and meat):					
Homemade	248	1 c	330	.7	2.45
Canned	250	1 c	260	.9	2.39
Spinach soufflé	136	1 c	218	.6	1.29
Taco, beef	78	1 ea	207	1.4	2.89
Taco, chicken	78	1 ea	172	.8	1.34
Tostada:					
W/refried beans	157	1 ea	212	.7	1.55
W/beans and beef	192	1 ea	332	1.1	3.57
W/beans and chicken	157	1 ea	249	.8	1.94
Tuna noodle casserole, recipe	202	1 c	251	.4	.966
Tuna salad	205	1 c	383	.3	1.15
Turkey pot pie, f/frzn	233	1 ea	416	.4	1.50
Veal Parmigiana, frzn entrée	205	7.25 oz	372	1.1	3.97
Waldorf salad	142	1 c	424	.2	.690
Nuts and Seeds					
Almonds, dried, whole	142	1 c	837	.5	4.15
Almond butter	16	1 T	101	.5	.488
Brazil nuts, dry (≈7)	28	1 oz	186	.7	1.30
Cashews, oil roasted	130	1 c	748	.8	6.18
Cashew butter	16	1 T	94	.9	.830
Chestnuts, roasted	143	1 c	350	.2	.815
Coconut:					
Fresh, grated	80	1 c	283	.3	.880
Packaged, flaked, sweet	74	1 c	351	.4	1.30
Dried, unsweetened	78	1 c	515	.3	1.57
Coconut milk, canned	226	1 c	445	.3	1.27
Coconut water, raw	240	1 c	46	.5	.240
Filberts (hazelnuts), whole	135	1 c	853	.4	3.24
Macadamias:					
Dried	134	1 c	940	.2	2.29
Oil roasted	134	1 c	962	.2	1.47
Mixed Nuts w/peanuts					
(cashews, peanuts, brazil nuts, filberts, almonds, pecans):					
Dry roasted	137	1 c	814	.6	5.21
Oil roasted	142	1 c	876	.8	7.22
Mixed Nuts w/o peanuts					
(cashews, almonds, brazil nuts, pecans, filberts):					
Oil roasted	144	1 c	886	.8	6.71
Peanuts:					
Dry roasted	146	1 c	855	.6	4.83
Oil roasted	144	1 c	837	1.1	9.60
Peanut butter	32	2 T	190	.4	.802
Peanut flour, defatted	60	1 c	196	1.6	3.06
Pecans, dried, chopped	119	1 c	794	.8	6.51
Pine nuts, dried pignola/ pinyon	28	1 oz	154	.8	1.22
Pistachio, dried, unshelled	128	1 c	739	.2	1.72
Pumpkin/squash seeds:					
Dry kernels	138	1 c	747	1.4	10.3
Roasted kernels	227	1 c	1185	1.4	16.9
Whole seeds, roasted	64	1 c	285	2.3	6.59
Sesame flour:					
High fat	28	1 oz	149	2.0	3.03
Low fat	28	1 oz	95	3.0	2.84
Part defatted	28	1 oz	109	2.8	3.04
***Nuts and Seeds** Continued*					
Sesame seeds:					
Dried kernels	150	1 c	882	1.7	15.4
Whole, dried	36	¼ c	206	1.4	2.80
Soybeans, roasted	86	½ c	405	.7	2.7
Sunflower seeds:					
Dried	36	¼ c	205	.9	1.82
Oil roasted	34	¼ c	208	.8	1.76
Tahini (sesame butter)	15	1 T	91	1.7	1.57
Walnuts, chopped:					
Black	125	1 c	759	.6	4.28
English	120	1 c	770	.4	3.28
Soups, Sauces, and Gravies					
Gravies:					
Beef, canned	233	1 c	124	1.9	2.33
Chicken gravy:					
From dry mix	260	1 c	85	.4	.320
Canned	238	1 c	189	1.0	1.91
Mushroom gravy:					
From dry mix	258	1 c	70	.5	.328
Canned	238	1 c	120	1.4	1.66
Onion gravy:					
Prepared from dry	261	1 c	78	.4	.287
Canned	241	1 c	57	1.1	.612
Sauces:					
Cheese sce f/mix w/milk	279	1 c	305	.3	.950
Hollandaise	160	1 c	867	.3	2.39
Spaghetti sauce, plain:					
Homemade	220	1 c	179	.3	.579
Canned	249	1 c	272	.2	.530
Spaghetti sauce w/meat:					
Homemade	248	1 c	297	.7	2.11
Canned	206	.8 c	220	.5	1.05
White sauce:					
Home recipe, med.	250	1 c	395	.3	1.05
From mix with milk	264	1 c	240	.5	1.15
Soups: soups are prep. from canned unless otherwise stated. RTS = ready to serve. For soups prepared with milk, assume whole milk.					
Bean w/bacon, w/water	253	1 c	173	.6	1.03
Beef bouillon	240	1 c	16	3.8	.600
Beef soup, chunky, RTS	240	1 c	171	1.5	2.64
Beef noodle	244	1 c	84	1.8	1.54
Celery, cream of:					
Prep with milk	248	1 c	165	.1	.196
Prep with water	244	1 c	90	.2	.151
Cheese, prep w/milk	251	1 c	230	.3	.688
Chicken broth, w/water	244	1 c	39	.6	.249
Chicken soup, chunky, RTS	251	1 c	178	.6	1.00
Chicken, cream of:					
Prepared with milk	248	1 c	191	.4	.675
Prepared with water	244	1 c	115	.5	.627
Condensed, undiluted	251	1 c	233	.5	1.26
Chicken gumbo	244	1 c	56	.7	.376
Chicken noodle:					
Prep with water	241	1 c	75	.7	.550
From dry	252	1 c	53	.4	.199
Chicken and rice	241	1 c	60	.4	.263
Chicken vegetable:					
Prep with water	241	1 c	74	.5	.366
From dry	251	1 c	49	.4	.208
Chicken vegetable, chunky, RTS	240	1 c	167	.2	.366
Chili beef soup	250	1 c	169	.8	1.40

APPENDIX 5. Zinc Content of Foods—mg per 100 kcal and Per Serving* *Continued*

	Wt (g)	Svg	Cal	Zinc (mg) 100 Cal	Zinc (mg) Svg
***Soups, Sauces, and Gravies** Continued*					
Soups *Continued:*					
Clam chowder, tom. base:					
Manhattan style	244	1 c	78	1.3	.976
Manhattan, chunky, RTS	240	1 c	133	1.3	1.68
Clam chowder, New England	248	1 c	163	.8	1.30
Minestrone soup	241	1 c	80	.9	.735
Mushroom, cream of:					
Prep with water	244	1 c	130	.5	.593
Prep with milk	248	1 c	205	.3	.640
Condensed, undiluted	251	1 c	257	.5	1.19
Oyster stew, prep w/ milk	245	1 c	134	7.7	10.3
Potato, cream of:					
Prep with milk	248	1 c	148	.5	.675
Prep with water	244	1 c	73	.9	.630
Shrimp, cream of, w/ milk	248	1 c	165	.5	.799
Split pea and ham	253	1 c	189	.7	1.32
Split pea, prep from dry	255	1 c	133	.4	.591
Tomato beef noodle	244	1 c	140	.5	.752
Tomato, cream of:					
Prep with milk	248	1 c	160	.2	.290
Prep with water	244	1 c	86	.3	.244
From dry	265	1 c	102	.2	.209
Tomato rice soup	247	1 c	120	.4	.514
Tomato noodle	244	1 c	69	.8	.583
Turkey	241	1 c	74	.8	.612
Turkey noodle, chunky, RTS	236	1 c	136	3.5	4.79
Vegetable, from dry	253	1 c	55	.3	.167
Vegetable, chunky, RTS	240	1 c	122	2.6	3.12
Vegetable beef:					
Prep with water	244	1 c	79	2.5	2.00
From dry	253	1 c	53	.5	.270
Vegetarian vegetable	241	1 c	70	.7	.460
Vegetables and Legumes					
Alfalfa sprouts	33	1 c	10	3.0	.304
Amaranth leaves:					
Fresh, chopped	28	1 c	7	3.6	.255
Boiled	132	1 c	28	4.3	1.21
Artichoke, globe, ckd (300 g whole)	120	1 ea	60	1.0	.588
Artichoke hearts:					
Cooked f/frozen	240	9 oz	108	.8	.864
Marinated	170	6 oz	168	.3	.540
Asparagus, pieces:					
Fresh, uncooked	67	½ c	15	3.1	.469
Ckd from fresh	90	½ c	23	1.9	.432
Ckd from frozen	180	1 c	50	2.0	1.01
Canned, drained	121	½ c	16	3.0	.484
Canned w/liquid	122	½ c	17	3.4	.573
Bamboo shoots:					
Cooked from fresh	120	1 c	15	2.1	.319
Canned	131	1 c	25	1.2	.300
Beans: see also garbanzo, lentils, soybeans.					
Baked (dry White beans with spices and sauce):					
Home prepared	253	1 c	382	.5	1.84
Canned, plain/vegetarian	254	1 c	235	1.5	3.55
Canned w/frankfurters	257	1 c	366	1.3	4.79
Canned with pork	253	1 c	268	1.4	3.69
***Soups, Sauces, and Gravies** Continued*					
Beans, baked *Continued:*					
Canned w/pork, swt sce	253	1 c	282	1.3	3.80
Canned w/pork, tom sce	253	1 c	247	1.1	2.60
Black beans, ckd f/dry	172	1 c	227	.8	1.92
Broadbeans, ckd f/dry	170	1 c	186	.9	1.72
Great northern, ckd f/dry	177	1 c	210	.7	1.55
Green (snap) beans:					
Fresh, uncooked	110	1 c	34	.8	.260
Ckd from fresh	125	1 c	44	1.0	.450
Ckd from frozen	135	1 c	36	2.3	.840
Canned, drained	135	1 c	26	1.5	.392
Canned w/liquid	240	1 c	36	1.3	.480
Hyacinth, ckd f/dry	194	1 c	228	2.4	5.53
Kidney beans, all:					
Ckd from dry	177	1 c	225	.8	1.89
Canned w/liquid	256	1 c	208	.7	1.41
Lima beans:					
Ckd from fresh	170	1 c	208	.6	1.34
Ckd from frozen:					
Large	85	½ c	85	.4	.370
Baby	90	½ c	94	.5	.500
Ckd from dry	188	1 c	217	.8	1.79
Canned, drained	170	1 c	164	1.0	1.60
Canned w/liquid	241	1 c	191	.8	1.57
Navy, ckd from dry	182	1 c	259	.7	1.93
Pinto beans:					
Cooked from dry	171	1 c	235	.8	1.85
Canned	240	1 c	186	1.0	1.66
Refried beans, canned	253	1 c	270	1.3	3.45
White beans, ckd f/dry	179	1 c	253	.8	1.96
Winged beans, ckd f/dry	172	1 c	252	1.0	2.48
Yardlong beans, ckd f/dry	171	1 c	202	.9	1.84
Yellow wax: see green beans.					
Bean sprouts (Mung beans):					
Fresh sprouts	104	1 c	31	1.4	.426
Boiled, drained	124	1 c	26	2.2	.580
Stir fried	124	1 c	62	1.8	1.12
Beets:					
Ckd f/fresh, whole	100	2 ea	31	.8	.250
Canned dices, drained	85	½ c	27	.7	.180
Canned dices w/liquid	123	½ c	36	.8	.283
Canned, pickled, slices	114	½ c	74	.4	.296
Beet greens, ckd fresh, drained	144	1 c	40	1.8	.720
Broccoli, chopped:					
Fresh, uncooked	88	1 c	24	1.5	.360
Ckd f/fresh	156	1 c	44	1.3	.592
Ckd f/frozen	184	1 c	51	1.1	.560
W/cheese sce	142	½ c	166	.2	.370
W/hollandaise sce	95	½ c	105	.3	.290
Brussels sprouts:					
Ckd f/fresh (1 sprout = 21 g)	156	1 c	60	.8	.500
Ckd f/frozen	155	1 c	65	.8	.550
Cabbages, chopped:					
Common, fresh	70	1 c	16	.8	.120
Common, cooked	150	1 c	32	.8	.240
Bok choy, fresh	70	1 c	9	3.2	.288
Bok choy, cooked	170	1 c	20	2.2	.432
Pe-tsai, fresh	76	1 c	11	1.5	.170

Table continued on following page

APPENDIX 5. Zinc Content of Foods—mg per 100 kcal and Per Serving* *Continued*

	Wt (g)	Svg	Cal	Zinc (mg) 100 Cal	Zinc (mg) Svg
Vegetables and Legumes *Continued*					
Cabbages, chopped *Continued:*					
Pe-tsai, cooked	119	1 c	16	1.4	.220
Red, fresh	70	1 c	19	.8	.150
Red, cooked	150	1 c	32	.7	.220
Savoy, fresh	70	1 c	20	1.3	.255
Savoy, cooked	145	1 c	35	.8	.263
Carrots:					
Fresh (7.5″ × 1-⅛″ dm.)	72	1 ea	31	.5	.14
Ckd f/fresh, sliced	78	½ c	35	.7	.234
Ckd f/frozen, sliced	73	½ c	26	.7	.175
Canned, drained	73	½ c	17	1.1	.190
Canned w/liquid	123	½ c	28	1.3	.357
Carrot juice	123	½ c	49	.5	.221
Cauliflower:					
Fresh, raw	50	½ c	12	.8	.090
Ckd fr/fresh	124	1 c	30	1.0	.298
Ckd fr/frozen	180	1 c	34	.7	.234
Celeriac (celery root) cooked	100	3.5 oz	25	1.2	.310
Celery stalk (7.5″ stalk = 40 g)	40	1 ea	6	.9	.052
Celery, cooked dices	150	1 c	27	.8	.21
Chard, Swiss:					
Fresh, chopped	36	1 c	7	2.3	.163
Ckd fr/fresh	175	1 c	35	1.7	.589
Collards:					
Fresh, chopped	36	1 c	11.2	.4	.047
Ckd fr/fresh	128	1 c	35	.4	.141
Ckd fr/frozen	170	1 c	63	.7	.460
Corn, kernels:					
Fresh uncooked	77	½ c	66	.5	.347
Cooked from fresh	82	½ c	89	.4	.394
Cooked from frozen	82	½ c	67	.4	.290
Canned, drained	82	½ c	66	.6	.381
Canned with liquid	128	½ c	79	.6	.460
Canned, vacuum pack	210	1 c	166	.6	.966
Corn, creamed, canned	128	½ c	93	.7	.678
Cucumber, 8″ × 2″ dm	301	1 ea	39	1.8	.690
Dandelion greens:					
Fresh chopped	55	1 c	25	2.5	.620
Ckd f/fresh	105	1 c	35	2.3	.800
Eggplant, ckd cubes	160	1 c	45	.5	.240
Endive, fresh, chopped	25	½ c	4	5.0	.200
Escarole, chopped, curly endive	50	1 c	9	4.4	.395
Garbanzo beans:					
Cooked f/dry	164	1 c	269	1.0	2.51
Canned w/liquid	240	1 c	285	1.0	2.53
Garden cress:					
Fresh, chopped	25	½ c	8	15.0	1.20
Ckd f/fresh	135	1 c	31	3.2	1.00
Kale, chopped:	67	1 c	33	.9	.295
Ckd f/fresh	130	1 c	42	.8	.312
Ckd f/frozen	130	1 c	39	.6	.234
Kohlrabi:					
Fresh slices	140	1 c	38	.8	.322
Cooked f/fresh	165	1 c	48	.7	.322
Leeks, chopped, fresh	104	1 c	32	.5	.165
Lentils, ckd f/dry	198	1 c	231	1.1	2.50
Lentils, sprouted:					
Fresh sprouts	77	1 c	81	1.4	1.16
Stir fried	100	3.5 oz	101	1.6	1.60
Lettuce, chopped:					
Butterhead	56	1 c	7.3	2.0	.144
Iceberg	56	1 c	7.3	1.8	.123
Loose leaf	56	1 c	10	1.8	.185
Vegetables and Legumes *Continued*					
Lettuce, chopped *Continued:*					
Romaine	56	1 c	9	2.1	.185
Mushroom:					
Fresh slices (1 avg ≈ 18 g)	35	½ c	9	3.4	.300
Cooked from fresh	78	½ c	21	3.2	.679
Canned, drained	78	½ c	19	3.0	.562
Mustard greens:					
Fresh, chopped	56	1 c	15	1.0	.144
Ckd f/fresh	140	1 c	21	1.4	.300
Ckd f/frozen	150	1 c	29	1.1	.300
Okra:					
Ckd f/fresh pods	85	8 ea	27	1.7	.468
Ckd f/frozen slices	92	½ c	34	1.7	.570
Onion:					
Fresh, chopped	160	1 c	61	.5	.304
Ckd f/fresh, chopped	105	½ c	46	.5	.22
Dehydrated flakes	14	¼ c	45	.6	.260
Spring chopped, all	50	½ c	16	1.3	.20
Parsley, fresh, chopped	30	½ c	10	2.2	.220
Parsnips:					
Fresh slices	133	1 c	100	.8	.785
Ckd f/fresh	156	1 c	125	.3	.400
Peas:					
Black-eyed peas:					
Ckd f/fresh	165	1 c	160	1.1	1.7
Ckd f/frozen	170	1 c	224	1.1	2.42
Ckd f/dry	171	1 c	198	1.1	2.20
Canned	240	1 c	184	.9	1.68
Green peas:					
Fresh, uncooked	145	1 c	118	1.5	1.80
Ckd f/fresh	160	1 c	134	1.4	1.90
Ckd f/frozen	80	½ c	63	1.2	.750
Canned, drained	85	½ c	59	1.0	.600
Canned w/liquid	124	½ c	61	1.4	.860
Green peas, edible-pods:					
Fresh, uncooked	145	1 c	61	1.0	.590
Ckd f/fresh	160	1 c	67	.9	.600
Ckd f/frozen	80	½ c	42	.9	.390
Split peas, ckd f/dry	196	1 c	231	.8	1.96
Peas, sprouted:					
Fresh sprouts	120	1 c	154	.8	1.26
Cooked from fresh	100	3.5 oz	118	.7	.780
Peas and carrots, ckd f/frzn	80	½ c	38	.9	.360
Peppers, Hot, chili peppers:					
Fresh, chopped	75	½ c	30	.8	.225
Canned, Jalapeno, chopped	68	½ c	17	.8	.130
Peppers, Sweet, green/red, chopped:					
Fresh	50	½ c	14	.4	.06
Ckd from fresh	68	½ c	19	.4	.082
Poi, two finger	240	1 c	269	.8	2.04
Potatoes:					
Baked in oven, 4.75″ × 2.3″:					
Flesh and skin	202	1 ea	220	.3	.650
Flesh only	156	1 ea	145	.3	.450
Potato skin	58	1 ea	115	.2	.280
Boiled, flesh only:					
Cooked w/o skin	135	1 ea	116	.3	.370
Cooked in skin	136	1 ea	119	.3	.410
Ckd f/frzn, small	70	1 ea	46	.4	.175
Canned, 1″ dm.	70	2 ea	42	.5	.200
Cottage fries, f/frzn	50	10 ea	109	.2	.210
Dehydrated flakes	200	1 c	722	.2	1.72

APPENDIX 5. Zinc Content of Foods—mg per 100 kcal and Per Serving* *Continued*

	Wt (g)	Svg	Cal	Zinc (mg) 100 Cal	Zinc (mg) Svg
Vegetables and Legumes *Continued*					
Potatoes *Continued:*					
French fried from frozen:					
Cooked in oil	50	10 ea	158	.1	.190
Oven heated	50	10 ea	111	.2	.210
Hash brown:					
Homemade	156	1 c	163	.1	.234
From frozen	156	1 c	340	.1	.500
Mashed:					
Prep w/milk	210	1 c	162	.4	.600
From instant	215	1 c	239	.2	.509
Potato puffs (tater tots), heated from frozen	62	½ c	138	.1	.190
Potato dishes, prepared:					
Au gratin, recipe	245	1 c	322	.5	1.69
Au gratin, from mix	245	1 c	228	.3	.588
Scalloped, recipe	245	1 c	210	.5	.980
Scalloped, from mix	245	1 c	228	.3	.613
Potato chips	28	14 ea	148	.2	.300
Potato pancakes	76	1 ea	237	.3	.680
Pumpkin:					
Ckd f/fresh, mashed	245	1 c	50	.9	.450
Canned	123	½ c	42	.5	.209
Radish, red	45	10 ea	7	1.8	.130
Radish seeds, sprouted	38	1 c	16	1.4	.213
Rutabaga, fresh cubes	140	1 c	51	.9	.480
Rutabaga, cooked	85	½ c	29	.9	.260
Sauerkraut, cnd w/liquid	236	1 c	44	1.0	.440
Seaweed:					
Irish moss, fresh	28	1 oz	14	4.0	.553
Kelp, fresh	28	1 oz	12	2.9	.349
Lavar, fresh	28	1 oz	10	3.0	.298
Soybeans, ckd f/dry	172	1 c	298	.7	1.98
Soybeans, sprouted:					
Fresh sprouts	35	½ c	45	.9	.41
Steamed	94	1 c	76	1.3	.98
Stir fried	100	1 c	125	1.7	2.10
Soybean Products: see tofu in this section; miso, natto, tempeh in Other; roasted soybeans in Nuts and Seeds; soy milk in Dairy; soy flour in Grains.					
Spinach:					
Fresh, chopped	56	1 c	12	2.4	.297
Ckd from fresh	180	1 c	41	3.3	1.37
Ckd from frozen, leaf	190	1 c	53	2.5	1.33
Canned, drained	214	1 c	50	2.0	.990
Squash, Summer, sliced:					
Crookneck, fresh	130	1 c	24	1.6	.380
Crookneck, ckd f/fresh	180	1 c	36	2.0	.710
Scallop, fresh	130	1 c	24	1.6	.380
Scallop, ckd f/fresh	90	½ c	14	1.6	.220
Zucchini, fresh	130	1 c	19	1.4	.260
Zucchini, ckd f/fresh	180	1 c	29	1.1	.324
Squash, Winter, mashed:					
Acorn, baked	245	1 c	137	.3	.418
Acorn, boiled	245	1 c	83	.3	.270
Butternut, baked	245	1 c	99	.3	.319
Butternut, ckd f/frzn	240	1 c	94	.3	.288
Hubbard, baked	240	1 c	120	.3	.360
Hubbard, boiled	236	1 c	70	.3	.220
Spaghetti, baked/boiled	155	1 c	45	.7	.310
Succotash:					
Ckd f/frzn	170	1 c	158	.5	.760
Canned w/liquid	255	1 c	161	.8	1.28

	Wt (g)	Svg	Cal	Zinc (mg) 100 Cal	Zinc (mg) Svg
Vegetables and Legumes *Continued*					
Sweet potato (whole ≈ 5″ × 2″):					
Baked in skin, flesh only	114	1 ea	118	.3	.330
Boiled w/o skin, flesh only	151	1 ea	160	.3	.400
Canned, mashed	128	½ c	129	.2	.270
Vacuum pack, mashed	255	1 c	233	.2	.460
Candied, recipe, 2.5″ × 2″	105	1 pce	144	.1	.160
Taro, ckd slices	132	1 c	187	.1	.240
Taro chips	23	10 ea	110	.3	.293
Tofu, soybean curd					
Firm, raw	126	½ c	183	1.1	1.98
Regular, raw	124	½ c	94	1.1	1.00
Tomatoes:					
Fresh, 2-⅗″ dm	123	1 ea	26	.4	.111
Fresh, chopped	180	1 c	38	.4	.162
Cooked from fresh	240	1 c	65	.4	.264
Canned, whole	240	1 c	47	.8	.380
Tomato juice, canned	244	1 c	42	.8	.342
Tomato paste, canned	262	1 c	220	1.0	2.10
Tomato purée, canned	250	1 c	102	.5	.540
Tomato sauce, canned	245	1 c	74	.8	.600
Turnips, cubes:					
Fresh cubes	130	1 c	35	.4	.156
Ckd from fresh	156	1 c	28	.6	.166
Turnip greens:					
Ckd from fresh	144	1 c	29	1.0	.290
Ckd from frozen	82	½ c	24	1.4	.340
Vegetable juice cocktail	242	1 c	46	1.1	.484
Vegetables, Combinations, cooked from frozen:					
Broccoli, mixed with:					
Carrots, pasta	95	⅔ c	88	.3	.300
Carrots, water chestnuts	91	⅔ c	32	.8	.258
Cauliflower and red pepper	95	⅔ c	25	.9	.230
Water chestnuts	95	½ c	33	.8	.273
Cantonese stir fry	95	½ c	53	.5	.257
Green beans and spaetzle	95	½ c	108	.2	.258
Japanese style	95	½ c	29	.8	.230
Mixed vegetables (corn, peas, carrots, green beans, and lima beans):					
Ckd from frozen	182	1 c	107	.8	.892
Canned, drained	163	1 c	77	.9	.668
Peas, mixed with:					
Cauliflower	95	½ c	118	.3	.397
Mushrooms	95	½ c	73	.8	.550
Onions	95	½ c	71	.7	.485
Onions, pasta	95	½ c	122	.4	.530
Onions, cheese sauce	142	½ c	165	.5	.750
Potatoes, cream sauce	76	½ c	140	.2	.260
Rice, mushrooms	66	⅔ c	108	.3	.340
Pasta, corn, cream sce	95	½ c	132	.5	.610
Spinach and water chestnuts	95	½ c	29	.8	.223
Water chestnuts, cnd slices	70	½ c	35	.8	.270
Yams, orange: see Sweet potatoes.					
Yams, white, cooked cubes	136	1 c	158	.2	.272
Zucchini: see Squash, summer.					

* From Hands ES: Food Finder, 2nd ed. Salem, OR, ESHA Research, 1988, p 202.

APPENDIX 6. Oxalate Content of Foods Per 100 Grams of Edible Portion*

Food	Oxalate (mg)
Cereal and Cereal Products	
Bread, white	4.9
Cake, fruit	11.8
Cake, sponge	7.4
Cornflakes	2.0
Crackers, soybean	207.0
Egg noodle (chow mein)	1.0
Grits (white corn)	41.0
Macaroni, boiled	1.0
Oatmeal, porridge	1.0
Spaghetti, boiled	1.5
Spaghetti in tomato sauce	4.0
Wheat germ	269.0
Milk and Milk Products	
Butter	0.0
Cheese, cheddar	0.0
Margarine	0.0
Milk	0.15
Meats and Eggs	
Bacon, streaky fried	3.3
Beef, canned corned	0.0
Beef, topside roast	0.0
Chicken, roasted	0.0
Eggs, boiled	0.0
Fish:	
Haddock	0.2
Plaice	0.3
Sardines	4.8
Ham	1.6
Hamburger, grilled	0.0
Lamb, roast	trace
Liver	7.1
Pork, roast	1.7
Vegetables	
Asparagus	5.2
Beans, green boiled	15.0
Beans in tomato sauce	19.0
Beetroot, boiled	675.0
Beetroot, pickled	500.0
Broccoli, boiled	trace
Brussels sprouts, boiled	0.0
Cabbage, boiled	0.0
Carrots, canned	4.0
Cauliflower, boiled	1.0
Celery	20.0
Chard, Swiss	645.0
Chive	1.1
Collards	74.0
Corn, yellow	5.2
Cucumber, raw	1.0
Dandelion greens	24.6
Eggplant	18.0
Escarole	31.0
Kale	13.0
Leek	89.0
Lettuce	3.0
Lima beans	4.3
Mushrooms	2.0
Mustard greens	7.7
Okra	146.0
Onion, boiled	3.0
Parsley, raw	100.0
Parsnips	10.0
Peas, canned	1.0
Pepper, green	16.0
Pokeweed	476.0
Vegetables *Continued*	
Potatoes, white boiled	0.0
Potatoes, sweet	56.0
Radishes	0.3
Rice, boiled	0.0
Rutabagas	19.0
Spinach, boiled	750.0
Spinach, frozen	600.0
Squash, summer	22.0
Tomatoes, raw	2.0
Turnips, boiled	1.0
Watercress, early fine curled	10.0
Fruits	
Apples, raw	3.0
Apricots	2.8
Avocado	0.0
Banana, raw	trace
Berries:	
Black	18.0
Blue	15.0
Dew	14.0
Green goose	88.0
Raspberries, black	53.0
Raspberries, red	15.0
Strawberries, canned	15.0
Strawberries, raw	10.0
Cherries:	
Bing	0.0
Sour	1.1
Currants:	
Black	4.3
Red	19.0
Fruit salad, canned	12.0
Grapes:	
Concord	25.0
Thompson seedless	0.0
Lemon peel	83.0
Lime peel	110.0
Mangoes	0.0
Melons:	
Cantaloupe	0.0
Casaba	0.0
Honeydew	0.0
Watermelon	0.0
Nectarines	0.0
Orange, raw	4.0
Peaches:	
Alberta	5.0
Canned	1.2
Hiley	0.0
Stokes	1.2
Pears:	3.0
Bartlett, canned	1.7
Pineapple, canned	1.0
Plums:	
Damson	10.0
Golden gage	1.1
Green gage	0.0
Preserves:	
Red plum jam	0.5
Strawberry jam	9.4
Prunes, Italian	5.8
Rhubarb:	
Canned	600.0
Stewed, no sugar	860.0
Nuts	
Peanuts, roasted	187.0
Pecans	202.0

APPENDIX 6. Oxalate Content of Foods Per 100 Grams of Edible Portion* *Continued*

Food	Oxalate (mg)	Food	Oxalate (mg)
Confectionery		***Juices*** *Continued*	
Chocolate, plain	117.0	Orange juice	0.5
Jelly, with allowed fruit	0.0	Pineapple juice	0.0
Marmalade	10.8	Tomato juice	5.0
Sweets, boiled (plain candies)	0.0	***Beverages, Alcoholic***	
Beverages, Nonalcoholic		Beer:	
Barley water, bottled	0.0	Bottled	0.0
Coca-Cola	trace	Draft	1.0
Coffee (0.5 g Nescafe/100 ml)	3.2	Lager draft, Tuborg Pilsner	4.0
Lemon Squash drink (lemonade)	1.0	Stout, Guiness Draft	2.0
Lucozade, bottled (soda)	0.0	Cider	0.0
Orange squash drink (orangeade)	2.5	Sherry, dry	trace
Ovaltine drink, 2 gm in 100 ml	10.0	Wine:	
Pepsi-Cola	trace	Port	trace
Ribena, concentrate (black currant drink)	2.0	Rosé	1.5
Tea, Indian:		White	0.0
2-min infusion	55.0	***Miscellaneous***	
4-min infusion	72.0	Cocoa, dry powder	623.0
6-min infusion	78.0	Coffee powder (Nescafe)	33.0
Tea, rosehip	4.0	Chicken noodle soup	1.0
Juices		Lemon juice	1.0
Apple juice	trace	Lime juice	0.0
Cranberry juice	6.6	Ovaltine, powder canned	35.0
Grape juice	5.8	Oxtail soup	1.0
Grapefruit juice	0.0	Pepper	419.0
		Tomato soup	3.0
		Vegetable soup	5.0

* Adapted from Ney DM et al: The Low Oxalate Diet Book for the Prevention of Oxalate Kidney Stones. San Diego, University of California, 1981, pp 19–23.

APPENDIX 7. Boys: Birth to 36 Months; Physical Growth NCHS Percentiles*

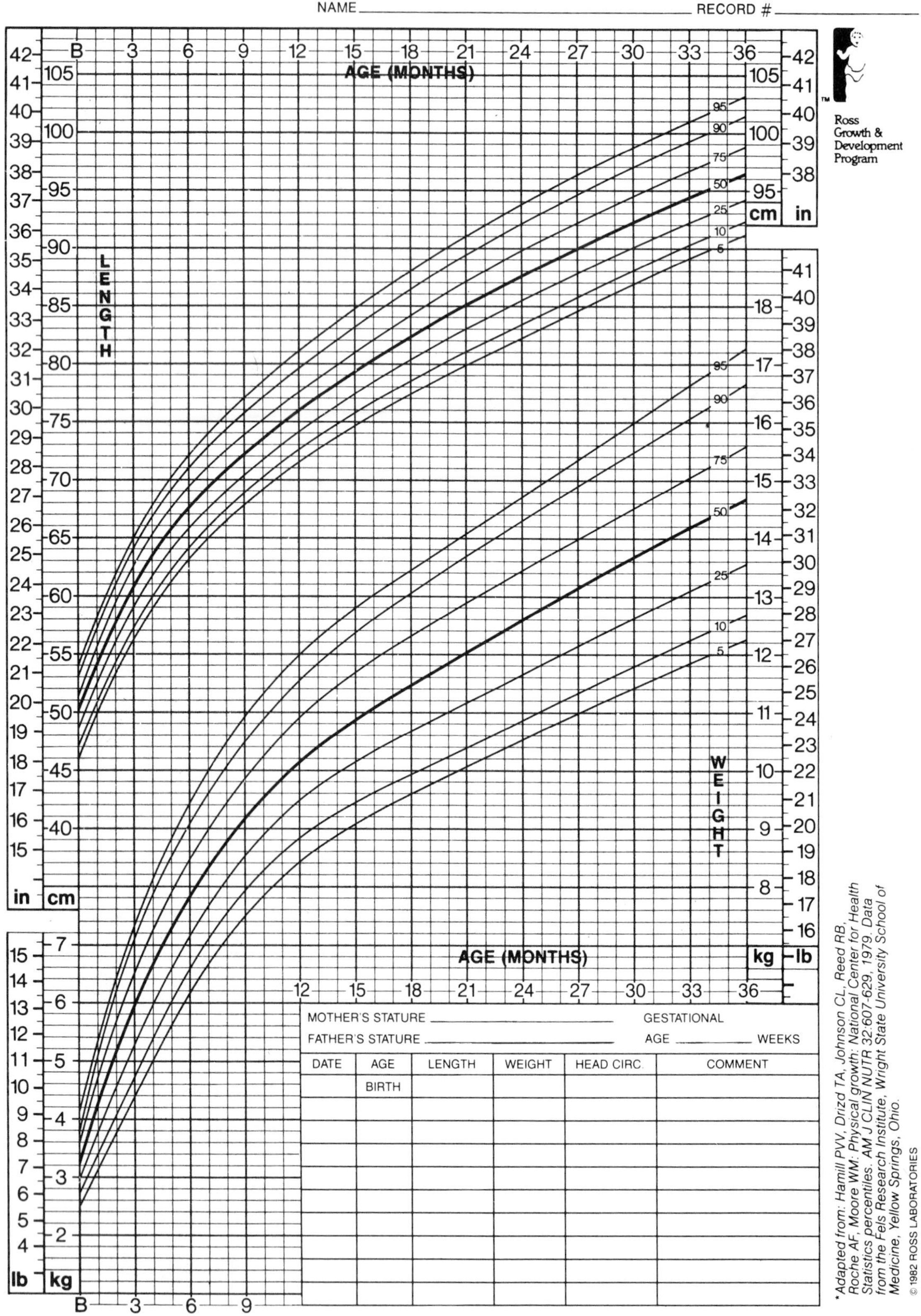

APPENDIX 8. Boys: Birth to 36 Months; Physical Growth NCHS Percentiles*

NAME ____________________ RECORD # ____________

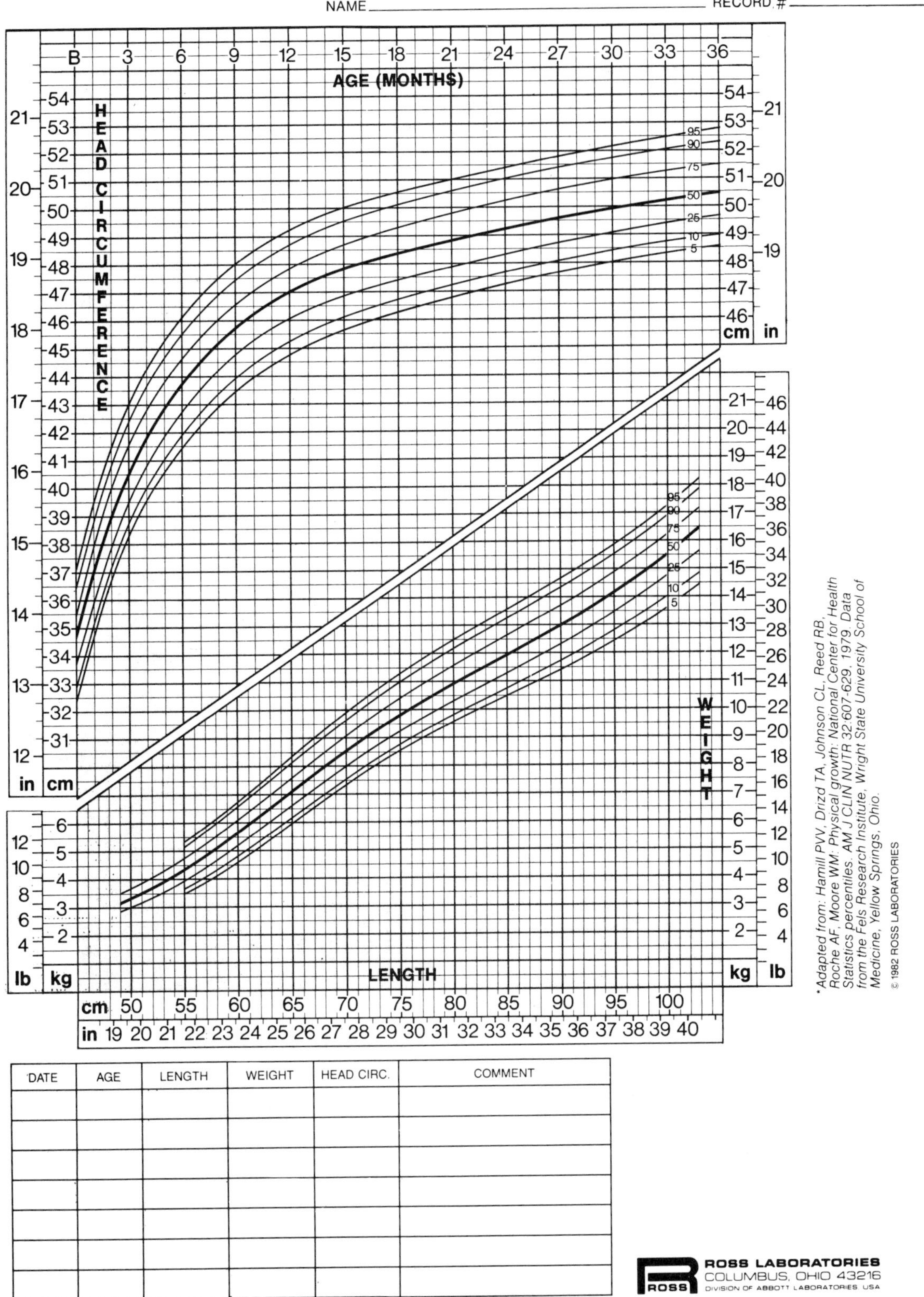

DATE	AGE	LENGTH	WEIGHT	HEAD CIRC.	COMMENT

*Adapted from: Hamill PVV, Drizd TA, Johnson CL, Reed RB, Roche AF, Moore WM: Physical growth: National Center for Health Statistics percentiles. AM J CLIN NUTR 32:607-629, 1979. Data from the Fels Research Institute, Wright State University School of Medicine, Yellow Springs, Ohio.

ROSS LABORATORIES
COLUMBUS, OHIO 43216
DIVISION OF ABBOTT LABORATORIES, USA

G105/DECEMBER 1982

APPENDIX 9. Boys: 2 to 18 Years; Physical Growth NCHS Percentiles*

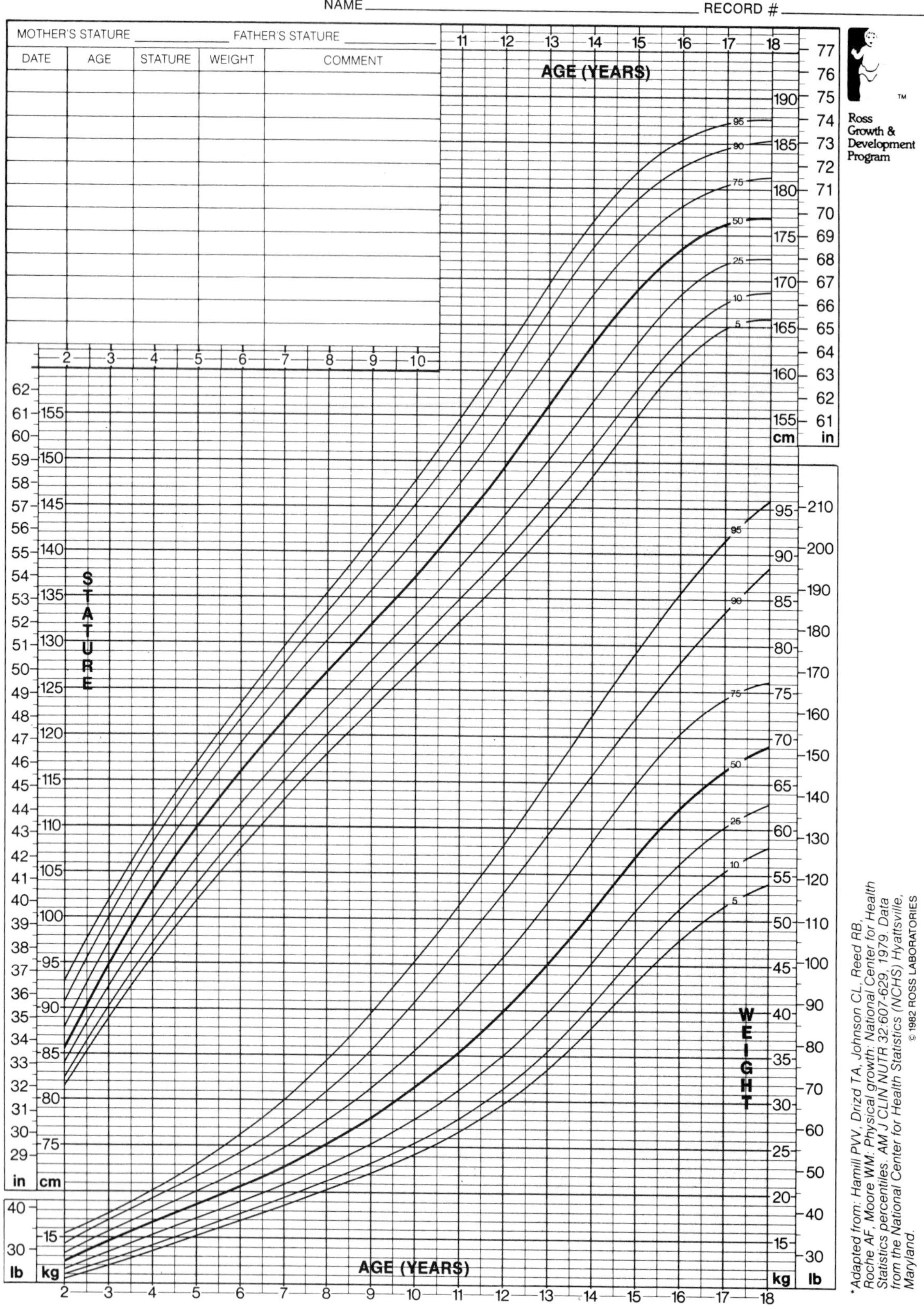

APPENDIX 10. Boys: Prepubescent; Physical Growth NCHS Percentiles*

NAME ____________ RECORD # ____________

DATE	AGE	STATURE	WEIGHT	COMMENT

*Adapted from: Hamill PVV, Drizd TA, Johnson CL, Reed RB, Roche AF, Moore WM: Physical growth: National Center for Health Statistics percentiles. AM J CLIN NUTR 32:607-629, 1979. Data from the National Center for Health Statistics (NCHS) Hyattsville, Maryland.

ROSS LABORATORIES
COLUMBUS, OHIO 43216
DIVISION OF ABBOTT LABORATORIES, USA

G107/DECEMBER 1982

APPENDIX 11. Girls: Birth to 36 Months; Physical Growth NCHS Percentiles*

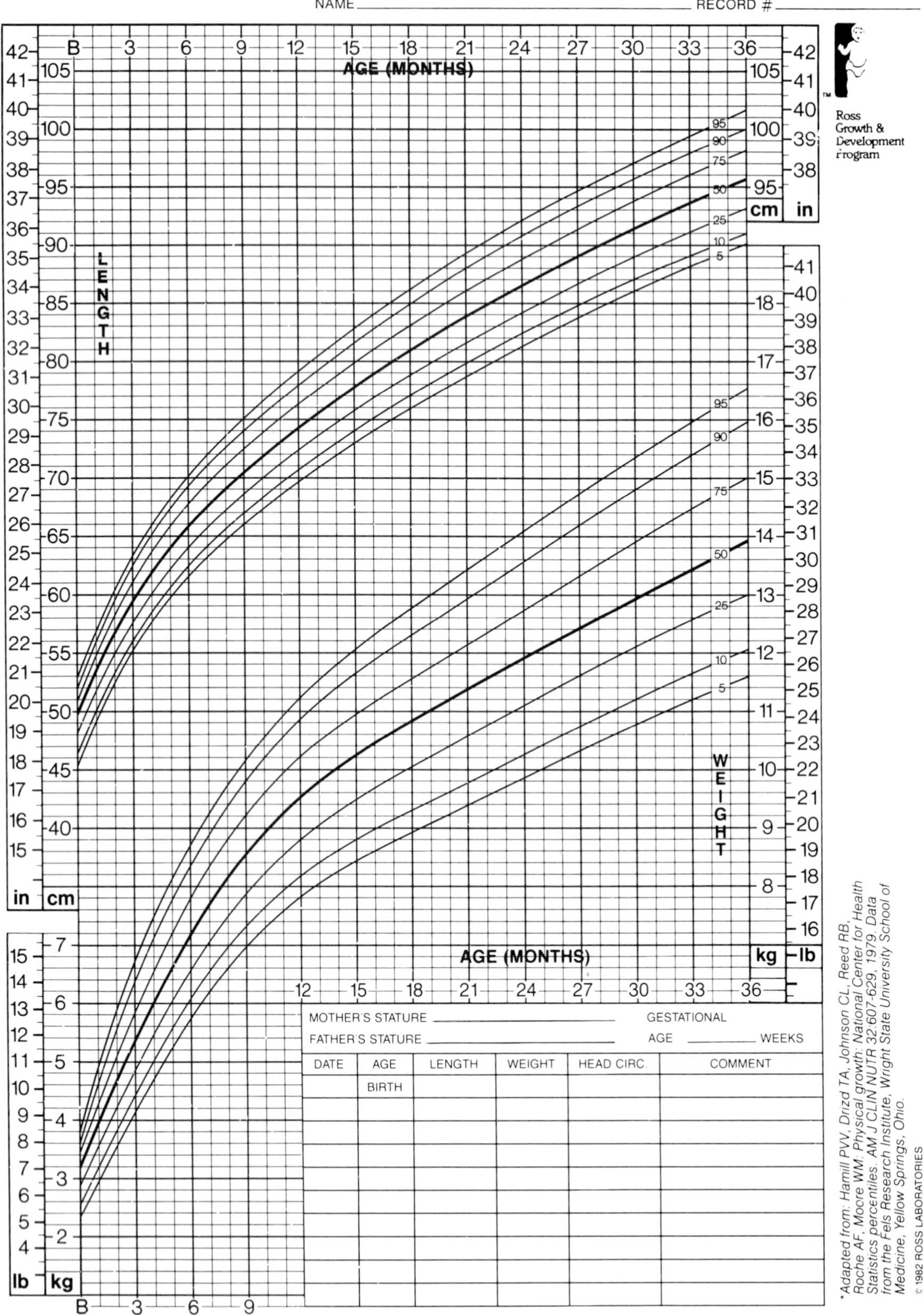

APPENDIX 12. Girls: Birth to 36 Months; Physical Growth NCHS Percentiles*

NAME ______________________ RECORD # ______________

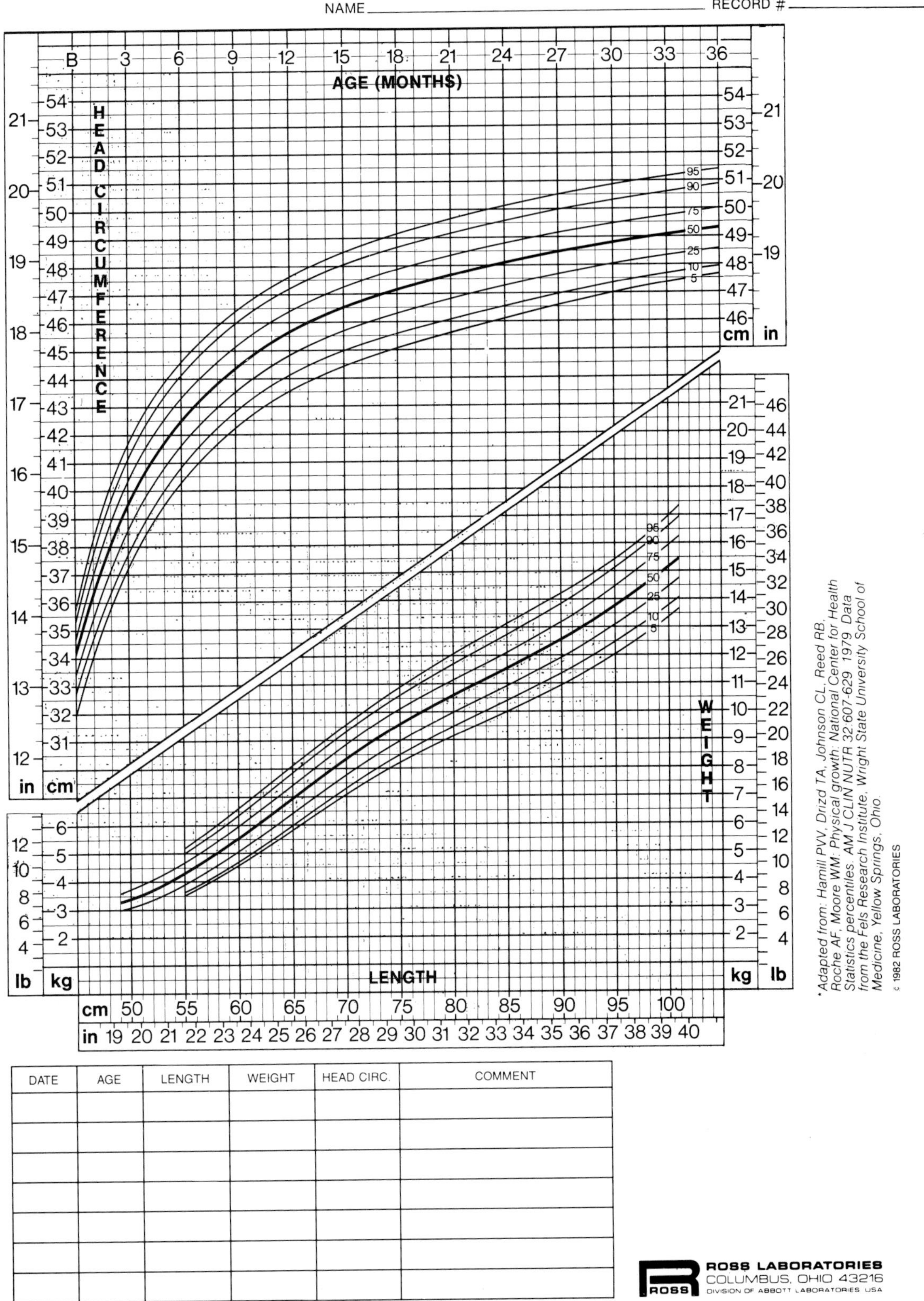

DATE	AGE	LENGTH	WEIGHT	HEAD CIRC.	COMMENT

ROSS LABORATORIES
COLUMBUS, OHIO 43216
DIVISION OF ABBOTT LABORATORIES USA

G106/DECEMBER 1982

APPENDIX 13. Girls: 2 to 18 Years; Physical Growth NCHS Percentiles*

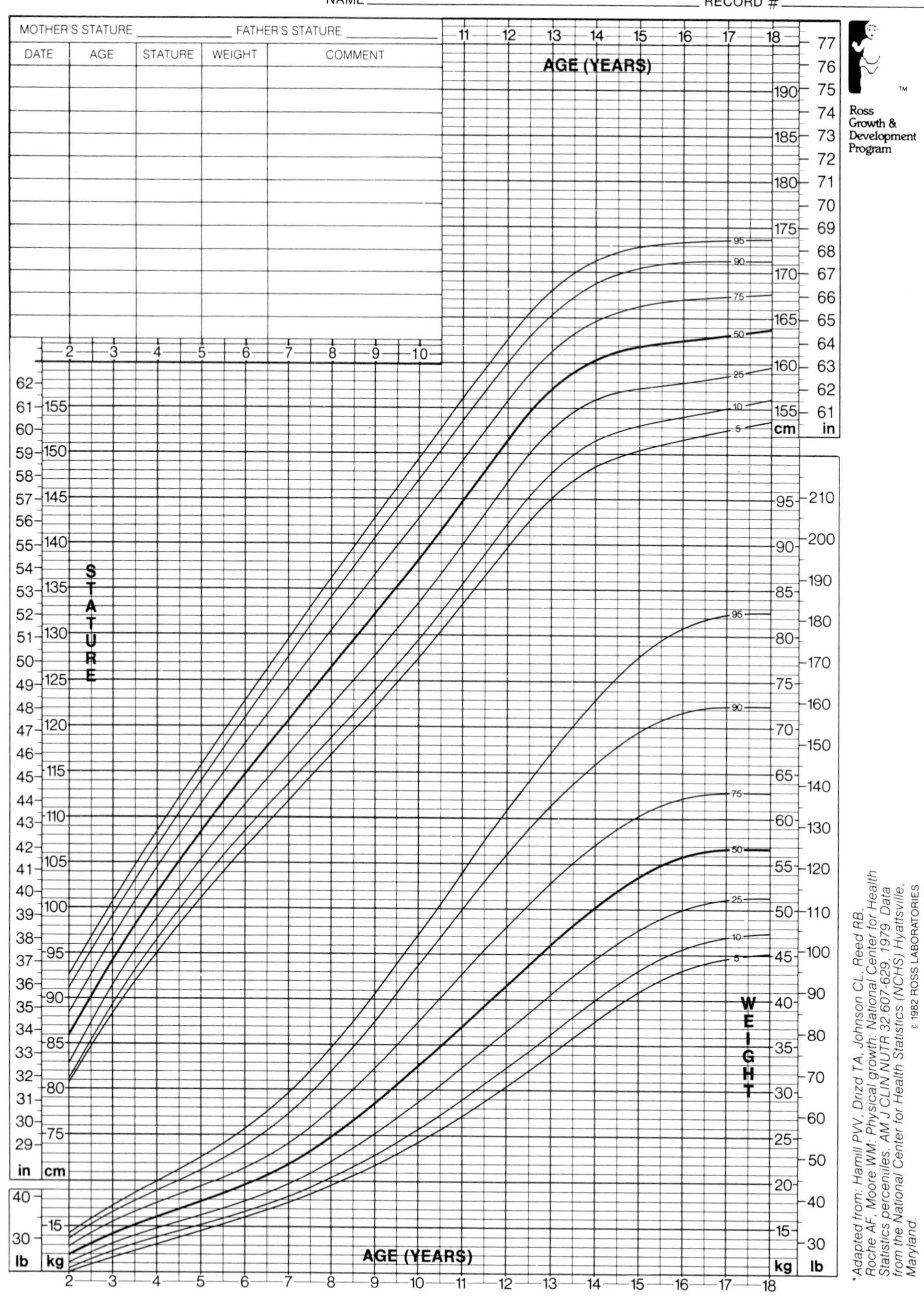

APPENDIX 14. Girls: Prepubescent; Physical Growth NCHS Percentiles

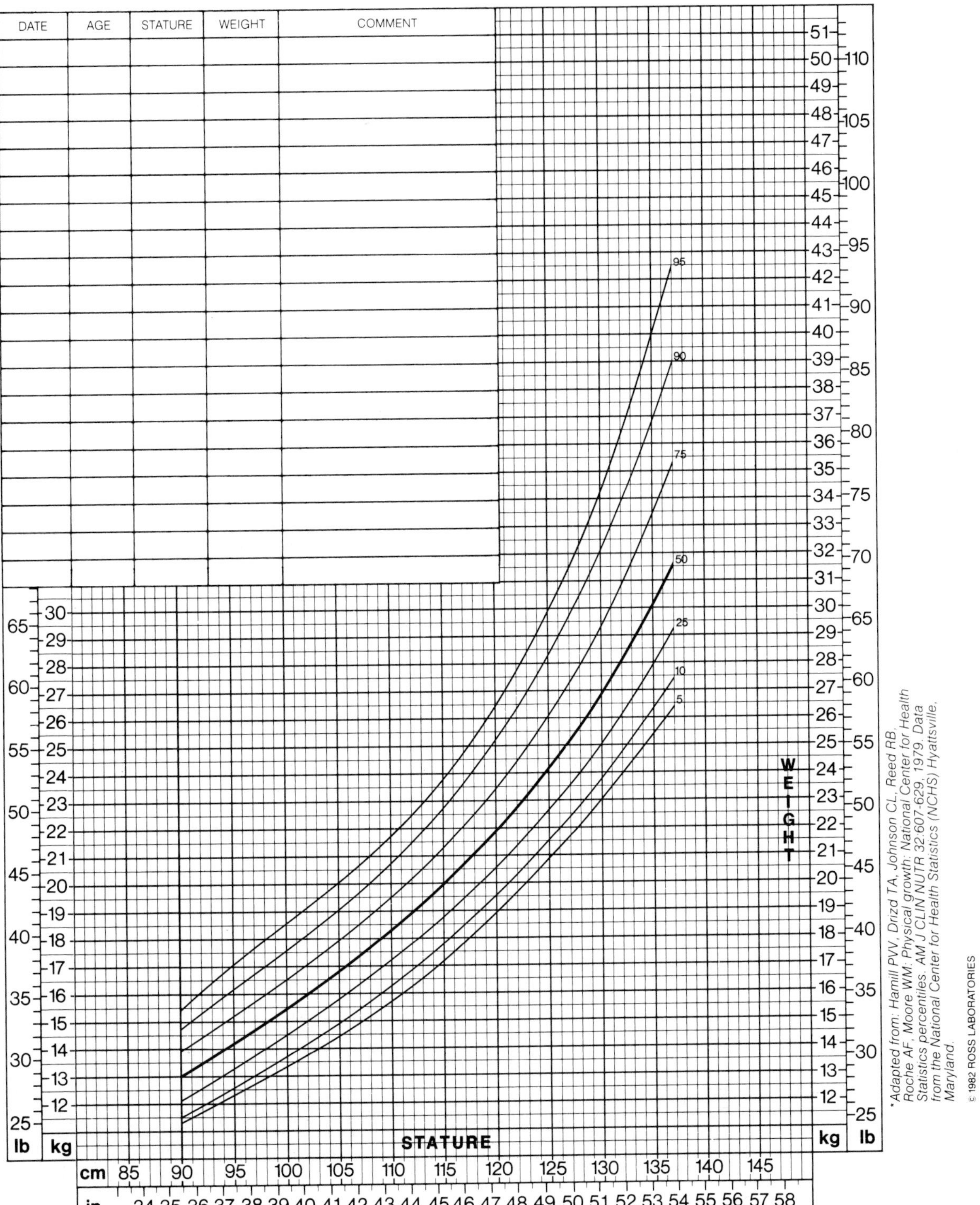

*Adapted from: Hamill PVV, Drizd TA, Johnson CL, Reed RB, Roche AF, Moore WM: Physical growth: National Center for Health Statistics percentiles. AM J CLIN NUTR 32:607-629, 1979. Data from the National Center for Health Statistics (NCHS) Hyattsville, Maryland.

ROSS LABORATORIES
COLUMBUS, OHIO 43216
DIVISION OF ABBOTT LABORATORIES, USA

G108/DECEMBER 1982

APPENDIX 15. Height in Centimeters of Youths Aged 12 to 17 Years*

Sex and Age	Average Age	n	N	$\bar{X}$	s	$s_{\bar{X}}$	Percentile 5th	10th	25th	50th	75th	90th	95th
Male							In Centimeters						
12 years	12.10	43	144	151.1	8.18	1.44	138.6	141.2	146.1	150.5	153.9	159.9	163.8
12¼ years	12.24	150	465	150.2	7.87	0.65	138.3	140.1	144.1	149.5	155.9	161.0	162.7
12½ years	12.50	187	577	151.5	8.33	0.87	138.0	140.4	145.9	152.6	156.8	161.2	165.1
12¾ years	12.76	184	589	154.3	7.48	0.62	142.3	146.1	149.6	153.7	158.0	164.4	167.6
13 years	12.99	165	520	154.7	9.37	0.67	136.9	143.0	148.1	155.4	161.4	166.6	170.3
13¼ years	13.25	154	511	158.9	8.55	0.82	146.2	148.5	153.0	157.8	164.9	171.1	174.4
13½ years	13.49	162	524	159.7	9.11	1.06	144.7	148.2	153.3	158.8	165.3	173.2	176.1
13¾ years	13.75	158	478	161.4	8.44	0.68	148.1	149.9	155.8	161.8	167.5	173.1	174.6
14 years	14.00	135	465	164.0	7.90	0.69	151.4	153.2	157.8	164.2	169.8	173.6	177.0
14¼ years	14.26	159	503	165.4	10.01	1.15	148.5	152.5	157.9	165.1	172.7	178.5	182.1
14½ years	14.50	155	487	167.5	7.96	0.79	153.5	156.6	161.5	169.4	173.0	176.5	178.7
14¾ years	14.76	151	467	167.1	8.46	0.99	152.7	155.2	162.3	167.7	173.5	176.5	180.8
15 years	15.00	155	489	169.4	7.59	0.59	156.3	158.7	163.7	169.4	174.8	178.1	181.4
15¼ years	15.25	169	511	171.4	7.57	0.62	159.2	160.8	166.5	171.7	176.5	180.5	183.1
15½ years	15.50	159	493	171.2	6.89	0.43	159.8	162.8	166.8	171.2	174.7	179.5	185.0
15¾ years	15.75	150	461	171.9	7.04	0.70	159.1	163.9	167.6	172.6	176.1	181.0	183.0
16 years	16.01	134	456	172.9	6.13	0.53	161.5	164.5	170.1	173.7	177.0	179.6	181.3
16¼ years	16.24	157	541	174.5	7.33	0.82	162.4	163.9	170.4	175.1	178.8	184.0	186.5
16½ years	16.50	135	413	174.3	6.56	0.44	165.1	166.8	170.5	173.9	178.4	182.4	184.5
16¾ years	16.75	122	401	174.7	6.78	0.66	164.6	166.1	169.8	174.4	179.6	183.1	185.4
17 years	17.00	136	479	175.1	6.94	0.61	163.2	166.4	170.5	175.6	179.7	183.7	186.3
17¼ years	17.26	125	435	176.4	6.97	0.71	162.6	167.5	172.1	176.7	181.3	184.3	188.0
17½ years	17.50	111	396	175.4	7.15	0.89	162.9	165.8	170.3	175.2	180.1	185.4	187.8
17¾ years	17.75	113	409	175.1	7.32	0.77	162.7	167.2	170.3	175.3	179.7	184.7	189.3
18 years	17.97	76	275	176.0	6.46	0.63	165.7	167.3	171.3	175.8	180.4	185.3	186.4
Female													
12 years	12.10	42	153	154.5	7.05	1.38	142.2	145.9	150.8	153.8	157.3	167.0	167.9
12¼ years	12.27	142	520	153.8	7.20	0.64	141.0	143.6	149.5	153.9	158.5	162.5	165.6
12½ years	12.50	140	511	155.6	7.69	0.60	141.8	145.4	151.7	155.5	160.4	164.6	168.3
12¾ years	12.75	147	517	156.0	6.82	0.57	143.6	147.5	151.8	156.3	160.5	164.5	166.6
13 years	13.01	166	578	157.1	7.30	0.43	143.8	148.3	152.5	157.3	162.7	166.7	169.2
13¼ years	13.25	144	461	158.1	7.54	0.73	145.3	146.8	152.6	158.6	163.4	167.7	169.5
13½ years	13.50	146	500	159.2	6.08	0.42	149.6	152.1	155.2	158.8	163.3	167.7	170.2
13¾ years	13.76	148	499	159.3	6.67	0.56	147.5	149.5	155.2	159.9	164.2	167.5	169.4
14 years	14.01	138	452	159.8	6.59	0.53	149.1	151.5	155.9	160.3	164.1	167.2	170.5
14¼ years	14.25	159	510	161.3	6.00	0.62	150.8	153.4	157.6	161.2	164.7	168.4	170.8
14½ years	14.51	137	415	161.2	6.66	0.63	150.3	152.6	157.1	161.2	165.4	170.3	172.2
14¾ years	14.76	130	457	162.5	6.43	0.69	153.6	154.7	157.7	162.9	167.2	170.0	174.1
15 years	14.99	133	449	161.3	5.73	0.53	151.7	154.6	157.5	160.7	164.8	169.4	171.4
15¼ years	15.25	135	479	162.2	6.68	0.58	151.3	153.2	157.3	163.2	166.7	170.3	171.8
15½ years	15.51	114	433	161.8	7.27	0.92	151.8	153.2	156.4	161.3	167.4	171.1	173.5
15¾ years	15.75	136	526	162.9	7.19	0.84	150.8	152.8	158.1	163.3	167.8	170.7	175.1
16 years	16.01	141	474	161.9	6.38	0.71	152.4	153.6	157.5	161.6	166.6	169.8	172.2
16¼ years	16.24	138	491	163.6	6.17	0.51	152.7	155.8	160.2	164.8	166.8	170.7	173.6
16½ years	16.50	112	341	161.5	6.51	0.70	151.3	153.0	157.2	161.8	166.1	170.2	172.2
16¾ years	16.76	135	450	162.9	6.52	0.52	151.5	154.0	158.6	162.8	167.3	171.7	173.0
17 years	17.00	135	477	163.0	6.48	0.71	151.5	154.5	158.9	163.4	167.0	171.1	173.3
17¼ years	17.24	125	461	162.7	6.62	0.52	151.5	153.8	157.8	164.2	166.9	171.3	173.6
17½ years	17.51	111	415	162.9	6.02	0.59	152.7	155.7	158.4	162.6	168.1	171.4	172.8
17¾ years	17.75	90	325	162.9	5.90	0.87	152.4	154.4	158.3	163.1	167.4	169.9	171.7
18 years	17.97	79	306	163.0	6.77	0.74	152.5	154.6	158.2	162.5	167.6	171.4	175.3

* From National Center for Health Statistics: Height and Weight of Youths 12–17 Years, United States. *In* Vital and Health Statistics, Series 11, no. 124. Health Services and Mental Health Administration. Washington, DC, US Government Printing Office, 1973.

NOTE: n = sample size; N = estimated number of youths in population in thousands; $\bar{X}$ = mean; s = standard deviation; $s_{\bar{X}}$ = standard error of the mean.

APPENDIX 16. Percentiles for Weight for Height of Youths Aged 12 to 17 Years*

(Weight in Kg of Youths Aged 12 Years at Last Birthday)

Sex and Height	n	N	$\bar{X}$	s	$s_{\bar{x}}$	Percentile 5th	10th	25th	50th	75th	90th	95th
						In kilograms						
Male												
Under 130 cm	5	15	*	*	*	*	*	*	*	*	*	*
130.0–134.9 cm	4	8	*	*	*	*	*	*	*	*	*	*
135.0–139.9 cm	34	111	32.50	3.741	0.727	26.6	27.6	30.2	31.6	34.7	37.7	39.4
140.0–144.9 cm	80	241	34.28	3.635	0.601	28.1	30.0	31.8	34.1	36.5	38.6	40.7
145.0–149.9 cm	123	386	39.27	6.243	0.615	32.1	33.2	35.7	38.2	40.9	46.1	52.5
150.0–154.9 cm	156	513	42.90	6.314	0.480	34.9	36.1	38.2	42.1	46.0	51.6	56.3
155.0–159.9 cm	135	432	47.35	7.551	0.769	38.3	39.4	41.9	46.2	50.5	57.4	61.9
160.0–164.9 cm	65	201	50.82	8.735	1.388	42.1	42.7	44.9	48.4	56.0	61.1	67.1
165.0–169.9 cm	29	88	55.75	8.811	2.031	43.3	46.4	49.0	54.4	59.9	68.3	76.6
170.0–174.9 cm	8	21	62.37	4.503	1.993	54.0	58.1	60.1	61.0	66.0	69.1	69.5
175.0–179.9 cm	3	10	*	*	*	*	*	*	*	*	*	*
180.0–184.9 cm	1	2	*	*	*	*	*	*	*	*	*	*
185.0–189.9 cm	–	–	–	–	–	–	–	–	–	–	–	–
190.0–194.9 cm	–	–	–	–	–	–	–	–	–	–	–	–
195.0 cm. and over	–	–	–	–	–	–	–	–	–	–	–	–
Female												
Under 130 cm	–	–	–	–	–	–	–	–	–	–	–	–
130.0–134.9 cm	3	10	*	*	*	*	*	*	*	*	*	*
135.0–139.9 cm	12	44	29.41	3.372	0.914	25.0	25.0	26.4	28.9	32.1	34.1	34.2
140.0–144.9 cm	32	116	38.30	7.314	1.194	28.8	30.6	33.3	36.8	41.4	49.2	55.1
145.0–149.9 cm	72	258	39.78	6.205	0.975	31.8	32.8	35.5	38.5	42.8	48.3	50.6
150.0–154.9 cm	147	517	44.00	7.421	0.677	34.4	35.8	38.9	42.8	47.4	52.9	57.4
155.0–159.9 cm	144	525	48.74	8.369	0.714	37.9	39.2	43.0	46.8	53.8	60.7	63.5
160.0–164.9 cm	95	336	53.06	8.010	0.658	42.5	43.9	47.2	51.1	57.2	65.6	69.6
165.0–169.9 cm	31	117	54.89	7.022	1.384	43.9	47.1	50.4	53.1	59.7	64.5	71.3
170.0–174.9 cm	11	42	63.66	14.501	6.214	48.7	50.1	50.8	56.7	82.2	86.0	86.1
175.0–179.9 cm	–	–	–	–	–	–	–	–	–	–	–	–
180.0–184.9 cm	–	–	–	–	–	–	–	–	–	–	–	–
185.0–189.9 cm	–	–	–	–	–	–	–	–	–	–	–	–
190.0–194.9 cm	–	–	–	–	–	–	–	–	–	–	–	–
195.0 cm. and over	–	–	–	–	–	–	–	–	–	–	–	–

* From National Center for Health Statistics: Height and Weight of Youths 12–17 Years, United States. *In* Vital and Health Statistics, Series 11, no. 124. Health Services and Mental Health Administration. Washington, DC, US Government Printing Office, 1973.

NOTE: *n* = sample size; *N* = estimated number of youths in population in thousands; $\bar{X}$ = mean; *s* = standard deviation; $s_{\bar{x}}$ = *standard error of the mean.*

Table continued on following page

APPENDIX 16. Percentiles for Weight for Height of Youths Aged 12 to 17 Years* *Continued*
(Weight in Kg of Youths Aged 13 Years at Last Birthday)

Sex and Height	n	N	$\bar{X}$	s	$s_{\bar{x}}$	Percentile 5th	10th	25th	50th	75th	90th	95th
Male						In kilograms						
Under 130 cm	–	–	–	–	–	–	–	–	–	–	–	–
130.0–134.9 cm	2	5	*	*	*	*	*	*	*	*	*	*
135.0–139.9 cm	6	25	32.62	5.624	7.716	27.2	27.6	28.9	31.0	34.9	43.1	43.2
140.0–144.9 cm	18	56	36.54	5.852	1.607	30.0	30.5	32.1	36.1	39.2	41.7	53.2
145.0–149.9 cm	65	204	39.03	5.270	0.662	32.4	33.9	36.1	37.9	41.2	44.5	46.4
150.0–154.9 cm	99	312	42.58	6.724	0.865	34.8	36.2	37.9	41.0	45.5	49.4	61.0
155.0–159.9 cm	131	421	47.27	7.482	0.717	37.8	39.2	41.7	45.8	51.1	58.7	61.7
160.0–164.9 cm	125	393	53.01	9.324	0.916	41.5	43.7	46.9	50.4	58.2	64.4	72.5
165.0–169.9 cm	91	285	55.92	8.560	0.833	46.3	47.5	49.3	53.6	59.4	69.0	75.0
170.0–174.9 cm	63	215	62.01	10.362	1.033	51.2	51.6	53.7	60.1	67.0	76.0	85.0
175.0–179.9 cm	19	68	67.92	12.085	3.428	56.3	57.9	60.1	63.3	70.3	88.3	89.0
180.0–184.9 cm	5	15	*	*	*	*	*	*	*	*	*	*
185.0–189.9 cm	–	–	–	–	–	–	–	–	–	–	–	–
190.0–194.9 cm	–	–	–	–	–	–	–	–	–	–	–	–
195.0 cm. and over	–	–	–	–	–	–	–	–	–	–	–	–
Female												
Under 130 cm	–	–	–	–	–	–	–	–	–	–	–	–
130.0–134.9 cm	1	3	*	*	*	*	*	*	*	*	*	*
135.0–139.9 cm	–	–	–	–	–	–	–	–	–	–	–	–
140.0–144.9 cm	15	51	37.13	7.317	2.259	26.6	27.5	30.5	36.7	40.1	44.5	56.1
145.0–149.9 cm	47	165	42.23	6.880	0.888	34.7	35.6	38.2	40.5	44.2	53.6	57.6
150.0–154.9 cm	98	329	44.32	7.029	0.787	35.6	36.5	39.2	42.9	47.3	53.7	57.9
155.0–159.9 cm	152	499	49.75	8.757	0.699	39.1	39.9	43.8	48.4	53.8	61.0	65.9
160.0–164.9 cm	156	515	53.16	8.399	0.522	41.2	43.9	47.7	52.2	57.0	63.8	68.5
165.0–169.9 cm	86	284	58.17	9.125	0.921	46.2	47.4	52.2	58.1	61.5	69.3	76.2
170.0–174.9 cm	24	87	58.11	13.209	2.343	46.2	47.1	48.4	52.9	65.3	68.6	96.8
175.0–179.9 cm	3	10	*	*	*	*	*	*	*	*	*	*
180.0–184.9 cm	–	–	–	–	–	–	–	–	–	–	–	–
185.0–189.9 cm	–	–	–	–	–	–	–	–	–	–	–	–
190.0–194.9 cm	–	–	–	–	–	–	–	–	–	–	–	–
195.0 cm. and over	–	–	–	–	–	–	–	–	–	–	–	–

* From National Center for Health Statistics: Height and Weight of Youths 12–17 Years, United States. *In* Vital and Health Statistics, Series 11, no. 124. Health Services and Mental Health Administration. Washington, DC, US Government Printing Office, 1973.

NOTE: n = sample size; N = estimated number of youths in population in thousands; $\bar{X}$ = mean; s = standard deviation; $s_{\bar{x}}$ = *standard error of the mean.*

APPENDIX 16. Percentiles for Weight for Height of Youths Aged 12 to 17 Years* *Continued*
(Weight in Kg of Youths Aged 14 Years at Last Birthday)

Sex and Height	n	N	$\bar{X}$	s	$s_{\bar{x}}$	5th	10th	25th	50th	75th	90th	95th
						Percentile						
						In kilograms						
Male												
Under 130 cm	–	–	–	–	–	–	–	–	–	–	–	–
130.0–134.9 cm	–	–	–	–	–	–	–	–	–	–	–	–
135.0–139.9 cm	2	7	*	*	*	*	*	*	*	*	*	*
140.0–144.9 cm	3	13	*	*	*	*	*	*	*	*	*	*
145.0–149.9 cm	11	42	40.51	1.829	0.644	36.9	38.6	39.6	40.6	42.0	42.5	42.7
150.0–154.9 cm	45	135	43.63	6.277	1.182	36.2	37.0	39.0	41.4	48.0	51.7	55.3
155.0–159.9 cm	83	261	47.42	7.822	0.872	37.7	38.7	41.8	46.1	51.2	58.0	62.7
160.0–164.9 cm	96	299	52.28	6.785	0.584	42.5	44.0	47.5	52.1	56.3	61.5	65.1
165.0–169.9 cm	134	432	58.07	9.416	1.054	47.7	49.3	51.6	55.4	62.3	70.6	75.7
170.0–174.9 cm	144	435	62.37	11.516	1.095	49.7	51.0	55.0	59.4	65.6	79.2	86.3
175.0–179.9 cm	71	228	65.54	9.704	1.306	50.9	55.1	58.5	64.7	69.9	74.5	84.0
180.0–184.9 cm	25	81	72.44	13.014	2.298	59.6	60.0	65.1	69.4	77.0	83.0	94.3
185.0–189.9 cm	3	9	*	*	*	*	*	*	*	*	*	*
190.0–194.9 cm	1	3	*	*	*	*	*	*	*	*	*	*
195.0 cm. and over	–	–	–	–	–	–	–	–	–	–	–	–
Female												
Under 130 cm	–	–	–	–	–	–	–	–	–	–	–	–
130.0–134.9 cm	–	–	–	–	–	–	–	–	–	–	–	–
135.0–139.9 cm	1	2	*	*	*	*	*	*	*	*	*	*
140.0–144.9 cm	2	6	*	*	*	*	*	*	*	*	*	*
145.0–149.9 cm	17	52	42.00	5.879	1.683	32.0	35.3	36.3	42.3	47.5	49.5	51.1
150.0–154.9 cm	64	196	48.26	6.797	0.926	37.7	39.2	42.5	47.9	53.3	55.9	58.8
155.0–159.9 cm	157	508	51.35	7.705	0.520	41.2	43.4	46.3	49.6	55.6	62.2	64.3
160.0–164.9 cm	186	603	54.59	8.810	0.707	43.0	45.0	48.4	53.0	59.7	66.7	70.7
165.0–169.9 cm	114	372	58.46	10.185	0.955	45.9	47.5	52.1	56.8	61.8	70.5	76.4
170.0–174.9 cm	36	121	64.37	15.821	2.814	49.2	52.1	56.2	59.8	70.5	72.9	99.4
175.0–179.9 cm	7	28	61.33	5.496	2.620	51.7	52.0	57.7	59.8	64.6	70.2	70.6
180.0–184.9 cm	2	7	*	*	*	*	*	*	*	*	*	*
185.0–189.9 cm	–	–	–	–	–	–	–	–	–	–	–	–
190.0–194.9 cm	–	–	–	–	–	–	–	–	–	–	–	–
195.0 cm. and over	–	–	–	–	–	–	–	–	–	–	–	–

* From National Center for Health Statistics: Height and Weight of Youths 12–17 Years, United States. *In* Vital and Health Statistics, Series 11, no. 124. Health Services and Mental Health Administration. Washington, DC, US Government Printing Office, 1973.

NOTE: *n* = sample size; *N* = estimated number of youths in population in thousands; $\bar{X}$ = mean; *s* = standard deviation; $s_{\bar{x}}$ = *standard error of the mean.*

Table continued on following page

APPENDIX 16. Percentiles for Weight for Height of Youths Aged 12 to 17 Years* *Continued*
(Weight in Kg of Youths Aged 15 Years at Last Birthday)

Sex and Height	n	N	$\bar{X}$	s	$s_{\bar{x}}$	5th	10th	25th	50th	75th	90th	95th
						Percentile						
Male						In kilograms						
Under 130 cm	–	–	–	–	–	–	–	–	–	–	–	–
130.0–134.9 cm	–	–	–	–	–	–	–	–	–	–	–	–
135.0–139.9 cm	–	–	–	–	–	–	–	–	–	–	–	–
140.0–144.9 cm	–	–	–	–	–	–	–	–	–	–	–	–
145.0–149.9 cm	1	2	*	*	*	*	*	*	*	*	*	*
150.0–154.9 cm	10	30	45.72	8.582	3.550	35.7	39.2	42.6	44.7	46.0	48.7	76.1
155.0–159.9 cm	34	99	52.81	10.552	1.695	40.3	43.1	46.7	49.2	56.7	69.6	76.3
160.0–164.9 cm	71	206	53.01	8.417	0.986	42.7	44.1	46.9	51.5	56.3	65.3	68.8
165.0–169.9 cm	132	404	57.72	8.503	0.819	48.0	48.8	53.1	56.4	61.3	67.1	73.3
170.0–174.9 cm	176	574	62.88	8.464	0.633	51.6	53.4	56.7	61.9	67.2	72.9	78.1
175.0–179.9 cm	118	374	65.80	9.457	1.045	53.1	55.6	59.7	64.3	69.5	80.2	89.2
180.0–184.9 cm	51	144	72.00	11.928	1.724	54.6	60.3	64.4	70.2	78.4	84.4	96.6
185.0–189.9 cm	14	48	74.21	15.035	5.200	58.3	58.5	62.9	70.7	84.6	92.4	110.8
190.0–194.9 cm	6	15	83.39	16.431	10.332	66.4	66.7	69.6	73.8	103.0	105.7	106.2
195.0 cm. and over	–	–	–	–	–	–	–	–	–	–	–	–
Female												
Under 130 cm	–	–	–	–	–	–	–	–	–	–	–	–
130.0–134.9 cm	–	–	–	–	–	–	–	–	–	–	–	–
135.0–139.9 cm	–	–	–	–	–	–	–	–	–	–	–	–
140.0–144.9 cm	2	5	*	*	*	*	*	*	*	*	*	*
145.0–149.9 cm	15	51	47.91	7.875	3.623	36.0	39.4	42.1	45.4	52.7	55.7	66.3
150.0–154.9 cm	69	242	49.69	8.895	1.190	39.1	40.6	44.3	48.1	52.8	60.5	68.3
155.0–159.9 cm	111	400	51.52	8.473	0.934	41.4	43.5	46.3	50.8	55.1	59.8	65.2
160.0–164.9 cm	137	509	57.03	10.828	0.875	45.1	47.3	50.2	55.0	60.2	71.7	77.7
165.0–169.9 cm	109	398	60.71	10.357	1.053	47.5	49.3	55.1	58.4	65.7	74.1	81.0
170.0–174.9 cm	49	188	65.27	10.730	1.880	49.7	53.6	57.2	61.2	71.6	85.3	86.4
175.0–179.9 cm	7	23	63.30	8.872	4.807	49.7	49.9	53.8	62.4	71.1	71.9	79.2
180.0–184.9 cm	3	26	*	*	*	*	*	*	*	*	*	*
185.0–189.9 cm	1	3	*	*	*	*	*	*	*	*	*	*
190.0–194.9 cm	–	–	–	–	–	–	–	–	–	–	–	–
195.0 cm. and over	–	–	–	–	–	–	–	–	–	–	–	–

* From National Center for Health Statistics: Height and Weight of Youths 12–17 Years, United States. *In* Vital and Health Statistics, Series 11, no. 124. Health Services and Mental Health Administration. Washington, DC, US Government Printing Office, 1973.
NOTE: n = sample size; N = estimated number of youths in population in thousands; $\bar{X}$ = mean; s = standard deviation; $s_{\bar{x}}$ = *standard error of the mean.*

APPENDIX 16. Percentiles for Weight for Height of Youths Aged 12 to 17 Years* *Continued*
(Weight in Kg of Youths Aged 16 Years at Last Birthday)

Sex and Height	n	N	$\bar{X}$	s	$s_{\bar{x}}$	5th	10th	25th	50th	75th	90th	95th
						Percentile						
Male						In kilograms						
Under 130 cm	–	–	–	–	–	–	–	–	–	–	–	–
130.0–134.9 cm	–	–	–	–	–	–	–	–	–	–	–	–
135.0–139.9 cm	–	–	–	–	–	–	–	–	–	–	–	–
140.0–144.9 cm	–	–	–	–	–	–	–	–	–	–	–	–
145.0–149.9 cm	1	1	*	*	*	*	*	*	*	*	*	*
150.0–154.9 cm	4	12	*	*	*	*	*	*	*	*	*	*
155.0–159.9 cm	11	33	49.89	7.323	3.572	42.0	42.2	44.7	46.8	54.4	59.8	67.2
160.0–164.9 cm	32	108	53.09	6.459	1.273	44.2	44.9	48.2	51.4	58.0	60.9	66.1
165.0–169.9 cm	87	275	59.39	9.178	0.981	48.5	49.8	52.7	58.0	63.9	69.3	75.9
170.0–174.9 cm	166	552	62.66	7.556	0.629	51.6	53.8	57.5	61.6	67.1	73.1	78.0
175.0–179.9 cm	149	511	67.33	9.018	0.856	56.3	58.2	61.0	65.4	72.5	80.1	83.8
180.0–184.9 cm	72	227	72.38	12.485	1.993	58.3	59.3	64.4	68.9	76.5	90.2	96.9
185.0–189.9 cm	29	95	81.06	14.268	3.265	63.7	66.6	69.7	78.4	90.3	97.0	111.4
190.0–194.9 cm	3	10	*	*	*	*	*	*	*	*	*	*
195.0 cm. and over	2	7	*	*	*	*	*	*	*	*	*	*
Female												
Under 130 cm	–	–	–	–	–	–	–	–	–	–	–	–
130.0–134.9 cm	–	–	–	–	–	–	–	–	–	–	–	–
135.0–139.9 cm	–	–	–	–	–	–	–	–	–	–	–	–
140.0–144.9 cm	2	5	*	*	*	*	*	*	*	*	*	*
145.0–149.9 cm	10	33	52.58	8.198	3.191	43.9	44.1	44.9	51.0	54.5	72.0	72.1
150.0–154.9 cm	57	178	51.79	10.457	1.053	41.4	42.0	45.8	48.9	54.1	61.5	83.3
155.0–159.9 cm	117	354	53.20	7.766	0.734	44.0	45.6	48.4	51.6	56.4	61.9	69.0
160.0–164.9 cm	160	547	57.71	11.129	1.246	46.1	47.3	51.5	55.5	61.2	69.5	75.1
165.0–169.9 cm	122	450	61.72	11.998	0.802	47.1	48.8	53.3	59.1	67.3	78.7	86.7
170.0–174.9 cm	53	170	63.61	8.734	1.126	52.9	53.8	58.1	62.1	66.8	73.8	84.2
175.0–179.9 cm	14	45	72.55	15.012	5.224	58.6	58.8	61.7	65.9	80.6	99.1	105.5
180.0–184.9 cm	1	2	*	*	*	*	*	*	*	*	*	*
185.0–189.9 cm	–	–	–	–	–	–	–	–	–	–	–	–
190.0–194.9 cm	–	–	–	–	–	–	–	–	–	–	–	–
195.0 cm. and over	–	–	–	–	–	–	–	–	–	–	–	–

* From National Center for Health Statistics: Height and Weight of Youths 12–17 Years, United States. *In* Vital and Health Statistics, Series 11, no. 124. Health Services and Mental Health Administration. Washington, DC, US Government Printing Office, 1973.

NOTE: n = sample size; N = estimated number of youths in population in thousands; $\bar{X}$ = mean; s = standard deviation; $s_{\bar{x}}$ = *standard error of the mean.*

Table continued on following page

APPENDIX 16. Percentiles for Weight for Height of Youths Aged 12 to 17 Years* *Continued*
(Weight in Kg of Youths Aged 17 Years at Last Birthday)

Sex and Height	n	N	$\bar{X}$	s	$s_{\bar{x}}$	5th	10th	25th	50th	75th	90th	95th
						Percentile						
Male						In kilograms						
Under 130 cm	–	–	–	–	–	–	–	–	–	–	–	–
130.0–134.9 cm	–	–	–	–	–	–	–	–	–	–	–	–
135.0–139.9 cm	–	–	–	–	–	–	–	–	–	–	–	–
140.0–144.9 cm	–	–	–	–	–	–	–	–	–	–	–	–
145.0–149.9 cm	–	–	–	–	–	–	–	–	–	–	–	–
150.0–154.9 cm	1	3	*	*	*	*	*	*	*	*	*	*
155.0–159.9 cm	11	39	54.63	9.397	3.414	43.8	46.4	48.2	49.7	57.8	69.9	73.2
160.0–164.9 cm	25	81	57.75	6.503	1.355	49.7	51.1	52.5	56.9	61.6	70.1	70.8
165.0–169.9 cm	63	248	62.57	8.344	1.224	50.2	53.2	56.4	61.5	66.9	72.7	77.3
170.0–174.9 cm	115	396	67.06	11.163	0.704	53.3	55.5	59.5	64.6	71.9	80.9	91.6
175.0–179.9 cm	151	537	68.37	9.907	0.831	56.9	58.9	61.5	66.5	73.6	79.4	88.4
180.0–184.9 cm	80	297	73.31	12.454	1.335	59.6	61.0	65.1	71.2	78.4	91.8	102.7
185.0–189.9 cm	36	133	76.03	9.171	1.301	62.4	66.3	70.5	75.3	80.8	90.3	92.9
190.0–194.9 cm	7	25	81.40	10.985	7.588	62.9	62.9	67.8	87.3	90.3	90.6	90.6
195.0 cm. and over	–	–	–	–	–	–	–	–	–	–	–	–
Female												
Under 130 cm	–	–	–	–	–	–	–	–	–	–	–	–
130.0–134.9 cm	–	–	–	–	–	–	–	–	–	–	–	–
135.0–139.9 cm	–	–	–	–	–	–	–	–	–	–	–	–
140.0–144.9 cm	2	5	*	*	*	*	*	*	*	*	*	*
145.0–149.9 cm	8	26	43.49	3.939	1.604	38.6	38.8	40.1	45.1	45.7	51.1	51.2
150.0–154.9 cm	43	151	49.96	6.508	0.827	41.6	42.3	44.6	48.9	53.5	59.2	64.1
155.0–159.9 cm	103	385	54.71	9.903	0.775	44.4	45.5	48.7	53.2	57.7	61.6	76.2
160.0–164.9 cm	133	506	57.79	10.620	1.028	46.8	48.0	50.2	55.4	61.5	72.3	82.3
165.0–169.9 cm	116	433	60.63	10.117	1.182	47.9	50.3	55.1	59.3	65.1	69.4	71.6
170.0–174.9 cm	51	186	62.18	9.132	1.407	50.6	52.9	55.5	60.2	65.7	76.1	82.7
175.0–179.9 cm	12	47	65.76	8.405	2.229	54.9	56.7	60.1	61.7	75.2	75.9	83.0
180.0–184.9 cm	1	2	*	*	*	*	*	*	*	*	*	*
185.0–189.9 cm	–	–	–	–	–	–	–	–	–	–	–	–
190.0–194.9 cm	–	–	–	–	–	–	–	–	–	–	–	–
195.0 cm. and over	–	–	–	–	–	–	–	–	–	–	–	–

* From National Center for Health Statistics: Height and Weight of Youths 12–17 Years, United States. *In* Vital and Health Statistics, Series 11, no. 124. Health Services and Mental Health Administration. Washington, DC, US Government Printing Office, 1973.

NOTE: n = sample size; N = estimated number of youths in population in thousands; $\bar{X}$ = mean; s = standard deviation; $s_{\bar{x}}$ = *standard error of the mean.*

APPENDIX 17. 1983 Metropolitan Height and Weight Tables*

Men					Women				
Height					*Height*				
Feet	Inches	*Small Frame*	*Medium Frame*	*Large Frame*	Feet	Inches	*Small Frame*	*Medium Frame*	*Large Frame*
5	2	128–134	131–141	138–150	4	10	102–111	109–121	118–131
5	3	130–136	133–143	140–153	4	11	103–113	111–123	120–134
5	4	132–138	135–145	142–156	5	0	104–115	113–126	122–137
5	5	134–140	137–148	144–160	5	1	106–118	115–129	125–140
5	6	136–142	139–151	146–164	5	2	108–121	118–132	128–143
5	7	138–145	142–154	149–168	5	3	111–124	121–135	131–147
5	8	140–148	145–157	152–172	5	4	114–127	124–138	134–151
5	9	142–151	148–160	155–176	5	5	117–130	127–141	137–155
5	10	144–154	151–163	158–180	5	6	120–133	130–144	140–159
5	11	146–157	154–166	161–184	5	7	123–136	133–147	143–163
6	0	149–160	157–170	164–188	5	8	126–139	136–150	146–167
6	1	152–164	160–174	168–192	5	9	129–142	139–153	149–170
6	2	155–168	164–178	172–197	5	10	132–145	142–156	152–173
6	3	158–172	167–182	176–202	5	11	135–148	145–159	155–176
6	4	162–176	171–187	181–207	6	0	138–151	148–162	158–179

* Source of basic data *1979 Build Study,* Society of Actuaries and Association of Life Insurance Medical Directors of America. Courtesy of the Metropolitan Life Insurance Company, 1983.

Weights for adults aged 25 to 59 years based on lowest mortality. For determination of frame size see Appendix 18. Weight in pounds according to frame size in indoor clothing (5 pounds for men and 3 pounds for women) wearing shoes with 1-inch heels.

APPENDIX 18. Determination of Frame Size

Method 1*

Height is recorded without shoes on.

Wrist circumference is measured just distal to the styloid process at the wrist crease on the right arm using a tape measure.

The following formula is used:

$$r = \frac{\text{Height (cm.)}}{\text{Wrist circumference (cm.)}}$$

Frame size can be determined as follows:

Males	*Females*
$r > 10.4$ small	$r > 11.0$ small
$r = 9.6–10.4$ medium	$r = 10.1–11.0$ medium
$r < 9.6$ large	$r < 10.1$ large

Method 2†

The patient's right arm is extended forward perpendicular to the body, with the arm bent so the angle at the elbow forms 90° with the fingers pointing up and the palm turned away from the body. The greatest breadth across the elbow joint is measured with a sliding caliper along the axis of the upper arm, on the two prominent bones on either side of the elbow. This is recorded as the elbow breadth. The following tables give the elbow breadth measurements for medium-framed men and women of various heights. Measurements lower than those listed indicate a small frame size; higher measurements indicate a large frame size.

Men		*Women*	
Height in 1" Heels	**Elbow Breadth**	**Height in 1" Heels**	**Elbow Breadth**
5'2"–5'3"	2½"–2⅞"	4'10"–4'11"	2¼"–2½"
5'4"–5'7"	2⅝"–2⅞"	5'0"–5'3"	2¼"–2½"
5'8"–5'11"	2¾"–3"	5'4"–5'7"	2⅜"–2⅝"
6'0"–6'3"	2¾"–3⅛"	5'8"–5'11"	2⅜"–2⅝"
6'4"	2⅞"–3¼"	6'0"	2½"–2¾"

* From Grant JP: Handbook of Total Parenteral Nutrition. Philadelphia, WB Saunders, 1980, p 15.

† From Metropolitan Life Insurance Co, 1983.

APPENDIX 19. Determination of Body Mass Index (BMI)

Body Weights in Pounds According to Height and Body Mass Index*†‡

Height (in)	Body Mass Index (kg/m²)													
	19.0	*20.0*	*21.0*	*22.0*	*23.0*	*24.0*	*25.0*	*26.0*	*27.0*	*28.0*	*29.0*	*30.0*	*35.0*	*40.0*
	Body Weight (lb)													
58.0	90.7	95.5	100.3	105.0	109.8	114.6	119.4	124.1	128.9	133.7	138.5	143.2	167.1	191.0
59.0	93.9	98.8	103.8	108.7	113.6	118.6	123.5	128.5	133.4	138.3	143.3	148.2	172.9	197.6
60.0	97.1	102.2	107.3	112.4	117.5	122.6	127.7	132.9	138.0	143.1	148.2	153.3	178.8	204.4
61.0	100.3	105.6	110.9	116.2	121.5	126.8	132.0	137.3	142.6	147.9	153.2	158.4	184.8	211.3
62.0	103.7	109.1	114.6	120.0	125.5	130.9	136.4	141.9	147.3	152.8	158.2	163.7	191.0	218.2
63.0	107.0	112.7	118.3	123.9	129.6	135.2	140.8	146.5	152.1	157.7	163.4	169.0	197.2	225.3
64.0	110.5	116.3	122.1	127.9	133.7	139.5	145.3	151.2	157.0	162.8	168.6	174.4	203.5	232.5
65.0	113.9	119.9	125.9	131.9	137.9	143.9	149.9	155.9	161.9	167.9	173.9	179.9	209.9	239.9
66.0	117.5	123.7	129.8	136.0	142.2	148.4	154.6	160.8	166.9	173.1	179.3	185.5	216.4	247.3
67.0	121.1	127.4	133.8	140.2	146.5	152.9	159.3	165.7	172.0	178.4	184.8	191.1	223.0	254.9
68.0	124.7	131.3	137.8	144.4	151.0	157.5	164.1	170.6	177.2	183.8	190.3	196.9	229.7	262.5
69.0	128.4	135.2	141.9	148.7	155.4	162.2	168.9	175.7	182.5	189.2	196.0	202.7	236.5	270.3
70.0	132.1	139.1	146.1	153.0	160.0	166.9	173.9	180.8	187.8	194.7	201.7	208.6	243.4	278.2
71.0	135.9	143.1	150.3	157.4	164.6	171.7	178.9	186.0	193.2	200.3	207.5	214.6	250.4	286.2
72.0	139.8	147.2	154.5	161.9	169.2	176.6	183.9	191.3	198.7	206.0	213.4	220.7	257.5	294.3
73.0	143.7	151.3	158.8	166.4	174.0	181.5	189.1	196.7	204.2	211.8	219.3	226.9	264.7	302.5
74.0	147.7	155.4	163.2	171.0	178.8	186.5	194.3	202.1	209.9	217.6	225.4	233.2	272.0	310.9
75.0	151.7	159.7	167.7	175.6	183.6	191.6	199.6	207.6	215.6	223.5	231.5	239.5	279.4	319.4
76.0	155.8	164.0	172.2	180.4	188.6	196.8	205.0	213.2	221.4	229.5	237.7	245.9	286.9	327.9

Body Weights in Kilograms According to Height and Body Mass Index†‡

Height (cm)	Body Mass Index (kg/m²)													
	19.0	*20.0*	*21.0*	*22.0*	*23.0*	*24.0*	*25.0*	*26.0*	*27.0*	*28.0*	*29.0*	*30.0*	*35.0*	*40.0*
	Body Weight (kg)													
140.0	37.2	39.2	41.2	43.1	45.1	47.0	49.0	51.0	52.9	54.9	56.8	58.8	68.6	78.4
142.0	38.3	40.3	42.3	44.4	46.4	48.4	50.4	52.4	54.4	56.5	58.5	60.5	70.6	80.7
144.0	39.4	41.5	43.5	45.6	47.7	49.8	51.8	53.9	56.0	58.1	60.1	62.2	72.6	82.9
146.0	40.5	42.6	44.8	46.9	49.0	51.2	53.3	55.4	57.6	59.7	61.8	63.9	74.6	85.3
148.0	41.6	43.8	46.0	48.2	50.4	52.6	54.8	57.0	59.1	61.3	63.5	65.7	76.7	87.6
150.0	42.8	45.0	47.3	49.5	51.8	54.0	56.3	58.5	60.8	63.0	65.3	67.5	78.8	90.0
152.0	43.9	46.2	48.5	50.8	53.1	55.4	57.8	60.1	62.4	64.7	67.0	69.3	80.9	92.4
154.0	45.1	47.4	49.8	52.2	54.5	56.9	59.3	61.7	64.0	66.4	68.8	71.1	83.0	94.9
156.0	46.2	48.7	51.1	53.5	56.0	58.4	60.8	63.3	65.7	68.1	70.6	73.0	85.2	97.3
158.0	47.4	49.9	52.4	54.9	57.4	59.9	62.4	64.9	67.4	69.9	72.4	74.9	87.4	99.9
160.0	48.6	51.2	53.8	56.3	58.9	61.4	64.0	66.6	69.1	71.7	74.2	76.8	89.6	102.4
162.0	49.9	52.5	55.1	57.7	60.4	63.0	65.6	68.2	70.9	73.5	76.1	78.7	91.9	105.0
164.0	51.1	53.8	56.5	59.2	61.9	64.6	67.2	69.9	72.6	75.3	78.0	80.7	94.1	107.6
166.0	52.4	55.1	57.9	60.6	63.4	66.1	68.9	71.6	74.4	77.2	79.9	82.7	96.4	110.2
168.0	53.6	56.4	59.3	62.1	64.9	67.7	70.6	73.4	76.2	79.0	81.8	84.7	98.8	112.9
170.0	54.9	57.8	60.7	63.6	66.5	69.4	72.3	75.1	78.0	80.9	83.8	86.7	101.2	115.6
172.0	56.2	59.2	62.1	65.1	68.0	71.0	74.0	76.9	79.9	82.8	85.8	88.8	103.5	118.3
174.0	57.5	60.6	63.6	66.6	69.6	72.7	75.7	78.7	81.7	84.8	87.8	90.8	106.0	121.1
176.0	58.9	62.0	65.0	68.1	71.2	74.3	77.4	80.5	83.6	86.7	89.8	92.9	108.4	123.9
178.0	60.2	63.4	66.5	69.7	72.9	76.0	79.2	82.4	85.5	88.7	91.9	95.1	110.9	126.7
180.0	61.6	64.8	68.0	71.3	74.5	77.8	81.0	84.2	87.5	90.7	94.0	97.2	113.4	129.6
182.0	62.9	66.2	69.6	72.9	76.2	79.5	82.8	86.1	89.4	92.7	96.1	99.4	115.9	132.5
184.0	64.3	67.7	71.1	74.5	77.9	81.3	84.6	88.0	91.4	94.8	98.2	101.6	118.5	135.4
186.0	65.7	69.2	72.7	76.1	79.6	83.0	86.5	89.9	93.4	96.9	100.3	103.8	121.1	138.4
188.0	67.2	70.7	74.2	77.8	81.3	84.8	88.4	91.9	95.4	99.0	102.5	106.0	123.7	141.4
190.0	68.6	72.2	75.8	79.4	83.0	86.6	90.3	93.9	97.5	101.1	104.7	108.3	126.4	144.4
192.0	70.0	73.7	77.4	81.1	84.8	88.5	92.2	95.8	99.5	103.2	106.9	110.6	129.0	147.5
194.0	71.5	75.3	79.0	82.8	86.6	90.3	94.1	97.9	101.6	105.4	109.1	112.9	131.7	150.5
196.0	73.0	76.8	80.7	84.5	88.4	92.2	96.0	99.9	103.7	107.6	111.4	115.2	134.5	153.7
198.0	74.5	78.4	82.3	86.2	90.2	94.1	98.0	101.9	105.9	109.8	113.7	117.6	137.2	156.8
200.0	76.0	80.0	84.0	88.0	92.0	96.0	100.0	104.0	108.0	112.0	116.0	120.0	140.0	160.0

Age Group (yr)	Body Mass Index (kg/m²)
19–24	19–24
25–34	20–25
35–44	21–26

Age Group (yr)	Body Mass Index (kg/m²)
45–54	22–27
55–64	23–28
65+	24–29

* From Bray GA and Gray DS: Obesity. Part 1: Pathogenesis. West J Med 149:431, 1988.

† Each entry gives the body weight in kilograms (kg) for a person of a given height and body mass index.

‡ Desirable body mass index range in relation to age.

APPENDIX 20. Nomogram for Determining Abdominal/ Gluteal Circumference Ratio (Waist/Hip Ratio)

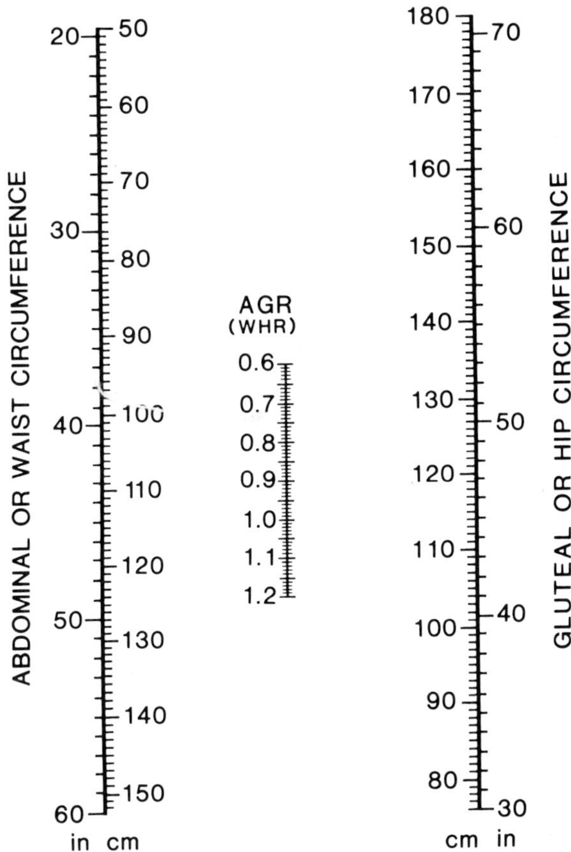

Nomogram for determining the ratio of abdominal (waist) circumference to gluteal (hips) circumference. Place a straight edge between the column for waist circumference and the column for hip circumference and read the ratio from the point where this straight edge crosses the AGR or WHR line. The waist or abdominal circumference is the smallest circumference below the rib cage and above the umbilicus, and the hips or gluteal circumference is taken as the largest circumference at the posterior extension of the buttocks. (From Bray GA: Overweight is risking fate. Definition, classification, prevalence and risks. Ann NY Acad Sci 249:14, 1987. (Copyright 1988, George A. Bray, M.D. Used with permission.)

APPENDIX 21. Arm Anthropometry for Children*

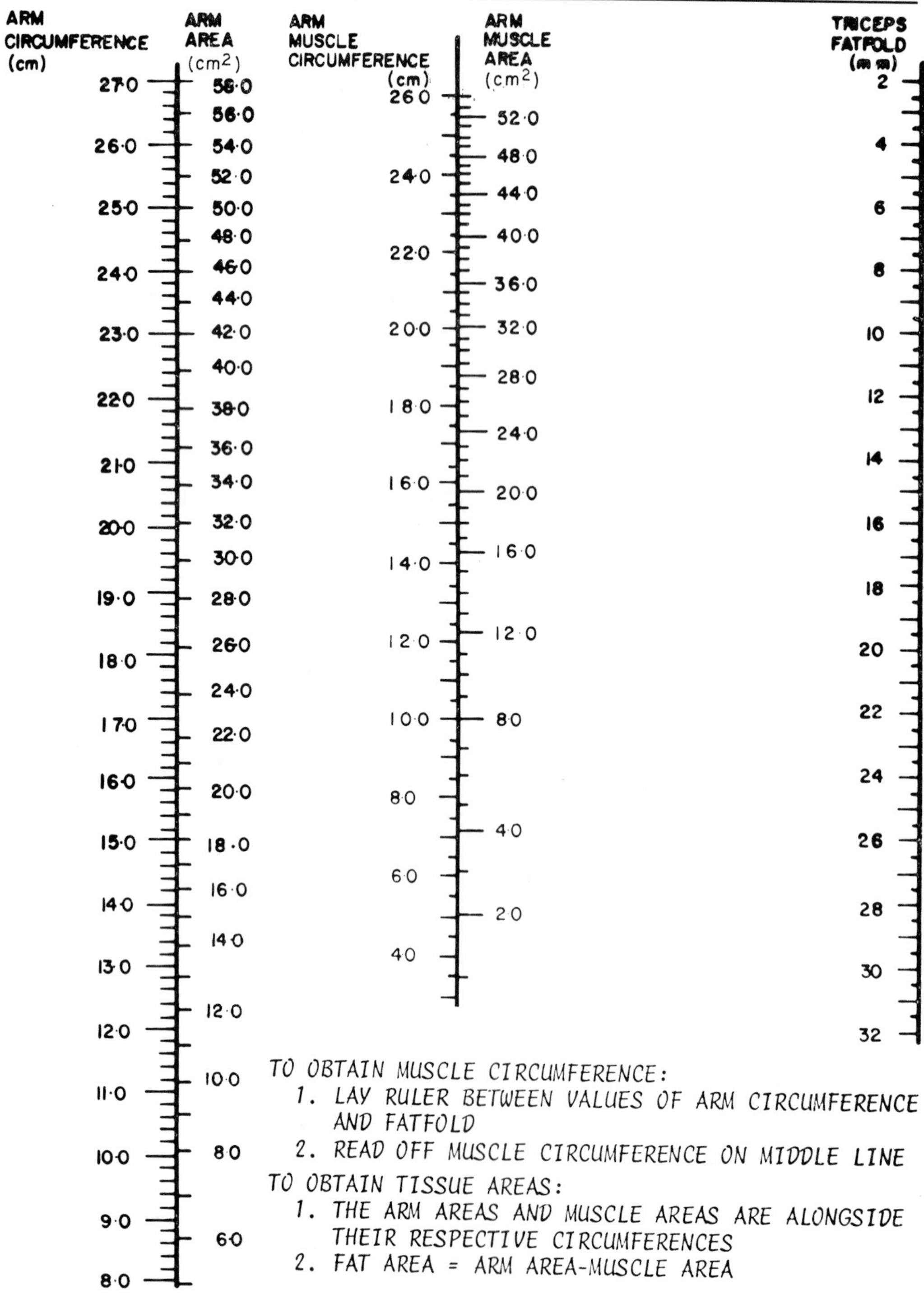

* From Gurney JM and Jelliffe DB: Arm anthropometry in nutritional assessment: Nomogram for rapid calculation of muscle circumference and cross-sectional muscle fat areas. Am J Clin Nutr 26:913, 1973.

APPENDIX 22. Arm Anthropometry for Adults*

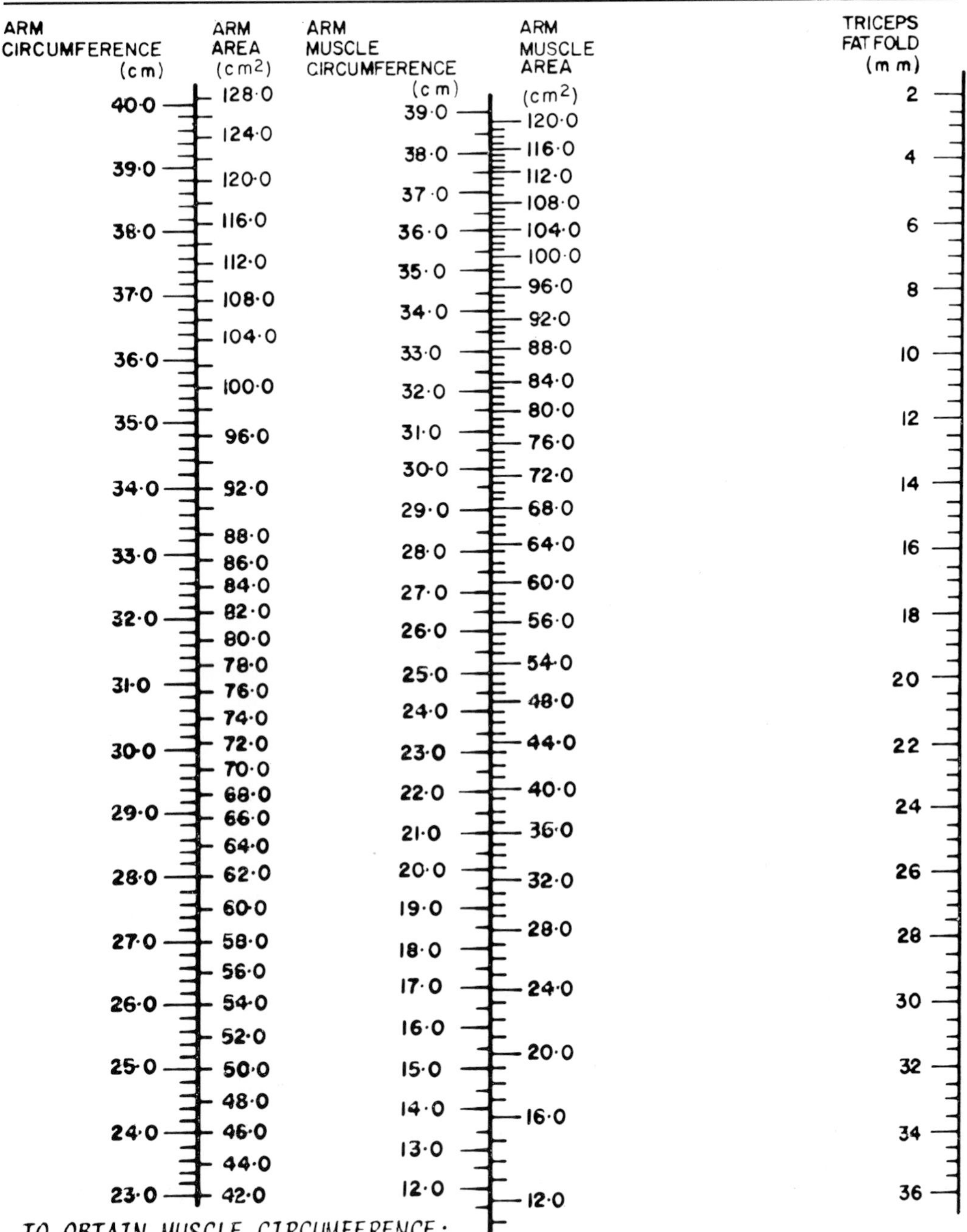

TO OBTAIN MUSCLE CIRCUMFERENCE:

1. LAY RULER BETWEEN VALUE OF ARM CIRCUMFERENCE AND FATFOLD
2. READ OFF MUSCLE CIRCUMFERENCE ON MIDDLE LINE

TO OBTAIN TISSUE AREAS:

1. THE ARM AREA AND MUSCLE AREA ARE ALONGSIDE THEIR RESPECTIVE CIRCUMFERENCES
2. FAT AREA = ARM AREA-MUSCLE AREA

* From Gurney JM and Jelliffe DB: Arm anthropometry in nutritional assessment: Nomogram for rapid calculation of muscle circumference and cross-sectional muscle fat areas. Am J Clin Nutr 26:913, 1973.

APPENDIX 23. Triceps Skinfold Thickness: Youth, 1–17 Years, United States: 1971 to 1974*

Race and Age in Years	No. in Sample	Estimated Population in Thousands	Mean	Standard Deviation	Percentile								
					5th	*10th*	*15th*	*25th*	*50th*	*75th*	*85th*	*90th*	*95th*
					Triceps Skinfold in Millimeters								
					Males								
White													
1	211	1,402	10.7	3.0	7.0	7.0	7.5	8.0	10.0	12.0	14.0	15.0	16.5
2	217	1,461	9.9	2.6	6.0	6.5	7.0	8.0	10.0	12.0	12.5	13.0	14.7
3	226	1,536	9.9	2.6	6.5	7.0	7.0	8.0	10.0	11.0	12.5	13.5	14.5
4	229	1,547	9.6	2.4	6.0	7.0	7.0	8.0	10.0	11.0	12.0	12.5	14.0
5	207	1,319	9.8	3.2	6.0	6.5	7.0	7.5	9.0	11.0	12.5	13.5	15.0
6	126	1,343	8.9	3.1	5.5	5.6	6.0	7.0	9.0	10.0	12.0	12.5	14.0
7	125	1,718	9.1	3.5	5.0	6.0	6.0	7.0	8.0	10.5	12.0	13.5	17.0
8	116	1,644	9.1	3.3	5.0	5.5	6.0	7.0	8.5	10.5	12.0	13.0	16.0
9	117	1,636	11.1	4.8	5.5	6.5	6.5	7.5	10.0	14.0	17.0	17.0	19.0
10	148	1,909	11.1	4.2	5.5	6.0	7.0	8.0	10.0	14.0	15.5	17.0	19.5
11	132	1,823	12.5	6.5	6.0	6.0	7.0	8.0	10.0	15.0	19.0	20.5	24.5
12	152	1,970	12.4	6.1	6.0	6.0	7.0	8.5	11.0	14.0	18.0	21.0	27.0
13	129	1,697	11.7	6.7	5.0	5.0	6.0	7.0	10.0	14.0	19.0	22.0	25.5
14	134	1,730	10.9	6.4	4.0	5.0	6.0	7.0	9.0	13.0	18.0	20.0	24.0
15	124	1,728	10.2	6.1	4.0	5.0	6.0	6.0	8.0	12.0	15.0	19.0	24.0
16	128	1,752	10.1	5.2	4.0	5.0	5.0	6.5	9.0	12.5	15.0	17.0	22.0
17	139	1,831	9.3	5.4	4.5	5.0	5.5	6.0	7.5	11.0	13.0	15.0	19.0
Black													
1	72	280	9.4	3.4	4.5	6.0	7.0	8.0	8.0	11.0	12.0	13.0	15.0
2	77	267	10.1	3.2	4.5	6.0	6.5	8.0	10.0	12.0	14.0	15.0	15.0
3	72	212	9.1	2.6	6.0	6.5	6.5	7.0	9.0	10.5	12.0	12.0	13.0
4	74	260	8.0	2.6	5.0	5.0	5.0	6.5	7.0	9.0	10.0	10.5	15.0
5	64	226	7.7	3.4	4.5	5.0	5.0	5.0	7.0	9.0	10.0	12.0	15.5
6	52	321	7.1	1.8	4.0	4.0	5.0	6.0	7.0	8.0	9.0	9.0	9.0
7	38	253	7.5	3.2	4.0	4.0	4.0	5.0	6.5	9.0	11.5	13.0	15.0
8	33	203	7.8	3.4	4.0	5.0	5.0	6.0	6.5	10.0	11.0	11.0	12.5
9	52	383	8.2	3.9	3.5	4.0	4.5	6.0	7.0	8.0	12.0	13.0	18.0
10	33	251	9.1	5.3	5.0	5.0	6.0	6.0	7.5	10.0	13.0	15.0	20.0
11	43	313	8.0	5.0	4.0	4.0	5.0	5.0	6.0	8.5	11.0	12.0	15.0
12	47	316	9.4	7.0	4.0	4.0	4.5	6.0	7.5	10.7	11.0	15.0	24.0
13	45	281	8.2	4.4	4.0	5.0	5.0	5.0	7.0	8.5	11.0	19.0	19.0
14	39	282	6.6	2.6	3.5	3.5	3.5	5.0	6.5	7.0	8.0	9.0	12.0
15	43	310	8.9	6.1	4.0	4.5	5.0	5.0	6.5	9.0	10.0	21.0	21.0
16	41	267	7.2	4.8	4.0	4.0	4.0	5.0	6.0	7.5	8.0	11.0	15.0
17	35	235	8.7	5.8	3.5	3.5	5.0	5.0	7.0	10.5	12.0	12.0	23.2

APPENDIX 23. Triceps Skinfold Thickness: Youth, 1–17 Years, United States: 1971 to 1974* *Continued*

Race and Age in Years	No. in Sample	Estimated Population in Thousands	Mean	Standard Deviation	Percentile								
					5th	*10th*	*15th*	*25th*	*50th*	*75th*	*85th*	*90th*	*95th*
					Triceps Skinfold in Millimeters								
					Females								
White													
1	189	1,328	10.2	2.8	6.0	7.0	7.0	8.0	10.0	12.0	13.0	13.5	15.5
2	203	1,434	10.6	2.6	7.0	7.5	8.0	9.0	10.0	12.0	13.5	14.0	15.0
3	211	1,438	11.1	2.6	7.0	8.0	8.5	9.0	11.0	13.0	13.5	14.0	15.0
4	204	1,339	10.8	2.6	7.5	8.0	8.0	9.0	10.5	12.0	13.0	14.5	16.0
5	224	1,416	10.7	3.7	6.0	7.0	8.0	8.5	10.0	12.0	13.0	15.0	17.5
6	125	1,445	10.6	3.3	6.5	7.0	7.5	8.0	10.5	12.0	13.0	14.0	16.0
7	122	1,507	10.9	4.2	4.0	6.0	7.0	8.0	11.0	12.0	15.0	15.5	17.5
8	117	1,507	12.4	4.7	7.0	8.0	8.0	9.0	11.5	15.0	16.5	18.0	22.0
9	129	1,751	13.6	4.6	7.5	8.0	9.0	10.0	13.0	16.0	18.0	20.0	22.0
10	148	1,855	13.4	4.8	7.5	8.0	8.5	10.0	12.5	15.5	19.0	20.0	23.0
11	122	1,569	14.9	6.1	8.0	8.5	9.0	10.0	13.0	17.5	20.5	24.5	28.5
12	128	1,506	15.2	5.6	8.0	9.0	10.0	11.0	14.0	18.5	20.0	23.0	26.0
13	153	1,886	16.2	6.8	7.0	8.0	10.0	11.5	15.0	20.0	24.0	25.0	28.5
14	132	1,731	17.8	7.3	9.0	9.5	10.5	13.0	16.7	21.0	24.0	28.5	33.0
15	125	1,752	17.7	6.7	9.0	10.5	11.0	13.0	17.0	21.0	24.0	25.0	28.5
16	141	1,933	18.2	6.6	10.0	10.5	12.5	14.0	17.0	21.0	24.0	26.0	32.1
17	117	1,549	19.8	8.0	10.0	12.0	12.5	13.5	19.0	24.0	26.5	29.5	35.0
					Females								
Black													
1	73	257	10.0	3.0	5.5	5.5	7.0	8.0	10.0	12.0	13.0	14.0	15.0
2	66	261	10.0	2.3	7.0	8.0	8.0	8.0	10.0	11.0	12.0	14.0	15.5
3	78	245	9.7	2.9	6.0	7.0	7.0	8.0	10.0	11.0	12.0	13.0	14.0
4	73	246	8.8	2.7	5.0	6.0	7.0	7.0	8.0	10.5	12.0	13.0	14.0
5	88	265	9.4	3.9	5.0	5.0	6.5	7.0	8.0	10.0	12.0	13.5	17.0
6	50	336	9.0	3.1	5.5	6.0	6.0	8.0	8.0	10.0	11.5	12.0	13.0
7	46	241	10.1	4.0	5.0	6.0	7.0	7.5	9.0	11.0	17.5	18.0	18.0
8	35	293	11.5	5.1	5.0	6.5	7.0	8.0	10.0	13.5	18.0	18.0	23.0
9	41	247	10.2	5.1	5.5	6.0	6.0	6.5	8.0	12.0	18.0	18.0	20.0
10	48	303	11.7	5.6	6.5	6.5	7.0	7.5	10.0	16.0	18.0	19.0	24.0
11	42	315	12.7	6.4	4.0	5.0	6.5	7.5	10.0	18.0	22.0	23.0	23.0
12	47	284	13.6	7.6	5.5	6.0	6.0	7.5	12.0	17.0	22.0	25.0	30.0
13	44	287	16.1	7.0	7.0	8.5	10.0	11.0	14.0	18.0	24.0	24.0	33.5
14	50	265	15.9	6.7	8.0	8.0	9.0	10.5	14.0	20.5	24.0	24.5	24.5
15	46	411	14.0	7.6	6.5	6.5	8.0	10.0	12.5	16.0	16.5	20.0	32.8
16	33	203	18.9	8.0	8.0	8.0	10.0	12.0	19.0	24.0	24.5	33.0	33.1
17	39	239	16.9	6.6	7.5	9.0	11.0	12.0	14.5	20.0	24.0	28.0	31.0

* From the National Center for Health Statistics, Department of Health and Human Services. Health and Nutrition Examination Survey I, 1971–1974.

APPENDIX 24. Triceps Skinfold Thickness: Adults, United States: 1971 to 1974*

Race and Age in Years	No. in Sample	Estimated Population in Thousands	Mean	Standard Deviation	Percentile								
					5th	*10th*	*15th*	*25th*	*50th*	*75th*	*85th*	*90th*	*95th*
					Triceps Skinfold in Millimeters								
					Males								
White													
	4,344	54,694	12.2	5.8	5.0	6.0	6.5	8.0	11.0	15.0	18.0	20.0	23.0
18–19	203	3,206	11.3	5.9	5.0	5.5	6.0	7.0	9.0	15.0	18.0	20.0	23.0
20–24	423	7,094	11.5	6.0	4.0	5.0	6.0	7.0	10.0	15.0	18.0	21.0	23.0
25–34	672	11,594	12.7	6.2	5.0	6.0	6.5	8.0	12.0	16.0	18.5	21.0	24.0
35–44	569	9,516	12.6	5.4	5.0	6.0	7.0	9.0	12.0	15.5	17.5	20.0	23.0
45–54	628	10,039	12.6	5.9	5.5	6.5	7.0	8.5	11.0	15.0	18.0	20.0	26.0
55–64	505	8,275	11.7	5.0	5.0	6.0	7.0	8.0	11.0	14.0	16.5	18.0	21.0
65–74	1,344	4,970	12.0	5.4	5.0	6.0	7.0	8.0	11.0	15.0	17.0	19.0	22.0
Black													
	847	5,753	10.6	7.0	3.5	4.0	4.5	6.0	8.5	13.0	16.0	20.0	23.0
18–19	52	404	8.9	6.7	2.0	4.0	5.0	5.1	7.0	8.0	12.0	21.0	24.0
20–24	80	866	10.0	7.9	3.0	4.0	4.0	6.0	8.0	11.0	13.0	18.0	24.0
25–34	119	1,232	11.8	8.4	4.0	4.0	4.0	5.0	10.0	15.0	20.0	22.0	23.0
35–44	87	1,005	11.3	6.5	4.0	4.5	5.0	7.0	10.0	14.0	17.0	18.4	22.0
45–54	130	1,057	10.0	5.1	4.0	4.0	5.0	6.0	10.0	12.5	14.0	16.0	20.0
55–64	85	703	10.7	7.2	3.0	4.0	4.5	5.0	8.0	14.0	20.0	22.0	26.0
65–74	294	486	9.7	5.4	4.0	4.5	5.0	6.0	9.0	12.0	14.0	15.0	19.5
					Females								
White													
	6,757	59,923	22.9	8.1	11.0	13.0	14.5	17.0	22.0	28.0	31.0	34.0	37.0
18–19	208	3,159	18.9	6.6	9.5	12.0	13.0	14.5	18.0	22.5	24.0	26.5	33.5
20–24	956	7,972	19.8	7.7	10.0	11.0	12.0	14.0	19.0	24.0	27.9	30.5	34.0
25–34	1,539	12,161	21.8	8.0	11.0	12.5	14.0	16.0	20.5	26.0	30.0	33.0	36.5
35–44	1,302	10,111	23.7	8.3	12.0	14.0	15.9	18.0	22.5	29.0	32.0	35.1	38.5
45–54	705	10,879	25.3	8.1	13.0	15.0	17.0	20.0	25.0	30.0	33.5	35.5	39.5
55–64	551	9,037	24.6	7.9	11.5	14.5	16.0	19.0	24.0	30.0	33.0	34.1	38.0
65–74	1,496	6,603	23.3	7.3	12.0	14.0	16.0	18.0	23.0	28.0	31.0	33.0	35.5
Black													
	1,557	7,302	23.7	10.3	9.0	11.0	12.0	15.5	23.0	30.5	34.0	36.6	41.0
18–19	70	504	16.2	7.3	8.0	9.0	9.0	11.5	14.0	20.0	25.0	29.0	32.0
20–24	259	1,073	19.3	8.7	9.0	10.0	11.5	12.5	17.0	24.5	28.6	32.0	36.0
25–34	335	1,646	22.5	9.6	8.5	10.0	12.0	14.0	22.0	30.0	32.6	34.1	40.0
35–44	334	1,318	25.8	9.2	11.5	13.0	16.0	20.0	25.5	32.0	35.0	36.5	41.0
45–54	126	1,237	26.8	9.8	12.0	14.0	17.0	20.0	26.0	34.0	37.1	40.0	42.2
55–64	115	871	28.2	12.9	10.0	11.0	13.0	19.0	28.0	34.0	40.0	45.0	51.5
65–74	318	652	23.8	9.0	7.5	11.5	15.0	17.5	24.0	30.0	32.2	35.5	40.0

* From the National Center for Health Statistics, Department of Health and Human Services, Health and Nutrition Examination Survey I, 1971–1874.

APPENDIX 25. Percentiles for Upper Arm Circumference and Estimated Upper Arm Muscle Circumference of Whites in the United States Health and Nutrition Examination Survey I, 1971 to 1974*†

	Arm Circumference (mm)							Arm Muscle Circumference (mm)						
Age Group	***5***	***10***	***25***	***50***	***75***	***90***	***95***	***5***	***10***	***25***	***50***	***75***	***90***	***95***
							Males							
1–1.9	142	146	150	159	170	176	183	110	113	119	127	135	144	147
2–2.9	141	145	153	162	170	178	185	111	114	122	130	140	146	150
3–3.9	150	153	160	167	175	184	190	117	123	131	137	143	148	153
4–4.9	149	154	162	171	180	186	192	123	126	133	141	148	156	159
5–5.9	153	160	167	175	185	195	204	128	133	140	147	154	162	169
6–6.9	155	159	167	179	188	209	228	131	135	142	151	161	170	177
7–7.9	162	167	177	187	201	223	230	137	139	151	160	168	177	190
8–8.9	162	170	177	190	202	220	245	140	145	154	162	170	182	187
9–9.9	175	178	187	200	217	249	257	151	154	161	170	183	196	202
10–10.9	181	184	196	210	231	262	274	156	160	166	180	191	209	221
11–11.9	186	190	202	223	244	261	280	159	165	173	183	195	205	230
12–12.9	193	200	214	232	254	282	303	167	171	182	195	210	223	241
13–13.9	194	211	228	247	263	286	301	172	179	196	211	226	238	245
14–14.9	220	226	237	253	283	303	322	189	199	212	223	240	260	264
15–15.9	222	229	244	264	284	311	320	199	204	218	237	254	266	272
16–16.9	244	248	262	278	303	324	343	213	225	234	249	269	287	296
17–17.9	246	253	267	285	308	336	347	224	231	245	258	273	294	312
18–18.9	245	260	276	297	321	353	379	226	237	252	264	283	298	324
19–24.9	262	272	288	308	331	355	372	238	245	257	273	289	309	321
25–34.9	271	282	300	319	342	362	375	243	250	264	279	298	314	326
35–44.9	278	287	305	326	345	363	374	247	255	269	286	302	318	327
45–54.9	267	281	301	322	342	362	376	239	249	265	281	300	315	326
55–64.9	258	273	296	317	336	355	369	236	245	260	278	295	310	320
65–74.9	248	263	285	307	325	344	355	223	235	251	268	284	298	306
							Females							
1–1.9	138	142	148	156	164	172	177	105	111	117	124	132	139	143
2–2.9	142	145	152	160	167	176	184	111	114	119	126	133	142	147
3–3.9	143	150	158	167	175	183	189	113	119	124	132	140	146	152
4–4.9	149	154	160	169	177	184	191	115	121	128	136	144	152	157
5–5.9	153	157	165	175	185	203	211	125	128	134	142	151	159	165
6–6.9	156	162	170	176	187	204	211	130	133	138	145	154	166	171
7–7.9	164	167	174	183	199	216	231	129	135	142	151	160	171	176
8–8.9	168	172	183	195	214	247	261	138	140	151	160	171	183	194
9–9.9	178	182	194	211	224	251	260	147	150	158	167	180	194	198
10–10.9	174	182	193	210	228	251	265	148	150	159	170	180	190	197
11–11.9	185	194	208	224	248	276	303	150	158	171	181	196	217	223
12–12.9	194	203	216	237	256	282	294	162	166	180	191	201	214	220
13–13.9	202	211	223	243	271	301	338	169	175	183	198	211	226	240
14–14.9	214	223	237	252	272	304	322	174	179	190	201	216	232	247
15–15.9	208	221	239	254	279	300	322	175	178	189	202	215	228	244
16–16.9	218	224	241	258	283	318	334	170	180	190	202	216	234	249
17–17.9	220	227	241	264	295	324	350	175	183	194	205	221	239	257
18–18.9	222	227	241	258	281	312	325	174	179	191	202	215	237	245
19–24.9	221	230	247	265	290	319	345	179	185	195	207	221	236	249
25–34.9	233	240	256	277	304	342	368	183	188	199	212	228	246	264
35–44.9	241	251	267	290	317	356	378	186	192	205	218	236	257	272
45–54.9	242	256	274	299	328	362	384	187	193	206	220	238	260	274
55–64.9	243	257	280	303	335	367	385	187	196	209	225	244	266	280
65–74.9	240	252	274	299	326	356	373	185	195	208	225	244	264	279

* From Frisancho AR: New norms of upper limb fat and muscle areas for assessment of nutritional status. Am J Clin Nutr *34*:2540, 1981.

† Percentiles are not yet available for the black population for upper arm circumference or arm muscle circumference.

APPENDIX 26. Percentiles for Estimates of Upper Arm Fat Area and Upper Arm Muscle Area of Whites in the United States Health and Nutrition Examination Survey I, 1971 to 1974*†

	Arm Muscle Area Percentiles (mm²)							Arm Fat Area Percentiles (mm²)						
Age Group	*5*	*10*	*25*	*50*	*75*	*90*	*95*	*5*	*10*	*25*	*50*	*75*	*90*	*95*
							Males							
1–1.9	956	1,014	1,133	1,278	1,447	1,644	1,720	452	486	590	741	895	1,036	1,176
2–2.9	973	1,040	1,190	1,345	1,557	1,690	1,787	434	504	578	737	871	1,044	1,148
3–3.9	1,095	1,201	1,357	1,484	1,618	1,750	1,853	464	519	590	736	868	1,071	1,151
4–4.9	1,207	1,264	1,408	1,579	1,747	1,926	2,008	428	494	598	722	859	989	1,085
5–5.9	1,298	1,411	1,550	1,720	1,884	2,089	2,285	446	488	582	713	914	1,176	1,299
6–6.9	1,360	1,447	1,605	1,815	2,056	2,297	2,493	371	446	539	678	896	1,115	1,519
7–7.9	1,497	1,548	1,808	2,027	2,246	2,494	2,886	423	473	574	758	1,011	1,393	1,511
8–8.9	1,550	1,664	1,895	2,089	2,296	2,628	2,788	410	460	588	725	1,003	1,248	1,558
9–9.9	1,811	1,884	2,067	2,228	2,657	3,053	3,257	485	527	635	859	1,252	1,864	2,081
10–10.9	1,930	2,027	2,182	2,575	2,903	3,486	3,882	523	543	738	982	1,376	1,906	2,609
11–11.9	2,016	2,156	2,382	2,670	3,022	3,359	4,226	536	595	754	1,148	1,710	2,348	2,574
12–12.9	2,216	2,339	2,649	3,022	3,496	3,968	4,640	554	650	874	1,172	1,558	2,536	3,580
13–13.9	2,363	2,546	3,044	3,553	4,081	4,502	4,794	475	570	812	1,096	1,702	2,744	3,322
14–14.9	2,830	3,147	3,586	3,963	4,575	5,368	5,530	453	563	786	1,082	1,608	2,746	3,508
15–15.9	3,138	3,317	3,788	4,481	5,134	5,631	5,900	521	595	690	931	1,423	2,434	3,100
16–16.9	3,625	4,044	4,352	4,951	5,753	6,576	6,980	542	593	844	1,078	1,746	2,280	3,041
17–17.9	3,998	4,252	4,777	5,286	5,950	6,886	7,726	598	698	827	1,096	1,636	2,407	2,888
18–18.9	4,070	4,481	5,066	5,552	6,374	7,067	8,355	560	665	860	1,264	1,947	3,302	3,928
19–24.9	4,508	4,777	5,274	5,913	6,660	7,606	8,200	594	743	963	1,406	2,231	3,098	3,652
25–34.9	4,694	4,963	5,541	6,214	7,067	7,847	8,436	675	831	1,174	1,752	2,459	3,246	3,786
35–44.9	4,844	5,181	5,740	6,490	7,265	8,034	8,488	703	851	1,310	1,792	2,463	3,098	3,624
45–54.9	4,546	4,946	5,589	6,297	7,142	7,918	8,458	749	922	1,254	1,741	2,359	3,245	3,928
55–64.9	4,422	4,783	5,381	6,144	6,919	7,670	8,149	658	839	1,166	1,645	2,236	2,976	3,466
65–74.9	3,973	4,411	5,031	5,716	6,432	7,074	7,453	573	753	1,122	1,621	2,199	2,876	3,327
							Females							
1–1.9	885	973	1,084	1,221	1,378	1,535	1,621	401	466	578	706	847	1,022	1,140
2–2.9	973	1,029	1,119	1,269	1,405	1,595	1,727	469	526	642	747	894	1,061	1,173
3–3.9	1,014	1,133	1,227	1,396	1,563	1,690	1,846	473	529	656	822	967	1,106	1,158
4–4.9	1,058	1,171	1,313	1,475	1,644	1,832	1,958	490	541	654	766	907	1,109	1,236
5–5.9	1,238	1,301	1,423	1,598	1,825	2,012	2,159	470	529	647	812	991	1,330	1,536
6–6.9	1,354	1,414	1,513	1,683	1,877	2,182	2,323	464	508	638	827	1,009	1,263	1,436
7–7.9	1,330	1,441	1,602	1,815	2,045	2,332	2,469	491	560	706	920	1,135	1,407	1,644
8–8.9	1,513	1,566	1,808	2,034	2,327	2,657	2,996	527	634	769	1,042	1,383	1,872	2,482
9–9.9	1,723	1,788	1,976	2,227	2,571	2,987	3,112	642	690	933	1,219	1,584	2,171	2,524
10–10.9	1,740	1,784	2,019	2,296	2,583	2,873	3,093	616	702	842	1,141	1,608	2,500	3,005
11–11.9	1,784	1,987	2,316	2,612	3,071	3,739	3,953	707	802	1,015	1,301	1,942	2,730	3,690
12–12.9	2,092	2,182	2,579	2,904	3,225	3,655	3,847	782	854	1,090	1,511	2,056	2,666	3,369
13–13.9	2,269	2,426	2,657	3,130	3,529	4,081	4,568	726	838	1,219	1,625	2,374	3,272	4,150
14–14.9	2,418	2,562	2,874	3,220	3,704	4,294	4,850	981	1,043	1,423	1,818	2,403	3,250	3,765
15–15.9	2,426	2,518	2,847	3,248	3,689	4,123	4,756	839	1,126	1,396	1,886	2,544	3,093	4,195
16–16.9	2,308	2,567	2,865	3,248	3,718	4,353	4,946	1,126	1,351	1,663	2,006	2,598	3,374	4,236
17–17.9	2,442	2,674	2,996	3,336	3,883	4,552	5,251	1,042	1,267	1,463	2,104	2,977	3,864	5,159
18–18.9	2,398	2,538	2,917	3,243	3,694	4,461	4,767	1,003	1,230	1,616	2,104	2,617	3,508	3,733
19–24.9	2,538	2,728	3,026	3,406	3,877	4,439	4,940	1,046	1,198	1,596	2,166	2,959	4,050	4,896
25–34.9	2,661	2,826	3,148	3,573	4,138	4,806	5,541	1,173	1,399	1,841	2,548	3,512	4,690	5,560
35–44.9	2,750	2,948	3,359	3,783	4,428	5,240	5,877	1,336	1,619	2,158	2,898	3,932	5,093	5,847
45–54.9	2,784	2,956	3,378	3,858	4,520	5,375	5,964	1,459	1,803	2,447	3,244	4,229	5,416	6,140
55–64.9	2,784	3,063	3,477	4,045	4,750	5,632	6,247	1,345	1,879	2,520	3,369	4,360	5,276	6,152
65–74.9	2,737	3,018	3,444	4,019	4,739	5,566	6,214	1,363	1,681	2,266	3,063	3,943	4,914	5,530

* From Frisancho AR. New norms of upper limb fat and muscle areas for assessment of nutritional status. Am J Clin Nutr 35:2540, 1981.
† Percentiles are not yet available for the black population for arm fat areas.

APPENDIX 27. Arm Anthropometry for the Elderly*

Percentile Norms for a Cincinnati Population

Sex and Age (yr) Group	No. in Sample	Mean	Percentile 5th	10th	25th	50th	75th	90th	95th
Triceps Skinfold Thickness (mm)									
Women									
60–89	496	25.2	12.5	14.4	18.5	24.0	30.8	38.1	43.6
60–69	146	27.2 ± 10.2†	13.0	14.7	20.7	26.2	33.0	40.3	47.2
70–79	239	25.1 ± 9.3	13.0	15.0	18.0	23.7	31.0	38.3	41.5
80–89	111	23.3 ± 9.7	10.9	12.9	16.7	21.8	27.5	34.6	43.4
Men									
60–89	250	22.5	5.7	7.6	11.5	20.4	31.8	42.1	45.8
60–69	86	21.9 ± 13.6	4.9	6.9	10.8	18.0	31.9	45.1	49.3
70–79	115	23.5 ± 13.3	6.3	7.9	12.0	22.0	32.7	41.8	45.4
80–89	49	21.6 ± 11.0	5.8	8.0	11.5	21.0	29.6	37.5	40.5
Mid-Upper Arm Circumference (cm)									
Women									
60–89	496	30.0	23.3	25.1	27.0	29.7	32.7	35.9	38.1
60–69	146	31.1 ± 4.8	23.5	25.6	27.7	30.6	33.7	37.5	39.9
70–79	239	30.0 ± 4.1	23.5	25.5	27.1	29.5	32.5	35.5	37.8
80–89	111	28.8 ± 4.6	22.5	23.5	26.0	28.8	31.6	34.5	36.4
Men									
60–89	250	30.4	24.9	26.6	28.7	30.4	32.2	34.6	36.3
60–69	86	30.5 ± 3.0	25.1	27.3	29.0	30.5	32.4	34.2	35.7
70–79	115	30.7 ± 3.1	25.3	26.8	29.0	30.7	32.4	34.6	36.6
80–89	49	29.6 ± 3.5	23.4	24.9	27.6	29.6	31.5	35.3	36.5
Mid-Upper Arm Muscle Circumference (cm)									
Women									
60–89	496	22.0	16.7	17.7	19.8	21.9	24.3	26.9	28.3
60–69	146	22.6 ± 3.6	17.8	18.4	20.2	22.3	24.6	27.5	29.2
70–79	239	22.1 ± 3.5	16.7	17.8	19.8	21.9	24.2	26.7	28.2
80–89	111	21.4 ± 4.1	15.2	16.7	19.1	21.3	24.2	26.7	27.5
Men									
60–89	250	23.3	16.6	18.1	20.5	23.4	26.2	28.4	29.7
60–69	86	23.7 ± 4.4	16.1	18.0	20.5	23.7	26.7	28.9	31.7
70–79	115	23.3 ± 4.1	17.0	18.2	20.4	23.4	26.3	28.4	28.7
80–89	49	22.8 ± 3.3	16.6	18.2	20.7	22.8	24.9	27.3	28.6
Mid-Upper Arm Muscle Area (cm^2)									
Women									
60–89	496	39.9	22.2	25.0	31.1	38.0	47.1	57.7	63.8
60–69	146	41.6 ± 13.5	25.1	27.0	32.6	39.6	48.3	60.3	67.6
70–79	239	39.8 ± 12.7	22.1	25.1	31.2	38.0	46.7	56.6	63.2
80–89	111	37.9 ± 13.3	18.4	22.3	29.0	36.1	46.5	56.8	60.2
Men									
60–89	250	44.6	22.0	26.2	33.5	43.6	54.4	64.1	70.4
60–69	86	46.0 ± 16.5	20.7	25.8	33.4	44.8	56.8	66.7	79.7
70–79	115	44.6 ± 14.6	23.0	26.4	33.3	43.7	54.8	64.3	65.7
80–89	49	42.3 ± 11.8	21.9	26.5	34.2	41.5	49.4	59.1	64.9

* From Falciglia G, O'Connor J, and Gedling E: Upper arm anthropometric norms in elderly white subjects. J Am Diet Assoc 88:569, 1988.
† Mean ± standard deviation.

APPENDIX 28. Percentage of Body Fat Based on Four Skinfold Measurements*†

Sum of Skinfolds (mm)	Males (age in years)				Females (age in years)			
	17–29	*30–39*	*40–49*	*50+*	*16–29*	*30–39*	*40–49*	*50+*
15	4.8	—	—	—	10.5	—	—	—
20	8.1	12.2	12.2	12.6	14.1	17.0	19.8	21.4
25	10.5	14.2	15.0	15.6	16.8	19.4	22.2	24.0
30	12.9	16.2	17.7	18.6	19.5	21.8	24.5	26.6
35	14.7	17.7	19.6	20.8	21.5	23.7	26.4	28.5
40	16.4	19.2	21.4	22.9	23.4	25.5	28.2	30.3
45	17.7	20.4	23.0	24.7	25.0	26.9	29.6	31.9
50	19.0	21.5	24.6	26.5	26.5	28.2	31.0	33.4
55	20.1	22.5	25.9	27.9	27.8	29.4	32.1	34.6
60	21.2	23.5	27.1	29.2	29.1	30.6	33.2	35.7
65	22.2	24.3	28.2	30.4	30.2	31.6	34.1	36.7
70	23.1	25.1	29.3	31.6	31.2	32.5	35.0	37.7
75	24.0	25.9	30.3	32.7	32.2	33.4	35.9	38.7
80	24.8	26.6	31.2	33.8	33.1	34.3	36.7	39.6
85	25.5	27.2	32.1	34.8	34.0	35.1	37.5	40.4
90	26.2	27.8	33.0	35.8	34.8	35.8	38.3	41.2
95	26.9	28.4	33.7	36.6	35.6	36.5	39.0	41.9
100	27.6	29.0	34.4	37.4	36.4	37.2	39.7	42.6
105	28.2	29.6	35.1	38.2	37.1	37.9	40.4	43.3
110	28.8	30.1	35.8	39.0	37.8	38.6	41.0	43.9
115	29.4	30.6	36.4	39.7	38.4	39.1	41.5	44.5
120	30.0	31.1	37.0	40.4	39.0	39.6	42.0	45.1
125	30.5	31.5	37.6	41.1	39.6	40.1	42.5	45.7
130	31.0	31.9	38.2	41.8	40.2	40.6	43.0	46.2
135	31.5	32.3	38.7	42.4	40.8	41.1	43.5	46.7
140	32.0	32.7	39.2	43.0	41.3	41.6	44.0	47.2
145	32.5	33.1	39.7	43.6	41.8	42.1	44.5	47.7
150	32.9	33.5	40.2	44.1	42.3	42.6	45.0	48.2
155	33.3	33.9	40.7	44.6	42.8	43.1	45.4	48.7
160	33.7	34.3	41.2	45.1	43.3	43.6	45.8	49.2
165	34.1	34.6	41.6	45.6	43.7	44.0	46.2	49.6
170	34.5	34.8	42.0	46.1	44.1	44.4	46.6	50.0
175	34.9	—	—	—	—	44.8	47.0	50.4
180	35.3	—	—	—	—	45.2	47.4	50.8
185	35.6	—	—	—	—	45.6	47.8	51.2
190	35.9	—	—	—	—	45.9	48.2	51.6
195	—	—	—	—	—	46.2	48.5	52.0
200	—	—	—	—	—	46.5	48.8	52.4
205	—	—	—	—	—	—	49.1	52.7
210	—	—	—	—	—	—	49.4	53.0

* From Durnin JVGA and Wormersley J: Body fat assessed from total body density and its estimation from skinfold thickness: measurements on 481 men and women aged from 16–72 years. Br J Nutr 32:77, 1974.

† Measurements made on the right side of the body, using biceps, triceps, subscapular and suprailiac skinfolds.

APPENDIX 29. Expected 24-Hour Urinary Creatinine Excretion for Men and Women*

Expected 24-Hour Urinary Creatinine Excretion for Men

Height		*Small Frame*		*Medium Frame*		*Large Frame*	
in	cm	kg	mg/24°	kg	mg/24°	kg	mg/24°
61	154.9	52.7	1212	56.1	1290	60.7	1396
62	157.5	54.1	1244	57.7	1327	62.0	1426
63	160.0	55.4	1274	59.1	1359	63.6	1463
64	162.5	56.8	1306	60.4	1389	65.2	1500
65	165.1	58.4	1343	62.0	1426	66.8	1536
66	167.6	60.2	1385	63.9	1470	68.9	1585
67	170.2	62.0	1426	65.9	1516	71.1	1635
68	172.7	63.9	1470	67.7	1557	72.9	1677
69	175.3	65.9	1516	69.5	1598	74.8	1720
70	177.8	67.7	1557	71.6	1647	76.8	1766
71	180.3	69.5	1599	73.6	1693	79.1	1819
72	182.9	71.4	1642	75.7	1741	81.1	1865
73	185.4	73.4	1688	77.7	1787	83.4	1918
74	187.9	75.2	1730	80.0	1846	85.7	1971
75	190.5	77.0	1771	82.3	1893	87.7	2017

Expected 24-Hour Urinary Creatinine Excretion for Women

Height		*Small Frame*		*Medium Frame*		*Large Frame*	
in	cm	kg	mg/24°	kg	mg/24°	kg	mg/24°
56	142.2	43.2	778	46.1	830	50.7	913
57	144.8	44.3	797	47.3	851	51.8	932
58	147.3	45.4	817	48.6	875	53.2	958
59	149.8	46.8	842	50.0	900	54.5	981
60	152.4	48.2	868	51.4	925	55.9	1006
61	154.9	49.5	891	52.7	949	57.3	1031
62	157.5	50.9	916	54.3	977	58.9	1060
63	160.0	52.3	941	55.9	1006	60.6	1091
64	162.5	53.9	970	57.9	1042	62.5	1125
65	165.1	55.7	1003	59.8	1076	64.3	1157
66	167.6	57.5	1035	61.6	1109	66.1	1190
67	170.2	59.3	1067	63.4	1141	67.9	1222
68	172.7	61.4	1105	65.2	1174	70.0	1260
69	175.2	63.2	1138	67.0	1206	72.0	1296
70	177.8	65.0	1170	68.9	1240	74.1	1334

* From Pemberton CM: Mayo Clinic Diet Manual, 6th ed. Philadelphia, BC Decker, 1988, p 558.
Average creatinine excretion = 23 mg/kg IBW for men.
Average creatinine excretion = 18 mg/kg IBW for women.

APPENDIX 30. Normal Physiologic Values*

Blood or Serum Values	Normal Ranges	
Ascorbic acid (vitamin C)	0.6–2.0 mg/dl	
Bleeding time—Simplate	3–11 min	
Calcium, total	8.9–10.1 mg/dl	
Carotene	48–200 μg/dl	
Chloride	100–108 mEq/l	
Copper	0.75–1.45 μg/ml	
Erythrocyte count	M, 4.5–6.2 × 10^6/μl	
	F, 4.2–5.4 × 10^6/μl	
Ferritin	Newborn: 25–200 μg/l	
	1 mo: 200–600 μg/l	
	2–5 mo: 50–200 μg/l	
	6 mo–15y: 7–142 μg/l	
	M, 20–300 μg/l	
	F, 20–120 μg/l	
Folate (serum)	2–20 μg/ml	
Glucose, fasting	70–100 mg/dl	
Glycosylated hemoglobin	4.0–7.0%	
Hematocrit	M, 38.6–48.0%	
	F, 34.5–43.9%	
Hemoglobin	M, 12.9–16.6 g/dl	
	F, 11.6–14.9 g/dl	
Iron	M, 75–175 μg/dl	
	F, 65–165 μg/dl	
Iron binding capacity, total	240–450 μg/dl	
Iron binding capacity, % saturation	18–50%	
Lipids		
Cholesterol	<200 mg/dl = desirable	
	200–239 mg/dl = borderline high	
	≥240 mg/dl = high risk	
HDL cholesterol	<35 mg/dl = high risk	
	40–55 mg/dl = mod. risk	
	>50 mg/dl = low risk	
LDL cholesterol	<130 mg/dl = desirable	
	130–159 mg/dl = borderline high	
	>160 mg/dl = high risk	
Triglycerides	Male (mg/dl)	Female (mg/dl)
upper 95th percentile	6 yr: 102	76
	10 yr: 103	121
	15 yr: 124	122
	20 yr: 137	97
	25 yr: 157	100
	30 yr: 171	106
	35 yr: 182	110
	40 yr: 189	117
	45 yr: 193	122
	50 yr: 195	128
	55 yr: 197	134
	60 yr: 198	140
Magnesium	1.7–2.1 mg/dl	
Osmolality	275–295 mOsm/kg	
Phosphorus	2.5–4.5 mg/dl	
Potassium	3.6–4.8 mEq/l	
Prealbumin	16.6–40.2 mg/dl	
Protein, total	6.3–7.9 g/dl	
Protein electrophoresis		
Albumin	3.1–4.3 g/dl	
Alpha-1 globulin	0.1–0.3 g/dl	
Alpha-2 globulin	0.6–1.0 g/dl	
Beta-globulin g/dl	0.7–1.4 g/dl	
Gamma globulin	0.7–1.6 g/dl	
Prothrombin time	10.9–12.85	
Sodium	135–145 mEq/l	
Urea	M, 17–51 mg/dl	
	F, 13–45 mg/dl	
Uric acid	M, 4.3–8.0 mg/dl	
	F, 2.3–6.0 mg/dl	
Vitamin A	360–1,200 μg/l	
Vitamin B_{12}	190–765 ng/l	
Vitamin E	5.5–17.0 mg/l	
1,25 Dihydroxy vitamin D	15–60 pg/ml	
25-hydroxy vitamin D	Winter 14–42 ng/ml	
	Summer 15–80 ng/ml	
Zinc	0.66–1.10 μg/ml	

APPENDIX 30. Normal Physiologic Values* *Continued*

Urine Values	Normal Ranges
Ammonia	36–86 mEq/24 hr
Calcium	M, 25–300 mg/24 hr F, 20–275 mg/24 hr
Chromium	<8 μg/24 hr
Creatinine clearance	M (20y), 90 ml/min/SA F (20y), 84 ml/min/SA (decreased by 6 ml/min/decade)
Osmolality	300–800 mOsm/kg <100, mOsm/kg overhydrated >800 mOsm/kg dehydrated
Oxalate	M, 20–60 mg/24 hr F, 20–55 mg/24 hr
Potassium	30–90 mEq/24 hr
Protein, total	M, 0–150 mg/24 hr F, 27–93 mg/24 hr
Renal clearance—standard	
Glomerular filtration rate (inulin or iothalamate^{125}I)	90–130 ml/min/surface area† at age 20 (decreased by 4 ml/min/decade)
Effective renal plasma flow (PAH)	400–700 ml/min/surface area† at age 20 (decreased by 17 ml/min/decade)
Filtration fraction	18–22%
Renal clearance—short	
Glomerular filtration rate (iothalamate^{125}I)	110 ml/min/surface area† at age 20 (decreased by 4 ml/min/decade)
Glomerular filtration rate (creatinine)	See creatinine clearance
Sodium	40–217 mEq/24 hr
Uric acid	<750 mg/24 hr
Zinc	300–600 μg/24 hr

Miscellaneous Values	Normal Ranges
Basal metabolism rate	−10 to +10%
Stool examination	
Fat, quantitative	2–7 g/24 hr
Fat, percentage	0–20%
Nitrogen	1–2 g/24 hr
Vitamin B_{12} absorption (Schilling test)	≥8% excretion

* Adapted from Pemberton CM et al: Mayo Clinic Diet Manual, 6th ed. Philadelphia, BC Decker, 1988, p 543.
† Surface area is a standard measure of body surface area; 1.73 m^2.

APPENDIX 31. Physical Signs and Nutritional Terms Associated with Malnutrition*

GENERAL APPEARANCE

APATHY. Unreactive, unresponsive, disinterested, and inattentive to surroundings.

CLINICAL MARASMUS. Evidence of pronounced wasting of subcutaneous fat without edema. Significant apathy may be present. Frequently the face and eyes of the child may appear unusually bright due to the combination of wasting and prominence of the eyes. The child is usually considerably underdeveloped in relation to age, and there may or may not be associated hair changes such as dyspigmentation, thinness, ease in plucking, or signs of avitaminosis.

IRRITABILITY. Hyperresponsive; excessive or overreaction to minor stimuli, particularly manifest through crying or unusual indication of fear as a result of minor or relatively insignificant happenings.

KWASHIORKOR. Pitting edema at least on the pretibial region; underweight, undersize, underdeveloped for age. Muscular wasting may be present but masked by edema. Apathy of some degree is present. Changes in the hair are usually noted, such as thinning, easily pluckable with dyspigmentation or flag sign, and change in texture to silken, sparse hair. Dermatosis with desquamation of the so-called flaky paint type, with or without hyperpigmentation. In severe cases the dermatosis may resemble a relatively severe burn but lacks erythema.

PALLOR. Paleness and loss of color of skin, nail beds, mucosa, and lips.

PRE-KWASHIORKOR. An underweight, undersized, underdeveloped child, without the evident pronounced wasting present in marasmus. Child is thin and undersized but has relatively normal body proportions and rather poor muscle tone, and hair changes may be present. Not apathetic, although would not be described as alert.

HAIR

DRY STARING. Dry, wire-like, unkempt, stiff hair, often brittle, sometimes may exhibit some bleaching of the normal color.

DYSPIGMENTATION. Definite change from normal pigment of the hair, most usually evident distally and best seen by carefully combing hair strands upward and viewing the orderly array of hair in good light. Dyspigmentation includes both change of pigment (usually lightening of color) and depigmentation. Not to be confused with dyed or tinted hair. Dyspigmentation is often bandlike in character and usually is associated with some change in texture of hair in the depigmented band. In some ethnic groups, particularly among negroid groups, the pigment may be slightly red. In others, especially among straight black-haired peoples, the bandlike depigmentation ("flag sign") is common.

EASILY PLUCKABLE. Easily pluckable hair is that in which the shafts are readily removed with minimum tug when a few strands are grasped between the finger and thumb and gently pulled. In such cases there is a lack of reaction of the child, indicating a lack of pain associated with removing of the hair.

SKIN

CRACKLED SKIN. Definite scales larger in size than those seen in xerosis. It is often congenital and is most prominent in cool weather. It is non-nutritional in origin.

DEPENDENT EDEMA. The presence of abnormally large amounts of fluid in the intercellular tissue spaces of the body; usually applied to demonstrable accumulation of excessive fluid in the subcutaneous tissues that is dependent upon position and gravity.

SKIN *Continued*

DERMATITIS WITH DESQUAMATION, OR CRAZY-PAVEMENT TYPE. Under this heading should be recorded those desquamating changes of the skin, usually with increased pigmentation, that occur on the extremities, especially legs, thighs, and buttocks, but may occur over the trunk in association with kwashiorkor. (These have been termed "flaky-paint" dermatoses.) Small, circumscribed bleb-like lesions are sometimes seen in association with kwashiorkor and may occasionally precede the desquamation. In addition, any "crazy-pavement" type of lesions observed should be noted. These are characterized by a thin-appearing epithelium marked by striations usually resembling in outline the microscopic picture of epithelial cells. Not to be confused, however, with ichthyosis (scaly skin).

FOLLICULAR HYPERKERATOSIS. This lesion has been likened to the "gooseflesh" that is seen on chilling, but it is not generalized and does not disappear with brisk rubbing of the skin. Readily felt, as it presents a "nutmeg grater" feel. Follicular hyperkeratosis is more readily detected by the sense of touch than by the eye. The skin is rough, with papillae formed by keratotic plugs that project from the hair follicles. The surrounding skin is dry and lacks the usual amount of moisture or oiliness. Differentiation from adolescent folliculosis can usually be made through recognition of the normal skin between the follicles in the adolescent disorder. It is distinguished from perifolliculosis by the ring of capillary congestion that occurs about each follicle in scorbutic perifolliculosis.

PELLAGROUS DERMATITIS. Symmetrical lesions typical of acute or chronic, mild or severe pellagra are observed; lesions are usually red, often swollen or blistered like sunburn, pigmented, scaly over exposed areas, clearly demarcated from normal skin.

PURPURA OR PETECHIA. Small localized extravasations of blood, red or purplish in color, depending on time elapsed since formation. Usually distributed at sites of pressure, and may be perifollicular.

XEROSIS. Xerosis is a clinical term used to describe a dry and crinkled skin that is accentuated by pushing the skin parallel to its surface. In more pronounced cases it is often mottled and pigmented and may appear as scaly or alligator-like pseudoplaques, usually not greater than 0.5 cm in diameter. Nutritional significance is not established. Differential diagnosis must be made from changes due to dirt and exposure and ichthyosis.

SKELETAL

BOWLEG. An outward curve of one or both legs at or below the knee (genu varum).

COSTOCHONDRAL BEADING. Palpable and visible enlargement of the costochondral junctions.

CRANIAL BOSSING. Abnormal prominence or protrusion of frontal or parietal areas.

ENLARGED JOINTS. When the more obvious ends of long bones are enlarged; that is, the wrist, ankles, knees.

WINGED SCAPULA. A scapula having a prominent vertebral border.

MUSCLE

MUSCLE WASTING. Appearance indicates abnormal loss of muscle substance, as exhibited by unusual prominence of bony skeleton, undue degree of folding of the skin of the buttocks, or the abnormal flabby feel (sometimes described as jelly-like) of the child with poor muscle tone.

APPENDIX 31. Physical Signs and Nutritional Terms Associated with Malnutrition* *Continued*

EYES

Bitot's spots. Bitot's spots are small, circumscribed grayish or yellowish gray, dull, dry, foamy superficial lesions of the conjunctiva. They most often occur on the lateral aspect of the bulbar conjunctiva in the interpalpebral area. Do not confuse with pterygium.

Blepharitis. Inflammation of eyelids.

Keratomalacia. Softening of the cornea.

Thickened opaque bulbar conjunctivae. All degrees of thickening may occur. The blueness of the sclera may disappear and the bulbar conjunctivae develop a wrinkled appearance with increase in vascularity. The thickened conjunctivae may result in a glazed, porcelain-like appearance, obscuring the vascularity.

Xerosis conjunctivae. The conjunctivae, upon exposure by holding the lids open and having the subject rotate the eyes, appear dull and lusterless and exhibit a striated or roughened surface.

FACE

Angular lesions. Present bilaterally when mouth is held half open. May appear as pink or moist whitish macerated angular lesions that blur the mucocutaneous junction. Angular fissures are recorded when there is definite break in continuity of epithelium at the angles of the mouth.

Angular scars. Scars at the angles that, if recent, may be pink; if old, may appear blanched.

Cheilosis. Cheilosis is present when the lips are swollen, tense or puffy and, where it appears, the buccal mucosa extends out onto the lips. These lesions are also denuded. This category may be used to record vertical fissuring of the lips but not for lesions of the angles of the mouth only.

Nasolabial seborrhea. Definite greasy yellow scaling or filiform excrescences in the nasolabial area that become more pronounced on slight scratching with the fingernail or a tongue blade.

MOUTH

Filiform papillary atrophy. Filiform papillae exceedingly low or absent, giving the tongue a smooth appearance that remains after scraping slightly with an applicator stick. "Mild" involves less than one fourth of the tongue (tip and lateral margins only); "moderate" involves one fourth to three fourths of the tongue; "severe" involves over three fourths of the tongue.

MOUTH *Continued*

Glossitis. Glossitis is any increase in redness, fissuring or swelling with color change (break in lingual mucosa) or diffuse involvement of mucosa. Geographic tongue has the typical irregularly shaped and distributed areas of atrophy with irregular white patches resembling leukoplakia. Glossitis is usually associated with some sensation of pain or burning, particularly upon eating.

Magenta color. The color of alkaline phenolphthalein.

Swollen gums. Swollen, red interdental papillae, with more than one papilla involved.

TEETH

Carious teeth. Molecular decay of a bone, in which it becomes friable, thinned and dark and gradually breaks down, with the formation of pus.

Fluorosis. Opaque paper-white areas in the enamel of the tooth, ranging in size from a few flecks to entire enamel surface. In the latter case brown stain is a frequent accompaniment, as is attrition of opposing surfaces. The most severe forms of fluorosis include discrete or confluent pitting, with widespread brown staining and a general corroded appearance.

GLANDS

Parotid enlargement. Because of various types of facial configuration, parotid enlargement may be easily missed in certain populations. Check by palpation, moving the gland with fingers upward and backward toward the ear. Check if bilateral.

Thyroid enlargement. Thyroid enlargement occurs when a visually perceptible enlargement that is definitely palpable with or without swallowing is noted. It is preferable to examine the subject with his or her head slightly extended in order to detect thyroid enlargements.

ORGANS

Hepatomegaly. Liver edges more than 2 cm below the costal margin. (In children, the liver edge may normally be palpable.)

Splenomegaly. Spleen is palpable.

* From Christakis G (ed): Nutritional Assessment in Health Programs. Washington, DC, American Public Health Association, 1973, pp. 26–27.

APPENDIX 32. Effects of Some Drugs on Nutritional Status

Drug	Possible Mechanism	Nutritional Implication
Analgesics		
Alcohol	Toxic effect on intestinal mucosa Excessive loss of magnesium in stool and urine	Decreased absorption of thiamin, folic acid, vitamin B_{12} Hypomagnesemic tetany
Colchicine	Decreases activity of intestinal disaccharidases Damages gastrointestinal mucosa by blocking mucosal cell replication	Decreased absorption of vitamin B_{12}, fat, carotene, sodium, potassium, lactose, xylose, protein Possible megaloblastic anemia
Antacids		
Aluminum hydroxide	Decreases absorption of phosphate	Phosphate depletion
Sodium bicarbonate	Alkalinization of proximal small intestine	Decreased folate absorption
Others	Basic environment inactivates thiamin and prevents formation of ferrous from ferric iron	Inadequate amount of thiamin Decreased absorption of iron
Anticoagulants		
Coumarins	Interference with regeneration of vitamin K from inactive form	Increased prothrombin time
Anticonvulsants		
Phenobarbital	Increases turnover of vitamin D, may block hydroxylation of vitamin D	Decreased serum levels of 24-hydroxyvitamin D_3 and calcium and magnesium
Phenytoin	May increase biliary excretion of vitamin D	Possible osteomalacia or rickets
Primidone	May inhibit folate conjugase	Decreased serum levels of folate can cause megaloblastic anemia
Barbiturates	Accelerates inactivation of vitamin D Increases urinary excretion of vitamin C	Increased need for vitamin D with long-term use
Antidepressants		
Amitriptyline		Interference with riboflavin metabolism
Imipramine	May increase appetite and craving for carbohydrate	Possible weight gain
Lithium carbonate	Causes change in sodium distribution and hyperexcretion	Altered blood glucose Hyponatremia Increased toxicity with low sodium diet
Phenelzine and other MAOI drugs	MAO inhibitor Increases appetite and carbohydrate craving	Reactions with tyramine in foods Weight gain
Antifungals		
Amphotericin B	Nephrotoxicity Hepatotoxicity	Multiple side effects if kidney and liver damaged
Antihistamines		
Cyproheptadine	May increase appetite	Weight gain
Anti-Inflammatory Agents, Nonsteroidal		
Aspirin (salicylates)	Decreases leukocyte uptake of ascorbic acid and alters ascorbic acid distribution Damage to gastrointestinal tract; bleeding Malabsorption of vitamin B_{12}	Decreased plasma and platelet ascorbic acid levels Increased urinary loss of ascorbic acid Decreased absorption of glucose and vitamin B_{12}
Indomethacin	Gastrointestinal bleeding May cause fluid retention	Hyperkalemia Dyspepsia May cause anemia
Antimicrobials		
Cephalosporin	Inhibits prothrombin carboxylation	Increased prothrombin time Risk of vitamin K deficiency especially in elderly
Chloramphenicol	Decreases protein synthesis by blocking mRNA-ribosome bond	Possibly increased need for riboflavin, pyridoxine, and vitamin B_{12} Possible peripheral neuritis, optic neuropathy Decreased response to folate, iron and vitamin B_{12} therapy
Penicillins	Carry potassium with them into urine	Hypokalemia
Tetracyclines	Chelate divalent ions Decrease synthesis of vitamin K by intestinal bacteria	Net effect with minerals not clinically significant
Neomycin (Some of these changes also seen with kanamycin and paromomycin)	Causes mucosal injury resulting in decreased activity of disaccharidases and other enzymes	Decreased absorption of fat, MCT, carbohydrate, protein, fat-soluble vitamins A, D and K, vitamin B_{12}, calcium, and iron
Gentamicin	Nephrotoxicity	Increased urinary excretion of magnesium and potassium
Viomycin	Induces hyperaldosteronism	May cause hypomagnesemia, hypokalemia, hypocalcemia, alkalosis
Antineoplastics	Cytotoxic; damages intestinal mucosa	Extensive effects discussed in Chapter 36

APPENDIX 32. Effects of Some Drugs on Nutritional Status *Continued*

Drug	Possible Mechanism	Nutritional Implication
Antipsychotics		
Chlorpromazine	Hepatotoxic May affect insulin release	Can reduce physical activity Possible weight gain
Molindone	Decreases appetite	Possible weight loss
Antitubercular Agents		
Para-aminosalicylic acid	Causes intestinal injury	Decreased absorption of vitamin B_{12}, which may result in megaloblastic anemia
Isoniazid	Blocks conversion of tryptophan to niacin Inhibits pyridoxine-dependent enzymes Inhibits hydroxylation of vitamin D	Increased urinary excretion of pyridoxine Possible pyridoxine depletion May cause polyneuropathy, megaloblastic anemia Decreased serum folate
Cycloserine	Acts as a pyridoxine antagonist	May decrease serum folate, vitamin B_{12}, and pyridoxine
Antivitamins		
Methotrexate	Inhibits dihydrofolate reductase; decreases formation of active folate Causes gastrointestinal mucosal injury	Malabsorption of vitamin B_{12} and folate Weight loss, diarrhea, nausea, anorexia, vomiting, gingivitis, and stomatitis
Cardiac Drugs		
Propranolol	Suppresses normal sympathetic response to hypoglycemia	Masked signs of hypoglycemia
Digitalis glycosides	Inhibits glucose absorption	Diarrhea; cachexia; anorexia is early sign of toxicity Increased urinary excretion of potassium
Chelating Agents		
Penicillamine	Chelates with pyridoxine Chelates with zinc and copper	Increased urinary excretion of pyridoxine, zinc, and copper Peripheral neuritis, convulsions, mood changes Decreased taste acuity; unpleasant taste
CNS Stimulating Agents		
Dextroamphetamine	CNS effect on appetite	Weight loss
Methylphenidate	CNS effect on appetite	Decreased rate of growth in children due to decreased intake
Corticosteroids	Stimulate protein catabolism Depress protein synthesis Decrease calcium absorption	Decreased serum calcium Increased urinary excretion of potassium, zinc, and nitrogen Increased need for vitamin D Decreased bone formation
Diuretics		
Ethacrynic acid and furosemide	Anorexia and nausea	Decreased food intake Increased urinary excretion of calcium, magnesium, potassium Decreased serum magnesium and potassium
Spironolactone	Possible fluid and electrolyte imbalance May increase serum glucose	Decreased carbohydrate tolerance
Thiazides	May increase intestinal calcium absorption or increase bone resorption	Increased urinary excretion of potassium, magnesium, and sodium Possible potassium and magnesium depletion
Triamterene	Competitive inhibition of dihydrofolate reductase; reduces activation of folic acid	Decreased serum folate Possible increased calcium excretion Possible megaloblastic anemia
Hypocholesterolemics		
Cholestyramine	Binds bile salts and disrupts micelles Binds intrinsic factor at ileal pH Binds iron May bind calcium	Decreased absorption of cholesterol, vitamins A, D, K and B_{12}, folate, fat, medium-chain triglycerides (MCT), glucose, xylose, carotene, and iron Decreased calcium absorption Decreased serum calcium and vitamin B_{12} Increased urinary excretion of calcium
Clofibrate	May decrease activity of intestinal disaccharidases	Decreased taste acuity, unpleasant aftertaste Decreased absorption of carotene, glucose, iron, MCT, vitamin B_{12}, and electrolytes Possible anemia
Colestipol	Bile acid sequestrant	Reduced serum cholesterol Lowered plasma and serum levels of vitamins A and E

Table continued on following page

APPENDIX 32. Effects of Some Drugs on Nutritional Status *Continued*

Drug	Possible Mechanism	Nutritional Implication
Hypotensive Agents		
Hydralazine	Inactivates pyridoxine May chelate trace metals	Increased excretion of pyridoxine; pyridoxine depletion Possible peripheral neuritis
Diazoxide	Inhibits insulin release	Decreased tubular excretion of uric acid May cause weight gain
Reserpine	Increases gastrointestinal motility and secretion	May cause diarrhea
Sodium nitroprusside	Binds vitamin B_{12}	Increased urinary B_{12} excretion Decreased plasma B_{12}
Laxatives		
Mineral oil (Petrolatum, liquid)	Dissolves fat-soluble vitamins Increases intestinal motility May decrease absorption of vitamins A, E, and K	Decreased absorption of carotene, vitamin D, and calcium and phosphate
Phenolphthalein	Can cause intestinal hyperperistalsis May irritate intestine	Can cause steatorrhea Can cause intestinal calcium and potassium loss
L-Dopa (levodopa)	Antagonizes pyridoxine Decreases absorption of some amino acids	Possible polyneuropathy related to pyridoxine depletion Risk of pyridoxine deficiency less with carbidopa/ievodopa preparation
Oral Contraceptives	May increase catabolism, decrease absorption or alter tissue uptake of vitamin C May inhibit folate conjugase May increase transport proteins for vitamin A Estrogens increase the rate of conversion of tryptophan to niacin	Altered tryptophan metabolism Decreased serum vitamin C levels Possibly decreased serum vitamin B_{12}, folate, pyridoxine, riboflavin, magnesium, and zinc Increased hemoglobin, hematocrit, serum levels of vitamins A and E, total lipids, triglycerides, iron, total iron-binding capacity (TIBC), and plasma copper Possible polyneuropathy, peripheral neuritis, and megaloblastic anemia Altered glucose tolerance
Oral Hypoglycemic Agents		
Metformin	Decreases activity of maltase, isomaltase, and sucrase in jejunum Competitive inhibition of B_{12} absorption	Decreased absorption of glucose, xylose, vitamin B_{12} Decreased serum folate, vitamin B_{12}
Phenformin	May affect active transport mechanisms	Decreased rate of glucose absorption in human ileum Possible decreased absorption of vitamin B_{12}, fat, calcium, and amino acids
Potassium Supplements	Slow release of potassium chloride causes decrease of ileal pH (acidification)	Decreased absorption of vitamin B_{12}
Sedative-Hypnotics		
Glutethimide	Possibly increases inactivation of 25-hydroxy vitamin D_3	Increased vitamin D turnover Altered calcium need Increased bone resorption
Sulfonamides		
Salicylazosulfapyridine (Sulfasalazine)	Inhibits intestinal transport of folate Inhibits action of polyglutamyl folate conjugase	Decreased absorption of folate Decreased serum folate and serum iron Decreased response to folate supplement
Other sulfonamides	Decreased iron absorption	Possible anemia Peripheral neuritis Increased urinary excretion of ascorbic acid
Uricosuric Agents		
Probenecid	Alters renal excretion Decreases absorption of riboflavin and amino acids	Increased urinary excretion of riboflavin, calcium, magnesium, sodium, potassium, phosphate, and chloride Decreased urinary excretion of pantothenic acid
Urinary Germicides		
Nitrofurantoin	May inhibit intestinal folate conjugase	Decreased serum folate Possible megaloblastic anemia and peripheral neuritis

APPENDIX 33. Enteral Nutrition Products

Prepared by Sharon Feucht, R.D.

SPECIALLY DESIGNED FORMULA DIETS

Product *Source*	**Citrotein** *Sandoz*	**SLD** *Ross*	**Portagen** *Mead Johnson*	**Lonalac** *Mead Johnson*
FORM	Powder[2]	Powder[2]	Powder[1]	Powder[1]
KCAL/ml	.66	.7	1.0	1.0
PROTEIN (% of calories)	25	21	14	21
CARBOHYDRATE (% of calories)	73	78	45	30
FAT (% of calories)	2	1	41	49
PROTEIN (g/liter)	41	38.5	35.7	53
CARBOHYDRATE (g/liter)	122	140	115	75
FAT (g/liter)	1.6	.5	48	55.4
CAL:N	101	117	177	118
SODIUM (mEq/liter)	31	37.2	23.8	1.74
POTASSIUM (mEq/liter)	18.2	23.7	32.4	50.7
OSMOLALITY (mOsm/kg)	480	545	320	390[1]
VOLUME TO MEET 100% of RDA for vitamins and minerals (ml)	1100	1170	828[3] (see label)	Incomplete
PROTEIN SOURCE	Pasteurized egg-white solids	Egg-white solids	Sodium caseinate	Casein
CARBOHYDRATE SOURCE	Sucrose, maltodextrin	Sucrose, hydrolyzed cornstarch	Corn syrup solids, sugar	Lactose
FAT SOURCE	Partially hydrogenated soy oil	—	Medium chain triglycerides (MCT) and corn oils	Coconut oil
FLAVOR	Orange			
USE	Low residue, low fat, presurgical	Low residue, low fat, presurgical	Fat malabsorption	Severe sodium restriction

Product *Source*	**Travasorb Renal** *Clintec*	**Amin-Aid** *Kendall-McGraw*	**Hepatic-Aid II** *Kendall-McGraw*
FORM	Powder[2]	Powder[2]	Powder[2]
KCAL/ml	1.35	2	1.2
PROTEIN (% of calories)	7	4	15
CARBOHYDRATE (% of calories)	81	75	57
FAT (% of calories)	12	21	28
PROTEIN (g/liter)	23.1	19.4	44.1
CARBOHYDRATE (g/liter)	271	366	168.5
FAT (g/liter)	17.9	46.2	36.2
CAL:N	365	645	167
SODIUM (mEq/liter)	Electrolyte free	<15	<15
POTASSIUM (mEq/liter)	Electrolyte free	<6	<6
OSMOLALITY (mOsm/kg)	590	700	560
VOLUME TO MEET 100% of RDA for vitamins and minerals (ml)	Incomplete	Incomplete	Incomplete
PROTEIN SOURCE	Crystalline amino acids	Essential amino acids + histidine	Free amino acids, 46% branched chain amino acids (BCAA)
CARBOHYDRATE SOURCE	Glucose oligosaccharides, sucrose	Maltodextrin, sugar	Maltodextrin, sucrose
FAT SOURCE	MCT and sunflower oils	Soy oil	Soy oil
USE	Renal failure	Renal failure	Liver disease

Table continued on following page

[1] Mixed at 30 cal/fl oz.
[2] Per standard dilution.

APPENDIX 33. Enteral Nutrition Products *Continued*

Product *Source*	**Alterna** *Ross*	**Replena** *Ross*
FORM	Powder[3]	Liquid
KCAL/ml	0.33	2
PROTEIN (% of calories)	11	6
CARBOHYDRATE (% of calories)	51	51
FAT (% of calories)	38	43
PROTEIN (g/liter)	8.9	30
CARBOHYDRATE (g/liter)	42.6	256
FAT (g/liter)	14	96
CAL:N	N/A	427:1[5]
SODIUM (mEq/liter)	15.9	34.2
POTASSIUM (mEq/liter)	25.3	28.7
OSMOLALITY (mOsm/kg)	[4]	615
VOLUME TO MEET 100% of RDA for vitamins and minerals (ml)	N/A	950[6]
PROTEIN SOURCE	Whey powder, nonfat dry milk, sodium caseinate	Sodium and calcium caseinates
CARBOHYDRATE SOURCE	Corn syrup solids, sucrose	Hydrolyzed cornstarch, sucrose
FAT SOURCE	Soy oil	Hi-oleic safflower oil, soy oil
USE	Liver failure or renal failure	Liver failure or renal failure

Product *Source*	**Stresstein** *Sandoz*	**Travasorb Hepatic** *Clintec*	**Glucerna** *Ross*	**Impact** *Sandoz*
FORM	Powder	Powder[7]	Liquid	Liquid
KCAL/ml	1.2	1.1[7]	1	1
PROTEIN (% of calories)	23	11	16	22
CARBOHYDRATE (% of calories)	56	77	36	53
FAT (% of calories)	21	12	48	25
PROTEIN (g/liter)	70	29.1	41.8	56
CARBOHYDRATE (g/liter)	170	212.8	93.8[8]	132
FAT (g/liter)	28	14.5	55.7	28
CAL:N	108	236	150	112
SODIUM (mEq/liter)	28.3	10.12	40.3	47
POTASSIUM (mEq/liter)	28.2	22.4	40	33
OSMOLALITY (mOsm/kg)	910	600	375	375
VOLUME TO MEET 100% of RDA for vitamins and minerals (ml)	2,000	2,062	1,422	1,500
PROTEIN SOURCE	Free amino acids (44% BCAA)	Crystalline amino acids	Sodium and calcium caseinates	Sodium and calcium caseinates, L-arginine
CARBOHYDRATE SOURCE	Maltodextrin	Glucose oligosaccharides, sucrose	Hydrolyzed cornstarch, soy fiber, fructose	Hydrolyzed cornstarch
FAT SOURCE	MCT and soy oils	MCT and sunflower oils	Safflower and soy oils	Palm, sunflower and menhaden oils
USE	Sepsis, trauma, metabolic stress	Liver failure	Abnormal glucose intolerance	Sepsis, trauma, cancer, stressed immune system

[3] Mixed at standard dilution.
[4] 124.7 mOsm/l
[5] Manufacturer's data.
[6] Except for phosphorus, vitamins A and D (limited in renal diets).
[7] Mixed at 30 cal/fl oz.
[8] Contains 14.3 g dietary soy fiber per liter.

APPENDIX 33. Enteral Nutrition Products *Continued*

WHOLE PROTEIN FORMULA—LACTOSE-FREE, HIGH CALORIE, HIGH NITROGEN

Product *Source*	**Ensure Plus HN** *Ross*	**Pulmocare[9]** *Ross*	**Trauma Cal** *Mead Johnson*	**Two Cal HN** *Ross*
FORM	Liquid	Liquid	Liquid	Liquid
KCAL/ml	1.5	1.5	1.5	2
PROTEIN (% of calories)	16.7	16.7	21.7	16.6
CARBOHYDRATE (% of calories)	53.3	28.1	37.8	43
FAT (% of calories)	30	55.2	40.5	40.4
PROTEIN (g/liter)	61.7	62.6	82.4	83.7
CARBOHYDRATE (g/liter)	197	105.7	143.7	217
FAT (g/liter)	49.5	92	68.5	90.9
CAL : N	150	150	114	150
SODIUM (mEq/liter)	50.7	57	51.5	50
POTASSIUM (mEq/liter)	50	48.8	35.8	60
OSMOLALITY (mOsm/kg)	650	490	490	690
VOLUME TO MEET 100% of RDA for vitamins and minerals (ml)	946	946	1,964	946
PROTEIN SOURCE	Sodium and calcium caseinates, soy protein isolate	Sodium and calcium caseinates	Sodium and calcium caseinates	Sodium and calcium caseinates
CARBOHYDRATE SOURCE	Hydrolyzed cornstarch, sucrose	Sucrose, hydrolyzed cornstarch	Corn syrup, sugar	Hydrolyzed cornstarch, sucrose
FAT SOURCE	Corn oil	Corn oil	Soy and MCT oils	Corn and MCT oils
FLAVOR	Vanilla	Vanilla	Vanilla	

[9] Use for respiratory insufficiency

Table continued on following page

WHOLE PROTEIN FORMULA—LACTOSE-FREE, HIGH CALORIE

Product *Source*	**Nutren 1.5** *Carnation*	**Nutren 2.0** *Carnation*	**Resource Plus** *Sandoz*	**Sustacal HC** *Mead Johnson*	**Comply** *Sherwood Medical*	**Ensure Plus** *Ross*	**Isocal HCN** *Mead Johnson*	**Magnacal** *Sherwood Medical*
FORM	Liquid	Liquid	Liquid	Liquid	Liquid	Liquid	Liquid	Liquid
KCAL/ml	1.5	2	1.5	1.5	1.5	1.5	2	2
PROTEIN (% of calories)	15.7	15.6	15	16	16	14.7	14.8	14
CARBOHYDRATE (% of calories)	44.5	38	53	50	48	53.3	39.7	50
FAT (% of calories)	39.8	46.4	32	34	36	32	45.5	36
PROTEIN (g/liter)	60	80	54.9	60.9	60	54.2	74.8	70
CARBOHYDRATE (g/liter)	170	196	200	190.2	180	197	200	250
FAT (g/liter)	67.6	106	53.3	57.5	60	52.5	102	80
CAL : N	159	161	171	156	156	170	167	179
SODIUM (mEq/liter)	32.7	43.5	39.1	36.8	44.5	48.9	34.9	43.5
POTASSIUM (mEq/liter)	48.2	64	44.6	37.9	44.2	53.4	43.4	32.1
OSMOLALITY (mOsm/kg)	530	800	600	650	410	690	690	590
VOLUME TO MEET 100% of RDA for vitamins and minerals (ml)	1,400	1,000	1,600	1,183	1,060	1,425	986	1,000
PROTEIN SOURCE	Potassium-calcium caseinate	Potassium-calcium caseinate	Sodium and calcium caseinates, soy protein isolate	Sodium and calcium caseinates	Sodium and calcium caseinates	Sodium and calcium caseinates, soy protein isolate	Sodium and calcium caseinates	Sodium and calcium caseinates
CARBOHYDRATE SOURCE	Maltodextrin, sucrose	Maltodextrin, sucrose, corn syrup	Maltodextrin, sucrose	Corn syrup solids, sugar	Maltodextrin	Corn syrup, sucrose	Corn syrup	Maltodextrin, sucrose
FAT SOURCE	MCT and corn oils	MCT and corn oils	Corn oil	Corn oil	Corn oil	Corn oil	Soy and MCT oils	Soy oil
FLAVOR	Vanilla	Vanilla	Vanilla	Vanilla		Vanilla		

MILK-BASED OR DESIGNED TO BE MIXED W/MILK

Product / ***Source***	**Carnation Inst. Brk.** / ***Clintec***	**Nutri-Care** / ***Advanced Healthcare***	**Sustacal** / ***Mead Johnson***	**Sustagen** / ***Mead Johnson***	**Nonfat Dry Milk**
FORM	Powder	Powder	Powder	Powder	Powder
KCAL/ml	373	375	358	391	360
PROTEIN (% of calories)	21	23	25	24	40
CARBOHYDRATE (% of calories)	72	69	74	68	58
FAT (% of calories)	7	8	1	8	2
PROTEIN (g/liter)	20	21.9	22.8	23.5	36
CARBOHYDRATE (g/liter)	68.8	65.6	66.7	66.4	52
FAT (g/liter)	<2.9	3.1	0.49	3.5	0.9
CAL : N	119	106	98+	104	62.5
SODIUM (mEq/liter)	16.8	16.3	15	9.5	23
POTASSIUM (mEq/liter)	26.5	24	26	18	46
OSMOLALITY (mOsm/kg)	694[10]	661	1,000[11]	1,100	—
VOLUME TO MEET 100% OF RDA for vitamins and minerals (ml)	Vitamins added	800	700[12]	454 g[10]	Incomplete
PROTEIN SOURCE	Nonfat dry milk, whey, calcium caseinate	Whey protein concentrate	Nonfat milk	Nonfat milk, powdered whole milk, calcium caseinate	Nonfat dry milk
CARBOHYDRATE SOURCE	Sugar, maltodextrin, lactose	Sugar, maltodextrin, lactose	Sugar, corn syrup solids, lactose	Corn syrup solids, dextrose, lactose	Lactose
FAT SOURCE	Milk fat	Milk fat	Milk fat	Milk fat	
FLAVOR	Vanilla	Vanilla		Vanilla	

[10] When mixed as directed.
[11] 56 g powder (1 packet) mixed with 8 oz of whole milk.
[12] Mixed with water, can also be mixed with milk, but values will change.

Table continued on following page

APPENDIX 33. Enteral Nutrition Products *Continued*

WHOLE PROTEIN FORMULA — LACTOSE-FREE (<1.5 kcal/ml)

Product *Source*	**Newtrition Isotonic** *Knight Medical*	**Nutren 1.0** *Clintec*	**Osmolite** *Ross*	**Pre-Attain** *Sherwood Medical*	**Replete** *Clintec*	**Resource** *Sandoz*	**Resource** *Sandoz*
FORM	Liquid	Liquid	Liquid	Liquid	Liquid	Liquid	Instant Crystals[13]
KCAL/ml	1	1	1.06	0.5	1	1.06	1.06
PROTEIN (% of calories)	14	16	13.9	16	25	14	14
CARBOHYDRATE (% of calories)	54	50	53.9	48	45	55	55
FAT (% of calories)	32	34	32.2	36	30	31	31
PROTEIN (g/liter)	36	40	37.5	20	62.4	37.2	37.2
CARBOHYDRATE (g/liter)	136	127.2	145	60	112.8	145	145
FAT (g/liter)	36	38	38.4	20	33.2	37.2	37.2
CAL:N	176	158	178	156	100	178	178
SODIUM (mEq/liter)	26	21.7	28	14.8	21.7	29.9	37
POTASSIUM (mEq/liter)	25.6	32	26	14.7	40	28.6	40
OSMOLALITY (mOsm/kg)	300	340	300	150	350	430	450
VOLUME TO MEET 100% of RDA for vitamins and minerals (ml)	1,900	2,075	1,893	1,600	2,000	1,893	1,896
PROTEIN SOURCE	Sodium caseinate, soy protein isolate	Potassium-calcium caseinate	Casein, soy protein isolate	Sodium caseinate	Potassium-calcium caseinate	Sodium and calcium caseinates, soy protein isolate	Sodium and calcium caseinates, soy protein isolate
CARBOHYDRATE SOURCE	Maltodextrin	Maltodextrin and sucrose	Hydrolyzed cornstarch	Maltodextrin	Maltodextrin and sucrose	Maltodextrin and sucrose	Maltodextrin and sucrose
FAT SOURCE	Corn and MCT oils	MCT and corn oils	MCT, corn, and soy oils	Corn oil	Corn oil	Corn oil	Hydrogenated soy oil
FLAVOR		Vanilla				Vanilla	Vanilla

[13] Reconstituted following manufacturer's instructions.

WHOLE PROTEIN FORMULA—LACTOSE-FREE (<1.5 kcal/ml)

Product *Source*	**Pediasure [child]**[14] *Ross*	**Attain** *Sherwood Medical*	**Ensure** *Ross*	**Entralife** *Corpak*	**Entrition** *Biosearch*	**Isocal** *Mead Johnson*	**Isosource** *Sandoz*	**Newtrition** *Knight Medical*	**Nutrapak** *Corpak*	**Sustacal** *Mead Johnson*	**Travasorb MCT** *Clintec*
FORM	Liquid	Liquid	Liquid	Liquid	Liquid	Liquid	Liquid	Liquid	Liquid	Liquid	Powder
KCAL/ml	1	1	1.06	1	1	1.06	1.2	1	1.06	1	1[15]
PROTEIN (% of calories)	11.8	16	14	15	14	12.8	14	14	14	24	20
CARBOHYDRATE (% of calories)	43.6	48	54.5	55	54	49.8	56	54	54	55	50
FAT (% of calories)	44.6	36	31.5	30	32	37.4	30	32	32	21	30
PROTEIN (g/liter)	30	40	37.2	37	35	34.2	43	36	37.2	61.3	49.3
CARBOHYDRATE (g/liter)	110	120	145	138	136	133	170	136	145	139.9	122.8
FAT (g/liter)	50	40	37.2	33.6	35	44.4	41	36	37.2	23.2	33
CAL:N	220	156	178.8	170	179	195	174	176	178	104	125
SODIUM (mEq/liter)	16.6	30	36.8	31.3	30.4	23	31.7	26	36.7	40	15.2
POTASSIUM (mEq/liter)	33.6	30	40	25.6	30.8	33.6	43.6	25.6	40.1	53	25.6
OSMOLALITY (mOsm/kg)	325	300	470	300	300	300	360	450	450	620	312
VOLUME TO MEET 100% of RDA for vitamins and minerals (ml)	1,100	1,600	1,893	2,000	2,000	1,892	1,500	1,750	1,892	1,065	2,000
PROTEIN SOURCE	Sodium caseinate	Sodium and calcium caseinates	Sodium and calcium caseinates, soy protein isolate	Whey and soy protein	Sodium and calcium caseinates	Sodium and calcium caseinates, soy protein isolate	Sodium and calcium caseinates, soy protein isolate	Sodium caseinate, soy protein isolate	Sodium and calcium caseinates, soy protein isolate	Sodium and calcium caseinates, soy protein isolate	Lactalbumin, sodium and potassium caseinates
CARBOHYDRATE SOURCE	Hydrolyzed cornstarch and sucrose	Maltodextrin	Corn syrup and sucrose	Hydrolyzed cornstarch	Maltodextrin	Maltodextrin	Hydrolyzed cornstarch	Maltodextrin, sucrose and glucose	Corn syrup solids, sucrose	Corn syrup, sugar	Corn syrup solids
FAT SOURCE	Safflower, soy, and MCT oils	Corn oil	Corn oil	Corn and MCT oils	Corn oil	Soy and MCT oils	MCT and canola oil	MCT and corn oils	Corn oil	Partially hydrogenated soy oil	MCT and sunflower oils
FLAVOR			Vanilla					Vanilla		Vanilla	

[14] Use for children aged 1 to 6 years old.
[15] Can mix up to 2.0 kcal/ml.

Table continued on following page

APPENDIX 33. Enteral Nutrition Products *Continued*

WHOLE PROTEIN FORMULA—LACTOSE-FREE, HIGH NITROGEN (1–1.28 kcal/ml)

Product *Source*	**Ensure HN** *Ross*	**Entrition HN** *Biosearch*	**Isocal HN** *Mead Johnson*	**Isosource HN** *Sandoz*	**Isotein HN** *Sandoz*	**Newtrition HN** *Knight Medical*	**Osmolite HN** *Ross*	**Entralife HN** *Corpak*
FORM	Liquid	Liquid	Liquid	Liquid	Powder	Liquid	Liquid	Liquid
KCAL/ml	1.06	1	1.06	1.2	1.2[16]	1.2	1.06	1
PROTEIN (% of calories)	16.7	18	16.4	17	23	20	16.6	17
CARBOHYDRATE (% of calories)	53.2	46	45.7	53	52	52	52.6	53
FAT (% of calories)	30.1	36	37.9	30	25	28	30.8	30
PROTEIN (g/liter)	44.3	44	44	53	68	60	44.4	42
CARBOHYDRATE (g/liter)	141	114	122.6	160	156	152	141	133
FAT (g/liter)	35.5	41	45.2	41	34	36	36.8	34
CAL:N	150	143	152	142	111	125	150	150
SODIUM (mEq/liter)	40.4	36.7	40.4	31.7	27	26	40	40
POTASSIUM (mEq/liter)	40.1	40.5	41.2	43.6	27.4	20.5	40	32
OSMOLALITY (mOsm/kg)	470	300	300	330	300	300	300	300
VOLUME TO MEET 100% of RDA for vitamins and minerals (ml)	1,329	1,300	1,183	1,500	1,770	1,250	1,330	1,250
PROTEIN SOURCE	Sodium and calcium caseinates, soy protein isolate	Sodium and calcium caseinates, soy protein isolate	Sodium and calcium caseinates, soy protein isolate	Sodium and calcium caseinates, soy protein isolate	Delactosed lactalbumin, sodium caseinate	Sodium caseinate, soy protein isolate	Sodium and calcium caseinates, soy protein isolate	Sodium and calcium caseinates
CARBOHYDRATE SOURCE	Corn syrup, sucrose	Maltodextrin	Maltodextrin	Hydrolyzed cornstarch	Maltodextrin, fructose	Maltodextrin	Hydrolyzed cornstarch	Maltodextrin
FAT SOURCE	Corn oil	Corn oil	Soy and MCT oils	MCT and canola oils	Soy and MCT oils	MCT and corn oils	MCT, corn, and soy oils	Corn and MCT oils
FLAVOR	Vanilla							

[16] Prepared per manufacturer's directions using one 2.9-oz packet.

DEFINED FORMULA DIETS

Product *Source*	**Criticare HN** *Mead Johnson*	**Peptamen** *Clintec*	**Pepti-2000** *Sherwood Medical*	**Precision Isotonic** *Sandoz*	**Precision HN** *Sandoz*	**Precision LR** *Sandoz*	**Reabilan** *O'Brien Pharmaceuticals*	**Reabilan HN** *O'Brien Pharmaceuticals*
FORM	Liquid	Liquid	Powder	Powder	Powder	Powder	Liquid	Liquid
KCAL/ml	1.06	1	1[17]	1[17]	1.05[17]	1.1[17]	1	1.33
PROTEIN (% of calories)	14	16	16	12	17	10	13	18
CARBOHYDRATES (% of calories)	83	50	75	60	82	89	52	47
FAT (% of calories)	3	34	9	28	1	1	35	35
PROTEIN (g/liter)	38	40	40	29	43.9	26	31.5	58
CARBOHYDRATES (g/liter)	222	127	189	144	216	248	131.5	157.7
FAT (g/liter)	3.4	39	10	30	1.3	1.6	39	51.9
CAL:N	176	156	157	215	150	267	199	144
SODIUM (mEq/liter)	27.6	21.8	29.6	33.5	42.6	30.4	30.4	43.4
POTASSIUM (mEq/liter)	33.6	32	29.5	24.6	23.3	22.6	32	42.3
OSMOLALITY (mOsm/kg)	650	260	490	300	525	530	350	490
VOLUME TO MEET 100% of RDA for vitamins and minerals (ml)	1,893	2,000	1,600	1,560	2,850	1,710	2,250	2,494
PROTEIN SOURCE	Enzymatically hydrolyzed casein	Hydrolyzed whey proteins	Hydrolyzed lactalbumin	Egg-white solids	Egg-white solids	Egg-white solids	Hydrolyzed whey and casein	Hydrolyzed whey and casein
CARBOHYDRATE SOURCE	Maltodextrin, modified cornstarch	Maltodextrin, starch	Maltodextrin	Glucose oligosaccharides, sucrose	Maltodextrin, sucrose	Maltodextrin, sucrose	Dextrin maltose, tapioca	Dextrin maltose, tapioca
FAT SOURCE	Safflower oil	MCT and sunflower oils	MCT and corn oils	Soy oil	Soy oil	Soy oil	MCT, primrose, and soy oils	MCT, primrose, and soy oils
FLAVOR			Vanilla			Vanilla		

[17] Diluted as directed.

Table continued on following page

APPENDIX 33. Enteral Nutrition Products *Continued*

DEFINED FORMULA DIETS

Product *Source*	**Tolerex** *Norwich Eaton*	**Traum-Aid HBC** *Kendall-McGraw*	**Travasorb STD** *Clintec*	**Travasorb HN** *Clintec*	**Vital HN** *Ross*	**Vivonex T.E.N.** *Norwich Eaton*
FORM	Powder	Powder	Powder	Powder	Powder	Powder
KCAL/ml	1[18]	1[18]	1[19]	1[19]	1[18]	1[18]
PROTEIN (% of calories)	8	22	12	18	16.7	15
CARBOHYDRATE (% of calories)	91	67	76	70	73.6	82
FAT (% of calories)	1	11	12	12	9.7	3
PROTEIN (g/liter)	20.6	56	30	45	41.7	38.2
CARBOHYDRATE (g/liter)	226	166	189.9	174.9	184.7	206
FAT (g/liter)	1.5	12.4	13.5	13.5	10.8	2.8
CAL:N	303	112	209	139	150	164
SODIUM (mEq/liter)	20.4	23	40	40	20.3	20
POTASSIUM (mEq/liter)	30	30	30	30	34.2	20
OSMOLALITY (mOsm/kg)	550	760	560	560	500	630
VOLUME TO MEET 100% of RDA for vitamins and minerals (ml)	1,800	3,000	2,000	2,000	1,500	2,000
PROTEIN SOURCE	Free amino acids	Free amino acids (50% BCAA)	Hydrolyzed lactalbumin	Hydrolyzed lactalbumin	Protein components (partially hydrolyzed whey, meat, soy), amino acids	Free amino acids
CARBOHYDRATE SOURCE	Glucose oligosaccharides	Maltodextrin	Glucose oligosaccharides	Glucose oligosaccharides	Hydrolyzed cornstarch, sucrose	Maltodextrin
FAT SOURCE	Safflower oil	Soy and MCT oils	MCT and sunflower oils	MCT and sunflower oils	Safflower and MCT oils	Safflower oil

[18] Diluted per manufacturer's directions.
[19] At standard dilution.

APPENDIX 33. Enteral Nutrition Products *Continued*

WHOLE PROTEIN FORMULA — LACTOSE-FREE WITH FIBER

Product *Source*	**Enrich** *Ross*	**Jevity** *Ross*	**Newtrition Isofiber** *Knight Medical*	**Pro Fiber** *Sherwood Medical*	**Sustacal w/Fiber** *Mead Johnson*	**Fibersource** *Sandoz*	**Fibersource HN** *Sandoz*
FORM	Liquid	Liquid	Liquid	Liquid	Liquid	Liquid	Liquid
KCAL/ml	1.1	1.06	1.2	1	1.06	1.2	1.2
PROTEIN (% of calories)	14	15.9	17	16	17	14	17
CARBOHYDRATE (% of calories)	57	54.4	54	50	53	56	53
FAT (% of calories)	29	29.7	29	34	30	30	30
PROTEIN (g/liter)	39.7	44.4	48	40	45.7	43	53
CARBOHYDRATE (g/liter)	162	152	152	132	139.5	170	160
FAT (g/liter)	37.2	36.8	36	40	35	41	41
CAL:N	173	149	141	156	145	174	142
SODIUM (mEq/liter)	36.8	40.4	36.7	32	31.2	37.8	37.8
POTASSIUM (mEq/liter)	43.4	40.1	32.5	32	35.8	46	46
OSMOLALITY (mOsm/kg)	480	310	310	300	450	390	390
VOLUME TO MEET 100% of RDA for vitamins and minerals (ml)	1,392	1,324	1,250	1,500	1,391	1,500	1,500
PROTEIN SOURCE	Sodium and calcium caseinates, soy protein isolate	Sodium and calcium caseinates	Sodium and calcium caseinates, soy protein isolate	Sodium and calcium caseinates	Sodium and calcium caseinates, soy protein isolate	Sodium and calcium caseinates	Sodium and calcium caseinates
CARBOHYDRATE SOURCE	Hydrolyzed cornstarch, sucrose	Hydrolyzed cornstarch	Maltodextrin, soy polysaccharide	Hydrolyzed cornstarch	Maltodextrin, sugar	Hydrolyzed cornstarch	Hydrolyzed cornstarch
FAT SOURCE	Corn oil	MCT, corn, and soy oils	MCT and corn oils	Corn oil	Corn oil	MCT and canola oil	MCT and canola oil
FIBER SOURCE	Soy fiber — 14.4 g total dietary fiber per liter	Soy fiber — 14.4 g total dietary fiber per liter	Soy fiber — 14 g total dietary fiber per liter	Soy fiber — 12 g total dietary fiber per liter	Soy fiber — 5.9 g total dietary fiber per liter	Soy fiber — 10 g total dietary fiber per liter	Soy fiber — 6.8 g total dietary fiber per liter

Table continued on following page

APPENDIX 33. Enteral Nutrition Products *Continued*

MILK-BASED WHOLE PROTEIN FORMULA

Product *Source*	**Meritene**[20] *Sandoz*	**Meritene** *Sandoz*
FORM	Powder	Liquid
KCAL/ml	1.06	0.96
PROTEIN (% of calories)	26	24
CARBOHYDRATE (% of calories)	45	46
FAT (% of calories)	29	30
PROTEIN (g/liter)	69.2	57.6
CARBOHYDRATE (g/liter)	119	110
FAT (g/liter)	33.8	32
CAL:N	96	104
SODIUM (mEq/liter)	47.8	38.3
POTASSIUM (mEq/liter)	71.8	41
OSMOLALITY (mOsm/kg)	690	505
VOLUME TO MEET 100% of RDA for vitamins and minerals (ml)	1,040	1,250
PROTEIN SOURCE	Nonfat dry milk, calcium caseinate	Concentrated sweet skim milk, sodium caseinate
CARBOHYDRATE SOURCE	Sucrose, corn syrup solids, fructose	Corn syrup solids, sucrose
FAT SOURCE	Milk fat from added whole milk	Corn oil
FLAVOR	Vanilla	Vanilla

BLENDERIZED TUBE FEEDINGS

Product *Source*	**Compleat Regular** *Sandoz*	**Compleat**[21] **Modified** *Sandoz*	**Vitaneed**[21] *Sherwood Medical*
FORM	Liquid	Liquid	Liquid
KCAL/ml	1.07	1.07	1
PROTEIN (% of calories)	16	16	16
CARBOHYDRATE (% of calories)	48	53	50
FAT (% of calories)	36	31	34
PROTEIN (g/liter)	42.8	42.8	40
CARBOHYDRATES (g/liter)	128	141.2	128
FAT (g/liter)	42.8	36.8	40
CAL:N	156	156	161
SODIUM (mEq/liter)	55.7	43.5	29.6
POTASSIUM (mEq/liter)	35.9	35.9	32.1
OSMOLALITY (mOsm/kg)	450	300	300
VOLUME TO MEET 100% of RDA for vitamins and minerals (ml)	1,500	1,500	1,500
PROTEIN SOURCE	Beef purée, nonfat dry milk	Beef purée, calcium caseinate	Beef purée, sodium and calcium caseinates
CARBOHYDRATE SOURCE	Maltodextrin, puréed foods	Maltodextrin, puréed foods	Maltodextrin, puréed foods, soy fiber
FAT SOURCE	Corn oil	Corn oil	Corn oil

[20] Prepared with whole milk.
[21] Lactose-free.

MODULAR COMPONENTS FOR ENTERAL FEEDING—PROTEIN

Product *Source*	**Casec** *Mead Johnson*	**Nutrisource Protein** *Sandoz*	**Pro-Mix R.D.P.** *Corpak*	**Pro Mod** *Ross*	**Propac** *Sherwood Medical*	**Nutrisource Amino Acids** *Sandoz*	**Nutrisource Amino Acids—High Branched Chain** *Sandoz*
FORM	Powder	Powder	Powder	Powder	Powder	Powder	Powder
KCAL/ml	370	400	360	424	400	380	380
PROTEIN (% of calories)	95	75	84	71	77	100	100
CARBOHYDRATE (% of calories)		6	6		5		
FAT (% of calories)	5	19	10		18		
PROTEIN (g/liter)	88	75.8	75.2	75.8	0.77	97.1	97.1
CARBOHYDRATE (g/liter)		6.9	5		5.2		
FAT (g/liter)	2	8.5	4		8		
CAL:N	26	33.6	30		33	25	25
SODIUM (mEq/liter)	6.5	11.6	10	9.9	10		
POTASSIUM (mEq/liter)	0.26	14.4	21.2	25.3	13.3		
OSMOLALITY (mOsm/kg)	[22]			[23]			
VOLUME TO MEET 100% of RDA for vitamins and minerals (ml)	Incomplete	Incomplete	Incomplete	Incomplete	Incomplete	Incomplete	Incomplete
PROTEIN SOURCE	Calcium caseinate	Delactosed lactalbumin, egg-white solids	Whey protein	Whey protein concentrate and soy lecithin	Whey protein	Free amino acids	Free amino acids (44% BCAA)*
CARBOHYDRATE SOURCE	—	—	—	—	—	—	—
FAT SOURCE	—	—	—	—	—	—	—

[22] 40 g of Casec or less added to any liquid equals liquid's osmolality.
[23] 5 g of protein = ~30 mOsm.

Table continued on following page

APPENDIX 33. Enteral Nutrition Products *Continued*

MODULAR COMPONENTS FOR ENTERAL FEEDING—CARBOHYDRATE

Product *Source*	**Moducal** *Mead Johnson*	**Polycose** *Ross*	**Pure Carbohydrate Supplement** *Corpak*	**Sumacal** *Sherwood Medical*	**Karo Syrup** *Best Foods*	**Liquid Carbohydrate Supplement** *Corpak*	**Nutrisource Carbohydrate** *Sandoz*	**Polycose** *Ross*
FORM	Powder	Powder	Powder	Powder	Liquid	Liquid	Liquid	Liquid
KCAL/ml	380	380	400	380	3	2.5	3.2	2
PROTEIN (% of calories)								
CARBOHYDRATE (% of calories)	100	100	100	100	100	100	100	100
FAT (% of calories)								
PROTEIN (g/liter)								
CARBOHYDRATE (g/liter)	95	94	100	95	75	62.5	80	50
FAT (g/liter)								
CAL:N								
SODIUM (mEq/liter)	3	4.8	0.7	4.4	6.5	2.7	<1	3
POTASSIUM (mEq/liter)	13	0.26	Unknown	<1	Unknown	0.48	<1	0.15
OSMOLALITY (mOsm/kg)	99[24]	[25]			Unknown	Unknown	Unknown	900
VOLUME TO MEET 100% of RDA for vitamins and minerals (ml)	Incomplete	Incomplete	Incomplete	Incomplete	Incomplete	Incomplete	Incomplete	Incomplete
PROTEIN SOURCE	—	—	—	—	—	—	—	—
CARBOHYDRATE SOURCE	Maltodextrin (glucose polymers)	Hydrolyzed cornstarch, glucose polymers	Maltodextrin or glucose polymers	Maltodextrin	Corn syrup, high fructose corn syrup	Glucose polymers	Deionized corn syrup solids	Glucose polymers from hydrolyzed cornstarch
FAT SOURCE	—	—	—	—	—	—	—	—

[24] 30 g of Moducal in 250 ml of distilled water.
[25] Same osmolality as liquid to which is added.

APPENDIX 33. Enteral Nutrition Products *Continued*

MODULAR COMPONENTS FOR ENTERAL FEEDING — FAT (POWDER)

Product / ***Source***	**High MCT Supplement** / ***Corpak***
FORM	Powder
KCAL/ml	6.12
PROTEIN (% of calories)	3
CARBOHYDRATE (% of calories)	27
FAT (% of calories)	70
PROTEIN (g/liter)	4.9
CARBOHYDRATE (g/liter)	40.4
FAT (g/liter)	47
CAL : N	
SODIUM (mEq/liter)	
POTASSIUM (mEq/liter)	
OSMOLALITY (mOsm/kg)	Unknown
GRAMS TO MEET 100% OF RDA for vitamins and minerals (g)	Incomplete
PROTEIN SOURCE	—
CARBOHYDRATE SOURCE	Dried corn syrup
FAT SOURCE	Coconut oil

MODULAR COMPONENTS FOR ENTERAL FEEDING — FAT (LIQUID)

Product / ***Source***	**Vegetable Oil**	**MCT Oil** / ***Mead Johnson***	**Microlipid** / ***Sherwood Medical***	**Nutrisource Lipid-long-chain Triglycerides** / ***Corpak***	**Nutrisource Lipid-medium-chain Triglycerides** / ***Corpak***
FORM	Liquid	Liquid	Liquid	Liquid	Liquid
KCAL/ml	8	7.67	4.5	2.2	2
PROTEIN (% of calories)					
CARBOHYDRATE (% of calories)					
FAT (% of calories)	100	100	100	100	100
PROTEIN (g/liter)					
CARBOHYDRATE (g/liter)					
FAT (g/liter)					
CAL : N					
SODIUM (mEq/liter)					
POTASSIUM (mEq/liter)					
OSMOLALITY (mOsm/kg)	Unknown	Unknown	60	Unknown	Unknown
VOLUME TO MEET 100% of RDA for vitamins and minerals (ml)	Incomplete	Incomplete	Incomplete	Incomplete	Incomplete
PROTEIN SOURCE	—	—	—	—	—
CARBOHYDRATE SOURCE	—	—	—	—	—
FAT SOURCE	Depends on selection	MCT oil	Safflower oil	Soy oil	Coconut oil
FLAVOR SOURCE	—				

APPENDIX 34. Calculation of the Caloric Distribution of a Diet

To calculate the number of grams of carbohydrate, protein, and fat needed to make up a diet that has a particular distribution of calories:

Total kcal in the diet $\times$ % of kcal desired from a particular nutrient = number of kcal to come from that nutrient

$$\frac{\text{number of kcal from nutrient}}{\text{number of kcal per g of that nutrient}} = \text{grams of nutrient required}$$

For example, to calculate the required number of grams of protein, carbohydrate, and fat for this diet:
total kcal = 2400
20% of kcal = protein
50% of kcal = carbohydrate
30% of kcal = fat

2,400 kcal $\times$ 20% = 480 kcal from protein

$$\frac{\text{480 kcal from protein}}{\text{4 kcal/g of protein}} = \text{120 g of protein}$$

2400 kcal $\times$ 50% = 1,200 kcal from carbohydrate

$$\frac{\text{1200 kcal from carbohydrate}}{\text{4 kcal/g of carbohydrate}} = \text{300 g of carbohydrate}$$

2,400 kcal $\times$ 30% = 720 kcal from fat

$$\frac{\text{720 kcal from fat}}{\text{9 kcal/g of fat}} = \text{80 g of fat}$$

The final diet contains 120 g protein, 300 g carbohydrate, and 80 g fat.

To calculate the caloric distribution of a diet of known composition:
g protein in diet $\times$ 4 kcal/g protein = number of kcal from protein
g carbohydrate in diet $\times$ 4 kcal/g carbohydrate = number of kcal from carbohydrate
g fat in diet $\times$ 9 kcal/g fat = number of kcal from fat
kcal from protein + kcal from carbohydrate + kcal from fat = total kcal in the diet

$$\frac{\text{kcal from nutrient}}{\text{total kcal in the diet}} \times 100 = \text{\% of total kcal from nutrient}$$

For example, to calculate the caloric distribution of a diet that contains 100 g fat, 100 g protein, and 300 g carbohydrate:
100 g protein $\times$ 4 kcal/g protein = 400 kcal from protein
300 g carbohydrate $\times$ 4 kcal/g carbohydrate = 1,200 kcal from carbohydrate
100 g fat $\times$ 9 kcal/g fat = 900 kcal from fat
400 kcal + 1,200 kcal + 900 kcal = 2,500 kcal = total kcal in diet

$$\frac{\text{400 kcal from protein}}{\text{2,500 total kcal in diet}} \times 100 = \text{16\% of kcal from protein}$$

$$\frac{\text{1,200 kcal from carbohydrate}}{\text{2,500 total kcal in diet}} \times 100 = \text{48\% of kcal from carbohydrate}$$

$$\frac{\text{900 kcal from fat}}{\text{2,500 total kcal in diet}} \times 100 = \text{36\% of kcal from fat}$$

APPENDIX 35. Milliequivalents and Milligrams of Electrolytes*

To Convert Milligrams to Milliequivalents

1. Divide milligrams by atomic weight and then multiply by the valence

$$\frac{\text{Milligrams}}{\text{Atomic weight}} \times \text{valence} = \text{milliequivalents}$$

Mineral Element	Chemical Symbol	Atomic Weight	Valence
Chlorine	Cl	35.4	1
Potassium	K	39	1
Sodium	Na	23	1
Calcium	Ca	40	2
Magnesium	Mg	24.3	2
Sulfur	S	32	
Sulfate	SO_4	96	2

To Convert Specific Weight of Sodium to Sodium Chloride

1. Multiply by 2.54
Example: 1,000 mg sodium = 1,000 × 2.54 = 2,540 mg sodium chloride (2.5 g)

To Convert Specific Weight of Sodium Chloride to Sodium

1. Multiply by 0.393
Example: 2.5 g sodium chloride = 2.5 × 0.393 = 1,000 mg sodium

Milligrams	Sodium Values (Milliequivalents)	Grams of Sodium Chloride
500	21.8	1.3
1,000	43.5	2.5
1,500	75.3	3.8
2,000	87.0	5.0

* Adapted from Mayo Clinic Diet Manual, 4th ed. Philadelphia, WB Saunders, 1971.

APPENDIX 36. Energy Expenditure During Various Activities (kcal/min) for People of Various Weights*†‡

Activity / Person's Weight (kg) (lb)	50 110	53 117	56 123	59 130	62 137	65 143	68 150	71 157	74 163	77 170	80 176	83 183	86 190	89 196	92 203	95 209	98 216
Archery	3.3	3.4	3.6	3.8	4.0	4.2	4.4	4.6	4.8	5.0	5.2	5.4	5.6	5.8	6.0	6.2	6.4
Badminton	4.9	5.1	5.4	5.7	6.0	6.3	6.6	6.9	7.2	7.5	7.8	8.1	8.3	8.6	8.9	9.2	9.5
Bakery, general (F)	1.8	1.9	2.0	2.1	2.2	2.3	2.4	2.5	2.6	2.7	2.8	2.9	3.0	3.1	3.2	3.3	3.4
Basketball	6.9	7.3	7.7	8.1	8.6	9.0	9.4	9.8	10.2	10.6	11.0	11.5	11.9	12.3	12.7	13.1	13.5
Billiards	2.1	2.2	2.4	2.5	2.6	2.7	2.9	3.0	3.1	3.2	3.4	3.5	3.6	3.7	3.9	4.0	4.1
Bookbinding	1.9	2.0	2.1	2.2	2.4	2.5	2.6	2.7	2.8	2.9	3.0	3.2	3.3	3.4	3.5	3.6	3.7
Boxing																	
in ring	6.9	7.3	7.7	8.1	8.6	9.0	9.4	9.8	10.2	10.6	11.0	11.5	11.9	12.3	12.7	13.1	13.5
sparring	11.1	11.8	12.4	13.1	13.8	14.4	15.1	15.8	16.4	17.1	17.8	18.4	19.1	19.8	20.4	21.1	21.8
Canoeing																	
Leisure	2.2	2.3	2.5	2.6	2.7	2.9	3.0	3.1	3.3	3.4	3.5	3.7	3.8	3.9	4.0	4.2	4.3
Racing	5.2	5.5	5.8	6.1	6.4	6.7	7.0	7.3	7.6	7.9	8.2	8.5	8.9	9.2	9.5	9.8	10.1
Card playing	1.3	1.3	1.4	1.5	1.6	1.6	1.7	1.8	1.9	1.9	2.0	2.1	2.2	2.2	2.3	2.4	2.5
Carpentry, general	2.6	2.8	2.9	3.1	3.2	3.4	3.5	3.7	3.8	4.0	4.2	4.3	4.5	4.6	4.8	4.9	5.1
Carpet sweeping (F)	2.3	2.4	2.5	2.7	2.8	2.9	3.1	3.2	3.3	3.5	3.6	3.7	3.9	4.0	4.1	4.3	4.4
Carpet sweeping (M)	2.4	2.5	2.7	2.8	3.0	3.1	3.3	3.4	3.6	3.7	3.8	4.0	4.1	4.3	4.4	4.6	4.7
Circuit training																	
Hydra-Fitness	6.6	7.0	7.4	7.8	8.2	8.6	9.0	9.4	9.7	10.2	10.5	10.9	11.4	11.7	12.1	12.5	12.9
Universal	5.8	6.2	6.5	6.9	7.2	7.5	7.9	8.3	8.6	8.9	9.3	9.6	10.0	10.3	10.7	11.0	11.4
Nautilus	4.6	4.9	5.2	5.5	5.8	6.0	6.3	6.6	6.8	7.1	7.4	7.7	8.0	8.2	8.5	8.8	9.1
Free Weights	4.3	4.5	4.8	5.0	5.3	5.5	5.8	6.1	6.3	6.6	6.8	7.1	7.4	7.6	7.9	8.1	8.4
Cleaning (F)	3.1	3.3	3.5	3.7	3.8	4.0	4.2	4.4	4.6	4.8	5.0	5.1	5.3	5.5	5.7	5.9	6.1
Cleaning (M)	2.9	3.1	3.2	3.4	3.6	3.8	3.9	4.1	4.3	4.5	4.6	4.8	5.0	5.2	5.3	5.5	5.7
Climbing hills																	
will no load	6.1	6.4	6.8	7.1	7.5	7.9	8.2	8.6	9.0	9.3	9.7	10.0	10.4	10.8	11.1	11.5	11.9
with 5-kg load	6.5	6.8	7.2	7.6	8.0	8.4	8.8	9.2	9.5	9.9	10.3	10.7	11.1	11.5	11.9	12.3	12.6
with 10-kg load	7.0	7.4	7.8	8.3	8.7	9.1	9.5	9.9	10.4	10.8	11.2	11.6	12.0	12.5	12.9	13.3	13.7
with 20-kg load	7.4	7.8	8.2	8.7	9.1	9.6	10.0	10.4	10.9	11.3	11.8	12.2	12.6	13.1	13.5	14.0	14.4
Coal mining																	
Drilling coal, rock	4.7	5.0	5.3	5.5	5.8	6.1	6.4	6.7	7.0	7.2	7.5	7.8	8.1	8.4	8.6	8.9	9.2
Erecting supports	4.4	4.7	4.9	5.2	5.5	5.7	6.0	6.2	6.5	6.8	7.0	7.3	7.6	7.8	8.1	8.4	8.6
Shoveling coal	5.4	5.7	6.0	6.4	6.7	7.0	7.3	7.7	8.0	8.3	8.6	9.0	9.3	9.6	9.9	10.3	10.6
Cooking (F)	2.3	2.4	2.5	2.7	2.8	2.9	3.1	3.2	3.3	3.5	3.6	3.7	3.9	4.0	4.1	4.3	4.4
Cooking (M)	2.4	2.5	2.7	2.8	3.0	3.1	3.3	3.4	3.6	3.7	3.8	4.0	4.1	4.3	4.4	4.6	4.7
Cricket																	
Batting	4.2	4.4	4.6	4.9	5.1	5.4	5.6	5.9	6.1	6.4	6.6	6.9	7.1	7.4	7.6	7.9	8.1
Bowling	4.5	4.8	5.0	5.3	5.6	5.9	6.1	6.4	6.7	6.9	7.2	7.5	7.7	8.0	8.3	8.6	8.8
Croquet	3.0	3.1	3.3	3.5	3.7	3.8	4.0	4.2	4.4	4.5	4.7	4.9	5.1	5.3	5.4	5.6	5.8
Cycling																	
Leisure, 5.5 mph	3.2	3.4	3.6	3.8	4.0	4.2	4.4	4.5	4.7	4.9	5.1	5.3	5.5	5.7	5.9	6.1	6.3
Leisure, 9.4 mph	5.0	5.3	5.6	5.9	6.2	6.5	6.8	7.1	7.4	7.7	8.0	8.3	8.6	8.9	9.2	9.5	9.8
Racing	8.5	9.0	9.5	10.0	10.5	11.0	11.5	12.0	12.5	13.0	13.5	14.0	14.5	15.0	15.5	16.1	16.6
Dancing (F)																	
Aerobic, medium	5.2	5.5	5.8	6.1	6.4	6.7	7.0	7.3	7.6	7.9	8.2	8.5	8.9	9.2	9.5	9.8	10.1
Aerobic, intense	6.7	7.1	7.5	7.9	8.3	8.7	9.2	9.6	10.0	10.4	10.8	11.2	11.6	12.0	12.4	12.8	13.2
Ballroom	2.6	2.7	2.9	3.0	3.2	3.3	3.5	3.6	3.8	3.9	4.1	4.2	4.4	4.5	4.7	4.8	5.0
Choreographed	8.4	8.9	9.4	9.9	10.4	10.9	11.4	11.9	12.4	12.9	13.4	13.9	14.4	15.0	15.5	16.0	16.5
"Twist," "wiggle"	5.2	5.5	5.8	6.1	6.4	6.7	7.0	7.3	7.6	7.9	8.2	8.5	8.9	9.2	9.5	9.8	10.1

Activity																	
Digging trenches	7.3	7.7	8.1	8.6	9.0	9.4	9.9	10.3	10.7	11.2	11.6	12.0	12.5	12.9	13.3	13.8	14.2
Drawing (standing)	1.8	1.9	2.0	2.1	2.2	2.3	2.4	2.6	2.7	2.8	2.9	3.0	3.1	3.2	3.3	3.4	3.5
Eating (sitting)	1.2	1.2	1.3	1.4	1.4	1.5	1.6	1.6	1.7	1.8	1.8	1.9	2.0	2.0	2.1	2.2	2.3
Electrical work	2.9	3.1	3.2	3.4	3.6	3.8	3.9	4.1	4.3	4.5	4.6	4.8	5.0	5.2	5.3	5.5	5.7
Farming																	
Barn cleaning	6.8	7.2	7.6	8.0	8.4	8.8	9.2	9.6	10.0	10.4	10.8	11.2	11.6	12.0	12.4	12.8	13.2
Driving harvester	2.0	2.1	2.2	2.4	2.5	2.6	2.7	2.8	3.0	3.1	3.2	3.3	3.4	3.6	3.7	3.8	3.9
Driving tractor	1.9	2.0	2.1	2.2	2.3	2.4	2.5	2.6	2.7	2.8	3.0	3.1	3.2	3.3	3.4	3.5	3.6
Feeding cattle	4.3	4.5	4.8	5.0	5.3	5.5	5.8	6.0	6.3	6.5	6.8	7.1	7.3	7.6	7.8	8.1	8.3
Feeding animals	3.3	3.4	3.6	3.8	4.0	4.2	4.4	4.6	4.8	5.0	5.2	5.4	5.6	5.8	6.0	6.2	6.4
Forking straw bales	6.9	7.3	7.7	8.1	8.6	9.0	9.4	9.8	10.2	10.6	11.0	11.5	11.9	12.3	12.7	13.1	13.5
Milking by hand	2.7	2.9	3.0	3.2	3.3	3.5	3.7	3.8	4.0	4.2	4.3	4.5	4.6	4.8	5.0	5.1	5.3
Milking by machine	1.2	1.2	1.3	1.4	1.4	1.5	1.6	1.6	1.7	1.8	1.8	1.9	2.0	2.0	2.1	2.2	2.3
Shoveling grain	4.3	4.5	4.8	5.0	5.3	5.5	5.8	6.0	6.3	6.5	6.8	7.1	7.3	7.6	7.8	8.1	8.3
Field hockey	6.7	7.1	7.5	7.9	8.3	8.7	9.1	9.5	9.9	10.3	10.7	11.1	11.5	11.9	12.3	12.7	13.1
Fishing	3.1	3.3	3.5	3.7	3.8	4.0	4.2	4.4	4.6	4.8	5.0	5.1	5.3	5.5	5.7	5.9	6.1
Food shopping (F)	3.1	3.3	3.5	3.7	3.8	4.0	4.2	4.4	4.6	4.8	5.0	5.1	5.3	5.5	5.7	5.9	6.1
Food shopping (M)	2.9	3.1	3.2	3.4	3.6	3.8	3.9	4.1	4.3	4.5	4.6	4.8	5.0	5.2	5.3	5.5	5.7
Football	6.6	7.0	7.4	7.8	8.2	8.6	9.0	9.4	9.8	10.2	10.6	11.0	11.4	11.7	12.1	12.5	12.9
Forestry																	
Axe chopping, fast	14.9	15.7	16.6	17.5	18.4	19.3	20.2	21.1	22.0	22.9	23.8	24.7	25.5	26.4	27.3	28.2	29.1
Axe chopping, slow	4.3	4.5	4.8	5.0	5.3	5.5	5.8	6.0	6.3	6.5	6.8	7.1	7.3	7.6	7.8	8.1	8.3
Barking trees	6.2	6.5	6.9	7.3	7.6	8.0	8.4	8.7	9.1	9.5	9.8	10.2	10.6	10.9	11.3	11.7	12.1
Carrying logs	9.3	9.9	10.4	11.0	11.5	12.1	12.6	13.2	13.8	14.3	14.9	15.4	16.0	16.6	17.1	17.7	18.2
Felling trees	6.6	7.0	7.4	7.8	8.2	8.6	9.0	9.4	9.8	10.2	10.6	11.0	11.4	11.7	12.1	12.5	12.9
Hoeing	4.6	4.8	5.1	5.4	5.6	5.9	6.2	6.5	6.7	7.0	7.3	7.6	7.8	8.1	8.4	8.6	8.9
Planting by hand	5.5	5.8	6.1	6.4	6.8	7.1	7.4	7.7	8.1	8.4	8.7	9.0	9.4	9.7	10.0	10.4	10.7
Sawing by hand	6.1	6.5	6.8	7.2	7.6	7.9	8.3	8.7	9.0	9.4	9.8	10.1	10.5	10.9	11.2	11.6	12.0
Sawing, power	3.8	4.0	4.2	4.4	4.7	4.9	5.1	5.3	5.6	5.8	6.0	6.2	6.5	6.7	6.9	7.1	7.4
Stacking firewood	4.4	4.7	4.9	5.2	5.5	5.7	6.0	6.2	6.5	6.8	7.0	7.3	7.6	7.8	8.1	8.4	8.6
Trimming trees	6.5	6.8	7.2	7.6	8.0	8.4	8.8	9.2	9.5	9.9	10.3	10.7	11.1	11.5	11.9	12.3	12.6
Weeding	3.6	3.8	4.0	4.2	4.5	4.7	4.9	5.1	5.3	5.5	5.8	6.0	6.2	6.4	6.6	6.8	7.1
Furriery	4.2	4.4	4.6	4.9	5.1	5.4	5.6	5.9	6.1	6.4	6.6	6.9	7.1	7.4	7.6	7.9	8.1
Gardening																	
Digging	6.3	6.7	7.1	7.4	7.8	8.2	8.6	8.9	9.3	9.7	10.1	10.5	10.8	11.2	11.6	12.0	12.3
Hedging	3.9	4.1	4.3	4.5	4.8	5.0	5.2	5.5	5.7	5.9	6.2	6.4	6.6	6.9	7.1	7.3	7.5
Mowing	5.6	5.9	6.3	6.6	6.9	7.3	7.6	8.0	8.3	8.6	9.0	9.3	9.6	10.0	10.3	10.6	11.0
Raking	2.7	2.9	3.0	3.2	3.3	3.5	3.7	3.8	4.0	4.2	4.3	4.5	4.6	4.8	5.0	5.1	5.3
Golf	4.3	4.5	4.8	5.0	5.3	5.5	5.8	6.0	6.3	6.5	6.8	7.1	7.3	7.6	7.8	8.1	8.3
Gymnastics	3.3	3.5	3.7	3.9	4.1	4.3	4.5	4.7	4.9	5.1	5.3	5.5	5.7	5.9	6.1	6.3	6.5
Horse-grooming	6.4	6.8	7.2	7.6	7.9	8.3	8.7	9.1	9.5	9.9	10.2	10.6	11.0	11.4	11.8	12.2	12.5
Horse-racing																	
Galloping	6.9	7.3	7.7	8.1	8.5	8.9	9.3	9.7	10.1	10.6	11.0	11.4	11.8	12.2	12.6	13.0	13.4
Trotting	5.5	5.8	6.2	6.5	6.8	7.2	7.5	7.8	8.1	8.5	8.8	9.1	9.5	9.8	10.1	10.5	10.8
Walking	2.1	2.2	2.3	2.4	2.5	2.7	2.8	2.9	3.0	3.2	3.3	3.4	3.5	3.6	3.8	3.9	4.0
Ironing (F)	1.7	1.7	1.8	1.9	2.0	2.1	2.2	2.3	2.4	2.5	2.6	2.7	2.8	2.9	3.0	3.1	3.2
Ironing (M)	3.2	3.4	3.6	3.8	4.0	4.2	4.4	4.5	4.7	4.9	5.1	5.3	5.5	5.7	5.9	6.1	6.3
Judo	9.8	10.3	10.9	11.5	12.1	12.7	13.3	13.8	14.4	15.0	15.6	16.2	16.8	17.4	17.9	18.5	19.1
Jumping rope																	
70 per min	8.1	8.6	9.1	9.6	10.0	10.5	11.0	11.5	12.0	12.5	13.0	13.4	13.9	14.4	14.9	15.4	15.9
80 per min	8.2	8.7	9.2	9.7	10.2	10.7	11.2	11.6	12.1	12.6	13.1	13.6	14.1	14.6	14.6	15.6	16.1
125 per min	8.9	9.4	9.9	10.4	11.0	11.5	12.0	12.6	13.1	13.6	14.2	14.7	15.2	15.8	16.3	16.8	17.3
145 per min	9.9	10.4	11.0	11.6	12.2	12.8	13.4	14.0	14.6	15.2	15.8	16.4	16.9	17.5	18.1	18.7	19.3

Table continued on following page

APPENDIX 36. Energy Expenditure During Various Activities (kcal/min) for People of Various Weights*†‡ *Continued*

Activity — Person's Weight (kg) / (lb)	50 110	53 117	56 123	59 130	62 137	65 143	68 150	71 157	74 163	77 170	80 176	83 183	86 190	89 196	92 203	95 209	98 216
Knitting, sewing (F)	1.1	1.2	1.2	1.3	1.4	1.4	1.5	1.6	1.6	1.7	1.8	1.8	1.9	2.0	2.0	2.1	2.2
Knitting, sewing (M)	1.2	1.2	1.3	1.4	1.4	1.5	1.6	1.6	1.7	1.8	1.8	1.9	2.0	2.0	2.1	2.2	2.3
Locksmith	2.9	3.0	3.2	3.4	3.5	3.7	3.9	4.0	4.2	4.4	4.6	4.7	4.9	5.1	5.2	5.4	5.6
Lying at ease	1.1	1.2	1.2	1.3	1.4	1.4	1.5	1.6	1.6	1.7	1.8	1.8	1.9	2.0	2.0	2.1	2.2
Machine-tooling																	
Machining	2.4	2.5	2.7	2.8	3.0	3.1	3.3	3.4	3.6	3.7	3.8	4.0	4.1	4.3	4.4	4.6	4.7
Operating lathe	2.6	2.8	2.9	3.1	3.2	3.4	3.5	3.7	3.8	4.0	4.2	4.3	4.5	4.6	4.8	4.9	5.1
Operating punch press	4.4	4.7	4.9	5.2	5.5	5.7	6.0	6.2	6.5	6.8	7.0	7.3	7.6	7.8	8.1	8.4	8.6
Tapping and drilling	3.3	3.4	3.6	3.8	4.0	4.2	4.4	4.6	4.8	5.0	5.2	5.4	5.6	5.8	6.0	6.2	6.4
Welding	2.6	2.8	2.9	3.1	3.2	3.4	3.5	3.7	3.8	4.0	4.2	4.3	4.5	4.6	4.8	4.9	5.1
Working sheet metal	2.4	2.5	2.7	2.8	3.0	3.1	3.3	3.4	3.6	3.7	3.8	4.0	4.1	4.3	4.4	4.6	4.7
Marching, rapid	7.1	7.5	8.0	8.4	8.8	9.2	9.7	10.1	10.5	10.9	11.4	11.8	12.2	12.6	13.1	13.5	13.9
Mopping floor (F)	3.1	3.3	3.5	3.7	3.8	4.0	4.2	4.4	4.6	4.8	5.0	5.1	5.3	5.5	5.7	5.9	6.1
Mopping floor (M)	2.9	3.1	3.2	3.4	3.6	3.8	3.9	4.1	4.3	4.5	4.6	4.8	5.0	5.2	5.2†	5.5	5.7
Music playing																	
Accordion (sitting)	1.6	1.7	1.8	1.9	2.0	2.1	2.2	2.3	2.4	2.5	2.6	2.7	2.8	2.8	2.9	3.0	3.1
Cello (sitting)	2.1	2.2	2.3	2.4	2.5	2.7	2.8	2.9	3.0	3.2	3.3	3.4	3.5	3.6	3.8	3.9	4.0
Conducting	2.0	2.1	2.2	2.3	2.4	2.5	2.7	2.8	2.9	3.0	3.1	3.2	3.4	3.5	3.6	3.7	3.8
Drums (sitting)	3.3	3.5	3.7	3.9	4.1	4.3	4.5	4.7	4.9	5.1	5.3	5.5	5.7	5.9	6.1	6.3	6.6
Flute (sitting)	1.8	1.9	2.0	2.1	2.2	2.3	2.4	2.5	2.6	2.7	2.8	2.9	3.0	3.1	3.2	3.3	3.4
Horn (sitting)	1.5	1.5	1.6	1.7	1.8	1.9	2.0	2.1	2.1	2.2	2.3	2.4	2.5	2.6	2.7	2.8	2.8
Organ (sitting)	2.7	2.8	3.0	3.1	3.3	3.4	3.6	3.8	3.9	4.1	4.2	4.4	4.6	4.7	4.9	5.0	5.2
Piano (sitting)	2.0	2.1	2.2	2.4	2.5	2.6	2.7	2.8	3.0	3.1	3.2	3.3	3.4	3.6	3.7	3.8	3.9
Trumpet (standing)	1.6	1.6	1.7	1.8	1.9	2.0	2.1	2.2	2.3	2.4	2.5	2.6	2.7	2.8	2.9	2.9	3.0
Violin (sitting)	2.3	2.4	2.5	2.7	2.8	2.9	3.1	3.2	3.3	3.5	3.6	3.7	3.9	4.0	4.1	4.3	4.4
Woodwind (sitting)	1.6	1.7	1.8	1.9	2.0	2.1	2.2	2.3	2.4	2.5	2.6	2.7	2.8	2.8	2.9	3.0	3.1
Painting, inside	1.7	1.8	1.9	2.0	2.1	2.2	2.3	2.4	2.5	2.6	2.7	2.8	2.9	3.0	3.1	3.2	3.3
Painting, outside	3.9	4.1	4.3	4.5	4.8	5.0	5.2	5.5	5.7	5.9	6.2	6.4	6.6	6.9	7.1	7.3	7.5
Planting seedlings	3.5	3.7	3.9	4.1	4.3	4.6	4.8	5.0	5.2	5.4	5.6	5.8	6.0	6.2	6.4	6.7	6.9
Plastering	3.9	4.1	4.4	4.6	4.8	5.1	5.3	5.5	5.8	6.0	6.2	6.5	6.7	6.9	7.2	7.4	7.6
Printing	1.8	1.9	2.0	2.1	2.2	2.3	2.4	2.5	2.6	2.7	2.8	2.9	3.0	3.1	3.2	3.3	3.4
Racquetball	8.9	9.4	10.0	10.5	11.0	11.6	12.1	12.6	13.2	13.7	14.2	14.8	15.3	15.8	16.4	16.9	17.4
Running, cross-country	8.2	8.6	9.1	9.6	10.1	10.6	11.1	11.6	12.1	12.6	13.0	13.5	14.0	14.5	15.0	15.5	16.0
Running, horizontal																	
11 min, 30 s per mile	6.8	7.2	7.6	8.0	8.4	8.8	9.2	9.6	10.0	10.5	10.9	11.3	11.7	12.1	12.5	12.9	13.3
9 min per mile	9.7	10.2	10.8	11.4	12.0	12.5	13.1	13.7	14.3	14.9	15.4	16.0	16.6	17.2	17.8	18.3	18.9
8 min per mile	10.8	11.3	11.9	12.5	13.1	13.6	14.2	14.8	15.4	16.0	16.5	17.1	17.7	18.3	18.9	19.4	20.0
7 min per mile	12.2	12.7	13.3	13.9	14.5	15.0	15.6	16.2	16.8	17.4	17.9	18.5	19.1	19.7	20.3	20.8	21.4
6 min per mile	13.9	14.4	15.0	15.6	16.2	16.7	17.3	17.9	18.5	19.1	19.6	20.2	20.8	21.4	22.0	22.5	23.1
5 min, 30 s per mile	14.5	15.3	16.2	17.1	17.9	18.8	19.7	20.5	21.4	22.3	23.1	24.0	24.9	25.7	26.6	27.5	28.3
Scraping paint	3.2	3.3	3.5	3.7	3.9	4.1	4.3	4.5	4.7	4.9	5.0	5.2	5.4	5.6	5.8	6.0	6.2
Scrubbing floors (F)	5.5	5.8	6.1	6.4	6.8	7.1	7.4	7.7	8.1	8.4	8.7	9.0	9.4	9.7	10.0	10.4	10.7
Scrubbing floors (M)	5.4	5.7	6.0	6.4	6.7	7.0	7.3	7.7	8.0	8.3	8.6	9.0	9.3	9.6	9.9	10.3	10.6
Shoe repair, general	2.3	2.4	2.5	2.7	2.8	2.9	3.1	3.2	3.3	3.5	3.6	3.7	3.9	4.0	4.1	4.3	4.4
Sitting quietly	1.1	1.1	1.2	1.2	1.3	1.4	1.4	1.5	1.6	1.6	1.7	1.7	1.8	1.9	1.9	2.0	2.1
Skiing, hard snow																	
Level, moderate speed	6.0	6.3	6.7	7.0	7.4	7.7	8.1	8.4	8.8	9.2	9.5	9.9	10.2	10.6	10.9	11.3	11.7
Level, walking	7.2	7.6	8.0	8.4	8.9	9.3	9.7	10.2	10.6	11.0	11.4	11.9	12.3	12.7	13.2	13.6	14.0
Uphill, maximum speed	13.7	14.5	15.3	16.2	17.0	17.8	18.6	19.5	20.3	21.1	21.9	22.7	23.6	24.4	25.2	26.0	26.9

Activity																	
Skiing, soft snow																	
Leisure (F)	4.9	5.2	5.5	5.8	6.1	6.4	6.7	7.0	7.3	7.5	7.8	8.1	8.4	8.7	9.0	9.3	9.6
Leisure (M)	5.6	5.9	6.2	6.5	6.9	7.2	7.5	7.9	8.2	8.5	8.9	9.2	9.5	9.9	10.2	10.5	10.9
Skindiving, as frogman																	
Considerable motion	13.8	14.6	15.5	16.3	17.1	17.9	18.8	19.6	20.4	21.3	22.1	22.9	23.7	24.6	25.4	26.2	27.0
Moderate motion	10.3	10.9	11.5	12.2	12.8	13.4	14.0	14.6	15.2	15.9	16.5	17.1	17.7	18.3	19.0	19.6	20.2
Snowshoeing, soft snow	8.3	8.8	9.3	9.8	10.3	10.8	11.3	11.8	12.3	12.8	13.3	13.8	14.3	14.8	15.3	15.8	16.3
Squash	10.6	11.2	11.9	12.5	13.1	13.8	14.4	15.1	15.7	16.3	17.0	17.6	18.2	18.9	19.5	20.1	20.8
Standing quietly (F)	1.3	1.3	1.4	1.5	1.6	1.6	1.7	1.8	1.9	1.9	2.0	2.1	2.2	2.2	2.3	2.4	2.5
Standing quietly (M)	1.4	1.4	1.5	1.6	1.7	1.8	1.8	1.9	2.0	2.1	2.2	2.2	2.3	2.4	2.5	2.6	2.6
Steel mill, working in																	
Fettling	4.5	4.7	5.0	5.3	5.5	5.8	6.1	6.3	6.6	6.9	7.1	7.4	7.7	7.9	8.2	8.5	8.7
Forging	5.0	5.3	5.6	5.9	6.2	6.5	6.8	7.1	7.4	7.7	8.0	8.3	8.6	8.9	9.2	9.5	9.8
Hand rolling	6.9	7.3	7.7	8.1	8.5	8.9	9.3	9.7	10.1	10.6	11.0	11.4	11.8	12.2	12.6	13.0	13.4
Merchant mill rolling	7.3	7.7	8.1	8.6	9.0	9.4	9.9	10.3	10.7	11.2	11.6	12.0	12.5	12.9	13.3	13.8	14.2
Removing slag	8.9	9.4	10.0	10.5	11.0	11.6	12.1	12.6	13.2	13.7	14.2	14.8	15.3	15.8	16.4	16.9	17.4
Tending furnace	6.3	6.7	7.1	7.4	7.8	8.2	8.6	8.9	9.3	9.7	10.1	10.5	10.8	11.2	11.6	12.0	12.3
Tipping molds	4.6	4.9	5.2	5.4	5.7	6.0	6.3	6.5	6.8	7.1	7.4	7.6	7.9	8.2	8.5	8.7	9.0
Stock clerking	2.7	2.9	3.0	3.2	3.3	3.5	3.7	3.8	4.0	4.2	4.3	4.5	4.6	4.8	5.0	5.1	5.3
Swimming																	
Back stroke	8.5	9.0	9.5	10.0	10.5	11.0	11.5	12.0	12.5	13.0	13.5	14.0	14.5	15.0	15.5	16.1	16.6
Breast stroke	8.1	8.6	9.1	9.6	10.0	10.5	11.0	11.5	12.0	12.5	13.0	13.4	13.9	14.4	14.9	15.4	15.9
Crawl, fast	7.8	8.3	8.7	9.2	9.7	10.1	10.6	11.1	11.5	12.0	12.5	12.9	13.4	13.9	14.4	14.8	15.3
Crawl, slow	6.4	6.8	7.2	7.6	7.9	8.3	8.7	9.1	9.5	9.9	10.2	10.6	11.0	11.4	11.8	12.2	12.5
Side stroke	6.1	6.5	6.8	7.2	7.6	7.9	8.3	8.7	9.0	9.4	9.8	10.1	10.5	10.9	11.2	11.6	12.0
Treading, fast	8.5	9.0	9.5	10.0	10.5	11.1	11.6	12.1	12.6	13.1	13.6	14.1	14.6	15.1	15.6	16.2	16.7
Treading, normal	3.1	3.3	3.5	3.7	3.8	4.0	4.2	4.4	4.6	4.8	5.0	5.1	5.3	5.5	5.7	5.9	6.1
Table tennis	3.4	3.6	3.8	4.0	4.2	4.4	4.6	4.8	5.0	5.2	5.4	5.6	5.8	6.1	6.3	6.5	6.7
Tailoring																	
Cutting	2.1	2.2	2.3	2.4	2.5	2.7	2.8	2.9	3.0	3.2	3.3	3.4	3.5	3.6	3.8	3.9	4.0
Hand-sewing	1.6	1.7	1.8	1.9	2.0	2.1	2.2	2.3	2.4	2.5	2.6	2.7	2.8	2.8	2.9	3.0	3.1
Machine-sewing	2.3	2.4	2.5	2.7	2.8	2.9	3.1	3.2	3.3	3.5	3.6	3.7	3.9	4.0	4.1	4.3	4.4
Pressing	3.1	3.3	3.5	3.7	3.8	4.0	4.2	4.4	4.6	4.8	5.0	5.1	5.3	5.5	5.7	5.9	6.1
Tennis	5.5	5.8	6.1	6.4	6.8	7.1	7.4	7.7	8.1	8.4	8.7	9.0	9.4	9.7	10.0	10.4	10.7
Typing																	
Electric	1.4	1.4	1.5	1.6	1.7	1.8	1.8	1.9	2.0	2.1	2.2	2.2	2.3	2.4	2.5	2.6	2.6
Manual	1.6	1.6	1.7	1.8	1.9	2.0	2.1	2.2	2.3	2.4	2.5	2.6	2.7	2.8	2.9	2.9	3.0
Volleyball	2.5	2.7	2.8	3.0	3.1	3.3	3.4	3.6	3.7	3.9	4.0	4.2	4.3	4.5	4.6	4.8	4.9
Walking, normal pace																	
Asphalt road	4.0	4.2	4.5	4.7	5.0	5.2	5.4	5.7	5.9	6.2	6.4	6.6	6.9	7.1	7.4	7.6	7.8
Fields and hillsides	4.1	4.3	4.6	4.8	5.1	5.3	5.6	5.8	6.1	6.3	6.6	6.8	7.1	7.3	7.5	7.8	8.0
Grass track	4.1	4.3	4.5	4.8	5.0	5.3	5.5	5.8	6.0	6.2	6.5	6.7	7.0	7.2	7.5	7.7	7.9
Plowed field	3.9	4.1	4.3	4.5	4.8	5.0	5.2	5.5	5.7	5.9	6.2	6.4	6.6	6.9	7.1	7.3	7.5
Wallpapering	2.4	2.5	2.7	2.8	3.0	3.1	3.3	3.4	3.6	3.7	3.8	4.0	4.1	4.3	4.4	4.6	4.7
Watch repairing	1.3	1.3	1.4	1.5	1.6	1.6	1.7	1.8	1.9	1.9	2.0	2.1	2.2	2.2	2.3	2.4	2.5
Window cleaning (F)	3.0	3.1	3.3	3.5	3.7	3.8	4.0	4.2	4.4	4.5	4.7	4.9	5.1	5.3	5.4	5.6	5.8
Window cleaning (M)	2.9	3.1	3.2	3.4	3.6	3.8	3.9	4.1	4.3	4.5	4.6	4.8	5.0	5.2	5.3	5.5	5.7
Writing (sitting)	1.5	1.5	1.6	1.7	1.8	1.9	2.0	2.1	2.1	2.2	2.3	2.4	2.5	2.6	2.7	2.8	2.8

* Data from Bannister EW and Brown SR: The relative energy requirements of physical activity. In Falls HB (ed): Exercise Physiology. New York, Academic Press, 1968; Howley ET and Glover ME: The caloric costs of running and walking one mile for men and women. Med Sci Sports 6:235, 1974; Passmore R and Durnin JVGA: Human energy expenditure. Physiol Rev 35:801, 1955.

† Adapted from McArdle WD, Katch FI, and Katch VL: Exercise Physiology, 2nd ed. Philadelphia, Lea & Febiger, 1986, pp 642–649.

‡ Values include the energy cost of rest for 1 minute; these values are not in addition to resting values.

Note: Symbols (M) and (F) denote experiments for males and females, respectively.

APPENDIX 37. Approximate Conversions To and From Metric Measures

Approximate Conversions to Metric Measures*†

When You Know	*Multiply By*	*To Find*
Length		
Inches	2.5	Centimeters
Feet	30	Centimeters
Yards	0.9	Meters
Miles	1.6	Kilometers
Area		
Square inches	6.5	Square centimeters
Square feet	9.09	Square meters
Square yards	0.8	Square meters
Square miles	2.6	Square kilometers
Acres	0.4	Hectares
Mass (weight)		
Ounces	28	Grams
Pounds	0.45	Kilograms
Short tons (2,000 lb)	0.9	Tonnes
Volume		
Teaspoons	5	Milliliters
Tablespoons	15	Milliliters
Fluid ounces	30	Milliliters
Cups	0.24	Liters
Pints	0.47	Liters
Quarts	0.95	Liters
Gallons	3.8	Liters
Cubic feet	0.03	Cubic meters
Cubic yards	0.76	Cubic meters
Temperature		
Fahrenheit	5/9 (after subtracting 32)	Celsius

Approximate Conversions from Metric Measures*†

When You Know	*Multiply By*	*To Find*
Length		
Millimeters	0.04	Inches
Centimeters	0.4	Inches
Meters	3.3	Feet
Meters	1.1	Yards
Kilometers	0.6	Miles
Area		
Square centimeters	0.16	Square inches
Square meters	1.2	Square yards
Square kilometers	0.4	Square miles
Hectares (10,000 m^2)	2.5	Acres
Mass (weight)		
Grams	0.035	Ounces
Kilograms	2.2	Pounds
Tonnes (1,000 kg)	1.1	Short tons
Volume		
Milliliters	0.03	Fluid ounces
Liters	2.1	Pints
Liters	1.06	Quarts
Liters	0.26	Gallons
Cubic meters	35	Cubic feet
Cubic meters	1.3	Cubic yards
Temperature		
Celsius	9/5 (then add 32)	Fahrenheit

* From Pemberton CM: Mayo Clinic Diet Manual, 6th ed. Philadelphia, BC Decker, 1988, p 577.

† From United States Department of Commerce, National Bureau of Standards: Metric Conversion Card (NBS Special Publication 365). Washington, DC, Government Printing Office, 1972.

APPENDIX 38. Abbreviations in Medical Terminology

Along with the specialized vocabulary that is employed in the medical, dietetic, and nursing fields, there are acceptable forms of abbreviations. Here is a list of abbreviations commonly used.

aa: Gr. *ana;* of each
ac: L. *ante cibum;* before meals
ad, add: L. *adde, addatur,* or *addantur;* add or added
ad lib: L. *ad libitum;* at pleasure, as desired
aq: L. *aqua;* water
aq dest: L. *aqua destillata;* distilled water
bid, bis in d: L. *bis in die;* twice a day
c: L. *cum;* with
c: cup
cc: cubic centimeter
Cent; cent; C: centigrade, Celsius
cm: centimeter
dilut: L. *dilutus;* dilute
div: L. *divide;* divide
fac: make
g: gram
gr: L. *granum;* grain
gtt: L. *guttae;* drops
hs: L. *hora somni;* at hour of sleep
IU: international unit
kcal: kilocalorie
kg: kilogram
kJ: kilojoule
lb: pound
μg: microgram
mcg: microgram
μU: microunit
mEq: milliequivalent
mg: milligram
mil or ml: milliliter
mM: millimole
mOsm: milliosmole
oz: ounce
prn: L. *pro re nata:* may be repeated according to instructions
pt: pint
pulv: L. *pulvis;* powder
qd: L. *quaque die;* every day
QID, qid: L. *quater in die;* four times daily
q3h: every three hours
qs: L. *quantum satis;* a sufficient quantity
qt: quart
RE: retinol equivalent
s: L. *sine;* without
sol: solution
ss: L. *semis;* half
stat: L. *statim;* immediately
t, tsp: teaspoon
T, tbsp: tablespoon
tid: L. *ter in die:* three times a day

APPENDIX 39. Cultural Food Practices

The dietary patterns of a number of countries are given in the tables at the end of this appendix. These should help the student obtain a better understanding of various foreign-born individuals and families who may need aid in meal planning, food budgeting, and dietary instruction.

It is a very large undertaking to provide food and nutritional care for persons who immigrate to the United States under conditions of stress. The rapid influx of Cubans to Florida and Vietnamese, Laotians, and Cambodians to California, for example, has led to crowded conditions, linguistic problems, and unfamiliar foods for the newcomers.

Rapid change is taking place in all countries, and it should be kept in mind that, although the dietary patterns listed here consist of typical native foods and customs, what is typical today may not be in a few years.

Dietary Patterns of Southeast Asians

Andrea Carlson, M.S., R.D.

During the past few years the number of Southeast Asian refugees has increased dramatically worldwide. By the beginning of 1982, 567,000 refugees from Laos, Cambodia, and Vietnam had entered the United States (Tripp, 1982). Among these refugees are numerous groups, each with a distinct language, culture, and food habits. From Laos, Cambodia, and Vietnam come the native ethnic groups, as well as Moslems and ethnic Chinese. From Laos, Thailand, and Southern China come the nomadic hill people, the Hmong, and the Mien. There are both urban and rural people whose lifestyles differ considerably, even though they might come from the same country. In order to understand the refugees it is important to appreciate their tremendous diversity as well as recognize their common characteristics.

Southeast Asia is a humid and tropical area with a primarily agricultural economy. Outside of the cities, most people earn their living by fishing or raising crops and livestock (Whitmore, 1979). A family raises enough food for its own consumption, with occasionally some left over to sell. Foods are usually produced and consumed locally. In addition to cultivation, the rural and highland people also obtain food by hunting and gathering such foods as deer, rabbit, snake, monkeys, mushrooms, bamboo shoots, watercress, and bananas.

Rice is the main crop and dietary staple, providing over 60% of the calories in Southeast Asian diets (Chang, 1977). In difficult times this percentage goes even higher. White, unenriched rice is very common. However, rice bran is sometimes added to fish pastes and pickled vegetables, thus increasing the nutritive value of the diet.

In cities and villages, food shopping is done once or twice daily, because fresh foods are preferred. Canned or refrigerated foods are expensive and available only in the cities. Sometimes salt is the only food purchased by the Hmong and Mien. In rural areas there is no refrigeration, and cooking is done over open fires. Drying, salting, pickling, and smoking are the most common methods of food preservation.

Lack of refrigeration prevents the widespread use of fresh cow's milk and other dairy products. Therefore, the calcium intake is generally low. Alternate native sources of calcium are tofu (soybean curd), fish pastes made from small whole fish, and soups or other dishes made from bones and vinegar. Unfortunately, these foods contain variable amounts of calcium and are not reliable sources. Soybean drinks do not contain significant amounts of calcium or protein. Lactose intolerance has been reported to be a problem in many Southeast Asians (Anh et al, 1957). However, most children accept milk readily, and many adults are able to drink it in small amounts without any discomfort.

Newly arriving refugees are at nutritional risk for a variety of reasons. They come from countries with limited food supplies caused by long histories of war and political strife. They may have spent as much as 5 years in refugee camps where food supplies were also limited. Poor sanitation has led to an increased incidence of parasites and therefore to an increase in anemia. General malnutrition, hypertension, dental caries, and iron-deficiency anemia have been identified as problems among incoming refugees (Kaufman, 1957).

After refugees arrive in the United States, other factors contribute to their nutritional problems. They are thrust into a foreign country that has a completely new language, culture, and society. They are faced with unfamiliar foods, food storage and food-buying habits. Many familiar foods are difficult or impossible to obtain. Low income limits their access to food, and they are susceptible to misleading food advertising.

Pregnant and lactating women, infants, and children are at greatest risk because of their increased nutritional needs. Multiple pregnancies and extended periods of lactation are common in Southeast Asia. A pregnant woman is less concerned about her prenatal diet than her postpartum diet. However, in the third trimester of pregnancy weight gain is often restricted in order for the woman to have a small baby and easy delivery. Foods such as fruits, vegetables, and certain meats are sometimes eliminated in the first postpartum month. A woman might lactate for as long as 2 years or until the next child is born. These practices, coupled with a low calcium intake, place great demands on a woman's nutritional stores.

Although in Southeast Asia most infants are breast-fed, in the United States infants of refugee women are usually fed formula. This alone does not constitute a problem, but it can lead to other problems. Improper dilution or unsanitary preparation and storage of formula are potential hazards. Misuse of the bottle, such as filling it with sweetened liquids, giving it to the infant at night, and using it as a frequent pacifier during the day can lead to baby bottle tooth decay (see Chapter 23). This serious dental problem is frequently seen in refugee children.

Rice-and-water soup is a common first food for infants. The introduction of other solid foods is often limited, and weaning is delayed. At about 1 year of age formula is replaced with cow's milk. Iron-deficiency anemia easily develops in the refugee children who drink large amounts of milk and eat few iron-rich foods.

Southeast Asian refugees are often shorter and lighter than their Western counterparts (Peck et al, 1981). Among children, weight for age, height for age, and weight for height, when plotted on National Center for Health Statistics growth charts (Appendix Tables 7 to 14), are below the fifth percentile more frequently than for the reference population. The use of these measurements in nutritional assessment is discussed in Chapter 17. At present there are no reliable standards with which to evaluate the growth of refugee children. Both genetic and environmental factors affect growth. Chronic undernutrition, especially low protein, calcium, and energy intakes, could contribute to poor growth in this population. In the countries of resettlement, improved diet and appropriate nutrition counseling to correct or prevent problems may improve the growth rates of refugee children and the health status of all refugees.

DIETARY RESTRICTIONS AND PATTERNS OF RELIGIOUS GROUPS

Jewish Food Customs and Dietary Laws

The Jewish dietary laws are biblical ordinances codified and interpreted into rules regarding food (Kaufman, 1957). The rules pertain chiefly to the selection, slaughter, and preparation of meat. Animals allowed to be eaten for food are the quadrupeds having a cloven hoof that chew a cud, specifically cattle, sheep, goats, and deer; they are considered "clean." Permissible fowl are chicken, turkey, goose, pheasant, and duck. All animals and fowl must be inspected for disease and killed by a ritual slaughterer according to specific rules. Only the forequarter of the quadruped may be used, except when the hip sinew of the thigh vein can be removed, in which case the hindquarter is also allowed.

Blood is forbidden as food, because blood is synonymous with life. Thus, the traditional process of "koshering" the meat and poultry removes all blood before cooking. Koshering involves soaking the meat in water, salting it thoroughly, allowing it to drain, and then washing it three times to remove the salt.

Meat and milk cannot be combined in the same meal. Milk or milk foods may be eaten immediately before the meal but not with the meal. After meat has been eaten, 6 hours must elapse before milk products may be used. Because of the rule of separating meat and milk products, traditional orthodox Jewish homes must keep two completely separate sets of dishes, silver, and cooking equipment—one for meat meals and one for dairy meals.

Fish allowed are only those having fins and scales. This bars all shellfish and eels. Fish may be eaten with either dairy or meat meals.

Eggs, too, may be used with either meat or milk. However, any egg yolk containing a drop of blood may not be used, because the blood is considered to be chick embryo or a sign of a new life.

Fruits, vegetables, cereal products, and all of the other foods that make up a diet may be used without restriction. Bakery products and prepared food mixtures must be produced under acceptable kosher standards.

APPENDIX 39. Cultural Food Practices *Continued*

Holiday Observance. The most important of the holy days is the Sabbath, or day of rest, observed on Saturday. The meal on Friday night is the nicest of the week and usually includes both fish and chicken. No food is allowed to be cooked or heated on Saturday, thus all food eaten on the Sabbath is cooked the previous day and is either kept warm in the oven or eaten cold.

The festival holidays are Rosh Hashanah, the New Year, in September; Succoth, the fall harvest holiday; Chanukah, the feast of lights, in midwinter; and Purim, a joyous holiday in spring. Each holiday has delicacies associated with it.

Yom Kippur, or the Day of Atonement, occurs 10 days after Rosh Hashanah and is a day of fasting, with abstinence from all food and drink, including water, from sundown on the eve of the holiday to sundown on the holiday. Pregnant women and those who are ill do not fast.

Passover, a spring commemorative festival lasting 8 days, requires special dietary consideration. During this period, leavened bread or cake is prohibited. Matzo, an unleavened bread, is eaten and all cake and baked products are made from flour of ground-up matzo or potato starch, leavened only with beaten egg whites. No salt is allowed in traditional Passover matzo. Variations of fried matzo or matzo meal pancakes are prepared with generous amounts of fat.

Muslim Religious Dietary Code

The following dietary restrictions are followed by the Muslims:

1. Pork and pork products such as gelatin are prohibited.
2. Alcoholic beverages and alcohol products (e.g., vanilla extract) are prohibited.
3. All meat used for food must be slaughtered according to ritual letting of blood and while speaking the name of God. This may be done by anyone, because there is no special person designated for this function. Muslims use kosher meat products because they know they have been slaughtered in the proper manner.
4. Although all foods not specifically prohibited are allowed, certain foods are recommended: milk, dates, meat, seafood, sweets, honey, and vegetable oil, especially olive oil.
5. Fasting is practiced during the month of Ramadan every year, which varies with the Islamic lunar calendar. Muslims fast completely from dawn to sunset and eat only twice a day—before dawn and after sunset. They are also encouraged to fast 3 days of every month. Menstruating, pregnant, or lactating women are not required to fast but must make up the fasting days at some other time.
6. Muslims are advised not to eat to capacity and always to share food.

CITED REFERENCES

Anh NT et al: Lactose malabsorption in adult Vietnamese. Am J Clin Nutr 5:676, 1957.

Chang KC (ed): Food in Chinese Culture. New Haven, Yale University Press, 1977.

Kaufman M: Adapting therapeutic diets to Jewish food customs. Am J Clin Nutr 5:676, 1957.

Peck RE et al: Nutritional status of Southeast Asian refugee children. Am J Pub Health 71:1144, 1981.

Tripp RR: World refugee survey 1982. New York, US Committee for Refugees, 1982

Whitmore JK (ed): An Introduction to Indochinese History, Culture, Language, and Life. Ann Arbor, MI, Center for South and Southeast Asian Studies, 1979.

TABLE 39A. Spanish-American-Mexican Dietary Habits*

Foods	Preparation
Meats: Chicken, pork chops, wieners, cold cuts, and hamburger.	Used only once or twice a week.
Other proteins: Eggs, beans.	Eggs used frequently and usually fried. In rural areas, chickens are kept for their eggs. Beans usually eaten mashed and refried with lard.
Vegetables: Potatoes, red and green chilies, fresh and canned tomatoes, pumpkin, corn, field greens, onions, carrots.	Potatoes are basic item, usually fried; may be used three times a day. Chilies are popular at each meal. Fresh tomatoes are very popular. Other vegetables used frequently.
Fruits: Bananas, melons, peaches, canned fruit cocktail, oranges, apples.	Oranges, apples used occasionally as snacks. Others are the more popular fruits.
Cereals and breads: Oatmeal, enriched white flour, packaged breakfast cereals, macaroni, white bread, tortillas, sweet rolls.	Sugar-coated packaged cereals are popular; oatmeal used occasionally. Macaroni is fried and served with beans and potatoes. Tortillas are homemade daily. Both purchased and homemade breads are used frequently. Purchased sandwich bread is a status symbol.
Milk: Limited availability, expensive.	
Cheese: Limited amounts used.	
Fats: Lard, salt pork, bacon fat.	Used liberally. Most foods are fried.
Beverages: Soft drinks; other sweets very popular.	

* Adapted from Cultural Food Patterns in the U.S.A. Chicago, American Dietetic Association, 1976.

TABLE 39B. Cuban Dietary Habits

Foods	Preparation
Meats: Beef, pork, lamb, veal, poultry, sausages.	Pork is either roasted or fried. Beef and chicken are used in soups, stewed, roasted, broiled, or barbecued. The sausages are used with beans.
Fish: All varieties of fish (fresh, salted, smoked, and canned).	Fried, boiled, marinated, roasted, or grilled.
Other proteins: Beans (black, red, kidney, navy, yellow, lima, green); split peas; eggs.	Black beans with rice and roast pork is a favorite dish and is eaten on Christmas day. Eggs are eaten daily: fried, scrambled, or in dessert.
Vegetables: Native tubers such as *yuca, ñame, malanga* (white and yellow), *boniato* (white yams), *chayote, berenjena,* plantain, potatoes, lettuce, tomatoes, carrots.	The tubers are boiled and served with *mojo* (made with sour orange, crushed garlic, sliced onions and hot oil), or mashed with butter and milk. Fried ripe or green plantains are a favorite side dish.
Fruits: Anona, *mamey, guanābana, chirimoya,* papaya, banana, *zapote, marañón,* mangoes, grapefruit, oranges (sweet and sour), coconuts, *caimito.*	Eaten fresh, in juice, or in desserts such as pastes, jellies, puddings.
Cereals: Rice, cornmeal, cornstarch, imported breakfast cereals, such as oatmeal, corn flakes.	The favorite is white (long grain) steamed rice; sometimes *bijol* is added to make it yellow as in *arroz con pollo* (yellow rice with chicken). White rice is eaten daily for dinner and supper.
Milk: Fresh cow's milk (whole, skimmed), condensed, evaporated, dry; sour cream; goat's milk for the sick, usually.	Adults use it in coffee; children use as beverage. Also used in cream sauces, gravies, desserts, etc.
Cheese: Gouda, cream, *queso de mano.*	The native cheese is *queso de mano* (hard cheese) made from milk, lactate of calcium, and salt, which looks like compressed cottage cheese; usually eaten with guava paste.
Fats: Pork lard, olive oil, peanut oil, soy oil, butter, margarine, and shortening.	Pork lard is most popular. Oil is used in salads and beans.
Desserts: Fruits, ice cream, cakes, pies, custards, puddings; guava, prune and mango pastes; *morón* cookies, *terrejas, boniatillo, buñuelos, cafiroleta.*	Eaten after each meal and also as snacks. *Raspadura* is very sweet and the most typical native dessert.
Seasonings: Oil, vinegar, cumin, oregano, *bijol,* salt, pepper, garlic, onion, green peppers.	
Beverages: Coffee, beer, wines, tea, carbonated beverages.	Dark strong coffee served demitasse, with or without sugar.

TABLE 39C. Greek Dietary Habits

Foods	Preparation
Meats: Lamb is main meat. Some beef, goat, mutton, pork products; poultry is popular.	Meat is either cut into small pieces or ground. Poultry is cooked into broth. Lamb is cooked on skewers or cut up and browned in oil or fat with rice or flour and vegetables.
Fish: Salt-water fish (fresh, smoked or salted), shellfish, smoked roe, squid, and octopus.	Fish is fried or steamed with vegetables. Used frequently.
Other proteins: Eggs, white beans, and legumes.	Legumes are boiled, mashed or stewed and eaten either hot or cold. Soup made of dried beans, onions, celery, and carrots is a national dish. Eggs are popular.
Vegetables: Cabbage, cauliflower, cucumbers, eggplant, greens, okra, onions, peppers, some potatoes, vine leaves, zucchini, tomatoes, salad greens.	Vegetables are boiled or fried in a small amount of olive oil and served hot or cold. Many vegetables are stuffed. Potatoes or vegetables are cooked with meat or fish. Lemon juice is used to dress salads and cold foods.
Fruits: Apricots, cherries, dates, oranges, lemons, figs, grapes, melons, nuts, plums, peaches, pears, quinces, and raisins.	Fruits in season are eaten raw, grapes are pressed into wine or dried as raisins. Fruit for dessert.
Cereals and breads: Maize, rice, and wheat.	Maize is used in polenta; rice is an ingredient for *pilawi* and stuffing for vegetables; wheat is made into bread. Bread used abundantly, and white is preferred.
Milk: Cow's, goat's, and sheep's milk.	Milk is boiled for children. Fermented milk or *yaourti* is eaten as dessert or with pastry.
Cheese: Soft and mild, hard and dry cheeses.	Cheese is popular.
Fats: Olive oil, seed oils, salted black olives, and little butter.	Olive oil is used to dress salads and hot or cold vegetables and in cooking.
Seasonings: Caraway and pumpkin seeds, herbs, honey, nuts (hazel, pignolia, and pistachio), and sesame.	Seeds are eaten between meals, and nuts are served as dessert.
Beverages: Coffee and wine.	Coffee (American) is the beverage served in the mornings. At other meals it is made and served Turkish style. Wine is served at meals.

TABLE 39D. Japanese Dietary Habits

Foods	Preparation
Meats: The Buddhist tradition of not eating meat conforms with the physical necessities of agriculture. The Japanese consume very little meat, except beef. Since World War II, however, protein intake has steadily increased.	Quantity is small. Usually cut into small pieces and served mixed with vegetables and cereal products.
Fish: Liked and one of the staple foods.	Prefer fish, shellfish, and other marine life to meats of all types. Certain kinds of raw fish are considered great delicacies. Others cooked or dried.
Other proteins: Soybean preparations used freely. Eggs used when available.	Variety of soybean preparations.
Vegetables: Prefer plants such as seaweed, bamboo shoots, onions, large radishes, dried mushrooms (*shiitake*), and beans. Potatoes and others when available.	Pickled is the favorite form. Others cooked with meat or fish.
Fruits: Principal fruit is *nasi* (tastes somewhat like pear, shaped like an apple; yellow, rough skin). Some persimmons and mulberries. Tangerines in mountain regions. Postwar increase in variety.	Dessert.
Cereals and breads: Rice is main food. Some barley, oats, and rye.	Rice is mixed with barley by farmers and the poorer classes. Wheat bread, especially in urban communities.
Milk: Enjoy when available; mainly import evaporated or dry milk powder.	Mostly for children.
Cheese: Very little.	
Fats: Soy oil. Rice oil. Suet when available. Practically no butter or cream.	Used in cooking.
Seasonings: Salt, *sake* (liquor distilled from rice).	
Beverages: Tea, *sake.*	Tea freely used when affordable.

TABLE 39E. Chinese Dietary Habits

Foods	Preparation
Meats: Pork (favorite), lamb, goat, and poultry. Entire animal is eaten, including organs, brain, spinal cord, skin, and coagulated blood.	Quantity is small and is usually cut into small thin slices about 2 inches long and cooked in sesame or peanut oil with soy sauce, spices, and a little water and served mixed with vegetables. Many methods for preserving and drying. Sweet and pungent pork or duck is a favorite (meat cubes rolled in batter and fried in oil, then simmered in sauce made of pineapple, green peppers, molasses, brown sugar, vinegar, and seasonings).
Fish: Fish and shellfish liked.	Fish is frequently baked with native spices or prepared in sweet-and-sour dishes. Many dried.
Other proteins: Hen, duck, and pigeon eggs in abundance when affordable; soybean products; legumes.	Eggs are preserved and dried; also combined with chicken, mushrooms, and bean sprouts and served with soy sauce (looks like vegetable omelet), termed *egg foo yong.* Egg roll served at beginning of meal is made of shrimp or meat and chopped vegetables rolled in thin dough and fried in deep fat. Soybeans used as sauce, as milk for infants in China, and in many products. Legumes as substitute for meat.
Vegetables: Many plants such as carrots, onions, leeks, peas, cabbage, white turnips, corn, cucumbers, green and yellow beans, squash, shepherd's purse, radish leaves, sprouts (bean, bamboo, etc), some white but more sweet potatoes.	Cut into uniform pieces and simmered or steamed with eggs or meat or added to meat and widely used in soups.
Fruits: Kumquat is favorite.	Preserved dessert.
Cereals and breads: Rice used freely. Some wheat, barley, corn, and millet seed. Noodles are popular. Rice is main dish; others are side dishes.	Rice is used as main dish, plain or fried. Millet seed is made into cakes or used in a gruel. Noodles are small and fried. Steamed bread is eaten at breakfast.
Milk: Very little and generally not used. Given to children and invalids.	
Cheese: Little used.	
Fats: Chief oil is peanut oil. Some soy oil, rice oil, sesame oil, or lard. Practically no butter or cream.	Used in cooking.
Seasonings: Sesame seed, salt, ginger, garlic, fresh herbs, red pepper.	
Beverage: Tea is the national beverage.	Beverage at all meals, when affordable.

TABLE 39F. Laotian Dietary Habits*

Foods	Preparation
Meats: Pork, beef, chicken, rabbit, wild pig, buffalo, deer, snake, and elephant.	Eaten fresh, dried, or salted. Prepared by frying, boiling, baking, or broiling, mixed with vegetables and spices. Hmong and Mien might also eat monkey and bear.
Fish: Numerous varieties of freshwater fish and shellfish. Saltwater fish available in cities.	Eaten fresh, fermented, dried, or salted. *Padek,* a fermented fish paste made from small whole fish, salt, and rice bran, is frequently eaten by lowland Lao but not by the Hmong and the Mien.
Other proteins: Eggs, peanuts, black-eyed peas, kidney beans.	Soybean products not eaten by the Lao. Soybean curd (tofu) sometimes eaten by Hmong. Legumes often used in desserts.
Vegetables: Wide variety of vegetables, including pumpkin, squash, squash blossoms and young shoots, tomato, cabbage, spinach, green papaya, bamboo shoots, mushrooms, watercress, cucumber, and corn. See also Vietnamese vegetables.	Eaten raw, as juice, or cooked with meat or fish. Preserved by drying or pickling.
Fruits: See Vietnamese fruits. Wide variety consumed.	Usually eaten fresh or as juice. Tamarinds sometimes salted and eaten as a snack.
Cereals and breads: Glutinous (sticky) rice, wheat, rice or bean thread noodles, French bread.	Sticky rice is rinsed several times and then soaked overnight. The soaking water is discarded, and the rice is steamed. It is eaten with the fingers at meals or as a snack. The Hmong eat regular rice. Bread is eaten plain, with paté or coconut milk.
Milk: Sweetened condensed milk.	Sometimes diluted and used as infant formula. Also as a beverage for adults.
Fats: Lard.	
Seasonings: Padek, chili, lemon grass, coconut milk, coriander, tamarind, curry, monosodium glutamate, red and black pepper, salt, fish sauce, browned ground rice, mint.	*Padek* and chilies are characteristic seasonings of the lowland Lao.
Beverages: Soybean drink, sugar cane drink, tea, coconut juice, fruit or vegetable juice, beer, wine.	

* Developed by Andrea Carlson, M.S., R.D.

TABLE 39G. Vietnamese Dietary Habits*

Foods	Preparation
Meats: Pork, beef, chicken, sausage, chicken feet, ox tails, liver, stomach.	Pork is most common. Chicken is consumed only on special occasions. Meats are usually cut into small pieces and fried, boiled, or steamed. (See also Chinese Dietary Habits.)
Fish: Numerous types of freshwater and saltwater fish and shellfish.	Eaten fresh, dried, salted, or fermented. Chinese like to steam fish, while Vietnamese like it fried and dipped in fish sauce.
Other proteins: Eggs, soybeans, peanuts, other legumes.	Soybeans eaten in processed forms such as soy sauce, soybean milk, and soybean curd (tofu). Peanuts eaten in soups or as a snack. Legumes eaten in desserts (Chinese influence) or in soups.
Vegetables: Wide variety of vegetables, including bamboo shoots, bok choy, broccoli, carrots, cauliflower, napa cabbage, mustard greens, bittermelon, wintermelon, green beans, eggplant, corn, water chestnuts, (see also Laotian vegetables).	Eaten fresh, dried, or pickled. Usually eaten with meat or fish. Vietnamese eat raw vegetables more often than Chinese-Vietnamese.
Fruits: Wide variety of fruits, including bananas, mangoes, papayas, pineapples, melons, oranges, pears, grapefruit, longans, and tamarinds.	Usually eaten fresh. Sometimes cook pear or papaya to make a sweet soup for dessert.
Cereals and breads: Short-grain, long-grain, and glutinous rice (See Laotian Dietary Habits), bean thread, wheat and rice noodles, French bread.	Rice is often eaten with every meal. It is rinsed several times before steaming. Bread eaten plain or with pork, paté, or sweetened condensed milk.
Milk: Sweetened condensed milk.	Served in coffee, with hot water, or on bread. Also sometimes used as infant formula.
Fats: Lard, peanut oil.	
Seasonings: Oyster sauce, soy sauce, monosodium glutamate, black pepper, ginger, garlic, green onion, coriander, sesame oil (Chinese influence), curry (Indian influence), mint, dill, red pepper, lemon grass, vinegar, lemon, *nuoc mam* sauce.	Vietnamese food tends to be hotter than Chinese food. *Nuoc mam* sauce is a fish sauce, a thin extract made from fermented fish and salt.
Beverages: Tea, coffee, soft drinks, soybean milk, sugar-cane drink, beer, and wine.	Tea is the most common beverage. Beer and wine are only for the men.

* Developed by Andrea Carlson, M.S., R.D.

TABLE 39H. Cambodian Dietary Habits*

Foods	Preparation
Meats: Pork, beef, chicken, deer, wild pig, buffalo, rabbit.	Eaten fresh, dried, or salted. Prepared by frying, boiling, baking, with spices. Not eaten as frequently as fish. Pork and chicken are expensive.
Fish: Numerous types of freshwater and saltwater fish and shellfish.	Very common food. *Prahoc,* a salted fermented fish paste, is a characteristic Cambodian food eaten with rice and raw vegetables. Fish also eaten fresh, smoked, or dried.
Other proteins: Eggs, peanuts, soybeans, other legumes.	Eggs are expensive and thus are not eaten often. Soybeans eaten only by Chinese Cambodians. Legumes eaten in desserts.
Vegetables: See Laotian and Vietnamese vegetables.	Eaten raw with *prahoc* or cut up small and cooked with other protein foods.
Fruits: See Vietnamese fruits.	Eaten raw as dessert or snack.
Cereals and breads: Long-grain, short-grain, glutinous (see Laotian Dietary Habits), and black, sweet rice; rice and egg noodles, French bread.	Glutinous and black, sweet rice used in desserts. French bread found mostly in cities.
Milk: Sweetened condensed milk.	Sometimes eaten on bread or used as infant formula.
Fats: Lard.	
Seasonings: Prahoc, red pepper, vinegar, garlic, ginger, curry salt, monosodium glutamate, lemon, coconut milk, and coriander.	*Prahoc* is a characteristic seasoning. Food is generally not as hot as Laotian food.
Beverages: Tea, coffee, soft drink, beer, soybean drinks, sugarcane drink.	

* Developed by Andrea Carlson, M.S., R.D.

APPENDIX TABLE 40. Provisional Table on the Content of Omega-3 Fatty Acids and Other Fat Components in Selected Foods (100 Grams Edible Portion)

Dashes (—) denote lack of reliable data for nutrient known to be present.
Tr = trace (less than 0.05 grams per 100 grams of food.)

Food Item	Total Fat (g)	Fatty Acids: *Total Saturated (g)*	*Total Monounsaturated (g)*	*Total Polyunsaturated (g)*	*18:3 (g)*	*20:5 (g)*	*22:6 (g)*	Cholesterol (mg)
Finfish								
Anchovy, European	4.8	1.3	1.2	1.6	—	0.5	0.9	—
Bass, freshwater	2.0	0.4	0.7	0.7	Tr	0.1	0.2	59
Bass, striped	2.3	0.5	0.7	0.8	Tr	0.2	0.6	80
Bluefish	6.5	1.4	2.9	1.6	—	0.4	0.8	59
Burbot	0.8	0.2	0.1	0.3	—	0.1	0.1	60
Capelin	8.2	1.5	3.8	1.5	0.1	0.6	0.5	—
Carp	5.6	1.1	2.3	1.4	0.3	0.2	0.1	67
Catfish, brown bullhead	2.7	0.6	1.0	0.8	0.1	0.2	0.2	75
Catfish, channel	4.3	1.0	1.6	1.0	Tr	0.1	0.2	58
Cisco	1.9	0.4	0.5	0.6	0.1	0.1	0.3	—
Cod, Atlantic	0.7	0.1	0.1	0.3	Tr	0.1	0.2	43
Cod, Pacific	0.6	0.1	0.1	0.2	Tr	0.1	0.1	37
Croaker, Atlantic	3.2	1.1	1.2	0.5	Tr	0.1	0.1	61
Dogfish, spiny	10.2	2.2	4.2	2.7	0.1	0.7	1.2	52
Dolphinfish	0.7	0.2	0.1	0.2	Tr	Tr	0.1	—
Drum, black	2.5	0.7	0.8	0.5	Tr	0.1	0.1	—
Drum, freshwater	4.9	1.1	2.2	1.2	0.1	0.2	0.3	64
Eel, European	18.8	3.5	10.9	1.4	0.7	0.1	0.1	108
Flounder, unspecified	1.0	0.2	0.3	0.3	Tr	0.1	0.1	46
Flounder, yellowtail	1.2	0.3	0.2	0.3	Tr	0.1	0.1	—
Grouper, jewfish	1.3	0.3	0.3	0.4	Tr	Tr	0.3	49
Grouper, red	0.8	0.2	0.1	0.2	—	Tr	0.2	—
Haddock	0.7	0.1	0.1	0.2	Tr	0.1	0.1	63
Hake, Atlantic	0.6	0.2	0.2	0.1	Tr	Tr	Tr	—
Hake, Pacific	1.6	0.3	0.3	0.6	Tr	0.2	0.2	—
Hake, red	0.9	0.2	0.3	0.3	—	0.1	0.1	—
Hake, silver	2.6	0.5	0.7	0.9	0.1	0.2	0.3	—
Hake, unspecified	1.9	0.5	0.6	0.5	—	0.1	0.4	—
Halibut, Greenland	13.8	2.4	8.4	1.4	Tr	0.5	0.4	46
Halibut, Pacific	2.3	0.3	0.8	0.7	0.1	0.1	0.3	32
Herring, Atlantic	9.0	2.0	3.7	2.1	0.1	0.7	0.9	60
Herring, Pacific	13.9	3.3	6.9	2.4	0.1	1.0	0.7	77
Herring, round	4.4	1.3	0.8	1.5	0.1	0.4	0.8	28
Mackerel, Atlantic	13.9	3.6	5.4	3.7	0.1	0.9	1.6	80
Mackerel, chub	11.5	3.0	4.7	3.0	0.3	0.9	1.0	52
Mackerel, horse	4.1	1.2	1.4	0.9	Tr	0.3	0.3	41
Mackerel, Japanese horse	7.8	2.5	2.4	2.3	0.1	0.5	1.3	48
Mackerel, king	13.0	2.5	5.9	3.2	—	1.0	1.2	53
Mullet, striped	3.7	1.2	1.1	1.1	0.1	0.3	0.2	49
Mullet, unspecified	4.4	0.3	1.3	1.5	Tr	0.5	0.6	34
Ocean perch	1.6	0.3	0.6	0.5	Tr	0.1	0.1	42
Perch, white	2.5	0.6	0.9	0.7	0.1	0.2	0.1	80
Perch, yellow	0.9	0.2	0.1	0.4	Tr	0.1	0.2	90
Pike, northern	0.7	0.1	0.2	0.2	Tr	Tr	0.1	39
Pike, walleye	1.2	0.2	0.3	0.4	Tr	0.1	0.2	86
Plaice, European	1.5	0.3	0.5	0.4	Tr	0.1	0.1	70
Pollock	1.0	0.1	0.1	0.5	—	0.1	0.4	71
Pompano, Florida	9.5	3.5	2.6	1.1	—	0.2	0.4	50
Ratfish	1.2	0.3	0.4	0.1	Tr	Tr	0.1	—
Rockfish, brown	3.3	0.8	0.8	1.0	Tr	0.3	0.4	—
Rockfish, canary	1.8	0.4	0.5	0.6	Tr	0.2	0.3	34
Rockfish, unspecified	1.4	0.2	0.3	0.6	Tr	0.2	0.3	—
Sablefish	15.3	3.2	8.1	2.0	0.1	0.7	0.7	49
Salmon, Atlantic	5.4	0.8	1.8	2.1	0.2	0.3	0.9	—

Data for the following omega-3 fatty acids are included in this table:
18:3 linolenic acid
20:5 eicosapentaenoic acid (EPA)
22:6 docosahexaenoic acid (DHA)

Mention of commercial products in this publication is solely for identification purposes and does not constitute endorsement by the U.S. Department of Agriculture over other products not mentioned.

APPENDIX 40. Provisional Table on the Content of Omega-3 Fatty Acids and Other Fat Components in Selected Foods (100 Grams Edible Portion) *Continued*

		Fatty Acids						
Food Item	**Total Fat (g)**	***Total Saturated (g)***	***Total Monounsaturated (g)***	***Total Polyunsaturated (g)***	***18:3 (g)***	***20:5 (g)***	***22:6 (g)***	**Cholesterol (mg)**
Salmon, chinook	10.4	2.5	4.5	2.1	0.1	0.8	0.6	—
Salmon, chum	6.6	1.5	2.9	1.5	0.1	0.4	0.6	74
Salmon, coho	6.0	1.1	2.1	1.7	0.2	0.3	0.5	—
Salmon, pink	3.4	0.6	0.9	1.4	Tr	0.4	0.6	—
Salmon, sockeye	8.6	1.5	4.1	1.9	0.1	0.5	0.7	—
Saury	9.2	1.6	4.8	1.8	0.1	0.5	0.8	19
Scad, Muroaji	8.7	2.8	2.2	2.6	0.1	0.5	1.5	47
Scad, other	0.5	0.1	0.1	0.1	—	Tr	Tr	27
Sea bass, Japanese	1.5	0.4	0.3	0.5	Tr	0.1	0.3	41
Seatrout, sand	2.3	0.7	0.8	0.4	Tr	0.1	0.2	—
Seatrout, spotted	1.7	0.5	0.4	0.3	Tr	0.1	0.1	—
Shark, unspecified	1.9	0.3	0.4	0.8	—	Tr	0.5	44
Sheepshead	2.4	0.6	0.7	0.5	Tr	0.1	0.1	—
Smelt, pond	0.7	0.2	0.1	0.3	—	0.1	0.2	72
Smelt, rainbow	2.6	0.5	0.7	0.9	0.1	0.3	0.4	70
Smelt, sweet	4.6	1.6	1.2	1.0	0.3	0.2	0.1	25
Snapper, red	1.2	0.2	0.2	0.4	Tr	Tr	0.2	—
Sole, European	1.2	0.3	0.4	0.2	Tr	Tr	0.1	50
Sprat	5.8	1.4	2.0	1.5	—	0.5	0.8	38
Sturgeon, Atlantic	6.0	1.2	1.7	2.1	Tr	1.0	0.5	—
Sturgeon, common	3.3	0.8	1.6	0.5	0.1	0.2	0.1	—
Sunfish, pumpkinseed	0.7	0.1	0.1	0.2	Tr	Tr	0.1	67
Swordfish	2.1	0.6	0.8	0.2	—	0.1	0.1	39
Trout, arctic char	7.7	1.6	4.6	0.9	Tr	0.1	0.5	—
Trout, brook	2.7	0.7	0.8	0.9	0.2	0.2	0.2	68
Trout, lake	9.7	1.7	3.6	3.4	0.4	0.5	1.1	48
Trout, rainbow	3.4	0.6	1.0	1.2	0.1	0.1	0.4	57
Tuna, albacore	4.9	1.2	1.2	1.8	0.2	0.3	1.0	54
Tuna, bluefin	6.6	1.7	2.2	2.0	—	0.4	1.2	38
Tuna, skipjack	1.9	0.7	0.4	0.6	—	0.1	0.3	47
Tuna, unspecified	2.5	0.9	0.6	0.5	—	0.1	0.4	—
Whitefish, lake	6.0	0.9	2.0	2.2	0.2	0.3	1.0	60
Whiting, European	0.5	0.1	0.1	0.1	Tr	Tr	0.1	31
Wolffish, Atlantic	2.4	0.4	0.8	0.8	Tr	0.3	0.3	—
Crustaceans								
Crab, Alaska king	0.8	0.1	0.1	0.3	Tr	0.2	0.1	—
Crab, blue	1.3	0.2	0.2	0.5	Tr	0.2	0.2	78
Crab, Dungeness	1.0	0.1	0.2	0.3	—	0.2	0.1	59
Crab, queen	1.1	0.1	0.2	0.4	Tr	0.2	0.1	127
Crayfish, unspecified	1.4	0.3	0.4	0.3	Tr	0.1	Tr	158
Lobster, European	0.8	0.1	0.2	0.2	—	0.1	0.1	129
Lobster, northern	0.9	0.2	0.2	0.2	—	0.1	0.1	95
Shrimp, Atlantic brown	1.5	0.3	0.3	0.5	Tr	0.2	0.1	142
Shrimp, Atlantic white	1.5	0.2	0.2	0.6	Tr	0.2	0.2	182
Shrimp, Japanese (kuruma) prawn	2.5	0.5	0.5	1.0	Tr	0.3	0.2	58
Shrimp, northern	1.5	0.2	0.3	0.6	Tr	0.3	0.2	125
Shrimp, other	1.3	0.4	0.3	0.3	Tr	0.1	0.1	128
Shrimp, unspecified	1.1	0.2	0.1	0.4	Tr	0.2	0.1	147
Spiny lobster, Caribbean	1.4	0.2	0.2	0.6	Tr	0.2	0.1	140
Spiny lobster, southern rock	1.0	0.1	0.2	0.3	Tr	0.2	0.1	—
Mollusks								
Abalone, New Zealand	1.0	0.2	0.2	0.2	Tr	Tr	—	—
Abalone, South African	1.1	0.3	0.3	0.2	Tr	Tr	Tr	—
Clam, hardshell	0.6	Tr	Tr	0.1	Tr	Tr	Tr	31
Clam, hen	0.7	0.2	0.1	0.1	—	Tr	Tr	—
Clam, littleneck	0.8	0.1	0.1	0.1	Tr	Tr	Tr	—
Clam, Japanese hardshell	0.8	0.1	0.1	0.2	—	0.1	0.1	—
Clam, softshell	2.0	0.3	0.2	0.6	Tr	0.2	0.2	—
Clam, surf	0.8	0.1	0.1	0.2	Tr	0.1	0.1	—
Conch, unspecified	2.7	0.6	0.5	1.1	Tr	0.6	0.4	141
Cuttlefish, unspecified	0.6	0.1	0.1	0.1	Tr	Tr	Tr	—

Table continued on following page

APPENDIX 40. Provisional Table on the Content of Omega-3 Fatty Acids and Other Fat Components in Selected Foods (100 Grams Edible Portion) *Continued*

Food Item	Total Fat (g)	Fatty Acids: *Total Saturated (g)*	*Total Monounsaturated (g)*	*Total Polyunsaturated (g)*	*18:3 (g)*	*20:5 (g)*	*22:6 (g)*	Cholesterol (mg)
Mussel, blue	2.2	0.4	0.5	0.6	Tr	0.2	0.3	38
Mussel, Mediterranean	1.5	0.4	0.4	0.3	—	0.1	0.1	—
Octopus, common	1.0	0.3	0.1	0.3	—	0.1	0.1	—
Oyster, eastern	2.5	0.6	0.2	0.7	Tr	0.2	0.2	47
Oyster, European	2.0	0.4	0.2	0.7	0.1	0.3	0.2	30
Oyster, Pacific	2.3	0.5	0.4	0.9	Tr	0.4	0.2	—
Periwinkle, common	3.3	0.6	0.6	1.1	0.2	0.5	Tr	101
Scallop, Atlantic deepsea	0.8	0.1	0.1	0.3	Tr	0.1	0.1	37
Scallop, calico	0.7	0.1	—	0.2	Tr	0.1	0.1	—
Scallop, unspecified	0.8	0.1	0.1	0.3	Tr	0.1	0.1	45
Squid, Atlantic	1.2	0.3	0.1	0.5	Tr	0.1	0.3	—
Squid, short-finned	2.0	0.4	0.4	0.7	Tr	0.2	0.4	—
Squid, unspecified	1.1	0.3	0.1	0.4	Tr	0.1	0.2	—
Fish Oils								
Cod liver oil	100	17.6	51.2	25.8	0.7	9.0	9.5	570
Herring oil	100	19.2	60.3	16.1	0.6	7.1	4.3	766
Menhaden oil	100	33.6	32.5	29.5	1.1	12.7	7.9	521
MaxEPA, concentrated fish body oils	100	25.4	28.3	41.1	0	17.8	11.6	600
Salmon oil	100	23.8	39.7	29.9	1.0	8.8	11.1	485
Beef								
Chuck, blade roast, all grades, separable lean and fat, raw	23.6	10.0	10.8	0.9	0.3			73
Ground, regular, raw	27.0	10.8	11.6	1.0	0.2			85
Round, full cut, choice grade, separable lean and fat, raw	17.5	7.4	7.8	0.7	0.2			66
Separable fat from retail cuts, raw	70.9	31.0	32.4	2.6	1.0			99
T-bone steak, choice grade, lean only, raw	8.0	3.2	3.4	0.3	Tr			60
T-bone steak, choice grade, separable lean and fat, raw	26.1	11.2	11.7	1.0	0.3			71
Cereal Grains								
Barley, bran	5.3	1.0	0.6	2.7	0.3			0
Corn, germ	30.8	3.9	7.6	18.0	0.3			0
Oats, germ	30.7	5.6	11.1	12.4	1.4			0
Rice, bran	19.2	3.6	7.3	6.6	0.2			0
Wheat, bran	4.6	0.7	0.7	2.4	0.2			0
Wheat, germ	10.9	1.9	1.6	6.6	0.7			0
Wheat, hard red winter	2.5	0.4	0.3	1.2	0.1			0
Dairy and Egg Products								
Cheese, Cheddar	33.1	21.1	9.0	0.9	0.4			105
Cheese, Roquefort	30.6	19.3	8.5	1.3	0.7			90
Cream, heavy whipping	37.0	23.0	10.7	1.4	0.5			137
Milk, whole	3.3	2.1	1.0	0.1	0.1			14
Egg yolk, chicken, raw	32.9	9.9	13.2	4.3	0.1			1,602
Fats and Oils								
Butter	81.1	50.5	23.4	3.0	1.2			219
Butter oil	99.5	61.9	28.7	3.7	1.5			256
Chicken fat	99.8	29.8	44.7	20.9	1.0			85
Duck fat	99.8	33.2	49.3	12.9	1.0			100
Lard	100	39.2	45.1	11.2	1.0			95
Linseed oil	100	9.4	20.2	66.0	53.3			0
Margarine, hard, soybean	80.5	16.7	39.3	20.9	1.5			0
Margarine, hard, soybean and soybean (hydrog.)	80.5	13.1	37.6	26.2	1.9			0
Margarine, hard, soybean (hydrog.) and palm	80.5	17.5	31.2	28.2	2.3			0

APPENDIX 40. Provisional Table on the Content of Omega-3 Fatty Acids and Other Fat Components in Selected Foods (100 Grams Edible Portion) *Continued*

Food Item	Total Fat (g)	Fatty Acids						Choles-terol (mg)
		Total Saturated (g)	*Total Monounsaturated (g)*	*Total Polyunsaturated (g)*	*18:3 (g)*	*20:5 (g)*	*22:6 (g)*	
Margarine, hard, soybean (hydrog.), and cottonseed	80.5	15.6	36.1	25.3	2.8			0
Margarine, hard, soybean (hydrog.), and palm (hydrog.)	80.5	15.1	32.0	29.8	3.0			0
Margarine, liquid, soybean (hydrog.), soybean, and cottonseed	80.6	13.2	28.1	35.8	2.4			0
Margarine, soft, soybean (hydrog.), and cottonseed	80.4	16.5	31.3	29.1	1.6			0
Margarine, soft, soybean (hydrog.), and palm	80.4	17.1	25.2	34.6	1.9			0
Margarine, soft, soybean, soybean (hydrog.), and cottonseed (hydrog.)	80.4	16.1	30.7	30.1	2.8			0
Mutton tallow	100	47.3	40.6	7.8	2.3			102
Rapeseed oil (Canola)	100	6.8	55.5	33.3	11.1			0
Rice bran oil	100	19.7	39.3	35.0	1.6			0
Salad dressing, comm., blue cheese, reg.	52.3	9.9	12.3	27.8	3.7			17
Salad dressing, comm., Italian, reg.	48.3	7.0	11.2	28.0	3.3			0
Salad dressing, comm., mayonnaise, imitation, soybean, w/o cholesterol	47.7	7.5	10.5	27.6	4.6			0
Salad dressing, comm., mayonnaise, safflower and soybean	79.4	8.6	13.0	55.0	3.0			59
Salad dressing, comm., mayonnaise, soybean	79.4	11.8	22.7	41.3	4.2			59
Salad dressing, comm., mayonnaise-type	33.4	4.7	9.0	18.0	2.0			26
Salad dressing, comm., Thousand Island, reg.	35.7	6.0	8.3	19.8	2.5			0
Salad dressing, home recipe, French	70.2	12.6	20.7	33.7	1.9			0
Salad dressing, home recipe, vinegar, and soybean oil	50.1	9.1	14.8	24.1	1.4			0
Shortening, household, lard and veg. oil	100	40.3	44.4	10.9	1.1			56
Shortening, household, soybean (hydrog.), and cottonseed (hydrog.)	100	25.0	44.5	26.1	1.6			0
Shortening, special-purpose, for bread, soy (hydrog.) and cottonseed	100	22.0	33.0	40.6	4.0			0
Shortening, special-purpose, for cake mixes, soybean (hydrog.), and cottonseed (hydrog.)	100	27.2	54.2	14.1	1.1			0
Shortening, special-purpose, heavy-duty, frying, soybean (hydrog.)	100	18.4	43.7	33.5	2.4			0
Soybean lecithin	100	15.3	10.9	45.1	5.1			0
Soybean oil	100	14.4	23.3	57.9	6.8			0
Soybean oil (hydrog.) and cottonseed oil	100	14.9	43.0	37.6	2.8			0
Soybean oil (partially-hydrog.)	100	14.9	43.0	37.6	2.6			0

Table continued on following page

APPENDIX 40. Provisional Table on the Content of Omega-3 Fatty Acids and Other Fat Components in Selected Foods (100 Grams Edible Portion) *Continued*

Food Item	Total Fat (g)	Fatty Acids						Choles-terol (mg)
		Total Satu-rated (g)	***Total Monoun-saturated (g)***	***Total Polyun-saturated (g)***	***18:3 (g)***	***20:5 (g)***	***22:6 (g)***	
Spread, margarine-like, about 60% fat, soybean (hydrog.) and palm (hydrog.)	60.8	14.1	26.0	18.1	1.6			0
Spread, margarine-like, about 60% fat, soybean (hydrog.), palm (hydrog.), and palm	60.8	13.5	24.1	20.4	1.6			0
Tomatoseed oil	100	19.7	22.8	53.1	2.3			0
Walnut oil	100	9.1	22.8	63.3	10.4			0
Wheat germ oil	100	18.8	15.1	61.7	6.9			0
Fruits								
Avocados, California, raw	17.3	2.6	11.2	2.0	0.1			0
Raspberries, raw	0.6	Tr	Tr	0.3	0.1			0
Strawberries, raw	0.4	Tr	Tr	0.2	0.1			0
Lamb and Veal								
Lamb, leg, raw (83% lean, 17% fat)	17.6	8.1	7.1	1.0	0.3			71
Lamb, loin, raw (72% lean, 28% fat)	27.4	12.8	11.2	1.6	0.5			71
Veal, leg round with rump, raw (87% lean, 13% fat)	9.0	3.8	3.7	0.6	0.1			71
Legumes								
Beans, common, dry	1.5	0.2	0.1	0.9	0.6			0
Chickpeas, dry	5.0	0.5	1.1	2.3	0.1			0
Cowpeas, dry	1.9	0.6	0.1	0.8	0.3			0
Lentils, dry	1.2	0.2	0.2	0.5	0.1			0
Lima beans, dry	1.4	0.3	0.1	0.7	0.2			0
Peas, garden, dry	2.4	0.4	0.1	0.4	0.2			0
Soybeans, dry	21.3	3.1	4.4	12.3	1.6			0
Nuts and Seeds								
Beechnuts, dried	50.0	5.7	21.9	20.1	1.7			0
Butternuts, dried	57.0	1.3	10.4	42.7	8.7			0
Chia seeds, dried	26.3	10.5	7.3	7.3	3.9			0
Hickory nuts, dried	64.4	7.0	32.6	21.9	1.0			0
Soybean kernels, roasted, and toasted	24.0	3.2	5.6	12.7	1.5			0
Walnuts, black	56.6	3.6	12.7	37.5	3.3			0
Walnuts, English/Persian	61.9	5.6	14.2	39.1	6.8			0
Pork								
Pork, cured, bacon, raw	57.5	21.3	26.3	6.8	0.8			67
Pork, cured, breakfast strips, raw	37.1	12.9	16.9	5.6	0.9			69
Pork, cured salt pork, raw	80.5	29.4	38.0	9.4	0.7			86
Pork, fresh, ham, raw	20.8	7.5	9.7	2.2	0.2			74
Pork, fresh, jowl, raw	69.6	25.3	32.9	8.1	0.6			90
Pork, fresh, leaf fat, raw	94.2	45.2	37.2	7.3	0.9			110
Pork, fresh, separable fat, raw	76.7	27.9	35.7	8.2	0.7			93
Poultry								
Chicken, broiler fryers, flesh and skin, giblets, neck, raw†	14.8	4.2	6.1	3.2	0.1			90
Chicken, dark meat, w/o skin, raw†	4.3	1.1	1.3	1.0	Tr			80
Chicken, light meat, w/o skin, raw†	1.7	0.4	0.4	0.4	Tr			58
Chicken, skin only, raw†	32.4	9.1	13.5	6.8	0.3			109
Turkey, flesh, with skin, roasted†	9.7	2.8	3.2	2.5	0.1			82

APPENDIX 40. Provisional Table on the Content of Omega-3 Fatty Acids and Other Fat Components in Selected Foods (100 Grams Edible Portion) *Continued*

		Fatty Acids							
Food Item	**Total Fat (g)**	***Total Saturated (g)***	***Total Monounsaturated (g)***	***Total Polyunsaturated (g)***	***18:3 (g)***	***20:5 (g)***	***22:6 (g)***	**Cholesterol (mg)**
Vegetables								
Beans, Navy, sprouted, cooked	0.8	Tr	Tr	0.5	0.3			0
Beans, pinto, sprouted, cooked	0.9	0.1	Tr	0.5	0.3			0
Broccoli, raw	0.4	Tr	Tr	0.2	0.1			0
Cauliflower, raw	0.2	Tr	Tr	Tr	0.1			0
Kale, raw	0.7	Tr	Tr	0.3	0.2			0
Leeks, freeze-dried, raw	2.1	0.3	Tr	1.2	0.7			0
Lettuce, butterhead, raw	0.2	Tr	Tr	0.1	0.1			0
Radish seeds, sprouted, raw	2.5	0.7	0.4	1.1	0.7			0
Seaweed, Spirulina, dried	7.7	2.6	0.7	2.0	0.8			0
Soybeans, green, raw	6.8	0.7	0.8	3.8	3.2			0
Soybeans, mature seeds, sprouted, cooked	4.5	0.5	0.5	2.5	2.1			0
Spinach, raw	0.4	Tr	Tr	0.1	0.1			0

* Data from Human Nutrition Information Service, USDA: Provisional Table on the Content of Omega-3 Fatty Acids and Other Fat Components in Selected Foods, HNIS/PT-103, 1988

† Contains trace amounts of 20:5, 22:5, and 22:6.

GLOSSARY

Abetalipoproteinemia: a familial lipoprotein deficiency caused by defective synthesis of apolipoprotein B; characterized by the presence of distorted red blood cells, hypocholesterolemia, progressive ataxic neuropathy, eye changes, and fat malabsorption

Acetoacetic acid: one of the ketone bodies composed of two molecules of acetyl-CoA; the end product of incomplete fatty acid oxidation, which may exist in starvation or in uncontrolled diabetes

Acetone: a dimethyl ketone with a pleasant ethereal odor that is the end product of unoxidized acetoacetic acid

Acrolein: a decomposition product produced by frying foods at excessive temperatures, which retards the flow of digestive juices

Actin: a protein of the myofibril; responsible for the contraction and relaxation of muscles

Adipocyte: fat cell

Alkaline phosphatase: an enzyme active in an alkaline environment that hydrolyzes monophosphoric esters with liberation of inorganic phosphate and that is present in blood, bone, kidney, mammary gland, spleen, lung, leukocytes, adrenal cortex, and seminiferous tubules

Alveolar: pertaining to a small sac-like dilatation; often referring to the alveoli of the lungs

Amenorrhea: absence or abnormal stoppage of the menses

Anabolism: any constructive process by which simple substances are converted by living cells into more complex compounds

Antibody: an immunoglobulin molecule that has a specific amino acid sequence, by virtue of which it interacts only with the antigen that induced its synthesis in B lymphocytes

Antidiuretic hormone: a hormone secreted by the posterior pituitary that is responsible for resorption of water by the distal portion of the kidney tubules, and thus the control of water excretion

Antioxidant: a natural or synthetic substance that prevents or delays the process of oxidation (the adding of oxygen to a molecule)

Articular: pertaining to joints

Asterixis: flapping or tremor of the hands when extended in front of the chest; characteristic of hepatic encephalopathy

Atopy: the genetic tendency to develop IgE-mediated reactions

Atrophy: a wasting away; diminution in the size of a cell, tissue, organ, or part

Autonomic nervous system: the portion of the nervous system concerned with regulation of the activity of cardiac muscle, smooth muscle, and glands

Beta-hydroxybutyric acid: a ketone body made up of unoxidized acetoacetic acid

Bioavailability: the degree to which a vitamin, mineral, drug, or other substance becomes available to the target tissue after administration

Bradycardia: slowness of the heart beat

Bruit: a sound or murmur heard in auscultation, especially an abnormal sound

Carcinogen: any cancer-producing substance

Catabolism: any destructive process by which complex substances are converted by living cells into more simple compounds

Cholinergic: stimulated, activated, or transmitted by choline (acetylcholine); a term applied to nerve fibers that liberate acetylcholine at a synapse when a nerve impulse passes (i.e., the parasympathetic nerve endings)

Chronic interstitial nephritis: a disease characterized by an inability to concentrate the urine and by mild renal insufficiency

Chylomicron: a lipoprotein containing 86% triglyceride in addition to cholesterol, phospholipids, and protein, which is in the intestinal lymphatics and blood after meals and is the form in which long-chain triglyceride and cholesterol are absorbed from the gastrointestinal tract and transported

Citric acid cycle: tricarboxylic acid or Krebs cycle

Coenzyme: molecule containing phosphorus and a vitamin that facilitates enzyme function, usually as donor or acceptor

Cruciferous vegetables: vegetables in the plant family Cruciferae that have four-petaled flowers, such as cauliflower, broccoli, Brussels sprouts, and cabbage

Cyanosis: a blue discoloration of the skin reflecting excessive concentration of reduced hemoglobin in the blood due to poor oxygenation

Cytochrome: any electron transfer hemoprotein

Cytochrome P-450 system: an enzyme system in the body that transforms drugs and other endogenous materials to water-soluble compounds so that they can be excreted

Denaturation: destruction of the usual nature of a substance; often used to refer to the change in the physical properties of proteins caused by extremes of temperature and pH

Diuresis: increased secretion of urine

Dysgeusia: alteration in taste sensation

Dysphoria: disquiet, restlessness, malaise

Dyspnea: difficult or labored breathing

Eicosanoid: any of the biologically active substances derived from arachidonic acid, eicosatetraenoic acid, and eicosapentaenoic acid, including the prostaglandins, thromboxanes, and leukotrienes

Emulsifying: converting two liquids into a suspension in which one liquid is distributed in small globules throughout the body of a second liquid, usually between an oil-based liquid and a water-based liquid

Endocytosis: the uptake by a cell of material from the environment by invagination of its plasma membrane

Endoenzyme: an intracellular enzyme; an enzyme that is retained in a cell and that does not normally diffuse out of the cell

Enteric: pertaining to the small intestine

Enterohepatic circulation: the recurrent cycle in which bile salts and other substances excreted by the liver pass through the intestinal mucosa and become reabsorbed by the hepatic cells and re-excreted

Epinephrine: a hormone secreted by the adrenal medulla

Erythroid: pertaining to the developmental series of cells ending in erythrocytes

Erythropoiesis: the production of red blood cells

Erythropoietin: hormone that stimulates the bone marrow to produce red blood cells

Esterify: to combine an acid and an alcohol with elimination of a molecule of water, forming an ester

Excoriation: any superficial loss of substance, such as that produced on the skin by scratching

Exfoliation: a falling off in scales or layers; a peeling

Exocytosis: the discharge from a cell of particles that are too large to diffuse through the wall; the opposite of endocytosis

Exoenzyme: an extracellular enzyme; an enzyme that functions outside the walls of the cells in which it originates

Extracellular: outside a cell or cells

Extravascular: situated or occurring outside the vessels

Fermentation: enzymatic decomposition of carbohydrates that is anaerobic and ends with the production of alcohol

Fibril: a minute fiber or filament; often a component of a compound fiber

Filament: a delicate fiber or thread

Glucocorticoids: any of the group of C21 corticosteroids predominantly affecting carbohydrate metabolism through promotion of gluconeogenesis and liver glycogen deposition and elevation of blood glucose levels

Glucogenic: giving rise to or producing glucose

Glucose polymers: chains of 5 to 9 glucose units linked together to form molecules of higher molecular weight, which when in solution result in solutions of lower osmolarity

Glutathione peroxidase: the enzyme responsible for the reaction that reduces toxic hydrogen peroxide formed within the cell

Glycogen: chief carbohydrate storage material made by and stored in the liver and to a lesser extent in the muscles

Glycogenolysis: the splitting up of glycogen in the body tissues, yielding glucose

Gravid: pregnant

Hematopoiesis: the formation and development of blood cells

Hemolysis: disruption of the integrity of the red blood cell membrane causing release of hemoglobin

Hemorrhagic disease of the newborn: prothrombin deficiency during the first few days of life as a result of poor placental transfer of vitamin K and failure to establish vitamin K-producing intestinal flora

Histamine: decarboxylation product of histidine found in all body tissues, particularly in mast cells; functions are to dilate capillaries, contract most smooth muscle tissue including that in the lungs, induce increased gastric secretion, and accelerate heart rate; it is implicated as the mediator of immediate hypersensitivity

Homeostasis: a tendency to stability in the internal environment of the organism; achieved by a system of control mechanisms activated by negative feedback

Homozygous: possessing a pair of identical alleles at a given locus on a gene

Hormone-sensitive lipase: an enzyme within the

adipose cell that catalyzes the release of free fatty acids from the cell

Hyperlipidemia: a general term for elevated concentrations of any or all of the lipids in plasma, including hyperlipoproteinemia and hypercholesterolemia

Hypertriglyceridemia: elevated level of triglycerides in the plasma

Hypogeusia: reduced acuity of taste sensation

Hypogonadism: a condition resulting from or characterized by abnormally decreased functional activity of the gonads, with retardation of growth and sexual development

Ideal body weight (IBW): the weight appropriate for an individual that results in a body mass index of between 20 and 25 in adults, results in a weight within 1 channel above and below the height gain channel and for a child

Idiopathic: self-originated; of unknown causation

Ileus: loss of intestinal peristalsis or lack of effective coordinated peristalsis

In utero: within the uterus

Indole: a compound produced by the decomposition of tryptophan in the intestines that is responsible in part for the peculiar odor of the feces

Infiltration: diffusion or accumulation in tissues or cells of substances abnormal in nature or quantity

Intermittent claudication: a complex of symptoms characterized by absence of pain or discomfort in a limb when at rest, and severely increasing pain during walking

Intracellular: situated or occurring within the cell

Intraluminal: within the opening of a tube; as of the intestinal tract

Intravascular: situated in or occurring within the blood vessels

Kernicterus: a condition with severe neural symptoms associated with high levels of bilirubin in the blood

Ketoacidosis: a pathologic condition resulting from the accumulation of acid accompanied by the presence of ketone bodies

Ketosis: a condition characterized by an abnormally elevated concentration of ketone bodies in the body tissues and fluids

Koilonychia: spoon-shaped nails sometimes associated with iron deficiency anemia

Kussmaul's breathing: deep sighing breathing, characteristic of acidosis

Kyphoscoliosis: backward and lateral curvature of the spine

Lacrimation: the secretion and discharge of tears

Lean body mass: the fat-free mass or that part of the body including all its components except neutral storage lipid

Leukopenia: reduction in the number of white blood cells in the blood to a count of 5,000 per cubic millimeter or less

Leukotriene: an eicosanoid whose function is the communication among the various types of cells involved in immunosurveillance, inflammation, protection against infection, and immune responses

Ligand: an organic molecule that donates the necessary electrons to form coordinate covalent bonds with metallic ions; for example, as oxygen is bound to the central iron atom of hemoglobin

Lingual papillae: the small nipple-shaped projections of the tongue

Lipolysis: the decomposition or splitting up of fat

Lipoprotein lipase: an enzyme located on endothelial cells lining the capillaries in the adipose tissue that hydrolyzes the constituent triglycerides of chylomicrons to permit entry into the adipocyle

Lymph: the clear watery liquid containing white blood cells and some red blood cells that travels through the lymphatic system, functioning to remove bacteria and certain proteins from tissues, to transport fat from the intestines, and to supply lymphocytes to the blood

Megacolon: colonic dilatation

Metabolic equivalent (MET): a multiple of the resting metabolic rate; a measure of oxygen consumed, thus energy expended; 1 MET is equal to 3.6 ml of oxygen/kg of body weight/min

Metabolism: the sum of all the physical and chemical processes by which living organized substance is produced and maintained (anabolism); also the transformation by which energy is made available for the uses of the organism (catabolism)

Metaphyseal: referring to the wider part at the extremity of the shaft of a long bone; during development it contains the growth zone and consists of spongy bone

Micellar: being of a submicroscopic aggregation of molecules such as a droplet in a colloidal system

Mitogen: a substance that induces blast transformation; DNA, RNA synthesis; and proliferation of lymphocytes

Multiparous: having had two or more pregnancies that resulted in viable fetuses

Mutagen: a chemical or physical agent that induces or increases genetic mutations by causing changes in DNA

Myenteric plexus: the part of the enteric network of lymphatic vessels, nerves, or veins in the tunica muscularis

Myoclonic: relating to or marked by shock-like contractions of a portion of a muscle, or group of muscles

Myopathy: any disease of the muscle

Myosin: the most abundant protein in muscle; the main constituent of the thick filaments of muscle fibers, which along with actin, is responsible for the contraction and relaxation of muscle

Neuropathy: noninflammatory lesions related to functional disturbances in the peripheral nervous system

Neutropenia: a decrease in the number of neutrophilic leukocytes in the blood

Neutrophil hypersegmentation: a granular leukocyte with a nucleus with more than five lobes

Nitrogen cycle: the continuous cycle of chemical reactions in which atmospheric nitrogen is compounded, dissolved in rain, deposited in the soil, assimilated and metabolized by bacteria and plants, and returned to the atmosphere by organic decomposition

Norepinephrine: a catecholamine; a neurohormone released by the postganglionic adrenergic nerves; also secreted by the adrenal medulla in response to splanchnic stimulation and stored in the chromaffin granules; released predominantly in response to hypotension

Organic: denoting chemical substances containing carbon

Pagophagia: ingestion of extraordinary amounts of ice, possibly due to an iron deficiency

Papilledema: edema of the optic disk, most commonly due to increased intracranial pressure, malignant hypertension, or thrombosis of the central retinal vein

Parasympathetic system: the craniosacral portion of the autonomic nervous system

Pepsinogen: a substance secreted by the chief cells, mucous neck cells, and pyloric gland cells that is converted into pepsin in the presence of gastric acid or of pepsin itself

Peptide bond: the joining of the carboxylic carbon of one amino acid with the nitrogen of another

Periconceptional: around the time of conception

Phagocytic: pertaining to or characterized by the taking of material into the cell in membrane-bound vesicles that originate as pinched off invaginations of the plasma membrane

Phenol: a generic term for any organic compound containing one or more hydroxyl groups attached to an aromatic or carbon ring

Phlebitis: inflammation of a vein; marked by infiltration of the coats of the vein and by the formation of a thrombus

Photophobia: abnormal visual intolerance of light

Pica: a compulsive eating of non-nutritive substances

Polycythemia: an increase in the total red blood cell mass of the body

Precursor: a substance from which another, usually more active or mature substance is formed

Pregravid: preceding pregnancy

Prostacyclin: a prostaglandin, PGI_2, synthesized by endothelial cells lining the cardiovascular system; a potent inhibitor of platelet aggregation, a powerful vasodilator, and thus a physiologic antagonist of thromboxane A_2

Proteolytic: promoting the splitting of proteins by hydrolysis of the peptide bonds with formation of smaller polypeptides

Pruritus vulvae: intense itching of the external genitals of the female

Puerperal: pertaining to the period of confinement after labor

Purpura: a small hemorrhage (up to about 1 cm in diameter) in the skin, mucous membrane, or serosal surface, which may be caused by various factors including blood disorders, vascular abnormalities, and trauma; may be associated with inflammation

Putrefaction: enzymatic decomposition of proteins with the production of foul-smelling compounds, such as hydrogen sulfide, ammonia, and mercaptans

Rancid: having a musty, rank taste or smell due to fats that have oxidized and decomposed with the liberation of fatty acids

Rectal prolapse: protrusion of the rectal mucous membrane through the anus

Reduced: altered by a chemical change involving a gain of electrons

Renal calculus: a mass formed by the coalescence of mineral salts, usually oxalates or urates, in the kidney

Renal tubular acidosis (RTA): a defect in tubular handling of bicarbonate owing to a defect in either the proximal or distal tubule

Reticulocytosis: an increase in the number of young red blood cells in the peripheral blood

Retrolental fibroplasia: a condition characterized by the presence of gliotic tissue behind the lens associated with detachment of the retina and arrest of growth of the eye due to excessively high concentrations of oxygen

Rhodopsin: visual purple; a photosensitive purple-red chromoprotein in the retinal rods that, when it is bleached to visual yellow by light, stimulates the retinal sensory endings

Rumen: the first of four stomachs of a ruminant or cud-chewing animal

Saponification: the process of hydrolyzing fats into soaps and glycerol by the addition of alkali

Sarcomere: the contractile unit of a muscle myofibril

Secretagogue: an agent that stimulates secretion

Serosal: pertaining to a serous membrane (a thin membrane containing, secreting, or resembling serum)

Sideroblast: a nucleated red blood cell containing granules of iron in its cytoplasm

Steatorrhea: excessive amounts of fat in the feces

Submucosal plexus: the part of the enteric plexus, a network of autonomic nerve fibers within the wall of the digestive tube, that is located in the tissues beneath the mucous membrane

Sucrose polyester: a sucrose molecule with 6 to 8 fatty acids attached that is formulated by heating soybean oil and sucrose in the presence of methyl alcohol

Sulcus: a groove, trench, or furrow

Sympathetic nervous system (SNS): the thoracolumbar portion of the autonomic nervous system as opposed to the parasympathetic nervous system, which is the craniosacral portion of the autonomic nervous system

Synthetic analogue: a chemical compound with a structure similar to that of the natural compound but differing function

Tachycardia: rapid heart rate, usually above 100 beats per minute

Tannin: an acid found in tea that is capable of reducing nonheme iron absorption

Thrombophlebitis: inflammation of a vein associated with thrombus formation

Thromboxane: an eicosanoid that is a potent inducer of platelet aggregation; also a vasoconstrictor, a physiologic antagonist to prostacyclin

Thyroxine: a crystalline iodine-containing hormone, L-3,5,3′,5′-tetraiodothyronine, secreted by the thyroid gland; its chief function is to increase the rate of cell metabolism

Turgor: condition of being swollen and congested; normal or other fullness

ABBREVIATIONS

ACTH adrenocorticotropic hormone
AD Alzheimer's disease
ADH antidiuretic hormone
ADI accepted daily intake
ALS amyotrophic lateral sclerosis
ARF acute renal failure
ATP adenosine triphosphate
BCAA branched chain amino acids
BEE basal energy expenditure
BHA butylated hydroxyanisole
BHT butylated hydroxytoluene
BMR basal metabolic rate
BPD bronchopulmonary dysplasia
BSA body surface area
BV biologic value
CAD coronary artery disease
CAPD continuous ambulatory peritoneal dialysis
CAVH continuous arteriovenous hemofiltration
CC cardiac cachexia
CCK cholecystokinin
CDC Centers for Disease Control
CHD coronary heart disease
CHF congestive heart failure
CHI closed head injury
CNS central nervous system
COPD chronic obstructive pulmonary disease
CPN central parenteral nutrition
CSII continuous subcutaneous insulin infusion
DAA dispensable amino acid
DCCT Diabetes Control and Complications Trial
DHA docosahexaenoic acid
DHEW Department of Health, Education, and Welfare
DHHS Department of Health and Human Services
DKA diabetic ketoacidosis
DNA deoxyribonucleic acid
EDTA ethylenediaminotetraacetate
EFA essential fatty acid
EPA eicosapentaenoic acid
EPO erythropoietin
ERT enzyme replacement therapy
ERT estrogen replacement therapy
ESRD end-stage renal disease
FAD flavin adenine dinucleotide
FFA free fatty acids
FIGLU formimino glutamic acid
FMN flavin mononucleotide
FPG fasting plasma glucose
GFR glomerular filtration rate
GIP gastric inhibitory polypeptide
GTF glucose tolerance factor
GVHD graft-versus-host disease
HA hyperalimentation
HAV hepatitis A virus
HBV hepatitis B virus
HCT hematocrit
HDL high-density lipoprotein
HE hepatic encephalopathy
HGB hemoglobin
HIV human immunodeficiency virus
HSL hormone-sensitive lipase
IBD inflammatory bowel disease
IBS irritable bowel syndrome
IBW ideal body weight
IDAA indispensable amino acid
IDDM insulin-dependent diabetes mellitus
IF intrinsic factor
IgE immunoglobulin E
IGT impaired glucose tolerance
IL-2 interleukin 2
INH isonicotinic acid hydrazide
IVH intravenous hyperalimentation
J joule
kcal (Cal) kilocalorie
kJ kilojoule
KS Kaposi's sarcoma
LBM lean body mass
LCT long-chain triglyceride

LDL low-density lipoprotein
LES lower esophageal sphincter
LNA alpha-linolenic acid
LPL lipoprotein lipase
MAOI monoamine oxidase inhibitor
MCH mean corpuscular hemoglobin
MCT medium-chain triglyceride
MCV mean corpuscular volume
MET metabolic equivalent
MFOS mixed-function oxidase system
MSG monosodium glutamate
MSUD maple syrup urine disease
NANB non-A, non-B hepatitis virus
NCEP National Cholesterol Education Program
NCJ needle catheter jejunostomy
NI nutritional index
NPU net protein utilization
NSAID nonsteroidal anti-inflammatory drug
NSP nonstarch polysaccharides
OC oral contraceptive
OGTT oral glucose tolerance test
OHA oral hypoglycemic agent
PAS para-aminosalicylic acid
PD Parkinson's disease
PEG percutaneous endoscopic gastrostomy
PEM protein energy malnutrition
PER protein efficiency ratio
PG prostaglandin
PHE phenylalanine
PKU phenylketonuria
PLP pyridoxal phosphate
PPN peripheral parenteral nutrition
PUFA polyunsaturated fatty acid
RAST radioallergosorbent test
RBC red blood cell
RDA recommended dietary allowance
RDS respiratory distress syndrome
REE resting energy expenditure
RMR resting metabolic rate
RNA ribonucleic acid
RQ respiratory quotient
RS resistant starches
RTA renal tubular acidosis
SCA sickle cell anemia
SCT short-chain triglyceride
SFA saturated fatty acid
SLE systemic lupus erythematosus
SMBG self-monitoring of blood glucose
TBSA total body surface area
TC total cholesterol
TEE total energy expenditure
TEF thermic effect of food
TG triglyceride or triacylglycerol
THFA tetrahydrofolate
TIA transient ischemic attack
TIBC total iron-binding capacity
TNF tumor necrosis factor
TPN total parenteral nutrition
TS transferrin saturation
UTI urinary tract infection
UWL unstirred water layer
VLCD very low calorie diet
VLDL very low density lipoprotein
VOD venous occlusive disease

INDEX

Note: Page numbers in *italics* indicate illustrations; numbers followed by a (t) or (b) refer to tables and boxed material, respectively.